Volume 2

A HISTORY OF MEDICINE

A HISTORY OF MEDICINE

ARTURO CASTIGLIONI

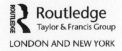

Routledge
Taylor & Francis Group

LONDON AND NEW YORK

First American Edition, published in 1941 by Alfred A. Knopf, Inc.
Second Edition, Revised and Enlarged, published in 1947 by Alfred A. Knopf, Inc.

This edition first published in 2019
by Routledge
2 Park Square, Milton Park, Abingdon, Oxon OX14 4RN

and by Routledge
52 Vanderbilt Avenue, New York, NY 10017

Routledge is an imprint of the Taylor & Francis Group, an informa business

British Library Cataloguing in Publication Data
A catalogue record for this book is available from the British Library

ISBN: 978-0-367-08576-6 (Set)
ISBN: 978-0-429-02312-5 (Set) (ebk)
ISBN: 978-0-367-02976-0 (Volume 2) (hbk)
ISBN: 978-0-367-02998-2 (Volume 2) (pbk)
ISBN: 978-0-429-01988-3 (Volume 2) (ebk)

Publisher's Note
The publisher has gone to great lengths to ensure the quality of this reprint but
points out that some imperfections in the original copies may be apparent.

Disclaimer
The publisher has made every effort to trace copyright holders and would welcome
correspondence from those they have been unable to trace.

also by

Arturo Castiglioni

ADVENTURES OF THE MIND

" Dr. Castiglioni, a distinguished medical historian . . .
has written a fascinating history of magic and its use
by both primitive and modern man."
— *New Republic*

This is a BORZOI BOOK
published in New York by ALFRED A. KNOPF

A HISTORY OF MEDICINE

ARTURO CASTIGLIONI, M.D.

Formerly Professor at the University of Padua
Research Associate in the History of Medicine at Yale University

A HISTORY

OF

MEDICINE

Translated from the Italian and Edited by
E. B. KRUMBHAAR, M.D., Ph.D.
Honorary President of the American Association of the History of Medicine

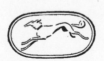

SECOND EDITION, REVISED AND ENLARGED

NEW YORK: ALFRED · A · KNOPF

1947

TO

the companion of my life and my work

this book

is affectionately dedicated

PREFACE TO SECOND EDITION

THE MANY important developments in medicine that have occurred during the eventful six years that have elapsed since the first appearance of this work in English would seem to have made a new edition necessary, even if it had not been required by the exhaustion of the first edition. The entire volume has been carefully amended, though changes were much greater in the modern than in the earlier periods. The amount of recent new material to be included has been so large that the chapter on the period since 1850 has had to be entirely rewritten. It has been divided into two chapters, one for the latter half of the nineteeenth century and one for the twentieth century — each longer than any other chapter in the book. It was found advisable to divide them into 23 and 27 sections respectively. The difficulties attending such a change are obvious: the writing of history always becomes more difficult the closer one approaches the present, and this is especially the case in the rapidly expanding fields of science and medicine. Additions to existing knowledge continue to be made ever more rapidly, so that it seems that more of significance has been learned about medical science in the past hundred years than in any previous period. No one or two individuals can hope to comprehend the new floods of knowledge in the various fields of medicine, much less evaluate the details properly and fit them into an efficient arrangement. For such reasons, some writers prefer to terminate their story at the end of some convenient period in the past. We have, nevertheless, perhaps too rashly, endeavoured in this edition to include in the narrative, however imperfectly, the latest important events — " history in the making," indeed. We hope that thus the chapters on modern medicine may bring the story up to date and at least serve as a useful reference source for those wishing factual details about medical leaders and their thoughts and discoveries. The effort has been maintained throughout the book to preserve a satisfactory balance between the history of medical ideas, of medical facts, and of medical personages. Especially in the last two chapters, much more factual

[i]

data have been given than in the first English edition; yet we have tried to avoid as far as possible mere cataloguing of events and disconnected items of brief biographical details. As much as feasible of the factual portions has been set up in smaller type.

Although we have closely collaborated on all the additions and changes in this edition, the senior author has in general been primarily responsible for most of the clinical sections and the sections on Public Health and on the History of Medicine of the last two chapters, and also the bibliography; his junior has written or supervised the basic science sections, the rest of the clinical and miscellaneous sections and the subject index. The Appendix (on the Rise of Universities and of Faculties of Medicine) has had to be regretfully abandoned in order to help keep the new volume to a reasonable size.

Our friends have been generous in their assistance. We are glad to acknowledge valuable help from the following on larger or smaller portions of the sections indicated: Dr. Hans Schlumberger (Philadelphia) — experimental embryology; Dr. Elizabeth Wilson (Philadelphia) — vitamins; Dr. D. L. Drabkin (Philadelphia) — biochemistry; Dr. M. Calabresi (New Haven) — cardiology; Dr. B. B. Crohn (New York) — gastrointestinal diseases; Dr. R. Nissen (New York) — surgery; Dr. J. Webster (New York) — plastic surgery; Dr. Edwin M. Jameson (Saranac Lake) — obstetrics and gynecology; Dr. A. Levinson (Chicago) — pediatrics; Dr. H. Friedenwald (Baltimore) — ophthalmology; Dr. C. L. Deming (New Haven) — urology; Dr. L. Goldman (Cincinnati) — dermatology; Dr. C. Proskauer (New York) — stomatology; Dr. G. Zilboorg (New York) — psychiatry; Dr. H. S. Martland (Newark) — legal medicine; Dr. A. Whittaker (Detroit) — occupational diseases. The rapidly progressing field of biochemistry has required a separate section in the last two chapters of this edition. Exigencies of space demand that the excellent monograph on the subject, prepared for us by Dr. Drabkin, unfortunately be greatly condensed. We have to thank also several friends, especially Dr. John R. Miner, for pointing out errors in the first edition. We shall be grateful to anyone helping us in the same way with this one. We also thank Dr. Curt Proskauer for his valuable help in making the name index and in the correction of the proofs.

At the Yale Historical Library, Miss Madeline Stanton, at the New York Academy of Medicine, Miss Gertrude Annan, and at the College of Physicians of Philadelphia, Mrs. Mary Elizabeth Shaffer have given freely of their expert assistance.

We believe that an appreciation of the value of the history of medicine is growing, especially in English-speaking countries and in Latin America.

The steadily increasing accumulation of the facts of medical science that the student, practitioner and investigator must possess has reached such a size that it has produced a greater realization of the need for preservation of its older sister, the art of medicine, and for learning from the past some of the pitfalls to be avoided in the future. In this country, the American Association of the History of Medicine and its constituent societies were never more vigorous; the intelligent lay reader is showing ever more interest in medical, as in other forms of scientific articles. It is our hope that this volume may be of use in promoting knowledge of this worthy discipline, as well as in serving as a useful book of reference and affording some pleasant reading.

A. Castiglioni
E. B. Krumbhaar

AUTHOR'S PREFACE

THE FIRST Italian edition of this book was published in 1927. At that time I was teaching the history of medicine at the University of Padua. Special attention to the historical factor in the evolution of medical thought was to be expected at this school, which has been one of the most ancient and glorious bulwarks of the freedom of learning, and has numbered among its scholars Dante and Albertus Magnus, Copernicus and Galileo, Fracastoro and Vesalius, Harvey and Morgagni.

I have been convinced that in the history of science as in that of any expression of human intelligence and emotion, the past is never past, but continues and is very active in every form and at every manifestation of the present. The close relation between the progress of medicine — connected more than any other science with the essential needs of life — and the advance of civilization is quite evident. It is perhaps not sufficiently appreciated that the modern art of healing not only is linked with old magical rites and religious creeds, with primitive opotherapy and classical Hippocratism, with dogmatic doctrines and revolutionary discoveries, but is also intimately associated with the economic, intellectual, and political condition of life of different nations at different times, with their wealth or their misery, their trade, their laws, their wars, their philosophy, their literature, and their art. Furthermore, medicine is one of the mightiest of all the suggestive agents active in the life of today: it affects both the individual and the group, constantly facing new threats and menaces, but offering also new promises opening unexpected horizons for the future.

The history of this evolution and these interferences I have tried to record. It has often been marked by the immortal touch of genius, illuminated by the flashing light of heroism and of sacrifice, and beautified by the radiant smile of poetry. Its progress has sometimes been darkened by superstition or by dogmatism, by hatred and intolerance. But from the most remote past up to our own time, medical thought, the noblest expression of human aspiration to deliver man from physical and moral evil, has maintained a striking historical unity, and only through a knowledge and a comprehension of the history of the past is it possible to understand or to judge the medicine of today.

At the time in which this book is presented to English-speaking readers a terrible war is raging through the world and the destruction of some of the most precious treasures of humanity is in progress. A grave crisis in the evolution of intellectual life and in the progress of science is likely to follow it in many countries and to have its repercussions everywhere. Many of the scientists who are referred to in the last chapter of this book have disappeared or are working no longer in the places where they were formerly active; many institutes are closed; many valuable traditions interrupted. This work is intended to give a picture of medicine at a time which perhaps marks the close of a historical period. It endeavours to express and teach through the example of the past that above all troubles, all wars, and all revolutions the precious treasure of humanitarian thought and of medicine as a science, as an art, and as an impetus to the will to live will not stop in its progress toward further conquests. If I have succeeded in my task, my work as scholar and as teacher will not have been in vain.

I feel it my duty to express here my gratitude first to the Dazian Foundation for Medical Research, whose valuable help made it possible for me to continue my studies in this country. I should like also to thank my American friends who have offered me so many proofs of their kindness and have given me a most hearty welcome to the United States. I want to cite especially the names of Dr. Henry E. Sigerist, who first invited me six years ago to deliver a series of lectures at the Johns Hopkins University and other medical schools; of Dr. Emanuel Libman of New York, who encouraged me in my work in the most friendly way; and Dr. John F. Fulton and Dr. Milton C. Winternitz of Yale University, to whom I owe the connection with the medical school where I am teaching today.

Finally, and most of all, I am deeply indebted to Dr. E. B. Krumbhaar, the eminent pathologist and historian of medicine at the University of Pennsylvania. He offered to assume the very difficult task of translating and editing my book; to every page he brought the valuable contribution of his comprehension and of his extensive knowledge. Almost the entire part which is dedicated to American medicine is due to his collaboration: and it is his merit that this work can be presented today to English speaking readers in this form. May it be accepted with the same confidence and good will with which I submit it to their attention and their judgment.

New Haven, Conn., Yale University, September 1940   ARTURO CASTIGLIONI

EDITOR'S PREFACE

THE STORY of medicine has become a long and complicated one, and continues to receive additions ever more rapidly. In spite of its importance and vital interest, then, we should not be surprised that general histories on the subject, especially in English, are not numerous. This book by Arturo Castiglioni, recognized as one of the world's leading medical historians, should have appeal as well as value. Its merit has already been recognized outside as well as inside of Italy, as is shown by the translations that have been made into French, Spanish and German.

English-speaking medical readers are seldom sufficiently aware of the leading part taken by Italy in the history of medicine through many centuries. It is chiefly for this reason that I turned to " Castiglioni " with special interest, and I was not disappointed. Written especially for Italian readers by the Professor of the History of Medicine at the University of Padua, the book naturally emphasizes the importance of Italy's role. It would be undesirable to remove this emphasis, not only because the author has a right to his own background, but also because desirable matter would thereby be lost which is not available in similar histories written in English. However, with the complete approval of the author, I have omitted many details of local Italian interest, and inserted new material, especially when dealing with the more important phases of American and British medicine. In a few cases where it appeared that statements might not coincide with Dr. Castiglioni's views, they have been placed in an editorial bracket. Though the author has seen the English text in fairly final form, he of course should not be held responsible for any statements that are not direct translations from the Italian.

No apologies need be offered the reader for a new volume in English on the history of medicine — a subject of both practical and recreational value. The erratic course that our profession has followed, its blind alleys and pitfalls, the methods of thought, observation, and experience that have proved profitable or fallacious in the past — comprehension of these should aid many of us today in recognizing the broader problems of the moment and in devising methods for their solution.

The history of medicine not infrequently has important bearings on the political history of a country or period in ways that are but little realized by the average reader, and not sufficiently appreciated even by some historians. The effect of malaria on the decadence of Greece and the eradication of the mosquito as a *sine qua non* of the Panama Canal are good examples. Many a decisive campaign, many a potentially important new colony, has been defeated by disease rather than by the more patent enemy, and many a section of a country retarded by factors inimical to the public health.

It is obvious that in a single volume on such a vast subject much that is important must be omitted, and equally obvious that matter that is less important has at times inevitably been included. Especially do these remarks apply to the period since 1850, which many writers would accept as including a majority of the greatest medical discoveries of all time. Even in the past decade, during which time no general history of medicine in English has appeared, many medical discoveries of prime importance have been made. Here the art of selection is especially difficult. The reader's indulgence is hoped for.

In the last chapter, where the different specialties contain subdivisions arranged by different countries, the order of the original text has sometimes been changed in an attempt to make the presentation more in accordance with the importance of the contributions of the various countries. Birth and death dates have been checked for each individual. When, as was not infrequently the case, different dates were given by the different authorities consulted and a primary source was not available, what appeared to be the most likely date was selected, with proper regard for that given in the original, especially in the case of Italians. It was seldom thought desirable to break the narrative with notice of individual differences, here as in the case of other factual conflicts. Greek script for Greek words has been abandoned with regret: few today can understand Greek or read Greek letters. Transliterated into the Latin alphabet, the words can at least be read and pronounced.

A number of references have been added to the bibliography, especially to works in English. For completing and checking all references I am much indebted to Mrs. Edith S. Moore. The help of W. B. McDaniel, 2d, the Librarian of the College of Physicians of Philadelphia, has been invaluable in many respects and has been correspondingly appreciated.

With due regard for the turmoil of the present political situation and for what may have happened between this writing and the appearance of the book in print, I believe that a work of this kind has its value, perhaps a special value today, for English-speaking readers. This is a puzzled world, indeed, for scientists as well as the man on the street, and both may with profit to themselves and to the world at large cultivate the "long view" by contemplating the progressive steps and the errors of the past as a possible guide for present action.

E. B. KRUMBHAAR

Philadelphia, October 1940

CONTENTS

CONTENTS

LIST OF ILLUSTRATIONS

A HISTORY OF MEDICINE

CHAPTER I

MEDICAL THOUGHT IN ITS

HISTORICAL EVOLUTION

1. Origins and Traditions of the History of Medicine

EVERY state of affairs at a given moment is in reality merely a phase of development, no matter how concise or static or how rigidly formed it may appear. Every one of the threads that make up the web of our knowledge goes back to distant and diverse origins and is also tied up with threads of other textures. No one can comprehend the present accurately and profoundly and look intelligently into the future who is not acquainted with the sources of knowledge or able to follow the roads along which knowledge of the truth has reached us. No one knows better than the physician the importance of this law as regards the biologic organization of the individual, and no one knows better than he the importance of the history of the individual and of living matter, without which it is not possible correctly to understand the functions of organs or their intimate nature. Now, what is true for the organization of the biologic individual applies equally to that complex but solidly constructed organism known as the sum of our scientific knowledge. The details of this knowledge interweave and overrun one another like the branches of a vigorous tree, which, however, all draw their nourishment from the same deep roots. He who follows the history of medical thought in its various branches will not find, as has been often and inaccurately stated, the continuous progress of a constantly ascending line. It is with strange interferences and marvellous spirals that this thought progresses from the demonism of the ancients to the suggestive

[3]

healing of our times, from Biblical organ therapy to recent glandular doctrines, from the humoral pathology of Hippocrates to modern immunology. Often the ideas of audacious and gifted predecessors appeared to be forgotten; or ancient errors which seemed permanently obliterated again came to light, and the discoveries which appeared to be the most assured of a rapid success met the most fierce opposition.

To follow the thread of medical thought in the whole marvellous texture of its history, as ancient as humanity itself, to consider in detail the associations of man and his pains throughout the centuries, realizing how they vary with the ages both in their essential being and in the way in which the individuality of the physician reacts upon them — there is the vast task which is laid before the medical historian.

The execution and documentation of such a difficult and complex task cannot be attained without profound and extensive research among ancient texts and the study of the past in the light of historical criticism. Such opportunity and ability is granted to but few; Italians have taken a worthy part in this work: Puccinotti and De Renzi were masters of this art and their monumental labours have conquered an eminent position in this field. They were among the first to initiate the renewal of medical historical studies in Italy which followed the intellectual pause which took place in that field during the Risorgimento, a development which is still under way. The zeal for historical study has always been great in Italy, because in that country is found the largest, most complete, and most beautiful historical documentation, both in its monuments, in the hygienic achievements of classical antiquity, in the creation of its great artists, and in the first medical books which saw the light in the famous Venetian presses. This flourishing condition is perhaps still to be found today in Italy, where medicine remains, on account of the very character of the people and the nature of its background, so closely bound to art and to philosophy. The art of medicine has had excellent representatives there from the most ancient times: the graphic and plastic arts represented physicians and sick people in all periods, preserving thus in the most eloquent manner the record of ancient legends, important events, and famous persons. Poetry and literature were closely related to Western medicine, and many great physicians held honoured positions in the history of Western literature. There the philosophy of medicine also has always been alive and vivid — not a sterile speculation fixed in scholastic disputes, but a live, deep, and continuous study of man, of his origin, of all the manifestations of his life, considered from the point of view of an objective, logical reasoning founded on experiment; a philosophy in the sense clearly defined by Hippocrates, of an inexhaustible love of study and research, and love of observation and reasoning, which cannot progress apart from each other.

In a period that is now fortunately distant an error was committed which might truly be called fundamental: that of wishing to construct the edifice of medicine exclusively on Aristotelian logic and on the force of dialectic, maintaining that speculative philosophy, when erected in the various systems, could give the definitive solution of all problems, including those of biology. When this edifice was undermined by the advent of experimental science, another was constructed, not less systematically founded, on the results of research into objective facts, an edifice whose solid and magnificent base no one today can deny. But there cannot and should not be lacking from this modern monument a close connection — now being painfully explored — with the origins and vital roots of our art — the expert observation of the patient. This almost universal return to biologic concepts and the Hippocratic method, even if not altogether a conscious one, shows that medicine, both in the free practice of its art and in the painstaking pursuit of its thought, cannot be bound exclusively to the test-tube or the microscope or be confined within the artificial bounds of any definitive system. By the very mutations to which the biological organism, whether individually or collectively, is subjected as a constantly evolving living unit, medicine itself is always in the process of change. Thus one accepts that there cannot exist problems with absolutely precise definition, or systems capable of completely providing for this or that chapter of medicine. There is perhaps no error which does not contain a grain of truth, and no truth, no matter how luminous and absolute it may appear, which does not contain a grain of error.

The changing successions of errors and victories constitute the very essence of our history, which leads us, by paths that are sometimes luminous and at other times barely discernible, to laws that today seem impregnable and yesterday seemed vague and distant; to doubts that yesterday were dogmas, to hypotheses that perhaps tomorrow will be truths. To study this process of evolution in medicine; to scrutinize the distant origins and structure of our knowledge, formed slowly and painfully through so many and such different paths; to recognize after strict analysis the part that was played in the formation of medical thought by instinct, fear, hope, and faith, and the influence on this thought of the great events of political and social history; to measure the effect of medicine, on its side, in determining the direction of the history of culture, art, politics, social life; to endeavour finally to tie the present logically and harmoniously to the past — this should be the program of the history of medicine. From it are easily derived the basic and directing forces which should guide our special discipline.

If the history of medicine on the one hand should study and teach what medicine was in the past, on the other hand it should range itself with the natural sciences as an experimental science, seeking for that which is permanent. It should, then, on the one side study the past and mark the route travelled, but on the other it should exert equal care in seeking out the laws that have guided the evolution of medical thought in the past and that will determine its development in the future.

It is the threefold history of ideas, facts, and persons that should above all determine and illumine what we might call the chief highway of our long course: namely, the reconstruction of the unity of medical thought in its origins and its limits. This historical unity should be reconstructed thread by thread. In recent times scientific research and analysis have placed in the hands of students the precious gift of many new discoveries, all of them, however, constantly introducing new problems; but there has not been maintained or taught or even appreciated the bond of unity without which all the individual parts are disconnected and none of the ways leads surely to the goal. Modern medicine, both in the schools and in life, in theory and in practice, is too often subdivided into branches and specialties, into technique and doctrine. We must not forget the common source of the original concept of medicine in the sufferings and fears of primitive man, perhaps even of animals, developing in ways that we cannot ignore. And no less often is forgotten the aim of this study: to diminish the pains of suffering humanity, making it stronger and more capable, an aim which is often lost from sight among our modern subtleties, yet one which can be taught objectively and successfully by the study of history.

2. The History of Ideas

Thus the origin of thought and its goal are the same; the plexus that exists in history is continuous and intimate in that nothing arises or disappears suddenly and without reason. In the history of literature and art the error has been repeated through many centuries of attributing a sudden and marvellous emergence of a high culture from a desert soil, like that of the Pharaohs in Egypt, the age of Pericles in Greece, and the Renaissance in Italy. Though contradicted by historical criticism, this error is strenuously maintained in medicine, where even cultured physicians frequently state that the history of medicine began but a few centuries ago. Historical research in recent times has shown that the history of medicine should logically be considered, like that of the history of all the sciences, as a slow but continuous accumulation and alternation of knowledge and of facts, some of which are forgotten over centuries and then come to light again. Up to the eighteenth century it was still maintained that the Hippocratic school should be regarded as a purely Grecian product flowering in the golden age of Greece; we know now that it is more correct to base the foundations of this school on influences from Babylon, Assyria, and Italy, and even from ancient Egypt. Today it is clear that the early medical knowledge of the Greeks, which until a few decades ago was regarded by historians as a first uncertain expression and childlike attempt at medicine, really represents results obtained from the fundamental concepts of antique civilizations, derived in their turn from phenomena occurring thousands of years earlier in the prehistoric period. A fine network, then, runs through the history of medicine from the thought of our most ancient ancestors up to the present time — a thought which, as I have indicated, exhibits truly interesting cycles. We know, for instance, to cite one among many eloquent examples, that throughout the first great period of civilization medicine was essentially Mediterranean, cultivated almost exclusively in the countries that touched this sea.

The tradition of the Vedas coming from holy India, the tablets of Niniveh, the papyri of Egypt, the Biblical records, and the bright light from the Ægean islands and Magna Græcia, all are from the Mediterranean littoral. Thence also are the products of the Greco-Roman civilization, followed in turn by the Arabs and again by the great epoch of the Italian Renaissance. Just as the Italian Renaissance renewed classic art in its Hellenistic and philosophic traditions, in its return to Greece by the way of the Arabs, and in the magnificent experiments of Galileo, so Western medicine reveals its noble inheritance from ancient Greece. In Italian universities the torch of knowledge was relighted, and just as students came from all Greece to Cos, so did they come from all Europe to hear the words of Italian masters. The study of epidemics was renewed with Fracastorius, who reaffirmed the contagious nature of phthisis, a concept that had been lost since the time of Plato. Morgagni, the founder of pathologic anatomy, was classic in his grandeur. The Italian governments toward the middle of the eighteenth century enacted some of the first public health laws against tuberculosis, just as four centuries earlier the Italian republics had created early public health laws against epidemics.

Thus a close bond is revealed between the work and thought of our most distant masters and that of their descendants. Thus the orientation of thought in the field of medicine, as in other fields of science and art, is bound closely to the land from which it sprang, to the background of its environment, and to the spirit of the race.

If we follow in its developments another of the more interesting concepts of medical history, we shall find other analogies which must appear striking even to those who are not familiar with the study of history. Let us observe how in very ancient times, and evidently in connection with the examination of secretions and excretions which impressed the imagination of primitive man, the concept of humoral pathology was born, and was elevated to the level of a scientific theory by the greatest of our ancient masters. It was Hippocrates who proclaimed the predominant importance of phenomena developing in the all-pervading humours in the blood, as compared with those located in single organs. Here is his striking statement about the functions of the glands: "The glands have the purpose of providing for the distribution of the humours in the body; if this does not happen regularly, they become inflamed and sick." Humoral pathology was definitely established by the work of Galen. It survived even the storm and stress that shook the basis of the entire Greco-Latin civilization, though it appeared to be forgotten and buried like the beautiful marble statues of the ancients and their classic poetry. The serene beauty of medical thought, analytical and above all critical, which drew its vital strength and laws from the ancient schools of philosophy, was forgotten; but the humoral theory survived in the scholastic tradition and dominated all of medicine for more than a millennium, until Virchow constructed the great modern edifice of pathologic anatomy on the basis of his cellular doctrine. The Latin school, supported by the philosophic and Hippocratic traditions, still defends humoral pathology even though Northern criticism severely shook its foundations, and cellular pathology temporarily occupied the entire field. It was the triumph of the exact research of the laboratory, with the clinic and the force of criticism too often laid aside as a useless hindrance. We still hear philosophic speculation and Neo-Latin romanticism spoken of disdainfully, forgetting Bassi, one of the great founders of bacteriology, and Spallanzani, who contributed so considerably to the foundation of modern bacteriology. With its doctrines of antigens and of immunity developed from the blood humours and its emphasis on the importance of clinical examination in connection with laboratory studies, modern medicine restores ancient humoral pathology to its honourable position. Today the limitations of cellular pathology have become more obvious and an "integrated pathology," which combines the truths of cellular and humoral theories and the knowledge obtained from both wards and laboratories, is making more and more deserved progress. From the distant concepts of Hippocratism is derived the modern edifice of the doctrine of the endocrine glands, and finally Hippocratic thought is born again and shines with increased strength in the modern studies of personality and of the individual constitution.

He who would follow attentively the story of the great conflict to which we have just referred will receive the impression of seeing such distant historical events as the schism of the Greek schools of Cos and Cnidus renewed again in the conflict between the French and German schools in the second half of the past century. Doubtless he will then be convinced that no scientific progress can be regarded as a sudden and autonomous formation, but that each of our achievements is closely allied to the past, without knowledge of which it cannot be understood.

3. The History of Facts

If what we have already said emphasizes the importance of the history of medicine as a study of the history of ideas, it is no less necessary to recognize the importance of the history of facts, examined according to their characteristics and essential nature. The experience of recent years has brought about a realization of the fact that the pathologic changes in the individual and collective constitution are not produced according to time and environment alone, but also that certain diseases have different characteristics at different times and under different circumstances. All who study, for example, the history of the great epidemics will note that their characteristics change at different periods and that such change is not entirely due to the modifications of the defence measures taken. The results obtained by modern hygienic measures and sanitary legislation, by governmental aid and laws of prevention, offer one of the most interesting problems for the historian or the hygienist. If we reflect on the valuable sanitary legislation of ancient times, we must recognize that the fact that it was later forgotten caused enormous preventable losses of human life. If we consider how Fracastorius in the sixteenth century illuminated the contagiousness of tuberculosis, we must admit that humanity today would be suffering much less from this terrible plague had the seed sown in those times been fertile. One could give a hundred other examples from the history of medicine to show how important it is to note and comprehend the facts of the past in order to illuminate the problems of the present. This was so well understood by eminent historians that they have not inappropriately given the name of historical pathology to this chapter of medicine. It is certain that at the present moment, when pathologic changes in the individual are being studied with such scientific fervour, this thought is worth our attention.

The social legislation of recent years, which marks great progress in the domain of preventive medicine, carries the marks of the medical thought that inspired it. The recognition of the relations that exist between pathology and economic and social conditions, the fight against occupational diseases, all the great organization of sanitary activities, the study of the connections between psychic affections and criminality, the proper evaluation of health statistics, and the protection of maternity and infancy — all these mark decisive steps in the activation of social legislation by medical thought. Here, then, in our own period a new concept of public health is emerging, one that has a larger scope and a field of action that is daily becoming greater and greater. Now we see medical thought, which was formerly confined to the halls of philosophy, the clinics, and the laboratories, making its triumphal entry into legislative chambers.

4. The Biographic History

Finally, although the history of medicine represents a history of facts and processes, it should also be in part a biographic history. This includes the history of the great pioneers and of those who made their indelible impression on medical progress; if it is to be accurate and alive it cannot be separated from the history of ideas. It is perhaps in these pages that the younger readers will be most keenly interested, because they tell of great battles fought not only against those who wished by every possible means to hinder free research; but also, the hardest battle of all, against the physicians themselves, who were hostile to new ideas or ready to exalt new errors. They recount the struggles against superstition and charlatanism, which throughout history are the same as they were in the time of Thessalus of Lydia, who called himself *Iatronicos*, the conqueror of physicians, announced that the medicine of the schools was nothing but a fraud, and promised to produce perfect physicians in six months. This is the part of history that shows eloquently and clearly that the identity of human suffering under all skies must create a solidarity both of science and of scientists. It shows that one cannot limit the free expansion of ideas nor erect barriers against them. Here, too, we may refer to Italian achievements, such as the wise course of the Venetian Republic in recognizing the powerful aid that the diffusion of culture could give to the State, and opening the hospitable doors of its university to students of every country and every creed.

It is this historical study that teaches us not to be precipitate in judgment and to be always and above all prudent. It is through the study of the history of medicine that we learn to evaluate with modesty the work of our own times, with reverence for the great ones of the past. It is this study that should guide the physician who speaks with devoted admiration of our immortal artists, poets, captains, and statesmen to recall also with pride the names of our greatest physicians. And if it is true that the work of great men can stimulate to great deeds, should we not perhaps believe that the younger generation will profit by the story of those who fought so strenuously for their ideals?

The attempt has been made here to summarize briefly, according to a single point of view, the characteristics, trends, and objectives of the history of medicine. The methods may differ from those which guided the historians of other periods, because today historical criticism follows rules which in the past have been ignored. It should probe carefully the facts of the past, examining them with a serene objectivity, and should follow the thread of medical thought through the centuries in its relations with religion, culture, philosophy, politics, and social progress. This study of the past should above all lead to reconstruction of the unity of medical thought from its origins to its final goal, and should demonstrate the continuity of its historical sequence. A national history of medicine should search out the particular features of medical science as they appear in its great men and its great concepts. A general medical history should record the progress of medical art in its great struggles and its great victories. Historical pathology should deal with the story of diseases, emphasizing the most useful and striking measures taken to protect against them.

From this historical edifice, which can and must be patiently constructed on the fundamentals laid down by our great masters, one can derive the laws that will determine the progress of the great and complex medical organism through the centuries.

Such are the general principles that should guide the historian. Girding himself for the high task, he should give close attention both to distant events and to the more recent facts which are connected with the past by so many more or less obscure threads. In the history of medicine, as in the history of art and philosophy, everything is dominated by an eternal and immutable rhythm. Everything, as Hippocrates says, is human and everything is divine. Thus there is no such thing as a modern truth or a modern error, an ancient ignorance or an ancient wisdom. There is only a single truth, immutable throughout the ages, a truth which is at the basis of all medicine, which is so human that it appears divine, and which in its aims is more and more pervaded with the spirit of human solidarity. Medicine is inextricably related by a thousand threads to this origin and this goal, as it is both an art and a science; and no physician, no matter how scientific, can be the perfect physician without being inspired by the flame of its art.

Born with the first expression of suffering and the first desire to alleviate this suffering, becoming scientific with the first need for an explanation of the phenomena manifested in the organism and the first laborious investigation of the human mind into the subject, medicine has for its supreme goal the task of rendering aid to those who suffer and of furthering the improvement both of the individual and of the race. Such is the truth revealed by the constant labour and marvellous effort that have been given with faith and enthusiasm by physicians from the most distant past up to our own times. The most illustrious scientists and their most humble followers alike have striven to defend man from everything that threatens his health and disturbs the fundamental harmony either of the individual or of the collective organism.

The teaching of the history of medicine should demonstrate this profound truth and should travel again over the pathways of the past. Thanks to this study, the physician of tomorrow, while solving the new problems posed for him by science, scrutinizing with serenity the new facts produced, and testing them without bias, will return for inspiration to the inexhaustible sources of the past. It will then often happen that he will hear a familiar voice from far distant times which will awaken in him the echo of ideas inherited from his ancestors. It is with profound emotion and the feeling of encouragement given to his work as scientist and artist that he will listen to the counsels and the teachings of those who have gone before.

CHAPTER II

THE ORIGIN OF MEDICINE IN PRE-HISTORY AND IN PRIMITIVE PEOPLES

EMPIRIC, DEMONISTIC, ANIMISTIC, MAGIC MEDICINE

1. Prehistoric Evidence of Disease

FROM the point of view of the chronologic and orderly relation of human facts and ideas, history is but a recent affair in relation to the environment in which it moves. Study of the earliest origins of medical thought and its developmental trends goes back to the most distant periods of the history of humanity, when man first appeared on the world stage, when his physical, psychological, and social individuality was slowly forming, when the characteristics of the race were scarcely apparent in their essential features.

But even in the period which preceded the appearance of man on the earth, the investigations of palæopathology (that is, scrutiny of the history of disease and its morbid manifestations in prehistoric periods) have demonstrated that almost synchronously with the first manifestations of life on the earth there are indubitable evidences of disease. In fact, in the palæozoic age there are numerous examples not only of fractures, but also of dental caries and parasitic diseases. One finds unquestioned evidences of bone lesions that correspond to the forms familiar to us, such as periostitis, necrosis, pyorrhœa alveolaris, arthritis, and perhaps also osteomyelitis in the dinosaurs and plesiosaurs and other animals of the Mesozoic period. Evidence of disease in prehuman times, for the study of which we owe much to E. J. C. Esper (1774), Rudolf Virchow, and Roy Moodie, is necessarily limited to fossilized bony lesions. One can assume, however, that bacteria — which are among the earliest of living types — and simple forms of animal life early became parasitized and pathogenic, in the Permian period according to some authorities. If the disease happened to be in soft parts, it would of course have left us no record. Garrison speaks of probable actinomycosis in a Miocene horse, and of a hemangioma in the bone in a Mesozoic dinosaur — probably the earliest tumour recorded. There is abundant proof of existence of such lesions in the relics of the Tertiary and Quaternary ages. As far as our researches extend, then — that is, through a period that includes hundreds of thousands of years — disease was the inseparable companion of the life of those far-distant precursors of the human race.

If we wish to summarize briefly the history of the human race, without entering into discussion of such problems as whether it descends from several different species or from a single trunk of animal ancestor, or whether the *Pithecanthropus erectus* belongs to the human species or to the anthropoids or to both, as its discoverer, Dubois, believes, we can say that the prehistory of man begins with the origin of anthropoid life in the Oligocene period, with the transformation of the anthropoid into man in the Pliocene, and the extinction of the great mammals in the Pleistocene or in the glacial period. The *Pithecanthropus erectus*, discovered at Trinil, Java, in 1891 by Dubois is still usually regarded as the oldest known representative of man on this earth (about a half-million years old). It is of interest that the femur of this very ancient specimen shows an exostosis that is undoubtedly pathologic. The recent discoveries in the caves of Chou-kou-tien, near Peking, may yet prove to be our oldest known ancestors; there is good evidence that they already knew the use of fire. Compared to them, the massive-brained Cro-Magnon man of 25000 B.C. was but of yesterday. Though there is no evidence that man has descended from any of the higher apes — the item that apparently is most obnoxious to many fundamentalists — there is good evidence that we, like them, descended from a common ancestor. The all-important accident or series of events that led our ancestors to function differently from their ape relatives still remains to be demonstrated.

Recent studies indicate that the most ancient type that lived in Europe was the Piltdown man (*Euanthropos Dawsoni*), whose relics were found in southern England some years ago. This was a type entirely different from the Heidelberg man and was followed in the last glacial period by the Neanderthal man. At the end of this period *Homo sapiens* appeared on the earth (the Grimaldi and Cro-Magnon types, and others).

For the history of those distant origins of primitive species, we find figures cut in the walls of caverns and on boulders, the forms of the first instruments, the positions in which dead bodies were buried, the character-

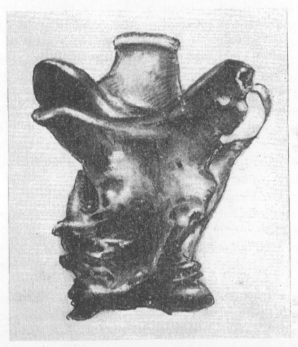

1. *Spondylitis deformans in the vertebra of a smilodont. California Pleistocene.*
(MUSEUM OF NATURAL HISTORY OF THE UNIVERSITY OF KANSAS.)

istic changes found in the bones (whether pathological or artificial). These constitute the earliest and inestimably valuable documentation of the first ideas of our distant ancestors. And just as the most ancient inscriptions that have come down to us show an already complete language — the result of a long formative period, certainly several thousands of years — in the same way these instruments, mural designs, and other evidences of activity represent an already advanced stage of a gradual evolution. In this process were accomplished the first two revolutions in the history of humanity: the first, in which man's ancestor removed the hand from the earth and began to use it as a most valuable instrument; the second, much later, in which the use of fire was discovered. The traces of these earliest events suggest the course followed in the formation of medical thought in the most distant times, just as the earliest lesions indicate the direction of the physical development of the race.

Just as in the normal infant we find expressions, gestures, and primitive ideas like those found in individuals of interrupted or abnormally slow development, so we find in the midst of primitive peoples today concepts and manifestations which may be presumed to be identical with those of the primitive races of distant epochs. And, as we shall see, this is also true in the history of medicine. So that when we write the history of medicine of the most ancient times, we are also writing that of the primitive peoples of every epoch. Further still, identical concepts are found in the popular medicine of all races, concepts of which we have sometimes lost the links that connect them with their far-distant origin. It is perhaps similar also in the case of certain languages, such as the Basque and the Etruscan, whose origins may go back to neolithic times. It is also true of certain beliefs or medical superstitions which may have had their origins in far-distant cultures that are now extinct.

Historical research has established that accounts of what are regarded as legends of antiquity, such as the Flood and the continent of Atlantis, most probably have a foundation in the occurrences of prehistory. The stories common to all the ancient races, of monstrous animals, for example, may in some cases merely represent the memory, changed by later events, of prehistoric realities.

It is for this reason that the study of prehistoric medicine presents problems which are of the greatest interest and yet difficult of solution. We must, then, in this general and necessarily incomplete history content ourselves with merely sketching the general lines of development.

2. Instinctive and Empirical Medicine

If we understand the term " medicine " to indicate the relief of pain by our own means or with the help of others, or the repair of damage produced by injury or disease, we should think first of all of its instinctive origin, much as the first expressions of pain are instinctive. Examples of this instinctive medicine are not infrequent even among animals, even without our having recourse to the legends of the ancient Greek and Latin writers, who in turn certainly borrowed from a much older tradition. There is no doubt that animals instinctively alleviate fever in cold water, skilfully hunt the parasites that torment them, and try to lessen the pain of their wounds by licking them. When a dog breaks a leg it trains itself to go on three legs, so that the broken bone is at rest and recovers with a minimum of shortening. Monkeys are capable of extracting foreign bodies, and undoubted examples have been seen in animals of intervention for the help of other sick animals.

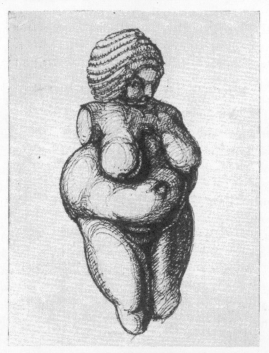

2. *The Venus of Willendorf, the earliest known sculpture of the human figure. A limestone statuette, 4⅜ inches high, from the Middle Aurignacian Period (c. 22,000 B.C.). To us an example of pathologic obesity, such females appear to have been the ideals of prehistoric man.*

Maternal solicitude, acting for the protection of the young, is one of the most obvious expressions of the instinct for the conservation of the race. In this category also is the help given to the pregnant or parturient woman, which perhaps represents the most ancient form of medical assistance.[1]

Such are the first recognizable traces of ideas that we can call instinctive, from which empirical medicine is soon derived and subordinated to the idea

[1] Veneration of the dead, a sentiment of which we seem to find a trace in the burial position of the Mousterian skeletons of Dordogne, lying on their side with the head raised on a pillow, dates from thousands of years before the historic period. The fact that the body is buried with the arm at the side suggests the possibility of the idea of the resurrection, of a life after death, which would thus be almost as old as man.

of a causal relation. This is immediately perceptible in the case of disease depending on external agents. The necessary and logical origin of the most ancient concept of the etiology of disease is to be found in the fact that in a great part of these diseases, such as wounds, surface lesions, and parasitic infections of the skin, one can easily discover the cause and often succeed in removing it. According to such a concept, it should be easy, or at least possible, to find for every disease the external and immediate cause. At the same time primitive man easily perceives the importance of the physiological fact of the secretions and of their relations to certain diseases. The marvellous phenomena of fertilization and birth, of the alternation of life and death throughout the whole organic world, suggest an explanation in a combination of factors that are not directly accessible to the senses and therefore supernatural, whether infinitely great or infinitely distant.

It is thus that is formed the concept that those manifestations of animal life or of disease where the cause is not visible, and therefore not attributable to demonstrable factors, must come from mysterious beings that bring about disease and death by their penetration into the body, like the parasites in man and animals that were well known to primitive people; or else that these manifestations are due to visible but far-distant agents whose phenomena primitive man could not explain, such as the stars or other heavenly or earthly bodies. Thus arose the conviction that the influence of certain stars could cause physical or pathological changes in the organism, especially in those instances where natural phenomena had an obvious element of periodicity, such as menstruation or intermittent fever. [The periodicity of menstruation is not always recognized by primitive people. Among the Australian aborigines, for example, menstruation is regarded as due to the bite of an insect or to a cold. *Ed.*]

This concept, which is common to all ancient peoples, would naturally also suggest systems of treatment. By removing the thorn, stone, or parasite, one got rid of the cause of the pain and of the lesion, and nature was allowed to go on to cure. In the same way arose the concept of the empirical removal of the visible or invisible cause of internal diseases, or, when physical removal is impossible, of casting spells that should lead to the cure of the disease. Searching in nature, in the action of the sun or moon, of the sea, thunder, or lightning, for the cause and the cure of his infirmities, man quickly learned to know the therapeutic value of natural forces: heat, the light of the sun, water. He observed the curative virtues of plants, perhaps led thereto by the example of animals, and found that some are poisonous and others produce certain more or less obvious results, while still others lessen the pain or cure the disease. It is thus that he came to regard as superior beings those majestic trees which spread their magnificent vegetation before his wondering eyes and still remain stupendous examples of a superhuman grandeur. This it is that proves how empirical medicine often is related to the magic concept, of which we find, at least in the case of plants, sure traces in the legends and traditions which are preserved in relatively late times, such as in the Biblical story of the tree of good and evil. We find the connection also in the rituals of ancient cults dedicated to trees, and in the custom, widespread in antiquity (such as among the Celts of ancient Scotland) but still met with in certain Nordic peoples, of hanging on trees clothes and objects belonging to the sick in order to obtain a cure. The tradition of " magic " plants to which was attributed a great healing power has been preserved in the frescoes of Pompeii and in our records of the Druids, essentially a medico-sacerdotal cult, and is kept alive even in our days.

3. Magic Medicine

Thus it is in empirical medicine that magic medicine, which is essentially empirical in its mode of thought, has its origin. If one believes that supernatural forces are the cause of disease, it is evident that to defend oneself against them or be cured, one must combat these malignant influences, whether they come from the stars or from unknown and distant forces, or whether they are caused by animals like the bird that flies at will through the air and seems to be a messenger of the celestial deities, or by the serpent that lives in the depths of the earth and thus is regarded as the bearer of the will of the dead. Beings that come from the infinite and unexplored regions of mystery have always stimulated belief in their importance by primitive races, and particularly in medical mythology do they play a most important role.

The aid of supernatural powers therefore becomes necessary, whether invoked directly or by means of deified and worshipped animals, or through men expert in the art of communicating with these superior beings and of exercising on them by prayers or threats a decisive effect capable of modifying the hostile act. And here we have in the thought of primitive man the idea of the struggle which takes place between the malignant and the good demon; here also the role of one or the other played by sacred animals or majestic trees; here also is the explanation of why primitive man seeks to avoid baleful influences by hiding from the sight of the evil demon. From this concept is derived the first origin of masks and of a whole series of rites, some of which are still preserved in popular superstitions. Such, for instance, is the symbolic chain placed about loved or holy individuals to guarantee preservation from harmful contacts (beads, phylacteries, etc.), or the rite of tabu, or changing the name of the patient in order to change his fate. Thence arises the power of those who have knowledge of the stars, of medicinal plants, of poisoned weapons (kinds of knowledge that have a special importance among primitive people), and who claim to possess means of triumphing over bad demons and of pacifying angry spirits and divinities.

Thus arise the first physician-magicians who know how to predict the future by observing the stars or natural phenomena or by examining the viscera of animals. They know, too, how to produce an effect on the human passions. Their power increases inordinately in times of epidemics or catastrophes which decimate entire populations, when the terror of the unknown makes the mind of man more than ever submissive to mystic influences. Thus arises suggestive therapy with its formulas and spells, as well as recourse to bones and ashes of the dead, to the claws and teeth of animals, carried about the neck. All such customs show the connection that existed in this ancient concept, and that is still preserved in many modern superstitions, between diseases and certain persons, animals, or things, to which is obviously attributed a notable role in producing disease or protecting against it.

To the same magic origin should be attributed the custom so widespread among primitive people of painting various designs of many colours on the skin. As a matter of fact, the underlying idea of the tattoo is probably none other than that of a form of defence against the evil demon, a sort of talisman. From this primitive medical concept many symbolic acts have found their way into the most ancient cultures. The religious dance — still in use among certain Oriental peoples — finds its origin in the characteristic movements of certain types of disease; the prayers written on scrolls of parchment and placed on the door of the house (*mezuzah*), prescribed by the Jewish religion, represent apotropaic rites — that is, they aim to turn away the evil demons. Many similar examples could be cited in all religions.

From the same order of ideas is derived an apotropaic concept that is widely diffused among primitive peoples: namely, that it is possible to substitute, figuratively or in reality, for the sick person, thus deceiving the evil demon and evading the danger. The substitution of one victim for another at the moment of sacrifice, as exemplified in the Biblical story of Isaac, but certainly of a much more ancient origin, is encountered in all the ancient mythologies. The change of name of the sick or dying person, the attempts to substitute for the sick one animals, plants, or other persons wearing masks, are still surviving customs which have their origin in this belief. On a similar basis are the beliefs of totemism, where the name or guise of an animal is assumed, and the individual is clothed in its skin in order to acquire its strength and courage and to place a whole group under its protection. It may be worth observing that the fundamental idea behind totemic practices is the establishment, in a symbolic way, of a blood kinship between the animals and the people of whom they are the ancestors. In order to commune with them the better, one dresses to resemble them. No less ancient is the therapeutic concept that believes it possible to utilize as medicine — swallowed or applied externally — the real or symbolic organs of animals or of enemies that have been killed. These are supposed to substitute for the deficiency of the sick organ or to augment its power.

Thus we meet, on the one hand, the custom of using certain organs to cure certain diseases; and on the other hand, the symbolic form of this concept in the use of amulets which simulate parts of the body, with the therapeutic aim of increasing the power of these organs. It is well known that the representation of the genital organs, which represent procreation and thus life itself, has been regarded from the most ancient times as a precious amulet, and that these symbols (to which we can attribute an apotropaic value) have been in general use throughout antiquity, and held their post of honour in the house. The origin of this idea can be attributed to the great role that sexual instinct plays in the life of primitive people, just as in the life of children. It dominates the manifestations of daily life and determines a complex series of actions which sometimes appear to us inexplicable just because they come from instincts that are submerged in the subconscious, and from primitive atavistic elements. It is to this complex of ideas that we owe (according to Freudian concepts) the phallic and, to civilized people, obscene pictures that are widespread among primitive people. The rites of the columns, of the huge stakes, of the monolithic monuments, sexual songs and dances that find their analogy in similar characteristic manifestations of some animals, will serve as examples. In the same way we must search in these instincts, which were much nearer the surface in our distant ancestors, for the origin of those mutilations and bloody rites which we shall speak of later.

It is an analogous mode of thought that selects as potent remedies those plants whose forms recall certain organs, a concept that we find in later centuries and even still existing in popular medicine (sympathetic magic, the law of signatures).

All these practices derive from the magic concept that we can regard as contemporary with or perhaps a little later than the empirical concept. The magic idea exists today in many places. Taylor has noted that the Malayans, for instance, attribute certain diseases to demons known as *bantu* and they believe that hemorrhage is caused by the flight of the demons from the body, an idea also found among more ancient peoples.

From this concept is logically developed in a later period the idea that at the moment of death the disembodied free spirit can abandon its mortal body, and that it can even temporarily leave its body during life, or have the spirit of another man or of a dead person or of a demon substitute for it or be subjugated to the other in its own body. This is undoubtedly suggested by such diseases as hysteria and epilepsy, during the attacks of which another spirit actually appears to have entered the body of the sick person. In another category are the impressions made on the imagination of man by dreams and those strange apparitions that are with difficulty separated from reality, duplications of the personality and similar occurrences that force consideration of a mysterious and unattainable world and of the interference that all this produces on the course of existence. These are phenomena to which are surely due the great importance attached to primitive religious practices, whether mystical or medical, and to the cult of the dead. These concepts establish a causal relationship between the wishes of the dead one and the living person whom he protects with his benedictions or persecutes with his imprecations.

It is in this atmosphere of mysticism and faith in which the life of ancient peoples is evolved, at the moment when vague superstitions are crystallized into precise customs and religious ideas, that there is born another concept, which has survived up to our time: namely, the persecution that the living and the dead can practise by the evil eye. What the origin of this belief may be it is difficult to determine. This interesting problem has been repeatedly the subject of extensive studies and we can perhaps accept the theory that the first origins of this idea are derived from the concept of the harmful influence exerted by evil spirits, whose presence in certain people is revealed by a particular colour or a certain expression of their eyes. It perhaps also has a relation to the very ancient concept that attributes to ill or perverse individuals the emanation of harmful humours that produce disease. Such a concept is the basis for a superstition, for example, that forbids women during the menstrual period to be near plants in flower. It is of considerable interest that modern physiological research has shown that menstrual blood contains substances that are harmful to plants and are not present in the blood at other times. Certainly the defence against the evil eye, to which has been attributed great malignant power since ancient times, constitutes one of the most important chapters in the therapy of primitive people. Amulets representing organs of man and of animals, especially eyes and genital organs, representations of animals, especially of insects, and of plants, these are the materials that have most frequently served for this purpose.

Magic medicine has been maintained practically unchanged almost up to our own day among people removed from their contact with civilization, as for instance in the Polynesian islands and in certain regions of central Africa and Australia. Particularly interesting, because better known and better documented, is the medicine of pre-Columbian America — Mayans, Aztecs, Incas, Araucanians. Scarification of the ears, lips, and tongue were prominent in their ritual, and the choicest of the race were offered as living sacrifices to the gods. Bloody rites played an important part with these people, and magic procedures were predominant. The artistic reproduction of pathological cases, and especially of skin lesions and destructive changes in the bones, appears to have been in use among the Incas living in ancient Peru. Such reproductions are often strikingly realistic, giving the impression that they have arisen from the desire for magical protection from terrible diseases. On the other hand, empirical medicine was well developed; its contribution to the therapeutics of the American Indians before the Spanish conquest is especially valuable. The anti-blenorrhagic property of pepper, the therapeutic virtue of yerba maté and of guarana, the stimulating effect of coffee, tea, cocoa, were all known to these peoples. They were acquainted with the twilight sleep of scopolamine and used the flowers of *Datura stramonium* (Jimson weed), which contains scopolamine as its active principle. The history of these peoples and the customs that are preserved in small groups of their descendants, who still exist in isolated parts of the American continent, give us a picture of the most obvious medical conditions in an early stage when magic and empiricism were completely dominant. Their magicians, too, possessed a gift of observation perhaps more profound than that possessed by us today, because it arose from a more acute sensibility as the result of long experience; this was an expressive and highly suggestive stock in trade and was linked with rational therapeutic procedures.

The Aztecs were skilled in the use of stone surgical instruments and employed rigid splints for fractures. The North American Indians, though living in the Stone Age as late as the nineteenth century, practised a medicine comparable to that of the great ancient civilizations. Demonistic in theory, and therefore often using charms and incantations — which were not without suggestive therapeutic value — their rational practices were numerous and efficient. They treated fevers with a liquid diet, purgation, diuresis, sweats (in special sweat lodges), and even with blood-letting. They used emetics, laxatives, carminatives, antispasmodics, and enemas, for digestive disorders; lobelia, flax, and other medicines, cupping and moxas, for respiratory disease, and so on. Stone lists 144 drugs used by the Indians for specific conditions, 59 of which are included in our modern

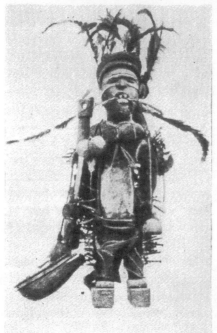 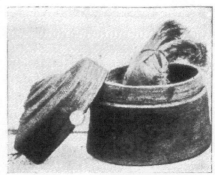

3a. *A figurine supposed to cause eczema and leprosy (South Africa).*
3b. *A box for magic implements and used to receive offerings.*
(CONGO MUSEUM OF TERVUEREN.)

pharmacopœia. Abdominal, and occasionally vaginal, manipulations were used in prolonged labour or to expel the placenta. The Indians were especially skilled in surgery, practising great cleanliness of wounds, and using sutures, cautery styptics, and poultices. They splinted fractures and reduced dislocations.

The medicine of the most ancient periods, then, was at first essentially empirical; on this basis was magic medicine then developed. Thus popular medicine stands in close relation to the observation of nature on one side and to magical beliefs on the other.

It is natural that those who practise medicine should be the same as those who know the virtues of plants and that animal poisons can cause the death of or damage to an enemy. These also are the ones who direct the sexual life of man and are in a position to predict the lot of the newborn or to ward off evil demons from him. It is they who can call forth or placate the shades of the dead, who teach the secret formulas of the conjurer and direct the religious dances. Thus, in order to guard their secrets, they quickly and necessarily constitute a separate or esoteric caste, bound by special rites and often by a secret and complicated system of initiations. Often secret, bloody rites are practised, because from the recognition of the importance of blood for life there is logically derived the idea of regarding it as the symbol of life itself and of a secret rite into which the profane must not penetrate. Customarily in primitive peoples, as in more ancient races, magicians loved to surround themselves with an appearance of mystery. The imposing colours of their vestments and implements, the skins of rare animals, sacred amulets, all contribute to give them the appearance of men different from others and therefore superior, and thus to give them the authority necessary for their calling.

But sometimes beneath this theatrical apparatus may be concealed real knowledge derived from the long continued study of nature, and beneath the clothing of the magician may be hidden the intelligent and expert physician. Search, then, among the mystic and symbolic practices that form the rich treasure of the primitive medicine of all people will often discover a kernel of truth, a foundation based on experience. One can say, without too much exaggeration, that at the bottom of all these practices, no matter how much they appear to be mere superstition, there exists some grain of truth. Among primitive peoples, too, there may be found customs and practices that have preceded the discoveries of scientific medicine. Experience has taught them from time immemorial the beneficent effects of drugs, the therapeutic value of which has scarcely been explored in recent times. The religious and mystic prescription of baths and of diet certainly has its origin in the recognition of the importance of these measures for certain diseases. The possibility of producing anesthesia by soporific potions was known, as is shown by the ancient use of mandragora. Certain ancient peoples, like primitive races today, attributed to certain colours a protective power against certain diseases. Thus the ancient Chinese, like the aborigines of New Zealand today, regarded the colour red as hostile to malignant spirits, and a red ribbon, necklace, or ring was worn as a sure defence against disease. We can perhaps find in early popular superstitions the germs of therapeutic concepts that are widely diffused today — not a cause for wonder when we realize that people of distant times vaccinated against snake-bite and anointed with the fat of poisonous animals.

Thus in the history of modern medicine we find, proved by scientific and clinical experiments, concepts and ideas that perhaps by intuition were familiar to men of ancient times.

4. Natural and Empirical Primitive Surgery

The surgery of primitive peoples possessed, even in the most ancient periods, an astonishing degree of technical efficiency. To be sure, the most ancient instruments were but sharpened stones that served to extract vari-

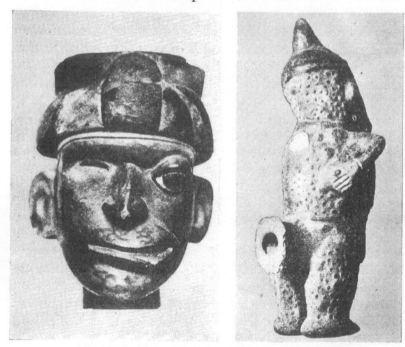

4. *Ancient Peruvian head showing facial paralysis and loss of an eye.*
From Holländer: Plastik und Medizin.
5. *An amphora of the Incas showing skin disease* (verruga peruana).

ous foreign bodies, to let blood, to open abscesses, to scarify; but they also served for more serious operations, such as trephining.

In 1875 Prunières and Brocard were the first to show that many millennia before our historic period, in the Neolithic period, trephining of the skull was frequently carried out — the most ancient operation of which we have objective evidence. It was easily established that trephining was performed — probably at first to remove splinters and fragments of the fractured skull and then perhaps for magical reasons — most frequently in the sincipital region, but also at times more frontally or in the occipital region. The operation was carried out with sharpened flints, moved rapidly in a circular fashion. Trephining was also practised on the cadaver, in order to remove from the skull of one previously trephined during life, who thus might have become thaumaturgic, small sections of bone (*rondelles*), which served as amulets. Such trephined skulls have been found in all parts of the world. This constitutes another example of the similarity of the medicine of ancient peoples with that of races living today in a lower stage of civilization. In fact, trephining by primitive methods was practised in

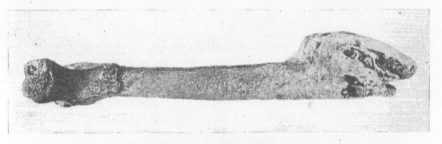

6. Prehistoric femur with healed fracture.

relatively recent times among certain tribes in the Bismarck Islands, in Bolivia and Peru, and was met by an English missionary, Ella, in 1874, in the practice among the inhabitants of the Loyalty Islands of making curious crosswise incisions of the skull along the coronary and sagittal sutures. Manouvrier found this same mutilation in a Neolithic skull and gave to it the name of the " sincipital T."

New growth of bone about the edges of the trephines shows that the operation was often followed by survival. Sometimes as many as five openings have been found in one skull, whether to secure amulets or to permit the escape of the demon in recurring convulsive states. In some instances squares of bone were removed by cross-hatched incisions. Modern students of this interesting subject have shown that the skull can be trephined in this way in little over a half-hour. The patient was usually, perhaps always, dulled or made unconscious with soporific potions. Trephining is still practised among many modern peoples — for instance, the Kabyles of northern Africa, the hill tribes of Dagestan, and people in many parts of Melanesia — and was practised in Europe among the Montenegrins.

All these operations owe their origin without doubt to a demonic or magic concept more than to the idea of therapy. It is in similar ideas that we should search for the origin of mutilations of the genital organs, operations that go back to the most distant times yet are still practised among uncivilized races. Ancient also is the use of infibulation, castration, and circumcision. The operation called *mica* (external urethrotomy), designed to imitate the female vulva and limiting procreation, is still in use among certain Australian people.

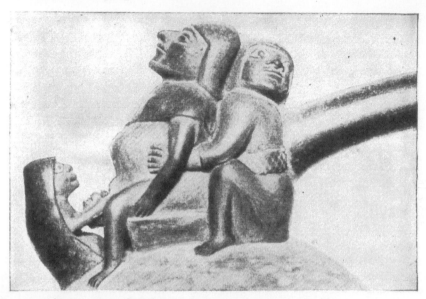

7. *Delivery, Peruvian Huaco.* (DAHLEM ANTHROPOLOGIC MUSEUM OF BERLIN.)

These mutilating operations sometimes replaced the human sacrifice that occurred among primitive people and they later assumed a symbolic significance. Circumcision is widespread in equatorial Africa, where it is called *ganza*. There it is almost always practised collectively, usually once a year, and separately for the two sexes. The young girls, usually fifteen or sixteen years old, are placed seated on the ground, thighs separated. The operator then removes the clitoris with a curved knife, but almost always mutilates the labia minora and sometimes the labia majora. In the region of Ubangi and Chari this ritual mutilation is widespread.

Surgery, then, followed the same lines that we have seen for medicine and therapeutics. Together with operations that had their origin in magic concepts, are to be found others that had a practical purpose. Thus in skeletons of very early periods one finds amputations and other evidences of rational operative intervention. Neolithic saws of stone and bone have been found with which limbs can be amputated in a few minutes. Knives, saws, files, and many other surgical implements were used in the Bronze Age.

The first and most ancient epoch of the history of medicine thus finds its parallel — we could almost say its faithful image — in the actual medicine of modern primitive races; and this should not astonish those who know that it is among these modern primitives that we can observe the forms of individual and social life of early man.

5. *Priestly Medicine*

From this primitive empirical and magical medicine priestly medicine was developed by logical necessity. With the development of religion in the satisfaction of a collective tribal need, castes were organized in which the practice of magical medicine was conserved as a traditional secret, possess-

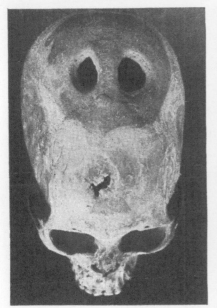 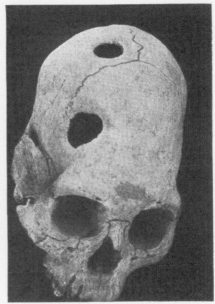

8. *Skull trephine.*   (ANTHROPOLOGIC INSTITUTE OF FLORENCE.)

ing the very great advantage of an assumed knowledge of superior benign or malignant forces. Perhaps ancient chiefs who had been victorious in their fierce struggles with the enemy and to whom popular opinion attributed unlimited power were the first to be regarded as capable of dominating natural forces, of foreseeing the future, and of curing diseases. Perhaps it was they who, invested with a mysterious power in the eyes of our distant ancestors, became the leaders of the first religions which appeared. Or perhaps, on the contrary, it was the priests of the earliest religions who, in the practice of their functions of mediating between man and the gods, naturally took to themselves also the greatest attribute of divinity in all times and places — namely, the power of life and death and hence the power of curing diseases.

Thus empirical medicine probably preceded magic and priestly medicine, but flourished along with them, sometimes relying on the power of men invested with supernatural gifts, sometimes growing in the shadow of mysticism. However this may be, when we study the history of religion — which is closely connected with the history of medicine, as religion and medicine strive essentially for the same end, the defence of the individual against evil — we note that as soon as religions began to take definite form, medicine changed from its first faltering footsteps and from daily contact with nature to enter the sanctuaries, which became for many centuries both its temples and its schools.

CHAPTER III

MESOPOTAMIAN MEDICINE

MAGIC AND PRIESTLY MEDICINE

1. Medical Concepts of the Most Ancient Civilizations

THE PERIOD of the pre-Hellenic culture of the eastern basin of the Mediterranean and of the plain between the Euphrates and the Tigris is usually regarded as going back to the fourth or fifth millennium before Christ. Obviously these dates cannot be regarded as definitely proved; but if, according to the calculations of Lepsius, we consider that in the last glacial epoch the greater part of Europe, Asia, and America situated above the latitude of 45° was extraordinarily cold, it is logical to think that the first civilization would be developed in its various manifestations especially in the great valleys where a temperate climate existed and the soil was more fertile and life easier. Actually we find the earliest civilizations along the Indus, the Euphrates, the Tigris, and the Nile, then spreading along the shores of the Mediterranean. To be sure, it is not possible to find definite documentation of the connections that undoubtedly existed between the most ancient peoples of Mesopotamia and of Egypt, between the oldest culture of central Africa and of the Nile, between the civilization of the Ægean and of the central plateaus of Asia. Perhaps when we become better acquainted with the medicine of regions which are still practically closed to our investigations, we can more easily evaluate the position of medicine in the Mediterranean civilization, which for five thousand years has been the scene of the most bloody wars, of political events of major importance, the

[31]

home of the monotheistic religions, the place where the arts and the sciences had their origin or at least their most intensive development. We can fix approximately the dates of the evolution of medical thought in its salient phases. We observe that in the fourth millennium before Christ there had begun to be formed in the people of southern Mesopotamia a systematic medical concept from which is derived Assyro-Babylonian medicine. In the second millennium Egyptian medicine attained an advanced development, at the same or almost the same epoch in which the maximum development of the Minoan civilization, of which we possess but few medical traces, was reached. A definite medical concept was formed by the people of Israel about 1500 B.C.; to Homeric medicine may be assigned the approximate date of 1000 B.C. The most recent studies of the civilization of the Hittites, of the inhabitants of the plateaus of Asia, and of central and southern America — especially Peru and Mexico — have shown us everywhere the existence of a primitive medical civilization surprisingly rich in pathologic observations, strikingly portrayed. But they have taught us nothing, however, that can throw light on prehistoric and primitive medicine. They represent transient forms, having many common characteristics, to be sure, of medical concepts more ancient than those that were crystallized in the civilization of the Mediterranean and Oriental peoples, which we shall consider more in detail.

Certainly the chronology that I have outlined is not only approximate but also tentative; because hardly a day goes by without new archæological discoveries that open new horizons for the history of medicine. The excavations undertaken in these regions show with certainty that two millennia before the golden age of Greece great civilizations that were far advanced in art, legislation, and forms of government had already flourished in the basin of Mesopotamia, on the banks of the Nile, and on the islands of the Ægean — civilizations that had many common basic characteristics for all the peoples of that period. This demonstrates, on the one hand, the frequent connections that early existed between these different peoples, and, on the other hand, the identical origin of certain fundamental ideas which obviously reached these civilizations from still more distant sources.

The material necessary for all these studies is still barely accessible to those who have not had special preparation. It is scattered in distant museums, published in reviews that are hard to obtain by scientists who are not specialists in archæology, and almost always offers many difficulties in interpretation.

The historical edifice, therefore, especially as regards medicine, is far from perfect; but at least it corresponds to the truth in its principal lines.

All memory of these great civilizations that have been engulfed by the march of time was already lost in the periods that followed soon after. But their medical thought left in its traditions, perhaps preserved by various colonies, traces which penetrated into Hippocratic medicine, which, though it seemed to be sudden and marvellous apparition, certainly was more or less directly attached to these ancient civilizations.

2. Astrologic Concepts

If we consider the medicine of ancient Mesopotamia, which is perhaps the most ancient of which we have thus far any clear knowledge, we see that it was dominated by a concept that was essentially magical and by a practice predominantly priestly. Astronomy was at that time the subject of intense study. In it we find the expression of a scientific medical principle, in the study of the relations which exist between the movements of the stars and the seasons and between these and the manifestations of certain diseases. The assumption of such relations between physiological facts and celestial phenomena contributed to the birth and development of the idea of the influence of periods, seasons, and stars on human life. We must not forget that the life of these peoples was pastoral and agricultural, and that it was passed on the banks of great rivers which flooded and periodically fertilized the neighbouring land. From this arose the great importance attributed to the sun, the first source of the fertility of the earth and the origin of every form of life. Here also is to be found the most obvious motive for the very important part attributed to water in religions and medical concepts — sometimes fertile and beneficent, but perhaps threatening and devastating. It is now easy to understand how, together with these early religions which had a basis on solar myths, astrologic medicine arose and flourished and even today, with various modifications, has not completely ceased to exist.

A comparison between the microcosm and the macrocosm suggested itself to these intelligent peoples, who were forced by the very conditions of their life to the observation of nature, an observation that was made accurate and penetrating by the custom of observing the most insignificant events that went on about them in the intense light that flooded those broad plains. It is obvious that an analogy should have been suggested to them between the waters that fertilized the earth and those that they had observed as having extreme importance in the life of vegetable and animal organisms. If it had not already been transmitted by vague, distant, primitive ideas coming from the time when man was more closely bound to the earth, it was at this epoch that was born the concept of an intimate union between man, plants, and animals, which found expression in the myths of metamorphoses which are to be found among almost all ancient peoples. These myths should seem less strange to those who are familiar with the modern doctrines of ontogenesis. In the same way arose from close contact with nature the idea of the resurrection of the individual, analogous to that of nature, and of life in another form after the death of the body. The impor-

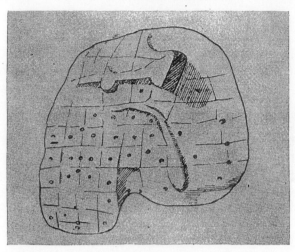

9. *Clay model of liver used by Babylonian priests to teach the art of the haruspex. Small pieces of wood were introduced into the holes. The superiority of this model (which should be compared with the Etruscan liver of Piacenza, Chapter xi) over mediæval representations of the liver should be noted.*

tant effects that rapid or violent alterations in natural phenomena produce in plants suggest that similar consequences might be expected in man; thus is born a pathologic concept according to which all phenomena of human life are regarded as parallel to those of nature. The study of the cuneiform tablets which have thus far been gathered, catalogued, and patiently studied has shown, even in the most ancient historical documents that we possess, a belief that the concourse of the stars determines the lot of man from birth onward. Just as an irregularity in the movement of the stars was regarded as of prognostic significance, so any modification in the birth processes was interpreted as an important augury, and the birth of monsters was taken as a precursor of great misfortunes. Jastrow (*Babylonian-Assyrian Birth-Omens*, New York, 1914) has shown that an unusually large organ or an anomaly of the right side indicated future strength or success, the same on the left side predicting weakness, failure, and disease. The influence of right-handedness or of the larger size of the right lobe of the liver here comes into consideration.

The first people that we meet in the history of civilization in Mesopotamia are the Sumerians, of whose racial origin we still are ignorant but who are found first established in Babylonia. According to the studies of Jastrow, it seems probable that they came to the plains between the Euphrates and the Tigris from some distant mountainous region. Their culture belongs in the fourth and perhaps the fifth millennium B.C.; their greatest expansion lasted until about 2500 B.C., at which period their civilization was supplanted by that of the Akkadians. Thus it is probable that the Sumerian civilization antedated the oldest hieroglyphic civilization of the Egyptians. The language of the Sumerians at first employed a writing that was purely ideographic. Figures and words were arranged in vertical lines proceeding from right to left. Shortly after, following the more general use of tablets of clay and stylets, it was changed into cuneiform writing composed of lines that went from top to bottom and from left to right. From the primitive ideographic writing can be drawn interesting conclusions about the concept that determined it. Representations of parts of the body to indicate single words are frequent. The breast and the abdomen are combined to indicate the pregnant woman; a method, as has been recently demonstrated, that is also met in later forms of writings.

These tablets, many of which have been interpreted by Oefele, may present entire medical works in serial form. One such composition, made up of twelve tablets, details a series of remedies of magic medicine. It begins with the words: " When the conjurer enters the house of the sick one "; an obstetrical book, which is made up of twenty-five tablets, begins with the words: " When the woman is sick."

These very interesting studies were important in guiding the interpretations of the tablets belonging to the celebrated Kuyunjik Collection in the British Museum, which contains the remains of the great library of King Ashurbanipal (668–626 B.C.) at Nineveh. Consisting of about twenty-five thousand tablets, this collection constitutes the chief source of our knowledge of Babylonian medicine. It now appears that the earliest medical tablets come from those distant times in which the kingdom was divided into two parts, a northern called Akkad, and a southern called Sumer. At the extreme north was Assur, and between the mouths of the rivers, Chaldea.

It is difficult to form an exact concept of the fundamental ideas of Sumerian medicine, which were from time to time adopted from the peoples which successively conquered the Assyro-Babylonian empire. It is fundamental, however, that medicine was essentially magic and that the most important role was attributed, as in all ancient magic concepts, to the blood as the carrier of every vital function. According to this concept, the liver, the organ in which all the blood is received, is the seat of the essential life processes. This concept was held by many Oriental peoples, who, attributing the most important role to the liver, hunted in its two lobes for the signs of destiny. In sacrificial animals the liver was examined first of all, to derive divinations and auspices from its form, position, and any irregularities that it might possess. This concept passed intact to Assyro-Babylonian medicine and to peoples even closer to us, especially the Etruscans, and evidence of it is found in Biblical texts. Thus Ezekiel says (xxi, 21): "For the King of Babylon stood at the parting of the ways, at the head of the two ways, to use divination; he made his arrows bright, he consulted with images, he looked in the liver." The central organ of the will is the ear which receives the commands and brings them to accomplishment.

More than forty of these tablets are concerned with the interpretation of dreams; some of them also contain therapeutic prescriptions as to the measures to be taken against the consequences of evil dreams. The physician designated under the name of *a-zu* — that is to say, " He who knows the waters " (water playing a preponderant role in incantations) — is at the same time an expert in interpreting dreams; but for the most ancient period of this civilization it has not yet been proved that the physician was also the priest. It is interesting to note that according to this concept the continuation of life is due to the renewal of blood by nourishment. Respiration, which assumes great importance in the medicine of ancient Egypt, is not even named. This need not cause astonishment if one remembers that the humours, their movements through the body, the results of disturbing this movement by loss of a precious fluid which is regarded as the seat of life or by interference with its course, were for these people the most notable phenomena of life. Thus medicine created a system of therapy essentially based on practices in which water and fire had the greatest importance, with prescriptions which certainly had a symbolic value, but which also had the support of success based on experiments. This is also true of baths, the application of hot and cold compresses, ablutions in rivers, all procedures that were connected at least in the first period with rites dedicated to the goddess Ea, who lived in the depths of the waters on which the earth floated like a balloon. To these prescriptions were added others purely ritual, accomplished with the aid of special prayers. Thus it was prescribed that in certain cases the patient should be bound or unbound while certain special formulas were being pronounced, so that he could be delivered from his disease. In the same way grains of wheat were scattered to be picked up with special ceremonies. Many prescriptions for this or that diseased organ are followed by indications to the physician of the measures to be followed with the patient. The command may be to abstain from all treatment when the intervention of the physician is hopeless.

3. Babylonian and Assyrian Medicine

The Babylonian and Assyrian conquerors of Mesopotamia inherited from the Sumerians their customs, laws, and doctrines, and to them we owe a great development of science and art. Babylonia, the centre of the Chaldean civilization, and Nineveh, already called the divine city in their ancient texts, were the homes of famous schools, which had their greatest development during the most splendid political, social, and commercial epoch in Mesopotamia. About the year 2000 B.C. the land between the Euphrates

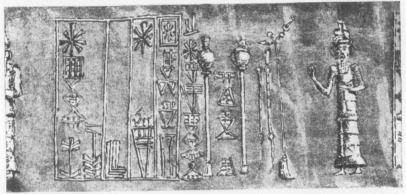

10. *Seal of the Babylonian surgeon Urlugaledin, about 2300 B.C. (enlarged).*
(LOUVRE MUSEUM.)

and the Tigris represented the centre of Mediterranean civilization. At this time, characterized by a firm and rigid administration of civil and military powers and governed by a powerful monarchy, medicine was entirely in the hands of a priestly cast.

Babylonia became the centre of a religious cult which attributed the greatest power to a triad of Heaven, Earth, and Water and to about twelve other lesser gods. The most ancient medical god of Mesopotamia was Sin, the god of the moon, who governed the growth of medicinal herbs, some of which for this reason should not be exposed to the rays of the sun. Plants had a close connection with divinity, as is shown by a number of tablets of the series *Maklu* (published by Tallqvist), in which the power of destroying malignant demons is attributed to plants. This concept of plants picked by moonlight and used to prepare medicines and magic philtres is met in other ancient races and also in modern popular medicine. To the greater divinities were attributed the most important functions in the lives of man and animals. Istar, the goddess of grace, is also the fecund Venus, the creator of libido in man and woman. In the cuneiform accounts of the deluge, she says that she will cause man to perish. Without her aid the fetus dies before birth. In the Semitic tradition she bears the name Jeledeth and much later appeared in the Greek pantheon under the name Eileithuia.

In a later period Babylonian medicine, which was taught under the auspices of Nabú, the god of the sciences and of the healing art for the Assyrians, or of Marduk, the god who healed the diseases of the Babylonians, was based on a magic symbolism. Signs and evil prophecies dominated human life completely. Marduk had the power to overcome disease and was the lord of the magicians; a large number of their incantations has been preserved in the Babylonian tablets. The procedure so closely recalls much more recent practices that this chapter of medicine well demonstrates how certain concepts, because they are indissolubly connected with the instincts and ideas that exist in the subconscious, have been preserved almost without change through the centuries.

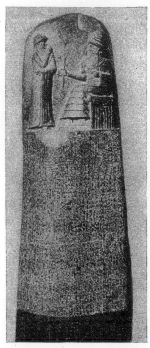

11. *Stele with the code of Hammurabi.* (LOUVRE MUSEUM.)

Ea was the special divinity of medicine, but an important part in medical mythology was also played by the goddess Ninchursag, to whom were related eight other divinities, each able to cure a special disease. The god Ninurta had the special rank of *azugallûtu*, chief of physicians, and was accompanied by his wife, Gula; another medical god was Ninazu, the lord of physicians, and his son Ningischzida; their attribute was the rod and serpent. The serpent Sachan was venerated as a symbol and as a healing god.

In Babylonia and in Assyria the practice of medicine was thus confided to a special caste, as is also shown by some seals of physicians that have been preserved. A seal attributed to the period of the King Gudea bears the representation of the god of health, Ninurta (or Adar), who holds in his hand a cupping instrument, while two other cups are placed on two columns. In the centre is a double scourge with two pieces of curved wood attached to straps for applying the cups. In the seal of Gudea the second name is that of the physician, while the first is that of the scarifier or operator, who ranks as a slave of the physician. This shows that already in those times the surgeon was regarded as belonging to a caste inferior to that of the physician and dependent on him. No less interesting is another seal of the same period in which is contained the name of the physician and the representation of his instruments.

The Assyrian and Babylonian physicians were often called into consultation as far as Egypt and were well repaid. Herodotus to the contrary notwithstanding, there were certainly specialists and popular physicians, some of whom treated the poor gratuitously. Some of the most renowned of these physicians are known to us, such as the famous Arad Nanai, who lived about 681 to 669 B.C. Many of his writings have been preserved, including prescriptions and letters of advice to the King, in one instance concerning a royal Prince with epistaxis, in another prescribing for one with severe ophthalmia. These physicians were neither magicians nor simple empiricists.

In various medical texts were described different fevers, apoplexy, phthisis, and the plague called by the name of *mûtânu* (pestilence). Mental diseases were distinguished, which were thought to be due either to wounds or to demons. There are descriptions of diseases of the eyes and the ears, of rheumatism, tumours, and abscesses, diseases of the heart and skin, and various venereal diseases. Toothache was thought by the Assyrians, as by the Egyptians, to be due to the gnawing of a worm, a common belief in Europe up to the time of John Hunter. Jaundice was attributed to the demon *axaxazu*, " who makes the body yellow and the tongue black." The demon *asakku* was regarded as the cause of consumption. Interesting are such descriptions of symptoms as this: " When a man has pains in the intestines and his food is not retained, is rejected from the mouth, and the stomach is as if perforated, and the flesh is macerated, and the wind moves hither and thither, and he cannot open his intestines, then the physician shall say . . ." The prescriptions are often very detailed. There is preserved a medical compendium written on clay tablets in cuneiform characters in which the text is divided into three columns; in the first is the name of the disease, in the second the drug, and in the third the method of using it.

The symptomatology of pulmonary tuberculosis is described with marvellous exactness: " The sick one coughs frequently, his sputum is thick and sometimes contains blood, his respirations give a sound like a flute, his skin is cold but his feet are hot, he sweats greatly, and his heart is much disturbed. When his disease is extremely grave his intestines are frequently opened. . . ." Even the idea of focal infection was considered: the physician to Ashurbanipal is said to have prescribed removal of the royal teeth to cure pains occurring in distant parts of the body.

These texts also contain descriptions of diseases of the extremities, of the tendons (*saggalu*), of the genital organs.

The drugs most frequently prescribed are the fruit, leaf, flower, bark, and roots of various plants: the lotus, olive, laurel, myrtle, asphodel, garlic, etc.; various parts and organs of animals; but also mineral substances such as alum, copper, iron. Many kinds of filth were prescribed, as is frequently the case among early peoples, perhaps so to disgust the demon that he will leave the body of the patient. Various preparations were used: pills, powders, enemas, etc.;

there were instruments to introduce medicines into the vagina or the rectum. Medical gymnastics and massage were frequently prescribed.

Among the most interesting documents are those which contain reports of the great physicians, about the diseases seen, the requests for drugs, concessions to special favourites or reproofs to individual physicians. The physician on his visits carried with him his case (*takâltu*), which contained his bandages (*sindu*), medicines, instruments, and so on. Thus one sees that Assyro-Babylonian medicine, however much dominated originally by magic concepts, from which it was never entirely freed, was eventually organized so that lay physicians conducted medical practice according to generally accepted standards.

The importance of the surgeon in ancient Mesopotamia is shown by the Code of Hammurabi, dating from about 1900 B.C., in which are contained certain very significant statements that regard the physician strictly as a professional and that show how frequently surgical procedures were carried out by these professionals. These statements have a very great historical value, because they established for the first time the concept of the penal and civil responsibility of the physician.

Concerning the wounds resulting from operations it is written: " If a physician shall produce on anyone a severe wound with a bronze operating knife and cure him, or if he shall open an abscess with the operating knife and preserve the eye of the patient, he usually shall receive ten shekels of silver; if it is a slave, his master shall usually pay two shekels of silver to the physician.

" If a physician shall make a severe wound with an operating knife and kill him, or shall open an abscess with an operating knife and destroy the eye, his hands shall be cut off.

" If a physician shall make a severe wound with a bronze operating knife on the slave of a free man and kill him, he shall replace the slave with another slave. If he shall open an abscess with a bronze operating knife and destroy the eye, he shall pay the half of the value of the slave.

" If a physician shall cure a diseased bone or a diseased organ, he shall receive five shekels of silver; if it is a matter of a freed slave, he shall pay three shekels of silver; but if a slave, then the master of the slave shall give to the physician two shekels of silver."

In this same code are indicated with a particular exactness the diseases of the slave which can annul the validity of a lay contract; two of these are cited frequently under the names of *bennu* and *siptu*, identified by some as epilepsy and leprosy, but by others as referring to other diseases, but always such as would prevent the patient from working. The expulsion of the lepers from the community — " Nevermore shall he know the ways of his abiding place " (Sudhoff) — indicates that the Babylonians were aware of the contagiosity of leprosy and took measures to combat it. Stone privies have been discovered in the relics of most of the early Mediterranean civilizations, while large stone drains suggest that the Babylonians used sewage systems.

The study of the Babylonian tablets shows that ancient civilization attributed to some small animals the character of carriers of disease and therefore of divinity. Thus, in Babylonian mythology, in which there is always a profound symbolic significance, the god of pestilence and destruction appears in the form of an insect with the name Nergal. It therefore may be maintained that even in those distant times, and starting from a magic ideation, the important part that insects played in the spread of infectious diseases had been observed or predicted.

4. Medical Concepts and the Practice of Medicine

This collection of laws, which contains regulations indicating far-advanced legal and penal concepts, shows that the practitioner of medicine in ancient Babylon was regulated by law, and that individuals and particularly surgeons practised the profession without belonging to the priestly caste. This is a very different state of Babylonian medical practice from that described by Herodotus (I, 80): " They bring out their sick to the market-place, for they have no physicians; then those who pass by the sick confer with him about the disease, to discover whether they have themselves been afflicted by the same disease as the sick person or have seen others so afflicted. . . . And they are not allowed to pass by a sick person in silence, without inquiring the nature of his distemper." One must remember that their medicine was bound to a cult, as is shown by many cuneiform texts in which prognosis and soothsaying bound to astrological facts had the greatest importance. Certainly, however, among these people culture had reached a high grade — the Babylonians had two well-developed astrological systems and several planetary systems; they knew the periodicity of eclipses, they were acquainted with the rising and the setting of the planets and their position relative to the sun. They calculated astronomical periods and the phases of the moon; they observed meteors and were well versed in mathematical studies (the divisions of the circle, mensuration by the sexagesimal system. the indications and names of the figures of the zodiac, the division of the months and the weeks, and the value of the connection between gold and silver based on the relation of the sun and the moon; all these are of Babylonian origin).

The Babylonian tongue was the diplomatic language of the eastern basin of the Mediterranean about 1500 B.C. The Babylonian culture, and especially mathematics, architecture, and sculpture, had reached a high grade of development.

People who had penetrated deeply into the secrets of the movements of the stars, who had divined the periodical laws that ruled the heavens in their various phases and were repeated on earth, necessarily formed an

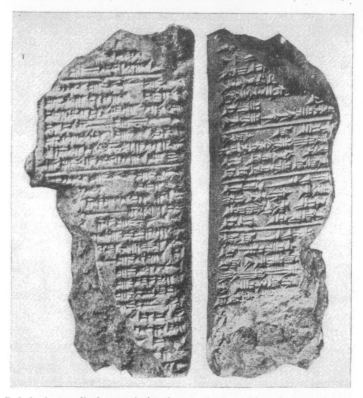

12. *Babylonian medical prescription in cuneiform writing.* (BRITISH MUSEUM.)

astronomical and mathematical concept of the universe and of the powers that governed it. From this concept comes the great importance attributed to numbers which was spread through the whole Orient. The number 7, closely related to the phases of the moon, became the centre of metaphysical speculations and symbolic practices, preserving the same character and the same importance in all the Oriental religions.

The Babylonian religion and philosophy culminated in the acceptance of unique and supreme laws which regulated both macrocosm and microcosm and were manifest in all, even the most minute forms of life. These laws were ineffaceably written in that great book of nature, the firmament, in which it therefore became possible to decipher the laws that governed living beings on the earth.

Thus from the simple concept of the causal relations between celestial phenomena and the manifestations of organic life, we arrive at a philosophic concept from which arose a form of religion which was closely connected with study of the heavens. In the same way, naturally, are related the

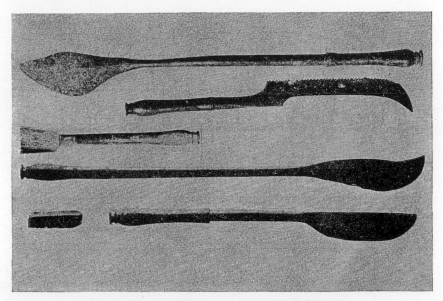

13. *Babylonian surgical instruments of bronze from Nineveh.*
(Collection of Prof. Meyer-Steineg.)

phenomena which develop in the human organism. Thence we have the alternation of health and disease, the appearance of pathologic phenomena at certain periods. Such factors point Babylonian medicine both to astrology and to the religion connected with it; but at the same time the empirical concept transmitted from prehistoric times is guarded solidly on what we might call its terrestrial basis.

The nature, then, of Assyro-Babylonian medicine is above all magical and empirical; everything depends on metaphysical forces represented or symbolized by the stars; but on the other hand, just as the stars exert their effect on the forces of nature, just as the tides depend on the changes of the moon, so the movements of the humours of the human body, in which life resides, also depend on the influence of the stars. Later a caste of lay physicians and surgeons is formed which practises the profession according to determined laws.

The barbarian invasions that destroyed the kingdom at the beginning of the seventh century B.C. removed all traces of the ancient civilization and marked with the destruction of Nineveh the end of the glorious period of Assyro-Babylonian history. Most of the monuments of that magnificent civilization disappeared also, a civilization characterized by the particular development of the mathematical discipline. But, as we shall see, the fundamental ideas and the most important progress made by the Assyro-Babylonian civilization are to be found in the medicine of adjacent peoples, or those who had the most frequent contacts with Babylon.

Certainly Babylonian medicine represents a closed system, organically constructed on concepts that were partly erroneous, but justified by the environmental conditions in which it arose. It appears to be an eloquent proof of the advanced stage of civilization of a people skilled in calculation and observation, who were skilful merchants and shrewd speculators. Its fundamental note is the comprehension of the close relations between man and the universe; but if, as we shall see, it is less scientific in the search for objective facts than the Egyptian civilization and less far advanced in its legislative regulations than the Jewish, it nevertheless represents an extremely interesting period of development. In the story of the peoples who lived between the Euphrates and the Tigris we see the slow evolution of demonic medicine into priestly and lay medicine, with a persistent retention of empirical medicine. We observe a notable enrichment of drug therapy and we see arise from an exact evaluation of natural phenomena the first and important concepts of hygiene and social medicine. These were the first people who concerned themselves with human anatomy as well as with that of animals, and who first codified the responsibility of the physician. Thus even in much later civilizations, we find the traces of the ancient *a-zu*, he who knows waters and the stars, the plants and the organs of animals, master of the art of exorcizing demons, but also an intelligent and sharp observer of nature.

CHAPTER IV

OLD EGYPTIAN MEDICINE

PRIESTLY MEDICINE, ORIGINS OF THE
PHILOSOPHIC CONCEPT

1. The Origins of Egyptian Medicine

WHILE a great civilization was becoming established in Mesopotamia, parallel to it and perhaps independently was developed the civilization of the people that inhabited the valley of the Nile. In this civilization were two main influences: one that came from the people of Nubia and other regions in central Africa, who were conquered in long wars during the first dynasty; the other from the Orient, and therefore not only from Mesopotamia but also from other Oriental countries that had frequent commercial relations with ancient Egypt. Examining the development of medical culture in Egypt we should remember above all that the period of this development includes five or six millennia, that the early documentation is very scanty and mostly on papyrus — a very fragile material and that the medical knowledge that we find in the oldest texts certainly represents the product of several previous millennia. On the other hand, considering the political history of ancient Egypt, long divided into two kingdoms often at war one with the other, dominated successively by sovereigns belonging to different races, governed in provinces some of which had acquired considerable autonomy, influenced by seasonal phenomena that often changed from easy to miserable circumstances, it is evident that one cannot speak of a precise evolution of medical thought in Egypt, with an orderly advance as to both time and form. Just as in various provinces and cities of the kingdom different divinities were worshipped, different laws were in force, and different dialects were spoken, so the differences in medical knowledge and in the practice of the art are no less noteworthy at various

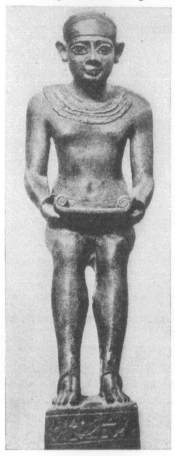

times and places. Certainly Egyptian medicine was predominantly mystic and priestly in those times in which the Oriental influence prevailed and in those parts of Egypt that had the most frequent contact with the Orient. It was chiefly empirical and realistic in those places where the contact with nature persisted longest and where the influence of the most ancient African civilizations was longest felt. For this reason the medical history of ancient Egypt must be limited to collecting the most important events and characteristic phases of a long and complex process of evolution, reconstructing merely the general outlines from the documents that are preserved for us.

In Egyptian mythology, which underwent constant and noteworthy changes according to different times and places, the gods concerned with health had an important place. The control of health was attributed more or less to all the gods. The most important position belonged to Thoth, who, according to the ancient legend, cured Horus from the sting of a scorpion, and in the struggle between Horus and Set treated the wounds of both. In the medicine of the Alexandrian epoch he became identified with Hermes Trismegistus, the master of the ancient mysteries. He is the most ancient of the healing gods and a specialist for the commonest

14. *Imhotep, the Egyptian God of Medicine.* (CAIRO MUSEUM.)

of all Egyptian diseases, ophthalmia. No less frequent are the invocations to Isis, the great enchantress who cured Ra; her word "brings to life him who was no longer living." The goddess Sechmet has a special power in curing diseases of women, and a physician of the King Schurè of the old kingdom had the attribute "*Sechmetua' e ônch* (Sechmet is for me life)," perhaps because he was a specialist for women's diseases. For the God Set, who was the special incarnation of the malignant spirit, was reserved the function of spreading and also healing epidemic diseases. But the special god of medicine is Imhotep, the son of Ptah, of whom we find many bronze statuettes. He was probably a king or a priest, expert in medicine, who lived at the time of the third dynasty. Temples, sanctuaries, and probably sanatoria bearing his name were erected to him at Memphis, which seems to have been the most important site of his cult, attaining to particular splendour in the period of the Ptolemies. The Hermetic literature attributes to him the highest healing powers, and compared to his, the cult of Serapis is of lesser importance. It is probable, as Maspero supposes, that the Ebers Papyrus belonged to one of his sanctuaries. A surprising number of details have come down to us about the earthly existence of this god of medicine, whose cult anteceded (2850 B.C.) that of Æsculapius by many centuries. Thus Hurry (Jamieson B. Hurry: *Imhotep*, 2nd ed., 1928, Oxford University Press) gives the place, day, and month (but only the approximate year, 3000 B.C.) of his birth, the names of his parents, and details of his activities as Grand Vizier, architect, chief lector priest, sage and scribe, astronomer, magician-physician. Apparently Imhotep was first worshipped as a medical demigod, as was Æsculapius also, a process that for Imhotep began within a few centuries of his death. His apotheosis as a full deity occurred about 525 B.C., when Egypt became a Persian province. At this time he replaced Nefertem, to form with Ptah and Sechmet the great triad of Memphis. The name Imhotep (I-em-hetep) signifies: " he who cometh in peace."

The kings of the ancient dynasties also appear to have been closely connected with the practice of medicine. According to tradition the son of King Menes, the founder of the first Egyptian dynasty, was the author of anatomical books. The Ebers Papyrus (CI, I) and the Brugsch Papyrus (XV, I) suggest that in the reign of Casti, the fifth king of the first dynasty, the anatomy of the veins may have been studied. King Zoser, of the third dynasty, bore the name *Sa* (healer) and in the inscriptions of the temple was given the title of " Divine Physician." The earliest king to appear in the full light of history was Snofru, the first king of the fourth dynasty, to which historians assign the period of *c.* 2830–2530 B.C., the period of the old kingdom, in which the construction of the Pyramids was begun. Though no texts of the old kingdom have been preserved, a tomb inscription (2600 B.C.) already speaks of a chief physician and his medical chest; and about 2400 a certain Iri was named as chief of the court physicians, with the quaint title of " Shepherd of the Rectum." Already such specialties as diseases of the eye and abdomen were recognized, and teeth were being held together with gold bands.

The accurate study of Egyptian mummies, which we owe especially to the careful work of Sir Armand Ruffer, with a technique which permitted the accurate diagnosis of pathologic changes and the confirmation of the diagnosis by microscopic studies, has furnished interesting information about Egyptian palæopathology. Thus it has been possible to establish the existence of arteriosclerosis in the mummies of the twenty-first dynasty (*c.* 1000 B.C.); in the kidneys of other mummies of the same period have been found ova of bilharzia. Ruffer supposes that the relative rarity of this disease in ancient Egypt was due to the ibis, which fed on the small mollusks that harbour the larva of bilharzia. In the prehistoric necropolis of Rhodes there was found the skull of a young

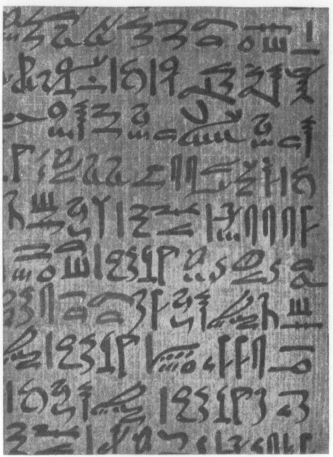

15. *Part of the Ebers Papyrus.*
(MUSEUM OF THE UNIVERSITY OF LEIPZIG.)

woman that showed a serpigenous ulceration with perforation of the bone. Loret claims that this is a luetic lesion, but this hypothesis has been bitterly contested. Often tuberculous lesions of the vertebræ are found; in some places with such frequency that the idea is suggested that the burial places belonged to sanitaria. In 1908 Elliot Smith found the mummy of a woman who had died a few days after having had a fracture of the forearm. This had been treated with a splint composed of strips of wood held together with twine.

Although medical texts belonging to the period of the Pyramids have not been found, it is certain that the earliest extant texts (1500–2000 B.C.), from their length and the medical knowledge that they contain, can be regarded as deriving from this period.

The sources for the history of Egyptian medicine are found in a number of medical papyri, the three most important of which are: the Ebers Papyrus, the Brugsch Papyrus, and the Edwin Smith Papyrus. Another important papyrus is the Kahun Medical Papyrus, discovered in 1889 by Sir Flinders Petrie in the Faiyum. Ascribed to the twelfth or thirteenth dynasty (c. 2000–1800 B.C.), its legible fragments show that it dealt entirely with gynæcology. The date at which the Ebers Papyrus was written can be reckoned from its astronomical systems as being between 1553 and 1550 B.C. It is a collection of medical texts, twenty metres in length, in a perfect state of preservation. It was discovered by Ebers at Luxor in 1873 and is now in the museum of the University of Leipzig. The date just given is the one at which it was committed to writing. Its contents certainly belong to a much more ancient period, and the role of the writer was to compile zealously a collection of the best-known texts of his time. It is one of the six medical writings that Clement of Alexandria notes among the forty-two Hermetic books of the Egyptians. The Brugsch Papyrus, at the Berlin Museum, is regarded by Hearst as having been written about 1200 B.C.

This papyrus and the Edwin Smith Papyrus, which is to be regarded as earlier than the Ebers Papyrus but more limited in content, and certain other smaller papyri have served to give us an excellent picture of Egyptian medicine as it was conceived and practised in the second millennium. To be sure, certain parts of these documents obviously reflect foreign influences, but this does not detract from their importance; in fact, they contain the most ancient and valuable documents that have come down to us from that ancient civilization. Religion and magic, astrology and incantations, charms and demonological writings are found here mixed with clear indications for surgical operations, with shrewd diagnostic observations, with rational prescriptions, and good hygienic regulations; so that Oefele supposes, probably correctly, that in these papyri, and especially in the Ebers Papyrus, are gathered together the writings that appeared on the walls of the temple of Heliopolis, which was also a great sanatorium.

2. Medicine and Surgery according to the Ancient Texts

The Egyptian concept of life differs from that of Assyro-Babylonia in that, while the latter regarded the liver as the centre of the blood supply and the seat of life, the Egyptian found the most important and most characteristic vital function in respiration. The Egyptians believed that the cessation of respiration preceded the failure of the blood, and thus they attributed to respiration the most important vital role. Thence arose the pneumatic concept which is characteristic of Egyptian medicine. The blood, however, was of great importance to the Egyptians. *The Book of the Dead* tells how the gods Hu and Lia arose from the blood that fell from the penis of the sun god, Ra, when he mutilated himself. Mummies were painted red to confer on them the strength of blood, and amulets of reddish stones, typifying the blood of Isis, were used for the same reason.

The anatomical knowledge of the Egyptians was perhaps less superficial than appears from the study of documents, which, being dedicated exclusively to the practice of medicine, did not take notice of theoretical concepts. It is true, to be sure, that mummification, from which it would be logical to expect that much anatomical knowledge would be derived, was generally done by technicians and not by physicians. But nevertheless we must accept that these procedures, repeated through thousands of years and carried out with a special care on the bodies of the rich or socially prominent, and the frequent dissection of animals for religious purposes, must have offered a sure foundation for anatomical knowledge. The heart was recognized in the Ebers Papyrus as the centre of the blood supply, as was also the fact that " there are vessels attached to it for every member of the body." Dawson points out that it is also stated that the motion of the heart can be detected not only in the region of the heart itself, but by placing the fingers on the head, the hands, the arms, and the legs. The noteworthy progress in the field of surgery shows that the distribution of the most important vessels was known to Egyptian surgeons, also the anatomy of those organs which were most frequently submitted to operation. In spite of the untold opportunities for the *taricheutes* to examine human viscera, however, Egyptian knowledge of anatomy was based mostly on that of animals — thus the hieroglyph for " uterus " was bicornate; for " heart," one shaped like that of a cow; for " throat," the head and windpipe of cattle.

The concept of the causation of disease was essentially a parasitic one, and is easily understood when one thinks of the importance of parasites in the etiology of diseases of tropical countries. It is even met in legends. Thus Ra, the god of the sun, falls sick because a worm, born from his sputum, bites him in the heel; Horus, the son of Osiris and Isis, was stung by a scorpion. In Egyptian pathology the animal becomes the symbol of disease; so that in those diseases in which the parasite is not visible, an invisible worm is imagined. It is to expel the parasites from the body that various magic procedures and spells are utilized.

The importance that worms, insects, and other parasites have in Egyptian pathological concepts is also shown by the fact that graphic reproductions of these animals are common in mural paintings and comprise an essential part of some hieroglyphs that indicate disease. Biological knowledge was considerable; the Egyptians knew of the evolution of insects from larvæ and were familiar with many phenomena of animal life. Swellings were described by at least six different words. Though we do not know their exact significance today, some obviously referred to boils and carbuncles, and to bilharzia infection, which is still prevalent in Egypt. Diseases of the eyes and skin appear, from the number of prescriptions preserved, to have been of great importance. Mastoid disease, alopecia, various fevers, and rheumatoid affections were also prescribed for. Uterine disorders such as dysmenorrhœa and prolapse, vaginal disease, and scanty lactation are treated in the Ebers and the Kahun papyri. Syphilis was not recognized; even its existence in ancient Egypt is denied by some. Dental caries appears to have been uncommon until the luxurious times of the Pyramid age. The poorer people of the earliest periods are found with worn teeth, exposed pulp, and alveolar abscesses, due to the coarse food, admixed with sand. Chronic arthritis has been found in mummies and poliomyelitis represented in sculpture. A case of Pott's disease with psoas abscess, examples of arteriosclerosis and calcification, gall-stones, appendicial and pleural adhesions, and achondroplasia indicate that human disease has not essentially changed since the earliest times.

Diagnosis already appears to have reached a fairly advanced position among the physicians in the periods from which documents have been preserved. They distinguished various abdominal affections, diseases of the heart, menstrual disturbances, diseases of the tonsils, a number of diseases of the eye, various tumours, and especially those of the spleen and the liver, which were indicated by differential symptoms, with considerable precision. The Egyptian physician not only knew of the importance of the examination of the pulse, of palpation and inspection, as is clearly shown in plastic reproductions, but he also appears to have been acquainted with auscultation, as may be seen in the phrase from the Ebers Papyrus; " Here the ear hears beneath. . . ."

As to therapeutics, we find, as in the medicine of all ancient peoples, a mixture of mystic and rational therapy. There is reason for believing that the rational therapy is the more ancient and represents the basis of Egyptian medicine, while probably the symbolic rites and magic treatment represent later interpolations.

The papyri that have been mentioned contain an enormous number of prescriptions. The Ebers Papyrus alone contains almost a thousand, the components of which are not yet all known to us. We find that among the remedies most used by the Egyptians were: honey, beer of various kinds, yeast, oil, dates, figs, onions, garlic, flaxseed, fennel, and so forth. Other medicines often prescribed were myrrh, aloes, lettuce, crocus, opium, and various lead preparations; parts of organs of various animals were often used (the fat, the brain, excrement, blood): of the hippopotamus, croco-

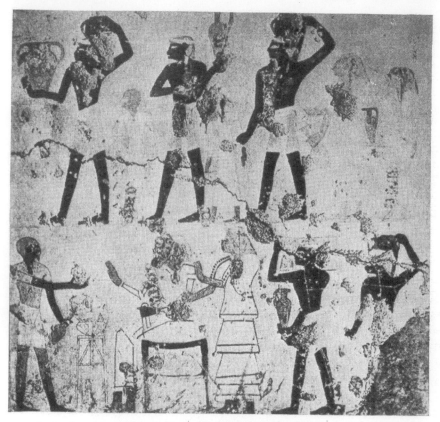

16. *An Assyrian ruler consults an Egyptian physician. Painting on the tomb of Nebamon, Royal Physician of Amenofis II (fifteenth century B.C.). The physician is offering the ruler the medicine which he has poured from a bottle into a cup. Slaves are carrying gifts for the physician.*

dile, gazelle, deer, numerous birds, reptiles, fish, and so forth. Minerals, such as salt, alum, antimony, copper, sodium carbonate, and others not yet identified were also utilized. Dawson describes the use of castor oil (*degam* or, later, *kiki*, according to Herodotus, Dioscorides, Oribasius, and others) for the scalp, as an ointment for foul sores, and as a temple illuminant, as well as for its purgative action. Medicines were prescribed in all the forms still in use today, in pills and in suppositories, whose form and function were accurately indicated, both to provoke evacuations and to lessen pain.

They were also introduced into the vagina for therapeutic purposes. There are many directions for the preparation of emetics, enemas, poultices, and ointments. Mention is made of a metal instrument heated white hot to stop hemorrhage. " Cure him with the knife and then burn him with fire so that he will not bleed too much " (CVIII, p. 192). Vaginal irrigations are also advised (XCV, p. 174).

The Ebers Papyrus begins as follows: " Here begins the book of the preparation of medicines for all parts of the body of a person. I was born in Heliopolis with the priests of Het-Aat, the lords of protection, the kings of eternity and of salvation. I have my origin in Sais with the maternal goddesses who have protected me. The Lord of All has given me words to drive away the diseases of all the gods and mortal sufferings of every kind. There are chapters for this my head, for this my neck, for these my arms, for this my flesh, and for these my limbs, to punish the supreme beings who allow disease to enter into this my flesh, placing a spell on these my limbs, so that [disease] enters into this my flesh, into this my head, into these my arms, into this my body, into these my limbs, whenever Ra has taken mercy and has said: ' I protect him against his enemies.' It is his guide Hermes who gave him the word, who created the books and gave glory to those who know everything and to the physicians who follow him to decipher that which is dark. He whom the god loves is made alive; I am the one whom the god loves, me he makes alive, to pronounce words in the preparations of medicine for all parts of the body of a person who is sick. As it should be a thousand times. This the book of the healing of all diseases. May Isis heal me as she healed Horus of all his pains which his brother Set inflicted on him because he killed his father, Osiris. O Isis, thou great enchantress, heal me, deliver me from all wicked, evil, typhonic influence, from the demonic and mortal diseases and impurities at all times which are precipitated upon me, just as thou didst free and save thy son Horus " (after H. Joachim's translation, Berlin, 1890).

We include certain examples of medical prescriptions and indications for intervention of the physician:

" If you examine a person who suffers from pains in the stomach and is sick in the arm, the breast, and the stomach, and it appears that it is the disease *uat*, you will say: ' Death has entered into the mouth and has taken its seat there '; you will prepare a remedy composed of the following plants: the stalks of the plant *tehua*, mint, the red seeds of the plant *sechet;* and you will have them cooked in beer; you will give it to the sick person to drink, then you will put your hands on the sick person and his arm will be easily extended without pain, and then you will say: ' The disease has gone out from the intestine through the anus, it is not necessary to repeat the medicine.' "

" If you examine a person who suffers in the region of the stomach (*ro-áb*) and vomits frequently, and you find a protuberance in the anterior parts, and his eyes are tired and the nose is stopped, then say to him: ' It is a putrefaction of the excrement, the excrements are not passing through the intestines'; prepare for him: wheat bread, absinthe in large amounts, add to it garlic steeped in beer, give the patient to eat of the meat of a fat beef and a beer to drink composed of various ingredients, in order to open both his eyes and his nose and to create an exit for his excrement " (XXXIX).

" To drive away inflammation of the eyes have ground the stems of the juniper of Byblos, have them steeped in water, and apply it to the eyes of the sick person and he will quickly be cured " (LVIII).

" To cure granulations of the eye you will prepare a remedy of collyrium, verdigris, onions, blue vitriol, powdered wood; you will mix it all and apply it to the eyes of the sick person " (LVIII) (from the translation by Joachim).

We are able to construct a fairly exact picture of the history of Egyptian surgery on account of the numerous documents that we possess. Among the surgical instruments used, first of all comes the knife, which probably was made of stone in the earliest times, then of bronze or of iron. Iron was believed to have been used in Egypt as early as 1600 B.C. Knives were used to cut hair, to open abscesses — those near the ear, for example — and to extirpate tumours. In the chapter that treats of wounds, the method of dressing them is exactly prescribed: a bandage of linen is used, impregnated with myrrh and honey, and is left on for four days. Numerous remedies are prescribed for burns. There are exact prescriptions for the treatment of tumours, and especially for tumours of the neck, which were apparently more frequent and better known. They were treated with the knife.

Circumcision was in use among the Egyptians, Ethiopians, and Copts, even in the most ancient times, as is shown also by the fact that in many monuments the virile organ is represented without the prepuce. In the prehistoric cemetery of Naga-adder, one hundred miles north of Luxor, Elliot Smith found that all the male corpses, which dated from about the fifth millennium B.C., were circumcised.

According to the Ebers Papyrus, circumcision was performed at the age of fourteen. It is represented in a figure in the little Temple of Khons at Karnak, which belongs to the period of Rameses II, of the nineteenth dynasty (about 1392 B.C.).

The studies of Peyron on the Greek papyri in the British Museum show that circumcision of girls also was in general use in Egypt. In one of the six papyri is contained a complaint by the Egyptian citizens living in the Serapeion of Memphis against a mother who had not had her daughter circumcised although she had reached the proper age according to Egyptian custom. The circumcision of girls consisted in excision of the prepuce of the clitoris.

The Edwin Smith Papyrus is not only the oldest known medical writing but also the most complete and important treatise on surgery of all antiquity. Acquired at Luxor in 1862, it was given to the New York Historical Society by Smith's daughter in 1906. In 1920 Breasted began his careful study of the document, which culminated in a magnificent publication (1930) with the collaboration of Dr. Arno B. Luckhardt, who paid particular attention to the interpretation of the words indicating diseases and their treatment. It was

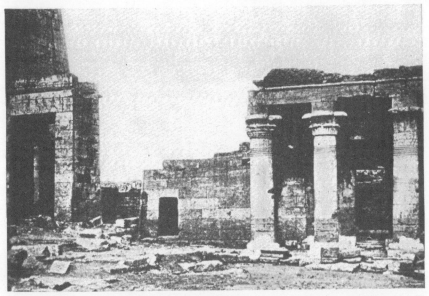

17. *The Temple of Imhotep on the island of Philæ. The entrance is between the columns on the right. From J. B. Hurry:* Imhotep (*Oxford, 1928*).

written about 1700 B.C. and was evidently a copy of a much more ancient manuscript written about 3000 B.C., and thus more or less contemporaneous with the great Pyramids.

The papyrus, which has been completely reproduced in beautiful plates that carry the translation at one side, is an account of forty-five traumatic lesions and of some surgical diseases of the thorax. It constitutes a most valuable and unique book in the history of surgery. All the cases are accurately described in more or less the same form, beginning with the result of the objective examination and passing to diagnosis, prognosis, and treatment. In most cases the favourable prognosis is expressed with the words: " I [the physician] will cure this disease "; if the prognosis is doubtful: " Nothing can be done in this case "; or if unfavourable: " The patient will die."

The systematic arrangement of the book shows that it was evidently intended to be a textbook of surgery; fortunately a great part of the text has been preserved. Though the papyrus contains no clue as to the author's name or position, Breasted believes (p. 9) that there is good evidence that this surgical treatise was written in the Old Kingdom (3000–2500 B.C.) and presumably in the earlier part of that remote age. He even suggests that it may have been written by Imhotep himself and that it may be the "Secret Book of the Physician" quoted in the Ebers Papyrus. The document is imperfect in that, starting with injuries of the head, it stops with an uncompleted account of a sprain

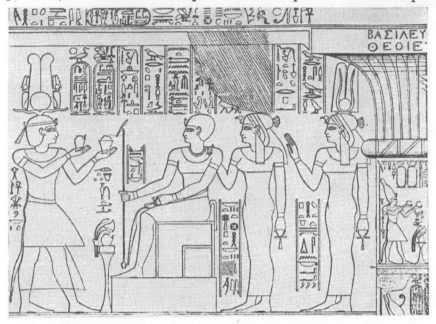

18. *The Pharaoh Ptolemy V worships Imhotep and other divinities. From the Temple of Philæ. From J. B. Hurry:* Imhotep *(Oxford, 1928).*

of the spinal column, omitting all consideration of abdomen and lower limbs. The clinical observations are so accurate and clear that it does not appear possible to the physician who reads these pages today that five thousand years have passed from the time in which an acute observer and expert operator collected the results of his rich experience to serve him in teaching. If the supposition of the great American Orientalist is true, or even if the period in which the original text was written will have to be brought forward by several centuries, we must accept in any case that this medical work presupposes the long preparation of many centuries, perhaps of millennia, before such a clear concept of pathologic symptoms could be reached or such an exact estimation of prognosis arrived at.

It is worth noting that often it is prescribed to sound the wound; frequently operative intervention is indicated. Medical applications are limited to the use of ointments, astringent substances, and dietary prescriptions. Bandages for fractures and dislocations are accurately described; in the case of a depressed fracture of the skull, the need for removing the bony fragments with an elevator is stated. Interesting also are the directions that the edges of the wounds should be closely applied to each other and that they should be so bandaged that they are held closely in place. For dislocations the procedure of reduction is accurately given; thus in the case of dislocation of the clavicle and the scapula the patient lies on a bed and the proper position is obtained by movements of the arm, the details of which are explained. The author notes that in wounds of the œsophagus water issues from the wound when the patient drinks. He notices paralysis of the bladder and of the intestines in lesions of the spinal cord. It is in this book that the brain is mentioned for the first time in history, its convolutions and meninges, showing clearly that it was recognized as the site of mental functions. It is with profound wonder that we recognize the knowledge of the suture of wounds and of the possibility of improving the appearance of old people with plasters which remove the wrinkles of the forehead. It is to be noted also that throughout this very ancient and valuable surgical text the employment of magic is spoken of only once, while there is frequent mention of the art of the physician.

The truly exceptional importance of this book is derived not only from the fact that it accurately described a series of surgical cases, outlining the proper diagnosis, prognosis, and treatment, but also from the obvious deduction that even in this remote period there already existed organized schools of medical practitioners, well versed in surgery, independent of the priestly castes, and not without some anatomical knowledge.

3. Hygienic Legislation

In the field of hygiene Egyptian medicine reached a high degree of progress and it may be stated that there existed a true social medicine, even if in rudimentary form.

Detailed regulations were in force for the burial of the dead; strict rules prescribed methods for cleaning dwellings, for normal diets, for sexual relations; so that the entire daily life of the Egyptians was regulated by precise laws clothed in the form of religious regulations. There is in Egyptian medicine, as in ancient Babylonian medicine, a combination of empirical rationalism with mysticism, which constituted a valuable basis for the further development of medical science.

In Egyptian medicine, also, it is often difficult to distinguish between hygienic and religious regulations. Certainly many rules which appear to have a profound hygienic purpose are in reality derived from magic concepts and apotropaic practices.

An example is the Egyptian regulation about the use of animals killed for eating-purposes; they were first examined by priests to decide if they were fit for sacrifice; if the flesh was not in the proper state for sacrifice, it would also be unsuitable as food.

Egyptian priestly regulations were very strict in providing for the bodily cleanliness of the priests, who had to bathe twice each day and twice

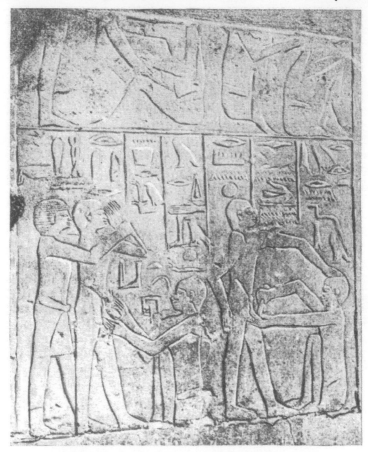

19. *Circumcision. Bas-relief of the Necropolis of Sakkara.*

each night, and cut their hair every third day; and in the representations of the third kingdom they appear regularly with the head completely shaved.

The priest had to wear nothing but white clothes and to avoid certain foods, especially pork and beans; only boiled or filtered water could be drunk. Egyptian law punished artificial abortion and exposure of infants severely. Sexual relations during menstruation were prohibited and in *The Book of the Dead* onanism was mentioned as a shameful vice.

Worth mentioning is the care that the ancient Egyptians gave to the hygiene of infancy. The newborn was wrapped in large white linen cloths, but not bandaged. After weaning, it was given cow's milk, then vegetables. Up to the age of five, children wore no clothes and played healthy games (ball games, rolling hoops, etc.); in the Egyptian museums are found a large number of toys from the ancient tombs for use in games. For older children detailed exercises were prescribed. The cosmetic art attained a high degree of perfection; excavations in the tombs demonstrate that there was knowledge and frequent use in ancient Egypt not only of perfumes but also of dyes for the hair and nails, rouge for the face, and so on.

The cult of the dead, which was widespread in ancient Egypt and derived from the belief in life after death, demanded the preservation of the dead body in the best possible way. To this is due the great development in the technique of embalming. Embalming was practised by men (Greek: *taricheutes*) belonging to a special, revered caste who were dedicated exclusively to this work. The incision was made by the *paraschistes* with a stone knife in the left flank; having made the incision, he fled, while those present performed the symbolic act of assailing him with stones (Diodorus Siculus). According to Herodotus, the brain was removed with hooks inserted through the nose, and the brain cavity washed out with drugs. The viscera were sometimes thrown into the Nile; at other times, as has been found in the tombs, they were preserved in precious alabaster vases (canopic jars). From the twenty-first dynasty on, the organs were wrapped in linen and replaced in the body. The heart was seldom detached from the great vessels. The corpse was then carefully wrapped in bandages of linen impregnated with bituminous substances, thus obtaining an excellent degree of preservation.

4. Professional Practice

The practice of the medical profession in ancient Egypt was controlled by special regulations. The position of the physician in the social system and in the State was clearly defined, even though for reasons already discussed there occurred in various times and places changes of titles and duties that reveal a long and slow process of evolution. It is well established that among all the peoples of antiquity the Egyptians enjoyed the reputation of being excellent physicians. Thus Homer extols (*Odyssey*, IV, 231) Egyptian medicine (" Each is a physician with knowledge beyond all men ") as the best of all, and Herodotus says (II, 84): " The art of medicine is thus divided: each physician applies himself to one disease only and not more.

All places abound in physicians; some are for the eyes, others for the head, others for the teeth, others for the intestines, and others for internal disorders." (See Hurry, Garrison, and also Dawson, in *Annals of Medical History*, 1924, VI, 183). Diodorus Siculus (I, 82) states that "in expeditions and journeys from the country all [the sick] are taken care of without giving pay privately. For the physicians receive support from the community, and they provide their services according to a written law compiled by many famous physicians of ancient times. And if after following the laws read from the sacred books they cannot save the patient, they are let go free from all complaint, but if they act contrary to what was written they await condemnation to death, since the lawmaker thinks that few men would have knowledge better than the method of treatment observed for a long time and prescribed by the best specialists."

It is evident, then, that in ancient Egypt physicians constituted a caste with special attributes. The fact that they were frequently given titles belonging to priests is not sufficient to prove that they were really priests; rather should we suppose that these titles derive from ancient times and that physicians had enjoyed the favours and privileges that were accorded to the more eminent ranks. The medical schools of Sais and Heliopolis were administered independently from the great temples to which they were annexed. The director of the School of Sais, traces of which are already to be found in the period of the third dynasty (about 4000 B.C.), bore the title "the Greatest of Physicians" and was at the same time the chief priest of the goddess Neith, the special divinity of Sais. The School of Osiris at Heliopolis, to which a sanatorium is known to have been annexed, had as director a physician who bore the title "the Great Seer."

Among the tombs of the most ancient physicians of this school is that of the physician Hwy, to whom was given the title, "The Greatest of the Seers." He is recorded in the Ebers Papyrus, written many centuries later, as the author of a remedy for the disease of the eye. The inscriptions that are found on the funereal monuments (steles) indicate to us other functions attributed to physicians bearing priestly titles. Thus among the constructions of the builders of the great Pyramids we find the tomb of a functionary designated by the title "Superintendent of the Secrets of Health in the House of the God Thoth"; and on another, "the Superintendent of the Palace for Sanitary Fumigation in the House of the God Thoth." Similarly, we find in the period of the fourth and fifth dynasties "the Chief of Physicians," "Consulting Physician of the Palace"; in the time of the eleventh and twelfth dynasties (about the middle of the third millennium), "the Great Physician of the House," a title which was also found two millennia later under the twenty-sixth dynasty. No less accurately were medicinal preparations supervised, as is shown by the existence of a "Superintendent of the Office for Measuring Drugs." Indications to oculists are frequent, and already about the middle of the fourth millennium we find a chief medical specialist, Ypy, who bears the title "Consultant of the Palace to Heal the Sight."

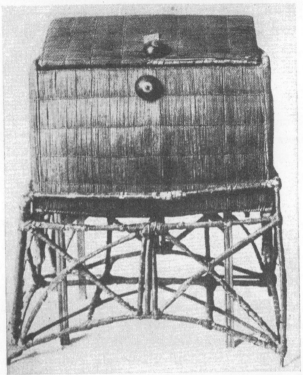

20. *The pharmacy and perfume box of the Queen Mentuhotep, eighteenth century* B.C.   (EGYPTIAN MUSEUM OF BERLIN.)

Thus we find for the first time in Egypt a perfectly organized medical caste. In the more ancient periods this probably was dependent on the high priests, but later it assumed an autonomous position in the medical schools, where were preserved the Hermetic books with their collections of the canons of medicine, in the sanatoria connected with the temples, to which ancient people flocked from every side, and in the administration of public health. The fact that physicians bore priestly titles on the funereal inscriptions has no greater significance, we may suppose, in proving that the physicians belonged to the priesthood than do the honorary titles and positions given in some countries to physicians of today, if taken literally.

In the period when Egypt passed under the domination of Persia the decadence of the arts and sciences was accompanied by a deterioration of medicine also. Even though the new conquerors tried to preserve the ancient traditions, and even though later, in the period of the Ptolemies, there are found traces in medical practice of these ancient traditions, nevertheless Egyptian medicine deteriorated and became merely a trade of sorcerers, drug vendors, and charlatans who preserved only the mystic vestments of the ancient medicine. The centre of the Oriental school of medicine, which in the last stages of the empire was transported to Memphis, lost all importance; only a part of the ancient magic medicine and the ancient traditions passed to the medicine of the Copts, concerning which there is some evidence in the Coptic papyri preserved in Naples and Turin. But the more important and vital part of Egyptian medical thought was transmitted later to Hippocratic medicine.

5. Characteristics of Egyptian Medicine

Study of medical culture among the Egyptians shows that when we are confronted with a collection of medical texts, like those of the Ebers and Smith papyri that I have quoted, we should accept that the sum of this knowledge represents the result of many centuries of observation and study. Even if the origins of the first and already complex medical concepts cannot be found, no one need suppose that they were created at one stroke by the genius of a single man or by the labour of a single people, even if extended over centuries. Evidently this complicated and magnificent construction, which reveals deep psychologic knowledge and extensive ideas of social relations, represents the results of the learning of distant generations, whose work has left no other traces.

The impression left by Egyptian culture on civilization is deeper than that of the Babylonian culture, probably because the monuments of the Egyptian culture were better preserved. But in the one civilization as in the other it is clear that medicine forms part of the complex of an architectural, religious, and political unity. It is also apparent that various sources and various epochs have contributed to the formation of this cultural edifice, which today more than ever — because better known — compels our admiration. Egyptian culture, through its geographical position exposed to the influence of neighbouring peoples and of the distant peoples with whom they had traffic, through its climate and the conditions of its fertile soil, bears the indubitable traces of all these currents. The development of the medical thought, also, that on the one hand shows a marked freshness

and originality of observation, but on the other a tendency to the codification of its precepts into a rigid ritual, is to be explained in the same way.
We can imagine that probably this process is derived from the Egyptian
mentality, which, as far as we can judge, was devoted on the one hand to
ardent speculations, freedom of research, depth of observations, but on the
other tended jealously to preserve and to transmit intact the conquests of

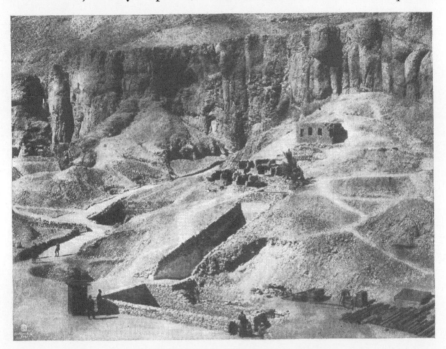

21. *Tombs of the Kings at Thebes.*

the mind, confided to a select aristocracy and veiled by traditions, mystical
practices, and mysterious rites that constituted their safeguard.

   Like the features of the kings and the warriors that are faithfully represented on the columns of the temples and even show characteristic ethnic
types, but yet are placed side by side without any consideration of the
laws of perspective, enclosed in rigidly stylized lines; like the mummies
hidden in their magnificent and stupendous tombs, just so does the medicine
of ancient Egypt appear in its complex ensemble: exact, often gifted in the
observation of details, far-sighted and shrewd in the promulgation of hygienic laws, wise and profound in the construction of social measures, but
rigid in enclosing all the treasures of their knowledge within barriers which
only experts with a pure body and enlightened mind can penetrate.

CHAPTER V

THE MEDICINE OF THE PEOPLE

OF ISRAEL

THEURGIC MEDICINE. CANONICAL CODIFICA-
TIONS OF SANITARY LAWS

1. Fundamental Concepts of Jewish Medicine

THE MEDICINE of the ancient people of Israel has essential characteristics deriving from the evolution of this ethnic unit, whose origins are not yet established with certainty, and from the social and political events that determined it. The medicine of Israel, or at least that official part of it that has come down to us in the canons of the books that were confined to the care of the priests, was dominated by the theocratic principle that guided the moral, social, and political legislation of the people. It is, nevertheless, easy to understand how this small people, which was submitted during the centuries to the influence of many races, at one time as conqueror and at another as conquered, should exhibit also in the history of their medicine the traces of neighbouring influences. We should not forget that the history of Hebrew medicine, as found in the Biblical and Talmudic records of their vicissitudes, legends, traditions, and laws, covers a period of almost two millennia, and that it is therefore natural that we should meet concepts and practices, some coming from very ancient sources, that were constantly

[64]

being modified by the historical events that upset the whole life of this people. But the fact that is particularly noteworthy and that makes the history of Hebrew medicine perhaps more interesting than that of other peoples of antiquity is that one can often establish how and by what ways concepts and traditions, customs and ideas that have come from outside, have been absorbed and, so to speak, filtered through the moral and legislative system of Judaism. Of prime importance, also, is the effect that the monotheistic concept, in which the function of healing belongs to divinity

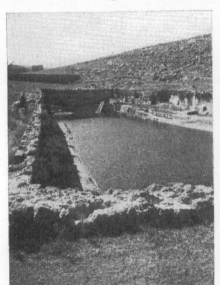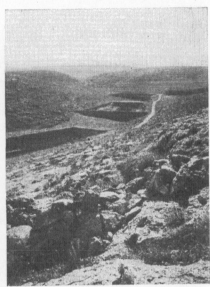

22. *The pools of Solomon near Jerusalem.*

alone, had on this process of assimilation and elaboration. This concept, in which the medicine of the Jews differs from that of every other ancient people, recognizes that in the one God is the source of health, but also of all diseases, which just because they come from God can be interpreted only as the deserved punishment for our sins. Thus teleologic concepts and religious training tend to subordinate the animistic concept, the idea of malignant demons, and therefore the magic practices and superstitions.

The Jewish concept of pathology, nevertheless, is essentially demoniacal and directly derived from that of primitive peoples. Humbert states correctly that the origin of disease was equally attributed by the Jews to the will of God or to a human malediction or to a fault committed by ancestors (as in the threat of divine punishment up to the third and fourth generation).

In primitive medicine the origin of disease is attributed to individuals, against whose evil deeds prayers and spells were used as defences. The studies of Mo-winckel and Lods have demonstrated that many of the invocations of the Psalms are to be regarded as simple incantations and that the curses to be read there ("Let their eyes be blinded that they see not. . . . Let them be wiped out of the book of the living . . .") (lxix, 23, 28), are to be regarded as magic procedures analogous in their form and scope to those which are preserved in the Assyro-Babylonian texts. According to the earliest ideas, it is not always God who strikes. It is much later that one meets the name of *Elohim*, representing a concentration of all the divine faculties, and its last syllable indicating the plural-ity of divinity in the original concept. Also in the sacred books, in which are found indubitable evidences of diverse origins, one notices the contrast between the monotheistic tendency (*Yahwist*) and the pluralistic (*Elohist*). The former is clearly of Sumerian origin, including the humoral concept that tends to attribute the greatest importance to the blood and in general a preponderant role to the humours; the latter suggests the influence of the Egyptian pneumatic concept of the spirit as the centre of life and of incense as an agent for improv-ing the quality of the air (see Genesis vii, 22: "in whose nostrils was the breath of life"). Disease comes from the divinity immediately and directly as a means of punishment and education: by His will God makes leprosy come and go (Exodus iv, 6). The plague is carried by an angel of God who strikes 185,000 Assyrians in one night (II Kings, xix, 35). The "destroyer" smites down the firstborn of Egypt (Exodus xii, 23), and the "adversary," one of the *Benè-elohim*, inflicts malignant ulcers on Job. Angels and malignant demons appear here and there in the sacred books; one of these demons devours the limbs of the dead ("the strength of his skin," Job xviii, 13).

In this concept there is a manifest tendency, clearly revealed to those who have studied the sacred sources, to concentrate all authority and power, and thus also the power of healing, in the hands of the priestly caste that is the depositary and intermediary of the will of the one God. When King Asa consulted physicians, instead of the one God through his priests, he promptly "slept with his fathers" (II Chronicles, xvi, 12, 13). Later Jesus, the son of Sirach (180 B.C.) said: "Honour a physician according to thy need of him with the honours due unto him, for verily the Lord hath created him."

It is from the one God that the people of Israel demand the cure of their ills, and to Him the sick one prostrates himself to invoke salvation. This concept, which we might call unitarian, prohibits believers from practising magic, without succeeding in abolishing it entirely. It is in it that we find the cause of the great development that sanitary legislation had among the ancient Hebrews, which we can properly call the first codification of hygienic regulations. When the principle has once been asserted that the one God is the dispenser of good and evil, that it is his will that decides health and disease, that those who call on other gods will be severely punished, it is natural that the ground will be swept of all superstitions and animistic and magic concepts. Or, if it is impossible to extirpate deeply rooted ideas completely from the minds of the people, such an idea at least hinders their spread and forbids the frequent obscene and cruel customs that flourished in other countries. It is logical to see derived from this concept the necessity of following divine precepts with no less scrupulous precision than was used by other nations in the case of magical prescriptions, and of carrying out all religious practices that have an element of sanitation with the same exact observance and fervid faith. It is in this, I believe, that lies the importance that the monotheistic concept had on the evolution of medicine in Israel; and it is for this reason that allusions to physicians and drugs are somewhat sparse in the sacred books and seem to have been included indirectly, often metaphorically. Those medical practices that we find described in ancient Egyptian and Babylonian texts are magic practices or the religious rites of strange gods and thus forbidden to the people of Israel. The reason that medicine is poorly represented in the earliest Jewish medical literature is that whenever the magic medicine of Babylonia and Egypt had access to ancient Judea, it was severely proscribed and destroyed. Thus it happens that we must search for the history of medical thought in the ancient people of Israel among their religious laws.

2. Sanitary Legislation

In the Biblical concept of medicine the priests, who have the high function of supervising all religious practices and acting as interpreters of the divine will, are the only ones to whom medical functions are officially allocated. They are the guardians of the purity of the people, and because physical purity is put on a par with moral purity and it is not admissible that the heart and mind can be pure without cleanliness of the body, it is evident that hygienic regulations have the characteristics of religious precepts and in part also of religious ceremonies.

Thus it is evident that the aim of Jewish hygiene customs is the purity of the body before God and it is for this reason that it was imposed upon the Hebrews. It should be noted here that certain traces of this concept can be found in Egyptian and Assyro-Babylonian medicine. But in Biblical law the religious and the hygienic concepts approach each other more and more closely and often merge; the distinction between pure and impure in religious ceremonies is extended as much to moral as to physical purity. Whoever becomes impure (*tamè*) for whatever reason, whether he has committed an evil deed or has become sick of a contagious disease, can become pure (*tahòr*) with the help of ceremonies. We have an exact description of some of these in the purification of lepers; here the bath plays an important role. All the customs concerning contact with corpses, the regulations for women in the menstrual period and in the puerperium, for those having gonorrhœa and leprosy, thus arise from a purely religious concept.

This mystic apparatus that accompanies all sanitary practices gradually becomes the principal element, transforming the purifying bath into the symbolic baptism. Thus especially in earlier times it characterizes the evolution of Jewish medical thought. Among the Jews it has this essential feature, however: that these practices are no longer limited to the priests alone or to a small number of initiates or adepts for whom it represents the advancement to a superior stage of knowledge, as among the ancient Egyptians, but are extended and imposed on the entire people without distinction. Circumcision, the prohibition of certain foods, ablutions before prayer, are rules that are met among other Oriental peoples, but only for the priestly caste, which in the period of the Middle Kingdom in Egypt had probably accepted the monotheistic concept as a late contribution to knowledge. In Judaism, in which the entire people, according to repeated statements in the sacred books, appear as a people of priests, a chosen people, in which every difference of caste is suppressed, all the religious and sanitary regulations (which, as we have seen, had the same significance as the former) were equally imposed upon everyone.

The priests, who served as an example to the people in the attainment of the highest moral precepts, were the custodians of the civil as well as the penal laws, and it is natural that from them should be required the most scrupulous observance of all the regulations about baths and ablutions. There were regulations that were generally practised, as the texts show, for cold bathing of the face, hands, and feet in the morning, and of the hands and feet in the evening. The importance that was attributed in ancient times to the bath is shown by an interesting interpretation given by Gruenwald in his classic work, *Die Hygiene der Juden*, published for the Hygienic Congress at Dresden in 1911. The verse of Jeremiah in exile (Lamentations iii, 17): "Thou hast removed my soul far off from peace; I forgat prosperity," is interpreted, according to the Talmud (Shab, 25), as due to the fact that in the Babylonian exile the Hebrews were not able to enjoy the baths to which they had been accustomed in their own country.

The rules about baths that one should offer to guests are mentioned as of the greatest importance in various places in the sacred books; Abraham's nephew, Lot (Genesis xix, 2), offered ablutions to his guests, but the Egyptians and the Gibeonites also practised this hospitable duty (Judges xix, 21). To demonstrate how these laws were understood even in a much later period,

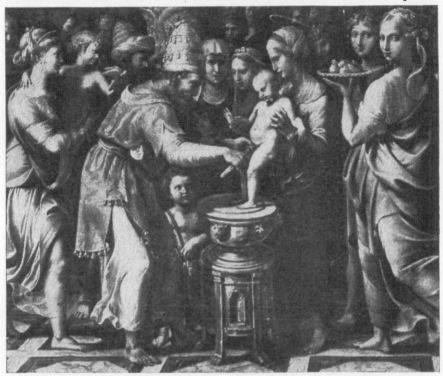

23. The circumcision of Jesus, by Bartolomeo Ramenghi, 1484–1542.
(LOUVRE MUSEUM.)

it is interesting to note the Talmudic regulation (R. Hunà, A.D. 216–296) that the wife, even when possessed of a dowry that permits her to have four servants and to direct the household seated, had the duty of washing the face, hands, and feet of the husband (Bab. Talmud, Ketuboth 61, A and V, 30). Ablutions before meals are strictly and repeatedly prescribed. The fact noted by Preuss is not without interest: namely, that washing the hands before the meal is regarded as a religious duty, while washing them after the meal is regarded as a duty of respect to other persons or things and thus not strictly of a religious nature.

According to Biblical law, no Jew could enter the Temple without being pure — that is to say, without having taken a bath if he had been in contact with impure persons or things, or if he had done anything that caused an impurity of his body. Even before beginning the study of the law, which was regarded as a daily duty by every Jew, a bath should be taken, which was also prescribed after every ejaculation.

Woman's impurity during menstruation constituted, according to strict Biblical law, an absolute hindrance not only to the performance of her religious duties in the Temple, but also to all relations with her husband. Similarly the Babylonians prohibited man from having contact with the menstruating woman; after menstruation an expiatory sacrifice was ordained, while the Bible decreed the pain of death for the man who approached a woman " as long as she is put apart for her uncleanness " (Leviticus xviii, 19). And if there are reasons for believing that this draconian measure was not actually put into practice, still it is an eloquent indication of the importance given to laws that undoubtedly had their origin in magic concepts.

The impurity did not stop with the hemorrhage. Purification could not be acquired without a ritual bath. This ritual bath, which throughout the social history of the Jewish people had great importance, was regarded as such an essential regulation that after the destruction of the Temple and the dispersion of the Jews, there was no religious community, no matter how small, that did not construct beside its synagogue a ritual bath, which was decreed also for the neophytes who wanted to embrace the religion of Israel. The law ordained that the entire body should be immersed in water, that before bathing all the vestments and ornaments should be removed, and that before the ritual bath the body should be carefully cleaned (Mikv, ix, 2). From similar concepts are derived the laws concerning contact with all impure things. Whoever entered a house in which there was a dead person was regarded as impure for seven days and should be washed on the third and seventh day with the *water of purification,* a ceremony in which some authors have seen a true disinfection, while for others it is more easily regarded as a remnant of magic procedure. A red cow was burned with a certain quantity of cedar wood, vinegar, and a thread of purple. From these ashes mixed with spring water was prepared the water of purification. In addition, the impure one should wash his clothing and take a bath. The regulations in Deuteronomy as to how soldiers should prevent the danger of infection coming from their excrement by covering it with earth constitute a most important document of sanitary legislation. It is even ordained that the soldier should take with him to camp an instrument with which to dig a hole in the ground to bury the fæces and cover them with plenty of earth; certainly a primitive measure, but an effective one, which indicates advanced ideas of sanitation.

To the same ideas are due the measures against epidemic diseases. The knowledge that we have of the spread of these diseases in Biblical times shows that the idea of contagion, its dangers and the necessity of fighting them with isolation, was known to the Semitic peoples, who derived this knowledge, like a great part of their culture, from the Babylonians. In the story (I Samuel, v,

1–2) of the capture of the ark of the covenant by the Philistines, who carried it to the Temple of Dagon, is found the description of an epidemic of bubonic plague; and when the Philistines decided to return the ark, they offered at the same time, to the God of Israel, a gift of five golden buboes and five golden rats. Here is remarkable evidence of the importance attributed to rats in the spread of plague in very ancient times. Aschoff's supposition that the rat merely symbolized the form of the bubo is contradicted, as Klebs recognizes, by the fact that the Philistines offered as their votive gift five figures representing the buboes and five others for the rats.

In another epidemic, cited in II Kings (xix, 35), there is mention of the mortality spread by the angel of the Lord, who killed 185,000 soldiers of Sennacherib (705–681 B.C.). In the story of this pestilence, which is also mentioned by Herodotus (II, 151), the rat plays an important part. In fact, according to the Egyptian tradition, the Assyrian army was decimated by the god Ptah, who was represented in the temple of Thebes with a rat in his hand. Apollo Smyntheus, who inflicted the plague on the Greeks at Troy, was the god of rats.

Study of Biblical texts appears to have demonstrated that the ancient Semitic peoples, in agreement with the most modern tenets of epidemiology, attributed more importance to animal transmitters of disease, like the rat and the fly, than to the contagious individual. This concept presumably also had a magic origin.

The ancient Hebrews, like the Babylonians, attributed great importance to flies, gnats, and other insects. Ekron, the most important site of the Philistines, had a temple dedicated to the god Baal-Zebub, which signifies " the lord of flies." This temple was so famous for its oracles that when Ahaziah, King of Israel, became sick he sent to it for consultation. This Baal-Zebub, who much later became a deity of the lower regions, was none other than the god who gave protection against the dangers of flies, like the Babylonian god Nergal and the Greek god Zeus Apomuios.

The laws against leprosy in Chapter xiii of Leviticus may be regarded as the first model of a sanitary legislation. These also may have been inspired by the Babylonian model, as some scholars believe that Leviticus had its source in the Babylonian exile of the Jewish people. The interesting discussion as to whether these laws were derived from a magic concept of the origin of disease or from an intuitive but accurate etiologic concept does not detract from the historical importance of the above facts.

Returning to Biblical regulations, the great importance of the laws for repose on the Sabbath cannot be disregarded from the point of view of hygiene. Some have wished to assign their origin to the Assyrian-Babylonian belief in unpropitious days; others, like Mahler, perhaps more correctly wish to interpret them as derived from the astronomical concept of the lunar phases. At any rate, when the Semitic lawmaker established this command as a divine decree, he codified for the first time in history a hygienic law of first importance, establishing definitely the need for physical repose at determined intervals. Some regulations of a strictly religious character, such as those forbidding certain foods and those detailing steps necessary for the slaughter of animals, may not necessarily have had a

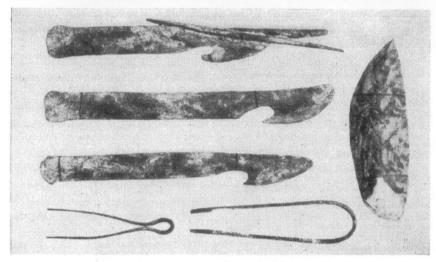

24. *Flint instruments used for circumcision.*
(WELLCOME MUSEUM, LONDON.)

hygienic basis in the intention of the old lawmakers. It seems more probable that these laws, like the law of circumcision, whose origin and practice are found in much earlier civilizations, form a part of all that complex of priestly laws which, for motives that we have given, were extended among the little people of Israel to the whole community. It is certain, though, that in their consequences and in their applications they had, as we shall see later, an importance from the medical point of view that cannot be neglected.

3. Medical Practice and Therapeutics

The art of healing was reserved for the one God. The priests were the interpreters and fulfillers of his laws and of the will of God. Thus the people of Israel did not have professional physicians, though an empirical medicine naturally flourished beside the priestly medicine. There was no question of a physician properly so called (*rophè*), even on such occasions as that of embalming the body of Jacob, when Joseph spoke of having embalming physicians come from Egypt. For the reasons given, and also because medicine does not appear in the Bible as a distinct science or art, but only as determining certain hygienic laws or giving comparative terms for moral punishments, the information that we can derive about medical cures and medicines from the ancient sacred texts is rare.

The Jewish word for leprosy was *zaraàth*. This is a good example of the fact that a Jewish term often was used for several modern clinical entities; it probably included psoriasis, eczema, and various inflammations of the skin, perhaps even syphilis. [That the Jews themselves apparently did not regard *zaraàth* as the equivalent of today's leprosy is indicated by the degrees of uncleanness that were recognized (Leviticus xiii, 2–46). The word *lepra*, which earlier meant a scaly disease, is said to have been given its specific connotation by Constantinus Africanus. *Ed.*] The leprosy miracles would then be more easily explained on rational grounds. Another skin disease is described in the Bible — the one that struck Job, indicated by the name *schehin:* " Satan smote Job with sore boils from the sole of his foot unto his crown " (Job ii, 7). "My skin is broken and become loathsome " (Job vii, 5); a terrible itch tormented him. Some commentators suppose that the disease was elephantiasis or smallpox; others, and among them Preuss, with more probability think that the disease was an *eczema universalis*. The King, Hezekiah, suffered from the same disease as did the Egyptians when stricken by the sixth plague. Among the most frequent diseases in Biblical times, in addition to the epidemic diseases mentioned, were dysentery, dropsy, apoplexy, and mental diseases such as that of Saul and of King Nebuchadnezzar, described in the Book of Daniel (iv, 25, 32–34). That certain venereal diseases were common in old Judea is apparent from the strict hygienic regulations for those with an issue (gonorrhœa?). He who is affected by a urethral issue is impure and everything that he touches becomes impure; whoever touches his couch or has had contact with him must wash his clothing and take a bath and remains impure until evening. After the flow has stopped, seven days must elapse before he is regarded as pure. During the sojourn in the desert those afflicted with gonorrhœa had to stay at a distance from the camp (Numbers v, 2). According to certain historians the Biblical account of the plague of Baalpeor should be regarded as giving the history of an epidemic of syphilis due to the fact that the Hebrews had frequented the brothels of the Midianites and had contracted a terrible disease that had killed twenty-four thousand. This view, however, is not generally adopted by critics.

At this period the origin of epidemics was attributed by tradition to the most diverse causes. The census-taking, for example, was thought to be a cause of epidemics.

In treatment a very important part is given to ritual ceremonies, it being granted that to some people supernatural powers were accorded. A man of god could transfer leprosy from one person to another (I Kings v, 27). With a number of charms the priest could "dry up the thigh and swell the stomach" of the sinful woman, by making her drink water in which had been immersed a curse written on parchment. Remedies were essentially divine or magic. In epidemics one could obtain relief by the sacrifice of the sinful person (II Samuel xxi, 5–6). By magic one could obtain the resurrection of the dead, as is told by the prophet Elijah (I Kings xvii, 21–22), who brought a child back to life by blowing into its mouth with a rite which, according to Daiches, is similar

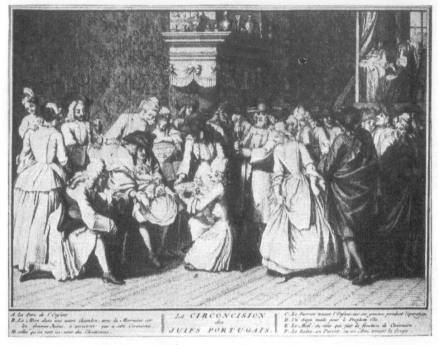

25. *The circumcision of Portuguese Jews.* (*French print, seventeenth century.*)

to a Babylonian practice. Naaman was healed of leprosy by dipping himself seven times in the Jordan (II Kings v, 10–14). The practices of the priests were for the most part founded on analogous concepts, witness the proceedings described in Leviticus xiv and the ceremony of the blood of the pascal lamb.

In the Biblical story we find traces of such very ancient ideas as that which attributes great importance to the serpent, which in all Oriental medicines appears as an infernal deity or as a mysterious protector of the occult and the symbol of all rebirth. In Genesis the serpent is the lord of mysteries, and figures as a demon (Num. xxi, 8–9) when God commands Moses to make a bronze serpent to heal the people. The Semites of Syria, Phœnicia, and even Palestine worshipped a god of health, Esmun (see Baudissin: *Adonis et Esmun*). He was similar to Æsculapius, who was always represented with a snake. Æsculapius is usually represented with a single snake, wound about a column. Mercury, the

Greek god of commerce and of thieves, is represented with two snakes entwined on his staff. The latter as the emblem of the United States Army Medical Corps was, therefore, not an altogether happy choice. Such figures have been frequently found in the country near the Jordan. It is probable, then, that the ancient Jewish traditions had some connection with this cult of the serpent.

In the same way other practices, such as that of the phylacteries, should be regarded as springing from ancient apotropaic rites. It is essentially an apotro-

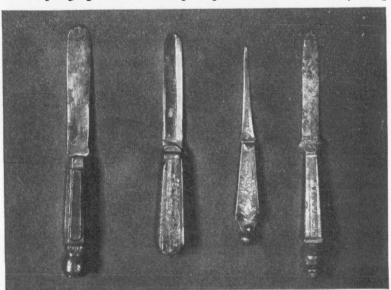

26. *Knives for circumcision, fifteenth and sixteenth centuries.*
(CLUNY MUSEUM.)

paic concept to kill an animal as a substitute for the guilty one, or to sacrifice a human victim to placate the irate god. This concept appears in the story of the sacrifice of Isaac and may be seen even today in the custom of sacrificing an animal to protect one's own life or one's dear ones. It is to be found also in other ancient religions (*Zeus Melichios* or *Apotropaios*).

Circumcision, about which there has been much discussion, and which, according to recent authors, should be regarded as practised by the Jews among the first, was certainly familiar to many ancient peoples, even though it was not performed according to precise rules. In early times it was done with a sharp stone, a practice continued even when bronze instruments were in use, perhaps because as a sacred law it was important to preserve the forms of the ancient rite.

Beside magic and priestly medicine there also flourished an empirical medicine. Thus it is reasonable to suppose from a passage in Genesis (xxxi, 14–15) that mandrake was used as an aphrodisiac; we see from a passage in II Kings (xx, 7) that for King Hezekiah, when afflicted with a grave plague, God advised, through the mouth of the prophet Isaiah, a plaster of dried figs. The preparation of medicinal unguents appears to have been customary, as in Exodus (xxx, 22–25), where an oil for holy unction is ordained, it is expressly stated that this should be prepared by the art of the apothecary. The treatment of wounds was *secundum artem*, as is seen in a passage of Isaiah (i, 6): "your wounds have not been bound up, neither mollified with oil." And in the same Isaiah are the words of God: "I have broken the arm of Pharaoh, King of Egypt, and he has not been cured by the application of medicines or the applying of splints to bind and strengthen it."

4. The Medicine of the Talmud

The medicine of the Talmud contains important information about the medical thought of the people of Israel in later times, and shows the influence of the peoples and the currents with which Judaism was in contact. The Babylonian Talmud (fifth century of our era) is a collection of tales and discussions that contains interesting anatomic and physiologic data: the œsophagus, the larynx, the trachea, the lungs, meninges, and the genital organs are well described, and the spleen, kidneys, heart, liver, intestines, and other viscera are often mentioned. The blood constitutes the vital principle. The Talmud recognized 248 (252) bones in the human body. One of these, *luz*, placed somewhere in the vertebral column, was thought to be the nucleus from which the body was reconstructed for the resurrection of the dead. Garrison[1] points out that this belief, which modern rabbis think originated in the Egyptian rite of burying the spinal column of Osiris, was exploded by Vesalius in a striking passage in the *Fabrica*. Many diseases, and especially the epidemic diseases, are accurately described with their symptoms. Diseases of the liver, and particularly jaundice, appear to have been common. Hemophilia is mentioned in the Talmud (tract Jebamot, p. 64b) as a hereditary disease which permits the omission of circumcision. Together with these observations, the Talmud contains traditions and popular legends which show that the magic concept has not entirely disappeared.

In the Talmud are found many malignant demons, either masculine (*scedim*) or feminine (*lilith*). From them come such diseases as insanity and angina, which was thought to be due to a malignant spirit attacking the child in the throat, while asthmatic attacks are caused by another malignant spirit. Certain magic words, passing by certain places, the look of certain persons, can cause

[1] *New York Medical Journal*, XCII, 149–51 (1911).

serious illness and even death. On the other hand, disease may be cured by the application of pieces of parchment containing Biblical verses or some magic formulas. The prophets cure by placing their hands on the head, and there are numerous cases of magic cures, like the resurrection of the child by the prophet Elijah.

The anatomical knowledge that we meet in these books is that which was common in the fifth century of our era to all the Mediterranean peoples and comes from the teaching of the various Greek schools. But it is to be noted that certain religious prescriptions, particularly of the Hebrews, are based on special anatomical knowledge; such as, for example, those concerning the examination of meat, according to which even the meat of animals slaughtered for food cannot be accepted as pure when pathologic changes are found after slaughtering. We know from the Talmudic laws in this respect that caseous degeneration, tumours of the lung, cirrhosis of the liver, and many parasites were accurately identified. One of the hygienic laws of the Talmud shows that diphtheria (*askarà*) was especially feared by the Jews, who regarded it as the most infectious of diseases. The first case found in a community was announced to the people by sounding the horn (*shofar*), while for all other infectious diseases this was done only after the third case (Preuss).

As regards surgery, we find in the Talmud the operation of anal fistula, reduction of dislocations, and Cæsarean section. Blood-letting is often mentioned, leeches and cups were in common use, also a sleeping-potion before operations.

After the period that follows the destruction of the Temple and the Jewish government, the medicine of the people of Israel no longer had any special independence, but followed the lead of the people among whom the Jews lived in exile. There was no special medical education until the Alexandrian period, and Jewish physicians did not become prominent in history until the Middle Ages. But, just as the basic ideas remained unchanged in the thought and consciousness of this people, so also their medical mode of thought, according to which the healing power is regarded as a special attribute of divinity, remained preserved through centuries. And it is precisely because of this fact that the hygienic and religious laws, even when their hygienic character was lost through changing interpretations, remain always essentially a lasting element of the moral legislation of the Jewish people.

5. Jewish Medicine as Essentially Theurgic

The conclusions to be drawn from what has been said are evident: the ancient Biblical texts show that the medical culture of the people of Israel obviously reflects Egyptian medicine on one side and Assyro-Babylonian medicine on the other. Hygienic laws, the fundamental lines of which are evidently drawn from other people, evolve and become perfected with a more accurate codification and with a greater accentuation of the religious side. This constitutes the most interesting and noteworthy element in the medicine of Israel.

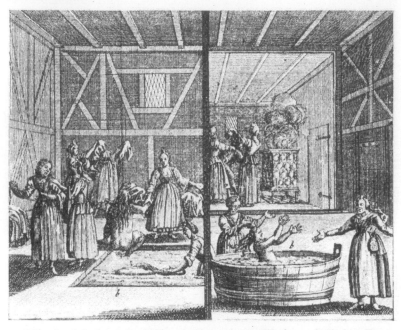

27. *The ritual bath of the Hebrews. From C. T. Kirchner:* Jüdisches Ceremoniel (*Nürnberg, 1726*).

Little trace is found in the Biblical texts of the physicians, methods of treatment, spells, and incantations to which the people continued to recur — as is shown by certain passages in the Bible where God sometimes threatens and sometimes strikes the Jews. This is because the holy books of this period that have come down to us have had removed from them all that might seem contradictory to the strict principle of monotheism, as seen in the very words of divine revelation: " It is I alone, the Lord, who am thy physician." Therefore, although there are frequent allusions in the canonical books to suppressed or forbidden cults, although at certain times even the priests of the one God returned to practices evidently derived from Assyro-Babylonian medical concepts (like the episode of the bronze serpents that Moses made to heal the people from the bites of serpents), the care of the lawmaker to suppress even the memory of that which would recall the people of Israel to the ancient foreign cults and give it confidence in the healing power of the deities of their people is very evident. Whenever Israel is unfaithful to the laws of its God, and its misery and suffering make it seek other gods, its punishment is immediate. When other people, like the Philistines in Samuel's story, outrage the cult of the God of Israel and steal the ark of the covenant, punishment quickly follows the crime in the terrible form of a plague. Only faith can provide healing and the salvation of mind and body.

It is in the same way that many centuries later Christianity turned from empirical and philosophic medicine to return to the pure virtue of the faith that heals. This, in the minds of the early Christians, tended to tear from the hearts of the people their faith in magic and occult practices, and to turn them to the earliest Jewish concept, according to which there is no salvation without faith, no cure without prayer and purification of the mind and body.

Thus the essentially theurgic nature of Jewish medicine arose on ground prepared by other civilizations in a people which grew through great difficulties and lengthy internal struggles to the superior ethical concept of monotheism and held to it throughout the centuries. It brought a very precious contribution to medicine — the essential basis of all social hygiene (and this, as Neuburger has said, constitutes the chief glory of Biblical medicine). In this people, in which for the first time in history was asserted the right of all individuals to legislative protection and the equal duty for all to obey strictly the moral laws, there arose also for the first time the concept of sanitary legislation, understood as a limitation of the rights of the individual, sacrificed to a superior idea and the interests of the community. Thus the just but severe rule of the law, which constitutes the fundamental character of the Jewish religion and regulates the political and social life of the people, appears manifest even in the evolution of medical thought.

CHAPTER VI

THE MEDICINE OF ANCIENT

PERSIA AND INDIA

SYSTEMATIC THEORIES

1. Oriental Civilizations and Their Migrations. The Medicine of Ancient Persia

ACCORDING to Elliot Smith's view of the migrations of primitive civilizations, culture with distinct characteristics migrated into the Mediterranean basin between the third and first millennia B.C. Then it pushed on toward India, about the tenth century B.C., by means of Phœnician navigators, whence it extended to Malaysia and Polynesia. It eventually reached the shores of America, taking on various modifications from the countries through which it passed.

This so-called heliolitic culture had as special attributes the adoration of the sun and its symbols, megalithic monuments and gigantic stone images, the custom of mummification or embalming the dead (which is also found among the North American Indians), tattooing, massage, circumcision, and so on.

This characteristic culture, whose typical manifestations can hardly be imagined to have arisen spontaneously in places so distant from each other, had influenced the first Minoan civilization about 2800 B.C. It was spread by the Phœnicians about 900 B.C., while in another direction Polynesia served as a connecting link between the Asiatic and American continents.

According to this hypothesis, which seems to have much to support it, the most ancient Persian and Indian civilizations were directly or indirectly connected with the Babylonian.

The history of Persian medicine is divided into two great epochs: the first is that included in the ancient books of the *Zendavesta;* the other be-

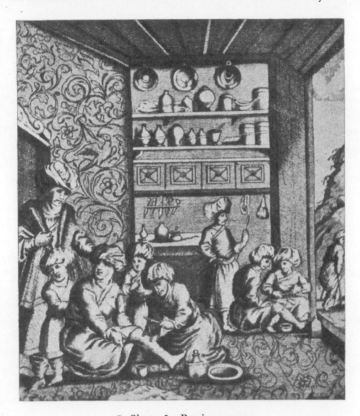

28. *Shop of a Persian surgeon.*

longing to Arabian and Mohammedan culture, which had a great development in Iran. The Arabian physicians of Persian origin, who brought an important contribution to this civilization, were among the most illustrious standard-bearers of Arabian medical science (see Chapter xiii).

But the ancient Persian medicine, which is an interesting feature in the study of Oriental civilization, flourished in the period in which the great empire extended its power from the Mediterranean to the shores of the Indus, from the Caucasus to the Indian Ocean. Of this civilization and medical culture but few traces are left today.

The religion of ancient Persia is essentially dualistic: two creators and two creations exist side by side and each of the superior gods has a large following of lesser divinities who translate their masters' plans into action. Ahura Mazda, Ormuzd, is the god of light, god of good, and creator of every good thing, supported by the six holy Amesha Spentas, who represent piety, goodness, and justice. Opposed to them is Angra Mayniu or Ahriman, spirit of evil, ignorance, and darkness, accompanied by six malign and diabolic spirits, who struggle for possession of the world. In this mythology medicine plays a notable role: it arises from the garden of Ameretap, the goddess of long life, in which garden grow thousands of health-giving plants. The goddess created the tree of all seeds which grows in the centre of the lake, Vourukasha. Near it grows the miraculous tree of Gaokarena, which cures all ills, the tree that gives immortality — enemy of the malignant spirit. A series of ritual ceremonies grew out of this legend, similar to the cult of the tree among primitive people. The gods of healing are Thrita, Thraetona, and Ahriman, who is regarded in the *Avesta* as the chief god of health. The divinity Mithra is very important in this very ancient mythology. He derives with certainty from the prehistoric solar myths, in which there are many symbolic customs such as the bloody rites, baptism, and communion with bread and wine. The cult of Mithra as a god of health, which was widespread in Rome and Greece during the Empire, afforded a notable contrast to the advance of Christianity.

To know the medicine of ancient Persia one must turn to the books of the *Avesta* and especially to the sixth book, the *Vendidad*, which treats of the purification ritual necessary to remove the malign demon. In this book are preserved the traditions, laws, and rites of the people that inhabited the plateaus of Persia when they still lived a simple pastoral life, close to the soil, and worshipped Ahura Mazda. Even after the coming of Zarathustra, a legendary character with no certain factual support, these traditions persisted, later to be transformed into the religion of Mithra. Eventually the faith was crystallized into one formula, fire-worship, and practices dictated by a high idealism became simple expressions of caste law. But it is in the ancient texts that we must look for exact information about the origin of medical concepts.

In consequence of the concept of impurity, there were severe laws for keeping lepers far from habitations, even though we may not be sure that the disease referred to by a term indicating " white spot " was really that which we know as leprosy. Purification of the body as well as of the mind is prescribed in the *Vendidad*, just as it was in the Bible.

All these rites of purification, ordered for those who have had contact with the bodies of dead men or animals, are connected with the magic concept that attributes disease to malignant spirits. The cure of disease is confided to Ahura Mazda and to his divine word: prayer, rites, invocation of the divine name, repetition of formulas, constitute the essential basis of every cure. The Dakmas, the places where the dead are deposited, are the places where malign spirits assemble and threaten man with contamination and disease. Against these causes of evil only the invocation of divine aid avails; nothing else will put them to flight. One may conclude, then, that the ancient medicine of the *Avesta* corresponds in its origins and general lines to the Jewish medical concept: it has as its basis the demonistic origin of all ills and a magical concept of healing that gradually changes into a religion ideation.

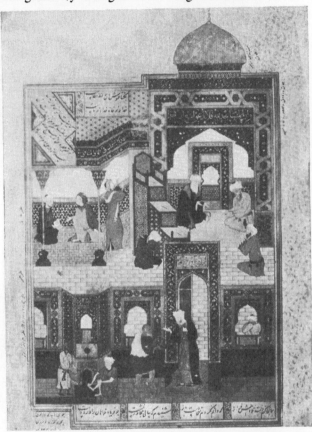

29. *Above: a medical consultation; below: a bath. From a Persian miniature of the fifteenth century.*

As regards the practice of medicine, we know that it belonged exclusively to the worshippers of Mazda — that is, to the elect. The *Vendidad* codifies the penalties for the physician who commits wrong in his medical practice, also his honoraria (varying according to the patient) and the tests to which he must submit before being admitted to practice. One must infer, then, that, as it is not possible to establish the date at which the *Avesta* was reduced to writing, this codification of the standards of the medical profession is of a fairly late origin in the history of this people, when its geographical location was settled and its civilization well advanced. It was prohibited to bury or cremate the dead, who were exposed to the air and to the sun to be consumed by vultures — a practice still observed by the Parsees, followers of the ancient religion of Zoroaster, which also had followers in India. This law, which was strictly observed, came from the idea that burial of the corpse made the earth unclean and that cremation was an offence against the purity and sanctity of fire. Herodotus (I, 138–40) describes the Persian practice of segregating the sick, especially lepers, and of exposing the dead to be devoured by crows and other scavengers.

Firdausi's *Shah Nameh*, completed A.D. 999, though fiction, contains some valuable traditions of early Persian medicine. It includes many references, for instance, to those who in ancient Persia healed with the knife, as well as to the healers with herbs or with the holy word. The rules for the care of women in pregnancy and childbirth were elaborate. Miscarriages were treated with cow's urine, both orally and as a douche. Abortifacients were known and criminal abortions were severely punished. Sexual intercourse with a woman during menstruation and in late pregnancy was forbidden. Cæsarean section for obstructed labour, after " bemusing " the lady with wine, is described in the *Shah Nameh:*

> His birth could not be natural;
> So willeth He who bringeth good. Bring thou
> A blue steel dagger, seek a cunning man;
> Bemuse the lady first with wine to ease
> Her pain and fear; then let him ply his craft
> And take the lion from his lair by piercing
> Her waist while all unconscious. Then imbruing
> Her side in blood, stitch up the gash.

Firdausi also gives a legendary account of the birth of Rustum by Cæsarean section: " A skilful Mobed arrived and intoxicated Rondabeh, the moon-faced beauty. Then he ripped open her side without her feeling it, and turning the child's head toward the opening, delivered it without harming the mother.

" She slept for a day and night. They sewed up the wound and gave her treatment for pain. When she saw the child she said: ' I am delivered (*Rustum*) and my pains are finished.' " (*Æsculape*, 1938, p. 168.)

2. Essential Features of Indian Medicine and the Various Stages of Its Development

The great difficulty in forming even an approximate estimate of Indian medicine comes above all from the fact that its history, like the history of the art, philosophy, social, political, and religious life of the people who inhabit the great land of India, is neither united, continuous, nor well established. One can only approximately evaluate the influences exercised by various invasions and foreign dominations. Knowledge of the ancient Indian medical texts is far from complete and the English translations thus far published are not to be regarded as entirely accurate. Besides which the very number of medical, surgical, and pharmacological texts, the complete uncertainty about their origin and compilation, the sparse information that we have about the lives of the most famous medical writers, together with a general legendary atmosphere, all these circumstances greatly hinder study of the subject. The lack of any positive facts about the relations between Indian and Sumerian and Babylonian civilizations and between Indian and Greek medicine, and about the relations between Indian and foreign physicians, are also stumbling-blocks to research. The historical indications, then, even though one takes account of the valuable studies that exist in this field, are vague and for the most part insecure. And this is because Indian historiography, in general, is so involved with legend that it is extremely difficult to extract the true facts from the available texts.

The characteristic note of Indian medical thought, of which we possess only documents that are relatively recent, is found in medicine as in philosophy in a systematic edifice in which every pathologic concept has its place. Every disease is entered in a certain category. Every medical prescription is expressed in its most minute details, so that the Indian medical books that have come down to us constitute complete encyclopædias. In them we find documents valuable for the comprehension of Indian civilization, even if we may not be able to establish which concepts have come by unknown ways from the Assyro-Babylonian civilization and which were born on the soil of India. The study of ancient Indian medicine is made easier by the fact that, as Jolly observes in his masterly volume on the subject, the Indian medical literature holds closely even in recent times to the ancient models, so that books published toward the end of the last century may represent the writing of more than a thousand years ago. The ancient medical texts that we shall have occasion to speak of are still being reprinted and studied; and the *kaviraj*, local physicians, who stick strictly to tradition still enjoy the confidence of the people. This is not the place to recall the discussions that have taken place between philologists and historians about the precedence of one or the other culture or about the currents from various sources that may have influenced the development of Indian medicine or that may have issued from it to penetrate in their turn into the medicine of the Greeks and Arabs. We may state, however, that Indian medicine was developed even in very ancient periods in an original form, that Indian anatomy, different from the Greek, remained in a primitive stage on account of the prohibition by religious laws of contact with the

dead body. We should recognize, however, that in the field of materia
medica the contribution of Indian medicine is especially valuable and that
it furnished a number of drugs to the pharmacology of the Western peoples. If the later humoral concept appears to have been of Greek origin, as
is suggested by the great similarity of later texts to separate passages in the
Hippocratic writings, one should recognize on the other hand that all the

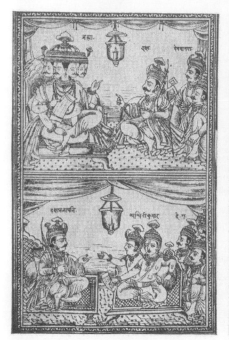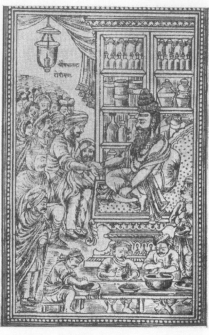

30. *Buddha teaching medicine.*   31. *The teaching of medicine by Susruta.*
From an Indian print of the eighteenth century.

hygienic and dietetic regulations (whose characteristics indicate an evident
relation to the climate, flora, and fauna of India) have found their origin
in a country where the sacred canonical books of medicine have the value
of law. Notable progress in the field of surgery, especially of rhinoplasty,
which derives evidently from a long evolution of ancient concepts, shows
how the medical thought of India for the most part has developed according
to the interests and traditions of that country, with rigid fidelity to ancestral
teaching.

The problem of Indian chronology, and therefore of the age to be attributed even approximately to the more important medical and surgical
texts that have been preserved, has given rise to long discussions which are
still far from being concluded.

According to the authoritative view of Jolly, the most important source for the history of ancient Vedic medicine is found in the *Atharvaveda*, published by Bloomfield, which contains, especially, magic formulas against demons and their human representatives. For many centuries medicine was almost wholly in the hands of the Brahmins, who had hospitals built for the care of the sick long before the Christian era. These appear to have disappeared, however, before the time of Susruta. Beside the Brahmin physicians there existed, even from ancient times, a caste of medical practitioners (*vaidya*). Medical information about the Buddhist period is to be found in the Bower manuscript, which was discovered in a Buddhist *stupa* (convent). This was published by Hoernle from 1893 to 1897, and dates from the fifth century B.C., a period in which Indian medicine appears completely systematized. The *Ayurveda*, the Veda of long life, contains the traditions transmitted from Brahma and treats of the various branches of medicine in eight parts.

The chief god of medicine in India was a minor deity, Dhanvantari, the physician of the gods. Perhaps originally a cloud deity, he was not mentioned in the Vedas, but appears in the epics and the Puranas. The Susruta Samhita (I, ii, 12, 16) calls him the divine physician who received the *Ayurveda* from Brahma and taught it to Susruta and his six colleagues. According to Jayne, he suffered the opposite from the more frequent process of deification: namely, he was demoted from the position of an independent deity to that of an avatar of Vishnu and finally of an earthly mortal, king and leech who died of snake-bite.

The book of *Charaka* is said to have been written by a physician of King Kaniska (A.D. 100); it probably, however, is one of the more ancient texts, because there is no mention in it of opium or of mercurial preparations, or of the examination of the pulse.

The basic text for Indian medicine is that of *Susruta*, which was translated by Hessler into Latin, in 1844, and published in an excellent English edition by Hoernle in 1897. It is very important for its anatomical and surgical content; it must have great age as it was already mentioned as an ancient book in the fifth century of our era. More recent books are the *Vagbhata* (published by Kuntz at Bombay in 1880, and in various later editions), the *Madhavanidana* (edition of Vidi, Calcutta, 1876), which is the most valuable text on pathology, and the *Bhava Prakasha*, written about 1550, which is a complete treatise of clinical medicine.

Under such conditions it is obviously difficult to distinguish the origin of medical concepts in their chronological order. Let us try, therefore, to study those which are especially worthy of interest as characteristic of this civilization.

In the Brahmin period we find a beginning of anatomic studies even though primitive. Sacred numbers had a great importance in Indian anatomy; according to Susruta, the body was composed of 300 bones, 90 tendons, 210 joints, 500 muscles, 70 blood vessels, 3 humours, 3 kinds of secretion, 9 sense organs. Both the blood vessels, which, according to the Indian concept, carried air, and the nerves started from the umbilicus.

The teaching of anatomy, according to Susruta, was very important. The corpse, in which the physician was directed to examine carefully every organ, was enclosed in a bag and exposed for seven days to a process of decomposition in river water. After this the internal organs could be disclosed without the use of a knife, which was strictly forbidden in religious laws, by mere friction of the soft parts. This is the only passage in Indian texts in which anatomical studies are mentioned (Susruta III, 5).

The formation of the embryo was the subject of long and accurate investigation in the Indian medical texts. The processes of development and all the phenomena that occur in uterine life were studied, especially those of the circulation. Minute indications are given to distinguish the various periods of pregnancy and no less detailed prognostic information on the influence of various phenomena on the fetus. The pregnant woman who was violent and bad-tempered would produce an epileptic; if she was addicted to alcoholic drinks, she produced a child that was always thirsty and had a weak memory. If her life was dissolute, the son was depraved and effeminate, and so on.

Indian pathology was founded on the fact that three chief elements, the spirit, the bile, and the phlegm, constituted essential, vital parts of the organism. Disease resulted from abnormal relations between these elements or between the lesser humours that derived from them. Disease origins (indicated by the word *nidana*) were ascribed to a disturbance of either the physical or the moral humours. The causes of disease were divided into several groups following the indications of a series of symptoms that the physician was directed to study accurately by means of his five senses. The greatest accuracy in medical observation was recommended. In all the texts the greatest importance was attributed to a careful diagnosis.

In regard to special pathology, we note the great importance that was attributed by all the medical texts to fever, which was called " the king of all the diseases." It was thought to arise from the anger of the god Siva. Various causes and forms of fever were distinguished: seven that resulted from disturbances of the humours, and one from wounds or other external causes. The prodromal signs of disease were enumerated with exactness: the most dangerous fever is that which is due to a disturbance of all the three fundamental humours. It became most dangerous on the seventh, tenth, or twelfth day. Intermittent fever was divided into five kinds, according to the interval between exacerbations. Tertian and quartan fevers were described in special detail.

Phthisis, which was very common in India from the most ancient times, was called the royal disease; it made itself known by eleven characteristic symptoms. The physician who had regard for his reputation should not undertake the care of a patient who had the three grave symptoms: fever, cough, and bloody sputum. If, however, the patient had a good appetite and digested well, and the disease was in its infancy, a cure might be hoped for.

Interesting are the descriptions of the infectious diseases and especially of smallpox, which was thought to come from the goddess Sitala, whose name is identical with that of the disease. The appearance of pustules was clearly described in the later texts. The treatment consisted in a series of ritual practices. The ceremonies propitiating the goddess and invoking her aid for sick children, which we have had the opportunity of seeing in the Temple of Sitala at Benares, are still practised with enthusiasm. There is some question as to whether or not inoculation against smallpox was practised (see Madras *Courier*, January 2, 1919). A celebrated passage in Susruta has been interpreted as indicating knowledge of the relation between mosquitoes and malarial fever; just as a warning to abandon a dwelling when its rats act queerly and die suggests knowledge of the spread of plague by rats.

The Indian physician made diagnostic use, not only of inspection, palpation, and auscultation, but also of smelling and tasting. Passages are to be found in the ancient medical texts that show that the appearance of the skin and of the tongue and the form and the extent of swellings were noted in diagnosis. Note was also made of the crepitus of fractured bones and of the sweet taste of diabetic urine (*madhumeha*). Prognosis arrived at a noteworthy point: the Indian authors were careful to indicate fatal symptoms exactly and all the prognostic phenomena that the patient presented, such as hallucinations, delirium, insomnia, sudden paralysis, and so on.

Among these prognostic signs, the accurate observation of which we must admire, there are others, to be sure, which are closely allied to magic practices. Thus it was regarded as a favourable sign if the messenger who was sent to the physician was dressed in white and belonged to the same caste as the patient, if he sat in a cart drawn by oxen, and so on. It was an unfavourable sign, on the other hand, if the messenger belonged to a caste higher than that of the sick, if it was a eunuch or a woman, if he wore worn-out clothing, if he came riding on an ass, and so on. If the physician met a virgin or a woman with a nursing infant, or two Brahmins, on his way to the patient, these were very favourable signs (Susruta I, 29).

The basis for therapeutic prescriptions was furnished by dietetics. Medicinal plants were known and commonly used. Blood-letting, cupping, and leeches were often prescribed. Indian therapy recognizes five kinds of remedies: emetics, purges, irrigations, oily enemas, and remedies that produce sneezing. Before the use of one of these remedies, applications of fat were prescribed. Fats played an important role in Indian therapy, whether for internal or external use.

In general, external applications were in special favour among the ancient Indians. Oil enemas, emetics, sneeze powders (which were thought to clear the head), ointments, and steam baths, applied in the most varied and ingenious forms, were all in common use. Medicinal inhalations and powders were prescribed; exact indications and contraindications for bloodletting were given.

Whether or not mercury was used in India before the time of the Arabian physicians is a problem that has not yet been solved. It is certain, however, that mercury eventually had an important part in Indian therapy.

3. Indian Surgery

The study of Indian surgical texts is particularly interesting, as Gurlt has shown in his monumental study of the history of surgery. In it we find proof of the priority of Indian to Hippocratic medicine. Indeed, operations are described in the Indian texts, such as that of anal fistula, which are not named in the Hippocratic writings. This is also true of the plastic operations which are characteristic of Indian medicine, and which did not come into use in the rest of the world until the late mediæval period.

In India many metals and methods for using them were known centuries earlier than in Europe; in this country also, inhabited by an intelligent people whose art, industry, and science even in early times had arrived at a high stage of development, surgery held a position of honour and was made the subject of careful study. This being the case, we must admit that Indian medicine, and especially its surgery, had a development in ancient times that was most probably quite independent of Greek medicine.

More than twenty-one books, in addition to those that have been mentioned, treat of medicine. Besides the four sacred Vedas, other books were concerned with medical practices and treatment, but the most important of the descriptions relative to surgery are to be found in the previously mentioned book of Susruta.

According to this book, the physician who undertook a surgical operation should be equipped with a number of blunt (*yantra*) and sharp (*sastra*) instruments that are accurately described. Among them were knives, cauterizers, cups, saws, syringes, scissors, hooks, forceps, trocars, catheters, specula, sounds, and needles for suturing. The incision for an abscess should be two fingers deep. Abscesses of various parts of the body are described accurately as to their form and are differentiated as to their degree of maturation. The incision should be made in the direction of the cavities. In certain specified regions, such as the eyelids, cheeks, temples, lips, axilla, the incision should be transverse; for the palms circular, and for the anus and the penis semicircular. After the operation the patient should be washed with hot water, the abscess should be pressed by the fingers for complete evacuation, then washed with an astringent solution. Into the opening of the abscess a strip of cloth impregnated with sesame (elecampane) and honey was inserted, after which the abscess was covered first with a poultice, then with a cloth neither too thick nor too thin, and bound. On the third day the bandage was removed and renewed. It was forbidden to remove the bandage on the second day unless it was indicated by violent pain.

The text indicates the formation of granulations and the whole process of healing.

We find in Chapter vii a list of 101 blunt instruments, of which the hand, according to the author, is the most important. There are described two forceps, to extract various bodies from the nose and ear; hollow instruments of various kinds; 28 varieties of sounds, of which the head might be turned like the head of a worm, which the physician used to explore abscesses or cavities.

There were 20 sorts of cutting instruments of various kinds: knives, razors, scissors, bistouries (an instrument which should have the form of a lily leaf), lancets for a single incision, needles, knives shaped like the leaf of the *kusa*, trocars of various kinds, forceps for extracting teeth, and so on.

In Chapter ix there is a series of instructions for the student about the use of instruments. He should practise the technique of operations on skin-covered sacs, or on bladders filled with water or mud. The opening of veins should be practised on animals; the passage of sounds tried on plants, and so on.

The exact list of the surgical operations, cited with many comments by Gurlt, shows that the Indian physicians knew the operations for anal fistula, tonsillectomy, and the extraction of the fetus in case of abnormal presentations; it shows further how the blood vessels were ligated with the fibres of plants; four sorts of sutures (hemp, flax, bark fibre, hair) were used, and three kinds of needles (round, triangular ones for the fleshy parts, and curved for the vital parts, such as the abdomen and the scrotum). Garrison states that " the Hindus apparently knew every important operative procedure except the use of the ligature " (of blood vessels?), checking hemorrhage with cautery, boiling oil, or pressure. They performed amputations, excised tumours, repaired hernias, and couched for cataract.

A special chapter in this book is dedicated entirely to the pathology and treatment of fractures, in which crepitation of the bone was indicated as a characteristic sign. The directions for amputations are precise. The treatment of dislocations is described with great accuracy and skill, also the method which should be employed for each separate dislocation. Dislocation of the humerus should be reduced by pulling downward on the bone and holding it to the side of the body after a pillow or piece of material has been placed in the axilla. A figure-8 bandage was then placed around the shoulder and the neck.

The pathology of vesical calculi, which have always been common in India, is exactly described. The operation, regarded as necessary when internal treatment has not sufficed, is minutely described according to the technique that was in use in Europe up to the end of the sixteenth century. The patient was

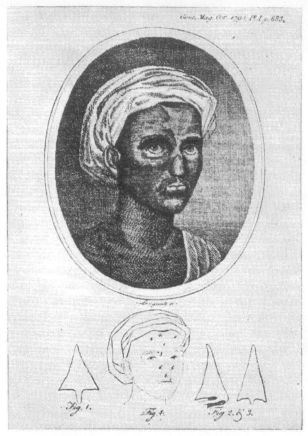

32. *Indian rhinoplasty, showing details of the technique and wax models. From the* Gentleman's Magazine of Calcutta, *October 1794.*

placed with the limbs spread apart and tied down separately. The incision was made over the stone in the left part of the perineum, and about two fingers' breadth from the anus. The opening was then enlarged according to the size of the stone, which was removed with an iron forceps. Care had to be taken not to break the stone or to leave fragments inside the body; it was important to avoid injury to the seminal vessels, or the spermatic cord, and the rectum. If the seminal vessels were cut, it was thought that the patient became impotent.

The rules for the same operation on the woman are no less exact, as are also those which deal with post-operative care.

In addition, we have exact indications for the operation on tumours of the neck, for the incision for dropsy, for removal of the tonsils, which is done with a semicircular knife after the tonsils have been seized with forceps and pulled downward. Directions are also given for the treatment of prolapse of the rectum.

An especially interesting item in the history of Indian medicine is the growth of a popular surgery, in which the operation of rhinoplasty is especially worthy of note. This often became necessary in India, where the nose was amputated as a punishment or in revenge.

According to the laws of Manu, amputation of the nose was the punishment decreed for adultery. Rhinoplasty is of very ancient origin in India. The modern European practice is probably derived from it through unknown paths, as was also that of the Brancas and of Tagliacozzi. In the book of Susruta it is prescribed that the physician should take the leaf of a tree, cut from it a piece of the size of the missing nose, apply it to the cheek, and so cut a piece of skin of the same size. This bit of tissue was applied to the stump of the nose, which had been scarified, and was sewed there. Two tubes were introduced into the nostrils to facilitate respiration. If the nose was made too big, it was recommended to cut it off and begin again; and if too small, to enlarge it. In the same way to make a new lobe of the ear it was recommended to take a piece of the skin of the cheek (Susruta I, 16).

The first publication about rhinoplasty is an engraving published by Wales at Bombay in 1794 which reproduces a portrait that he has made of this operation on an Indian, on whose amputated nose a local physician had constructed a new nose with a piece of skin from the forehead.

The journal which reported the procedure said that this operation was frequent in India, and gave a good description of it, as may be seen from the illustration. Information from physicians and other sources showed that it had been practised in India from time immemorial, exclusively by the caste of the potters and always successfully. Almost always the operators transmitted their art from father to son; the operation was done with a razor and lasted about an hour and a half.

Lithotomy, as is shown by various reports, was practised successfully in India up to very recent times by Mohammedan natives. It is strange that only these two operations have been preserved in the medicine of the Indian people and that the very people who performed these operations with great skill are not in a position to practise even the most simple procedures of other surgical operations.

4. Hygiene. Indian Medicine as a Systematized Discipline

Hygiene plays a most important role in Indian medicine. According to the laws of Manu, strict hygienic regulations and frequent ablutions form the basis of the religious cult. Only the flesh of animals killed for the purpose could be used as food; many vegetables, such as onion, garlic, and mushrooms, were prohibited. The principal food was rice and legumes. After every meal a generous ablution was required, and after various contacts, a bath. All excrement and also the bath water had to be immediately removed from the house. We find recommendation for frequent bathing of the eyes; the hygiene of women during the menstrual period and the puerperium was covered by severe rules.

Daily cleansing of the body was prescribed in detail. The teeth were to be cleaned with sticks made from the bitter astringent twigs of certain trees, the mouth rinsed with cold water, the face washed copiously, the eyes treated daily with an ointment of antimony. The body was to be anointed with a sweet-smelling oil; there were frequent regulations for massage and baths, but these are regarded as healthful only for the lower parts of the body and harmful for the upper parts. Other hygienic prescriptions deserve special mention. They are collected in the canonical books, which were first printed in recent times; but they come without any doubt from more ancient sources and reveal an early knowledge of fundamental facts. Thus, according to the laws of Manu, the priest who wished to marry should not take his wife from an unhealthy family — that is, where there was tuberculosis, epilepsy, white leprosy, or elephantiasis — even if this family was of high lineage and very rich. Indian law prescribed an almost exclusively vegetarian diet, ordained the cremation of the dead, and imposed severe laws for the abuse of spiritous and intoxicating liquors. There were three chief kinds of intoxicating drinks: that obtained from the residue of sugar, that extracted from milled rice, and that obtained from flowers of *madhuka*. All three were equally forbidden to Brahmins. The drunkard was punished with a mark of infamy on his forehead; if he was a *dwidja*, he had to undergo a year of penance in haircloth and wearing the hair long. A woman addicted to spiritous liquors was regarded as a leper and repudiated.

In view of the obscure chronology of ancient Indian medicine, it is to be expected that a much greater antiquity and importance has been claimed for it than is accorded here. Thus Muthu maintains that in the *Rigveda* (placed by him at about 4000 B.C.) over a thousand medicinal plants are given; water is praised as an all-healer; surgeons acted as accoucheurs; and an entire hymn is devoted to the description and treatment of phthisis. Already in Vedic medicine medical men were divided into surgeons (*shalya vaidyas*), physicians (*chisaks*), and magicians (*bhisag atharvans*). Three humours were recognized in the body — the earliest example of humoral pathology, antedating the Greeks by many centuries. They were *vayn* (nerve force), *pitta* (heat-production), and *kapha* (governing heat-regulation and the secretions). Charaka's book on medicine, of 120 chapters, deals with diseases of various parts of the body and how to treat them, the construction of hospitals, sterilization of bedding. Both Charaka and Susruta (dated by Muthu at 1000 B.C.) used wines " to produce insensibility to pain," and the fumes of Indian hemp were used for the same purpose. Muthu states that Susruta advocated the dissection of dead bodies as indispensable for the successful surgeon. With the advent of Buddhism (especially in the fourth century B.C.), anatomy and surgery declined; but State medicine (registry of births and deaths, reporting dangerous diseases, extermination of pests, medico-legal autopsies) and hospitals and schools flourished. The last great Hindu physician, Bhava Misra of Benares, flourished about A.D. 1550. He wrote an extensive work covering most branches of medicine and is said by Muthu to have mentioned the circulation of the blood and to have prescribed mercury for syphilis.

Considering thus the whole system of Indian medicine, as formed by different phases whose chronology is difficult to establish, we find two special characteristic facts: the exalted concept of hygiene in the morality of the priests and lawmakers of the Indian peninsula, and the great development of surgical technique. Indian medicine, like the medicine of other Oriental peoples, was first empirical and then predominantly priestly; finally, in a later period, while the priestly medicine was restricted by formulas and magic procedures, practical medicine underwent a great development and was manifested not only by important innovations in the field of pharmacology, but also by bold surgical operations. Considering the environment and the special conditions in which Indian medical thought developed through the centuries, it seems natural that the religious concept should be dominant, in which the individual suffers pain with a serene mind and goes tranquilly toward death, which is regarded not as a punishment but as the beginning of a new and better life. For this reason Indian medicine was directed chiefly toward the concept of the purification of the body, toward the endeavour to make man more deserving of his greater destinies. It was also motivated by the tendency toward a deep mysticism which accompanied almost every form of thought and action. The metaphysical medicine of India had the special feature that suggestion and all the psychic phenomena that accompany it have played an important role in the life of the people, even back to far-distant times.

The Ayurvedic system, according to those who have studied it carefully and appreciate its value, is important for its fundamental teaching. The theory of *thridosha* is a kind of humoral doctrine which even today, or perhaps especially today, affords great interest for students. It affirms the existence of three *doshas,* or essential principles, which pervade all the tissues, secretions, and excretions and determine health and disease. These are the vital principles on which foods, drugs, medicines, and experimental applications exercise an influence which is determined by their general effect (*veerya*), by their chemical constitution (*vipaka*), and by their physiological action (*guna*). A special causative factor of disease, which in Western medicine is called the constitutional factor, is recognized and described in Ayurvedic medicine under the name *prabhava.*

In the system of *Yoga* the faithful attained through successive grades to a state of concentration that is analogous to that of Christian mysticism, and joined to this domination an extensive knowledge of internal vital forces and nerve centres. Exact knowledge of these practices explains obscure phenomena established by many observations, and suggests to many students, among whom are Rele and recently Schulze, that it is a question of applying rules furnished by a vast and lasting experience with physical and psychological facts.

The picture that is presented today to the European physician who concerns himself with this problem and wishes to study it with the aid of less superficial criteria than those regarded as valid up to the end of the last century is a most interesting one. India offers all the attractions of a large and marvellous museum, in medicine as in other fields; the magic practices of primitive peoples, the cult of stones and trees, the dominance of healers, all are manifestations which are still found existing there. In this historical picture, in which all the stages of medical history are represented, Ayurvedic medicine plays an important part. Along the streets of the cities and villages are numerous doctors' signs bearing the name, in both Indian and Latin letters, *kaviraj*, often with the typical English suffix L.I.M. (i.e., Licentiate in Indian Medicine). In the crowded market-places of the great Indian cities, into which English trade is seldom allowed to penetrate, one sees here and there, and usually in the side streets, the booths of physicians — open rooms on the street — in which sit the servant or the assistant of the physician, awaiting patients. In some villages even the physician himself is there, rapidly treating the patients, who are often numerous. This exemplifies perhaps the most primitive form of the practice of medicine. It suggests that these empirical physicians, who often furnish the patient with the medicine that they have prepared themselves, which almost always is an infusion or decoction of herbs, represent but a slight and doubtful advance from the times of the ancient physician spoken of in the classic texts of Charaka and Susruta. They constitute the great majority of physicians who treat patients in the villages and the country as well as in the city. Rarely do the people have recourse to physicians who have studied in English universities; almost never to European physicians.

Thus Ayurvedic medicine, as practised by empirical physicians, is founded more on the letter than on the spirit of the ancient texts. The quotations that these practitioners repeat, with the respect that would be given to divine utterances, are often far from exact, according to the best students of Indian literature. Anatomical and physiological knowledge is rudimentary and the anatomical figures that are sometimes seen in the booths are puerile in design. In the large and best-arranged Ayurvedic schools, to be sure, the attempt is being made today to adapt the teaching of the classic texts, which are studied with great veneration, to the doctrines of Occidental medicine.

Indian medicine, after having been almost completely destroyed, and maintained today only by oral tradition and in the practice of popular empirical medicine, is studying ancient paths and reconstructing the new edifice on the old foundations. It is passing through a period of formation and new birth at a time when Western students are turning to the sayings of the ancient masters and re-establishing contact with the medicine of classic times.

CHAPTER VII

FAR EASTERN MEDICINE

SYSTEMS OF SCHOLASTIC MEDICINE

1. Origins and Characteristics of Chinese Medicine

THE HISTORY of Chinese civilization dates from many centuries before the period of the Emperor Fi, who reigned about 2800 B.C. In very ancient times, when a brilliant Chinese civilization raised the arts and sciences to a high level and produced discoveries which revealed not only the profound gifts of observation of this people but also its excellent methods of study, Chinese medicine also had a great development. But about A.D. 1000 we see a complete arrest of this progress; the respect for tradition, the veneration of the sayings of ancestors, the transformation and stylization of the love of knowledge and study into the adoration of the written word, all these factors determined the crystallization of the civilization of the Far East into forms which assumed an almost rigid aspect. Chinese medicine moved in the same way as Chinese art and literature: a reduction of ideas, perhaps excellent in their origin, into infinite, insignificant details, so that the more essential facts were totally obscured. But just as the acute observer of ancient Chinese works of art finds in them the marks of genius by considering them in the right light, so, if we know how to read sympathetically the old Chinese texts of philosophy and the literature, we find clear and living sources of great ideas. Thus scanning all the infinite forms and minute details in which was distilled through millennia the meticulous cunning of the Chinese physicians, we see how the original concept of Chinese medicine, which has characteristics independent of the other civilizations that we have examined, is truly of great interest and worthy of close attention.

The pantheon of the Chinese gods of medicine is a large one. Every author who has paid especial attention to this subject names several: The most ancient is Pan Ku, the god who formed the universe, according to a Taoist legend, after the division of chaos into its two principles *Yang* and *Yin*. Among the six greater divinities of medicine, first to be mentioned is Hua T'o, who appears to have been a great surgeon who lived about the second century of our era in the romantic Period of the Three Kings (Han dynasty). He was one of the great exponents of acupuncture and it was he who first prescribed physical exercises. Chinese medical historians say that he practised many important operations on the brain, abdomen, and other parts after producing unconsciousness in his patients. The Emperor Shen Nung, the second of the five legendary rulers, is also generally regarded as one of the chief gods of medicine. The others are Fu Hsi (the first of the legendary rulers), Pien Ch'iao (a contemporary of Hua T'o, more famous as a physician, but celebrated as another first to use anesthesia), Tsen Ren (who lived about A.D. 620, and published thirty volumes on medicine), and Chang Chung Ching (the "Chinese Hippocrates," who flourished about A.D. 170). But besides these six greater divinities, there are also many lesser gods of medicine, such as the God of the Eye, who is pictured with an eye in his hand, the God of Smallpox, the God of Measles, and so on. There are also seventy-two great physicians who are worshipped as holy. Thus we see that religion plays an important part in Chinese medicine; no other people so frequently gave their physicians the honour of being included among the gods.

China offers the history of a political unity of a nation of four hundred millions lasting over three thousand years. It is therefore of essential interest to consider the history of the thought of this people, which has undergone so many modifications in its ethnic constitution, yet whose origins and rise to civilization are unknown.

According to ancient legends, the origin of Chinese medicine is attributed to the Emperor Shen Nung, who is said to have lived about 2700 B.C. He is said to have taught his subjects the cultivation of plants and the use of agricultural implements. He is also said to have been the first to compile a herbal, in which more than a hundred remedies are mentioned. To him is attributed the technique of acupuncture. The most ancient as well as the greatest medical work, one which is still studied in China, is the *Nei Ching* (*Book of Medicine*), the author of which is said to be the Emperor Hwang-Ti (2698–2599 B.C.). If these statements were accepted, this would be the most ancient known medical book; but Chinese specialists generally maintain that its origin is much more recent and that, in the form in which we now have it at least, it does not go back further than the third century B.C. It is divided into two separate works: *Su Wen* (*Plain Questions*) and the anatomical treatise, *Ling Shu* (*Mystical Gate*).

Among other sources of Chinese medicine found in ancient books is the important encyclopædia, the *Golden Mirror*, a work in forty volumes, attributed to *I Ts'ong Chin Chien*, that is to say, the Imperial writer on the medical art. This book is still held in great esteem and was a text in use up to the most recent times in the Chinese Imperial medical college. It contains a compilation of the works of the ancient writers of the Han dynasty (206 B.C.–A.D. 220), made about 1700 by the Emperor K'ang Hsi of the Manchu dynasty and published for the first time in .1744. Sixteen volumes of the surgical part of this work have recently been translated into English by W. R. Morse.

Among other important medical texts are the famous *Book of the Pulse* (*Mei Ching*), a work by Wang Shu Ho (A.D. 280) in twelve volumes, which is accepted as a medical classic; and the anonymous *Mei Chueh, Secrets of the Pulse* (tenth century). There are also many other fragments from ancient authors that transmit the precepts preserved from oral tradition, with the addition of short comments. Wong and Wu's history of Chinese medicine (Tientsin, 1932) contains an invaluable account of this ancient literature.

The basis of Chinese medicine is to be found in a first stage of magic and demonic medicine, which is still predominant in those parts of China where the most ancient customs and superstitions are preserved analogous to the magic of the primitives. In a second period Chinese medicine is based on their philosophy and cosmology, while contemporaneously with it there was developed an empirical and popular medicine founded on expert knowledge of vegetable drugs.

The concept of the universe which forms the essential basis of all Chinese philosophy and medicine is that of the religion of Lao-tse: man is composed, like everything else in the world, of wood, fire, earth, metal, and water, and constitutes a microcosm in the macrocosm of the universe. In the Chinese philosophy the number five has the greatest importance. Corresponding to the five elements. there are five senses, five viscera, five colours, five tastes, and so on.

Another important element in macrocosmic combinations is the relation between masculine and feminine. The two opposing qualities are *Yang* (masculine) and *Yin* (feminine): The masculine represents heaven, the sun, light, force, hardness, heat, dryness, eyes, left side, and all positive qualities; the feminine or negative principle represents earth, the moon, darkness, weakness, moisture, cold, ears, right side, and all passive qualities. On the perfect equilibrium of these two principles, which continually ebb and flow, rest the foundations of health, tranquillity, and well-being. Everything is produced by union and perishes by decomposition. The alternation of these phenomena arises from the supreme laws which govern the universe.

This concept is different from those that we meet in other ancient civilizations, partly because the *Yang* in the Chinese concept is always dominant. Revulsive medicines are much used by the Chinese in order to excite the activity of the *Yang*. Psychic cures are also probably directed toward this end. The fundamental importance of the masculine generative fluid is demonstrated by a statement of the philosopher Wankh'Ung, who wrote in the first century of our era. Without this fluid, *Yang,* the body cannot live, but without the body the fluid loses its vitality.

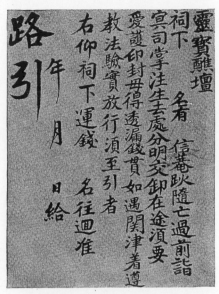

33. *A magic pass issued to the soul of the dead, which is to be delivered at the entrance into the Kingdom of Death.*

According to Chinese anatomy, the human body is composed of five important organs that store nourishment: heart, lungs, kidney, liver, and spleen, on which five other "viscera" that eliminate are dependent: small intestine, colon, gall bladder, bladder, stomach. Each of the important viscera corresponds to an element, a plant, a color, a season, and so on, and has a particular relation to one or other of the organs. Thus the heart, the most important of all, has the liver as its mother, the stomach as its son, the kidney as its enemy. It corresponds to the element fire and to the planet Mars. The circulation owes its motor principle to *Yang* and is completed fifty times in twenty-four hours.

In the several organs the vital substance, formed by the union of the two principles and the blood, *Ke,* is diffused through channels of communication.

The concept of Chinese pathology is derived from the two main principles, *Yang* and *Yin*: the chief cause of all diseases is a disharmony in their equilibrium or an arrest of their flow. These two principles create and destroy, personify energy and dissolution; and the effluvia or humours are the result of a disturbance in the balance of these two cosmic forces.

Chinese anatomy is described in many ancient texts, among the most noteworthy of which is the *Ling Shu*, the second part of the *Nei Ching*. It is almost entirely fanciful, being constructed on a purely theoretical doctrine and system of natural philosophy. Dissection is said to have been first mentioned in the *Ling Shu* (*c.* 1000 B.C.?) and was occasionally practised on criminals at the time of the Sung dynasty (tenth to thirteenth cen-

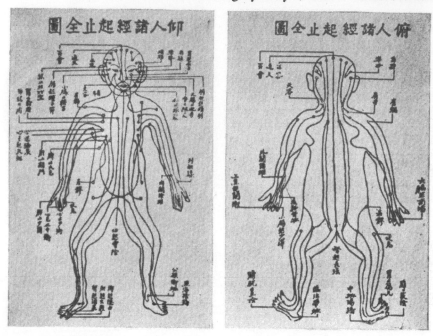

34. *Anatomical figures showing the course of the blood vessels. From the book of I Ts'ong Chin Chien.*

tury). Anatomical studies are based on ideas of natural philosophy without regard for actualities; the teaching of Confucius, according to which the body is sacred and cannot be touched, has hindered the study of anatomy up to our own time.

Nor was the knowledge of physiology any less fanciful, various intellectual and moral qualities being ascribed to various viscera. (On the other hand, even the *Nei Ching* seems to have come close to such an important concept as the circulation of the blood, as may be seen in passages quoted by Wong [2nd ed., p. 35]: " The heart regulates all the blood in the body. . . . The blood current flows continuously in a circle and never stops.")

Diagnosis is dominated by the theory of the pulse in a very complicated way. The human body is likened to a chord instrument, of which the different pulses are the chords. The harmony or discord of the organism can be recognized by examining the pulse, which is thus fundamental for all medicine. On it depend diagnosis, prognosis, and therapy. It is examined in eleven different places. Each pulse should be examined three times separately: first with light pressure, second with slightly more pressure, and third with strong pressure.

Chinese medicine takes account of two hundred kinds of pulses, and not less than twenty-six indicate approaching death. With this premise it is evident that according to the Chinese the examination of the pulse alone lasts several hours. The Chinese physician attributes no importance to the history and makes his diagnosis without consulting it. Morse, however, states that the better-class Chinese physicians inquire about the patient's family history and present condition, inspect the body, but not the excreta, and listen to voice changes. Palpation is limited to the pulse only. Observation is ranked highest among the physician's methods.

A treatise on *The Art of Acquiring a Long and Healthy Life* recommends, first of all, dietetic and hygienic measures, physical exercise, and daily labour according to a regular system. All medical prescriptions are regulated according to the laws of *Yang* and *Yin*, as they affect not only the human body but also the appropriate planet, element, colour, and taste. Organ therapy has been used in China since ancient times, because it is thought that certain organs of certain animals possess a great quantity of vital spirit. The lungs, the liver, the testicles, and other parts of animals were regarded as potent in China from the most ancient times. Soldiers and wrestlers drank blood or ate the liver of the tiger, and in more ancient periods it was customary to tear the liver from the dying, to increase the courage of him who ate it. " The key to treatment," according to Morse, " is in the production or depletion of Yang and Yin in the body, or parts of the body, through the action of suitable remedies and this secures equilibration of the flow of these cosmic forces."

Among the best-known diseases in China is smallpox, of which there have been great epidemics. Inoculation against smallpox was known from ancient times, but probably was not of Chinese origin. The crust of a pustule was pulverized and introduced into the nose or was insufflated with a bamboo tube; for boys the inoculation was made in the left nostril, for girls in the right.

Syphilis, with its primary, secondary, and tertiary stages and also in its hereditary form, was frequently described. The Chinese writers maintained that it was brought into China at the beginning of the sixteenth century by a vessel from Europe touching at the port of Canton.

The most important part of Chinese medicine is found in its materia medica. The principal work, *Pen Ts'ao Kang Mu*, composed in the six-teenth century and contained in fifty-two volumes, is the accepted standard for Chinese doctors today. It is based on a very ancient book attributed to the Emperor Shen Nung. In it are described almost two thousand prescriptions. It recognizes the use of iron for anæmia, of arsenic for skin diseases and intermittent fever, and mercury for syphilis. It prescribes rhubarb, the

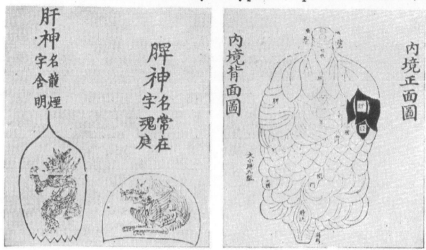

35. *From an anatomical treatise of the Sung dynasty. Mythical animals are shown in the liver and spleen.*
36. *Anatomical figure of the viscera. From* Nei-Ching, *composed toward the middle of the fourteenth century.*

use of which went from China to Europe, and sodium sulphate as purgatives; the root of pomegranate against worms; and opium as a narcotic.

Surgery flourished in ancient China. Ancient texts speak of the great surgeon Hua T'o and describe many operations. In the third century B.C. there were already in use practical methods for the treatment of wounds; in the ninth century the operation for hare-lip was frequently and skilfully performed. However, Chinese surgery made no progress after the Tang dynasty (619–907); no books were written on the subject, and the surgeon has always occupied a position inferior to the physician, performing a few crude operations with the aid of crude instruments.

Castration was mentioned before 1000 B.C. and was performed by specialists, in order to produce eunuchs for the Imperial court. The number of eunuchs at the time of the greatest splendour of the Chinese Empire reached several thousand. The operation was done by making the genitalia anesthetic, perhaps with secret medicines, and then binding together the penis and scrotum with silk bandages. Then the operator amputated the organs in front of the pubis with scissors or a semicircular knife. An astringent powder, composed of alum and various resins, was applied to the wound and pressure was exerted until the hemorrhage was stopped. Then a sort of wood or metal catheter was introduced into the urethra. Healing generally took place after the third month. Mortality was probably very high; some author calculated that about fifty per cent died, while according to others it did not rise above two per cent.

The excised parts were preserved by eunuchs in alcohol and after their death were buried with them, because according to the religious beliefs of the Chinese it is not possible for a person who enters the kingdom of the dead with a mutilated body to be reunited with his ancestors.

Another important surgical procedure used by the Chinese was the deformation of the feet, which began in the seventh year by means of a bandage applied according to special rules, so that the toes were compressed and the heel raised.

Acupuncture plays a most important part in Chinese therapy. It consists in introducing into the skin a number of thin needles, either cold or heated, made of silver, gold, steel, or iron, and of various lengths (from one to ten inches). The aim is to penetrate one or more of the imaginary canals called *chin* which contain no blood but are the channels for the two vital principles. These twelve canals are thought to occupy a profound relation to the vital organs. Puncturing them is thought to remove obstruction and allow the escape of bad secretions. Connected with them are the, also imaginary, three burning spaces, situated in specified parts of the abdomen, which are regarded variously as storage spaces for *Yang* and *Yin* and as a drainage system from the twelve canals into the bladder. Elaborate charts and details for the performance of acupuncture have been in existence since ancient times. Acupuncture began about 2700 B.C. and has been preserved almost without change up to our own day. It can be accompanied by the application of *moxa* — that is, burning on the skin the powdered leaves of mugwort (*Artemisia vulgaris*), to which a little incense may be added. This form of treatment, like acupuncture, is widespread through the Far East and is used for all diseases. In recent times this practice, which has such a remote origin, has been attentively studied in the West, and particularly in France. Some authors do not hesitate to attribute great benefit to it as a counter-irritant.

2. The Practice of Medicine — Spread of Chinese Medicine through Korea to Japan

The conditions of the medical profession in China have been maintained up to now through centuries without important changes. The teaching of medicine was always confided to a superior college of physicians. Under the Than dynasty the career of the court physician was stabilized, and to him was given the task of instructing students in the canonical books of medicine. The Emperor Kublai of the Mongolian dynasty, who ruled about the end of the thirteenth century, was the first to introduce detailed rules for the medical examination, and the Ming dynasty (fourteenth to

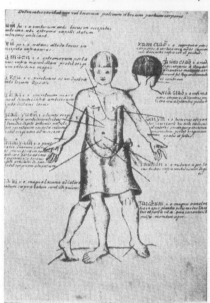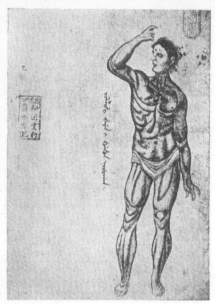

37. *Indications of the pulse in various parts of the body. From the* Specimen Medicinæ Sinicæ, *1682.*
38. *A sheet of the Manchu anatomy. From Johnson:* Anatomie Mandchoue (Copenhagen, 1927).

seventeenth century) instituted a complicated system of study for medical students. It was this dynasty that founded the medical college of Peking, to which was confided the instruction of the court physicians, while the physicians that conducted the ordinary practice of medicine were mostly empirical and self-taught. The physician, called *I-Sheng* (Sir physician), belonged to the second class of the people, while only the court physicians and those of the supreme medical college belonged to the first class. In China, as perhaps in few other countries, we are enabled by the state of medicine today to arrive at a fairly exact judgment of its condition in the flourishing period of Chinese civilization.

If we consider the principal characteristics of Chinese medicine, we note that it consists in a rigid, closed system, which has undergone but few modifications through the centuries. The essentially dogmatic Chinese medicine avoids anatomical observation and experiment, being jealous only of traditional doctrines and faithful to the most minute and extreme exactness of the letter rather than the sense of the ancient texts. These traits have left but few traces in the evolution of medical thought, in the history of which they represent a branch detached from the great tree of life. The greatest obstruction to any scientific element in Chinese medicine has been that when the observed structure or behaviour of the body did not conform to traditional metaphysical belief, purely hypothetical structures and functions were invented to bring it into conformity.

The above description of native Chinese medicine should today be supplemented by some notice of the marked advances that have been made by the Chinese in the application of modern (Occidental) medical science. Together with the gradual penetration of foreign missionaries into China through the nineteenth century, European and American medical hospitals and medical schools were established, which have slowly taught scientific medicine to Chinese students and accustomed the people to the new methods. Today almost every province has its modern hospi-

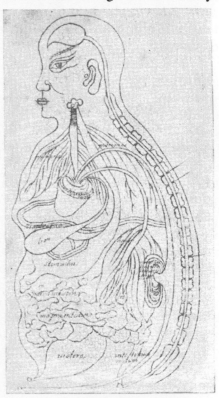

39. *The circulation of the blood. From a Chinese print of the eighteenth century.*

tal (unless it has been destroyed in the present war), even though small. More than a score of modern medical schools, founded chiefly by foreign influence and teachers, have laboured to spread rational medical knowledge, the oldest and best-known being the University of Pennsylvania's Medical School of St. John's University (St. Luke's Hospital), Shanghai; the Hunan-Yale Medical School; the Peking Union Medical College (founded by the Rockefeller Foundation); the West China Union University of Hong Kong; and that of Lingnan University, Canton. The terrific Manchurian epidemic of plague (1910–11) stimulated the newly formed Republic to support a National Quarantine Service, which, at least up to 1937, was expanding rapidly and performing efficient sanitary service. A National Medical Association was formed in 1916, with the *National Medical Journal of China* (the former *Chinese Medical Journal*) as its official organ. Naturally, the surface of the problem has been merely scratched — there are but a few thousand trained physicians for the hundreds of millions of population; but the foundations have been so well laid that the establishment of scientific medicine in ageless China may now be said to be only a matter of time.

The influence of Chinese medicine was early extended to Japan. For many centuries Japan was entirely dominated by Chinese civilization, which completely supplanted the original autochthonous Japanese medicine. As far as can be learned from the old legends, this ancient medicine possessed rudimentary anatomical knowledge. About the fourth century after Christ the Chinese civilization penetrated into Japan through Korea; Chinese physicians were called to the court; and Chinese schools were rapidly created that acquired a great importance. The conservative system of social life in Japan divided even the physicians into various categories. The physicians of the Mikado and the aristocracy belonged to the nobility, and wore a sword and a dress with long sleeves, while the physicians of the people belonged to the lower classes of the population. About the seventh century of our era Chinese medicine was still entirely dominant. The first Japanese hospital was built, A.D. 758, by the Empress Komyo.

In the medical book *I Shinho,* written by YASUYORI TAMBA in 982, smallpox hospitals are already described. The entire system of Chinese therapy had a great vogue, especially acupuncture, which was practised on a large scale and was always the treatment recommended by the Japanese physicians.

Toward the end of the fifteenth century there were certain Japanese physicians of importance who tried to free medicine from the bondage of Chinese science. Among these should be mentioned the great physician TOKUHON NAGATA (1512–1630), who was regarded as one of the best of the reformers.

With the arrival of the Portuguese in 1542, European medicine began to penetrate slowly into Japan. Later certain Dutch physicians were highly regarded and brought to Japan the teaching of the great Flemish physicians. Paré's works were translated into Japanese in the seventeenth century. Boerhaave, van Swieten, Heister, and others followed in the eighteenth century. In 1857 the Dutch physicians founded a medical school at Yeddo, from which the present University of Tokyo later sprang. In the second half of the past century Japanese medicine was entirely under German influence, but toward the end of the century it freed itself from this dependence and brought important original contributions to the progress of medicine. European methods of teaching were introduced into all the medical schools of Japan.

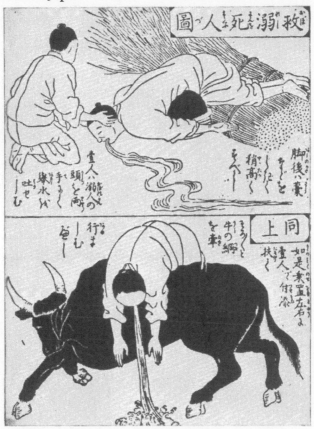

40. *Treatment for reviving the drowned. Japanese print.*

Thus after a first, mystic period, during which Japanese medicine was exclusively magic, and a second period in which Chinese medicine predominated, there followed a period called Yeddo (1616–1867) during which European medicine penetrated slowly into Japanese schools. In the last historical period, called Meiji (from 1868 to our own days), Japanese medicine made great progress and the medical schools were organized on European models. During this modern period many illustrious Japanese scientists have rendered a noteworthy contribution to the progress of medicine. It is sufficient here to cite the names of SHIBASABURO KITASATO (1852–

1931), studies on plague and tetanus; KIYOSHI SHIGA (1870–   ), dysentery bacillus; HIDEYO NOGUCHI (1876–1928), *Treponema pallidum*, Oroya fever; S. Hata (1873–   ), treatment of syphilis; Katsusaburo Yamagiwa (1863–1930), production of tar cancer.

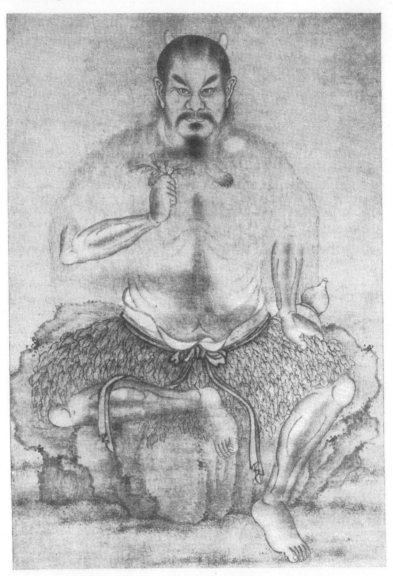

41. *Shen Nung, one of the major gods of medicine, second of the legendary Emperors.*
(*From an original painting now in the* JOHNS HOPKINS DEPARTMENT OF MEDICINE.)

It is an interesting phenomenon that with the sharp awakening of Japanese nationalism in all walks of life, there has also been very recently a manifest tendency to return to the ancient doctrines and practices of Japanese medicine. The ancient medical texts are being studied again, especially as regards the clinic and therapeutics.

Thus while on the one side universities, scientific institutions, hospitals, laboratories, medical societies, are developing rapidly and according to Western ideas, on the other hand the study and practice of acupuncture and the use of ancient drugs and of practices that were in vogue in distant times are returning to a position of honour.

Medical science and practice in Japan has made great advances in this century and today compares favourably with that of world leaders. Nine universities (Tokyo, Kyoto, Tohoku [Sendai], Kyushu, Hokkaido, Keijo, Taiwan, Osaka, Nagoya), six government medical colleges, and twelve medical academies, organized on modern lines, well equipped, and staffed mostly by Japanese, provide a satisfactory medical education and conduct extensive and valuable studies in all fields of medical investigation. Most schools are on the university (*daigaku*) standard; that is, they require three years of pre-medical education, followed by four years of the regular course, leading to the

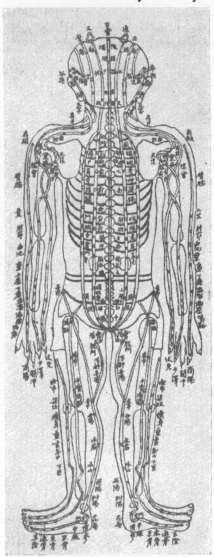

42. *Table showing the lines for acupuncture. Chinese print.*

title of *Igakushi*. Postgraduates completing a satisfactory medical thesis receive the degree *Igaku-hakushi* (Doctor of Medical Science). The more than a thousand hospitals, especially those attached to the schools, are usually well equipped and there are several well-known institutes of specialized research. There are over fifty medical journals — varying greatly in excellence, here as elsewhere — and numerous medical societies, general and specialized. The scientific output today is characterized more by worthy size than by brilliancy. However, in addition to the outstanding discoveries

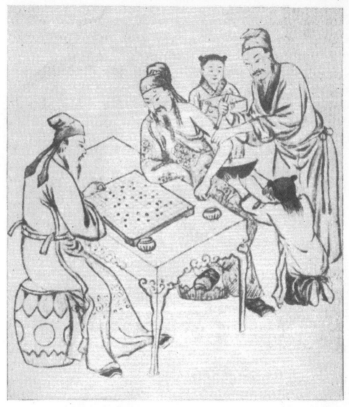

43. *The surgeon Hua T'o amputating the arm of the hero Quan Kung, who continues his game. Ancient Chinese print.*

mentioned above, the following important contributions should be mentioned: discovery of *Schistosoma japonicum* (Katsurada and Fujinami, 1904) and its intermediate host (Miyairi and Suzuki); the hosts of *Clonorchis sinensis* (Kobayashi, 1911) and *Paragonimus westermannii* (Nakagowa, 1914); the discovery of *Leptospira icterohæmorrhagica* (Inada, Ito, et al., 1914); of *Spirochæta morsus muris* (Futaki et al.). The inaccessibility of the Japanese language is mitigated by frequent abstracts in English or German and by the laudable custom of the National Research Council of publishing in English reports of studies in the various special fields.

CHAPTER VIII

THE MEDICINE OF ANCIENT GREECE

THE TEMPLES AND CULT OF AESCULAPIUS —
THE GRECO–ITALIAN SCHOOLS — THE
DAWN OF SCIENTIFIC MEDICINE[1]

1. Origin of Greek Medicine

THE HISTORY of medicine in ancient Greece offers an extremely complex problem because of the difficulty of distinguishing chronological periods and of indicating, at least approximately, the moment at which Hellenic medicine began to possess sufficient knowledge to constitute a particular system. Also, in the case of Greece it is more difficult to separate medicine from the rest of a culture to which it is closely connected than it is in the case of many peoples who preceded the Greeks in history. It would be wrong to regard the Greek medicine of its Golden Age, as has been done for centuries, as an autochthonous growth in Hellas. It grew out of the past just as did art, philosophy, music, and politics; it reflects the influence of peoples who, for different reasons and in different ways, had their effect on the Hellenic culture that inherited from them treasures both of ideas and of practical facts.

From the historical point of view the medicine of ancient Greece is but one phase of medical thought through the centuries. But this phase of de-

[1] On account of the greater familiarity of English-speaking readers with the Latinized forms of the names of Greek divinities, " Æsculapius " is used instead of the more correct " Asclepios," and so also with other proper names.

velopment manifests in their full strength orientations which in the preceding civilization were merely budding germs. It is on the soil of Hellas that perhaps for the first time in history we find men attempting, not as individuals, but with disciples gathered about them, to search freely, beyond the bond imposed by any cult, for the profound reasons of existence.

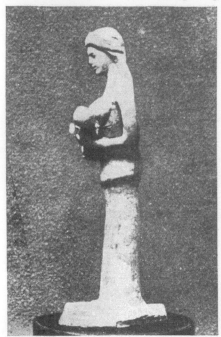

44. *A Cretan woman nursing. Terracotta of sixth century* B.C.

All the knowledge that Oriental medicine had collected, all that the different civilizations had contributed to the people inhabiting the shores of the Mediterranean in the pre-Hellenic period, all this was collected and fused in the crucible of the Ægean. It is as conquerors that the pre-Hellenes appear to have entered the region of the Greek islands, free from any chains of ancient traditions; as if these islands, the centre of the early Ægean civilization, had, in detaching themselves from the Continent, left behind their ancient bonds. While absorbing the treasures of Oriental knowledge, of medicine as of philosophy, of astronomy as of mathematics, they examined these subjects in the light of an agile, independent criticism unhindered by prejudices.

Already in the period of the Minoan civilization (fourth to second millennia B.C.) medicine had reached a grade of development that was not inferior to that described later in the Homeric period. This is apparent in the remains of the Palace of Cnossus, where such hygienic equipment as latrines, water conduits, etc., are found as indications of an advanced civilization. It is also shown by the fact that Egyptian medical books often attribute formulas to the *kefti* (the people of the sea or of the islands), the name that they gave to the Cretans, who had made their little country the centre of Mediterranean life. The arts had reached a high degree of cultivation in a favourable and temperate climate. The reputation that certain remedies of Cretan origin enjoyed in Egypt shows that in this island both empirical medicine and the priestly medicine of the mystical serpent goddess were successfully practised. We may hope that further investigation, which is steadily unveiling new evidence of this civilization, may eventually establish for it a satisfactory documentation.

The characteristic note that dominates all Grecian civilization is already evident. The first factor in it is that the forms of art are free from any traditional rigidity, so that the figures of the Cretan frescoes appear active and alive as compared with the Babylonian and Egyptian monuments. In the same way philosophic thought proceeded to abandon the stylistic lines of mystic dogmatism and to enter into the dominion of free thought, in which no speculation is too bold, no hypothesis too hazardous or subversive of established ideas. Finally, medical thought slowly sloughed off magic concepts and priestly dogmatism and established its basis on observation and a constant study of nature and of man in his relation to animals — a biologic study that brings an essentially new note into medicine. Tempered by criticism, also an eminently Hellenic trait, this produced, perhaps for the first time in history, a medicine that was both an art and a science.

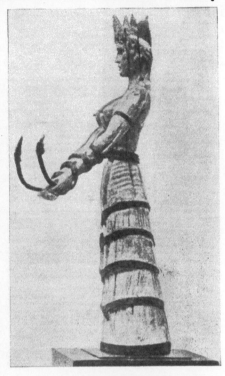

45. *The serpent goddess of the Palace of Cnossus.*

To judge properly the process of formation of Hellenic medicine, it is necessary to consider the influences to which Greece was exposed through centuries and those which Greece in its turn exerted on adjacent and distant peoples. We must think of the colonies which from the Nile to the Black Sea, from Sicily to the Northern coast of Africa, established and brought to fruition, often in very diverse environments, the fortunes and thought of the home country. We must think, too, of a great international commerce, through which navigators, traders, and adventurers brought back from their long voyages, which often seem to us legendary, knowledge of other and foreign cultures. We must consider the effect produced by those Hellenic outposts in Asia Minor which ensured the constant contact of Greece with Egypt and the Orient.

These strains, mixed with indigenous Phœnicians who were in contact with Lydia and Phrygia, knew the Babylonian culture and had been the creators of a poetry that was epic, lyric, and elegiac. This people of clever merchants and navigators, in whom commerce with agricultural products, constant use of money, and diligent observation of weights and measures had developed an extremely critical faculty, was the one that was to initiate the era of scientific research.

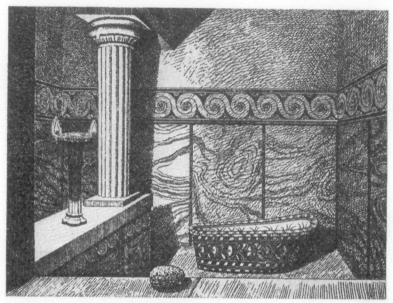

46. *Reconstruction of a bathroom in the Palace of Cnossus of the second Minoan Period. From Sir Arthur Evans's account of the excavations.*

The material advances of the ancient civilizations were thus assembled in a country well favoured by nature climatically, and one that was master of the seas through both its navigation and its commerce. It was also a country enriched by the rapid exchange of its products with surrounding peoples, and accustomed, as has always been the case with maritime races, to distribute freely its material and intellectual riches. This almost necessarily made Greece the theatre of one of the most important and most interesting phenomena of the history of evolution: namely, the stimulation of the ancient seed by contact with new energies.

The history of medicine in early Hellenic culture cannot be separated from the history of its philosophy. It is born with the philosophy

of the school of Thales, takes form in the *Theogony* of Hesiod, is expressed in the dicta of the Pythagoreans and the school of Croton, and

freely and securely grows from
these strong roots to its climax in
the ethical heights of the Hippocratic
school.

Why do we find in Hellenic culture this freedom of thought, of observation and investigation which
alone can guarantee to medicine the
possibility of development, and without which — as we are taught by the
history both of the most ancient times
and of those much nearer to us — there
cannot be any true progress of science? The answer is found in the critical but speculative Greek mentality
and in the political and religious life of
the Greeks. In Greece there was
never a closed priestly caste; religion
was a poetical myth, never a political
edifice, and it never dominated critical thought. Ideas therefore could develop freely, contradictions with and
discussions of the most venerable traditions could flourish; culture, without established boundaries or dog-

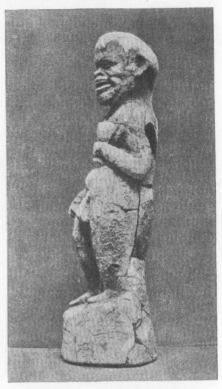

47. *Figure of an erotic alcoholic.
Theban terracotta.*

matic laws, offered to the Greeks assistance to their imagination unhindered
by the fear of punishment.

2. Homeric Medicine

The most important documents bearing on the evolution of Greek medical
thought and professional practice in the early times are the Homeric poems,
which furnish copious facts and indications.

The medicine of the time of Homer was a noble art; the illustrious
heroes who knew the art of war were expert in medicine; but already there
is mention of lay physicians whose aid was sought for the cure of the sick.
The physician was held in great honour, because, according to the poet, he
was "a man who was worth more than many others."

Anatomical knowledge was primitive, but fairly exact as regards the bones, muscles, and joints. Life resides in the breath, which is the transmitter of every vital activity and of all the passions. The seat of life is the diaphragm. The soul, which abandons the body with the last breath, or escapes with the blood of wounds, continues its existence in Hades. Very realistic are the descriptions of the traumatic lesions of man and horse as produced by spear or arrows (*Iliad,*

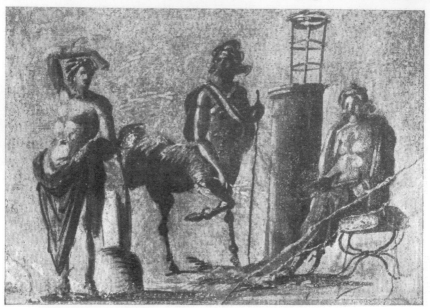

48. *Apollo, Chiron, and Æsculapius.*   (NAPLES MUSEUM.)

VIII, 80). The poet described the use of medicines to alleviate pain, of bandages, and of stimulating drinks.

The severe injury of Æneas is described in the *Iliad* (V, 294 et seq.) in the following verses, which give the clinical picture of fracture of the femur:

> With this stone he smote Æneas on the hip,
> Where the thigh joins its socket. By the blow
> He broke the socket and the tendons twain,
> And tore the skin with the rough jagged stone.
> (translation of William Cullen Bryant)

In Book XI of the *Iliad* (lines 754–61), Nestor takes the wounded Machaon into his tent to treat him and Eurypilus, wounded in the thigh by an arrow, calls on Patroclus to extract the arrow head, to wash off the blood with warm water, and to apply the balms about which Achilles has taught him, which he in turn learned about from the centaur Chiron (*Iliad,* XI, 740–4).

Patroclus tells (*Iliad,* XVI, 28) how the most illustrious of the Greek heroes were treated by physicians wise in medicines; but in addition to the physicians, nurses are named, not only for mortals (*Iliad*, XI, 652; XIV, 6) but also for the gods of Olympus (*Iliad*, V, 894).

In the Homeric poems 140 wounds are described, some superficial, some penetrating. (The mortality averaged 77.6 per cent, being highest in the sword and spear thrusts and lowest in the wounds from arrows, according to Fröhlich.) The extraction of foreign bodies is mentioned; the method of stopping

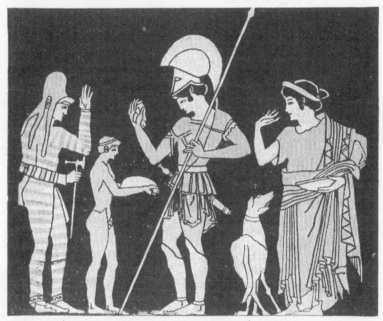

49. *Adrastus leaving for the Theban war consults the liver of a victim.*
From Gerard: Auserlesene griechische Vasenbilder.

hemorrhage is indicated, also the application of compresses or of powdered roots, and the use of bandages.

Magic medicine is also named in the Homeric poems, even though a minor role is attributed to it, and especially in the *Odyssey*, which was reduced to writing at a later period than the *Iliad*. Incantations aid healing; Circe, Agamedes, and the Egyptian Polydamna knew philtres and medicaments. It is to Egypt that Hellas owes the knowledge of many remedies; among them *nepenthe*, which, brewed in wine, made one forget pain (*Odyssey*, IV, 220). Physicians already in the *Iliad* were known as professionals and were servants of the public (*Iliad*, XVI, 28).

In Oefele's interesting studies of the excavations of Troy he notes four embryos of the sixth month which could hardly have been born except by Cæsarean section or as the result of abortion. In the *Iliad* (XIX, 114) also is given the description of a premature birth in the seventh month.

It is evident, then, that Greek medicine was not predominantly magic or priestly, even though the *Iliad* speaks of Apollo as the avenger and the spreader of plague (Apollo Loimios) and other contagious diseases, and even though there are frequent references to the gods as healers of disease and they are invoked in the prayers of the wounded or dying. Evidently in the Homeric concept medicine is decidedly an independent art, practised by experts who are dedicated especially to this art and who are paid for their work. This suggests that perhaps in an earlier distant period of Greek culture medicine was empirical and practised by laymen, while it was only in later times that it became more mystical and priestly.

3. Mythical and Priestly Medicine — the Cult of Æsculapius

In the post-Homeric literature we find with increasing frequency incantations, superstitions, signs, demons, and so forth. The increase of the mystic current reflects the Oriental influence, which was felt more and more in Greek culture. At first all the gods possessed healing attributes or could cause disease; but soon particular powers were attributed to some among them.

The inventor of the healing art is Apollo, " who chases away all ills " (*Alexikakos*), sometimes identified with Pæon, the physician of the gods. Artemis was the protectress of women and children, who in a later period was identified with the Egyptian goddess Istasp, and probably with the " great mother " of the Cretan Olympus, known under the name of Eileithyia. Hygiea was the goddess of health and sometimes was represented with Æsculapius. Panacea was the healer of all ills; Pallas Athene, goddess of science and art, was the protectress of life and lawmaker of hygiene. But other gods were also venerated as healers, among these Aphrodite, the protectress of sexual life, Pan, Juno, Neptune, Bacchus, Mercury, and the chthonic deities — Pluto, Proserpine, Hecate, and even Cerberus and the Fates; they could also cause or avert disease. It should not be forgotten, too, that, as Walter Pater has pointed out, the Greeks had not a religion, but religions. Cults varied in different parts of the country and were constantly undergoing change.

The centaur Chiron was generally regarded as the founder and master of medicine, or perhaps especially of surgery. The most famous of the Greek heroes were his pupils in the chase and in the healing art. Finally, Asclepios — in Latin, Æsculapius — the pupil of Chiron, became in Grecian mythology the son of Apollo and the god of medicine.

According to the hypothesis of Rohde, the origin of the Æsculapius myth is to be sought in the transformation through the centuries of a number of Greek divinities, especially of the lower regions.

To this origin should be attributed, above all, the tradition of the serpent; which, in all chthonic mythology, has the greatest importance; the serpent being regarded, as we have already seen, in the most ancient Biblical myths as

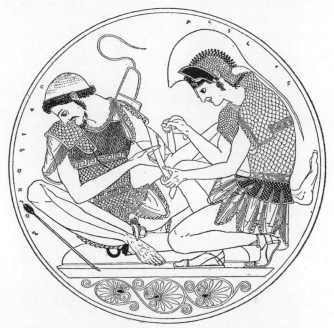

50. *Achilles binds Patroclus' wound. Note the spica bandage.*
(*The bowl of Sosia, fifth century* B.C., *in the* BERLIN MUSEUM.)

a representative of subterranean forces and therefore of the gods of the lower regions. The serpent plays an important part in the most ancient magic medicine. Thus already among the Babylonians it was attributed to the healing god and figured in the *ex votis* offered to give thanks for the cure that had been obtained. The Semitic peoples of Syria, Palestine, and Phœnicia worshipped the god of healing Esmun (see Baudissin: *Adonis et Esmun*), who was often represented as holding a rod in his hand about which are twined two serpents. Other figures of bronze and stone serpents have been discovered in the excavations of Canaan, Gezer, and other parts of Palestine and Transjordania. Certainly this is the cult that produced the Biblical episode of the bronze serpent. Originally, in Thessaly, Æsculapius was probably worshipped as a god of the lower regions; in Homer he was a chief who was taught the healing powers of plants by Chiron. Stricken to death by Jupiter, who was jealous of his success, he was taken to Olympus and transformed into a god (Pindar). He returned later as a hero among mortals and chief of the race of Asclepiads. But we may suppose that originally he was a god of the lower regions, or at least that the cult of an infernal divinity was closely connected with his own. In more ancient times he appeared in the form of a serpent and the votive offerings from the sick were presented to this serpent.

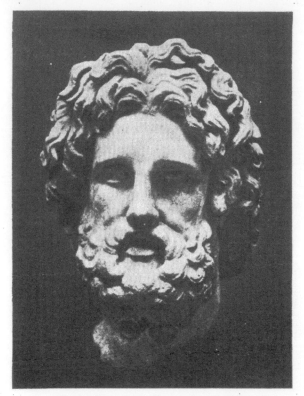

51. *Marble head of the Æsculapius of Melos.*

In any case it is certain that the cult of Æsculapius originated in Thessaly. The Thessalian legend says that he was born at Trikka and names Ischys, the son of King Elatos, as his father, and Coronis, the daughter of Phlegyas, as his mother.

The most ancient centre of the cult of Æsculapius in the Peloponnesus is at Titanos near Sicyon, where the Thessalian serpents live. The founder of this temple was Alexander, the son of Machaon, or of Æsculapius. A different parentage is attributed to Æsculapius in Argolis and Messenia, where he is regarded as the son of Apollo and Arsinoe. The Temple of Epidaurus in Argolis became the centre of the cult of Æsculapius, but it quickly spread throughout the whole Mediterranean basin.

The titles given to Æsculapius in the ancient Greek literature are: *Iatros* (physician), *Orthios* (healer), and *Soter* (saviour). He is represented always by the serpent, which is the symbol of the god and his healing power, and sometimes by the omphalos, a dog, a goat, a cupping instrument, a bowl

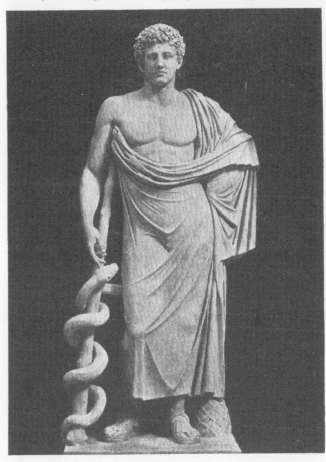

52. *Æsculapius.*   (*Antique statue in the* VATICAN MUSEUM.)

of medicines, a book or staff. Often with him is a boy, Telesphorus, to whom healing powers were later attributed.

In Athens the cult of Æsculapius was introduced about 429 B.C. The priests of Epidaurus, which, as we have seen, was the centre of the cult, sent the serpent, the symbol of the god, to those cities where new sanctuaries were to be established. Thus in 293 B.C., when the plague raged in Rome, messengers were sent to Epidaurus to bring back a sacred serpent, and a temple to Æsculapius was erected on the island of the Tiber.

The temples of Æsculapius were usually built in places where the position and natural beauties of the surroundings made them particularly suitable as places to treat the sick. They were very often built near the sea, with its refreshing breezes; they were architectural masterpieces and were adorned with works of art by the finest masters (Lund).

The ruins of his temple still stand on the southern slopes of the Acropolis. Though not prominent until historic times, the cult undoubtedly had been in existence for centuries, perhaps even before the Homeric period, when it is not mentioned. The various stages of its development may be pictured as: first, an outstanding physician of Thessaly who taught his art to two distinguished sons; next, glorified as an earth demon or cave spirit associated with the serpent cult; eventually deified as the son of Apollo (or Jupiter) and honoured throughout Greece and later by the Romans as the chief god of healing.

The indispensable accessory was a spring of pure water; often the temples were erected in places where there were baths of mineral waters. Later, about the spring and the primitive sanctuaries, were erected magnificent theatres, gymnasia, stadia, and even hippodromes. Here the chronic patients were treated with gymnastic exercises, baths and inunctions; there were also living-quarters for the patients.

All those who came to the sanctuary to invoke the intervention of the god underwent a preliminary treatment, purgative in every sense of the word, which consisted in a series of baths, and abstinence from wines and certain sorts of food. It was only after this preliminary period that they were allowed to enter the temple and begin a strict dietary regime that lasted several days. Then the sick persons were admitted to the ceremonies of the cult, with suggestive prayers by the priest, accounts of former cures, and so on. Finally the patients spent one or more nights in the *abaton* of the temple at the feet of the statue of Æsculapius, awaiting the healing dream. The history of the sanctuaries of Æsculapius and of the treatment in use there, as can be deduced from the votive tablets (*stele*) and the indications of contemporary literature, reveals in a first period a direct personal intervention of the priest, who appeared during the night in the mask of the god, accompanied by the priestess, and accomplished various medical treatments. In later times it seems that the treatment was limited to advice or suggestions that come during the dream, or in the interpretation of the dream. After the treatment, it was the custom to dedicate to the god an *anathema*, a plastic representation in gold, silver, or marble of the part that was cured, or money was thrown into the sacred spring.

Certainly in different sanctuaries, and according to the tendencies of the inhabitants of the different countries, different treatments were practised with a greater or lesser tendency to mysticism or empiricism.

The essential part of all practices, however, was the dream or the hyp-

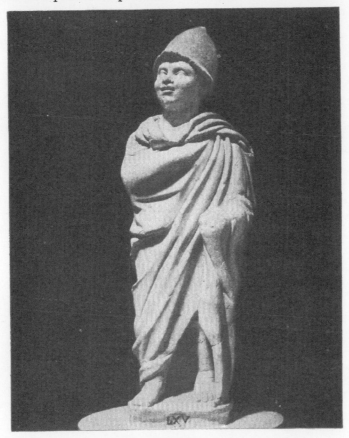

53. *Telesphorus.*
(*Copy of a Hellenistic original in the* BORGHESE GALLERY, ROME.)

notic state, during which the cure was produced. The dream, in sacred places, is still today regarded as highly curative in various Oriental countries, and this is easily understood when one considers the specially favourable conditions that the dream and the hypnotic state offer for suggestion therapy.

Often the faithful compared Æsculapius to Jupiter in his power; his features, also, as handed down by the ancient sculptors, are like those of Jove. Pausanias, who made his famous journey to Greece in the second century of our era, in his description of the sanctuary at Epidaurus, which was still flourishing, states that Æsculapius had been regarded as a god from the most ancient times. In the excavations at Epidaurus steles have been found which were already mentioned by Pausanius, who, however, states that he had seen only six that were preserved intact. On them were written the

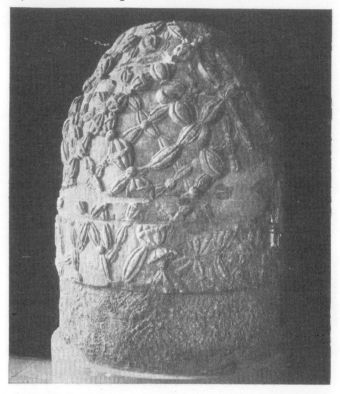

54. *Marble Omphalos.*   (MUSEUM OF DELPHI.)

names of those who had been cured by Æsculapius and also the names of the diseases they had suffered from and the method of treatment.

The Greek Archæological Society, under the direction of Cavvadias, to whom we owe especially intensive study in this field, has been able to find at Epidaurus many inscriptions and tablets dating from ancient times. There are forty-four tablets from the fourth century B.C. — that is, the period in which the *abaton* was constructed. They evidently served the purpose of offering to those who came to the sanctuary for treatment the opportunity of drawing encouragement from perusal of the accounts of famous cures.

It is certain that some of these inscriptions come from very ancient times and perhaps take the place of even more ancient tablets that had been destroyed. To give an idea of them, two of the most significant may be translated: " Aristagora of Troixenes: she has a worm in her body. She slept in the temple of Æsculapius at Troixenes and the god appeared to her in a dream. She dreamed that the sons of the god, while the god was at Epidaurus, cut off her head, but that, not being able to attach it again to the body, they sent a messenger to Æsculapius inviting him to come to Troixenes. The next morning the priests found that actually [and no longer in a dream] the head of Aristagora was separated from the body. When night came again, the patient had a second dream: it appeared to her that the god, who in the meantime had arrived from Epidaurus, had put her head back on her neck, then had opened her belly, taken out the worm, and sewed it up. Then the woman was healed."

Another narration is particularly instructive: " Hermo of Pasos: the god cured him of his blindness, but when he refused to pay the honorarium to the sanctuary, the god made him blind again as a punishment. When he returned again and slept once more in the temple, the god healed him again."

From these stories we see for example that the priests of Epidaurus, jealous of the crowds attracted to Troixenes, relate how their colleagues of the rival town committed an error of diagnosis, evidently believing that the worm was in the neck instead of in the belly, and had to have recourse to the authentic sanctuary to correct the mistake.

A very interesting contribution to the history of the sanctuaries of Æsculapius is given in the *Plutus* of Aristophanes, a comedy produced in Athens in 388 B.C. Here we find in burlesque a subtle, witty satire on the cult of Æsculapius and the treatments practised in his temples.

The god of riches, who is blind, helps a good old man who, in gratitude, has him led by his slave to the temple of Æsculapius. The story of the treatment in the sanctuary is especially interesting as all the procedures are described in satiric form. First the blind god is given a cold bath; then, accompanied by the slave, he goes to the temple to place his offering on the altar of the god. There, according to custom, the patient is placed on a couch near several other patients, who, like him, are awaiting cure. The servitor of the temple puts out the lights and tells everyone to go to sleep and not to move even if they should hear a noise. But the slave, Charyon, cannot sleep because he is disturbed by the penetrating odour from a stew that was the offering of one of the old patients.

He opens his eyes and sees the priest go from one altar to another, take all the offerings, and put them in his bag. Then Æsculapius appears accompanied by Jason and Panacea; Æsculapius goes from bed to bed examining the patients. Behind him comes a slave with a stone mortar and boxes of drugs. In the mortar the slave prepares ointments composed of onions from Tenos, the juice of figs and resin, on which he casts the vinegar of Sphectos. Then he opens the eyelids of Neocleides, another patient, who complains of poor sight and is a famous busybody, and he applies the ointment to them. The patient runs away, uttering cries. Then the god approaches Plutus, touches him on the head, then wipes his eyelids with linen. The daughter of the god, Panacea, she who cures everything, places a red bandage on the head; then the god whistles and two great serpents appear on the stage. They go beneath the red bandage and lick

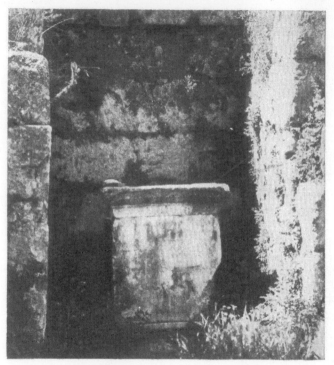

55. *The sacred spring of the Temple of Æsculapius at Cos.*

the eyelids of the patient: "Before you can find time to drink ten glasses of wine, the blind god Plutus is cured and goes away in perfect health."

The satiric form in which the temple treatment is described, the irreverent and even obscene terms used in the verses of the poet, and the lack of esteem that Aristophanes shows for the practices of the sanctuary are characteristic of the intelligent criticism of the Greeks. It also proves that even in those times independent persons understood the superstitions and tricks used in these treatments. The comedian could speak in this way before the Athenian public without fear of shocking the sensibilities.

Nevertheless, priestly medicine spread with great success throughout Greece about the fifth century B.C., and continued to be in common practice up to the fourth or fifth century of our era. A short and graceful poem by Herondas, a poet who lived at Cos two centuries after Hippocrates, was called " The Women Who Sacrificed in the Temple of Æsculapius " (published by the humanist Otto Crusius, in Leipzig, 1928). It brings an interesting contribution to the history of the cult of Æsculapius. The women Cinno and Cocale enter the temple, describe it, and give detailed descriptions of the works of art to be found there. They speak with the sacristan, invoke the god, and present their offerings. This delicate and graceful poetry makes us live again in one of the most famous centres of the ancient cult of Æsculapius. The Neo-Platonist Proclus, who lived in Athens A.D. 410–485, declared himself a convinced and faithful follower of Æsculapius. St. Jerome deplored the imbecility of those who sought for safety in the sanctuaries of the pagan god, and about A.D. 500 we find the cult of Æsculapius (*Soter*) often mingled in strange combination with the cult of Christian saints.

Thus, the more recent historical investigations show that, if Homeric medicine was practised by the laity, the medicine of the sanctuaries of Æsculapius was practised exclusively by priests, and the cures were regarded as miraculous. The treatment, in addition to suggestion and magic practices which contributed in a very important way to its success, consisted in dietary measures, baths, and massage. A very important aid to treatment was conferred by the marvellous situation of the temples and by the conveniences by which the patients were surrounded. In Epidaurus one still sees the remains of the magnificent Propylæum, constructed by Polycletus in the fourth century B.C., which was certainly one of the most magnificent in Greece, and of a theatre in which there were marble seats for more than ten thousand spectators. In the centre of the sanctuary was the space allotted to the sleepers, the *abaton*. Near it stood the magnificent chryso-elephantine (gold and ivory) statue of the god.

4. The Dawn of Scientific Medicine — Early Philosophic Schools

The origin of scientific medicine is contemporary with the emergence of Greek philosophy, when for the first time in history we see an attempt to construct on the basis of speculative reflection a system capable of explaining the phenomena of nature and establishing its laws. Before this period medicine was variously instinctive, empirical, magical, priestly, or religious. But even if in certain periods and countries, as we have seen, it attained a high degree of practical knowledge and technical perfection, it is revealed as purely and directly utilitarian, applied entirely to the immediate purpose of stopping the pains of the sick person or of prolonging his life. As the mathematics and astronomy of the Assyro-Babylonians, the Egyptians, and the ancient Indians pursued a practical purpose, so also their medicine was aimed at practical results, without being concerned with the discovery of fundamental causes, and above all without arranging in logical sequence the cause and effect of observed phenomena. The ancient Orient had ac-

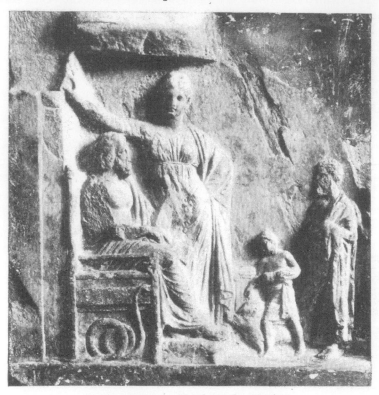

56. *An offering to Æsculapius by a patient.*
(*Bas-relief in the* ATHENS MUSEUM.)

cumulated, through millennia, an extremely rich store of observations diligently studied and preserved, and had deduced from them regulations for practical life. But the Greek philosopher applied to their knowledge a critical thought based on observation and experience. There is no doubt that some of the great philosophers of the pre-Socratic school were also physicians; and that indirectly the fertility of the most ancient philosophic thought proceeded from medical knowledge and from the accumulated wisdom of the Orient. It is from the observation of nature and the vicissitudes of human life and its accompanying phenomena that the first philosophic speculations arose. These first philosophers were in fact naturalists and biologists who passed from the study of the individual to that of the cosmos; and, regarding the cosmos as a unit, returned to the study of the individual and thus established that line of philosophic thought that will never again be abandoned.

Of the great pre-Socratic schools of philosophy, the Ionian school of Miletus was probably the most ancient. Founded by Thales of Miletus (639–544 B.C.), who was regarded by Plato and Aristotle as the initiator of philosophy, it concerned itself above all with mathematical problems, regarded from the cosmic point of view. It is to this school that we probably owe the concept of nature as *physis*, a concept that was later so wisely developed by Aristotle. There exists, according to Thales, a substance that is the original principle of everything in the cosmos and of the cosmos itself. This principle is the origin of all generation, the eternal element of every form of life and nature, the *physis* in the sense of Thales. This original substance, according to the philosophy of Thales, is water. But it is not water in the sense of a divine substance, as it was considered in the ancient cosmogony, but water regarded as an essential fundamental substance, and — what is more valuable — logically demonstrable in every living thing. From water, or from one of its transformations, everything is derived: the fertility of seeds, the life of plants, the life of animals and man. All life ends in water, because everything that is corrupted or dies is transformed into liquid — that is, water. Perhaps, if we can rightly interpret the words of Aristotle, Thales thought of the spirit as a motive force and made a distinction between it and the body. In any case, however, it is not the results of the philosophy of this school that chiefly interests us, but the method of its reasoning. This system was followed by Anaximander, of Miletus (c. 600 B.C.), who speaks of a cyclical rhythm of generation and corruption, and by Anaximenes, also of Miletus (570–500 B.C.), who believed that the essential substance was not water but air, and that from the condensation or rarefaction of air are derived the most important phenomena of life. The Ionic school, as we have seen, applied itself to an explanation of those basic facts whose comprehension was indispensable for the creation of a biologic system. It is interesting to note that Huxley thought the activity of this school to be but one of several manifestations of a " mental ferment over the whole area comprised between the Ægean and northern Hindustan," spread, according to Elliot Smith, by the Phœnician navigators. Jonathan Wright, also, has pointed out (*Scientific Monthly*, New York, 1920, XI, 131) that Zoroaster, Confucius, Buddha, Thales, and Pythagoras were active along the 35th degree of north latitude at almost the same time.

5. *Biologic Concepts and Medicine of the Greco-Italic School: Pythagoras, Alcmæon, Philolaus, Heraclitus, Empedocles, and Their Pupils*

It was the great philosophic school to which Aristotle gave the name of Italic that became the most important basis of scientific medicine. If it reflected Ionic influences, because Pythagoras (580–489 B.C.), its founder, was of Ionic origin, it quickly took on a special character oriented toward medicine and biology. The displacement of the seat of this philosophic

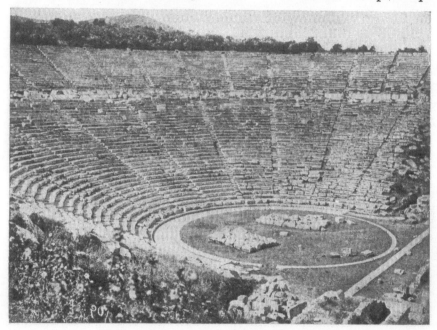

57. The theatre of the Temple of Æsculapius at Epidaurus.

school and the reasons that it found its most important and flourishing centres in southern Italy have been differently explained by those who have concerned themselves with this question, and have given rise to various conjectures. Certainly one must admit that even before Pythagoras arrived at Croton there was an important and flourishing school of medicine there; and that, if not in its shadow, at least it was near this school that Pythagorism had its first development. The figure of Pythagoras is largely legendary. All the writings attributed to him are of uncertain origin, so that to form an opinion of Pythagorean activities we must trust to the testimony of the ancient biographers and philosophers who have described his doctrines. This is not the place to look into the relations that exist between the ancient Orphic associations and the Pythagorean sect, or to study the problem, no matter how interesting it is for the history of medicine, of the significance of the catechism of the " Acousmatics," in which are exposed in mystic form the dominant ideas of the Pythagorean schools. We note only that Pythagoras was certainly a physician, a penetrating and deep

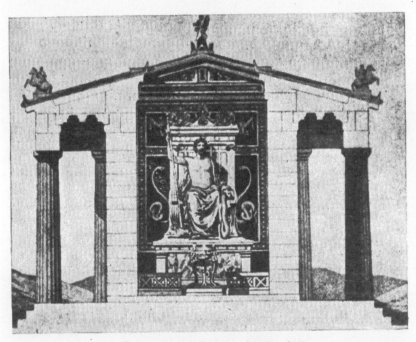

58. *Restoration of the statue of Æsculapius in the Temple of Epidaurus.*

observer of the animal organism, particularly curious about the phenomenon of procreation, and that from him may be derived in its essential principles that doctrine of numbers which constitutes one of the bases of Pythagorean philosophy and has a very great importance for Hippocratic medicine. Pythagoras was perhaps the first to note the relations between musical pitch and the weight of the hammer and the length of the cord, and to establish the doctrine of perfect numbers. It is from this theory of numbers, which perhaps more justly should be called the theory of harmony, that is derived the concept of the universe as in perfect numerical harmony, and also the Hippocratic concept of the crisis, the critical days, and the healing power of nature.

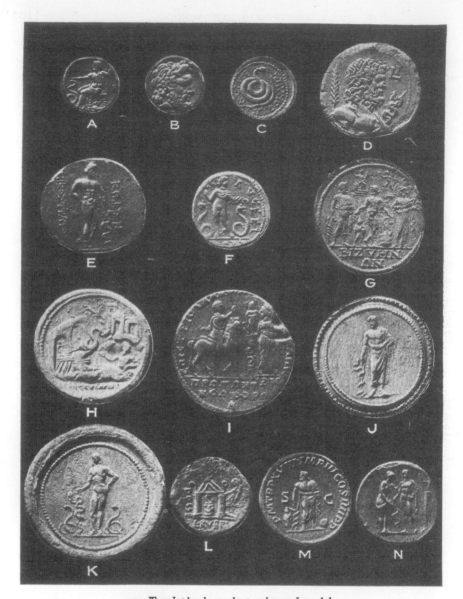

59. *Æsculapius in ancient coins and medals.*

A, Coin of Cos of the first century B.C. *B, C*, Silver coin of Epidaurus with the head of Æsculapius and the sacred serpent. *D*, Bust of Æsculapius, on a bronze coin of Alexander Severus (A.D. 222–35). *E*, Tetradrachma of Cos with the standing figure of Æsculapius leaning on the staff with the serpent. *F*, The Phœnician Æsculapius, Esmun, with two serpents, on a bronze medal of Heliogabalus (A.D. 218–22). *G*, Copper coin of Thrace of the third century, showing Apollo, Omphalos, Hygeia, and Telesphoros. *H*, A bronze medal of Antoninus Pius recording the arrival of the Æsculapian serpent at Rome and the

The biological and medical concepts of the Pythagoreans certainly derived, as I have said, from relations that they had with the medical school of Croton. ALCMÆON, who was perhaps a pupil of this medical school and who certainly was closely connected with the Pythagorean school, was the most distinguished physician of the pre-Hippocratic period. His book *On Nature*, of which only traces have been preserved in later writings, was the fundamental text for pre-Hippocratic medicine. The theory advanced by De Renzi, and supported by recent studies, that some of the books of the *Corpus Hippocraticum* are derived from this eminent Pythagorean does not seem improbable. It is certain that in the doctrine of the Pythagorean numbers we find the principle of the Hippocratic doctrine of crises, and in the book of Alcmæon a doctrinal basis for the school of Cos.

Alcmæon of Croton, who lived about 500 B.C., was a contemporary of Pythagoras, though somewhat younger. Tradition states that he was the first to practise anatomic dissections, and to him we owe important anatomical discoveries. Certainly he was an enthusiastic investigator, who made experiments on animals. To him is owed the idea that medical investigation is happily combined with philosophic reasoning; whence comes the concept of *Isonomia:* that is, the perfect harmony of all the substances that compose the human body. According to this concept, health consists in a state of perfect harmony; disease is nothing but an expression of a disturbance of this harmony. Cure consists in the return from the disturbed to the harmonious state. From this line of thought, as we shall see, came the later studies of Empedocles, and it is essentially on it that was based the principle of humoral pathology, which for more than twenty centuries was the basis of all pathology.

According to Alcmæon, it is not in the heart, as had been hitherto asserted, but in the brain that the seat of the senses and the centre of intellectual life should be sought. Alcmæon was the first to study the course of the optic nerves and he recognized the necessity of three substances for vision: external light, the internal fire of the eye, and the liquid contained in the eye, as a means of transmission. He is said to have discovered the Eustachian tube (in goats). To this great physiologist we owe also the first indications regarding the circula-

---

construction of the temple on the island in the Tiber. *I*, Bronze medal of Caracalla (A.D. 211–17). The Asclepieion of Pergamos. Caracalla on horseback worships the statue of the god. *J*, Æsculapius. A bronze medal of Hadrian (A.D. 117–38). *K*, The Æsculapius of Thrace with two serpents. Medal of Marcus Aurelius. *L*, The statue of Æsculapius on the altar of a temple. Gold coin of Caracalla. *M*, Æsculapius with Telesphoros. Bronze coin of Caracalla. *N*, Æsculapius and the goddess Salus. Bronze coin of Hadrian. *Courtesy of Dr. M. Bernhardt of St. Moritz, Switzerland.*

tion, as he distinguished the veins from the arteries. To him we owe the first researches on the functional disturbances caused by lesions of the brain and also an explanation of the origin of sleep, which he thought was due to an exodus of blood from the brain to the vessels. He explained death in a similar way.

In the work of Alcmæon we also find the first ideas of the concept of the individual constitution and of the influence that this can have on the occurrence of diseases. If the elements are combined two by two — for example, wet and

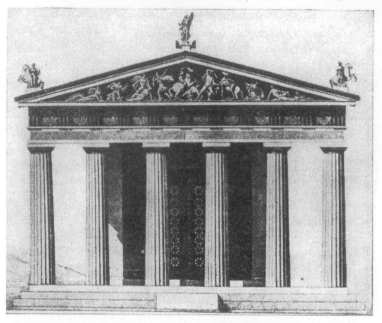

60. Reconstruction of the front of the Temple of Æsculapius at Epidaurus.

dry, cold and hot, bitter and sweet — and if disease, as has been said, is caused by the predominance of one element over the other, or of one pair over another pair, such circumstances as irregular nutrition, or such external causes as climate, environment, or topographical character of the country where the sick person lives, can produce, according to Alcmæon, a disturbance of the reciprocal relations among the elements, and thus be a cause of disease. Among the fundamental principles of the doctrine of Alcmæon are: that animal life is a movement and subordinate to a movement of the blood, which, even if not always uniform, is continuous; that sensation and thought are subordinate to the invisible and unnoticed movement of the brain, and that as movement is the essential factor to life, so diseases arise from a movement that disturbs the normal harmony of life.

The doctrine of Alcmæon is set forth in the *Phædo* of Plato. In the words put into the mouth of the dying Socrates, the concept is announced that " the brain furnishes the sensations of hearing, sight, and smelling, from which memory and judgment are born, and from these sensations, once established, wisdom also is born."

From what we have seen above, it is evident that in the work of this Crotonian physician there are to be found the beginnings of the fundamental doctrines of the Hippocratic school. To Pythagoras, as head of this school, may be awarded the merit of having established its basis, although, as we have seen, his figure has been largely enveloped in mystery and become legendary, and even though, rightly or wrongly, he has been connected with important brotherhoods which took his name and became politically predominant at Sybaris, Reggio, Catania, and Agrigentum. To Alcmæon, however, belongs the greater merit of having been a magnificent initiator in the field of biology and medicine, who always turned to practical experience to support the truth of his thinking.

To the school of Alcmæon belongs another important physician, PHILOLAUS of Tarentum, who lived about the middle of the fifth century B.C. According to Franck (1923) and Howard, of Zurich (1924), Philolaus is one of the most important pre-Platonic Pythagoreans, in whom is to be found the fundamental origin of Platonism. According to Philolaus, who should really be regarded as the head of a school, there is a complete analogy between the world and the individual: " As the former has its central fire, so the human body has its essence in heat: the heat of the seed and of the uterus are the origin of all life; the body attracts to itself the external air on account of its desire that heat should be tempered by cold and thus restores itself in respiration." This exchange acts on the blood, on the phlegm, and on the yellow and black bile, and it is the alterations that may occur in the interchange of these humours that produce diseases. Thus animal life is to be regarded as a harmony, an accord of contrary factors. This is the belief that we see maintained by the Theban Simias, a pupil of Philolaus, in the *Phædo* of Plato. The thesis of Simias is evidently of Pythagorean origin; it maintains that the accord in the microcosm is determined by the spirit, that the body is comparable to a lyre whose chords are properly stretched when the unity of all the factors is maintained; if tension is relaxed or becomes excessive, harmony vanishes, which signifies the death of the spirit, even before the destruction of the body. This thesis, which according to Plato had the support of Echecrates, who belonged to the school of Philolaus, is compared with other beliefs in this same dialogue.

In the *Timæus* of Plato the Pythagorean doctrine is exposed at length, probably according to the ideas of Philolaus. The anatomical and physiological concepts are still fairly vague: the liver is regarded as the mirror in which is reflected the thought of the intelligent spirit, which, as the case may be, is disturbed by bitterness (excess of bile) or calmed by sweetness. Thus, according to Plato, the liver has an almost moral position subordinate to the intellect. The spleen is designed to collect in itself, as in a sponge, the impurities of the liver.

As to diseases: " the manner in which they are formed can be clear to anyone. The body is composed of a mixture of four elements: earth, fire, water, and air. The abundance or lack of these elements beyond the natural (*contra naturam*); or a change of place, making them go from their natural position to another that

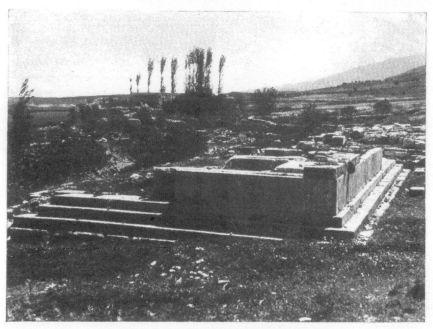

61. *Ruins of the Temple of Æsculapius at Cos.*

does not suit them; or the fact that one of them is forced to receive a quality that is not proper for it but suitable for another kind (for there are different qualities for every kind): all these and other similar factors are the causes that produce disturbance and diseases. There is also another kind of disease that must be regarded as having three different origins: one from the air that is breathed, another from the phlegm; a third from the bile " (*Timæus*, Chs. xxxix, xl).

To the school of Alcmæon is attributed, especially by those historians who have been recently concerned with this question, a fairly important part in the origin of Hippocratic thought. Thus Wellmann (1930) attributes to a pupil of Alcmæon the book *On Ancient Medicine*, and maintains that the old physicians referred to by the author as the founders of medicine are the Pythagoreans, whom he defends as opposed to the pupils of the school of Cnidus. Deichgräber (*Hermes*, 1933) has the same opinion. Wellmann (1929) also attributes the book *On the Sacred Disease* to a physician of the school of Croton. Finally, Roscher (Paderborn, 1913) believes that the treatise *On the Weeks*, the origin of which has been much discussed, is of Ionic origin. In the work of Olivieri (Naples, 1917), of J. Soury (Paris, 1899), of D. B. Roncali (Naples, 1929), and in Golgi's lecture at the meeting in Padua of the Italian Society of Science (1909), there is the same tendency to attribute more and more importance to the doctrines of the school of Alcmæon.

In the basic teaching of the Pythagorean school, as was already noted in ancient times, three main principles stand out: the immortality of the soul, the passage of the soul into animals of different species in various periods, and the relationship of all animal beings.

Aristotle speaks of the Pythagorean doctrine and maintains that an intimate relationship unites all living beings on the earth. It was this essentially spiritual doctrine that created in Magna Græcia the ideal frame for a religious sect which later became a political body teaching its believers the pure life of the body and soul and the philosophic principle that there are simple and intelligible laws for all natural phenomena. From this was doubtless derived the conscious search for a supreme law founded on the harmony of opposite principles.

It is important to follow the medical thought thus vigorously maintained in the studies of Alcmæon and Philolaus through the philosophic doctrines of other schools and the philosophic speculations of HERACLITUS of Ephesus (*c.* 556–460 B.C.), down to the Eleatic school of Parmenides, according to whom the essence of life consists in heat and living beings are born from mud by means of heat.

Heraclitus was the first, as Hegel has stated, to conceive of philosophy in its speculative form. Among the pre-Socratic philosophers, no one more than he exercised a deeper influence on Greek philosophy. Even though, according to Bodrero, the complexity of his philosophic synthesis is such that it is impossible to connect it with a given school, still it appears that his system suggests Oriental mysticism as well as revealing fundamental principles of philosophic Hellenism. Heraclitus believed that a single element, fire, was the basis of matter. He maintained that death is for man the principle of rebirth, immortality consisting in placing the individual in a universal current. Philolaus was the first philosopher who explicitly substituted the knowledge of the universal absolute for the knowledge of a particular and individual absolute. He stated that what appears to be difference is really but a single phenomenon: development coming from continuous contrasts. Diverse appearances are nothing but single aspects of the constant change of matter. From Heraclitus comes the famous aphorism: *Panta rhei* (everything flows), which is the clearest expression of the concept of development.

EMPEDOCLES of Agrigentum (504–443 B.C.) is regarded by some philosophers as belonging to the Pythagorean school. Others, and especially the more recent ones, such as Robin, called him the founder of a new school which felt the influence of both the Pythagorean and the Eleatic schools. The figure of Empedocles is without doubt one of the most interesting and complex of this period. The fervent admiration of his pupils and of his followers has surrounded his personality with a legend attributing to

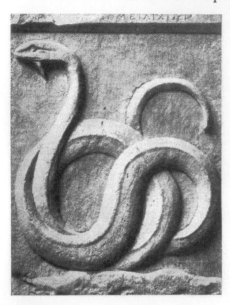

62. *Bas-relief of the healing serpent.*
(ATHENS MUSEUM.)

him not only the invention of rhetoric but also supernatural powers. Among the most important of his works was a didactic poem *On Nature*, dedicated to the physician Pausanias, a book of dietary prescriptions in six hundred verses. The few remaining fragments of his work have been published by Karsten (Amsterdam, 1838). They suffice to demonstrate a powerful vision of the laws of the universe.

Empedocles regarded the world as composed of four elements which he called the roots of everything: fire, water, ether (air), and earth. These are substances without formation and indestructible, the elements from which comes everything that was and is and is to be. They are equal among themselves and of the same age, each of them possessing its own character and from time to time dominating or being dominated by the others. The human body, like all living beings, is composed of these four elements, and health comes from their harmony, just as their disturbance or disharmony causes disease.

The union of the elements which determine generation and every other form of life, the proper mixture and proportions among them, is due to two principles: the one, exterior, is discord; the other, internal, is accord. This is the dynamic basis of the physiology of Empedocles: by the action of accord the various elements unite and constitute a unity; by the action of discord, unity itself is broken up into its elements. Thus the two essential motive forces are antagonistic in the passage of time. Adjacent and similar things attract each other by analogy and by accord. Through the pores of the body the emanations of exterior things penetrate into the organism: air penetrates into the lungs and into the pores; thus respiration, according to Empedocles, occurs not only through the lungs but also through the skin. The blood is the carrier of animal heat; the heart is the first organ to be formed in the fetus. Biological phenomena are explained according to this doctrine, which makes the play of well-defined substances depend on the dynamics of motor forces.

The fundamental principle of Empedocles consists in the opposition and the accord of various parts of nature, in dualism, therefore, and equilibrium (Bodrero). In his doctrine are to be found the methods of the philosophers who preceded him and the germs of thought of those who followed him. He is an eminent figure in the history of Greek philosophy, the constructor of a philosophic system based on a natural philosophy. He gives for the first time a complete, rational, and totally new doctrine of the world, imagining it as oscillating between two extreme principles, containing them and contained by them.

Stripping from the figure of Empedocles those supernatural and marvellous attributes that his contemporaries and followers ascribed to him, we may still recognize in him a great master in the field of biology. This we may do even though we regard as insufficiently proved the position as hygienist and conqueror of epidemics accorded him for his freeing the city of Selinuntum from a severe pestilence by draining swamps and delivering his native city of Agrigentum by ordaining widespread fumigation. Among the thinkers of the pre-Socratic period and the physicians who paved the way for the Hippocratic school, a most honourable position should be reserved for this great Sicilian, who had a clear vision of the most varied problems of physiology.

His admirers find in some of his concepts the germs of very modern ideas. Thus, in his belief that living beings are composed of single organs that successively unite and can be maintained alive and reproducing only when perfectly combined, Neuburger sees the germ of the Darwinian theory of the survival of the fittest. The Empedoclean theory, according to which the exchange between external substances and the organism was accomplished by the passage of minute particles through the pores, appears to Puccinotti as similar to the quite modern doctrine of endosmosis.

The Sicilian medical school, thanks especially to the work of Atron and Philistion, progressed rapidly. ANAXAGORAS (500–428 B.C.) of Clazomene, a contemporary of Empedocles, brought to Athens the teaching of philosophy. He created the theory of *Homoiomeria*, countless minute particles that were separated or aggregated by *Nous* (the mind) as the ruler of the universe. In the field of medicine his name is celebrated because he was supposed to be the first to dissect animals; he maintained the dependence of most diseases on the bile.

Of later Greek philosophers, there should be noted HIPPO of Reggio and ARCHELAUS of Athens, who elaborated the theories of Anaxagoras; also DEMOCRITUS of Abdera (460–360 B.C.), founder of the atomic theory, zoologist, and eager investigator, who was particularly concerned with the study of the causes of epidemic diseases.

The influence on the evolution of medical thought exercised by the pre-Socratic schools of philosophy, led by the school of Pythagoras, may be said to have been twofold. On the one hand was elaborated the doctrine of the four cardinal elements, to which the four basic humours correspond, a concept which dominated all pathology for many centuries. On the other hand, there was introduced into medicine, and this is without doubt of much greater importance, the study of nature, of philosophic reasoning, of investigation of the causalities and finalities of life. Thus in these schools, to which southern Italy brought such an important contribution, we find the essential foundations of Hippocratic medicine.

6. Medical Schools and the Practice of Medicine — Their Development Independently of Priestly Medicine

While in southern Italy and Sicily medical schools developed adjacent to and under the influence of philosophic schools, and in turn had their effect on the orientation of philosophy, other schools of great historical importance flourished in Cyrene, Rhodes, Cnidus, and Cos. The most ancient of these schools seems to have been that of Cyrene, already honourably mentioned by Heraclitus, who states that from Cyrene come excellent physicians (III, 131). Here was a famous temple of Æsculapius, whose cult is said to have been brought to Cyrene about 429 B.C. Cnidus, a Lacedemonian colony in Asiatic Doris, had a medical school which obviously reflected the influence of Mesopotamian and Egyptian culture. The physicians of Cnidus schematized a series of morbid types and collected in the so-called " Cnidian maxims " the most important medical prescriptions. The theory of numbers still dominated this school, and pathology was strictly localized in the different parts of the body.

Anatomy is almost unknown to the Cnidian school, so that it was guided by an obvious a priori tendency. It possessed important knowledge in the field of practical medicine and gynæcology. Among the physicians of this school should be noted above all Ctesias, contemporary of Hippocrates, and Euryphon, who was said by Galen to be the author of the Cnidian maxims. Neuburger states that Euryphon recognized that the arteries contained blood as well as the veins, as they bled when cut. The arteries received their name because they contained air when examined after death, an error that persisted for centuries. When bleeding from a cut artery was admitted, it was rationalized as a mixture of pneuma and blood that had percolated through from the neighbouring veins.

The school of Cos, which gave the world the master physician of all times, arose, contrary to the statements of the ancient historians, well before the foundation there of the temple of Æsculapius. This temple, which had great renown throughout Greece, was erected about the fifth or fourth century B.C., as is shown by excavations and by the architecture of the temple. All hypotheses that the physicians of the school had learned the art of medicine from the priests of the temple are entirely without foundation. This is demonstrated by the fact that in all the Hippocratic writings there is no mention of miraculous cures nor of the practice of medicine by priests. The divinity did not act either as the producer of disease or as its healer.

The medicine of the school of Cos is founded much more than that of Cnidus on direct observation. It is concerned — and this is one of its principal characteristics — not so much with disease as with the patient, not so much with subtle discussions of diagnosis and explanations of the causes of disease as with the prognosis of the individual patient.

Another important characteristic of this school is that pathology in it for the first time became general; in other words, it is the first time in history that disease was recognized as a general affection and not limited to this or that organ. This concept, derived directly from the philosophic schools that I have mentioned, guided students to a correct estimate of the place of man in the macrocosm.

The studies of the school of Cos were directed especially to those diseases which are most striking on account of their acute manifestations — those which by the rhythmicity and constancy of their symptoms suggested more easily a relation to other phenomena of nature.

Thus is formed the doctrine of the crisis and of the critical days — old Babylonian astrological concepts — which are useful in the field of prognosis. From this concept arose the principle of the three stages of disease (prodromal, fastigium, and decline). It also suggested humoral pathology, based chiefly on the principle of a harmonious and reciprocal influence of the various elements.

Thus we see how a number of factors act simultaneously, even if with different intensity, to form the main features of Greek medical thought: they are the ancient traditions of an empirical, lay medicine, on the one hand; and, on the other, the mathematical and astronomical knowledge of the Assyro-Babylonians and the sanitary regulations of ancient Egypt and Judea, which under the stimulating effect of Greco-Italic philosophy and criticism combined to form the foundation of the magnificent edifice that we are accustomed to call Hippocratic medicine.

It was these schools that impressed a special character on Greek medicine and determined its development. In them began critical discussions which had never happened up to that time. It was in these early schools of the practice of medicine that scientific thought had its birth.

Besides the schools, at the same time there were formed organizations of physicians. The so-called Oath of Hippocrates, which perhaps constitutes the most ancient historic document that codifies the ethics of a professional corporation, comes from this same period.

Priestly medicine, as we have seen, was at this time well organized and prosperous in the sanctuaries, with exact regulations for the payment of honoraria. While it was developing an activity that assumed more and more the character of a real practice of medicine, in which suggestion, diet, and drugs were wisely combined, a practical form of lay medicine continued to be developed in the hands of specialists. The fact, however, that the name of Asclepiads was given to the pupils of the non-priestly medical schools does not prove that they were in connection with the sanctuaries. In reality, the Asclepiads existed before the time of priestly medicine; and in the *Iliad* (II, 645–8) probably written in the tenth century B.C., Podalirius and Machaon, the sons of Æsculapius, are cited as worthy physicians and leaders of the people.

> The men of Tricca and Ithome's hills
> And they who held Œchalia and the town
>   of Eurytus the Œchalian had for chiefs
> Two sons of Æsculapius, healers both,
> And skilful — Podalirius one, and one
>   Machaon.

It was the descendants of Podalirius and Machaon who constituted in early times the family of the Asclepiads — that is, of the physicians initiated into the secrets and practice of the art.

Lay physicians, then, from ancient times practised their art intelligently. *Periodeuteis*, travelling physicians, went from city to city to examine patients. However, at the same time we know of physicians of chieftains and princesses, like Democedes of Croton, quoted by Herodotus (III, 125), who was the physician of Polycrates of Samos and later of Darius. He received a very large salary. Certain foreign physicians also practised in Greece, such as Thales of Gorchina. There were physicians paid from the public exchequer in the large and small cities, such as Herodicus of Leontium, a brother of Gorgias, named by Plato (*De Legibus*, VIII). Of these physicians the *periodeutes* seemed to be held in less esteem than the others; they were perhaps the empirical practitioners who also made and sold their own drugs. Even today in the villages and market-places of Greek cities

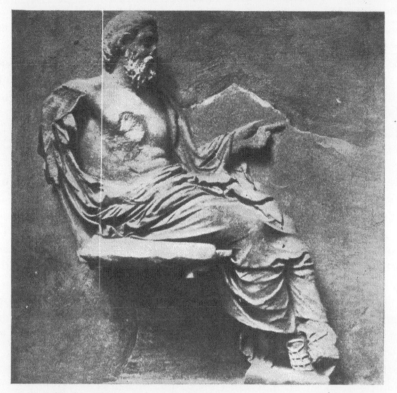

63. *Marble bas-relief of the healing god.*   (ATHENS MUSEUM.)

this strange type of ambulant physician can be met, probably stemming directly from the very ancient type. The *periodeutes* were generally lithotomists and frequently damaged the spermatic cord. It is perhaps for this reason that the physician was obligated in the Oath of Hippocrates not to practise this operation.

All the literature of the period shows that these physicians were not dependent on a sanctuary, but lived in close intimacy, like adopted sons, with their masters and families. Thus it is evident that already before the Hippocratic period there existed large and flourishing Greek schools of medicine. It is particularly interesting that they arose in the great centres of commerce in the islands and coastal cities. From these schools, which probably had both a patriarchal and an initiate organization, medical physicians went out who practised their art in the courts, the cities, and the armies, independent of priestly medicine, which in its turn continued to flourish quietly in the shadow of the sanctuaries.

The physician, *iatros* (Ionic, *ietros*), belonged to the class of " *demiurgoi*," the workers useful for the people; sometimes he was classified as a *technites*, or artificer. The teaching in the more ancient times was patriarchal from father to son. A little later schools were formed, which always preserved the familial trait. In Athens the physicians who were candidates for public office had to state to the *ecclesia* the name of their school and their master, before being nominated by the assembly. The *iatreion* was the place where they received, examined, and treated the sick. Even in pre-Hippocratic times their compensation was paid in money. Xenophon speaks also of military physicians.

Along with the physicians, there is early evidence of the existence in Greece of others concerned with health. Physicians ordinarily prepared medicines themselves, but often had them prepared by the rhizotomist (cutter of roots), who was regarded as the assistant of the physician. The rhizotomist collected the roots and prepared them after drying and pulverizing. Later the rhizotomists became pharmacists and also prepared other drugs.

Midwives are mentioned by the ancient writers and even in early times there are found requests for illicit help, often for abortifacients or aphrodisiacs and even for lewd services. We note that the mother of Socrates was a midwife, and there is still preserved a textbook for midwives.

Such is the picture that is presented by Greece before the fifth century B.C. The books of the *Hippocratic Corpus*, in which are collected the standards for the practice of the profession, should not be regarded as collections of original precepts derived from the teaching of the master of Cos, but as a confirmation of a state of affairs that was already firmly organized and known to all.

This first period of Hellenic medicine, in which we see medical thought becoming more and more developed and improved, and the essential elements of scientific medicine being prepared, thus constitutes one of the most interesting epochs in the history of medicine. It is the moment in which is fixed the principle of that secular movement whereby the unrestricted studies of the philosophers broke new ground and passed beyond the experiences of civilizations that had existed for millennia. The essentially Grecian trait of the harmonious development in the individual of all the human faculties had become manifest in health matters, as in thought, education, and the arts. Wilfully repressed in the early Christian era and throughout the Middle Ages, it is only in modern times that this ideal has again become appreciated and sought for. It is from free observation and investigation, vitalized by the stimulating force of reasoning, by the passionate desire for knowledge, and by the evident necessity of looking into the deepest mysteries of existence, that scientific medicine was born.

CHAPTER IX

THE GOLDEN AGE OF GREEK

MEDICINE

HIPPOCRATIC MEDICINE — A BIOLOGIC AND SYNTHETIC CONCEPT

1. Hippocrates — Biographical Data — The Hippocratic Writings

In that glorious age of Greece when Pericles gave new impulse to the arts, and Herodotus and Thucydides wrote the immortal pages of their histories; when Phidias carved in marble the pure forms of ideal Hellenic beauty, and Sophocles and Euripides stirred the souls of the common crowd, and it seemed as if an impulse to grandeur and glory and a striving for liberty and beauty pervaded all Greece, there arose also a physician who was both the wisest and the greatest practitioner of his art. Just as these great men indelibly stamped their individuality on their country's history and art, so HIPPOCRATES, the physician and master, dominated the schools and physicians of his time. He stands above priestly medicine as he does above empirical medicine, and includes in his person, idealized through the centuries, the sum of the knowledge of the past. Advancing to new investigations and new concepts, he established himself as the most important and most complete medical personality of antiquity.

The biographical data on Hippocrates are taken from the biography written by Soranus in the second century after Christ. They are derived rrom information coming from the third century B.C., and from evidence contained in the writings of other Greek authors, especially Plato (*Protagoras*, Ch. 311, Par. B; *Phædrus*, Ch. 270, Par. C–E). The date of his birth has given rise to much discussion, but historians are now generally agreed in accepting the statements of Soranus, according to which he was born in

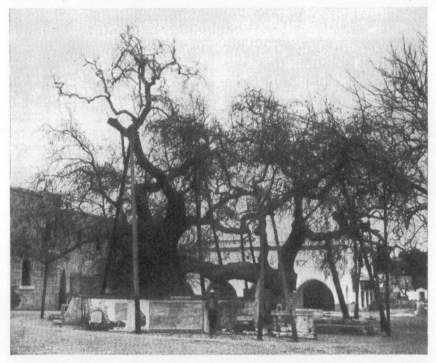

64. *The plane tree of Hippocrates at Cos. On the marble tablets at its base is inscribed the Oath of Hippocrates.*

460 or 459 B.C., on the small island of Cos. He is said by some to have died in 355 B.C., at the advanced age of a hundred and four; according to others, in the ninety-fifth year of his age; certainly, and here all biographers are agreed, at a very advanced age. At Cos recent excavations have brought to light the remains of an ancient temple of Æsculapius and also a very beautiful statue of the fourth century B.C., which may be properly regarded as the most ancient representation of Hippocrates that has been preserved.

About the genealogy of Hippocrates the data are uncertain or even legendary. According to Soranus, he belonged to the twentieth generation of Asklepiads; Jourdain says that he was the second of seven of the same name. His father was the physician Heracleides; his mother was Praxitela,

the daughter of Phenaretis. He was the pupil of his father and perhaps studied philosophy under Democritus and Gorgias Siculus. He made frequent
voyages, and we know from his writings that he was certainly on the island
of Thasos and in Thessaly, in Thrace, and in the Propontis. According to
some authors he travelled also in Egypt, Libya, and Scythia. There is no
evidence that Hippocrates ever was in Athens; neither Thucydides nor
Plato mentions his presence there.

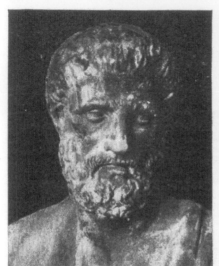 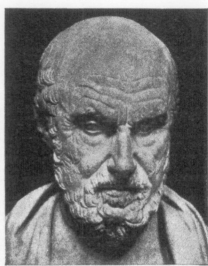

65. *Hippocrates* (?). *Statue of the fourth century* B.C. *discovered on the island
of Cos.*
66. *Hippocrates* (?). *Marble bust in the* British Museum.

Many biographical statements that we find about him in the ancient texts
have a legendary character. For example, Varro and Pliny tell us that he
destroyed the temple and the archives of the sanctuary of Æsculapius in
Cos, in order to assure for himself the glory of the discovery of medicine.
Even in ancient times myths formed about his figure. Thus ancient stories
narrate that bees formed their hives on his tomb, and that their honey cured
the thrush of infants. It is stated that he was initiated into the Athenian
mysteries and was admitted into the Prytaneum, that he treated the madness
of Democritus and was active in fighting the plague of Abdera. He appeared to his contemporaries and to posterity surrounded by an aureole of
glory. Plato compared him in the *Protagoras* to Polycletus and Phidias;
Aristotle in his *Politica* called him " Hippocrates the Great "; Apollonius of
Chito called him " the Divine "; Erotian regarded him as the equal of Homer; Galen, as " the divine — the wonderful inventor of all that is beauti-

ful "; Alexander of Tralles, as " the ancient sage," " the absolutely divine ";
while the Middle Ages generally regarded him as the father of medicine.

What brought about this reputation, which began to be formed when he
was alive and grew progressively from the beginning of the fourth century
B.C.? The writings that constitute the *Corpus Hippocraticum* are without
doubt those with which the name of the great sage is connected. Historical
criticism has been able in recent times to distinguish in this great collection
of medical writings some that obviously come from authors in different
periods and schools, others that should be attributed to Hippocrates himself, or to those, such as his son-in-law, Polybus, who were very close to
him. He was certainly, and about this there is no shadow of doubt, not
only the best-known physician of his time, but also the most profound investigator and acute observer; he was the head of the most flourishing
medical school of his age, who gathered about him many pupils and
spread his teaching throughout the Greek world and even beyond. If one
is bold enough to estimate the chief contribution of this greatest physician
of all time, it would seem to be that he established the facts that disease
was a natural process, that its symptoms were the reactions of the body to
the disease, and that the chief function of the physician was to aid the
natural forces of the body.

The number of writings that are ascribed to Hippocrates differs considerably according to the criteria used. Littré, who certainly was the most authoritative of the students and interpreters of Hippocrates, counts 53 subjects in 72
books and later historians have for the most part adhered to this classification.
Lund includes 76 treatises. The definitive editing and combination of all these
writings under the name of Hippocrates dates from the third century B.C., when,
at the command of the Egyptian *diadochi*, they were collected for the Library
of Alexandria. Before that, they had been spread through all Greece, carefully
copied and carried overseas.

They are written in the Ionic dialect, which at that time was the literary
language of Greece. They present marked differences of style; in the better
works, those that are attributed to Hippocrates himself, the form is simple,
distinguished, and clear; in the nobility of its incisive eloquence the diction can
be compared to that of the best of the classic authors. The most ancient manuscripts (tenth to twelfth century) that we possesses, none of which contains
the entire *Corpus*, are in the State libraries of Vienna, Paris, the Laurentian in
Florence, the Vatican in Rome, and St. Mark's in Venice. There are preserved
many other codices, written between the twelfth century and the middle of
the fifteenth, when printing was invented.

Among the oldest editions are the *editio princeps* of the *Opera Omnia* in
Latin, printed in Rome in 1525; the Greek *editio princeps*, published by Aldus

in Venice in 1526; the Basel edition of Cornarius in 1538 from the Froben Press, the Greco-Latin edition of Mercurialis published by Giunta in 1588 in Venice.

Of the modern editions, the clearest and most valuable is that of the complete works, in ten volumes, published with a French translation by Littré (Paris, 1839–61).

Among the other numerous translations, we note that in Italian by M. G. Levi (Venice, 1838), in French by Daremberg (Paris, 1843), in German by R. Fuchs (Munich, 1897), Ilberg and Kuhlewein (Teubner, Leipzig, 1894–1902), and R. Kapferer (Hippocrates Verlag, Stuttgart, still appearing in fasciculi); in English by F. Adams (Sydenham Society Publications, London, 1849); and in English with the Greek text by W. H. S. Jones and E. T. Withington (four volumes, Loeb Classical Library, London, 1923–31). A few of these are bilingual, some being complete, some limited to the so-called "genuine works," others including those rejected from the *Corpus* by most commentators.

The commentaries on Hippocrates date from ancient times; the most famous of the commentators were Galen and Herophilus, while Erotian's selections have been useful to modern students (A.D. 50). All the great authors of later times, and especially the Arabs and the great Italian physicians of the Renaissance, wrote full commentaries on his work. From the beginning of the eighth century one could say that a great part of medical publications appeared in the form of comments on one or other of the Hippocratic works. The discussion about the authenticity of Hippocratic texts and their authorship has lasted now for nearly twenty centuries, as even Galen tried a critical selection of the authentic versus the doubtful works. But in the absence of unequivocal indications, philologists and historians, basing their opinions on different criteria, attribute writings that bear the name of Hippocrates to various authors and periods; and others, on the other hand, reaffirm the Hippocratic origin of repudiated books; so that it is practically impossible to form an accurate judgment on this perennial subject. Galen, in his extensive study of the problem, probably followed the indication of Quintus Romanus, who was his master, in distinguishing *The Aphorisms, The Book of Epidemics, On Prognosis,* and certain others from those merely attributed to the master.

There is no doubt whatever that in this collection there are works coming from authors of different periods and schools. In the editing and style there are manifest divergences and even opposite statements about the same subject in different Hippocratic texts. It is evident, then, even for one who is not expert in the examination of ancient texts, that, as has happened with many classical texts of antiquity, the books of Hippocrates, collected and codified at Alexandria, represent in reality an agglomeration of works coming from various sources, most of which reflect the direct influence of the individuality of Hippocrates and his school. This being the case, we need not be surprised if we meet discordant statements in the various texts. It has happened to Hippocrates as to Socrates, differing reports of whose activity were set down by his pupils.

But the fact that, even in times close to the man himself, he was regarded as the author or at least the inspirer of important medical texts is shown by the praise given him by his contemporaries, especially Plato.

The Hippocratic writings that are really worthy of the name — that is, those which most probably come directly from the school of Cos and the period of Hippocrates — include: *On the Physician, On Honourable Conduct, Precepts, On Anatomy, On the Nature of the Bones, On the Humours, On Crisis, On Critical Days, On the Use of Liquids, On Fractures, On the Seventh-Month Fetus, On the Eighth-Month Fetus, On Dentition.*

Genuinely Hippocratic, so far as one can judge today, are the books: *On Diet, The Prognostics, The Coan Prænotions,* the book *Of Prænotions, Of Prorrhetics,* the second book *Of Prorrhetics,* the famous book of *The Aphorisms, The Physician's Establishment, On Wounds and Ulcers, On Hemorrhoids, On Fistulas, On Injuries of the Head, On Fractures, On Reduction of Dislocation,* two of the seven books *On Epidemics,* and the book *On Airs, Waters, and Places.* These can be stated with certainty to have come from Hippocrates himself or from pupils very close to him.

As to the other books of the *Hippocratic Corpus,* some are of Cnidian origin, among them the three books *On Diseases,* the book *On Affections,* and almost certainly all the gynæcological books.

Some writings show without doubt the influence of the Sophist school and are thus of later origin, such as the famous book *On the Sacred Disease,* that *On Aliment, Regimen of Persons in Health, On Dreams, On the Nature of Man,* and the famous book *On Winds.*

Other books are important for Hippocratic ethics, such as *On Ancient Medicine, On the Law,* about the origin of which there are heated discussions, some even urging an Egyptian origin, and the discourse *On Art.* These are regarded by some historians as coming from the Iatro-Sophist school. De Renzi believes that the book *On Ancient Medicine* should be attributed to Alcmæon, but Del Gaizo offers strong backing for its authorship by Hippocrates. Many of the latest critics, however, are today returning to De Renzi's idea. Jones dates this work at about 430–420 B.C. — that is, in the prime of Hippocrates' lifetime.

2. *The Ethical Books of the Hippocratic Corpus*

The first of these works is the *Oath of Hippocrates,* which, even if attributed to an earlier period, is inextricably bound in spirit to the Hippocratic school and period.

The text of the *Hippocratic Oath* is as follows: " I swear by Apollo the physician, and Æsculapius, and Hygeia, and Panacea, and all the gods and goddesses, that, according to my ability and judgment, I will keep this Oath and this stipulation — to reckon him who taught me this art equally dear to me as my parents, to share my substance with him, and relieve his necessities if required; to look upon his offspring in the same footing as my own brothers, and to teach them this art, if they shall wish to learn it, without fee or stipulation, and that by precept, lecture, and every other mode of instruction, I will impart a knowledge of the art to my own sons, and those of my teachers, and to disciples bound by a stipulation and oath according to the law of medicine, but to none others. I will follow that system of regimen which, according to my ability and judgment, I consider for the benefit of my patients, and abstain from whatever is deleterious and mischievous. I will give no deadly medicine to anyone if asked, nor suggest any such counsel; and in like manner I will not give to a woman a pessary to produce abortion. With purity and holiness I will pass my life and practise my art. I will not cut persons labouring under the stone, but will leave this to be done by men who are practitioners of this work.[1] Into whatever houses I enter, I will go into them for the benefit of the sick, and will abstain from every voluntary act of mischief and corruption; and, further, from the seduction of females or males, of freemen and slaves. Whatever, in connection with my professional practice, or not in connection with it, I see or hear, in the life of men, which ought not to be spoken of abroad, I will not divulge, as reckoning that all such should be kept

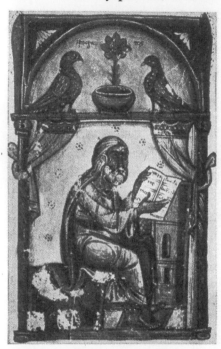

67. *A mediæval representation of Hippocrates.*
(*From Codex 16, XIII,* LAURENTIAN LIBRARY, FLORENCE.)

[1] Dr. Savas Nittis has suggested (*Bull. Hist. Med.*, 1939, VII, 719) a new interpretation of this passage, wherein *temeo* is translated as " castrate " rather than " cut." The sentence would then literally and grammatically be translated: " I will not castrate, indeed not even sufferers from the stone, and I will keep apart from men engaging in this deed," which was regarded as an abomination.

secret. While I continue to keep this Oath unviolated, may it be granted to me to enjoy life and the practice of the art, respected by all men, in all times! But should I trespass and violate this Oath, may the reverse be my lot! "

This oath shows to what ethical heights the concept of professional

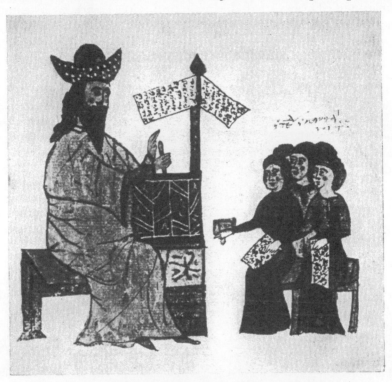

68. *A mediæval representation of Hippocrates teaching his pupils.*
(*A thirteenth-century Codex in the* VATICAN LIBRARY.)

practice had reached even in the times of the early medical schools of Greece. The hieratic character of this oath, and the clear allusion to medical art as a doctrine of the initiated, all show how it was derived directly from the rites of the Pythagoreans, the Orphics, and other sects of initiates. But in its essence, in the clear intention of elevating the cure of the patient to be the chief aim of medical art, without having recourse in any way to priestly rites or to divine aid, it is evident that those who took this oath were physicians who practised their art in freedom and taught it in freedom. It is therefore correct to state that this precious document constitutes the undoubted proof of the existence of a medical sect, governed by fixed laws and independent of the priestly caste, even in the times before Hippocrates. Especially worthy of note are three precepts that appear in this oath: first, the prohibition to the physician of practising abortion; second, the clearly expressed duty of the physician not to allow, advise, or commit any act that may prejudice the health of his patient; and finally, the obligation, for the first time codified in an oath, to maintain professional secrecy. The injunction not to perform lithotomy was probably due to an agreement that such an operation should be practised only by specialists, or perhaps arose from the known danger of producing sterility (functional castration) by this operation.

The second of the books of the ethical group, called *On the Physician*, is predominantly deontologic, containing a series of interesting precepts concerning the behaviour of the physician, the arrangement of his office, his instruments, poultices, and war surgery. An analogous book is that *On Honourable Conduct*. In it the unity of philosophy and medicine is maintained and advice is given about the knowledge necessary to the physician, how he should enter the patient's room, how he should conduct the examination of the patient, and so on.

The importance of three other books of the *Corpus Hippocraticum* (*On the Law, On Art, On Ancient Medicine*) is beyond question (even if critical study indicated that they are predominantly under the influence of the Sophist school), because they collect in their essential canons the ethical principles of professional practice. The first is the book *On the Law*, a collection of precepts about the practice of medicine which contain excellent advice about medical ethics.

" The art of medicine is the most beautiful and noble of all the arts, but on account of the inexperience of those who practise it, on the one hand, and the superficiality of those who judge physicians, on the other hand, it is often ranked behind the other arts."

" He who wishes to acquire exact knowledge of the medical art should possess a natural disposition for it, should attend a good school, should receive instruction from infancy, should have the desire to work and the time to dedicate to his studies."

In the book *On Art*, which is an apologia of medicine, it is written: " As regards the art of medicine, I should state first of all what I believe to be its scope: to remove the sufferings of the patient, or at least to alleviate these sufferings. The fact that even those who do not believe in it can be cured by it is proof that this art exists and that it is a powerful one."

In the book *On Ancient Medicine*, the first in which the history of medicine is considered, it is stated: " Medicine has long had all its means to hand, and has discovered both a principle and a method, through which the discoveries made during a long period are many and excellent, while full discovery will be made, if the inquirer be competent, conduct his researches with knowledge of the discoveries already made, and make them his starting-point. . . . It is laborious to make knowledge so exact that only small mistakes are made here and there. And that physician who makes only small mistakes would win my hearty praise. Perfectly exact truth is but rarely to be seen. For most physicians seem to me to be in the same case as bad pilots; the mistakes of the latter are unnoticed so long as they are steering in a calm, but when a great storm overtakes them with a violent gale, all men realize clearly then that it is their ignorance and blundering which have lost the ship. So also when bad physicians, who comprise the great majority, treat men who are suffering from no serious complaint, so that the greatest blunders would not affect them seriously — such illnesses occur very often, being far more common than serious disease — they are not shown up in their true colours to laymen; if they meet with a severe, violent, and dangerous illness, then it is that their errors and want of skill are manifest to all" (Ch. ii and ix, W. H. S. Jones translation).

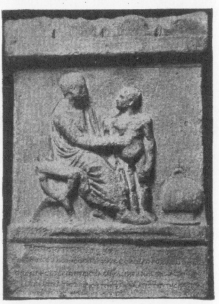

69. *The physician Jason palpates the epigastrium of a patient. (Greek bas-relief.)*

In the magnificent book entitled *On the Physician* there are various observations which on account of their freshness, vitality, and correctness deserve to be read and considered even today. "For the physician it is unquestionably an important point to have a fine appearance and to be well nourished, because the public believes that those who do not know how to take care of their own bodies are not in a position to think about the care of others. He should know how to be silent at the proper moment and should conduct a regular life, because this contributes much to his good reputation. His behaviour should be that of an honest man and as such he should appear gentle and tolerant before honest men. He should not act impulsively nor precipitately; he should maintain a calm and serene visage and should never be in a bad humour, but on the other hand should not appear too gay."

The books entitled *On Honourable Conduct* (*Decorum*) and *On Precepts* present the most perfect statement of medical ethics in all medical literature.

"The physician who is at the same time a philosopher is like the gods. There is not a great difference between medicine and philosophy, because all the qualities of a good philosopher should also be found in the physician: altruism, zeal, modesty, a dignified appearance, seriousness, tranquil judgment, serenity, decision, purity of life, the habit of brevity, knowledge of what is useful and necessary in life, reprobation of evil things, a mind free from suspicions, devotion to the divinity."

Certain precepts in regard to the practice of medicine are so apt today that it does not seem possible that they have existed for more than twenty centuries: " It is necessary to have simple remedies ready for an emergency or to carry on a voyage, because the physician at the last moment cannot

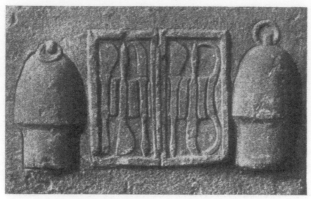

70. *A surgical case with various instruments and two cupping instruments.* (*Bas-relief from the* ASCLEPIEION OF ATHENS.)

select from many the one that is fitting. When the physician enters the room of the patient he should be attentive to the manner in which he sits down and the manner in which he comports himself; he should be well dressed, have a calm face, give the patient his entire attention, answer objections calmly and not lose patience, and be calm in the presence of difficulties that arise. The most important rule is to repeat his examinations frequently to avoid mistakes; he should keep aware of the fact that patients often lie when they state that they have taken certain medicines. . . . It is important to consider the couch of the patient; both the season and the kind of illness will make a difference as to its position. Noises and odours are to be avoided. All the directions of the physician should be made in a friendly, quiet manner. Naught should be betrayed to the patient of what may happen or of what may eventually threaten him, because many patients have been driven in this way to extreme measures." And finally: " Where there is love of man, there is also love for the art. There is no harm in the physician finding himself embarrassed before the patient. If on account of his insufficient experience he does not see the situation clearly, let him call other physicians in consultation, so that after a combined study the state of the patient can be made clear and he can be helped. . . . The physicians who are brought together in consultation should never have acrimonious disputes nor render each other ridiculous."

These medical books give obvious proof that along with priestly medicine, and in fact distinct from it, practical lay medicine had already reached considerable development. Here the author, seeking to codify the more important ethical and moral precepts, appears well acquainted with both the practical evils, abuses, and defects of bad physicians, and the virtues and good qualities of the physicians who are truly worthy of the name. He writes with a broad and serene knowledge that can be nothing but the result of mature reflection and long experience. A scorn for the applause of the crowd, an ardent and constant desire for the truth, and a continued urge to bring the individual problems into a supreme moral law, and finally a predominating thoughtfulness for the welfare of the patient, all these could not have arisen from the teaching or the practices of the temple of Æsculapius. They could only be the result of long and fervent study at the bedside of the patient.

3. Biology, Anatomy, Physiology
— the Doctrine of Humoral Pathology

Considering those directions which concern especially the practice of the art and which have an essentially ethical foundation, let us try to construct a concept of the positive knowledge of the physician of the Hippocratic school. We see first of all that a fundamental part of this doctrine is the truly biological point of view, which is fundamental to the mode of thought, decisions, and actions of the physicians of that school. It is a concept arising from the philosophic schools, fortified by the observation and experience that Hippocrates maintained as indispensable.

The Hippocratic doctrine, excluding every theological concept, regards the body as formed of four elements: air, earth, water, and fire, which unite in the composition of the single parts of the organism. Then as each of these four elements possesses its particular quality — cold, hot, dry, or wet — the single parts of the organism also possess their essential qualities.

The essential factor in life is heat; but because it pervades the entire body and maintains itself in equilibrium, it is necessary also that the *pneuma* constantly penetrate to it. Thus we see in Hippocratic physiology the combination of the two currents of Babylonian and Egyptian physiology. The seat of heat is the left heart; thanks to heat, the organs and the humours are formed from the nutritive substances. The blood, which is collected in the liver, carries the necessary heat to the left heart in a constant flow. The pneuma reaches the heart by way of the trachea or, according to some writers, through the arteries. This pneuma has its seat in the heart. It passes through all the veins of the body and to it is given the task of maintaining a proper balance, particularly in those organs which excrete liquid.

" The body of man," as is stated in the book *On the Nature of Man* (Ch. iv), " has in itself blood, phlegm, yellow bile, and black bile; these make up the nature of his body, and through these he feels pain or enjoys health. Now he enjoys the most perfect health when these elements are duly proportioned to one another in respect of compounding, power, and bulk and when they are perfectly mingled. Pain is felt when one of these elements is in defect or excess, or is isolated in the body without being compounded with all the others. For when an element is isolated and stands by itself, not only must the place which it left become diseased, but the place where it stands in a flood must, because of the excess, cause pain and distress. In fact, when more of an element flows out of the body than is necessary to get rid of superfluity, the emptying causes pain. If, on the other hand, it be to an inward part that there takes place the emptying, the shifting and the separation from other elements, the man certainly must, according to what has been said, suffer from a double pain, one in the place left, and another in the place flooded " (from Jones's translation).

This humoral concept does not stop, as is generally maintained by superficial observers and even by some historians, with the establishment of the four fundamental humours, but assumes the scope of an important generalization: namely, that of the reciprocal relations between various organs, the so-called sympathy arising from the humours. In the book *On Aliments* is written (xxiii): " Everything is founded on a united confluence of all the humours, a united concordance, and united sympathy." The dominance of the humours, according to the seasons and the effect that this changing dominance exercises on the origin of certain diseases, these form one of the most interesting chapters in humoral pathology. The tenets of the Hippocratic school on these questions have given rise to all the depurative and purgative treatments of spring and fall, and all those revulsive treatments that were in great favour almost uninterruptedly through twenty-five centuries, and that in our own times are again being seriously considered by physicians.

The anatomical knowledge of the Hippocratic school, as far as can be judged, is based on experience with animals. The evidence from which certain authors have wished to draw proof that human dissection was known and practised is wholly insufficient to prove this point. The scanty knowledge in all the fields of anatomy, except the bones, about which they had accurate information, as is shown by the marked development of bone surgery, proves that examination of the cadaver was almost unknown. Nerves and tendons were confused with muscles, often also with blood vessels; ideas about the thoracic and abdominal organs were vague, although these organs were named and sometimes even briefly described. The term

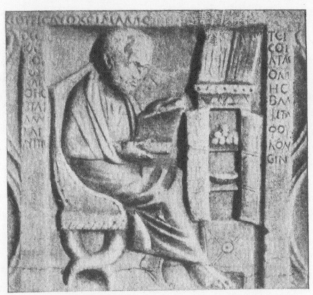

71. *Gravestone of a Greek physician. The physician studying a scroll; other scrolls are seen in the cabinet, above which is an instrument case.*

" artery (*arteria*) " is used chiefly for the trachea and the bronchi; it was adopted later for those vessels which were thought to contain air because it was observed that they were empty after death. By the word " veins (*phlebes*) " is meant those vessels which contain blood. Knowledge of the heart also, and of the part that it plays in the circulation, is uncertain; some Hippocratic books state that the veins carry the blood to the head.

Ideas about generation are derived from observations on animals and from pure speculation. According to the Hippocratic writers, the uterus is always bicornate; in the right side males are conceived, in the left side females. Fertilization is produced by the mixture of the male and female seed.

The centre of thought and of the will is the brain, which is almost always regarded as a gland that has the function of collecting the excess liquid from the body. The brain is regarded as the centre of sensation; sight is thought to occur from the formation of the image on the pupil; the bones of the ear carry the auditory sensations to the brain.

Hippocratic general pathology is essentially humoral. The attention of the physician is directed especially to the humours, and, corresponding to the division that has already been mentioned, there are four cardinal humours which form the fundamental elements of the organism and of life: the blood, which comes from the heart and represents heat; the phlegm, which, according to the major opinion, comes from the brain and is diffused through the whole body and represents cold; the yellow bile, which represents dryness and is secreted by the liver; and the black bile, which comes from the spleen and the stomach and represents wetness. For the Pneumatists and others blood represented the hot, moist humour; phlegm, the cold, moist humour; yellow bile, the hot, dry humour; black bile, the cold, dry humour.

When these four humours are properly mingled, the body is in a state of health; when there is a defect or an irregularity in the mixture, disease arises. Hippocratic pathology is thus founded on the concept of a disharmony or dyscrasia, which in its turn can be brought about by various factors, congenital, accidental, or determined by natural phenomena.

According to this concept, nature, which is nothing but the resisting force of the human body against the factors which tend to change the *crasis* (harmony), manifests itself with a special clearness in the acute diseases. The heat seeks to dominate the wet humour, by changing or eliminating its essence, and this is how the different stages of a disease are explained: in the first stage, the stage of crudity (*apepsis*), the *materia peccans* brings the humours into a raw or crude state; then, thanks to heat, nature brings the disease to coction or maturity (*pepsis*); next the morbid phenomena bring about a crisis (*crisis*) which is regarded as a decisive struggle between nature and the disease. The crisis, according to Hippocrates, is characterized by an increase of the secretions, by the passage from one form of fever to another (*metastasis*), and often by delirium.

In this doctrine the Pythagorean numbers have a special importance, forming the basis of the doctrine of the crisis, and determining the days or the periods in which it occurs. Ordinarily the periods were said to be of three or four days, but often changes or irregularities in the days of the crisis were recognized.

Besides these fundamental principles, we find in the Hippocratic books allusions to other theories which are in part contradictory. Thus the treatise *Of Regimen* speaks of fluxions, which may be of two kinds, caused by either heat or cold, and seven fluxions are distinguished. This doctrine is allied to the teaching of the school of Cnidus. In other places, as in the treatise *On Ancient Medicine*, diseases were attributed to errors in diet or to special meteorological conditions. However, this is not concerned with the direct cause of diseases, but with occasional predisposing factors.

Hippocratic pathology considered various types of diseases, which were generally classified according to the principal symptoms.

Among the febrile diseases, malaria was known, and quotidian, tertian, and quartan types were recognized.

Among the diseases of the respiratory tract are described: nasal catarrh, laryngitis, and pneumonia, which, however, is sometimes confused with pleurisy. The origin of pneumonia is attributed to the phlegm which, descending from the head, is transformed into pus and can cause empyema or clots of blood or phlegm, from which tumours (tubercles?) can be formed. The question as to whether the term *phymata* really indicates tubercles has been much discussed. But undoubtedly the Hippocratic writers knew tubercles and knew that cavities could be formed from them. Pleurisy is described as a disease coming from pneumonia and actually from contact of the lung with the costal pleura. With empyemata or pulmonary abscess are included any collection of pus in the thorax and therefore also tuberculosis.

Phthisis was generally regarded as the result of hemoptysis; its principal symptoms are described in a masterly way. The close connection between this disease of the lungs and disease of the larynx was known to the Hippocratic writers. The characteristic temperature, the appearance of the sputum, the loss of hair, and diarrhœa, which was regarded as a fatal symptom, are phenomena accurately described. The contagiousness of pulmonary consumption is explicitly mentioned in the Hippocratic writings.

Among the diseases of the intestinal tract are noted: diarrhœa, dysentery, ileus caused by masses of indurated fæces.

Cirrhosis of the liver, mumps, diphtheria, erysipelas, gout, puerperal sepsis, and cancer are among the many diseases recognized in the Hippocratic writings.

In the diseases of the nervous system, the origin of disease of the brain is found in a loss of phlegm from the brain, as a result of which the nerves become dry and can no longer have the proper amount of humidity. Thus are explained epilepsy, paraplegia, tetanus, apoplexy, convulsions, and so on. It is noteworthy that the superstition that epilepsy was a " sacred disease " was combated by the Hippocratic writers. All those diseases which were manifested by hallucinations or delirium were grouped under the term " phrenitis."

It is this branch of medicine especially that demonstrates that the Hippocratic writings should be regarded as a collection of all the medical knowledge known at that time.

As to the part that divinity played in the origin and course of disease, the

Hippocratic school did not maintain that it ever intervened directly, though it might influence the natural forces, which play a very important role. Thus the sun, shade, climate, the wind, waters and their exhalations, heredity, irregularity of the secretions, and so on, all had their importance in determining disease.

4. Constitutional Pathology

Let us consider now a chapter of Hippocratic knowledge that is especially deserving of study, because it contains the germs of original ideas which are only now after many centuries being justly appreciated.

The importance attributed by Hippocrates to the pathologic constitution in his book *On Airs, Waters, and Places* demands attention. This constitutes the first example known to us of a rational attempt by a man of genius, endowed with a deep power of observation, to put the phenomena of the macrocosm and the microcosm in direct causal relations.

Many authors have attributed to Hippocrates the authorship of this work. We maintain that it should be attributed without doubt either to him or to someone close to him who profited by his teaching.

The first part of this book is a true work on climatology. It considers the diseases that occur in a given locality in relation to its climatic position and to the seasons. The second part treats of the differences between Europe and Asia and without doubt constitutes one of the most interesting books that classical antiquity has transmitted to us. It is the first attempt to put external causes in direct connection with the origin of diseases, but also with the constitution of man and with the ethnic characteristics of nations. Let us look briefly at the content of the first part. According to this: "Whoever wishes to pursue properly the science of medicine must proceed thus. First he ought to consider what effects each season of the year can produce; for the seasons are not at all alike, but differ widely both in themselves and at their changes. The next point is the hot winds and the cold, especially those that are universal, but also those that are peculiar to each particular region. He must also consider the properties of the waters; for as these differ in taste and in weight, so the property of each is far different from that of any other. . . . Using this evidence he must examine the several problems that arise. For if a physician knows these things well, by preference all of them, but at any rate most, he will not, on arrival at a town with which he is unfamiliar, be ignorant of the local diseases, or of the nature of those that commonly prevail " (Ch. i and ii, Jones's translation).

He speaks at length of the diseases which are frequent in various regions and of their characteristics. He considers the waters and the effects that some of them may produce on the organism, and especially the water from swamps and stagnant places. Those that are too cold produce severe intestinal disturbance, and those that come from swamps often give rise to quartan fevers. The author then considers the importance of the seasons

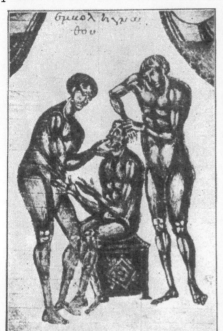 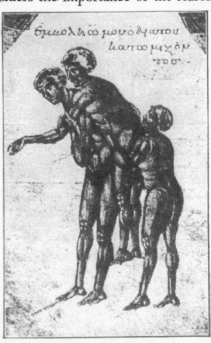

72. *Reduction of dislocations.*   (*From an ancient Greek codex.*)

and the diseases that occur most frequently in each, and he notes the greater frequency of the intermittent fevers in the summer months.

This part of the book is to be regarded, as has been observed by Hirsch, the first to write a historical geographical pathology, as the only attempt in two thousand years to make an intensive, careful study of medico-geographical facts.

The second part of this interesting treatise begins with the observation of the differences of the flora and fauna of Europe and Asia. He observes that the climate of Asia is milder, the character of the people softer, and the cause for this is to be found in the even temperature of the seasons. That part of Asia that is situated between the greatest heat and cold has better and more tasteful fruits, more beautiful trees, and more healthful waters. It is therefore natural that the products of the soil grow abundantly in all seasons. Animals prosper and reproduce frequently, and therefore, also, people are well nourished, tall, and handsome.

In such a climate, however, it is more difficult to find energy, courage, and quickness of decision. Instead, the thirst for pleasure usually dominates.

As regards the ethnic characteristics of the various peoples, he observes that some are macrocephalic. "This at first depended on the custom of compressing the head, but then nature formed it in this way." Thus we see that the author of the text believes that an acquired character could become hereditary.

Then examining the moral character of the Asiatics, Hippocrates states that this is due to the climate, in which there are no great changes, but always a mild and equal temperature. Therefore the people are not exposed to hard labour and privations, but are accustomed to remain idle for many hours, and thus they resign themselves to tyranny, remaining subjects of kings who dominate them completely, and do not develop their warlike virtues, even seeming to become unfit for war.

Other noteworthy observations concern the Scythians, and especially those races who live on the steppes, in regions where the atmosphere is always humid and the spring lasts for many months and often mists cover the land for many days. The animals are small and reproduce infrequently, the plants are scarce and vegetation poor, and the inhabitants are fat and weak, with poor musculature. The women are fat and not very fertile.

Masculine impotence is frequent in this race, and often men do the work of women and behave like women.

Thus in a series of acute and profound observations the author of this memorable work demonstrates the direct relation between the environment and the physical and psychic life of the inhabitants, thus laying the foundation of the concept of constitutional pathology.

Among the most valuable books that have come down to us are the seven books on *Epidemics*, of which the first and the third are without doubt by Hippocrates himself, according to the unanimous testimony of all the commentators since Galen.

The first is a chronological account of the three years that the author passed on the island of Thasos, an accurate nosological journal. The third is the chronicle of another year passed in the same place, accompanied also by various medical observations.

The other books are probably the work of scholars who followed the example of the master. Not only epidemic diseases are considered in these books, as might be supposed from the title. We find here, for the first time in history, the attempt to group together certain diseases according to their symptoms and characteristic phenomena, and to study the possible causal relationship between these diseases and the observed climatic conditions. These observations are supported by a series of clinical histories, and in the first two books appears the foundation of the concept of the " *genius epidemicus*," which was successfully maintained in medicine through later centuries. As Garrison has pointed out, the forty-seven clinical histories contained in the Hippocratic writings are the only ones worthy of the name to be found in medical literature for the next seventeen hundred years. It is significant too that sixty per cent of the cases ended fatally; in other words, Hippocrates was not interested, like Galen, in magnifying his own importance, but, in his own words, believed it " valuable to learn of unsuccessful experiments and to know the causes of their failure."

5. *Diagnosis and Prognosis — the Aphorisms*

The Hippocratic doctrines regard observation of the patient as the most fundamental obligation of physicians, giving very accurate directions to their followers as to how the examination of the patient should be made: " It is necessary to begin with the most important things and those most easily recognized. It is necessary to study all that one can see, feel, and hear, everything that one can recognize and use." The visit of the patient should be made in the morning, as then both patient and physician have more tranquil minds. First, the physician should closely examine the body of the patient and then learn about the evacuations; study the respiration, the sweat, the attitude of the patient, and the urine.

The temperature is estimated with the hand applied on the chest.

Statements about the hardness and size of the liver and spleen and about the lungs show that perhaps the art of percussion was known. Auscultation (of course without a stethoscope) was expressly prescribed, to be aided by shaking the chest. Gross bubbling râles were noted. The succussion splash was taken to establish the presence of pus, and it is directed to apply the ear to the thorax to listen for noises which are like snoring, when there is pus in the thorax (*On Diseases*, I, 17; II, 61; III, 16). In pleurisy it is stated that one hears a noise like that from rubbing a leather strap (*On Diseases*, II, 59). Finlayson calls attention to a description of Cheyne-Stokes respiration, " like that of a person recollecting himself," in the cases of Philiscus and of the wife of Dealces (*Epidemics*, I, 3, 13, first case; and III, 3, 17, fifteenth case).

The Hippocratic physicians attributed the greatest importance to prognosis, as can be seen in the books that are concerned with it. From the start, they teach that only a physician who knows how to make an accurate prognosis can acquire the confidence of the patient. Prognostic signs are closely related to the diagnostic signs; in fact, the term was used then in a much broader sense than now, including the collection and analysis of observations as well as the predictions about the course of the disease that logically followed. A good mixture of the humours is manifested in a good appearance, quiet sleep in a restful position, clear mind, abundant sweat in the critical days, mobility, and good humour; and these are signs of a favourable prognosis. Great prognostic importance in the unfavourable sense is to be attributed to such symptoms as: lying with the mouth and eyes open, with the legs spread apart, the sensation of great heat, sudden and unexpected changes in the morbid picture, insomnia, constant diarrhœa, and violent gestures.

Alarming prognostic phenomena are those of the so-called *facies Hippocratica:* " nose sharp, eyes hollow, temples sunken, ears cold and contracted with their lobes turned outwards, the skin about the face hard, tense, and dry, the colour of the face being yellow or dark." Other grave symptoms of imminent danger include a petechia surrounded by a livid aureole, cold sweats, painful swollen abdomen, the emission of foul pus, œdema after acute illness, unexpected chilling of the body, unexpected pallor of the hands and nails (*On Prognosis*, Ch. ii).

The book *The Coan Prænotions* is a collection of short directions or observations for scholastic use. Hirschfeld has maintained that these are derived directly from the inscriptions of the Temple of Cos; but for various good reasons this hypothesis appears to be incorrect. The two books *On Prognostics* are closely connected with this work; they contain prognostic statements that often indicate the name of the patient, and appear to be a series of notes for the use of students.

The Aphorisms, collected in seven books, were regarded up to the end of the Middle Ages, and even later, as the quintessence of Hippocratic medicine. They were regarded as undoubtedly by Hippocrates himself up to the end of the past century, and only recently has doubt been raised as to their authenticity. In this collection is found certain evidence of the work of a man of genius; observations that could not be composed except by the mind of a physician of the highest rank, of vast experience and deep knowledge.

This book is without doubt the most famous of all Hippocratic writings. For centuries it was regarded as the sum of all medical knowledge. Its title was customarily used, as for example by Dante, to indicate the study of medicine. Commentaries upon it began about 300 B.C. and have been made by hundreds in all nations. More than 140 Greek codices have transmitted the text, and hundreds of translations in Arabic, Latin, Hebrew, have come down to us from ancient times. No medical book had a greater success or more constantly enjoyed the favour of physicians. It may be, as Fuchs has very plausibly suggested, that the text has been changed, modified, and added to in later periods, but certainly in its deepest essence it should be regarded as the one most closely related to the person of Hippocrates. It is in this book that his personality and characteristics are outlined with the greatest clearness.

Let us quote here some of the most famous of the aphorisms. The first states: "Life is short, and the art long; the occasion fleeting; experience fallacious, and judgment difficult," and the last one concludes: "Those diseases which medicines do not cure, the knife cures; those which iron cannot cure, fire cures; and those which fire cannot cure are to be reckoned wholly incurable" (VII, 87). Garrison points out that this aphorism, which was responsible for so much damage, down to the time of Paré, was really pre-Hippocratic, being mentioned in Æschylus' *Agamemnon*, and that Baas has traced it to the ancient Hindus. "For extreme diseases, extreme strictness of treatment is most efficacious" (I, 6); "Old persons endure fasting most easily; next, adults; young persons not nearly so well; and most especially infants, and of them such as are of a particularly lively spirit" (I, 13); "Use purgative medicines sparingly in acute diseases, and at the commencement, and not without proper circumspection" (I, 24); "Persons who have a painful affection in any part of the body and are in a great measure insensible of the pain are disordered in intellect" (II, 6); "In acute diseases it is not quite safe to prognosticate either death or recovery" (II, 19); "Of two pains occurring together, not in the same part of the body, the stronger weakens the other"; "Pains and fevers occur rather at the formation of pus than when it is already formed" (II, 46; II, 47); "In old people [occur] dyspnœa, catarrhs accompanied with coughs, dysuria, pains of the joints, nephritis, vertigo, apoplexy, cachexia, pruritus of the whole body, insomnolency, defluxion of the bowels, of the eyes, and of the nose, dimness of sight, cataract (glaucoma?), and dullness of hearing" (III, 31); "In persons attenuated from any diseases, whether acute or chronic, or from wounds, or any other cause, if there be a discharge either of black bile, or resembling black blood, they die on the following day" (IV, 23); "In convalescents from diseases, if any part be pained, there deposits are formed" (IV, 32); "Sweat supervening in a case of fever without the fever ceasing is bad, for the disease is protracted, and it indicates more copious humours" (IV, 56); "When jaundice supervenes in fevers before the seventh day, it is a bad symptom, unless there be watery discharges from the bowels" (IV, 62); "Blood or pus in the urine indicates ulceration either of the kidneys or of the bladder" (IV, 75); "In those cases where there is a spontaneous discharge of bloody urine, it indicates rupture of a small vein in the kidneys "; " In those cases where there is a sandy sediment in the urine, there is calculus in the bladder (or kidneys) " (IV, 78; IV, 79); " Phthisis most commonly occurs between the ages of eighteen and thirty-five years " (V, 9); " In persons who cough up frothy blood, the discharge of it comes from the lungs " (V, 13); " Diarrhœa attacking a person affected with phthisis is a mortal symptom " (V, 14); " Diseases about the kidneys and bladder are cured with difficulty in old men " (VI, 6); " It is better not to apply any treatment in cases of occult cancer; for, if treated, the patients die quickly; but if not treated, they hold out for a long time " (VI, 38); " Upon severe pain of the parts about the bowels, coldness of the extremities coming on is bad " (VII, 26) (translation of Francis Adams).

Among the most remarkable of the Hippocratic observations is that concerning the effect that malaria has on certain diseases: " Those who are stricken with the quartan fever do not become sick of the great disease (epilepsy). But if they are first stricken with this disease and then take a quartan, they are then cured of the great disease " (*Epidemics*, VI, Sect. VI, 5). And in *The Aphorisms*: " Persons attacked with quartans are not readily attacked with convulsions, or if previously attacked with convulsions, they cease if a quartan supervene " (V, 70); and in another place: " Elcippus became sick with maniacal attacks; when an acute fever supervened the attacks stopped " (*Epidemics*, VI, 48).

Speaking of the exanthemata and distinguishing them from diseases of the skin: " Lichen and leprosy are not apostases, but a disease; when, on the other hand, an exanthem appears unexpectedly and widespread, this case is an apostasis (that is to say, a deposit of harmful substances that can be expelled) " (*Prorrhetics*, II, 43).

6. Surgery, Ophthalmology, Obstetrics

The surgical writings of the *Corpus Hippocraticum* give valuable information about the surgical knowledge and technique of the period.

Gurlt in an admirable *History of Surgery* has patiently collected the list of all the instruments and operations described in the *Corpus*. We see that the sound of lead or copper was known and it could be straight or curved, solid or hollow. The various kinds of knives were accurately indicated; the convex, concave, and pointed bistouries, the cautery, and the curette.

Trephines were used for trephining the skull. The vaginal speculum was used in hemorrhages and fistulas, also syringes and cannulas. Forceps for extracting teeth were described (odontagra).

The chapter that treats of fractures and dislocations is one of the most worthy of admiration in all the surgical writings of the Hippocratic school. It is evident that it represents the results of a long and profound experience.

The anatomy of the bones and joints, and, what is most interesting, the physiology of movement were well known and the descriptions rational and accurate. Simple and compound fractures were distinguished and the approximate time for the formation of bony callus indicated.

There are exact descriptions of bandages and the modes of applying them. The bandage should be left on for three days and then changed. About the seventh day, when the swelling had gone down, a new bandage should be applied more tightly. After the thirtieth day the fracture was regarded as cured. There are accurate indications for the positions in which fractured limbs should be placed. There are descriptions also of special apparatuses for the leg and a sort of neck bandage for fracture of the arm.

Dislocation of the humerus was reduced, with the aid of an assistant, by extension with the foot, shoulder, or hand of the physician, in the axilla, or with a stake, a ladder, or a branch. For the dislocated femur was used a wooden apparatus called " the bench of Hippocrates," on which the patient reclined so bandaged as to permit extension and counter-extension. A number of important directions are given for reduction of dislocations of the acromion, hands, fingers, and jaw. In certain cases of fracture of the jaw it is directed to bind together the teeth with gold wire.

Directions are given for the treatment of spondylitis, a treatment which, as Heussner has observed, was repeated twenty centuries later by Callot. Injuries of the head are described in detail. Trephining the skull should be so performed that the trephine does not penetrate quickly to the dura mater. One should, on the contrary, let the bone detach itself, and it is advised to plunge the trephine frequently in cold water to avoid overheating of the bone.

The operations on rectal disorders, and especially on rectal fistula and hemorrhoids, are described with especial exactness. In both cases the speculum was used. A sound was passed through the fistula, which was then treated with astringents or bandaged. Hemorrhoids were treated with suppositories, with cautery, or finally by excision. As to ophthalmology, odontology, rhinology, we merely record that in these fields also the knowledge of the Hippocratic surgeons had reached a notable stage.

Hirschfeld, in his work on the ophthalmology of Hippocrates, and Magnus, in his study of the history of cataract, have demonstrated that many of the more important operations were successfully practised by the Hippocratic surgeons. In the field of obstetrics in the time of Hippocrates it was ordinarily the midwife and not the physician who examined the pregnant woman. The writings that refer to these subjects are probably of Cnidian origin. The anatomy of the genital organs was fairly well known, although the position of the uterus was regarded as changeable. The clitoris was unknown, however, also the Fallopian tubes, which were briefly described by Aristotle. There is a fairly accurate description of leucorrhœal flow, which was treated by dietary measures, by bleeding beneath the nipple, and by the introduction of vaginal capsules containing astringents. Pessaries were indicated for prolapse, for cancer of the uterus, and for sterility, for the latter of which various treatments were recommended according to the different causes held responsible by the physicians of the period.

The entire chapter on the treatment of sterility, which contains an element of mysticism, shows how very vague were the ideas of the Hippocratic writers about the physiology of fertilization, even though this problem occupied them constantly. All the positions of the fetus were known and the difficulties in delivery of some of these cases. In the oblique position, for instance, rotation of the head was prescribed, after the use of various methods that are not clearly explained. There is no indication of Cæsarean section in the Hippocratic writings, in spite of the very ancient legends about the birth of Dionysos and Æsculapius in this way.

Hippocrates, like many other pre-Listerian surgeons, knew empirically the advantages of pure or boiled water or wine in the treatment of wounds, without of course having the remotest idea of asepsis. He knew, also, that dry wounds were better than wet ones and that greasy dressings should be avoided. The edges of clean wounds were kept as closely approximated as possible and healing " by first intention " sometimes obtained. He also described healing by second intention and knew the signs of suppuration and how to treat them.

7. Hippocratic Therapeutics. The Healing Power of Nature

Healing comes through the power of nature, whose effects are produced by means of the vital forces; therefore the aim that Hippocrates proposes for treatment is to aid nature in its healing powers. In the book On Epidemics (VI, 5) it is stated: " It is nature itself that finds the way; though untaught and uninstructed, it does what is proper." And in the book On Aliment (XXXIX): " Nature acts without masters."

The body, according to Hippocrates, has within itself the means of cure; the symptoms of disease, and especially fever, are merely expressions of the effort of the organism: the physis represents the capacity of the vital forces of the individual to react against disease.

Nature has been defined in the Hippocratic writings in different ways: at times it indicates the entire organism, at others the four qualities or the four cardinal humours, or essence or substance; sometimes also, as Neuburger has shown, it signifies dominating laws. Certainly the activity of nature is regarded as always necessary and corresponding exactly to individual requirements. In the Hippocratic concept, cure is closely connected with riddance of the materia peccans: fever is one of the means of obtaining cure. This is shown in many Hippocratic passages, but especially in that famous aphorism (V, 70), already quoted, that emphasizes the antagonism between convulsions and quartan fever. Also, in a frequently quoted passage from *On Epidemics* (III): " Quartan fever is the least dangerous, the lightest, and the longest of these diseases, but it often cures other dangerous diseases." (See the twentieth-century use of this principle by Wagner von Jauregg.)

Nouson physeis ietroi (*Epidemics* VI, 5), " the forces of nature " (literally, " the natures ") " are the physicians of disease." From the knowledge that nature often cures disease without the intervention of the physician, and always accomplishes the cure by an innate function, is derived the proof of the healing power of nature, and at the same time the method of Hippocratic treatment. Treatment should be deductive — that is, drawn from observation of the signs and symptoms — and should tend to aid and regulate the work of nature. The physician should intervene wisely at the proper moment, at times proceeding according to the principle: " *similia similibus*," aiming to produce results similar to the symptoms. If the physician co-operates with nature, thanks to the results that both produce, the patient is turned from disease to health. Thus that which produces strangury cures the strangury of disease; cough is caused and cured by the same agents. Veratrum provokes vomiting and diarrhœa; Hippocrates speaks of having given it to a cholera patient and cured him.

It is incorrect, however, to state, as is sometimes done both by ancient authors and by homœopathists, that the principle of *similia* was the only one used by the Hippocratists. In the *Aphorisms*, for example (II, 22), it is stated: " All diseases due to plethora should be treated with purgatives, and those due to excessive evacuations should be treated with repletion; in general also in other diseases one should employ contraries." And in the Hippocratic book *On the Places in Man* (Ch. xlii), one reads: " Pains can be cured with means that are contrary to their origin; every disease has its special remedy." Hippocratic therapeutics, then, were not bound by any fixed rules.

Great importance in treatment was attributed to diet, gymnastics, exercise, massage, sea bathing. We find in the book *On Diet* an interesting and valuable treatise on the preparation of a number of foods.

At the height of the disease nourishment should be lessened. In fevers a liquid diet is recommended, also in cases of wounds. Wine is allowed in small doses; among the approved beverages are a honey-vinegar, a paste of barley or flour. Milk in large amounts was prescribed by the Cnidian school.

Blood-letting was rarely prescribed by the Hippocratists, but often by the Cnidian school. In the works thought to be of Cnidian origin, there are exact directions as to how it should be carried out.

Cupping was often used, also scarification. The cups were of glass or metal. We know that the Hippocratic materia medica was large. Most of the drugs recommended, however, are included in those works thought to be Cnidian, where hundreds of drugs are listed. Many are undoubtedly of Egyptian origin.

Let us look at some of the more important. Among the purgatives are: milk, and especially large amounts of asses' milk, decoctions of melon, cabbage, and other plants, often mixed with honey; more drastic remedies were black helle-bore, castor oil, coloquinth.

As emetics were recommended hot water, white hellebore, hyssop, the root of thassia; as sudorifics, hot drinks; as diuretics, the juice of scilla, celery, parsley, asparagus, etc. As narcotics were used: belladonna, mandragora, *jusquiam*, opium; as astringents, oak bark, *sanguis draconis*, grenadine, etc.

Remedies for external use were: water, vinegar, olive oil, and wine, applied in compresses, irrigations, and in the treatment of wounds. Various fatty sub-stances were used for diseases of the eyes; various minerals, such as sulphur, asphalt, and alum, as fumigants in diseases of women; preparations of lead, cop-per, and arsenic for various diseases of the skin. Hippocrates recognized, how-ever, that the physician was but the servant of nature and that " If Nature resists, all measures are in vain."

8. *Essential Characteristics of Hippocratic Medicine*

Summarizing the chief features of Hippocratic medicine, we note first of all that it is constructed on a wide knowledge of the natural sciences, a pro-found experience in practical medicine, a clear and logical reasoning about the relations of cause and effect, and an ethical concept based on an ele-vated moral law. These fundamentals made possible the development of a medical system in which the almost total absence of anatomical knowledge was partially compensated for by accuracy of observation and profundity of reasoning. Actually, from the medical point of view, the *Corpus Hippo-craticum* represents the most precious document that we possess of an ad-vanced evolution of the medical art in a period in which science had hardly taken its first steps. In spite of the faulty knowledge of anatomy, physi-ology, and pathology, in spite of the poverty of animal investigations, sel-dom and but crudely attempted, Hippocratic medicine, founded essentially on bedside experience and philosophic reasoning, succeeded in rising to heights that have seldom been surpassed. This is one of the most interesting phenomena of history and perhaps the most significant of all, because it shows that valuable treasures of information can be gathered by empirical experience, practical observation, and accurate reasoning; but that they will be limited and sterilized without the fundamental aid of anatomy and physiology.

Nevertheless, or perhaps on account of it, the importance that the person and the school of Hippocrates have in the history of medicine was estimated at its correct value, even in ancient times. Hippocrates is not to be regarded, as has been stated erroneously, as the perfection of medical science, but he does determine the beginning of a decided trend in the history of medicine. In his work is to be found the union of threads that come from the most diverse origins. He has a vivid comprehension of human suffering, the first necessity of the art of medicine and one that should never be forgotten. He represents the philosophic thought of the wisest of his time and also the best traditions of a caste of physicians that undoubtedly influenced him and his school.

Just as philosophic concepts in the greatest Grecian epoch surpassed their moral and religious concepts after long travail, so also medicine shifted from a religious to a clinical point of view. During this transition period in the schools of philosophy, as in those early and glorious medical schools of which only the names have been preserved, only the general outlines of the work as a whole are known and the contributions of individuals are to be distinguished with difficulty. Only a few names, almost legendary, such as those of the Seven Wise Men, detach themselves from the general obscurity.

The Greek physician was neither prophet, priest, nor magician. He was not a depositary of divine secrets, but an independent agent, guided by his own critical thought, and animated by the impelling necessity of searching for a logical explanation of natural phenomena. To this he added knowledge of himself, that internal contemplation that is summarized in the formula of Thales: "Know thyself." Thus, in the history of medical thought, Hippocrates and his school ignored the sanctuary of the god and made clinical observation and critical reasoning their fields of activity. They recognized the need of hypotheses to explain natural phenomena and they created the masterly method of investigation and strict analysis of all knowledge.

Later, in the period of decadence, Oriental mysticism again exerted its influence on Greek philosophy and medicine. And then, in the dawn of the Christian era, the faith overturned classic thought. But Greek thought was victoriously to be born again. The problems that the ancient Greek thinkers posed are eternal and necessarily keep presenting themselves to the human mind.

The master who had such a profound concept of the art of medicine and who recognized that we should not neglect the precepts of ancient medicine, even if these were not entirely correct, who deemed worthy of praise those pupils who committed only minor errors, obviously carried within himself the precious heritage of a great past, of which both the triumphs and the defects were familiar to him. In the first and most celebrated of his *Aphorisms*, which should be taught in every school of medicine, even remembered at the patient's bedside, he recognized every state of being as but a phase in the process of development. For him the medicine of his day was indissolubly bound to the past, and in his concept of disease every organ was connected with all the others, and there was no morbid affection that did not involve the whole organism. So also in his concept of the art of medicine, he could not imagine one event disconnected from another, or an observation or deduction as anything but a link in an unbreakable chain.

A philosopher above all, if philosophy signifies the close study of nature combined with logical reasoning, he fought vain speculation vigorously. Like Socrates, who divorced philosophy from cosmic speculation and directed it toward ethics, so Hippocrates freed medicine from superstition, on the one hand, and from philosophic speculation on the other, and intelligently and deliberately directed it toward its immediate and only goal: the cure of the patient.

" The philosophic physician is like unto a god," said the sage of Cos, believing that reasoning should never be absent from the physician's task, which, following the old tradition of priestly medicine, he also calls divine. Speaking of the special characteristics of certain diseases, he adds: " It is a mistake to regard one disease as more divine than another, as all is human and all divine."

9. Hippocratic Medicine and Priestly Medicine

When pupils gathered together in the quiet shades of Cos and the torches of knowledge shed their brightest light on those little rocky islands of the Ægean, colonized probably in pre-Hellenic times, the temples of Æsculapius still maintained their fame and were frequented by thousands of the faithful. By means of dreams and oracles, the god still produced his miraculous cures. But in the Hippocratic works there is no trace of these cures, not even to condemn them. It is only in the rules imposed on those who practise the art of medicine that Hippocrates remains faithful to the tradition of the Asclepiads. But this tradition, through Hippocrates, and thanks to him, is now directed toward the free practice of the art, inspired with a high moral sentiment. The *Oath of Hippocrates*, which covers the duty of the physician to his teacher, his pupils, and his patients, clearly shows that a relationship existed between Hippocratic medicine and priestly medicine; but it raises medicine to a height and human dignity that assures it its own position as a science. From priestly medicine Hippocrates borrowed the forms that tend to give authority to the physician. The physician's bearing, according to the ethical precepts of the master, is elevated, direct, severe. He should be the true Socratic philosopher; all the best qualities of the philosopher should be found in him: disinterestedness, modesty, dignity, tranquil judgment, serenity, decision, knowledge of useful and necessary things, avoidance of evil, freedom from all superstition. We have read how details of conduct are carefully outlined, all leading to the enthusiastic study of the case. Substituted for the healing power of the gods is a sure faith in nature and love of the art, which, according to the Hippocratic concept, cannot be separated from love for the sick.

Joining the useful features of priestly practice to the observation of natural phenomena and the search for their causes, and mellowing all in a philosophy freed from dogmatism, the Hippocratic physician produces a new type of medicine, highly conceived, marvellously thought out, and raises it into an independent art. No longer studying the stars or the victims in the temples, but the patient and his ills, reasoning on the basis of facts rather than on abstract speculations, Hippocratic medicine is essentially individualistic. It is perhaps this very individualistic tendency that connects it with the characteristic aims, seventeen centuries later, of the Renaissance.

It seems as if every great period in which civilization attained to new heights had first to find its impetus and perhaps its very essence in an initial timid awakening; in the next phase it appeared as a vigorous manifestation of individual knowledge; and finally in a supreme surge toward beauty and glory. Thus it is in the Golden Age of Greece in all the manifestations of its art. The individual now issues from the dark shadows of history and advances to the footlights in the theatre of the human drama. Socrates shows man to himself as the aim and goal of all thought. In sculpture, representation of the human figure is the climax, and on the black background of those marvellous amphoras the artist portrays the human form with a sure hand, and signs the work of art with his name. In this first humanism the tendency to individualism is manifest most clearly in the thought of Hippocrates and his school. To study man as the end in itself, leaving aside the idea of any divine intervention in the affairs of men; to study all suffering with feeling; and to retain as a most important basis for action the axiom of *non nocere* — this is the principle that animates both the philosophy of Socrates and the medicine of Hippocrates.

Hippocrates constructs the edifice of medicine on the rock of experience and affirms the need for the study of nature. He recognizes, in spite of the scanty knowledge of anatomy, a dominating law by virtue of which all the phenomena that appear in the individual represent an attempt at the individual defence by which nature seeks to heal. According to this concept, humanistic in the fullest sense of the word, the physician emerges from the constricted precincts of the temple and proceeds with open eye and pure mind to consider the vast mystery of nature. He tries to read in the great book that is opened to him, wherein are written the immutable laws that govern all things that live on the earth. It is for this reason that to Hippocrates all is divine and all is human. Everything in nature tends to re-establish that perfect harmony that constitutes normal life. Every force in the individual tends to preserve a perfect equilibrium, and, if it has been disturbed, to re-establish order and harmony. Thus is indicated with absolute clarity the function of the physician according to the Hippocratic concept.

Not a ruler or violator of nature, following the will of or in the name of the gods, but with his own will and in his own name, he stands ready to aid the healing power that is inherent in nature. Acute observer of every disturbance, and convinced therefore that many diseases will be cured spontaneously if the forces of nature are wisely assisted; untiring student of the causes of disease, in order to keep them remote from the patient, in this sense the physician is also a philosopher. In treatment, the essential is to intervene at the right moment, as " the occasion is fleeting "; to assist all the forces that tend toward good and to combat every dangerous sign. And this is the final aim of Hippocratic therapy: to maintain, in whatever way possible, the energies of the individual, with proper diet, with hygienic measures, and with the prescriptions, individualized for each case, that the condition of the patient from day to day requires. To seek in quiet thought the causes of disease without losing sight of the immediate aim, to use reason and experience, free from preconceived ideas, superstitions, and *a priori* concepts, as the basis of every action — that is the fundamental program of Hippocratic medicine.

CHAPTER X

POST–HIPPOCRATIC MEDICINE

THE ALEXANDRIAN SCHOOL.
BEGINNINGS OF ANATOMICAL AND
PHYSIOLOGICAL STUDIES

1. Medicine after Hippocrates. Aristotle

AMONG the first direct inheritors of the doctrines of the Hippocratic school were the sons of Hippocrates, THESSALUS and DRACO, who later studied in Macedonia, his son-in-law POLYBUS, the famous scholar Diocles of Carystos, and Menon, a pupil of Aristotle. The school owed much of its prosperity to those who had learned the art directly from the master or from his pupils. To the school of Cos belonged Crytodemus, who was the physician of Alexander the Great and once saved his life by extracting an arrow from his body. Hippocrates IV, physician of Roxane, was a great-grand-son of the great master. For a long time the courts of the Orient preferred to choose their personal physicians from Cos. It appears that one of these physicians, Philotimus (third century B.C.), transmitted to the Alexandrian library the books *On the Epidemics*, together with the library of the medical school of Macedonia at Cos (Neppi Modona). In the course of time various ideas and systems, disciplines or hypotheses, detached themselves from the main trunk and gave rise to new lines of thought, more often to new speculations, sometimes to a more direct and immediate application of what the sage of Cos had thought.

[179]

At this time philosophy appeared to be more than ever in close relation to medicine and both disciplines closely studied nature. Plato, who in his *Phædo* speaks of Hippocrates as a master, laid the basis of biology. His philosophy reflects the work of Philolaus, one of the most illustrious physicians of the Sicilian school, just as Hippocrates had been deeply influenced by the doctrines of Gorgias Siculus. The school of Cnidus was still flourishing with Eudoxus and Chrysippus. Diocles of Carystus (*c.* 350 B.C.), son of the physician Archidamus, was a student of anatomy who was regarded by antiquity as the greatest physician after Hippocrates and was the author of a series of medical works in which he sought the causal connection between symptoms. According to his theory two factors are important in organic life: the pneuma and the elements. His successor and pupil Praxagoras of Cos belonged to the school of Dogmatists, who regarded pathological facts as links of a rigid chain derived from theoretical laws.

But now the fundamental lines of Hippocratic philosophy lived again in the work of a great philosopher. Aristotle (384–322 B.C.), however little was his effect on the physicians of his time, as Dante's " master of those who know," had an important influence on the history of civilized thought up to the sixteenth century and beyond. In the field of medicine also he was undoubtedly a great pioneer.

Born at Stagira, son of Nicomachus of Asclepiad stock, pupil of Plato, physician to the Macedonian court, he reflects in all his work the effect of the medical atmosphere in which his mental habits were formed and of his contact with the Hippocratic writings. His studies in the field of natural sciences, his method — in which apparently for the first time in history a master placed himself at the head of a school of pupils and gave them systematic instruction — his marvellous activity in the field of biology, his genius in collecting a vast material and organizing it with an invincible, critical spirit, all require that he be regarded as one of the most important factors in the historical evolution of medical thought.

The biological knowledge of Aristotle shows, especially in the field of zoology, the results of his profound studies. His *History of Animals*, with the classification that is in part still accepted today, is but one evidence of his intensive and long-continued research. His descriptions of plants and animals reveal an exactness of observation and anatomical study and a knowledge of muscular detail that is as striking as that seen in the celebrated Minoan goblet (sixteenth century B.C.). His observations on Cetacea, justly quoted by Singer (in *The Evolution of Anatomy*) as an example of clear description, and his masterly attempt at the classification of invertebrates, are further examples of his genius. Especially worthy of interest is the tree of nature which Aristotle constructed, extending from the lower plants through molluscs, arthropods, crustacea, reptiles, and mammals to man.

Differing from the concept maintained up to that time, that generation was due to the union of the masculine seed with an analogous substance from the female, Aristotle maintained the possibility of spontaneous generation and did not think that it was absolutely necessary for a male substance to fertilize the ovum (cf. J. Loeb's experiments in parthenogenesis). But Aristotle also accomplished interesting results in other fields of biology — witness his studies on the stomachs of ruminants, on which, to judge from his accurate descriptions, he had obviously performed post-mortem examinations; also those on the generative processes of cephalopods, with observations that have been confirmed only in recent years. Noteworthy also are his observations on the torpedo fishes and on the life of bees, while in the field of botany his studies were no less interesting and profound. Thus Darwin does not seem to have exaggerated when he stated that all modern biologists can only be regarded as pupils of Aristotle.

Kalthoff's book on *The Hygiene of Aristotle* (Berlin, 1934) collects from his writings his regulations for the administration of public health, social hygiene, and the care of the unfortunate. The chapters that treat of anatomy and heredity, psychiatry and prophylaxis also show that this great philosopher had a profound knowledge of the field of medicine and hygiene. Aristotle's " entelechies " have been used by Driesch in the modern revival of vitalism as a substitute for the " vital spirit."

From Aristotle are traced the beginnings of comparative anatomy; from him the investigative method of connecting cause and effect and of force closely bound with matter. To him we owe notable progress in embryology, and to him and his followers the beginning of the critical study of nature in which the position of man in the macrocosm was clarified. Thus is justified the very great authority that the Stagirite exerted for two millennia in the field of medicine.

Among the pupils of Aristotle, one of the most celebrated was Tirtanus, to whom Aristotle himself gave the name THEOPHRASTUS (370–285 B.C.), the divine orator. He was born at Eresos in the island of Lesbos, and was so dear to Aristotle that when the latter was preparing to leave Athens he arranged that Theophrastus should be his successor at the Lyceum, where Theophrastus taught until his death. He was the first to occupy himself scientifically with the natural history of plants; he was the most celebrated of the botanists of antiquity, unexcelled up to the time of the Renaissance. In the two works *The History of Plants* (9 books) and *The Causes of Plants* (6 books) he described all the plants known to his time, with pro-

fundity of observation and a clear and lucid vision of the facts of organic
life. This work, which was a classical botanical text for almost twenty centuries and contained valuable indications of the therapeutic value of many
plants, should be regarded as one of the great scientific monuments of antiquity. The first Latin edition of Theophrastus was published at Treviso in

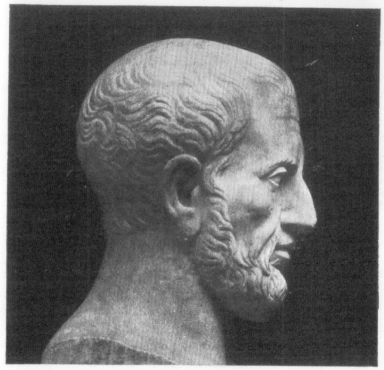

73. *Theophrastus.*   (*Marble bust from the* TORLONIA COLLECTION, ROME.)

1483, and the first Greek edition at Venice in 1497 (Aldus). A bilingual
Greek and English text by A. Hort appears in Loeb's Classical Library.

Slowly in the course of centuries, however, the Hippocratic idea lost
ground. Its practical and virile concepts became crystallized in the rigidity
of formulas and became the source of scholastic doctrines to which the
physicians of all times and nations adhered, without knowing how to interpret correctly the thought of the master. Often it remained a rigid
schema in which the myopic followers of the wise physician sought to incorporate unimportant ideas, substituting for the living spring of direct
observation, personal experience, and intelligent goodwill, the sterile discussion of the verbal interpretation of the text.

There happened to Hippocratic thought that which seems to be the destiny of many great and philosophic ideas: they are not able to live, flourish, or, much more, to progress when separated from their origin, but take on inferior forms and orientations according to subsequent times and events. Thus Hippocratic thought, with its profound yet simple statements and its clarity of vision, was transformed on the one hand into *a priori* ideas that sought explanation and support in philosophy rather than observation, and on the other hand into a formulation of dogmas which proposed theoretical considerations rather than rational experiences as the basis of medicine.

In this transformation, that part of the Hippocratic system which was merely an attempt at the explanation or application of a correct fundamental thought became the essence of medicine; and on the other hand that which constituted the central idea of Hippocratic medicine became merely an accessory. The change might be regarded as parallel to that of the Socratic philosophy, which in the philosophy of Plato and in the systems of its followers took on very different meanings and orientations. And just as the central idea of the Hippocratic system — which culminated in the characteristic that the essence of medical art consisted in giving direct and immediate aid to the sufferer — later degenerated into the speculative nonsense of its followers; so the Socratic concept of philosophy degenerated into textual and metaphysical speculations, and great schools dwindled into small sects.

2. Medicine of the Alexandrian Period. Herophilus, Erasistratus, the Empiric School

The extensive conquests of Alexander the Great and the resultant political changes brought about a great transformation in the entire culture of the period. Together with its political liberty, Greece lost its intellectual primacy in the civilized world; but Grecian civilization expanded rapidly in the path of the Macedonian conqueror whose dream of glory was to dominate and unite in a single State the peoples of the Orient and those of Grecian stock. Greek culture came into close contact with the ancient culture of the Orient when Alexandria, founded in 332 B.C., became the centre of Mediterranean trade. On this ever increasing richness and this magnificent political expansion, which under the Ptolemies attained to its greatest splendour, the science, philosophy, and art of ancient Greece bestowed its noble and beautiful characteristics. The city into which all the markets of the Orient poured their rare and valuable gifts, the trade centre in whose streets men of all races and tongues lived the tumultuous and febrile life of traffic and industry, aimed through the will of its leaders to take unto itself the traditional glory of Greece and by hard work and zealous study to show itself worthy of this proud position. Thus in the capital of the Ptolemies philosophers, physicians, artists, and poets flourished in the favourable regard of princes and populace. The cult of beauty, like that of scientific research, found its followers in the resplendent life of the Mediterranean metropolis. Here was gathered in its marvellous library a large collection of the classic works of the Greek philosophers.

From Persia, Mesopotamia, and even more distant countries flowed in the traditions of mystic and empiric medicine; all these different currents coming together to form the complex of Alexandrian medicine which so clearly reflected in itself the characteristics of its origin and period. On the one hand was the detailed investigation of the causes of being, of vital manifestations, and of diseases, which reflected the fervid studies of the Alexandrian philosophers and produced those first steps in anatomy and physiology whose genius still excites our admiration; on the other hand, the persistence of a dogmatism which accentuated more and more the formal and literary side of medical studies and substituted erudition for science. It was, to be sure, the glorious period when mathematics could boast of the names of Euclid and Archimedes; but at the same time philological discussions of the texts were becoming interminable. We observe a constant struggle between realism and mysticism, while beliefs oscillated between scepticism and superstition.

Medicine, as we have said, actively reflected these various tendencies. The Hippocratic writings were collected and codified in Alexandria, were the objects of close, continuous, and devoted study, and held the position of honor in the library. The interpretation of such and such a passage in the text might give rise to the most lively discussions. But at the same time it must be remembered that Erasistratus and Herophilus and their pupils were creating new foundations for anatomy and pathology; and Alexandrian medicine seemed about to make great advances in the investigation of new paths in science. When the kingdom of the Ptolemies became decadent, the political structure began to fall apart, and Oriental currents to predominate in social life, medicine also acquired the same tendencies: superstition and dogmatism corroded the living substance of the new medicine, so that toward the end of this period it dwindled into a sterile search of the written word, while the practice of medicine was almost exclusively in the hands of empiricists and charlatans.

Thus this brief splendour signalizes but a transient episode in the history of medicine; one, however, of which we shall later find traces in the medical history of the people who inherited the Hellenistic culture on the shores of the Mediterranean.

As if the need was felt for filling in gaps in the Hippocratic writings, it is to the study of anatomy, physiology, and experimental pathology that the Alexandrian school devoted itself with the greatest enthusiasm. Some of the physicians of this period are particularly worthy of note. The first of these is HEROPHILUS, who lived about 300 B.C. and was a pupil of Praxagoras and Chrysippus. He left but few writings, but we know from his contemporaries and followers that he was a tireless investigator in the field of anatomy. He was the first to study systematically the anatomy of the brain and spinal cord; to him is owed the differentiation between nerves and blood vessels, a point that was still vague in the Hippocratic writings. Herophilus knew that the nerves both carried sensations to the nerve centres and also determined movements. With exact statements that indicate studies on the cadaver, he observed and described the abdominal organs and the female genital organs, and distinguished the lymphatics, without, however, recognizing their origin or significance. He analysed respiratory movements and tried to solve the problem of the circulation. He was without doubt the first and most illustrious of the anatomists of his period. Clinician also, he was the founder of the doctrine of the pulse and counted its rate with a water clock and analysed its systole and diastole.

Galen states that Herophilus was the first to practise dissection of human and animal bodies; but Singer surmises that this signifies that he was the first to practise dissection in public. His observations on the anatomy of the nervous system are notable. To him we owe not only the clear statement that the brain is the central organ of the nervous system and the site of the intelligence, contrary to the doctrine of Aristotle, who placed this centre in the heart; but also he was the first to distinguish the cerebrum from the cerebellum, to describe the *torcular Herophili* and the *calamus scriptorius*, to name the duodenum, and to recognize pulsation as a phenomenon taking place in the vessels.

ERASISTRATUS (*c*. 310–250 B.C.), son of a physician and disciple of the school of Cnidus, followed the doctrines of this school in his pathological concepts. He abandoned the humoral theory and attributed the greatest importance in the origin of disease to the tissues and the vessels. He held that the blood provided the nourishment of the body, and that the pneuma was the substance necessary for life. He was perhaps the first to initiate the study of pathologic anatomy, searching for the anatomical causes of pleurisy and pericarditis. He recognized an association between ascites and hardening of the liver. He gave particular attention to the normal and pathological anatomy of the brain, which he regarded as the centre of psychic function. He regarded plethora of parts or organs as of prime importance in the development of disease.

Erasistratus was more physiologist and pathologist than anatomist; some historians have even regarded him as the founder of physiology. He maintained that every organ is supplied with three kinds of vessels: veins, arteries, and nerves. He believed that the air which entered the lungs penetrated even to the heart, where it formed the vital spirit that the arteries carried to different parts of the body. In the brain the vital spirit was transformed, probably in the ventricles, into the animal spirit, which was transmitted by the nerves to different parts of the body. Erasistratus' observations on the function of arteries and veins were important; he believed that the blood passed from the veins into the arteries through extremely small intercommunicating vessels. Thus he approached the concept of the circulation, but thought of it in a reverse direction. It is to him that we owe the discovery of the function of the tricuspid valve; he believed that the mitral valve had the function of preventing the vital spirit from leaving the heart except by the aorta.

These indications suffice to show that this Alexandrian scientist was a skilled investigator, free from prejudice, independent of any dogmatic doctrine, who thoroughly appreciated the importance of the observational method to which he dedicated his studies.

Thus one sees that medicine was tending to advance along lines that would supplement the Hippocratic system and give it a solid basis. But probably on account of the political situation of Alexandria and the events that determined the deterioration and finally the fall of the Kingdom, Alexandrian medicine rapidly became decadent. The disciples of these two great physicians and scientists became founders of two sects: the Herophilists and the Erasistratists, the first of which lasted until the first century after Christ, while traces of the second were to be found considerably later. But the pupils did not follow the paths outlined by their masters in persevering in their investigative work. Following the example of the commentators and the exegetes of the Alexandrian school, they gave all their attention to the examination and study of texts and carried medicine along the sterile path of dogmatism.

Contemporaneous with this latter school, and perhaps as a reaction to its dogmatism, there developed in Alexandria between 270 and 220 B.C. a third school which was to attain great importance. The school of the Empiricists was the only one to have any success in reviving the essentials of the Hippocratic concept. They detached themselves slowly from the assertions of the dogmatists, abandoned completely speculative and philosophic medicine, and maintained that it is only practice that can foster medical art, and that theoretical discussions can be nothing but harmful. They believed that dogmas and doctrines had no value in medicine, which must not be regarded as a science but as an art solely based on experience.

Founding their doctrine on experience, they utilized the observations of Hippocrates and regarded him as their master, especially in that part of his writings that treated of empirical medicine. They affirmed that the basis of all experience should be, first, personal observation, then the tradition of the observation made by others, and, last of all, analogy. These three elements were called the "tripod" and for the empiricists constituted the basis of all medicine and particularly of therapy.

The Empirical school had its greatest development in HERACLEIDES of Tarentum (second century after Christ), a celebrated physician surgeon, to whom is credited a number of writings, and especially an important commentary on Hippocrates. Of all his writings, however, only a few fragments have been preserved. We know that he was a pharmacologist of the first rank, and that he was one of the first to recommend opium, though carefully limiting its use.

In surgery and gynæcology, also, we know that the Empirical school attained a considerable degree of knowledge. The use of bandages, reduction of dislocations, operations for hernia, cataract, and removal of vesical calculi were well known. Materia medica was developed by CRATEUAS, physician to the court of Mithridates VI, a wise author of important works, especially on the use of poisons and antidotes. This constituted a subject of great importance, if only for the frequency with which in that period tyrants made use of poisons to eliminate their enemies and for their terror at the possibility of themselves being victims. History records that Mithridates VI, Eupator, King of Pontus, himself was addicted to these studies and acquired considerable experimental knowledge of poisons and their antidotes. The most famous of these antidotes (*Mithridaticum*) preserved the name of its inventor for many centuries. To Mithridates also tradition attributes the first attempts to immunize the organism with repeated administrations of poison, steadily increased from small doses.

Political catastrophe initiated the sterilization of this vigorous shoot from the ancient tree of scientific knowledge; the end of Egyptian independence signalized the end of Alexandrian medicine. Rome became the centre of the culture of the period and the inheritor of the science and art of medicine.

Thus Hippocratic medicine experienced a slow decadence, which was due especially to the diffusion of Alexandrian empirical medicine. We see the beginning of that pernicious system of local pathology which distinguishes diseases according to their local sites, completely losing contact with the concept of general pathology. To the same tendency should probably be attributed the growth of specialists of all sorts for all kinds of diseases. At the same time mysticism, occultism, and magic practices multiplied rapidly and invaded all the domains of scientific research. With the exhaustion of a soil formerly so fertile, Hellenistic civilization approached its end. But its most vital elements were reborn and flourished again in the civilization which was to inherit the grandeur of the Greek traditions. By various ways, some of which are known and others mysterious, this new civilization attracted to itself the riches and treasures of commerce, art, and science to complete a grandeur of its own.

CHAPTER XI

ROMAN MEDICINE

THE LATIN CONCEPT OF MEDICINE AND SANITARY LEGISLATION

~~~~~~

1. *Etruscan Medicine*

OUR knowledge of the medicine of the ancient peoples of Italy is vague and uncertain, just as all questions about the first inhabitants of the peninsula and of their origins still remain in the zone of mystery. Even the most recent historical investigations have not been able to decide for us where the Etruscans had come from when they arrived in Italy; or even whether they belonged, as certain authors supposed, to an Oriental race and were colonists arriving in Italy from Lydia, or from some other Oriental country, who were subjected by the continual contacts of commerce to the lasting influence of the more ancient Mediterranean civilization. Their culture reached them by lines of communication that are obscure but certainly different from those of the Greco-Sicilian civilization.

We find in the Etruscan culture ancient and indubitable traces of Oriental currents. Furthermore, the characteristically Greek influences are different from those that we find in Sicily.

In the Etruscan mythology, founded on a divine trinity and an infernal trinity, analogous to those of the Cretan and Mycenæan mythologies, demonology plays an important part. We borrow from the valuable book of Ducati on ancient Etruria the following facts that summarize all that is known about

Etruscan medicine. Ducati believes that the Roman theory of the Genius, which, according to the phrase of Horace (*Ep.* II, 187), accompanies each individual and guides his star, is of Etruscan origin. Etruscan mirrors of polished bronze have acquainted us with the existence of female aphrodisiac demons having the appearance of winged young women; sometimes they have the function of protecting women in labour, and in a mirror from Palestrina, which

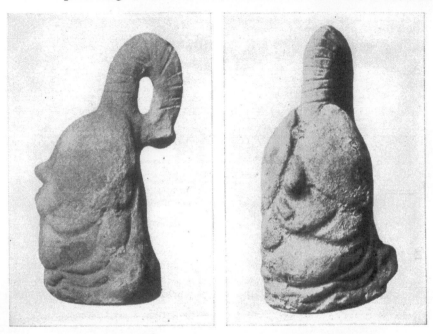

74. *Etruscan ex-voto showing the thoracic and abdominal organs.*
(ETRUSCAN MUSEUM, FLORENCE.)

is now in the British Museum, two such figures are to be seen, Ecthanova and Tharn, assisting at the birth of *Mnerva* (Minerva) from the head of Tinia. Their special name is *Lasa*. One often finds serpents belonging, as in other mythologies, to infernal gods. They are generally accompanied by the hammer with axe, symbolizing the force of death, like the scythe of Christian symbolism. Frequent also is the belief in " animal " gods — that is to say, in the deification of the *anima*, the soul. This belief probably came from the Orphic Pythagorean traditions.

The art of observing the viscera of animals, and especially the liver (*extispicium*), had great importance in divination, and in fact it seems that the Latin word *haruspex* comes from the ancient Chaldean word *har*, which means liver. There is no doubt that this rite originated in Chaldea. Perhaps, as Ducati supposes, its transmitters were the Hittites, who dominated a great part of Syria and Mesopotamia during the second half of the second millennium B.C. We know of clay models of livers with cuneiform inscriptions coming from Chaldea, and of others with Hittite inscriptions which were found at Bogaz-Kévi, the capital of the Hittite Empire. From this source, according to Ducati, comes the bronze of Piacenza of the third century B.C. that is an actual *templum*, having the form of a sheep's liver, divided into small compartments, each containing the name of a divinity, in full or abbreviated. It appears to have been

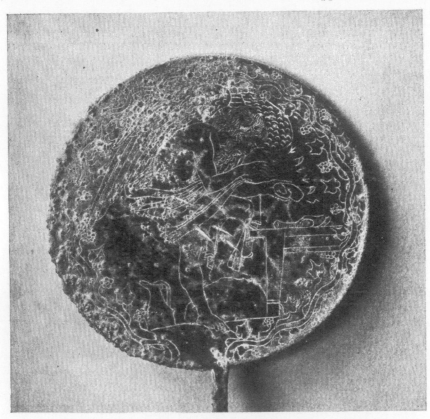

75. *Etruscan mirror showing the haruspex Kalkas examining the liver.*
(GREGORIAN MUSEUM, ROME.)

an instrument used for teaching the art of the haruspex, and each compartment of bronze corresponds exactly to each of the regions of the heavens inhabited by the corresponding divinity. There were in the liver, as in the celestial temple, a *pars familiaris* (propitious) and a *pars hostilis* (contrary), corresponding to the right and left of the observer. The *fissum* or *limes* was an incision limiting the parts; noteworthy also was the *caput jecinoris*, the protuberance found on the livers of sheep and cattle, and the *fibræ* (extremities or borders). Each of these parts had its special function. We know also that apotropaic and deprecatory rites were frequent among the Etruscans, not only from the leaden tablets of *devotiones* of Volterra and Monte Pitto and the leaden relic of Magliano in the museum of Florence, but by the magic formula against diseases which Varro translates from the book of the Etruscan Saserna:

<blockquote>
Terra pestem teneto
Salus hic maneto;
</blockquote>

that is to say, "May the earth keep the pest, and health remain with me." Ex-votos are often found representing parts of the human body, limbs or viscera, and expressing the gratitude of the cured to the divinity.

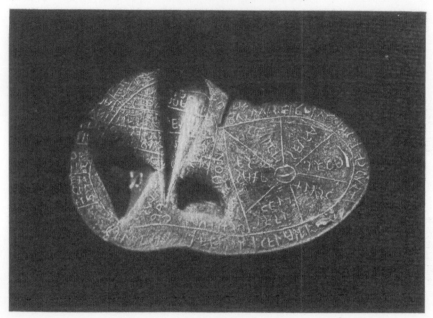

76. *The Etruscan liver of Piacenza with the divisions for the haruspex.*
(*Compare illustration of the Babylonian model.*) (CIVIC MUSEUM, PIACENZA.)

The Etruscans are said to have enjoyed a great medical reputation in antiquity. Theophrastus declares (*History of Plants*, IX, 15, 1): "Æschylus states in his elegies that Etruria is rich in medicines, and that the Etruscan race is one that cultivates medicine." One can also add the legend given in the *Theogony* of Hesiod, in which the sons of the sorceress Circe, expert in medicines, became Etruscan princes. It appears to be a fact that the thermal waters of ancient Etruria were known from very distant times; and we have definite proof of the existence of the art of surgery and especially of dentistry among the Etruscans. In the tombs of Tarquinia, Capodimonte, and Civita Castellana have been found teeth bound with gold wire (*dentes auro juncti*). These methods of treating the teeth passed from Etruria to Latium, where dentures containing gold work have been found at Palestrina and Conca, and also at Rome, where a regulation of the Laws of the Twelve Tables forbade placing gold in tombs, except where it is in the teeth of the dead person.

But just as Etruscan art quickly felt the Greek influence and the Greek alphabet became generally adopted (between 600 and 500 B.C.), so it is evident also that Greek medical concepts about this time made their way into Etruria. We find, for instance, the names and images of the gods of Grecian mythology on Etruscan *objets d'art*. We can reasonably suppose, then, that the cult of the healing gods was also imported into Italy from Greece.

Of great importance was the work performed by the Etruscans in excavating galleries and subterranean tunnels and levelling the hills of tufa, both in the city and in the country, in order to combat malaria, as noted by Celli. In a period that cannot now be dated, paludism destroyed entire populations of Latium and brought about the complete disappearance of a prosperous and flourishing countryside. The record of these occurrences was preserved up to the time of the Empire. Pliny stated: " *Ex antiquo Latio tres et quinquaginta populi interiere sine vestigiis* (In ancient Latium fifty-three populations perished without a trace)." Celli states that the history of these peoples shows that the region was inhabited from neolithic times by a strong race of agriculturists and that it was not until the second or third century of the Roman period that disease began to disseminate through the people and then to be spread in epidemic form. All the sanitary operations to which we have referred show that the Etruscans understood that the draining of swamps had become necessary and that they had immediately begun colossal works by way of defence.

The construction of the Cloaca Maxima, as legend states, by Tarquinius Priscus, a king of Etruscan origin, continued this program. It must be accepted that in the construction of this *receptaculum omnium purgamentorum urbis* Etruscans, accustomed to combat the dangers of maremma, played a most important role. This great work was a drainage system before it was a sewer; it was only when the aqueducts were constructed that it was given the function of draining the sewers of the city.

2. Roman Medical Mythology

The foundation of Rome and the extension of its power over a great part of the peninsula, the domination that it exercised on such ancient peoples as the Umbrians and Oscians, whose conquerors absorbed their re-

ligion, increase the difficulty of studying the origins of this or that tradition of Roman mythology, because they all belonged to indubitably older
myths.

One of the most ancient Roman goddesses of healing was Carna, protectress
of vital functions, as may be seen in a passage in Ovid (*Fasti*, VI, 182): "*Prima*

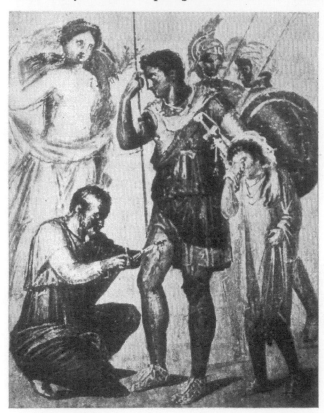

77. *Japyx treats the wound of Æneas with dittamy collected by Venus on
Mount Ida. (See Æneid, Bk. XII) (Pompeian mosaic.)*

dies tibi Carna datur, dea cardinis hæc est (The first day is given to thee, O
Carna, who art the goddess of the door-hinge [i.e., of family life])." She defended man against the *Strigæ*, greedy of blood. To her was consecrated the
first day of June, the *kalendæ fabariæ*, when beans and lard were offered to her
as the typical food, and thus symbolic, of the ancient people of Italy. The goddess *Salus* had a sanctuary on the Quirinal Hill, and the gate of the city was
called *Porta Salutaris*.

Apollo and Mars were regarded from very ancient times as protectors of
health. Castor and Pollux were also worshipped as health gods. Against the

fevers of the Roman Campagna the goddesses Febris and Mephitis were invoked. The former had her temples where patients made their offerings on the Esquiline, the Quirinal, and the Palatine; Mephitis, goddess of miasmas, had her sanctuary in a sacred wood on the Esquiline. In the Latin writers, and especially in Varro, Pliny, and Tacitus, are given the different places where the goddess Mephitis was worshipped, probably in those places where malaria was most prevalent. The temple of the goddess Minerva was near the Esquiline. The protection of pregnant women and of the newborn was confided to a number of deities. Ovid tells of Carmenta, in honour of whom were celebrated the feasts of the *carmentaria*, during which the *carmentarii* noted the oracles of the goddess. She was called Prorsa and Antevorsa when the fetus presented itself in the anterior position. Lucina was, above all, the protecting goddess of menstruation and delivery. To her were addressed the prayers of pregnant women. Her temple was near the Esquiline in the Forum Olitorium. A number of other deities protected virgins and exercised a beneficent influence on all the acts of sexual life.

Mutus-Tutunus was the god of conception and of masculine fecundation. To invoke him the young women and the modest matrons took their seats on the statue of Priapus. Women entered his temple in Rome only when veiled. Uterina, Cunina, Mena, and Rumina were the goddesses guiding the various events of sexual life. We know from monuments that are still in existence about the cult that Rome devoted from the most ancient times to Priapus, deified, who was represented in various forms.

But also foreign gods of healing acquired followers in Rome. The introduction of the cult of Æsculapius into Rome is told by Livy (X, 47), by Valerius Maximus (I, 82), and by Ovid (*Metamorphoses*, XV, 62). In the year 293 B.C. a severe epidemic was inflicted on Rome and it seemed impossible to find any way of checking its rapid and terrible spread. After consulting the Sibylline Books, it was decided to send a deputation to Epidaurus to seek the advice and aid of Æsculapius. At Epidaurus, while the Roman legates were being received ceremoniously, an important event happened: while they were in the temple a serpent made its way down the road, boarded the Roman vessel, and entered the cabin of the legate Ogulnius. It was clear to all that a miracle had happened: the god had entered the vessel, thus signifying his intention of going to the aid of the Romans. When the vessel arrived in the Tiber the serpent swam to the island which later was given the name of St. Bartholomew. In obedience to the sacred omen a temple was built there and Rome was freed from the epidemic. A beautiful bronze medallion was struck by Antoninus Pius (Figure 59, *H*) to illustrate this event: the serpent is seen passing from the vessel beneath the arch of the temple. To the right is seen Father Tiber extending his arm to the god and in the background the Aventine Mount. From then on Asclepios, called in Latin Æsculapius, became the god of health of the Roman people.

3. Roman Medicine in the Times of the Kings and of the Republic

In spite of the contacts which certainly were made in early times with the Greeks, and in spite of the proximity of such important centres for the development of medicine as the Sicilian schools, Roman medicine in its early periods was almost exclusively based on magic. To the gods alone were attributed the power of healing. To them alone the patient had recourse and not only was an infinite number of healing divinities venerated, but the aid of a special god was invoked for almost every single disease. Nevertheless, it appears that there were physicians in Rome from the fourth century B.C. Indeed, the *lex Aquilia*, formulated at this time, makes the physician who has been negligent in his operation responsible for the death of a slave, thus indicating the existence of practitioners.

Among the laws of the period of the kings we find several sanitary regulations, such as that which made it necessary to bury the dead outside the city. But it is certain that before the arrival of Greek physicians, Rome did not possess truly professional practitioners. The practice of medicine was regarded as a function of the *pater familias*. Cato (234–149 B.C.), the ardent defender of ancient Roman customs, who hated Greek refinements and thundered in the Senate against those who tried to introduce Greek customs into Rome, was one of the most violent enemies of Greek medicine. Pliny tells how Cato accused the Greek physicians of poisoning and killing the sick (Bk. XXIX, 1).

Rome, according to Cato, had no worse enemies than physicians. " The Greeks," he wrote to his son Marcus, " are a hard and perverse race. Believe me when I tell you that each time that this nation brings us some new knowledge it will corrupt Rome; but it will be much worse if it sends us its physicians; they have sworn to kill all the barbarians by means of drugs, and they call the Romans barbarians. Remember that I forbid physicians for you."

In spite of the statements of Pliny, then, that the Romans lived without physicians, or at least without Greek physicians, up to the time of Cicero, we have reason to believe that even before this period Greek physicians were practising in Rome. Cassius Emina states that in the year 219 Archagathus of the Peloponnesus, the son of Lysanias, established himself at Rome, where he acquired the rights of the city and of citizenship and had an office open to the public. His arrival was welcomed at first with joy; he was given the name *vulnerarius* and was regarded as a surgeon of value.

But soon, perhaps because of some mistake in treatment, he acquired a bad reputation and was given the name of *carnifex*.

There is also no doubt that at the same time as Archagathus, or shortly after, other Greek physicians appeared in Rome in spite of various prohibitions and of Cato's warnings. When a local man recognized cabbage as a universal and potent remedy and prescribed as a sure cure for dislocations the sacrifice of a swallow while reciting the (nonsense) words: *Huat hana huat ista pista sista domina damnaustra luxato*, he could not long count on the confidence of his followers. Especially would this be the case as the Romans had already been educated by the Greek masters to a freedom of criticism and a habit of scepticism and undoubtedly had recognized the superior knowledge of the Greek physicians on their first contact. When the Romans got to know the requirements of the Greek physicians for one wishing to enter their schools — including an oath taken before the masters — they could not but appreciate the difference between the Greek physicians and those to whom the care of the sick of Rome had hitherto been confided. It became evident, then, that only the Greeks could be regarded as physicians worthy of the name. Although the first disciples of Æsculapius who came to Rome were, like many pioneers arriving in a new country, far from ideal followers of the Hippocratic method and but little worthy of being regarded as his disciples, they nevertheless acquired the favour of the public.

The Greek physicians made no distinction between the practice of medicine and surgery. They performed phlebotomies and sold remedies, and in their infirmaries (*iatreia*, or *medicatrinæ*, as they were later called in Latin) they offered their services to all who asked. These physicians soon penetrated into the patrician houses and rapidly made their fortunes. Soon they were employed in the baths, the gymnasia, and the army. They became the physicians of gladiators and slaves; slaves themselves, they were often freed by their masters in recompense for their services. Recent historical studies seem to show that even toward the end of the Republic the physicians were almost all foreigners. Medicine continued to be regarded at Rome as a profession unworthy of a Roman citizen. The idea could not be accepted that a citizen in a toga could spend his time in a small shop prescribing ointments for gladiators, handing out love philtres for women of ill fame, or bleeding slaves — too frequent practices among the Greeks and without doubt the most profitable of all. But little by little things changed. Greek physicians coming to Rome were able to acquire the favour of the most eminent citizens, to be received in the houses of the consuls, to gain the protection of the Roman nobles, and to be treated on

a par with the most valiant soldiers and illustrious writers. Many of them
quickly acquired great wealth, and their elaborate way of life helped them
acquire high positions in Rome, where the primitive purity of customs had
already been corrupted by luxurious Greek habits and victorious wars.

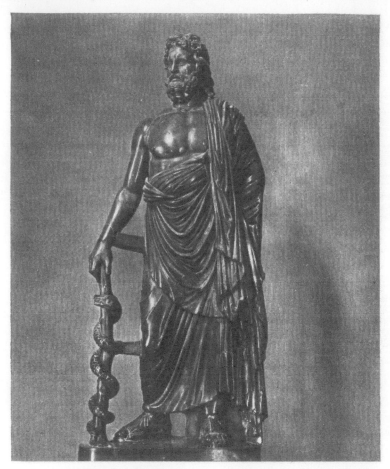

78. *An ancient statue of Æsculapius.*   (CAPITOLINE MUSEUM, ROME.)

Then one sees no longer the arrival of small country physicians hunting
fortunes, but the most illustrious physicians, attracted by the glory of the
great city which had become the capital of the civilized world. As it was
necessary to possess the title of Roman citizen in order to live and practise
one's profession with freedom in Rome and to occupy a worthy position,
they specially directed their efforts to this end. During the last period of
the Republic all the rights of citizens were granted to the physicians more

and more freely. Slaves, barbers, and phlebotomists who had assumed the title and role of physician continued to exercise their trade in secret and to make their living by all sorts of practices; but little by little the superiority of those who came from the Greek schools and had obvious medical knowledge became manifest. The situation of these physicians was defi-
nitely established in large part by a
man of great intelligence who came
from Bithynia to Rome about the beginning of the first century B.C.: As-
CLEPIADES of Prusa, who was called
the prince of physicians and was a
friend of Cicero, Crassus, and Mark
Antony. He was invited to the courts
of foreign kings and was sought after
by the richest and most powerful families of Rome.

Lucius Apuleius (*Florida*, Bk. IV,
Ch. 19) tells us how Asclepiades acquired
his great renown; it is worth repeating
despite its doubtful veracity because it
shows how attempts have been made in
all times to attribute marvellous cures to
the physicians who had the favour of the
public. One day while Asclepiades was
going to his villa, which generous honoraria had already permitted him to acquire in Rome, he met on the Via Sacra a
funeral procession composed of a great
number of persons who were weeping.
Tired from carrying the corpse, they
had set it down beside the road to rest.
The Greek physician drew near and in-

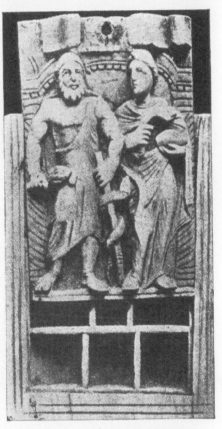

79. *Ivory medicine box showing
Æsculapius and Hygeia.*
(SION MUSEUM, SWITZERLAND.)

quired the cause of death, and as no one was able to give him sufficient information, he looked more closely at the corpse and thought that he saw traces of life.
He extinguished the fire which had already been lit and stopped the funeral
banquet for which the relatives and friends were assembling. His eloquence persuaded them to wait. He had the supposed corpse carried into a neighbouring
house, and after several minutes of manipulation they were astonished to see the
dead move and gradually come back to life. The news of this miraculous cure
spread through Rome with the rapidity of lightning. The Greek physician, who
was already known there for his great eloquence, his refinement of manner, and

his able methods of tending his patients, saw his success increase rapidly. A man of intelligence, who had studied rhetoric before he became a physician, he had a good understanding of Rome and the Romans and knew well how to exploit the situation for his profit.

The part that Asclepiades played in the history of medicine has been variously evaluated. We are told that he was born in Prusa in Bithynia about the year 124 B.C., and that he studied rhetoric, philosophy, and medicine in some of the best schools of his time. He was certainly a pupil in the medical school at Alexandria, whence he derived the most important of his doctrines. The judgment of his contemporaries and of posterity has undoubtedly been affected by Pliny, who regarded him as a charlatan who thought of nothing but accumulating the greatest possible number of patients and proclaiming his cures abroad. Recent studies, however, especially those of Neuburger and Wellmann, indicate that he played an important role in the evolution of the atomistic theory and in the intelligent interpretation of the doctrine of Hippocrates. While Neuburger regards Asclepiades as the first physician who opposed with the whole strength of his personality the doctrines taught under the banner of the Hippocratic school and the empiricism of the late Alexandrian school, Wellmann believes that he harks back to a much more ancient atomistic school of which Iginius the Eleatic was the master. None of his writings has come down to us complete; remnants are preserved for us in the quotations of Celsus, Galen, and other writers and in fragments that have been collected by G. Gumpert and published in Weimar in 1794.

His corpuscular theory, which is certainly closely connected with the atomistic theory of Epicurus, forms the basis of his pathological concepts. Asclepiades was a materialist who excluded metaphysical reasoning from his doctrines. He maintained that the combination of particles continuously moving one toward another was brought about by means of small canals or pores in which the atoms were constantly moving. These particles were divisible ad infinitum. It was from their movements and other subdivisions that all organisms were composed. The atoms which composed the soul were more perfect; heat and cold were due to the movements of the atoms.

Atoms in the atmospheric air penetrated into the body by means of respiration; and the air, together with the blood, was driven by the heart through the organism. *Anima*, according to Asclepiades, consisted in the movement of the psychic atoms, and this was constant and therefore constantly changing. Health was nothing but the normal movement of the atoms in the pores; disease came from any disturbance in this movement. Thus the pathological concept of Asclepiades is essentially mechanical and solidistic.

In the observation of the patient he shows an often surprising acuteness: he describes the malarial fevers accurately, clearly distinguishes between acute and chronic diseases, observes the rhythmic course of certain diseases but rejects the doctrine of the critical days. Denying the healing power of nature, he is in opposition to this part of Hippocratic doctrines, but utilizes a mechanico-physical, hygienic-dietetic therapy. Thus an important part of his treatment consists in fasting, dietetics, abstinence from meat, frequent walks, horseback riding, massage, hydrotherapy. He rarely prescribes drugs and avoids the use, which was then frequent, of drastic purges. It was Asclepiades who taught as a fundamental precept of the art of medicine that treatment should be given " *cito, tute et jucunde* (promptly, safely, and pleasantly)." Asclepiades was a close observer of mental disease, distinguishing between delusions and hallucinations. The latter, as they are promoted by darkness, he treated in daylight, instead of the darkness then in vogue. He is said to be the first to have mentioned tracheotomy. He is credited with at least one principle of the very highest importance: namely, that it is the method of investigation that is essential and determining.

Among his more notable pupils were THEMISON of Laodicea, CHRYSIPPUS, CLODIUS, and ANTONIUS MUSA, who was the personal physician of Augustus and cured the Emperor of a disorder of the liver by means of hydrotherapy.

The school of the METHODISTS followed that of Asclepiades and is thought by some to have been founded by THEMISON, celebrated physician to whom perhaps Juvenal alludes in one of his satires. Juvenal, who often joked about physicians and their cures, said that he could not count all the patients killed by Themison, and again " as many as Themison kills in one autumn." While accepting the atomistic pathology of Asclepiades, Themison's system tended to enclose medicine more and more in rigid doctrines. To him is owed the statement that diseases are divided into two fundamental forms: one a state of tension (*status strictus*) and the other a state of relaxation (*status laxus*). Both come from an abnormal state of the pores, too constricted in the former case, too dilated in the latter. Therapy, then, consists in restoring the pores to their normal condition, keeping in mind the acute or chronic state of the disease. He divided all remedies into those intended to combat tension or relaxation. This was a simple system adapted to the exigencies of practice, lent itself to facile explanations, and, as is always the case with simple concepts, acquired the favour of the common people. To these two states a *status mixtus* was later added, in which one or other of the conditions preponderated. Eventually surgical diseases were included in the same system. Though in therapy the Methodists did not neglect the importance of diets and of climate, their success was always explained by means of their theory.

4. Medicine during the Empire

The Methodists formed the most important school in Rome at the time of the greatest splendour of the Empire. Many of them were highly esteemed and cultivated by the Cæsars; among the most celebrated were PROCLUS, DIONYSIUS, ANTIPATER (author of a number of medical books), VETIUS VALENS (who was killed because he was accused of being the lover of Messalina), and JULIAN (author of a lengthy anti-Hippocratic work).

The most celebrated of the Methodist school was SORANUS of Ephesus, who was called the prince of the Methodists and who may be regarded as the founder of obstetrics and gynæcology. Soranus was a physician first in Alexandria and later in Rome, where he lived in the times of Trajan and Hadrian, about A.D. 100. His work on the diseases of women, dedicated especially to midwives and particularly valuable for the history of obstetrics, had a direct influence on this branch of medicine for many centuries.

Even though his anatomy of the female genital system may be obscure and inexact, it must be noted that Soranus knew the various changes in position of the uterus and the existence of the cotyledons, and that he maintained that the uterus opened during coitus and menstruation. On the other hand, he does not speak of the presence of the hymen, which fact, as Neuburger observes, throws an interesting light on the conditions of Roman life at this period.

Soranus advises blocking the orifice of the uterus with cotton, ointments, or fatty substances in order to avoid conception. He prohibits the performance of abortion by mechanical means. He indicates the signs of maturity in the fetus; he advises a double ligature of the umbilical cord before cutting it; is the first to prescribe bathing the eyes of the newborn with oil; lays down the rules for weaning the infant; states that nursing should not begin until the third day, and that for the first two days only boiled honey should be given. All the directions that he gives for nursing, weaning, diet, baths, care of the teeth, and of infantile diseases — especially diarrhœa — indicate that he was a good practitioner, a man of great experience, and a conscientious physician.

In a work of Soranus we find, perhaps for the first time, attempts at differential diagnosis. In these early indications for obstetrical intervention, we find measures for the protection of the perineum and emptying the bladder with a catheter before delivery. Retroversion is described accurately and embryotomy is advised only in urgent cases. Although his doctrines require Soranus to be regarded as a Methodist, he is nevertheless one of the most remarkable physicians of his time, whose teaching acquired a noteworthy importance through his study of anatomy, his exact observation of his cases, and his precise indications for dietetic and operative measures. Thanks to him, the medical knowledge of the Alexandrian school was clearly surpassed.

The writings of Soranus, among which the work quoted above is the most celebrated, were freely borrowed from by the writers of the fourth and fifth centuries and especially by AURELIANUS CÆLIUS, who probably lived much later. They were translated from the Greek into Latin by MOSCHUS (fifth or sixth century), who made a résumé in popular form.

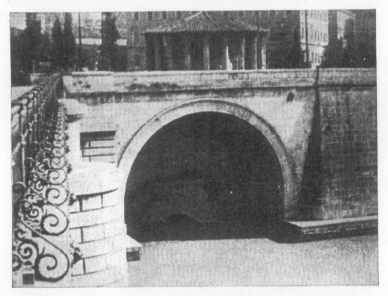

80. *Entrance to the Cloaca Maxima in Rome.*

In spite of the success of the Greek physicians in Rome, tradition forbade the Roman patricians to practise medicine, which was regarded as a profession worthy only for slaves, freedmen, or foreigners. Nevertheless, legislators and writers soon realized the importance of hygienic regulations. Vitruvius, in his book *On Architecture*, treats this subject at length, emphasizing the need for the sanitary location of dwellings and accurately describing the construction of aqueducts, to which he attributes great importance. He alludes to the diseases of workmen who handle lead, and he supposes that goitre, which was fairly frequent at this time in certain parts of Italy, was due to the water.

Marcus Terentius VARRO, one of the first encyclopædists (117–27 B.C.), who wrote at length on scientific and agricultural matters, outlined a series of hygienic regulations for the construction of houses, especially as to ventilation and the isolation of the sick. One of his works (Lib. I, Ch. xii,

Script. Rei Rust.) contains the masterly and prophetic statement: " Perhaps in swampy places small animals live that cannot be discerned with the eye and they enter the body through the mouth and nostrils and cause grave disorders. (*Advertendum etiam si qua erunt loca palustria, et propter easdem causas, et quod arescunt, crescunt animalia quædam minuta, quæ non possunt oculi consequi et per aër intus in corpus per os, ad nares perveniunt, atque efficiunt difficiles morbos.*) "

A contemporary of Varro was LUCRETIUS CARUS (95–55 B.C.), poet and philosopher, author of the most beautiful scientific work of classic Latinism, the *De rerum natura*, which discusses the mystery of life with the marvellous clarity of genius. In a period in which the most ferocious class and party struggles signalized the beginning of the political downfall of Rome, Lucretius sought beyond the confines of society for a satisfactory way of life. An Epicurean, he wanted to keep himself and others free from all superstition. The world, according to Lucretius, has no bounds. The atoms (the *primordia*) are invisible and insensible and they come in contact with one another in a constant movement, whether harmonious or discordant. Life and death follow each other in an eternal cycle in which there is neither beginning nor ending. Though Lucretius was not a physician, his famous work contains many advanced statements about anatomy and physiology, diet and hygiene and the effect of climate, while his sixth book gives the celebrated account of the Plague of Athens. All the most exalted and profound problems were the concern of the poet: the meaning of life, the contrast between the materialistic concept and free will, the mystery of the mechanism of the laws of matter, all the problems of the life of the body and of the spirit, of love and passion. The poetry of Lucretius is the highest and purest expression of the restless and tireless spirit of an investigator of the truth who can express his thought and teaching in noble verse.

5. Celsus and Pliny

The greatest of Latin medical writers was without doubt Aulus Cornelius CELSUS, who lived in Rome at the beginning of the Christian era, born of the patrician family of the Cornelii.

We shall not discuss whether or not Celsus was a physician, but shall regard as solved this problem which has occupied so many scholars; that is, we shall accept that Celsus belongs, like Varro and Pliny, to the group of encyclopædists who proposed to gather together everything that was known in their time about a given subject. Without being a practitioner, he was, however, a *philiatros*, a friend of physicians, a man of vast culture, learned in the natural sciences and in medicine, who rightly believed that he could express himself freely and with value on medical questions. Celsus is the first of the great encyclopædists of whom we have a basis for judgment in his works, because the works of Cato and Varro, who probably had the same fundamental concept, remain only in sparse fragments. The complete work of Celsus, called *De artibus*, included agriculture, the military art, rhetoric, philosophy, jurisprudence, as well as medicine. The book that treats of medicine is the sixth of the series, the first five being devoted to agriculture. It is thought that it was written in the reign of Tiberius, between A.D. 25 and 35. It is almost ignored by contemporary physicians, perhaps because nearly all of them as Greeks looked down on the work of a Roman. But also during the Middle Ages Celsus was but little known. It was Pope Nicholas V (1397–1455) who rediscovered Celsus' work on medicine. The *De re medica* of Celsus was the first book on general medicine to be printed; its *editio princeps* was published in Florence in 1478. There were many later editions, so that knowledge of it was widespread during the Renaissance.

A great merit of Celsus' work is that it constitutes the first attempt that we know of at an organic history of medicine. It is to Celsus that we owe a great part of our information on the medicine of the Hellenistic period and on Alexandrian surgery; it is in Celsus that we find the first translation of Greek medical terms into Latin; the Latin nomenclature created by him, or at least collected by him for the first time, has dominated medical science for two millennia.

Celsus is one of the great Latin classics. This is not the place to discuss whether he should be placed in the golden period of Latinity or whether, as some maintain, he belonged to the first decadent period of Roman letters. There is no doubt, however, that from the literary point of view his work is outstanding and that he deserves the title of the Cicero of medicine. Studies of Celsus were numerous, not only in the Renaissance, when his writings were most highly and widely cherished, but also in the past century, especially in Italy. The best edition, without doubt, is the Latin text with an Italian translation by Dr. Angelo del Lungo. A bilingual edition, in Latin and English, has recently been published by W. G. Spencer in the Loeb Classical Library (London: William Heinemann; Cambridge, Mass.: Harvard University Press; 1935–8). Worthy of mention are Daremberg's excellent edition (Leipzig, 1891) and the translation into German by E. Scheller (Braunschweig, 1906).

Celsus divides his work into three parts according to the various treatments used against disease: dietetic, pharmaceutical, and surgical. This division, which is also found in other writers of the period, has led certain historians to believe that the practice of medicine was sharply divided between physicians, surgeons, and pharmacologists, who were especially concerned with the use of drugs. This opinion is incorrect even though upheld by such authoritative writers as Sprengel. We know that in Rome, as in Alexandria, although certain physicians were particularly concerned with surgery, for the most part general medicine was practised. Celsus made this division in order to correspond to a practical necessity and to a Hippocratic tradition. Actually he did not belong to any of the schools then in vogue, and his book has the merit of impartiality. He noted the errors of both the Empiricists and the Methodists; for while the Empiricists on the one hand pretended to cure all diseases, as he states, by means of drugs, Asclepiades and his school, on the other hand, went to the other extreme, curing all diseases with diet and exercise.

In those diseases that can be helped by diet, Celsus' first category, after an introduction in which the efficacy of diet in general is discussed, he divides the subject into two main chapters: on general and on local diseases. For his second great category, diseases to be treated with drugs, after an introduction where he speaks at length about different remedies, he examines those diseases which need immediate treatment, diseases presenting acute or chronic manifestations, accidental or traumatic manifestations, diseases with external phenomena. Finally, in the last class of diseases, which we call surgical, Celsus made a new subdivision into the diseases of the bones and of the organs.

Celsus can be regarded as a Hippocratist in the sense that he is calm in his reasoning and accurate in his observations; occasionally he is far in advance of his times: ". . . *rationalem quidem puto medicinam esse debere; mortuorum corpora incidere discentibus necessarium* (I am of the opinion that the Art of Medicine ought to be rational . . . to open the bodies of the dead is necessary for learners)," (*De Medicina*, Proemium, Sect. 74). Thence come the usefulness of his book and the favour that it enjoyed even with celebrated physicians, who regarded it especially in Italy as the most important canon of medicine.

The anatomical indications in Celsus are certainly insufficient, partly perhaps because he did not believe it necessary to emphasize such matters in a book that was intended especially for the practitioner. The passage quoted above, however, shows that dissection was allowed in Rome at this time; without doubt he had occasion to attend autopsies. His anatomy of the head shows that he certainly knew the sutures of the cranium, which are exactly described;

he knew the semicircular canals of the ear, and seems to have understood the difference between arteries and veins, because he states that "the vein is in close proximity to the artery, and the nerve passes between the two." He observed also the important fact that the artery may spirt blood when cut ("*interdum etiam, ut sanguis vehementer erumpat, efficit*"); from which one must conclude that the error of the ancient Hippocratic concept that the arteries contained air was now appreciated (Bk. II, Ch. 10, Sect.15). Although some of the chapters are insufficient, one must conclude that Celsus recognizes the importance of anatomy in medicine. He insists particularly on this fact at the end of his introduction where he states that "medicine is connected to theories but should be based on visible causes: obscure causes should be excluded not only from medical thought but from its practice. I regard it as useless and cruel to open the living body, but it is necessary for those who study to see corpses, in order to learn to recognize the position and arrangement of the single parts, a thing that is seen much better in the cadaver than in the living body." His physiological knowledge comes entirely from the Alexandrian physicians.

Concerning pathological concepts and the etiology of disease, Celsus holds strictly to Hippocrates. In the preface of Book II he states: "I shall not hesitate to rely on the authority of the ancients and especially of Hippocrates." He takes into consideration the influence of the seasons, the weather, the patient's age and constitution. His symptomatology in its grand lines suggests the Hippocratic school. Fever, sweat, salivation, sensation of fatigue are regarded as precursors of grave diseases; importance also is attributed to a rapid and sudden increase of the weight of the body or of a sudden emaciation.

Special pathology is treated in the Hippocratic sense, but one also finds noteworthy observations that seem to come from other sources. Hemorrhage from the mouth is regarded as a symptom of laceration of the nose or œsophagus when it is not accompanied by fever, headache, or pain in the chest. A thick urine with a white sediment is regarded as a precursor of arthritic pain. Micturition, drop by drop, and hematuria with violent pains in the pubic region announce an affection of the bladder. Interesting also are the symptoms of kidney disease, in which, according to our author, there are noted: pains in the kidney region, polyuria, vomiting, and urine which is pale and watery, but may be foamy or bloody or contain gravel. The presence of foamy blood in the sputum indicates a disease of the lungs; Celsus maintains that the prognosis is favourable if the expectoration is whitish and of a consistency like mucus from the nose; but unfavourable if the sputum is purulent, accompanied by continued fever, and if the patient complains of thirst and continued loss of appetite. The end is near when frequent diarrhœas supervene.

Celsus' description of malaria is justly praised by Marchiafava and Bignami in their study of the æstivo-autumnal malarial fevers (Sydenham Society Publications, Vol. CL, 1894, p. 231): "Of fevers, one is quotidian, another tertian, a third quartan. At times certain fevers recur in even longer cycles, but that is seldom. . . . Now quartan fevers have the simpler characteristics. Nearly always they begin with shivering, then heat breaks out, and the fever having ended, there are two days free; thus on the fourth day it recurs. But of tertian fevers there are two classes. The one, beginning and desisting in the same way as a quartan, has merely this distinction, that it affords one day free, and recurs on the third day. The other is far more pernicious; and it does indeed recur on the third day, yet out of forty-eight hours, about thirty-six, sometimes less, sometimes more, are in fact occupied by the paroxysm, nor does the fever entirely cease in the remission, but it only becomes less violent. . . . Quotidian fevers are, however, variable and multiplex. For some begin straightaway with a feeling of heat, others of chill, others with shivering. . . . Again, some desist so that complete freedom follows, others so that there is some diminution of the fever, yet none the less some remnants persist until the onset of the next paroxysm; and others often run together so that there is little or no remission, but the attacks are continuous. Again, some have a vehement hot stage, others a bearable one; some are every day equal, others unequal, and the paroxysm in turn slighter one day, more severe another: some recur at the same time the day following, some either earlier or later; some take up a day and a night with the paroxysm and the remission, some less, others more; some set up sweating as they remit, others do not; and in some, freedom is arrived at through sweating, in others the body is only made the weaker " (Bk. III, Sect. 3; translation of W. G. Spencer, Loeb Classical Library, I, 227).

As well as the fevers, which are the diseases to which is attributed the greatest importance, Celsus regards insanity as a general disease, which may be manifested in the form of phrenitis accompanied by delirium. Another form of insanity is paranoia, which attacks the intellectual as well as the emotional part of the brain. Long and accurate descriptions are devoted to *lethargus*, a disease which is manifested by an invincible sleep and which rapidly goes on to death. Tabes (in Latin, a wasting away), a term·used to indicate tuberculosis as well as other forms of cachexia, is carefully described. Noteworthy is the advice to be careful of phthisis from the beginning, without which care therapy cannot be successful. Especially to be recommended are climatotherapy, sea voyages, a long sojourn in Egypt, moderate exercise, diet, with especial emphasis on milk, light massage, and warm baths. Turpentine and honey are regarded as a sovereign remedy for pulmonary phthisis (III, 22). Among the general diseases epilepsy is also mentioned. For this disease a strict diet, with abstinence from alcohol, and local revulsive cures (cauterization, inunction with counter-irritants, and so on) are advised.

Celsus pays particular attention to headaches, which he regards as having the most varied origins; for them he prescribes diet, bleeding, mustard plasters, and massage. For angina of the throat he advises bleeding and incision in case of abscess; for asthma and dyspnea, bleeding, purgatives, hot, wet compresses, emetics, diuretics, and so forth. For the treatment of pneumonia, which he describes accurately, he recommends bleeding, a light diet, frequently changed compresses, and frequent changes of air of the room (IV, 7). In acute diseases of the liver, manifested by vomiting and hiccups, treatment consists in giving laxatives, and incision in the case of abscess (IV, 8). The treatment of kidney diseases is extremely interesting. Frequent diuretics and hot baths are prescribed and strict prohibition of salty and stimulating foods (IV, 10).

Diseases of the stomach are considered at length. Treatment generally consists in a carefully arranged diet, massage, baths, suppositories. In the case of acute diarrhœa, an absolute fast is prescribed for several days, then astringent food and drugs.

The dietary and hygienic prescriptions which formed the basis of the therapeutics of Celsus are especially to be noted; here one should regard him as a faithful follower of Hippocrates. He recommends moderate exercise, frequent voyages, a sojourn in the country, moderation in coitus and drinking, abstention from violent exercise. All sudden changes in diet or in the method of living, or rapid change from one climate to another, are to be avoided. One finds exact prescriptions for reducing weight (a single meal a day, frequent purgation, less sleep, baths of salt water, gymnastics, and massage). These prescriptions are followed by detailed indications for the regime to be followed in certain diseases and especially in gout and rheumatism. Dietary therapy plays a considerable role; one half of the second book is devoted to this subject and one finds there a lengthy selection of the most nutritious and most desirable foods. Those that provoke stomach trouble are distinguished, also those that have a diuretic effect, narcotics, laxatives, astringents, stimulants, and so on. Hydrotherapy is treated at length and such great importance is attributed to it that one must accept the estimate of Marcuse, who regarded Celsus as the first to fix in an adequate way the proper indications for its use.

The pharmacology of Celsus divided all the remedies known to him into various groups according to their effects: purgatives, diaphoretics, diuretics, emetics, narcotics, and so on. Among the narcotics we find pills of opium, and, when a still more energetic action was required, the seeds of jusquiamus and the root of mandragora. It should be noted that the active principles of hyoscyamine and scopolamine are to be found in mandragora. As Kobert has stated, Celsus prescribed for painful affections of the eye the inunction of a substance containing mandragora, evidently in order to enlarge the pupil. Galen also knew of this effect, but it was then forgotten for two millennia.

In the diseases of the genital organs, he gives a clear description of phimosis (for which he prescribes a surgical operation), also of ulcers, both simple and purulent, on the glans or prepuce. The surgery of Celsus shows a notable advance from the time of Hippocrates. Devoting the seventh and eighth books to this subject, he also mentions various surgical conditions in the previous books. The treatment of fractures is accurately described. After reduction, immobilization is secured with bandages of various lengths and with the application of splints and a mixture of wax and starch to make the bandage rigid. This was to be renewed, when the swelling of the limb was diminished, on the seventh or not later than the ninth day. For open fractures he advised the resection of the protruding fragment. After the union of the broken bones, he recommended the prescription of frequent exercises, so that the patient should reaccustom himself to the normal use of the limb. In fractures of the humerus, elbow, and forearm, the methods of applying the bandages are carefully given.

Celsus concerned himself in detail with the treatment of wounds and their

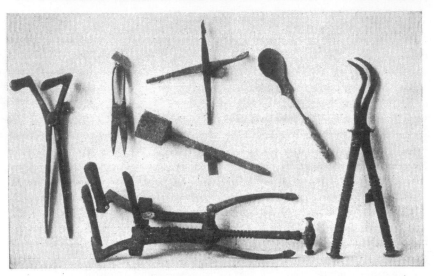

81. *Pompeian surgical instruments.*   (NAPLES MUSEUM.)

secretions, and indicated the methods of treating hemorrhage and the phenomena of inflammation. [His four cardinal signs: *Calor, Dolor, Rubor, Tumor* (Bk. III, Ch. 10) (to which Galen later added *Functio Læsa*) are still learned by every medical student. *Ed.*] He was acquainted with the complications that might follow wounds, and described erysipelatous and gangrenous forms. He paid particular attention to bites of animals.

Hemorrhage was to be stopped by means of linen soaked in cold water. When this did not suffice, vinegar was applied, after which the vessels were ligated. At that time a ligature included not only the vessels but also the surrounding tissue.

For head wounds, trephining is described accurately. For ascites, paracentesis is recommended with the introduction of a lead cannula with turned-back edges. For abdominal injuries, the procedure is exactly prescribed: suture of the intestine, when it is the large intestine that is damaged; but there is no hope of cure, according to Celsus, when the small intestine is damaged. The injured person should be placed on his back, the pelvis elevated, the wound enlarged, and the viscera carefully put back in place; those parts of the omentum that appear livid should be cut away with scissors; then the wound is sewed up, taking care to bring the margins of the peritoneum in contact, as well as those of the skin.

Celsus knew ulcers, fissures, atresia of the vulva, fleshy excrescences, abscesses, fistulas, and so on.

For cancer of the breast excision was recommended, but only when it was diagnosed early. For the advanced forms, Celsus maintained that surgical intervention only aggravated the situation. The chapter on the eye constitutes a summary of early knowledge in this field. Mention is made of the operations for pterygium, exophthalmus, and cataract.

Plastic surgery occupies an important place in Celsus' text, especially that of the nose and other parts of the head. He outlines the procedure for repair by using the skin of neighbouring parts. The indications that we find in Celsus about the bladder show that this branch of surgery had made considerable progress. There are exact indications for crushing stones (lithotripsy) with a description of the instruments used.

One can find in Celsus good descriptions of all the surgical instruments of the period. Of more than one hundred described, we may mention scalpels of different forms (*scalpri*), cups (*cucurbitæ*), sounds (*specilli*), hooks (*unci*), forceps (*forceps*), and a special tenaculum for the extraction of the roots of teeth (*rhissagra*), an instrument for removing the bone fragments after trephining, an iron in the form of the letter V to separate the sides of the wounds in the extraction of arrowheads, a catheter of lead, a lithotome, amputation saws, various trephines, a *meningophylax* (to hold back the meninges when the border of the trephine opening is being manipulated), also spatulas, compresses, special bandages for hernias, whalebone, leather straps, and so forth. The instruments excavated at Pompeii, now to be found in the museum of Naples, correspond exactly to those described in the surgery of Celsus.

We cite a passage from the first book of Celsus which shows how closely he had studied the history of medicine up to his time: " Those who take the name of Empirics from their experience, do indeed accept evident causes as necessary; but they contend that inquiry about obscure causes and natural actions is superfluous, because nature is not to be comprehended. That nature cannot be comprehended is in fact patent, they say, from the disagreement among those who discuss such matters; for on this question there is no agreement, either among teachers of philosophy or among actual medical practitioners. Why, then, should anyone believe rather in Hippocrates than in Herophilus, why in him rather than in Asclepiades? If one wants to be guided by reasoning, they go on, the reasoning of all of them can appear not improbable; if by method of treatment, all of them have restored sick folk to health: therefore one ought not to derogate from anyone's credit, either in argument or in authority. Even philosophers would have become the greatest of medical practitioners, if reasoning from theory could have made them so; as it is, they have words in plenty, and no knowledge of healing at all. They also say that the methods of practice differ according to the nature of localities, and that one method is required in Rome, another in Egypt, another in Gaul; but that if the causes which produce diseases were everywhere the same, the same remedies should be used everywhere; that often, too, the causes are apparent, as, for example, of ophthalmia, or of wounds, yet such causes do not disclose the treatment: that if the evident cause does not supply the knowledge, much less can a cause which is in doubt yield it. Since, therefore, the cause is as uncertain as it is incomprehensible, protection is to be sought rather from the ascertained and explored, as in all the rest of the Arts, that is, from what experience has taught in the actual course of treatment: for even a farmer, or a pilot, is made not by disputation but by practice. That such speculations are not pertinent to the Art of Medicine may be learned from the fact that men may hold different opinions on these matters, yet conduct their patients to recovery all the same. This has happened, not because they deduced lines of healing from obscure causes, nor from the natural actions, concerning which different opinions were held, but from experiences of what had previously succeeded" (Proemium 27–32, translation of W. G. Spencer, Loeb Classical Library).

To Celsus we owe valuable information about the Alexandrian school. We find in his writings a veneration for the great men of the past. In the introduction to his work we have an essay on the history of medicine. There he exposes with lucid judgment the part played by Hippocrates in the development of medicine, the system initiated by Asclepiades, the doctrine of the Methodists; and he clearly traces the evolution of medical art up to his own period. This picture is further illuminated by many quotations from the writings of contemporaries and of more ancient writers. About eighty physicians are mentioned in his book, belonging to different periods and to different schools. We know the names of some of them only through his book.

Celsus was surely the most powerful and intelligent mind in the medical history of classical Italy. His great intellect knew how to include all the desirable features of the enormous treasure of philosophic speculations and practical experiences that had accumulated in Greece, Egypt, and Rome. He was familiar with all the medical literature that existed before him. He was a calm critic and profound observer who took his stand outside of the schools and sects, making an admirable résumé of everything that seemed to him worth being saved in the accumulation of the current ideas of the time.

A worthy disciple of Hippocrates in the field of medical ethics, as well as in medical history, he recognized and loudly proclaimed that the physician should admit his errors, believing that " the simple avowal of an error committed is proper for a man of great intelligence " because thus he may be useful to those who follow and prevent others from being mistaken as he was mistaken.

Thus the honour in which Celsus was held, particularly in Italy during the Renaissance, does not seem unjustified. Perhaps at that period, when the renascent art and literature of the Latins was rekindling Italian racial pride, Italians realized that Celsus was the incarnation of the best Roman tradition in his nobility of style, elegance of form, clarity of exposition, and the practical nature of his recommendations. He might then be properly regarded as the leader of the new efflorescence of medical literature in the Occident.

Besides Celsus we must name another encyclopædist, as his work was a favourite medical text during centuries — we refer to the natural history of CAIUS PLINIUS SECUNDUS (A.D. 23–79), the greatest of the Latin naturalists.

The elder Pliny had a long military service in Germany, was Proconsul in Spain, then lived in Rome, and also at Misenum, where he commanded the Roman army. It is known that he died during the eruption of Vesuvius that destroyed Pompeii and Herculaneum, because he wished to observe the eruption more closely. The only one of his works that has come down to us is the *Historia naturalis* or *Historia mundi*, divided into thirty-seven books, which include many facts taken from many authors, some of whose writings have been lost to us. To many uncritical and worthless statements the author joins valuable personal observations, and although he declares himself openly hostile to scientific medicine and research, there are many important statements in his book that give us a good idea of the medical knowledge and the state of medicine of his time. The first edition of this work was printed in Venice in 1469 by Giovanni di Spira; throughout the Middle Ages he was one of the authors most frequently consulted and quoted by physicians. The work has been preserved in many manuscripts and passed through more than eighty editions. A quaint English translation is that of Philemon Holland (London, 1601).

In medicine, Pliny was certainly less versed than Celsus, but his knowledge of natural history, his wide culture, and his love of study made him one of the most interesting of the Golden Age of Latin writers. One of the greatest merits of his work consists in the citation of his sources, a habit unknown before him, greatly contributing to the value of his picture of the medicine of his time. Books XX to XXVII deal with drugs of vegetable origin; Books XXVIII to XXXII with those taken from animals and minerals; magic therapy is often mentioned and sometimes recommended. Observations on comparative physiology and pathology are scattered through the earlier books on zoology. Together with such false statements as that the speedy giraffe has no spleen, we find original references to atavism, an infant born with teeth, superfetation, change of sex, scurvy, narcotics, and possibly even to an eyeglass: " *Nero princeps gladiatorum pugnas spectabat smaragdo* (Nero, the prince, watched the contests of the gladiators with an emerald) " (*Bk.* XXXVII, Ch. 5). The word " *smaragdus* " was also used for some semi-precious stones; it is not clear if Pliny meant spectacles, a magnifying glass, or some other instrument. Without doubt he often appears naïve in his judgments and far too credulous; but one must not forget the period in which he lived and the absence of a valid critique for separating the true from the false in those times when superstition was rife in medicine and the author himself was a member of the collegium of the augurs. His work — as he states in the dedication to the Emperor Vespasian — is directed to the humble, the foreigners, the labourers. It should be regarded in the language of today as a popular encyclopædia.

A zealous compiler, an indefatigable reader, Pliny has left us a noteworthy monument of the culture of his time; an inexhaustible mine for those who wish to be informed about the traditions and practices of popular medicine and the forms of treatment current in Rome at that time. To give an idea of the profit that can be derived from the reading of ancient texts, we cite an example given by Neuburger. It was the reading of a passage in Pliny about the use of the juice of *anagallis* before the operation for cataract (Bk. XXV, Ch. 13, 92) that in 1800 gave the idea to Himly to investigate the action of jusquiamus and belladonna on the pupil.

6. The Pneumatic and Eclectic Schools. Rufus, Aretæus, Dioscorides

The school of the Pneumatists, whose doctrine is founded on the principle that the *pneuma* is the basis of health, flourished in Rome about the first half of the first century of our era, especially in the work of ATHENÆUS of Attalia. According to the Pneumatists, perfect health consisted in the perfect condition of the pneuma and of the *tonus* that it maintained, as recognizable by the pulse. Disease consisted in an abnormal state of the pneuma, and this in turn is caused by a dyscrasia of the elements. This concept was taken by the Pneumatic school from the humoral doctrine of Hippocrates. In the diagnosis and therapeutics of the Pneumatic school this concept predominated, hence the great importance of the doctrine of the pulse and of dietetic and physical therapy.

To this school belonged some of the most celebrated physicians of the period, such as AGATINUS of Sparta, APOLLONIUS of Pergamon, and the surgeon HELIODORUS, who lived in the time of Trajan. Opposed to them was the Eclectic school, which proposed as its program to free itself from the existing sects and select the best of each.

To RUFUS of Ephesus (A.D. 98–117) is owed an anatomical treatise and several important contributions on the pulse. He was the first to describe the human liver as having five lobes, the condition that exists in the pig, an error which was perpetuated until the time of Vesalius. In Rufus we find first descriptions of bubonic plague and traumatic erysipelas. His dietetics, in five books, was much studied and quoted, especially by the Arabian writers. He knew how to control hemorrhage by compression, styptics, cautery, torsion, and the ligature.

To the period of the Pneumatic and Eclectic schools belonged also ARETÆUS of Cappadocia, who is thought by some to have lived in Alexandria about the second half of the first century after Christ; by others in the time of Trajan (second century). Two of his works are noteworthy: *On the Causes and Signs of Acute and Chronic Diseases* and *On the Treatment of Acute and Chronic Diseases*, each in four volumes in the Ionic dialect. Aretæus is revealed as a Hippocratic physician in the true sense of the word, and among the Greek authors after Hippocrates, as Neuburger justly observes, he is the one who best exhibited the spirit of pure Hippocratism. With him there was a return to the observation of the patient, to bedside study, and the desire to be useful. He had a clear vision of the duty of the physician — the profession of medicine regarded as the pure and noble performance of an exalted purpose.

The first Greek edition of Aretæus was published in Paris in 1554; the first Latin edition in Venice in 1552. The French translation by Renaud appeared in Paris in 1834; the Italian by Puccinotti in Florence in 1838, and the Greek text with English translation by Francis Adams (London: Sydenham Society; 1856).

The descriptions of diseases, especially that of pleurisy, can be regarded as models. The cerebral paralyses are closely studied: one finds the observation that in a cerebral lesion the paralysis is crossed, which is not the case in a spinal lesion. Examination of the heart is the subject of a long and minute dissertation. The therapy of Aretæus is not very different from that of his contemporaries and consists almost entirely in dietetics and physiotherapy.

PEDANIUS DIOSCORIDES, born in Anazarbos near Tarsis in Cilicia, lived in the first century after Christ and was a contemporary of the elder Pliny. He assembled all the pharmacological ideas of his time in a work that was regarded for centuries as the leading text on the subject. In its five books one finds accounts of all the medicines taken from the animal, vegetable, and mineral kingdoms. In many of his descriptions Dioscorides is in almost literal agreement with Pliny, a fact which is to be explained by the supposition that they both borrowed from the same older sources, such as

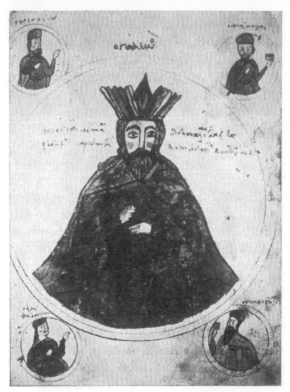

82. *Galen.*
(*From a miniature in Codex 3632, f. 26 r. XIV century*, VATICAN LIBRARY.)

the books of Theophrastus, Crateuas (physician of Mithridates VI), and others.

The descriptions of drugs are exact and frequently reveal a remarkable gift of observation; we often find in Dioscorides for the first time remedies that have not been mentioned in earlier authors, and particularly those of mineral origin, such as lead acetate, calcium hydrate, copper oxide, and other copper salts.

Dioscorides wrote in Greek; his style is weak and he himself warns the reader to pay attention rather to the substance than to the elegance of the style. His most important book is that on materia medica, *De universa medicina*, dedicated to Areios. It contains a list of the most important remedies with a description of their preparation. It is divided into five books, to which a sixth is added, *De venenis*, which contains a description of poisons and antidotes. In the Aldine editions this is followed by the two treatises *De venenatis animalibus*. The most important codex of the works of Dioscorides is the ninth-century manuscript in the French *Bibliothèque Nationale*. The first Greek edition was printed by Aldus in 1499, the first Latin translation by Collé in 1478; and the first Italian translation by Fausto di Longiano in 1542. The best translation is that of Mattioli, published in Venice in 1544 with a lengthy commentary; the best edition of this translation was published in Venice in 1568 by Valgrisi with magnificent illustrations. The modern authoritative Greek text was published by Max Wellmann in three volumes (1906–14). A seventeenth-century English translation, edited by R. T. Gunther, was published by the Oxford University Press in 1934.

7. Galen

In this period, in which study in the various fields of medicine, and especially pharmacy, was becoming more intensive, and the teachings of the Greek physicians were being carefully collected, there was, however, no fundamental progress in scientific concepts, which seemed to have been definitely arrested and rigidly encysted in the writings of the ancients.

The teaching of Hippocrates was shared by various schools, but in crystallized form. Hypotheses were maintained that had scanty support from uncertain anatomical knowledge. Dissections of animals were almost the sole source of anatomic study. It was rare that physicians made observations on the cadaver. Physiology was still in its infancy, and the explanations that were given of body functions were derived from the results of the vivisection of animals, which were then applied *in toto* to man. Therapeutics in the second century of our era was not much more advanced than at the time of Hippocrates. Although in certain operations a remarkable degree of technical perfection had been attained, surgery continued to be an art almost by itself, founded more on manual dexterity than on a pathological knowledge that was still vague and insecure.

The same uncertainties in the schools, the frequent discussions between disciples of different masters, the long theoretical controversies on which medical thought spent its energy, all these show how vague and uncertain medicine still was. A definitive pathological structure, of which the vision of Hippocrates had traced outlines, had not yet been attained.

The axiom of Hippocrates about the healing force of nature had given rise to the often chaotic therapy of the Herophilists, whose controversy with the Erasistratists seems characteristic of the history of medicine. It had already appeared in the two ancient schools of Cnidus and Cos, and will be found later as a controversy born from the opposition of the clinical to the localistic concept of disease. The discussions by Solidists, Atomists, Methodists, and Eclectics prevented the construction of any system which, while relying on the direct clinical observations of Hippocrates, could give true value and a proper proportion to the anatomical and experimental concept.

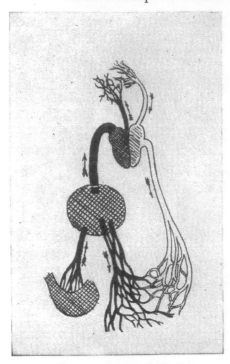

83. *The movement of the blood according to Galen.*

This is the task that was reserved for CLAUDIUS GALEN (A.D. 138–201), born at Pergamon in Asia Minor, where there was a famous temple of Æsculapius. We have exact information about his life in the accounts that he included in his writings. We know that when he was still young he studied first philosophy and then medicine, that he had as teachers of anatomy Satyrus and the Hippocratist, Stratonicus, that he devoted himself to practice and examined his patients with the greatest care, that he left his fatherland to acquire further knowledge, that he was the pupil of Pelops at Smyrna, that he studied anatomy at Alexandria, and that he was an indefatigable student of the rules of the art of medicine in the works of Hippocrates. After about ten years, when he was barely twenty-eight years old, he returned to Pergamon and his reputation was already assured.

He was appointed physician to the gladiators, a much sought-after position; but after several years, driven by the desire to live in a large city, he came to Rome, where in a short time he acquired an extraordinary reputation. He had as his friends the most illustrious men of his time, and, thanks to his constant, zealous labour as a practitioner, writer, and student, he attained a position such as no other physician had had before him.

His clientele in Rome grew constantly. The lectures that he gave in the public theatre, performing experiments on animals before a large audience, gave him a fame that soon passed beyond the boundaries of Rome. His fertility in writing secured for him an honourable place among the most prominent writers. But at the same time his success provoked such opposition among the Roman physicians that life in Rome soon became very difficult. In the clinical histories that he collected, he often magnified in exaggerated terms his diagnostic and therapeutic successes, and he complacently gave a miraculous appearance to his cures. In them one finds many polemical passages against his colleagues, while at the same time he dilates on the great rewards and immense popularity that he enjoyed.

One can easily imagine, then, how strenuously he would be opposed by other physicians who, at least according to his statement, so hated each other that they often resorted to poison. In 166, the year of the plague of Antoninus, he left Rome shortly before the epidemic made its appearance, to return to Pergamon. It has been supposed that the cause of his departure was his fear of the epidemic. The fact is that Marcus Lucius Verus and the Emperor Aurelius Antoninus soon recalled him from Aquileia, where he had spent the winter of 168. He returned to the Roman court and devoted himself assiduously to his writings. One should remember that through many long years he never stopped writing or dictating his works, which amounted to about four hundred, including some that were lost when the Temple of Peace was destroyed by fire. Remaining to us are eighty-three books that can certainly be attributed to him, nineteen doubtful ones, and fifteen commentaries on the Hippocratic text. Other writings of Galen have only recently been brought to light, having been found in Arabic translations. Of these works, published in the complete edition of Kühn, the most important are those On the Ideal Physician, On the Ideal Philosophy, On the Elements according to Hippocrates, On Anatomical Preparations or Encheirasis (this, the principal anatomical work of Galen, remained an authority for centuries), On Dissections of the Veins and Arteries, On the Movement of Muscles, On the Teachings of Hippocrates and Plato, On the Diseases' Places (his most important work on pathology), On the Use of the Parts of the Human body (seventeen books that contain all the physiological doctrines of Galen), On the Medical Art (this book, which is a summary, is generally indicated by the names of Microtechne, in Greek, Ars Parva, or Tegni in Latin, or Articella in the literature of the Middle Ages and later), On the Method of Treatment (the Megatechne or Ars Magna, in fourteen books). Besides these there are many other texts of dubious paternity, many writings falsely ascribed to Galen, and some fragments.

The first Latin translation of the complete works is that by Diomedes Bonardo, a physician of Brescia, published in Venice in 1490 by Filippo Pinzio da Caneto. The first edition in the original Greek is that of Aldus published in Venice in 1525 in five volumes, followed by the Basel edition of 1538, and the Latin translation of the Giunta Press of Venice in 1541. Many other editions followed; it can be safely said that up to the end of the eighteenth century Galen was the medical author who was most frequently consulted and the only one to be placed on a level with Hippocrates. The excellent French translation by Daremberg (two volumes, Paris, 1854–6) includes the anatomical and physiological writings and many valuable comments. A new complete edition of all the writings of Galen is in course of publication in the *Corpus Medicorum Græcorum* at Leipzig.

The writings of Galen mark a culminating point in the ancient history of medicine. On the one hand his work assembles the investigations of a gifted physician, who, relying on Hippocrates, utilizes his great experience and practical observations. On the other hand, he represents the speculations of a dogmatist, equipped with the highest opinion of his own value, sure of his scientific knowledge or rather of his infallibility, and constructing an extensive edifice of dogma on the basis of an Aristotelian philosophy.

Obviously, all this superstructure could not avoid damaging the useful and healthy part of his work. Each experimental observation had to be submitted to philosophic or rather teleologic proof. In his system everything has its purpose. Nature acts with perfect wisdom and does nothing uselessly. The organs therefore are made in a way that perfectly corresponds to their function, and every part of the organism corresponds to a pre-established purpose. There is therefore a perfect relation between the cause and the aim, and it is precisely this perfect relation that proves the omniscience of God. Galen, who proclaims himself a monotheist, obviously was influenced by Judaism, which at that time had numerous sympathizers in Rome, even in the higher social classes. Adapting all his experimental medicine to his teleologic dogmatism, he submitted to a vain philosophic speculation the valuable discoveries that he was the first to bring to medicine through his accurate anatomical and physiological researches. This course was apparently adopted by him in order to satisfy a vanity which his real successes, but poorly understood by the crowd, were not sufficient to appease.

Galen knows everything, has an answer for everything; he confidently pictures the origin of all diseases and outlines their cure. He is the incarnation, perhaps for the first time in history, of the physician who regards himself as omniscient and whose attitude of authority emanates from every act and every word.

The observations that he made on the anatomy of animals, in which field he was certainly better versed than any previous individual, were transferred by him without the least hesitation to human anatomy. His hypotheses in the field of physiology appeared justified whenever they coincided with the premises of Aristotelian philosophy. The *pneuma*, which is the essence of life, is of three kinds: the *pneuma psychicon* (animal spirit), which has its seat in the brain, the centre of sensation and movement; the *pneuma zoticon* (vital spirit), which mixes with the blood in the heart, the centre of the circulation and of the heat regulation of the body; and the *pneuma physicon* (the natural spirit), which comes to the blood from the liver, the centre of nutrition and metabolism. For Galen the body is but the instrument of the soul. One can easily see therefore the reason why his system, which corresponds in its essential features to Christian dogmatism, quickly received the support of the Church. His authority thus received important support. This explains how his system remained unchanged and impregnable up to the time of the Renaissance; how his anatomical observations were regarded as an absolute canon against which it was not even permissible to risk criticism or attempt an experiment; and how those who dared question the truth of his statements were treated as heretics. Galen assumed in medicine the same title of lord and master as Aristotle held in philosophy. At the same time his monotheistic system caused him to be cherished by the Arabic and Hebrew physicians; and his position remained unassailable for centuries.

His concept of the movement of the blood, which assumed communication between the two ventricles by invisible pores, remained supreme in anatomy even after the time of Vesalius.

This man, to whose authority we owe a perpetuation of fundamental errors which produced a long arrest in medical evolution, was nevertheless a student and experimenter of the highest quality, especially in anatomy and physiology. He was probably the first to produce cerebral lesions in animals, to establish a distinction between lesions of the cerebral lobes and those of the brain stem and cerebellum. He recognized seven of the twelve pairs of cerebral nerves and distinguished between motor and sensory nerves; in fact, he knew most of the gross structures of the brain as we know them today.

This is the kind of work which constituted his chief merit and made him worthy of the veneration in which he was held for centuries, and of the esteem of the impartial historian. Greater still were his achievements in experimental physiology, of which he undoubtedly is entitled to be called the founder. He might also be called the first exponent of the myogenic theory of the heart-beat, which he demonstrated in the excised heart — that is, separated from all nerve connections. He knew that arteries contained blood and was the first to show experimentally pulsations of the artery by introducing a feather into its lumen and observing the disappearance of the pulsation when it was ligated above the point of observation. The movement of the blood he errone-ously regarded as an ebb and flow, the arterial blood conveying vital spirits from the heart; the venous blood, natural spirits from the liver. The animal spirits moved in a similar way from the brain through hollow nerves, which became solid after death. He showed that when the fifth cervical nerve was cut, there followed a paralysis of the subscapular muscle, the dentatus magnus, the scalenus, and the pectoralis major. When the intercostal nerves were cut or the recurrent laryngeal ligated, the voice disappeared (*De administrationibus anatomicis*, I, vii). A lesion of the cerebral hemispheres damaged neither the sensory nor the motor faculties as long as the ventricles were not touched (*De Hippocratis et Platonis decretis*, I, vi). When the communication be-tween the nervous centre and the heart is broken by cutting the cervical nerves, the action of the heart is seen to stop, an observation that shows the error in the ancient concept that the nerves came from the heart, when in reality they come from the brain (*De Hippocratis et Platonis decretis*, I, vi, 6). He was also the first to ligate both ureters, together or one at a time, in order to demon-strate their function (*De facultatibus naturalibus*, I, iii).

We are indebted to him for the recognition of an important principle: every alteration of function corresponds to a lesion in an organ, and con-versely every lesion of an organ results in change of a function. He was the first to compose pathognomonic pictures of various diseases founded precisely on this principle.

He distinguished two fundamental kinds of disease: those that are simple or elementary, like the inflammations and the dyscrasias considered in relation to the tissues involved; and the organic diseases — that is to say, those classified according to the different organs' diseases and susceptible to changes of position, intensity, and duration. His authoritative support of the theory of coction in inflammation perpetuated almost to our day the appalling fallacy that suppuration was essential to healing and that the right kind of pus was therefore laudable. The causes of disease were: exciting (procatarctic), predisposing (proegumenic), or coincident (synectic). Given diseases gave certain signs and symptoms which were thus useful in both diagnosis and prognosis. Fevers were either ephemeral (in the spirits), putrid (in the humours), or hectic (in the solids). Continued fevers were in the blood; tertians in the yellow bile, quartans in the black bile and quotidian in the phlegm. Inflammations (e.g., phlegmons, erysipelas, cancer, œdema) were similarly distributed. He recognized that the patient's illness might be profoundly influenced by his disposition or constitution (diathesis) as well as by the disease itself (pathos).

Among the diagnostic observations of Galen, some are particularly interesting and strikingly acute. Thus he notes that when air escapes from a wound of the thorax, it indicates that the weapon has penetrated into the lungs. He distinguishes accurately between ulcerations of the bladder and the kidney by the appearance of the urine. Purulent affections of the bones are differentiated from simple lesions by the constitution of the pus. He differentiates traumatic from fusiform aneurysms (*Methodus Medendi*, Bk. V, f. 74b, Linacre, 1526 ed.) and recognizes the infectiousness of consumption.

Among all the works of Galen his anatomical, dietetic, and therapeutic writings are those that have been the most frequently read and studied. Throughout the Middle Ages, and even up to the seventeenth century, résumés of his important works, especially the *Microtechne*, were used as textbooks in the schools, particularly those dealing with the crises of diseases and the examination of the pulse.

An interesting work of Galen is that which treats of " pathomimes " – i.e., malingerers – from which we give a short extract: " People for many reasons may pretend to be ill; it is desirable, then, that the physician should be able to arrive at the truth in such cases. The ignorant imagine that it is impossible for him to distinguish between those who pretend and those who speak the truth." " The phlegmonous and cutaneous affections due to erysipelas or similar diseases, and the œdemas produced by the application of irritants, can be distinguished from each other by the diseased state of the rest of the body. One can distinguish also the bloody sputum that arises in the mouth from that coming from the respiratory organs. People can be found who cough voluntarily, spitting up blood at the end of the cough, because they can open a small vessel of the gum at will, suck blood from it with the tongue, and spit it out with their cough as if it had come from deeper parts. Some feign delirium or insanity or even try to make others appear insane. Now, even the ignorant are aware that the physician should discover such subterfuges and distinguish them from the true signs."

We also quote from Galen's text several medical definitions: " Hydrophobia is a disease that follows the bite of a mad dog and is accompanied by an aversion to drinking liquids, convulsions and hiccups. Sometimes maniacal attacks supervene " (Kühn, XIX; 418).

" Cholera is a very acute and severe disease, which rapidly depletes the patient with violent vomiting, diarrhœa, and abundant secretion. Colic then occurs and, shortly after, fever, like the fever of dysentery, with dangerous changes in the viscera " (XIX, 421).

" Tenesmus is a diathesis of the large intestine and especially of the rectum, which produces a frequent desire to evacuate, though the discharges are slight " (XIX, 422).

" Ozena is a severe ulceration of the nostrils, with emission of a foul odour " (XIX, 440).

" Scirrhus is a hard, heavy, immobile, and painful tumour; cancer is a very hard malignant tumour, with or without ulceration. Its name comes from the animal called the crab " (XIX, 442, 443).

We take as an example of Galen's cures one that caused a great stir in Rome: a Persian Sophist had a sensory paralysis of the fourth and fifth fingers of one hand and of half of the middle finger. The Sophist called some physicians of the Methodist school, who first applied emollients and then astringents. When he found that all these remedies were doing no good, he called Galen, who asked immediately if the patient had been hurt in the arm and then learned that he had fallen on a sharp stone so that he had received a blow between the shoulders. He had immediately felt a violent pain, but this soon lessened. Galen diagnosed it as an inflammation of the spinal cord, put his patient to bed, and ordered applications of soothing remedies to the dorsal region; and the patient recovered. Galen explained that he had been led to indicate the region of the seventh cervical vertebra as the seat of the trouble because he knew that every nerve has an origin distinct from the other nerves and then unites with those near it (brachial plexus), but nevertheless retains its special attributes; and because he did not forget that it is at the height of the seventh cervical vertebra that the cubital (ulnar) nerve begins which goes to the last two fingers and half of the middle finger. After the patient was cured, Galen says, this case gave rise to a violent discussion between the other physicians and himself as to the reason why there was only a paralysis of sensation. It was for him to explain to the physicians that there are distinct nerves for the muscles and for the skin and that in the affections of the former, movement is abolished; and in the affections of the latter, sensation is lost.

The basic concept of the therapy of Galen is contained in the formula: *contraria contrariis*, for instance, the application of heat for the diseases that come from cold, and vice versa; evacuation in case of plethoric diseases, and so on. The indications for the choice and modes of application of therapeutic measures are numerous and complex; drastic remedies could only be administered at the beginning and the end of an illness, and there are complications which can change therapy; for example, the dreams of the patient. The treatment consisted in diets and drugs; it made use of exercises, massage, and climatotherapy, prescribed in cases of phthisis; even violent gymnastic exercises were used for the constitutionally weak and for convalescents. Among the successes recorded by Galen was the cure by means of breathing-exercises, singing, and gymnastics of the arms of a young man afflicted with a deformity of the thorax. Bleeding held an important place in Galenic therapeutics. It was thought to exercise a revulsive action when practised on a part of the body distant from the diseased part, or a derivative action when used near the diseased organ. The medicinal therapy of Galen recognized a very large number of drugs, of which some were regarded as specifics: for instance, pepper for tertian and quartan fever, scammony for jaundice, parsley and celery for diseases of the kidneys. Thus in his therapeutics, as elsewhere, Galen followed a strictly rational line and repudiated the animal or human secretions used at the time, such as excrement, urine, spermatic fluid, and so on.

The surgery of Galen made use of operations that had not been previously described, such as resection of the ribs in empyema, and resection of the sternum (*De administrationibus anatomicis*, Bk. VII, Ch. 13).

The doctrine of Galen, when compared with that of Hippocrates, can be regarded as founded on a localistic rather than on a general pathology such as was taught by the master of Cos. His line of thought, instead of being the eminently synthetic reasoning of the Hippocratists, tending to reach conclusions through the proper consideration of universal laws, was analytical and systematized in rigid forms, as we have seen. The system of Galen is based on morphology rather than on the biologic concept that is the basic foundation of the teachings of Hippocrates and of Aristotle.

We see, then, that Galen really guided medicine to an orientation that would have brought about great progress if, on the one hand, it had not been confined in a teleologic doctrine, and, on the other hand, the decadence of the spirit of investigation at this time — a strange phenomenon of collective decrease of the critical faculties coming from the politico-social situation — had not made a *noli me tangere* of his system. This also deprived it of perhaps the greatest of its virtues, that of being an encouragement and guide along the route of experience.

Thus it came about that the seed sowed by him in such a masterly way in the field of experimental studies remained unfertile, just as the discerning biological observations of Aristotle and the doctrine of Ptolemy remained sterile.

It was a period in which people preferred to believe rather than to discuss, when dogma was accepted more easily than criticism, when it appeared easiest to borrow the dictates rather than the principles of the great masters. Thus the treasure of observations, still in its infancy in the work of Galen, was crystallized and became sterile, instead of giving rise to the efflorescence of observation and investigation which could logically have been expected. Throughout centuries his disciples followed the letter of his work rather than the spirit; they did not follow the ideas of the ob-

server, whose work was excellent, but of the philosopher, who was mediocre, and of the dogmatist, who gave to his personal observations the semblance of infallibility and to his hypotheses the appearance of immutable
precepts.

8. Public Hygiene

Hygienic measures, certainly inspired by very ancient laws and traditions, such as that of the draining of the swamps by the Etruscans, date
from the very earliest times of Rome. In the Cloaca Maxima, Tarquinius

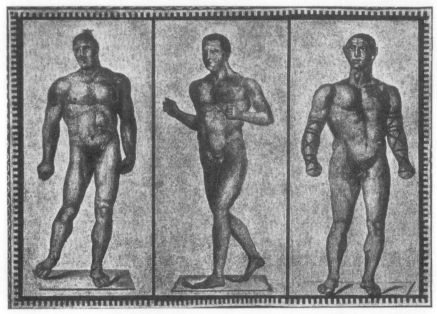

84. *Mosaics of athletes in the Baths of Caracalla.*   (LATERAN MUSEUM, ROME.)

Priscus had erected a monument eminently worth copying. The Lake of
Curtius had also been drained in early times. In Vitruvius we find exact indications for the selection of places suitable for the foundation of cities, for
the construction of houses, and for the improvement of the soil. The zeal
that the Romans showed for public hygiene is easily comprehensible by
those who study their laws and can still observe today the monuments that
have come down to us.

The Lex Aquilia provided supervision of physicians and held them responsible for negligence. The Lex Cornelia punished with deportation or
decapitation those who caused the death of a patient. The supervision of

prostitution was strict. The *lupanaria* only opened in the evening and had to be located outside the city (*sub mœnia*). The ædiles kept a register of the prostitutes, who were forbidden to use their family names. The law against abortion was also strict. Thus the Lex Cornelia prescribed that whoever gave an aphrodisiac beverage or caused an abortion should be punished with deportation and the loss of part of his goods. If the patient should die as a result of these practices, the guilty party was condemned to death.

The law of the Decemvirs fixed the term of pregnancy at ten months, and denied legitimacy to a child born in the eleventh month. The Lex Cornelia also provided that the existence of pregnancy should be established in the presence of five accoucheuses. The Roman legislation in the field of social hygiene shows that the legislators regarded the care of the public health as the most important of their duties. Even in the period of the kings, as we have seen, they had begun to arrange for the canalization of the swamps and a supply of drinking water. The Forum, on account of its low position near the river between the Palatine and the Aventine, was swampy and frequently flooded. In the period of the kings subterranean drains were built beneath it, which were enlarged by Tarquinius Superbus; they were so solidly constructed that they remain for the most part to this day. Throughout the periods of the Republic and the Empire the greatest care was given to this type of construction. We know that supervision of the drains was confided to special magistrates; house-owners were obliged to contribute to their upkeep.

Malaria, as Celli has shown in his exhaustive history of malaria in the Ager Romanus (1925), was known from the most ancient times, and it is certain that the first inhabitants of the peninsula preferred to live in elevated places on account of their greater healthfulness. According to Vitruvius, up to the time of Romulus the districts about Rome were regarded as pestilential — that is to say, swampy. Even in the time of the kings and of the Republic, when doubtless malaria had already ravaged the people, the Romans had not contented themselves with invoking the goddess Febris, who had her temple on the Palatine, but they had begun those marvellous hydraulic works of which the most important were the draining of the swamps situated within the city, and later the construction of the Cloaca Maxima. The obliteration of the small surface or underground bogs was brought about, according to Lanciani, by means of drains constructed either from small porous conduits or from dry stones. According to Manzi, Marcus Appius, the legate of Scipio Æmilianus, is said to have perpetuated on coins the memory of the marvellous work that he had accomplished in the sanitation of the Ager Romanus. Julius Cæsar excavated a lake and planted a forest on the right bank of the Tiber where the Codetan Swamp had previously existed. In 398 B.C. the subterranean outlet for the Alban Lake was constructed. All these works greatly diminished the unhealthfulness of the Campagna Romana in the Imperial epoch.

In the earlier times it was the censors who supervised the drainage work; but in the time of Augustus special magistrates were appointed, the *curatores alvei et riparum Tiberis*, to whom later was added a *comes cloacarum*. The supply of water by aqueducts was the object of special attention from the authorities of Rome from the earliest times. Up to the year 300 B.C. the people drank the water of the Tiber, but at that time the censor, Appius Claudius, constructed the aqueduct of the Aqua Appia, which brought to Rome water from the district of Præneste between the seventh and eighth milestones. It was only fifty years later that a second aqueduct was constructed, then that of Annius, which was begun by Curius and finished by Fulvius Flaccus. In 144 B.C. the city acquired a fourth aqueduct, which brought water from the Sabine Mountains and was called the Aqua Marcia after the prætor Marcius, its builder. The construction of this aqueduct cost not less than one hundred million sesterces, which corresponds to more than ten million dollars of today.

But even these aqueducts did not suffice for the enormous consumption of water by the Romans, and twenty years after the aqueduct of the Aqua Marcia, the aqueduct of the Aqua Tepula was built, which brought to Rome water from Frascati. In the Augustan period it was necessary to construct the aqueducts of the Aqua Julia, Aqua Augusta, and Aqua Virgo.

It was this Aqua Virgo that supplied the baths constructed by Agrippa, A.D. 27. It was regarded as the best and purest of all the waters of Rome; but the aqueduct deteriorated rapidly, and it was only some time later that Hadrian attempted its reconstruction. It can be calculated that in addition to the water employed for the baths in the time of Imperial Rome, the people had at their disposal over a hundred gallons of water per person daily, brought by fourteen aqueducts. No modern city has even approximated such figures.

The baths of Rome in the most ancient times consisted of the cold baths in the Tiber and in the great basins that had the name of the public pools (*piscinæ publicæ*). It was only later, when Greek and Oriental customs began to be introduced into Rome, that first private baths were built in the dwellings, and then the magnificent public baths constructed by the State or the emperors or rich citizens.

These *balnea*, whose number was small in the time of the Republic, increased enormously under the Cæsars. It is reckoned that there were more than eight hundred at the time of Diocletian. The first public *thermæ* were built by Agrippa, who was Ædile in the reign of Augustus. They were conceived and executed in that spirit of simple grandeur which is the characteristic of the Roman architecture of that period. After the Baths ôf Agrippa, there were constructed those of Nero, Titus, Caracalla, Alexander Severus, Constantine, and Diocletian, tô name only the most sumptuous and beautiful. In the writ-

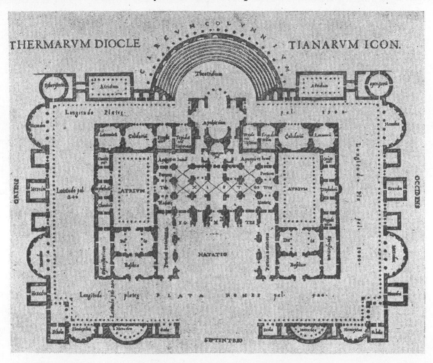

85. *Plan of the Baths of Diocletian.*
(*From* De Thermis Lacubus Balneis, *1571, by A. Bacci of Sant' Elpidio, 1524–1600*.)

ings of the times the frequent descriptions of these establishments show that their usefulness and hygienic efficiency have never been surpassed or even equalled. In the *thermæ* there were both hot and cold baths. From the atrium, where the bathers assembled, one passed to the *exedra*, which contained seats of marble and was covered by a cupola. From here one passed to the *apody-terium*, or dressing-room, thence to the cold bath (*frigidarium*), supplied by water from reservoirs connected with the aqueduct; or one might go to the *tepidarium* and the *calidarium*, which furnished the steam for a vapour bath from tubes passing between double walls. Finally came cold bathing in special rooms. Ventilation was obtained by means of openings in the ceilings. The *thermæ* also contained rooms for massage and for separate baths, for meetings and gymnastic exercises.

The architecture of the streets and of the houses was greatly improved by the reconstruction of the city after the conflagration of Nero. The ædiles at that time arranged for the straightening of the streets, which had previously been crooked and poorly kept up. They also supervised the street-cleaning, for which the house-owners were responsible, aided in this duty by the *quatuor viri viis purgandis*, who were especially responsible for this duty in each of the

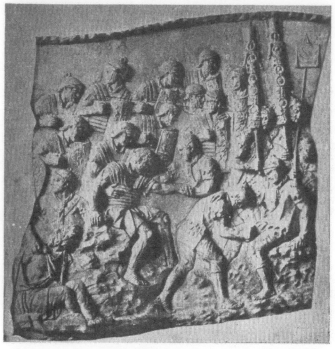

86. *First-aid treatment in the Roman army. A detail on Trajan's Column.*

quarters of the city. At the time of the Empire, Rome had public latrines. A topographic plan from the period of Constantine shows that there were no less than one hundred and fifty of these.

Control of the food supply fell to the ædiles, who supervised the markets and the foodstuffs offered there; they had the right to forbid the sale of spoiled articles and to impose fines on the vendors. Meats had to be sold in well-ventilated places. Wheat was kept in the granaries of the State, following the suggestion of Caius Gracchus; under the Empire there were more than three hundred of these in Rome. There was an enormous quantity of wheat kept in them — almost ten times as much as was necessary for a year's supply.

The provisioning of the wheat was confided to the *ædiles cereales*, later to the *curatores frumenti dandi*. It is known that every year on special occasions large quantities of grain were distributed gratis to the people, a custom that caused an enormous drain on the public treasury. Thus in the

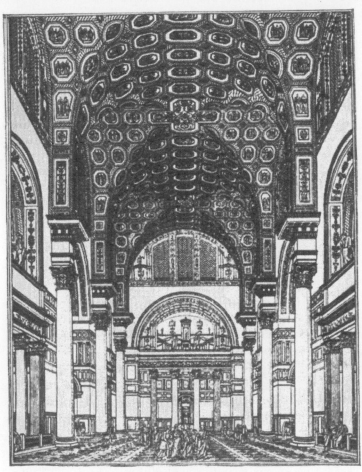

87. *The* Tepidarium
in the Thermæ of Caracalla, Rome.

time of Pompey these public distributions represented an expense of more than a million dollars in today's money.

The burial of the dead, according to the law of the Twelve Tables, was forbidden inside the walls of the city. For the ordinary rank-and-file citizen of Rome there was a cemetery on the plain beyond the Esquiline. In the time of Augustus, Mæcenas transformed this into a magnificent park.

At this period there were already societies in existence for the payment of funeral expenses of all those who had made a regular contribution. The burial places of the more prosperous were usually along the main roads, such as the Appian Way. The corpse was placed in a sarcophagus of metal or marble (*arca*), then buried in a walled-up chamber. But the practice of cremation soon became popular, and in the time of Sulla it was practised almost universally. It was carried out on the *ustrinæ* which were placed near the tombs, and on them a funeral pyre erected. When the pyre had burned out, some wine was poured on the ashes, after which they were collected and placed in an urn with spices. The urn, in its turn, was placed in a tomb, or, for the poorer people, in niches in the *columbaria*, huge stone chambers in which hundreds of compartments were cut to contain the urns.

Later, about the second century of our era, the burial of the dead became more common, and after the spread of Christianity cremation was entirely abolished.

9. *Professional Practice. Status of the Physician*

Medicine at Rome was at first, as we have seen, practised exclusively by foreigners. It was regarded as an ignoble profession to which no free man would devote himself. The first foreign physicians in Rome about whom we know anything were the Greeks.

These Greek physicians, among whom there were certainly adventurers and common speculators, used their title of physician and the meagre information that they had acquired in the schools of Greece and Alexandria solely as a source of gain. The hatred of those who saw in the Greek penetration a peril for the Roman customs was soon aroused against them. It was only later that one could begin to speak of real medical instruction in Rome. At the time of the Republic instruction seems to have been delivered privately and without any control by the State; medicine formed part of the general culture, as we have already observed in speaking of the writings of Varro, Vitruvius, and Pliny. Athenæus maintained that every cultivated man should concern himself with medicine, which was necessary for all professions. Galen wrote about the nobility conferred on the physician by the study of philosophy. By that he meant that the physician should possess all the necessary knowledge of life and its manifestations, and he estimated that a period of study of at least eleven years was necessary to attain this goal. His contemporary and enemy Thessalus, on the other hand, declared that six months was all that was necessary to make an excellent physician. In 46 B.C., when Julius Cæsar granted the rights of Roman citizenship to all physicians, this much sought-after privilege assured greatly increased dignity to the practice of medicine. It was at this time that it was begun to be thought necessary to organize medical studies, in view of the increasing danger from the invasion of adventurers and pseudo-physicians, who, though lacking in medical knowledge, had been attracted to Rome by the mirage of easy profit. The physician who had completed his regular studies was indicated by the name of *medicus a republica*.

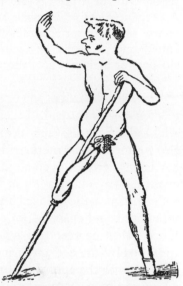

A great number of medical schools, among which the most celebrated outside of Italy were those of Marseille, Lyon, Saragossa, Antioch, without mentioning the Athenian and Alexandrian depositaries of the great traditions of antiquity, furnished physicians for the entire Roman Empire. But a true organization of medical study dates from the commencement of the third century, when Alexander Severus instituted special schools for the teaching of medicine. This teaching consisted largely in the anatomy of animals, especially of monkeys, and the examination of wounds. The study of medical botany was also emphasized.

88. *Prosthesis of the right leg. (From an Italic vase of the fourth century* B.C.*)*

Statements by Pliny inform us that there were in Rome large gardens, some belonging to physicians (Antonius Castor, for example), in which Pliny himself had carried out his studies. Clinical instruction probably took place in the *valetudinarii* and the *tabernæ;* often also in the house of the patient, whither the pupils accompanied their master, as we learn from the famous epigram of Martial against the physician Symmacus (V, 9). Martial complains of having had to undergo the visit of a hundred pupils who accompanied Symmacus in his visits and of having had in consequence to submit to the contact of one hundred cold hands. He says: " Before, I was doing well; after your visit, I have the fever."

We have information about the charlatans and the empiricists who practised in Rome at this time from the writers of the period, who tell us that the attacks led by Cato, and later by Celsus and the satirical poets, were far from being unjust. Antonius Musa himself, who, as a reward for curing Augustus with cold baths, had his statue erected beside that of Æsculapius, boasted of being the inventor of a secret remedy with which he claimed to be able to maintain Cæsar and Mæcenas in good health. He prescribed the excrement of dogs for angina, maintained that he was able to pulverize stones inside the bladder, and regarded the herb betony as a sovereign remedy for all diseases. At the time of the Empire we know that even famous physicians were subservient to the emperors and lent themselves to the preparation of poisons. A certain Crinas of Marseille treated his patient by astrology, regulating the course of treatment according to the stars. He succeeded in this way in accumulating a fortune of ten million sesterces, after having spent an equal amount for building the walls of his native city.

Toward the end of the Empire there was certainly public instruction in medicine. Physicians had their place in the Athenæum built by Hadrian. Alexander Severus (208–235) was the first Emperor to decree privileges also for medical instruction. Those who taught in Rome, even if they were not born there, enjoyed all the rights of citizens " as if they would teach in their own country (*ita ac si propria patria docerent*)." Valentinian, in his reforms of the Roman Gymnasium, ordained that students should be supervised, and chastised, or even expelled, if they did not attend the lectures. Julian decreed that whoever wished to practise medicine should be approved by the collegium and that he could only be granted a licence to practise with the approval of the best physicians. In the Temple of Peace, where the men of science and letters gathered, were the libraries where the most valuable books were preserved. We learn from Galen himself that there were among these some of his manuscripts that were destroyed in the conflagration. Private libraries were numerous; Cicero had one, also Julius Cæsar. Augustus founded a public library. Diocletian sent scholars to Alexandria to transcribe the classical authors; and Pompey, after he had conquered Mithridates, had the medical treasures of the King of Pontus searched in order to bring the best to Rome and make them public there. Thus Pliny wrote: " *Vitæ profuit non minus quam reipublicæ victoria illa* (Life itself profited from that victory no less than did the Republic)."

Soon, with the systemization of medical study, the social position of physicians was also regularized.

The Palatine Archiaters, who were true court physicians, many of whose names are known, played an important part in political life, having the title of *præsules spectabiles*. They were regarded as high functionaries, equal in dignity to the *comites*, and received enormous emoluments. It seems, however, that the title of Archiater was also used to designate celebrated physicians even when they were not directly connected with the court. It is clear that it was not a mere title, but that it carried with it various functions of an administrative character, including the duty of supervising all the physicians who practised in a town or a given province. The acceptance of a new physician was decided upon by a majority of the Archiaters sitting in conclave. This acceptance required also the approval of the Palatine Archiaters. In addition, *Archiatri Populares* selected by the municipalities had been instituted in the early days of the Empire. They

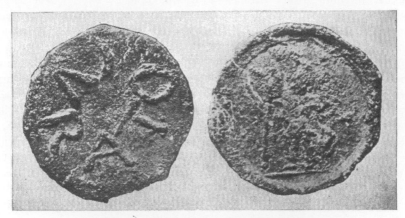

89. *Lead token used in a Gallo-Roman bath.*
(MUSEUM OF THE SCHOOL OF MEDICINE, ROUEN.)

were responsible for the free care of the poor. Besides these physicians, who had an official character, there were in Rome practitioners without a definite title but enjoying various privileges, such as exemption from all taxation and the right of naming to the judges those who refused to pay their honoraria. These honoraria were often considerable. We know that Galen received in a single case a payment equivalent to several thousand dollars today.

Thus as the decadence of the Empire became accentuated, improvement took place in the situation of the physicians, who in the days of the last emperors included in their ranks the most important members of the court. Their opinion had great weight not only in matters of hygiene but often also in the most important political problems.

CHARICLES, the physician of Tiberius, played an important role in the last illness of the Emperor. Tacitus and Suetonius speak of him as a physician of great renown whose opinions were held in high esteem. EUTERION, physician of Livia, the sister of Germanicus, was a member of the conspiracy to kill Drusus. VETIUS VALENS, the physician of Messalina, according to Tacitus, had great power at court and was one of the closest counsellors of the Empress. Thus, from what we can learn from the writers of the period, it is apparent that toward the end of the Empire the position of physicians at Rome was clearly established, not only by their standing at court, but also by the high rank that they occupied among the State officials.

According to the Code of Theodosius, dating from the year 368, the Archiaters of the People had the right to demand payment from rich clients. The posts of Archiaters of the People were instituted in all the quarters of Rome except those of the Porticos and of the College of the Vestal Virgins, for whom physicians were expressly designated. When a position of archiater became vacant, the election of his successor took place only after an examination and a decision had been given by the other physicians of the college. It was expressly stated that no outside influence should be exerted on the choice of the candidate. Occurrences were not infrequent, nevertheless, which gave rise to protest. A writer of the sixth century has preserved the account of one such for us: Symmacus recounts that a physician of a patrician family, having been named an archiater of Rome, thanks to the favour of the Emperor, instead of another named Epictetus, thus obtained a post superior to that which his record deserved. The matter was brought before the college after a protest had been registered, but discussion of an Imperial decision was not allowed according to the Code of Justinian, which declared it a sacrilege to doubt that a man chosen by the Emperor should be worthy of the choice (*Codex Justiniani*, Bk. IX, Tit. XXIX, 1–2).

The Theodosian Code recognized that the two quarters of Rome for which physicians could not be named after 368, mentioned above, were those which were most in need of an expert physician who was thoroughly aware of the importance of his function and responsibility. The functions of the physician of the Gymnasium were perhaps partly religious, for the practices there were in close relation to the religious cult. In addition, it was in the quarter of the Porticos that the athletes took their exercise, and when one realizes the importance that the Romans gave to physical exercise, it is easy to understand that the physician who was responsible for the care of athletes and perhaps even directed their daily life had an especially delicate task. It is doubtless for this reason that from ancient times physicians for this post were chosen with special care and according to special rules.

The dignity of the Vestal Virgins and the high rank that they occupied in Roman society, the particular privileges that they enjoyed, and the veneration in which they were held by the Romans sufficed, as Pliny tells us, to add great importance to the physician who had them in charge. Vestal Virgins who were slightly indisposed were treated in the interior of the Temple; but those who were attacked by severe disease were allowed to go out of the Temple and were confided to the care of some respectable matron.

We know that the schools of medicine founded under the early emperors each had their special secretary, *scriba medicorum,* and their professors also bore the title of Archiater. Thus we see that at the time of the Empire there was an extensive professional organization of the medical schools, with all the forms and defects of more recent organizations. Even the lesser sanitary professions, such as the *obstetricæ,* the *pharmacopoli,* and the *iatrolipti,* were strictly regulated.

The Latin satirical poets often speak of patients' diseases and physicians.

> *Eximit aut reficit dentem Cascellius aegrum,*
> *Infestos oculis uris, Hygine, pilos,*
> *Non secat et tollit stillantem Fannius uvam,*
> *Tristia servorum stigmata delet Eros,*
> *Enterocelarum fertur Podalirius Hermes.*
> (Martial, X, 56)

(Cascellius draws or repairs the diseased tooth.
You, Hyginus, burn the hairs that are dangerous to the eyes.
Fannius does not excise, but raises up the dropping uvula.
Eros removed the slaves' melancholy stigmata.
Hermes is called the Podalirius of hernias.)

Horace tells us that he suffered from rheumatic pains and gastric distress. He often speaks of physicians and drugs, and he tells of having obeyed Musa, the physician of Cæsar, who had recommended sulphur baths. Persius, speaking of an insane patient, says that it is too late for him to use hellebore. Juvenal speaks of physicians practising both medicine and surgery, and also selling drugs. Martial, who often scourged ignorant physicians and charlatans, speaks of a gladiator who was formerly an oculist:

> *Hoplomachus nunc es: fueras ophthalmicus ante:*
> *Fecisti medicus quod facis hoplomachus.*

(Now you are a gladiator; before you were an oculist
You did as a physician what you now do as a gladiator.)

From some of the passages in the Roman satirists, attempts have been made to infer that the physicians at that time already knew syphilis, and this hypothesis does not seem at all unlikely.

Military medicine had a remarkable development in Imperial Rome. Celsus touches upon it in a discussion of extraction of missiles from the body (Bk. VII, Ch. 5). With the formation of stationary armies the thought of a medical service arose. In the book on Tactics by Claudius Ælianus (A.D. 100–140) physicians are classified among the non-combatants; and, as Haberling shows, the physicians of the legions are cited in more than forty-six Latin inscriptions of the time of the Empire. Germanicus and Trajan were concerned with the medical treatment of the soldiers, and it is certain that in the time of Hadrian every legion and every warship had its physician. These physicians were regarded as *immunes;* that is to say, they were exempted as combatants and had the rank of *principales* (non-combatant officers). They took their orders directly from the commandant of the camp (*præfectus castrorum*) or, in his absence, from the tribune of the legions. Funereal inscriptions show us that the volunteers (*cohortes civium Romanorum*), the auxiliaries (*cohortes auxiliares*), the squadrons of cav-

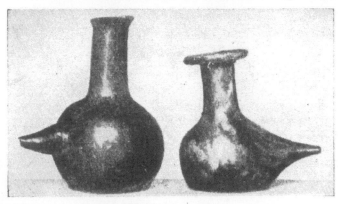

90. *Roman nursing vessels.*

alry (*alæ equitum*), and the triremes of the army had their medical personnel. The naval physicians were named *duplicarii,* indicating that they received double pay. The inclusion of bandages in the army baggage is shown by a passage in Tacitus concerning the loss of this material in the Teutoburg Forest. Dio Cassius related that the Emperor Trajan personally treated the wounded, and that, when bandages gave out, he did not spare his own clothing, but cut it in strips to bind the wounds of his soldiers. Military physicians enjoyed several privileges, such as the *jus restitutionis,* which gave the right to the physician of demanding an indemnity for all the material loss that he might incur by his absence from home during military service. The Justinian Code (X, 53, 1–6) notes that the physician of the legion is exempt from every civil obligation during his military service.

The discovery of Roman military hospitals near Vienna, at Bonn in Germany, and at Baden in Switzerland shows that the sanitary service was well provided for even in the provinces.

The arrangement of the hospitals, with rooms opening on corridors and a central rectangular court with excellent arrangements for water, kitchens, and pharmacies, has been revealed by the discoveries of Colonel von Droller, in 1904, in the ruins of the Hospice of Carnuntum on the Danube.

Just as there were hospitals for soldiers, so the slaves had hospitals, called *valetudinaria*, and a physician who had the title of *medicus commensalis* was charged with the care of the slaves.

There were other *valetudinaria* for the athletes and for the wounded gladiators, who were submitted to special treatment. *Frictores* and *unguentarii* were employed in their service. The physicians of athletes and gladiators, called *vulnerarii*, included well-known physicians, even Galen himself. There were even *valetudinaria* for the legions, which consisted of tents placed in the middle of camps.

Polybius relates that there were special commandants for the *valetudinaria* and that they accompanied the physicians of the legions on their visits to the wounded.

The number of physicians in Rome seems to have been considerable. Specialists were common. There were many oculists, among whom were especially mentioned Charmides and Uelpides, but there were also dentists, gynæcologists, otologists, specialists for the fistula, and so on. There were also women physicians, midwives, and many people abusing the practice of medicine, such as barbers, masseurs, and so on.

Nurses were called *censi, accensiti, optiores valetudinarii*. Soldiers who helped their sick comrades were called *contubernales*.

Real hospitals, in the modern sense of establishments designed to receive and treat all sorts of patients, were only instituted, as we shall see, much later.

10. Essential Characteristics of Roman Medicine

The problem which arises for all those who study ancient Roman medicine is to determine whether a decisive effect on the progress of medical sciences should be attributed to Roman civilization, as our older historians affirm; or whether one should not regard Roman medicine as essentially, or exclusively, Greek medicine; in other words, whether all that the Romans did and knew in the domain of medicine was not entirely the result of Greek teaching. Most recent historians, and especially historians in countries outside of Italy, are of this opinion. Some of them deny any initiative to the Romans in the field of medicine and affirm that anything worth while in ancient medical Rome, even in the progress of hygiene, is but a more or less faithful copy of the examples furnished by the Greeks. This is also true, they add, in the case of sculpture, architecture, and poetry, which are basically nothing but imitations, rarely reaching the heights of the immortal models of ancient Greece.

This would be a reversal of the judgment of the Renaissance, for which period everything that was great and beautiful was due to the Romans and for which Celsus became the most eminent medical author. Whoever observes calmly and judges impartially must recognize the merit in Roman medicine. In the domain of science, to be sure, Latin medicine did not register notable progress other than that due to the Greek physicians; and one must recognize that the Latin medical writers were diligent compilers and collectors of Greek texts often without great critical judgment. It is also true that medicine in the early centuries of Rome, as we have seen, was almost exclusively practised by strangers and had no glorious traditions nor flourishing scientific development. This victorious people applied itself especially to the military art and to the consolidation of its power by an admirable system of laws, and did all in its power to establish the strength of the city and of the State. Later, when great riches flowed in and the reviving breath of Greek art could be felt passing over Rome, civil war and internal strife predominated and there were but few who dedicated their studies to science. But, on the other hand, it cannot be gainsaid that in this field as in many others Romans played a distinguished role: namely, that of having codified in admirable form the rules that the Greeks had transmitted to them, that of having constructed from the hygienic laws of the ancient Babylonians and Egyptians, of the Greeks and of other Oriental peoples, the fundamental lines of a perfect system of hygienic legislation which has not been equalled in twenty centuries.

The city which provided its citizens with a perfect water system from fourteen aqueducts, thus furnishing to each inhabitant of Rome several times the amount of water demanded even by the hygiene of today; the city which, from the earliest times of the Empire, had instituted the curators of the Tiber and supervisors of the sewers; which had regulated by detailed and strict legislation all the problems of canalization; which had special functionaries for the conduct of the markets; which had constructed baths like those of Diocletian, with accommodations for several thousand bathers at a time; which had made the great parks of the Janiculum, instituted the free treatment of the poor, and made exemplary arrangements for the cremation and burial of the dead — such a city without any doubt deserves an eminent position in the history of medicine. These sanitary rules actually furnished a model for all that has since been done in this field; and Rome has stood as the great activator whose example has carried Latin hygiene into the most distant regions.

Finally, the Romans deserve credit in medical history for another reason: it was only in Rome that physicians constituted a class, protected by the law, to which the State accorded special guarantees. At the time of the Empire they enjoyed the esteem of the citizens, and the emperors confided to them the highest State dignities. For the first time in history, physicians attained to the more important public positions and took part in the political administration. Thus there arose a complicated sanitary organization governed by strict principles which guaranteed its proper functioning. The right to practise medicine was granted only after determined precautions had been taken, and for the first time one sees officially recognized by law the special position that the medical schools should occupy in society and in the State.

If, then, scientific medicine did not make decisive progress in Rome, we should not forget that it was there that the rules of hygiene were codified in a most admirable way, and that it is in Rome that we meet for the first time a legal medicine which constituted an important part of the marvellous Roman system of laws. It is in Rome that we find the constitution of a sanitary organization governed by wise regulations, and it is to Rome that we owe the systematization of medical teaching and the comprehension of its great importance. In fact, it was the Roman genius that snatched the physician from his humble and uncertain position, granted him the rights of citizenship, raised him to the top of the social ladder, and placed in his hands the supreme responsibility for public health, without which, according to the lofty Latin and Greek concept, it is not possible to picture a true grandeur for the State.

CHAPTER XII

THE DECADENCE OF MEDICAL

SCIENCE

CHRISTIAN DOGMATIC MEDICINE
THE BYZANTINE SCHOOL

1. The Political Decadence of the Empire. The Great Epidemics

THE WORK of Galen, contemporary with the greatest splendour of the Roman Empire and the greatest extension of the power of the Cæsars, marks the culminating point of Greco-Roman medicine — the decisive force in which all the currents of scientific thought seemed to have been united. At the same time it signalized the beginning of decadence.

This is not the place to trace the origin of this decadence, the part played therein by the great wars, the corruption of habits attributed to frequent contact with the Orient, the political contests and the misery of large classes of the population. This is a problem that has long been discussed by historians and solved in various ways. Here it is interesting to note how other factors can certainly be regarded as having played an important, perhaps determining, part in this decadence. They are extremely important factors for the hygienist and for the medical historian; yet they have been frequently overlooked by those concerning themselves with Roman history. There were terrible epidemics which destroyed entire cities, preceded or accompanied by inundation and earthquakes, which were frequent in Italy in the first centuries of our era, and often followed by famine and drought. Frightful epidemics of malaria desolated Rome in the later periods of the Empire, and literally decimated the population.

The special nature of these epidemics is not clearly indicated by the writers of the period. As Galen himself has stated, the Greek term *loimos*

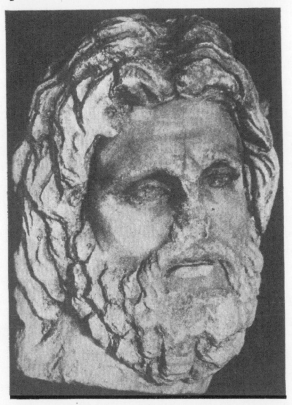

91. *Marble head of Christ adapted from the head of Æsculapius. Excavations of Jerasch, Palestine.*

indicates any severe disease with a high mortality that attacks a large number of people at the same time. The Latin words *pestis* and *pestilentia* have the same meaning, and like our English word " pestilence " were often used to indicate any sort of misfortune. It is therefore difficult or even impossible to identify the plagues of antiquity. The descriptions that have been preserved by physicians of the period are scarcely of sufficient accuracy to permit even an approximate estimate of the characteristics of the disease, much less a correct diagnosis. The opinions of historians vary about the epidemics of the early centuries, and especially about that which bears the name of Galen. Even though bubonic plague was without doubt one of the most frequent and destructive epidemics, it is probable that other serious contagious diseases were also often manifest in these centuries. Five great pestilences should be recorded: the first was that which followed the terrible eruption of Vesuvius A.D. 79, which destroyed Herculaneum and Pompeii. Immediately after this eruption a terrible pestilence spread through the Campagna, and the writers of the period relate that it destroyed tens of thousands of victims daily. The plague of Orosius began A.D. 125, after a frightful invasion of grasshoppers, which completely destroyed the crops. In Numidia more than eight hundred thousand people are said to have died; on the coast of Africa between Carthage and Utica, more than two hundred thousand. In Utica itself, thirty thousand Roman soldiers, who had been sent to Africa to defend the colony, were almost entirely destroyed. The pestilence called the Plague of Antoninus, or of Galen, which lasted A.D. 164–180, began on the eastern frontiers of the Empire and spread rapidly to its western boundaries. It was carried to Rome by the army which had been sent to Syria to suppress a revolt. It broke out in Rome in 166 and spread rapidly. Historians state that thousands of persons died daily in Rome. Soldiers were the most frequently attacked. From the accounts of contemporaries, it appears to have been an epidemic of exanthematous typhus, but perhaps of bubonic plague, though the diagnosis still remains doubtful. The fourth pestilence, that of Cyprian, lasted A.D. 251–266. It was probably smallpox, in view of its extremely contagious nature and the frequent involvement of the eyes.

Finally, in 312 there was another severe epidemic of smallpox. From the descriptions of contemporaries, which still leave a most profound impression, we can form some idea of the enormous destruction of human life and national wealth that these epidemics brought about. It is reasonable, then, to attribute to these destructive factors a more important role in the decadence of the Roman Empire than those played by destructive wars and a soft and luxurious mode of living. It is evident that these scourges paralysed the political and social life of the Empire, but especially hampered the progress of medical science.

2. Christian Dogmatic Medicine

The almost constant threat of death caused by these diseases, against which all methods of cure were useless, and which struck down the youngest and most robust, was demoralizing to the highest degree. The prostrate condition of the country following these epidemics necessarily gave free rein, as is always the case at the time of great scourges, to superstitions and credulities, especially among the ignorant elements of the population. It removed confidence in physicians; and, as a result of phenomena which were periodically repeated in their essential characteristics, led people toward a blind faith. It is precisely at this period that we see a new efflorescence of magic and mysticism. An anguished and fearful search for supernatural aid is a phenomenon common to children, sick people, and primitive races when they find themselves the victims of grave disasters.

Compared with the misery and the great physical and moral suffering of the time, the redeeming features of the religion of the humble appeared as a shining light; thus Christianity exercised an extremely important effect, whether direct or indirect, on the development of the medicine of this period. The faith, which spread more and more through a people whose mystic sensibility had been prepared by political and social events, overcame a philosophical speculation that was already undermined by scepticism. The passionate desire for penitence and salvation which spread through a suffering humanity found its expression once again in the fusion of medical with religious thought. The worship of Christ, regarded as the Saviour from all physical and moral ills, suppressed in the people the worship of Æsculapius Salvator, whose cult was widespread up to the fourth century of our era. We may even observe that in many classical representations of the early centuries of the Christian era the face of the Nazarene was obviously modelled on the traditional portrayal of Æsculapius. We know also that the statue of the Greek god was sometimes carried over to the Christian temple and honoured there as the image of Christ. It is thus that, from the union of various currents in an atmosphere of a dissolving civilization, medicine once again becomes theurgic. In the worship of the faithful, Christ is the physician both of the soul and of the body. The gospel concerns itself with the sick; there are frequent descriptions of cases of disease miraculously cured by the divine power. Furthermore, it was logical that Christianity should combat the kind of medicine practised in the first centuries of our era, where constantly increasing recourse was had to pagan and magic practices. Thus there was formed a Christian religious medicine in which prayer, the imposition of hands, unction with holy oil, were regarded as the most important remedies, those to which the faithful should have exclusive or almost exclusive recourse in seeking divine aid for the cure of bodily ills.

The Christian idea, then, exercised a determining influence on the development of medicine: it gives a different valuation of human life, a fraternal concept of equality and charity which imposed on all the faithful the most severe sacrifices in order to lessen the suffering of others. The example of the early Christians who during the epidemics of the early centuries were tireless in caring for the sick at the peril of their own lives is an admirable proof of the value and the justifying force of those humanitarian ideas which, as we shall see, brought about the creation of a series of institutions designed to care for the aged and the sick.

The influence of Christianity on the history of medicine of this period is also manifest in the fact that it attracted and held the most active minds and the most elevated intellects to such an extent that one can say that intellectual activity converged almost exclusively upon great religious problems and the ethical problems that derived from them. The practice of medicine was regarded as a work of charity; but concern about medical problems and investigations into the causes of disease seemed a useless and almost culpable study at a time when mystic sentiment predominated. At the beginning of the third century some Christians were accused by their coreligionists of venerating Galen. It was only later, as we shall see, that Galen was regarded almost as a canonical authority by the Christian Church itself.

The renewal of religious fervour on the one hand, and the influence of Oriental currents on the other, developed, along with the purely religious medicine, a popular medicine which followed ancient concepts in its recourse to the cult of the saints. It was at this time also that there were founded the sects that had great importance in the development of medical art. The sect of the Essenes or Therapeutists, based at first on a mystic-philosophic program of the adoration of God in a state of purity, on the renouncement of sexual life, on isolation from men in order to attain clear contact with God and His angels, was the first to affirm the necessity of curing disease by faith. This sect devoted all its efforts to study and to the mystic interpretation of ancient texts, and maintained that disease should not be treated except by the invocation of superior forces. Similarly, the sects of Simon Magus and Apollonius Tyanæus (c. 5 B.C.–c. A.D. 95) united the traditions of the ancient sanctuaries of Æsculapius, which were still patronized by the faithful, with those of the Orphic and Pythagorean myths, to create a renascence of magic medicine. Philostratus, who wrote the life of Apollonius, tells us that the latter succeeded in making himself invisible in the presence of Domitian and in appearing at Pozzuoli at the same moment. He also related that Apollonius resuscitated the daughter of a proconsul and gave her back to her husband, and that he controlled the winds when he travelled on the sea, and made the shade of Achilles come out of Avernus. Later the Neo-Platonists constructed, partly on the basis of the doctrines of Zoroaster and partly also on ancient Aristotelian theories invested with new Christian ideas, a system in which the world is conceived as being full of divine emanations and threatened by demons of various sorts which can only be combated in a special state of ecstasy. The lower demons are regarded as the causes of disease and can be expelled with sacrifices or exorcisms, symbols or mysterious formulas. Thus arose a mystic therapy formulated in detail. From it arose the idea of emanations, and this concept, translated to Christianity, created the idea of the potency of holy relics.

The schools of the Gnostics, formed at this time, considered as prophylactic measures of great importance the talismans with Gnostic diagrams and the mystic words *Abraxas* and *Abracadabra*.

Throughout this period, in which the minds of the people veered about in their search for safety in an atmosphere of terror and fright, of doubt and pain, the decadence of science and research was rapidly accentuated.

3. *Post-Galenic Medical Literature*

In the early centuries of our era, medical students and writers were numerous; but they were almost always mere compilers who were content to discuss the classical texts or write commentaries upon them.

Among the medical men of the period to be singled out for diligent work and vast knowledge is ANTYLLUS (second century), who was celebrated even among his contemporaries as a physician and surgeon of uncommon worth.

Of his works there are preserved for us only fragments and long quotations in the works of other physicians, especially Oribasius. His great work *On Medicaments*, in four books, contained a large section devoted to surgery. It was the inspiration of the great surgeons of the Pneumatic school, ARCHIGENES and HELIODORUS. The fame of Antyllus is chiefly due to his account of aneurysms, of which he described two kinds: those that come from a local dilatation of the artery and are in a cylindrical form, and those that come from the lesion of the vessel and are rounded. On the first type it is possible to operate with a longitudinal cut in the direction of the artery, exposing the artery and tying above and below the lesion with a needle and a double ligature.

The indications relative to plastic surgery for defects of the skin, and especially of the eyelids, forehead, nose, and cheeks, are accurate and show that the author was certainly a surgeon of wide experience and unusual ability. In the field of ophthalmology, Antyllus' knowledge was no less vast. He prescribed a number of collyria for ophthalmia; and a passage in Rhazes leads one to believe that Antyllus successfully practised the operation for cataract.

In other fields of medicine, also, Antyllus showed himself to be a careful observer and a wise clinician. He made valuable contributions to the prob-

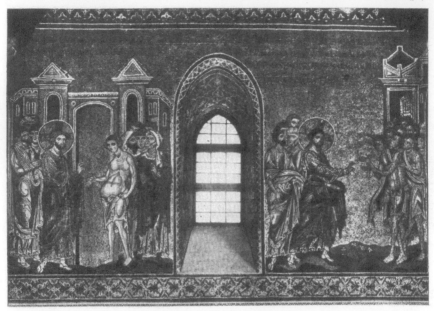

92. *Cure of the dropsical and of ten lepers. Twelfth-century mosaic from the Cathedral of Monreale, Palermo.*

lems of the hygiene of dwellings, diet, medical gymnastics, and economic aid to the sick.

We quote from Oribasius a passage taken from Antyllus in which he speaks of mineral waters and shows that the knowledge of the period in this field had progressed further than is generally recognized:

"The action of baths of natural mineral waters is much more efficacious than that of artificial waters. There are differences in the various mineral waters due to the nature of the soil of the ground through which they pass. Some are saline, others contain alum, others sulphur, others tar, others copper, and others iron; there are still others which contain various combinations of these materials. These mineral waters are not adapted to the cure of acute diseases, but rather to that of chronic diseases and especially those due to cold and humidity. The alkaline and saline waters are recommended for catarrhs of the head and rheumatisms of the chest, and also for those who have stomach trouble or are hydropic. They are useful in the œdemas and in the phlegmatic constitution. The alum baths are recommended for those who have bloody sputum, for those who are subject to vomiting and those who suffer from hemorrhoids; these mineral baths are very useful for women who have irregular or painful menstruation " (Bk. X, 3).

The fragments of the works of Antyllus were published for the first time by Sprengel (Halle, 1799), then in the edition of Oribasius prepared by Bussemaker and Daremberg (Paris, 1851–76).

Among the other surgeons of the period were the brothers PHILIGARIUS and POSEIDONIUS (the latter being especially concerned with the physiology and the pathology of the brain); also THEON of Alexandria, and ZENO of Cyprus, who was the master of Oribasius. Among the writers of the early centuries of our era was QUINTUS SERENUS (Samonicus), who lived in the fifth century and was the author of a medical poem in hexameters called *Liber medicinalis*. About the beginning of the fourth century appeared the so-called Herbarium of the Pseudo-Apuleius, *Herbarum vires et curationes*, a book which contains a clear account of the medicinal virtues of plants, borrowed in large part from Pliny. The problem of the sources of this book has been carefully studied by German historians, especially Henschel. Sigerist industriously collected all the existing information on the subject in manuscripts, from which he has drawn interesting conclusions about the lessons to be learned from it (Kongr. d. deut. Ges. d. Gesch. d. Med., 1924). R. Simonini has published a fragment of the Apuleius which was in the library of Modena, 1925, and a splendid edition of this work, with comments, has recently been published by F. W. Hunger (Leiden, 1935). Among the other writers of the fourth and fifth centuries, VINDICIANUS AFER, a friend of St. Augustine, had a certain importance; he wrote a book of prescriptions called *De expertis remediis*. Theodorus PRISCIANUS was the author of a medical treatise entitled *Rerum medicarum Libri IV*, which was published for the first time at Basel in 1532.

The most celebrated medical writer of the fifth century was AURELIANUS CÆLIUS, born at Sicca in Numidia. He was the author of *De morbis acutis et chronicis*, in which he closely followed Soranus. The books on chronic diseases were first published by Aldus, in 1547, in a collection entitled *Medici Antiqui Omnes*. The works of Cælius, written in barbarous Latin, were already regarded as a medical text by Cassiodorus, who recommended them warmly to his monks. Cælius can be regarded as the last of the medical writers of the western Roman Empire.

4. Byzantine Medicine. Oribasius, Alexander of Tralles, Paul of Ægina

With the growth of the Byzantine Empire and the transference of the centre of culture toward the east, Constantinople became the seat of the medical culture of Europe. The influence on the development of science exerted by the diffusion of the Christian doctrines and the Neo-Platonists' philosophy, imbued with mysticism, was of great importance. Science was placed under the authority of the Church. The Church Fathers became its guardians, and it is to them that we owe in great part the conservation of the traditions of ancient Greek medicine. Among the first Christian physicians, who were almost all Syrians, were the brothers Cosmas and Damian, who, according to legend, had studied medicine and then practised the medical art in Cilicia. They cured by means of faith and suffered martyrdom under Diocletian. From early times they became the protectors of physicians and pharmacists, and miraculous cures took place near their tombs. Justinian erected in honour of the two brothers a church which soon became a place of pilgrimage for the sick.

Special healing powers came to be attributed to many saints. St. Roch and St. Sebastian were invoked as protectors against pestilence, St. Job against leprosy, St. Anthony the Hermit against ergotism (called " St. Anthony's fire "), St. Anthony of Padua against various diseases, but especially fractures and diseases of the stomach and intestines. St. Apollonia was invoked for diseases of the teeth, St. Lucia had a great reputation for curing diseases of the eye. To many other saints were attributed miraculous cures at various times and places.

The medicine of the Church Fathers, like their philosophy, naturally closely followed Christian dogma. Tertullian (160–230), who called medicine the sister of philosophy, accepted the doctrines of the Stoics and of the Sicilian school and regarded the heart as the seat of the soul, and the soul as the seat of sensation and of knowledge. In accordance with Christian doctrine, he believed the instinct of self-preservation to be healthy and normal, but that the sexual instinct was sinful. Clement of Alexandria concerned himself with the physiology of childbirth and with dietetics. The plague, which sometimes was attributed to the machinations of the Christians and later, in the Middle Ages, of the Jews, was described by many of the Church Fathers, such as Cyprian, Dionysius, and Eusebius.

Among the medical writers of the Byzantine period, the one that deserves especial study is ORIBASIUS (325–403), born of a patrician family in Pergamon, a city that was already famous for having given birth to Galen and for having been the seat of a school of famous physicians. In Alexandria he was a pupil of Zeno, of Cyprus; in 355 he was called to the position of palace physician to the Emperor Julian, whom he accompanied on his voyages. His *Synagogæ medicæ* is an anthology, compiled by Julian's order, of the more important medical writings, in order to preserve the ancient texts in a complete medical treatise.

Oribasius was named by Julian, after his ascent to the throne, as Quæstor of Constantinople. Julian's successors, Valens and Valentinian, condemned Oribasius to exile; but his fame was so great that the two emperors were forced to recall him and restore his goods that had been confiscated.

The writings of Oribasius were first comprehensively collected and translated by Bussemaker and Daremberg, in a magnificent edition (Paris, 1851–6) comprising seventy books. The author closely follows Galen, but delves abundantly into the writings of Apuleius of Pergamus, Archigenes, Rufus, and Antyllus; Aristotle, Asclepiades, Soranus, and other writers are freely quoted from.

Some chapters, and especially those of an epitome bearing the name of *Synopsis*, that he wrote at the request of his son Eustachius, demonstrate his clarity of judgment; a good example is the chapter about diet in pregnancy, the choice of nurses, and diseases of children. Another work of Oribasius, the *Euporista*, is a small medical treatise addressed to the cultivated public. According to the author's statements in his preface, this book aimed to give the layman, while travelling or in the country and thus beyond the aid of the physician, some useful and practical advice on the treatment of disease or of unforeseen accidents.

First among later Byzantine writers was AËTIUS OF AMIDA, who lived in the early sixth century in Amida, a city on the banks of the Tigris. He studied in Alexandria, lived in Byzantium under Justinian, and wrote a medical compend in sixteen books, in which he quotes many of the Greek writers. The physicians of the Renaissance held Aëtius in great esteem. Cornarius regarded him as the greatest of medical writers. Boerhaave thought that the work of Aëtius should hold for the physician the same place that the Pandects of Justinian held for the lawyer. Among modern writers, however, Wellmann and Puschmann have judged him severely. As a matter of fact, he should be regarded chiefly as a compiler, though he must be allowed good critical sense in the choice of his material.

His *Tetrabiblos* (so called because in some manuscripts the text is divided and subdivided into four parts each), a work, in Greek, of sixteen books, is a compilation which constitutes the chief source of knowledge for the works of Rufus and Leonides in surgery, and of Soranus and Philumenus in gynæcology and obstetrics. Aëtius gives perhaps the best classical description of diseases of the eyes, ears, nose and throat, and teeth; he has good accounts of goitre, hydrophobia, an epidemic of diphtheria, and various surgical procedures, such as tonsillectomy, urethrotomy, and the treatment of hemorrhoids. He is said to have been the first to describe ligation above an aneurysm of the brachial artery. However, he does not hesitate to use charms, some based on the Bible, as an aid in various treatments. There is as yet no complete edition of the Greek text. A Latin translation of the entire work was published at Venice, 1534; a better one at Basel, 1542, the latter being several times reprinted.

ALEXANDER OF TRALLES (525–605?) is the Byzantine writer who has been most carefully studied in recent times. He probably practised, and may also have taught, in Rome. He enjoyed a great contemporary reputation among the most illustrious men of his time, and died at a ripe old age surrounded by many devoted pupils. His chief work was a pathology and therapy of internal disease in twelve books, in which he assembled the observations made in the course of a long life of practice, arranged to serve as a basis for instruction.

His writings were soon translated into the Arabic and Latin (*Libri duodecim de re medica*) and were quoted by all the great medical writers. A Latin translation was first published in 1504. The first Greek edition was printed in Paris in 1548; his first Greco-Latin edition in Basel in 1556; an excellent Greek edition with German translation was published by Puschmann (Vienna, 1878–9). The works of Alexander have recently been published in a French translation by F. Brunet (4 vols., 1933–7, Paris).

Alexander was a physician of wide experience, but he possessed scanty anatomical and physiological knowledge. He studied the diseases of the nervous system with great care. Phrenitis was regarded as a cerebral disease to be treated with narcotics, bleeding, warm baths, wine, and so on. Melancholia could change into mania, and represented an advanced stage of dementia. He devotes special attention to the treatment of diseases of the eye. Diseases of the respiratory tract are described clearly; for hemoptysis he prescribes absolute rest, potions of diluted vinegar, cold compresses on the chest, and strict diet, hot or cold soups, and, finally, bleeding for patients of a plethoric habit. For consumptives he strongly recommends change of air, sea voyages, easily digested food, and a milk cure, especially asses' milk.

The description of pleurisy and its treatment is clearly that of a master. In the domain of diseases of the stomach and the intestine also we find in Alexander a profound and exact observer. In one of his letters we find the names of various intestinal parasites with accurate differentiation of oxyuris, ascaris, and tænia, for which he prescribes the seeds of pomegranate, fern, and castor oil. For ascaris he especially prescribes a decoction of *artemisia maritima*, seeds of coryander, timianus. For oxyuris he prescribes enemas of ethereal oils.

In the chapter on the treatment of gout, or rather podagra, Alexander prescribes bleeding and strong purges (aloes) and coloquinth, diaphoretics, and diuretics.

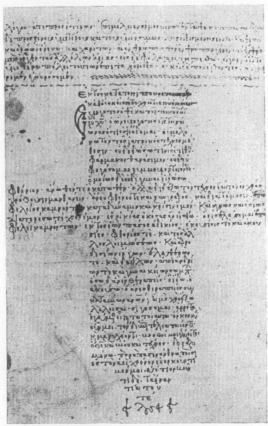

93. *The Oath of Hippocrates written in the form of a cross, a Byzantine manuscript of the twelfth century.* (VATICAN LIBRARY.)

We also find in his books the account of a cyclical dietetic cure, according to which the patient should live for a year on a strict diet, avoiding every excess, and taking purges regularly on determined days.

The last great Byzantine physician is PAUL OF ÆGINA, who belongs to the first half of the seventh century and who attained great fame even in his lifetime. He also studied at Alexandria and came to Rome. His works were early translated by the Arabs. The work *On Medicine*, in seven books, is the only one of his writings that has been preserved. The first book treats of dietetic hygiene; the second of general pathology; the third of diseases of the hair, brain, nerves, ears, eyes, nose, and mouth; the fourth of leprosy, skin diseases, burns, general surgery, and hemorrhage; the fifth is devoted to poisons; the sixth to surgery, and the seventh to pharmacology. The most noteworthy of these books is the sixth, devoted to surgery; we find descriptions in it that give us a clear idea of the progress made by surgery since the time of Celsus. It demonstrates that, in spite of scanty anatomical knowledge, the technical skill of the surgeons of the period had arrived at such a point that they could attain to notable success in difficult and delicate operations.

According to Paul, the most frequent site of cancer is the uterus and the breast. He regards operation on the former as useless, in view of the rapidity of recurrence. For cancer of the breast, he recommends extirpation, and advises against the cauterization that was recommended by some physicians.

For various internal infections, such as abscess of the liver and diseases of the spleen, he recommends the use of the cautery. Catheterization of the bladder with subsequent injection of various drugs is described with much exactness. Thus Paul indicates precisely the curves that the solid catheter must follow in the curvatures of the urethra.

In Chapter 60 there is a good description of lithotomy, indicating the proper position of the patient. He describes the way in which the lithotome should be introduced, and the procedures for avoiding hemorrhage. The operations for scrotal and inguinal hernia are accurately described. We quote here the radical operation for inguinal hernia, which was regarded as a classic up to the end of the seventeenth century: " One makes an incision the length of three fingers' width in the inguinal region above the swelling. One separates the skin and the fat and exposes the peritoneum and pushes aside the intestines with the tip of a sound. The bulges of the peritoneum, which are formed on two sides of the sound, are united with sutures, after the sound is withdrawn; one does not cut the peritoneum or touch the testicle, but one proceeds simply to the treatment of the wound."

Castration, designated under the name of eunuchism, is described with a technique which could be either the crushing of the testicle in a hot bath, a procedure that was always recommended in the case of children, or its extirpation.

In other chapters Paul of Ægina treats of the operation for condylomata of the female genitalia, and also for atresia, and describes the position to be assumed by the patient. The preparation of the genital organs is indicated in the following detail: " For the operation the woman is placed on a chair, turned backwards, with her limbs flexed against the stomach and the thighs open. The forearm should be placed against the knee and attached to it by a bandage fixed to the nape of the neck. The operator should be seated on the right side of the patient and proceed to her examination with the aid of a speculum, the size of which is proportionate to the age of the patient. If the speculum is larger than the vagina, compresses should be placed on the labia so as not to harm the patient. While the operator holds the speculum, the assistant turns the screw which separates the leaves of the speculum and thus makes possible the enlargement of the vulva."

The treatment of anal fistulas, hemorrhoids, anal condylomata, and varices is indicated in considerable detail. In the treatment of fractures Paul almost always follows the indications of Hippocrates and Oribasius. His descriptions, however, reveal a rich personal experience, and at times in quoting the opinion of Hippocrates on a given condition he advises: " Time, however, has shown that this procedure is not advisable."

The books of Paul of Ægina, and especially the book on surgery, bring valuable contributions to the history of medicine toward the end of the Eastern Empire. They show us that even though notable progress was accomplished in the field of scientific research in this century and that even though, as we have seen, dogmatism had become absolute, nevertheless practical medicine, and especially surgery, had not remained stationary.

Under Justinian the Eastern Empire was ravaged by a frightful pestilence which bears the name of this Emperor. It was preceded in the year 512 by a violent eruption of Vesuvius, which was followed by a series of earthquakes which devastated the Ægean Islands. In 526 a violent earthquake destroyed the city of Antioch, killing more than three hundred thousand people. In 542, for the first time, Constantinople was visited by the plague in epidemic form. The chronicles of the period state that many thousands of sick people died daily in Constantinople, and narrate that the epidemic was so violent that more than half of the Roman Empire of the East was destroyed and that many flourishing cities were left without inhabitants. This pestilence without question contributed greatly to the end of the Byzantine civilization.

5. Characteristics of Byzantine Medicine. The Decadence of Scientific Medicine

Byzantine medicine, then, should be regarded as the manifestation of a period of decadence, when the transmission of the Roman and Greek civilization to Byzantine Christianity felt the influence of the political and social conditions of a time of complicated intrigue, unbounded luxury, and relaxation of the moral sense. The philosophic mysticism of Roman decadence and the dawn of Christianity, together with the widespread belief in Oriental superstitions pervaded with magic and astrology, brought about a state of affairs in which the predominant authority of the Church was soon manifest.

The Church solemnly affirmed the principle that the canonical writings should be regarded as a supreme indisputable authority, not only in matters of faith but also in science. Medicine oriented itself rapidly in this direction. The first Christian physicians, among whom were many dignitaries of the Church, such as Theodore of Laodicea, Eusebius, Bishop of Rome, and Zenobius, priest of the Christian community at Sidon, practised medicine in this way. They preached the all importance of faith and recognized the complete authority of the Nazarene, whose gospel is addressed to suffering humanity awaiting salvation. Mysticism was already flourishing in decadent Rome, and had led the people, broken by long wars and frightful epidemics, to the cult of Æsculapius, which maintained its greatest splendour in the second and third centuries of our era. The people now turned passionately to Christianity as toward the Saviour of soul and body. Sufferers welcomed Christianity with a new faith, and it is for this reason that one sees the Church Fathers devoting themselves to the care of the sick with enthusiasm and infinite pity. The very fact that thousands who suffered in both body and soul turned to the new religion and its priests is sufficient explanation of the necessity for medicine becoming an important consideration to the ecclesiastics. Helping the sick especially assumed the greatest importance in Christian thought, even though modern historical criticism may refuse to admit that the first hospitals arrived with Christianity. The truly new and dominating concept is that hereafter the assistance of the sick is imposed as a duty on both the individual and the community — an ethical and religious duty from which no one is exempt. In the Epistle of St. James one reads: " Is any sick among you? let him call for the elders of the church; and let them pray over him, anointing him with oil in the name of the Lord " (v, 14). The supreme care of the sick is often confided to the bishop; on him are dependent the deacons and deaconesses who should assist the sick. Public hospitals prospered everywhere. The most ancient of these was founded at Cæsarea by St. Basil, A.D. 370; in 400 Fabiola constructed at Rome the first of the great hospitals; and it is about this time that the hospitals of the Empress Eudoxia were built in Jerusalem. These early structures bore the names of *xenodochion, nosocomium*, or *brephotrophium*.

Soon there were added hospices for travellers and pilgrims, and leprosaria, especially in southern Italy and Constantinople. The *parabolani* (male nurses) were charged with aiding the sick and bringing them to the hospital. There were many of them at Alexandria. Thus in the first flourishing period of Christianity medicine experienced the profound changes that the new political and social conditions and the arrival of Christianity determined throughout the civilized world, but especially in the basin of the Mediterranean. After having been successively empirical and priestly, after having risen to great heights of scientific research in the most brilliant period of Hellenism, after having become experimental and philosophic in the great schools of Alexandria, Sicily, and Asia Minor, after having played an extremely important role in the politics and hygiene of the State in the Roman Empire, medicine now returns again in the period of Roman decadence to shelter itself in the shadow of the Church. Under the influence and domination of Christianity, it becomes a dogmatic medicine, of which faith is the first article. Its essential aim is the assistance of the sick, regarded as a work of human and divine pity.

CHAPTER XIII

ARABIAN MEDICINE

LAY MEDICINE. RENAISSANCE OF CLASSIC DOCTRINES

1. Origins of Arabian Medicine

AT this time, when the lands that had been the great centres of civilization had been devastated by wars, depopulated by epidemics, and invaded by barbarian hordes that crossed the Alps and poured into Italy, the fall of the Roman Empire of the West marks a period of arrest in the history of civilization. Rigidified in a system of formulas and dominated by mysticism, medicine was forced to exist in a state of scholastic dogmatism, in which it is difficult to find any animating ideas. In Italy the traditions of recent grandeur, only too quickly forgotten, were kept alive solely by those who lived within the shadow of the church or cloister. The medical thought which was founded on analysis, criticism, and experience, established in its fundamental concepts by the Greek school, further developed in the school of Alexandria, and systematized by Galen, returned to the ancient paths of its distant origins. Syria, the theatre of eternal contests, a blood-stained land where the most ancient civilizations, Babylonian, Hittite, Egyptian, Persian, and Jewish, had left their profound traces, was now the country which gave shelter to Greek thought and especially to medicine. From the flourishing ancient medical schools of the Empire that had illuminated all the Mediterranean countries was born the school of the Nestorians. NESTORIUS, Patriarch of Constantinople in the beginning of

[258]

the fifth century, died in exile in Egypt in 440 — one of the many heresiarchs whose profoundly sectarian mind troubled the Christian Church in its early centuries. The Nestorians were the founders of the medical schools of Edessa and Nisibis, which attained great importance toward the end of the fifth century. It was these Christians of the Orient who brought the Greek civilization with them into exile, translated the Greek texts into

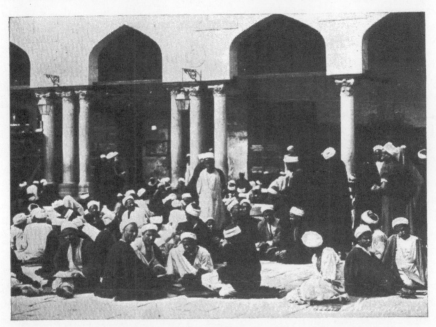

94. *The school in the mosque El-Azhar at Cairo.*

Syriac, and spread knowledge of them through the Orient from Syria to Mesopotamia. Expelled from home by religious persecution, they found refuge in Persia, and brought to the countries that received them in a spirit of tolerance the treasure of the great Persian school of Gondischapur (Jundi Shapur), in which all the arts and sciences were taught and the learning of Aristotle and Hippocrates was devotedly received. As Elgood has emphasized, Gondischapur was long the storehouse of Western medicine, until it was bled to death to vitalize the school of Bagdad. In the older school were trained the Bakhtîschû, Hunain, Meşue, and many other excellent physicians. The school disappeared in the ninth century, and Elgood says that on a recent visit he could find no trace of its ancient glory. When the last pagan philosophers, belonging to the latest Platonist school of Athens, were expelled by Justinian I in 529, they joined the Nestorian current. Thus Greek civilization assumed Oriental clothing, entering Persia by way of Mesopotamia with the aid of other ethnic groups, such as the Jews and the Hellenized Persians.

When the Arabs, united by the impulse of religious fanaticism, emerged beyond the boundaries of their own country and advanced to the conquest of Syria and Persia, they discovered these ancient schools and on their victorious way came in contact with this civilization, which actually was not entirely unknown to them. Already before the time of Mahomet certain physicians who had been brought up in the Hellenic school had brought their science to the Arabs. In quick succession the faithful of Islam occupied Damascus (635), Cæsarea (640), and Alexandria (643). Victory everywhere followed the banner of the Prophet. The dominion of Islam extended from the banks of the Indus to the Caucasus and included almost all of northern Africa and southern Spain, Sardinia, and Sicily. Bagdad was founded in 762 and became the capital of the caliphate.

During this century of furious strife and bloody victories the new conquerors felt the necessity of taking over the civilization of the conquered countries. The caliphs became the most ardent protectors of the schools of learning: first the school of Bagdad attained the greatest splendour; then at Samarkand, Ispahan, and Damascus there arose new and flourishing academies. They were housed in buildings crowded about the mosque, such as those one still sees in the Arabian universities that have been preserved. Teachers and pupils lived there; there were rooms for the libraries, but also for ambulatory and bed patients, and often there were hospitals. In these academies pupils from all parts received their instruction, a little in all the sciences, but especially in theology, philosophy, and medicine. The texts for the study of medicine were at first entirely translations from the Greek. In 765, the Caliph al-Mansûr (died A.D. 769), greatly developed the ancient school of Gondischapur; other caliphs, and especially the descendants of Harûn-al-Raschîd (763?–809), favoured the school of Bagdad, which became the principal centre of learning and certainly felt the influence of the currents of Indian thought. Nestorian physicians and Sabæans (star-worshippers, astronomers, and mathematicians from Harrân in Mesopotamia) were well received by the Arabs and translated the Greek texts, especially those of Galen. The Arabian passion for mathematics and physics and especially for chemistry brought about a new development in these studies, all of which was integrated with a wide practical experience and accurate observation at the bedside. Thus, in its new Oriental raiment, medicine began again to be Hippocratic — based on experience and logic — as if the contribution to science by this race of warriors was determined by a fresh and youthful concept and by a simple manner of reasoning (far removed from scholastic speculation), always ready to return to that Nature to which these people of nomadic origin were so closely bound.

To the great power of Islam was joined the splendour of Arabian scholarship in Spain. New and flourishing schools were being rapidly founded: at Cordova (founded in 960), which soon possessed a library of three hundred thousand volumes and became the centre of Spanish knowledge, at Seville, Toledo, and Murcia. At this period, in which Arabian domination attained its greatest heights, and art and poetry had their maximum development, medicine was regarded as the most precious of all forms of instruction. Thus the Arabs inherited all the medical patrimony of the past and became the faithful guardians of ancient medicine. When they and their relations disappeared from the theatre of their greatest exploits, and the fall of the Arabian domination of Spain marked the end of this historic period, the traces that they left were so remarkable that they remain highly significant of the role that the Arabs played in the history of civilization and of medicine.

This contribution of the Arabs to the history of medicine has been differently evaluated by historians. Some think that it is entirely due to Islam that the traditions of Hippocrates and Galen were not lost for ever in the night of the Middle Ages. Others, on the other hand, maintain that the contribution of the Arabs to the progress of medicine should be regarded as practically nil, because they merely became the depositaries of medical knowledge that at the same time was confided to the Fathers of the Church, handing it over at the time of the Renaissance without having contributed any notable additions. We believe that their contribution is indeed difficult to evaluate, short of examining all of the elements that contribute to the interesting phenomenon of the recurrent development of medical culture in the Mediterranean. It is, then, not a question of an isolated episode; in fact, one cannot even properly speak of an Arabian medicine as such. We must consider that after the fall of the Roman Empire of the East, the Mediterranean for several centuries came entirely or almost entirely under the power of Islam, because the Arabs dominated most of its shores, and its commercial traffic belonged to them. It was through the Arabian storehouses and harbours that the enormous current of Oriental products passed; the commercial expansion and growing richness of the Arab peoples were contemporaneous with their territorial expansion. These new masters came in contact in the recently conquered countries with peoples who were more highly developed and had a more advanced culture. Thus, as is always the case in history, feeling the necessity for understanding and absorbing this more cultured civilization, they sought contact with the philosophy, art, and medicine of the Greeks. The intermediaries of this exchange were above all the Syrians and the Jews, who were related by race and religion to the Arabs and were favourably received by them. It was the Syrians, imbued with Greek culture, who became the trans-

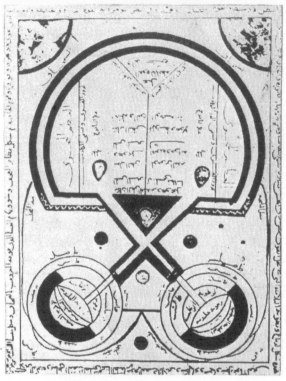

*95. Representation of the cerebrum with the optic chiasm and the eyes.
Arabian manuscript of the fifteenth century.*

lators of the Greek classics into Arabic, just as several centuries later the Jews were the translators of the Greek works from Arabic into Spanish. The Jews were the great intermediaries of the Mediterranean, through whose hands there passed for centuries all the material treasures of science as well as those of art and literature. The influence of the Jews on the Arabs was felt especially in medicine. Generally, Jewish physicians were philosophers and subtle reasoners, able practitioners, especially versed in the study of botany, and expert in diagnosis. Arabian medicine is in reality formed by various diverse currents which exercised their predominating influences according to the times and places in which they developed. Only a few of the writers and teachers of so-called Arabian medicine were native Arabs. The chief contribution of the Arabs to the history of medicine, then, was that of collecting and concentrating these various currents, with the further credit of adding a special impetus toward chemistry and the exact sciences in general, and a notable tendency to lay practice.

The truth doubtless lies between the two extreme views that we have just mentioned. It is not proper to deny, as writers such as Puccinotti and Daremberg have done, all credit whatever to the Arabs, because it is certain that many of the chief works of the Greeks would have been more or less lost if they had not been patiently preserved and commented upon and accurately translated by the Arabs. Furthermore, some of the great Arabian physicians have certainly made notable progress in the domain of practical medicine. Neither would it be in accord with the facts to regard them as the sole guardians of Greek medicine without whom the thread of the tradition of Greek science would have been completely severed.

When the Middle Ages were under consideration, too many historians have committed the error of exaggerating the sombre picture of the first centuries after the fall of the Roman Empire of the West, presenting them as a period in which every delicacy, every fine æsthetic tradition, and every manifestation of science was forgotten. Certainly at that time the flame of civilization did not burn high in a Europe devastated by wars, pestilences, famine, and general misery, when for years a renewed mysticism was dominant and the sum of scientific knowledge seemed to be enclosed within the walls of monasteries. But within these very walls humble but patient scholars whose names have rarely come down to us maintained as a slender flame, obscure but still alive, the light of the ancient tradition. At the same time, independently and under different conditions, the medicine of Hippocrates and Galen found refuge in the schools of Islam, where it could flourish and develop, thanks to the political and commercial prosperity of the people that dominated the culture of that era.

This historical period of Arabian medicine, which lasted more than seven centuries, coincided with the most flourishing period of Islam. It is particularly interesting, therefore, as it furnishes a characteristic example of certain laws which seemed to regulate the evolution of medical thought.

We can speak but briefly of the first period of Arabian medicine and only note that Mahomet already understood the importance of physical health and promulgated important hygienic rules. We find also in his writings certain medico-chirurgical indications which show that the concepts of the earlier times were not very different from those of other monotheistic peoples for whom the healing art is regarded as a supreme attribute of the Divinity.

Elgood speaks of a well-known work, *Tibb-ul-Nabbi* (*Medicine of the Prophet*), which claimed to be the very words of Mahomet. This collection of traditional sayings was committed to writing in the eighteenth

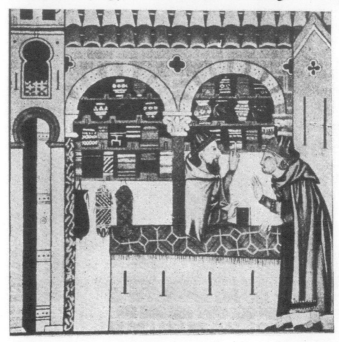

96. *An Arabian pharmacy. Miniature in a codex of the fourteenth century.*

century and cheap copies still circulate in the bazaars of the East, containing among the short epigrams and aphorisms many of a dietetic nature, such as: " The best food is bread and the second best meat. Nothing can replace milk both as a food and as a drink."

The Arabs soon came into contact with Oriental medicine, and especially with the schools of Alexandria and of Syria. In the Nestorian schools of Edessa and Nisibis, illustrious masters taught medicine, translating the ancient Greek classics into Syrian and Persian. Soon, under the protection of the Abbasids, actual schools were formed in which the Greek originals were translated and preserved with the greatest care as precious treasures. Of all the Greek writers, Aristotle was the most studied, the most translated and venerated by the Arabs. The works of the great Greeks such as Hippocrates, Dioscorides, Galen, Oribasius, Alexander of Tralles, and Paul of Ægina were often translated, widely commented upon, and diligently studied. But at the same time the Persian, Chaldean, and Indian currents influenced the culture of the Arabs, who as a primitive people were particularly sensitive to foreign influence. It is the valuable material from all these sources that became the precious edifice on which the Arabs based their knowledge.

2. First Period

The history of Arabian medicine and its literature can be divided into three great periods, of which the earliest (750–900) includes the first two or three centuries after the Hejira (622). It may be called a period of preparation influenced on the one hand by the current deriving from the ancient traditions of the Arab tribes and the fundamental regulations of the Koran, on the other hand by Greek medicine, which in the translations penetrated into the schools and academies. In this period also was felt the influence of Egyptian currents, magic and hermetic medicine, when alchemy began to develop. The Greek philosophers, notably Aristotle, were studied; astronomers and geographers, especially Hipparchus and Ptolemy, became familiar to students. All the great Greeks from Hippocrates to Paul of Ægina assumed Arabian raiment. In this first period there were but few writers who treated the subject from an original point of view; all seemed bound by the authority of the ancients. It is during this period that we find the names of authors who were the first representatives of the transition period: such as those belonging to the Nestorian family BAKHTÎSCHÛ (*Bokht-Ioko, Bukht-Yishu, Bakhtyashû*) — servants of Jesus — which produced famous physicians. No fewer than seven of them were court physicians, up to the eleventh century. The first of this dynasty of physicians, George (Jurjis), was the head of the hospital of Gondishapur and was called to Bagdad in 765 by the Caliph al-Mansûr, who received him with great honours. His son was the personal physician to the Caliph Harûn-al-Raschîd, and one of the outstanding representatives of Hippocratic medicine in Arabia. Bakhtîschû IV, of the seventh generation of this dynasty, was the physician of al-Muqtadir, who died A.D. 940.

Still another well-known family was that of QURRAH, a Sabæan from Harrân. The grandson, SINAN, was both a diligent translator and a competent physician who was given charge of epidemics by the caliphate and made president of a board of examiners that examined as many as 860 candidates at one time (see Elgood). In 918 he opened a hospital in Bagdad that was one of the first of a long series which Arabian medicine has to its credit.

Under the Omayyad caliphs of Damascus there lived a Jewish Persian physician, MASARGIAWAIH, who translated from Syrian into Arabic the *Pandectæ medicæ* of the Syrian Christian priest and physician Aharon. This was certainly the first work of Greek origin that fell into the hands of the Arabian physician and was often quoted by the authors of the later period and especially by Rhazes.

YÛHANNÂ O YAHYÂ IBN MÂSAWAYH (the Mesue of the Latin writers) was the first Syrian medical writer to use the Arabic tongue. He was of Christian origin and practised medicine in Bagdad; was physician of the Caliph al-Ma'mûn, who about 830 put him in charge of a school of translators to whom the Caliph gave the task of translating Greek manuscripts acquired in Asia Minor and Egypt. This outstanding physician of the first period is known in the literature of the Renaissance as Mesue the Older, and also as Johannes Damascenus, or JOHN OF DAMASCUS. He died in 857, leaving many works on dietetics and gynæcology, among which the most important was the *Aphorisms,* first published in Bologna in 1489, in a volume headed by the Aphorisms of Maimonides.

The best of the pupils of Mesue and the most illustrious of the translators was HUNAIN IBN ISHÂQ, known in the West as Johannitius (809–873), a Nestorian born at Hira in Mesopotamia. He was certainly the most profound student of the Greek language among the Oriental scholars, and to him is due the creation of the technical terms and the scientific language of the Arabs. All the Arabian scientific writers of later times used the terminology created by Hunain, who adapted many words from the Greek and Persian into Arabian forms when no equivalent Arab word was available. Many of these words then penetrated into Latin mediæval translations. Hunain made more than two hundred translations from the Greek into Syriac and Arabic; many of the former were later translated into Arabic by his pupils. He was the official translator of the Caliph al-Mutawakkil, translating into Arabic all the *Corpus Hippocraticum,* all the writings of Oribasius and Paul of Ægina and Dioscorides' classical text on pharmacology, the Dioscorides especially having an enormous influence on the Arabian writers. The translations of Hunain were regarded as classics and are today of the greatest importance for the textual criticism of the Greek writers and for the reconstruction of many ancient medical texts whose originals have been lost. Hunain also translated many of the works of Aristotle. He was for some time out of favour, but toward the end of his life he had the reputation of being the most illustrious physician and most famous scientist in all Islam. He left more than one hundred writings of his own, among the most famous of which is the *Quæstiones medicinæ,* a textbook in the form of questions and answers, and the *Ten Dissertations on the Eye,* which is preserved in Arabic and in a Salernitan edition in Latin by Constantinus Africanus.

Among his many pupils the most celebrated were his son Ishâq, who translated many important philosophic texts into Arabic, and his nephew Hubaisch, who translated into Arabic the Syrian translations of his uncle. Hunain's writings were so highly valued that he is said to have been paid for them by their weight in gold.

The most important Arabian medical works of the ninth century are entirely derived from Greek medicine. Yûhannâ ibn Sarâbiûn (the Serafion or Serapion of Western writers) was a Syrian Christian who wrote several works that were soon translated into Arabic and therefore regarded in the Renaissance as original Arabic writings. His principal work, called *Aphorisms*, in twelve books, was adopted by the Arabian schools as a textbook and can still be found today in all the great medical libraries of the East. Another of his works, called *Pandectæ*, in seven books, almost exclusively derives from Alexander of Tralles. It was translated into Latin by Gerard of Cremona, and first published in Venice in 1479. Serapion was frequently quoted by the medical writers of the Renaissance.

Alî ibn Rabban al-Tabarî, a Christian born in eastern Persia and converted to Islamism, wrote a medical treatise, called *Firdaus-ul Hikmat* (*The Paradise of Wisdom*), which was one of the first medical encyclopædias and enjoyed a great success. This book is especially interesting for a chapter on Indian medicine and its influence on Persian medicine.

3. The Flourishing Period of Arabian Medicine

In the second period, that of the greatest glory of Arabian medicine, writers showed some independence from their old masters. Although they derived the essentials of their doctrines from ancient medicine and cited Hippocrates and Galen with respect, we can also observe in their writings a spirit of observation and even of intelligent criticism, and a tendency to develop new lines, especially in the field of therapeutics.

In this period of Arabian medical splendour, the best-known writer, whose works were studied through centuries by physicians all over the world and cited as an indisputable authority, is Abû Bakr Muhammad ibn Zakariâ, called Rhazes (865–925), a Persian like most of the great physicians of the Arabian period. He was properly regarded as chief of the practical physicians of his time. After having studied medicine at the school of Bagdad, he became physician to the hospital of Raj (Ray) in Tabaristan, near Teheran, the part of Persia in which he was born. Later he moved to Bagdad, where he quickly acquired the reputation of a great physician and a worthy teacher. Al-Mansûr, ruler of Bokhara, maltreated him, according to the legend, because of the failure of some chemical experiments that he had promised to carry out, commanding that he be beaten with his own book till either the head or the book was broken. Rhazes is said to have lost his sight as a result. Later, wishing to regain his vision, he refused operation when he found that the surgeon was ignorant of the gross anatomy of the eyeball.

Rhazes' fame rests not only on his differentiation of smallpox from measles and other exanthemata, but also on the use of animal gut in sutures, and the introduction of various new remedies such as mercurial ointment. He is said to have been the first to describe *spina ventosa* and to show that the swelling caused by guinea worm was due to a parasite. In a treatise on anatomy he described the recurrent laryngeal nerve.

Rhazes died in want at an advanced age. He left more than two hundred books on medicine, philosophy, religion, mathematics, and astronomy. Of his books, three which have been preserved are of great importance: the first is a sort of encyclopædia of practical medicine and therapy bearing the Arabic name *al-Hâwî*, and known in Western literature under the title of *Liber Continens*.

This book is an enormous compilation that includes all the knowledge of the Mohammedan world at the beginning of the tenth century. Rhazes died before it was finished; but it was completed by his pupils. The *Continens* was translated by order of Charles of Anjou, King of Sicily, by the Jewish physician Farag ben Salem of Girgenti, who completed the work in 1279. In the complete manuscript in the Escorial the *Continens* is composed of twenty-four books. The *editio princeps*, printed by Jacobus Britannicus in folio (Brescia, 1486), is the largest incunabulum in existence, weighing about twenty-two pounds.

The second of Rhazes' important works is the *Liber medicinalis ad Almansorem*, dedicated to the Governor of Chorasan, al-Mansûr ibn Ishâq; it contains a compend of ten treatises on the most important medical subjects. Of these books, the worthiest of note are the seventh, on general surgery, and the ninth, on the treatment of all diseases, the latter called in Latin *Nonus Almansoris*. It was often read and commented upon in the Western universities, and was frequently printed separately or with the *Microtechne* of Galen. Frequently quoted in the Renaissance period also were the *Aphorisms* of Rhazes. One of the most celebrated of these states: " When Galen and Aristotle agree on a subject, the decision of physicians is easy; but when their opinions differ, it is very difficult to bring them into agreement." The most important book of Rhazes, from the point of view of the medical historian, is the work on smallpox, which was called *Liber de Pestilentia*, and was first published in Valla's Nicephori Logica collection (Venice, 1498).

This book can be regarded as certainly and completely original; it is founded on the experiences and personal observations of a physician who knows how to examine the patient completely and to draw from his observations the conclusions of a great intellect. This is the first accurate study that we possess of the infectious diseases. Rhazes distinguished two kinds: true smallpox and measles. Both forms are described in detail according to their signs and symptoms, with indications for differential diagnosis. In the prognosis of the course of the disease the author advises close attention to the action of the heart, the pulse, the respiration, and the excreta. He states that a warm temperature favours the appearance of the rash; he prescribes measures to protect the eyes, the face, and the mouth, and to avoid the occurrence of deep scars. The cosmetic section is thus treated with no less attention than the therapeutic portion.

We quote the most interesting passage of this famous description of smallpox: "As to any physician who says that the excellent Galen has made no mention of the Small-Pox, and was entirely ignorant of this disease, surely he must be one of those who have either never read his works at all, or who have passed over them very cursorily. . . . If, however, anyone says that Galen has not mentioned any peculiar and satisfactory mode of treatment for this disease, nor any complete cause, he is certainly correct; for, unless he has done so in some of his works which have not been published in Arabic, he has made no further mention of it than we have just cited (Ch. I). . . . I am now to mention the seasons of the year in which the Small-Pox is most prevalent; which are, the latter end of the autumn, and the beginning of the spring (Ch. II). . . . The eruption of the Small-Pox is preceded by a continued fever, pain in the back, itching in the nose, and terrors in sleep. These are the more peculiar symptoms of its approach, especially a pain in the back, with fever; then also a pricking which the patient feels all over his body; a fullness of the face, which at times goes and comes; an inflamed colour, and vehement redness in both the cheeks; a redness of both the eyes; a heaviness of the whole body; great uneasiness, the symptoms of which are stretching and yawning; a pain in the throat and chest, with a slight difficulty in breathing, and cough; a dryness of the mouth, thick spittle, and hoarseness of the voice; pain and heaviness of the head; inquietude, distress of mind, nausea, and anxiety; (with this difference, that the inquietude, nausea, and anxiety are more frequent in the Measles than in the Small-Pox; while, on the other hand, the pain in the back is more peculiar to the Small-Pox than to the Measles;) heat of the whole body, an inflamed colour, and shining redness, and especially an intense redness of the gums (Ch. III). . . . As to those white pustules which are very small, close to each other, hard, warty, and containing no fluid, they are of a bad kind, and their badness is in proportion to the degree of difficulty in their ripening. And if the patient be not relieved upon their eruption, but his condition continues unfavourable after it is finished, it is a mortal sign. And as to those which are of a greenish, or violet, or black colour, they are all of a bad and fatal kind; and when, besides, a swooning and palpitation of the heart come on, they are worse and still more fatal. And when the fever increases after the appearance of the pustules, it is a bad sign (Ch. XIV) . . . (Greenhill's translation, Sydenham Society Publications, 1848).

Interesting also are certain aphorisms that are found in the famous *Liber ad Almansorem:* " The truth in medicine is a goal that one cannot attain, and everything that is written in books is worth much less than the experience of a physician who reflects and reasons." And again: " He who interrogates many physicians will commit many errors."

Rhazes can be regarded as a Hippocratist in the true sense of the word. Opposed to every sort of charlatanism, he was the first of the Arabians to combat the exaggerated importance that was attached to the examination of the urine. This was the period in which physicians claimed to be able to diagnose pregnancy and almost any disease by examining the urine without seeing the patient.

A well-known physician who is often quoted in the literature of the early Renaissance is Alî ibn al-Abbâs al-Magûsî, known in the West as HALY ABBAS (died 994). He was born (year unknown) in Ahwaz, in southern Persia, near Gondischapur. The title " magus " signifies that he was descended from a Persian family of the faith of Zoroaster. He has left a book, in Arabic, which bears the title *The Perfect Book of the Art of Medicine;* it was translated into Latin by Constantinus Africanus, of Montecassino, about 1180, under the name of *Pantegni*, without Constantinus indicating in any way the name of the real author. A later Latin translation by Stephen of Antioch, about 1200, bore the name of *Liber Regius* (known to the Persians as *Kitab-I-Malikî* or *Kamil-ul-Sina*), which attained a great reputation. This translation was published in Venice in 1492, and in Lyon in 1523. Though soon superseded in popularity by Avicenna's Canon, the book was thought by many earlier generations to be superior to the Canon. Browne writes that in his opinion it was " far superior in style, arrangement and interest " to the Canon and contained admirable estimates of Haly's predecessors and a good description of pleurisy. He suggests that Haly Abbas was the first to suggest the existence of the blood capillary system, when he stated that there were pores between the pulsating and the non-pulsating vessels — that is, between the arteries and the veins.

The most illustrious physician of this golden age of Arabian medicine, without doubt, is AVICENNA (Abû Alî al-Hussein ibn Abdallâh ibn Sînâ) (980–1037), who was born in a little town near Bokhara in Persia. After studying the Koran, which he knew perfectly at the age of ten, then grammar and dialectics, geometry and astronomy, he dedicated himself to Aristotelian philosophy, and finally to medicine. The young physician was recognized by everyone as having a marvellous memory and a profound and

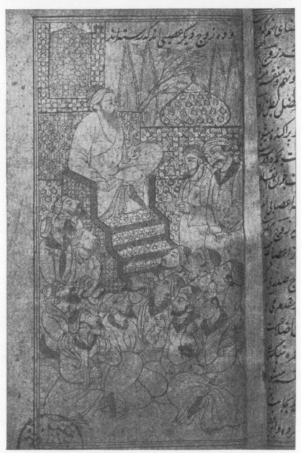

97. *Avicenna lectures on the anatomy of the cerebral nerves. (A Persian miniature of the seventeenth century, from a text on human anatomy.)*
(Courtesy of Dr. M. Meyerhof, Cairo.)

extensive knowledge of all the medical works of his time. At the age of sixteen he began medical composition and throughout his stormy life, which led him through many transitions and great sufferings to death in the fifties, he gathered personal experiences which resulted in his book of the Canon (*Q'anun*). For the Orient, and later for the Western world also, this constituted a statement of authoritative, scholastic dogmatism which was founded much more on an extremely wide culture, extraordinary diligence, and brilliant exposition than on profound knowledge arising from personal experience. The Canon may best be regarded as a magnificent attempt to co-ordinate systematically all the medical doctrines of Hippocrates and Galen with the biological concepts of Aristotle. It was translated for the first time by GERARD OF CREMONA (born at Cremona in 1114, died at Toledo in 1187).

The medical science of Avicenna is founded on the humoral doctrine of Hippocrates. He does not admit the slightest doubt. He legislates in medical matters with an absolute authority, as is shown in the title that he selected, the Canon, with the idea that it should constitute an immutable law. The clarity of the clinical histories, the accuracy of the therapeutic indications, constructed logically and without dangerous exaggerations, and the eloquence of his forcible style were sufficient to confer on this book up to the end of the seventeenth century an almost indisputable authority in the minds of the physicians of all countries. It also led to the publication of innumerable commentaries.

The Canon of Medicine of Avicenna is divided into five large books. The first concerns itself essentially with theoretical medicine; the second with simple medicaments; the third with diseases and their treatment, *a capite ad calcem* (in other words, he examines all diseases according to their locality); the fourth book treats of general diseases (that is, those which attack different parts of the body at once); the fifth is devoted to the composition and preparation of drugs. Each book is divided into treatises (*fen*), each of which in its turn is subdivided into chapters and paragraphs. The first book contains in the first *fen* the definition of medicine, the methods that it employs, and its fundamental doctrines, all borrowed in their principal lines from Hippocratic texts. The second *fen* treats of general diseases and especially their symptoms, with lengthy observations and detailed precepts about the pulse and the examination of the urine. In the third *fen* is contained a number of hygienic and prophylactic prescriptions which constituted the principal source for all books on hygiene for centuries. In the last *fen* the author considers general therapeutics and especially enemas, purges, bleeding, cautery, and so on. These two *fens* remained important standards of medical treatment up to the seventeenth century. The second book, which is based especially on the writings of Dioscorides, contains, however, information about many drugs unknown to the Greeks. The third is devoted to special pathology. For every disease there are long descriptions of symptoms; especially interesting are those of pleurisy, empyema, and intestinal diseases, and a short description of venereal diseases. In order to give an idea of the way in which the diagnostic part is treated, we quote the passage describing the symptoms of pleurisy: " The signs of simple pleurisy are clear: the fever is continuous, there is a sharp pain beneath the ribs which sometimes is only felt when the patient breathes strongly. . . . The third sign is a difficulty and frequency of respiration; the fourth sign is a rapid and weak pulse; the fifth sign is the cough, which at first is dry and then is accompanied by sputum; in this case it signifies it is also an affection of the lung." The fourth book, the first chapter of which treats of fever in its various forms, describes a number of epidemic diseases, such as smallpox and measles. The fifth *fen* is a treatise on surgery, in which fractures and dislocations are well described. The seventh *fen* is a meticulous consideration of cosmetics. Finally, the fifth book contains detailed directions about the preparation of drugs; in the field of materia medica it constituted the classic text, accepted everywhere up to the time of the Renaissance.

The first complete edition of the Canon was printed at Milan in 1473. In 1523 the Giunta Press published the works of Avicenna with comments by the most illustrious Italian masters of the period. Whoever examines these volumes cannot fail to be impressed with the authority that this prince of Arabian physicians enjoyed in Europe.

A contemporary of Avicenna was the Persian Abû Mansûr Muwaffaq, who, about 975, wrote in the Persian language a *Compendium of Simple Remedies*, which has considerable historical and philological importance. Like the second book of the Canon of Avicenna, it contains a number of new Oriental remedies.

Isaac Judæus (the elder), in Arabic Ishâq ibn Sulaimân al-Isrâ'îlî (880?–932?), of Qairawan in Tunisia, a contemporary of Rhazes, was the greatest physician of Western Islam. He was especially eminent as an oculist. After the fall of the Aglabitic ruler of Qairawan, he entered the service of the Fatimid, al-Mahdî (908). His writings *De elementis*, *De febribus* (looked upon by him as his chief work), and *De urina* were regarded as classics and were translated into Latin in the eleventh century by Constantinus Africanus. These works were printed under the title *Opera Omnia Isaaci* (Lyon, 1515), and were in widespread use throughout Christendom. A book by Isaac Judæus, called *The Guide of Physicians*, lost in Arabic but extant in Hebrew and translated into Italian by Soave (*Giornale Veneto di Scienze Mediche*, 1861), contains many important maxims about the behaviour of the physician in the presence of the patient. His treatise *De particularibus diætis* (Padua, 1487) is supposed to be the first separately printed work on the subject of diet.

A pupil of his was the Mohammedan physician Ibn al-Giazzâr (Jazzar) (*c.* 920–1009), of Tunisia, whose celebrated book *Zâd al-Musâfir* was translated by Constantinus Africanus under the name *Viaticum peregrinantis*, and later in Sicily into Greek under the name *Ephodia*.

The Arab dominion of lower Spain also developed a Moorish medicine that included famous names. In Abulcasis, Cordova produced the greatest surgeon of the Arabian school. ABULCASIS (Alsaharavius or Abu'l-Qâsim) (d. *c.* 1013) was the author of a surgical treatise which in surgery held the same authority as did the Canon of Avicenna in medicine.

Abulcasis, born in the caliphate of Abd al-Rahmân III, near Cordova, is the most important of the Arabian surgical writers, though it is interesting to observe that he was probably not himself a surgeon. Although his work was not entirely original, as many of his statements and prescriptions were borrowed from Paul of Ægina, it nevertheless possessed the merit, from the historical point of view, of including personal observations and statements that reveal to us not only an author who was familiar with the ancient texts but also a wise and skilful practitioner. It is also valuable in presenting a good account of the surgery of the period; and, in the numerous and invaluable illustrations that it contains, gives an excellent picture of the instruments used by the Arabian surgeons. The surgical treatise which forms the thirtieth chapter is part of an encyclopædic work called *Tesrif* (*al-Tasrif* or *Vade Mecum*), divided into three parts. It was translated into Latin by Gerard of Cremona, also into Provençal and Hebrew, and was the most valued surgical text throughout the West. It is largely based upon Paul of Ægina. From it all the great surgeons of the fourteenth century drew valuable information, and Fabricius of Acquapendente regarded its author as the greatest of ancient surgeons.

Especially interesting are the author's observations, in his introduction, on the reasons why surgery made but little progress among the Arabs. He attributes it to an inadequate study both of anatomy and of the classic writers, especially of Galen, to whom he constantly refers. The first part is particularly concerned with cautery, which is especially recommended in surgical disorders, but also in apoplexy, epilepsy, and dislocation of the shoulder. For arterial hemorrhage he recommends digital compression followed by the cautery. The second book treats of surgical operations and advises above all not to undertake any operation without an exact program and without knowing the cause of the malady. He recommends the surgeon never to forget that omnipotent God is watching his work and that he therefore should never operate merely for the sake of gain. Especially interesting are the indications for lithotomy, for herniotomy, for the treatment of abdominal wounds. For injuries of the intestine he recommends holding together the edges of the wounds and applying large ants.

He describes lithotomy with especial care, but also the other operations in use at the time, such as trephining, amputations, the operations for fistula, goitre, and aneurysm. There are interesting observations about disorders of the teeth; he recommends the use of artificial teeth made of beef bone. For disorders of the bladder he recommends the use of a silver catheter instead of the bronze catheter that had been used up to that time. Various sutures for wounds, and particularly the double suture, are carefully described; and all the instruments that the surgeon should use are specified in detail. In the third book the author is especially concerned with fractures and dislocations, recommending once more the study of anatomy in the works of Galen.

Chapters 28 and 29 of the encyclopædia, which are devoted to materia medica, were much studied and frequently quoted in both the Orient and the Occident.

A Jewish physician of Spain, HASDAI BEN SCHAPRÛT, was the minister of the Grand Caliph, Abd al-Rahmân III, of Cordova. This monarch had received in 948 as a gift from the Emperor of Byzantium, Constantine Porphyrogenetus VII, a precious Greek manuscript of the *Materia medica* of Dioscorides with marvellous illustrations. As no one in Cordova at this time knew much Greek, in 950 the Emperor sent along the monk Nicholas of Cordova, who, with the aid of Hasdai and other Mohammedan physicians and herbalists, and using Hunain's translation of Dioscorides, translated all the names of the plants and drugs into Arabic. The Spanish-Arabian physician IBN GOLGOL (IBN JULJUL), who gives the details of this story, twenty years later added important notes and corrections to this translation. The book had an extraordinary influence on the pharmaceutical studies of Mohammedan Spain.

Ibn Golgol, contemporary with Abulcasis, was physician to the Spanish Omayyad court, and was known to have written *Lives of the Physicians and Philosophers*, which unfortunately is completely lost. Among the most celebrated of the Spanish physicians of the eleventh century was IBN AL-WÂFID (997–*c*. 1074) of Toledo, known also in the West as Abenguefit. He was a Minister of State and also wrote a famous book on treatment. Another was AL-BAKRÎ, who flourished in Cordova and died at an advanced age in 1094. He was a geographer as well as the author of *Medical Experiences*, which contains important therapeutic advice. Two Jewish physicians of this period attained renown: IBN-GIANÂH, a great philosopher and grammarian, and IBN BUKLARISCH, the body physician of an Arabian Prince of Saragossa; both wrote famous books on drugs.

The most celebrated of the Egyptian physicians of the eleventh century was Alî ibn Ridwân (HALY RODOAM to the Occident), a Mohammedan who had a wide knowledge of Greek medicine and of the Egyptian medicine of his time. To him we owe a medical topography of Egypt with many interesting descriptions of the poor hygienic conditions of Cairo.

Among the great Arabian physicians of this golden period were Ibn Giazla (in the Occident, BINGEZLA), a Christian converted to Islam, author of a text of pharmacy; also Alî ibn Isâ (in the Occident, JESU HALY), author of a book on the eye, the *Tadhkirat* (memorandum book for eye doctors), which was the standard throughout Islam and Christendom and is still used by the Arabs. It was translated at least twice into Latin and once into Hebrew in mediæval times. A German translation was published by Hirschberg and Lippert (1904), and one in English by Casey Wood (1936). ALHAZEN (Abu Alî al-Hasan ibn al Haitham), of Basra (965–1039), was one of the most important figures in the whole study of optics. He taught that the visual rays passed from the object to the eye and not contrariwise, as had been earlier believed. His main work is *On Optics*, though he wrote many other treatises, largely made up of extracts from the Greek. He correctly stated so many principles of optics and so well understood the eye and its function that he is rightly regarded as a figure of the greatest importance in this field.

4. Period of Decadence of Arabian Medicine

The third period, from the twelfth to the seventeenth centuries, though containing some celebrated figures, is chiefly one of decadence, contemporary with the decline of the caliphate, which was threatened internally by strife among the Arab dynasties, and externally by the growing power of Christendom. The wars of the Orient and the Occident finished with the destruction of the empire of Islam. Eventually the Osman Turks by successful military invasion occupied a great part of the territories that had belonged to the Arabs in the East. The school of Bagdad began to decline in the twelfth century, its most illustrious scholars moving to places where rulers such as the Turkish Nûr-al-Dîn ibn Zengî in Damascus and the famous Saladin in Egypt still resisted their enemies. Both these rulers were founders of great hospitals and promoted the progress of medicine in every possible way.

In Mohammedan Spain of the twelfth century, in spite of the wars that were prevalent, there occurred a period of great scientific progress. MUHAMMAD AL-IDRÎSÎ (or Edrisi), of the family of the caliphs of Morocco, a scholarly ruler, who for political motives had to flee from Spain and find refuge at the court of the King of Sicily, wrote two important works on geography, and also an excellent work on drugs, of which the first part has only recently been found. He and the philosopher AL-KINDÎ (d. c. 873), who wrote on medicine and pharmacy among many other subjects, were among the best scientific writers of Arab blood.

Greatest of all the Spanish Mohammedan physicians of the time were Ibn Zuhr (Avenzoar), and his friend and pupil Ibn Rushd (Averroes).

AVENZOAR (1113–62), known as the "Famous Wise Man," opposed the philosophy of Avicenna and his dialectic speculations in medical matters. He dared even to express opinions contrary to Galen, and was an empiricist who attached the greatest importance to practice. He held surgery as unworthy of a physician, and even felt himself above preparing his own medicines. In this Arabian author we find clearly expressed the tendency that was to be manifest throughout the Middle Ages and the Renaissance: namely, the separation of medicine and surgery, a condition that did great harm to the progress of science in the centuries that followed, and gave rise to constant discussion and grave struggles between the medical and surgical castes and the lesser representatives of the profession, such as the barbers.

One of the most interesting figures in Arabian philosophy and medicine is Abû'l-Walîd Muhammad ibn Rushd, or AVERROES (1126–98), who was born at Cordova. Later Governor of Andalusia, he was a tireless worker who was perhaps a greater philosopher than physician, one of his epithets being the " Prince of Philosophy." He was the author of a work that Dante called the *Grand Commentary* (on Aristotle), which was regarded as a classic and was much studied in the early part of the Middle Ages. Its influence in the Occident gave rise to that great intellectual movement known as Averroism, which is one of the most interesting phenomena in the history of medical and philosophical thought of the fourteenth century. In the domain of medicine his most frequently quoted book is the *Colliget* (in Arabian, *Kitâb-el-Kollijat*), an encyclopædic work in which there are more Galenical discussions than medical observations.

A pupil of Averroes was the great MAIMONIDES, Abû Imrâm Mûsâ ibn Maimûn (1135–1204), born in Cordova, and often known under the abbreviation Rambam (Rabbi Moses ben Maimon). He was even more celebrated as a philosopher and Talmudist than as a physician. However, he has left works that demonstrate a wide medical knowledge, commentaries on the Aphorisms of Hippocrates and various letters on dietetics that can be regarded as one of the first models of those innumerable treatises *On Health* which constitute the model of most of the hygienic literature from the thirteenth to the fifteenth century.

The medical work of Maimonides is collected in his *Medical Principles*, or *Moses' Aphorisms* (*Fusul Musa*), written about 1190, translated into Hebrew and Latin; and in his *Regimen* (*Tadbir al Sihha*), dedicated to the melancholic eldest son of the Sultan Saladin, and published for the first time in Florence in 1480. In addition, Maimonides wrote various treatises, of which the treatise on sexual intercourse, *Ars Cœundi* (*Maqala fi-l-jima*), in nineteen chapters, dedicated to the Sultan of Hamàh, attained the greatest reputation in his own lifetime. His writings were frequently published and have been recently studied, notably by Steinschneider and Kroner. His *Treatise on Poisons* (1199) contains a number of valuable observations on rabies, venomous stings, and various poisons and their antidotes, with descriptions of clinical cases. It was translated into French by Rabbinowicz (Paris, 1865) and partially into German by Steinschneider (*Virch. Arch.*, 1873, LVII, 62). In all his writings Maimonides reveals an original, independent thought; often he criticizes Galen's statements and maintains a point of view that is contrary to the classic tradition. The celebrated Physician's Prayer, ascribed though without proof to Maimonides, attains a high ethical standard. Philosopher, rationalist, and Aristotelian, he underwent grave trials on account of his religious convictions. His tomb at Tiberias in Palestine is still regarded as a sanctuary to which the Hebrew makes his pilgrimage. Sick Jews of Cairo may spend the night in the crypt of the synagogue named after him — one of the many survivals of the ancient rite of incubation.

A younger contemporary of Maimonides was the physician ABD AL-LATÎF, who lived at Bagdad. He undertook a voyage to Cairo especially to meet Maimonides, and left a short but famous description of his voyage to Egypt and of the earthquakes and epidemics of the years 1201 and 1202.

Among the writers who belong to this century are many others who should be mentioned here: we note among the pharmacists MESUE THE YOUNGER, about whose personality there has been much discussion; also SERAPION THE YOUNGER, author of a book on simple drugs, of which we know only the Latin translation. Among the famous Arabian oculists, to whom Hirschberg has devoted an important study, should be noted MUHAMMAD AL-GHÂFIQÎ of Cordova (d. 1165), part of whose treatise on ophthalmology has been translated into French by Max Meyerhof (Barcelona, 1933). AHMAD AL-QÂISÎ (thirteenth century), "the Prince of the Egyptian Doctors," flourished in Cairo under the Sultan al-Salih. He wrote a treatise on the eye called *Result of Thinking on the Treatment of Troubles of Vision*, divided into fourteen chapters, according to the anatomical parts of the eye (see N. Kahil, Cong. de med. de Cairo, 1928).

The Arabian culture in Spain, after it was reconquered by the Christians, remained limited to the small territory of Granada. In Syria and in Egypt in the fourteenth century, however, Arabian medicine still flourished. We may note among the famous physicians who worked in the hospitals of Damascus and Cairo a new scientific impulse, due to a great clinician, MUHADDHIB AL-DÎN AL-DAKHWÂR, who at his death left his house and his library and a large bequest for the foundation of a school of medicine.

The most important of his pupils was Alâ'al-Din ibn al-Nafîs (al-Qurashî, ANNAFIS) (d. 1288), a Mohammedan who came from Damascus to Egypt and became chief physician there. He wrote numerous commentaries on the Hippocratic writings and on the Canon of Avicenna; his accurate summary of the Canon became a classical text in the Orient and especially in Persia and northern

India, where it was frequently republished with numerous commentaries. It is noteworthy that in one of his commentaries on the anatomical part of Avicenna's Canon, this author clearly affirms five times that, contrary to the opinion of Galen and of Avicenna, the ventricular septum is not permeable, and he describes the lesser circulation three hundred years in advance of Servetus and Realdus Colombus. His information is not founded on the study of the cadaver,

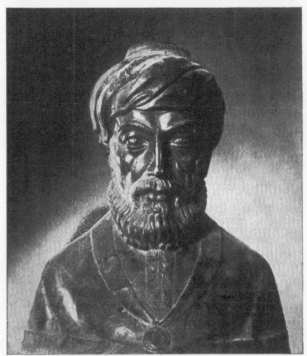

98. *Bust of Maimonides. In the hall of the Jewish University of Jerusalem.*

which was always strictly prohibited by the Arabs, but probably on observations made on animals and on theoretical considerations. Though this hypothesis had no influence in the Orient and was unknown in the Occident, if al-Nafîs' work is authenticated, it will constitute an important chapter in the history of the discovery of the circulation. The book was published in 1933 with a German translation and commentary by Meyerhof (*Quellen und Studien zur Geschichte der Naturwissenschaft und Medizin*, Vol. IV, Berlin, 1933; for résumé in English, see *Isis*, XXIII, 100, 1933).

In the field of materia medica the Arabians made considerable progress. They introduced into medicine a great number of drugs derived from both vegetables and chemicals; commerce in drugs in the Orient flourished greatly. The most authoritative writer in this field is IBN AL-BAITÂR (1197--

1248) of Malaga, an eminent botanist and worthy successor of Dioscorides. He travelled widely through the East in search of new medicines; he was the physician of the Egyptian emirs and taught in the school at Cairo.

His principal work, *The Corpus of Simples*, translated into French by Leclerc (Paris, 1877–83), is a complete materia medica, containing not only all the material earlier collected by Dioscorides and Galen, but also an enormous number of personal observations with critical notes based on long experience.

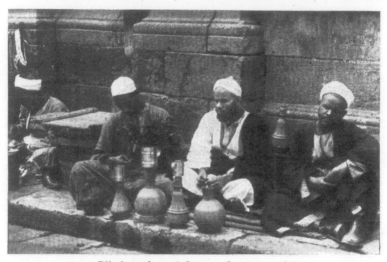

99. Blind vendors of drugs and syrups at Cairo.

This work is to be regarded as one of the most complete that we possess in the field of botany and materia medica. Leclerc calculates that more than fourteen hundred drugs are described, of which three hundred are met with for the first time in this work. Among the medicines introduced by the Arabs into materia medica are amber, musk, manna, cloves, various kinds of peppers, *sanguis draconis,* and *galanga* (Chinese ginger), betel nut, sandalwood, rhubarb, nutmeg, tamarind, camphor, senna, cassia, Croton oil, nux vomica, and many others. It is also noteworthy that the author indicates among the common names of plants the names that they bear also in Spain, Persia, and other Oriental countries, so that from the linguistic point of view, also, this book constitutes a valuable historical document.

The pharmaceutical book of AL-KÛHÎN-AL-ATṬÂR-AL-ISRÂ'ÎLÎ (translated: the Jewish druggist of priestly origin), who lived in Cairo about the middle of the thirteenth century, was regarded as the best text on the art of pharmacy. It gave not only good professional standards for the pharmacists, but also many directions about gathering simples, preserving them, and the preparation of drugs from them.

Pharmacy, one might say, began its scientific existence with the Arabians because of their special inclination to chemical studies and the great abundance of valuable drugs in the Orient. The Arabians were aided in attaining a high degree of perfection in their pharmaceutical preparations by the traditional lore of Persia in the preparation of perfumes and colouring materials. It is among the Arabians that we find the first real pharmacies. In the Hebrew codex of Avicenna in the library of the University of Bologna, and in many other important Arabian codices, one can find illustrations of these ancient pharmacies with their large jars of majolica arranged on the shelves.

From these Arabian and Persian pharmacies many drugs and medicines were imported into western Europe. In the early centuries after the year 1000 the commerce in Oriental drugs was very large and formed one of the chief sources of wealth of the Italian maritime republics. With the drugs were imported the Persian and Moorish jars that contained them, and it is perhaps in this way that the art of decorating faience ware reached Italy. These pharmacy jars are ordinarily called *albarelli* and are in a cylindrical form designed to preserve thick and viscid materials, and especially conserves of fruit, which in ancient therapeutics had a great importance. The body of the jar is usually constricted in the middle; the opening sometimes is larger and sometimes smaller, occurring above a neck on which are repeated the simple and characteristic designs found on the body of the jar. On these Oriental pharmacy jars are found many designs of fruits; they were reproduced in a number of Italian and Flemish pictures of the early Renaissance, and also in the materials, tapestries, and Oriental ceramics of the time.

In the history of medicine in the Arabian period, a valuable book must be mentioned which bears the Latin name of *Fontes relationum de classibus medicorum*, of which only single chapters have thus far been translated into French and German. The author of this book is IBN ABÎ USAIBIA, of Damascus (1203–70), a highly cultured physician who lived at the court of the Emir of Sarkhad, Syria, after having studied at Damascus and Cairo. This book contains the biographies of more than four hundred Arabian physicians, thus constituting probably the most important source for the history of Mohammedan medicine. Wüstenfeld and Leclerc have drawn largely from it. Another historian who deserves mention is ABÛL FARAJ (1226–96), born of a Jewish family and thus known in literature under the name of Bar Hebræus. He is the author of a book called the *History of the Dynasties*, in which he treats at length of the history of Arabian civilization and particularly its medicine.

When science was in full decadence among the peoples of Islam, two intelligent Spanish Mohammedan physicians had the courage at the time of the
terrible epidemic of plague in 1348 and 1349, to maintain the contagiousness
of the epidemic against the doctrine of the Koran. The first of these was IBN
AL-KHATÎB of Grenada (1313–74), a celebrated statesman, historian, and physician, who believed that the plague was spread by clothing, soiled linen, and
other objects in common use. He maintained the need for isolating those attacked by the plague. The second physician, IBN KHATIMÂ (d. 1369), described
the epidemic of plague of Almería and clearly stated the dangers of contagion.

The last of the Mohammedan physicians who deserve mention is DÂWÛD AL-
ANTÂKÎ of Antioch (died 1599), who lived in Egypt and was the author of
an important lexicon of medicines and drugs called *al-Tadhkira* (*The Memorial*),
which even today is frequently used and consulted by Oriental pharmacists.

5. The Teaching and Practice of Medicine

The teaching of medicine and the organization of sanitary services
showed rapid and marked progress. Already under the Caliph Harûn-al-
Raschîd a hospital was founded at Bagdad in the ninth century following
the model of Gondishapur. In the next century Rhazes lent his aid to the
hospital founded by the Caliph al-Muktadir at Bagdad; and in 970 the
powerful vizier Adud-al-Daula founded another and larger hospital, in
which twenty-five physicians worked and taught, examining pupils and
attesting to their proficiency. This hospital was preserved up to the destruction of the city in the year 1258. In all, there are records of about
thirty-four hospitals in the territory occupied by Islam. The most celebrated were those of Bagdad, and many physicians came from Persia and
Spain to study there; often they carried away with them new drugs and
valuable manuscripts on medicine and philosophy. It is important to note
that from early times it was obligatory for Mohammedan students to make
long voyages; and that the pilgrimages to Mecca and Medina, which the
faithful had to undertake at least once in a lifetime, often joined religious
with scientific aims.

The hospitals were generally well organized. In the hospital at Cairo,
founded in 1283, for example, there were special divisions for the wounded,
for eye patients, for those with fever — in whose rooms the air was re-
freshed with fountains — also rooms for women, kitchens, and so on. The
hospital was directed by a physician who had other, subordinate physicians
under him; he gave daily lessons to his pupils. There were male and
female nurses. A large library and an orphanage were annexed to the hos-

pital, which, as is usual in the Orient, was one of a number of edifices built about a mosque. After completing their lessons the pupils had to pass an examination given by the older physicians. One may accept, then, without being able to speak of a medical organization in the modern sense of the word, that the practice of medicine was none the less reserved to

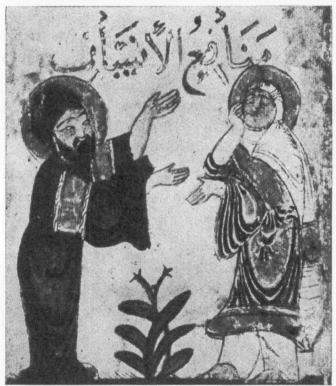

100. *A physician visiting a woman patient. Arabic miniature of the thirteenth century.*

those who had completed a course of studies. It was only in abuse of the system, just as happens today, that medicine was also practised by empiricists and charlatans.

Large libraries also were founded at this time, and medical works formed an important part of them. Especially famous were the libraries of Bagdad, Ispahan, Cairo, Damascus, and those of Mohammedan Spain, where there was a very large library founded by the Caliph al-Hakam II about 960. This library is said to have contained many hundreds of thousands of volumes. In the Escorial there are still to be found precious Arabian manuscripts written in this flourishing period of Mohammedan science.

An institution that had its first development in Bagdad but then became diffused rapidly throughout Islam was the *hisba,* or supervisory office of occupations and morals, at first a religious institution. The head of this office, the *muhtasib,* supervised among others the physicians, surgeons, druggists, and sellers of perfumes. He had the responsibility of determin-

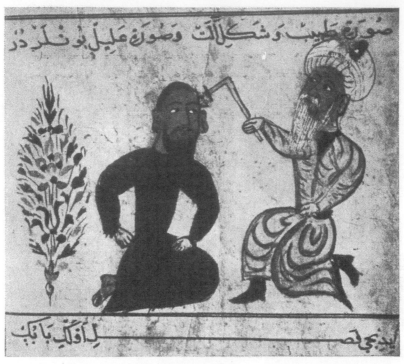

101. *A physician cauterizing a patient. Turkish manuscript of the fifteenth century.*

ing whether those who practised the health professions had sufficient knowledge of anatomy.

Surgery was generally regarded as unworthy of the physicians and was practised by a lower caste; practical anatomy, forbidden by strict religious regulations which, even in very recent times, have acted as a grave handicap, was not one of the studies of the faithful of Islam, so that the subject of anatomy was learned only from the texts. Special importance, on the other hand, was attributed to the study of chemistry and materia medica.

Modern historical research has not yet produced accurate biographical data about the famous chemist GEBER, or Giabir, who lived about the middle of the seventh century. It seems, for instance, that various discoveries — such as the preparation of mercuric chloride — attributed to him by some Arabian writers really were made by later scientists. Nevertheless, chemistry found adept investigators in the Arabian physicians, even though they were chiefly occupied in hunting for the elixir of life and potable gold. The concept of the transmutation of metals had inspired the belief that gold was capable of conferring eternal youth and of curing all diseases. But aside from these researches, in the practical field of materia medica the Arabian physicians obtained important successes. It is without

doubt to them that we owe the necessary information about the preparation of syrups, extracts of fruits, and the use of various narcotics that are named in such Arabian tales as *The Thousand and One Nights*.

The Arabians also made important progress in the mathematical sciences, and therefore also in mechanics and optics. Ophthalmology was one of the fields in which they were most active; so that we know of no less than thirty Arabian texts on the eye, of which the most celebrated was that of Alî ibn Isâ already cited.

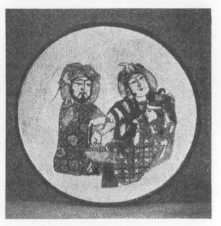

102. *Blood-letting.*
(*From an Arabian majolica bowl of the fifteenth century.*)

The practitioners received honoraria, which, according to Arabian texts, were often very large, especially for the best-known physicians and for those who attended the rulers. Thus one learns that Gabriel Bakhtîschû (Jibril ibn Bakhtyashû), a favourite of the Caliph Harûn-al-Raschîd, received a monthly honorarium of the equivalent of several thousand dollars, and an equal annual recompense " for bleeding and purging the commander of the Faithful." The total that he gained from his professional work amounted to over a million dollars. We know from Abu Nasr that he received a payment of the equivalent of almost fifty thousand dollars for having performed a lithotomy on a caliph.

Toward the middle of the thirteenth century the Arabian power began to decline. In 1236 Cordova fell to Ferdinand II of Castile, and in 1258 Bagdad was destroyed by the Mongols. Arabian civilization, chased out of Spain and destroyed in the Orient, seemed to disappear for ever from the Mediterranean, but not without leaving its indelible marks in history. If we wish to reach an equitable judgment on the role that it played in the history of medicine, we should not forget that we owe to it the preservation of the ancient traditions and the Greek texts which would have been otherwise largely lost, and that in the domain of surgery, and especially in ophthalmology, the contribution of the Arabians led to notable progress. Thanks to them, the number of useful drugs was greatly increased, so that we owe to this period of medicine valuable remedies which even today constitute an important part of modern therapeutics. Finally, and this seems to us extremely important for the history of medicine, we owe to this Arabian civilization the maintenance of a lay medicine at a time when in the West it had become largely a monopoly of the clerics. It is, however,

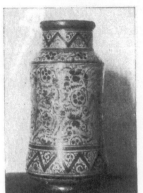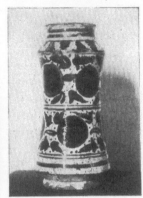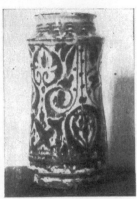

103. *Hispano-Moorish pharmacy jars. From the early fifteenth century.*
(Collection of A. Castiglioni.)

doubtful whether, as some authorities maintain, the great Arabian libraries and hospitals should be regarded as the first models of the universities which began to flourish in the West in the thirteenth century, because the Arabian schools themselves were modelled on the Greek schools of Alexandria and the Christian schools of Syria. Nevertheless, it cannot be denied that at this period, when teaching was confined exclusively to the Church in all Christian countries, in Spain, Egypt, and Syria on the contrary medical instruction was given by lay physicians, thanks to the intelligent and mighty rulers in these countries. And this teaching cannot even be regarded as exclusively dogmatic and scholastic; for, even if its theoretical part is founded on the philosophy and later on the canonical texts of Hippocrates and Galen, it is a remarkable fact that a practical instruction flourished beside this theoretical teaching. Anatomical knowledge, to be sure, was scanty on account of the strict prohibitions of Islam; but clinical instruction flourished in the Arabian schools, traces of which are to be found later in Western civilization. By accepting in their great academies the medical knowledge that came to them through the Nestorians, the Jews, the Greeks, and the Persian schools, by translating the ancient texts and preserving them in libraries, by improving clinical observation and increasing the store of knowledge in chemistry and materia medica, the Arabians proved themselves to be faithful guardians of Hippocratic thought. To be sure, they did not contribute greatly to its evolution by the addition of new observations and concepts, nor did they open new lines of medical study; but in a period of great trouble in the West, they were preservers of medical tradition, they nourished lay medical culture, and they were the intermediaries from whose hands the civilization of the West was to receive back a precious deposit.

CHAPTER XIV

MEDICINE IN THE CHRISTIAN WEST DURING THE FIRST CENTURIES OF THE MIDDLE AGES

FROM MONASTIC MEDICINE TO THE LAY MEDICINE OF SALERNO

1. Greco-Roman Traditions and Medicine of Western Europe

THE EARLY centuries of the Middle Ages may be regarded as a period in which western Europe, devastated by wars and epidemics and invaded by the barbarians, had preserved only the memory of its past grandeur, while the Greco-Roman civilization had completely disappeared, to reappear at first slowly and timidly, then with more strength and boldness. At the beginning of the Renaissance it might well have seemed that medical thought had disappeared with the Roman civilization, or that it had migrated to distant parts to return later with the medicine of the Arabians. As a matter of fact, however, even at the lowest ebb, although the classic civilization had been overthrown and mostly destroyed, and although the conquerors had changed the civil regime and pillaged the monuments of ancient grandeur, nevertheless civilization and accumulated knowledge were not entirely obliterated. The progress of letters, sciences, and arts had suffered a severe check; Christianity in its rapid spread had changed the direction of study and of literature and art; but at the same time it had fervently preserved the achievements of the ancients. The Goths and Lombards, whose arms reduced much of Italy to slavery, cut the marvellous flowers and trampled on the plants, but did not succeed in destroying the roots. Inconspicuously and little by little, at first in those parts of the Mediterranean that had escaped invasion and had preserved the Roman laws and customs under the nominal domination of the Empire of the East, then in Rome, which had become the capital of Christianity, and finally nearer the Alps — natural ramparts against the foreign invaders — a free and vigorous life sprang up, the ancient tradition became more alive and more aware of its past grandeur. Finally, after the wars had ceased, the invaders even began to adopt the customs of the conquered and to bow to that moral force which impregnated them with the grandeur of the Roman civilization. Theodoric said: " We are glad to live under the Roman law (*delectamur jure Romano vivere*) "; and Cassiodorus is cited by De Renzi as having emphasized that a certain Gaul whom he was recommending for the Roman Senate had lived in Italy and thus had the dignified attitude of a Roman rather than the coarseness of the barbarians.

Up to the time of the Roman conquest the medical culture of the Germans had been that of a primitive people; medicine was almost entirely magical and demonistic. Generally the physician (*lachner*) was no more than a sorcerer who expelled demons from the body by means of incantations and symbolic rites. The gods were appeased by bloody sacrifices, and the priest touched the patient with a finger dipped in the blood of the victim (*kedfinger*). Medicinal herbs were collected on special days and with magic rites. The runes, signs marked in red on staffs of wood, played an important part in these observances. Magic stones, magic phrases, magic plants, such were the mainstays of treatment; amulets of all sorts protected children and cured diseases.

Together with magic medicine, empirical medicine played a very important part. The marvellous virtues of the healing plants were exalted in traditions, legends, and popular songs and consecrated by innumerable ceremonies. The mistletoe had a prominent role in Germanic and Celtic medicine: beverages prepared with it protected against all poisons and made women fertile. A number of other plants, such as mandragora (*alraun*), plantain, verbena, sage, were regarded as magic remedies and were utilized with special practices and rites.

Especially worthy of note in ancient Germanic medicine is the part played by women, to whom recourse was had for treatment and aid for the sick. Tacitus writes of the ancient Germans: " *Ad matres, ad coniuges vulnera ferunt, nec illæ numerare et exigere plagas pavent* (They take their injuries to their mothers and wives, who do not fear to examine and treat their wounds)." Some of these women, the so-called *sagæ*, enjoyed the reputation of possessing supernatural powers. It was only much later that men began to busy themselves with medicine. Cure required above all a sacrifice, often of blood, in order to placate the gods. Wotan was worshipped as the god of healing. The medicine of the Gallo-Celts was almost exclusively priestly and was confided to the caste of the Druids, custodians of religion and of medicine no less than of science and of poetry.

The first contact of the northern peoples with Latin medicine came through the physicians of the Roman armies, who brought to these countries the theory and practice of medicine. When the Germans invaded Italy they found there the monuments of the ancient medical culture and soon comprehended their importance.

THEODORIC (*c.* 454–526), profound admirer of Roman culture, was one of the first to accept the sanitary administration as it had been preserved in the Empire. He, too, drained marshes to improve public health. Cassiodorus informs us that he enacted a law to re-establish the *comes archiatrorum* in his rights and duties, and stated the formula for his nomination. " Among the most useful arts that contribute to sustain frail humanity, none may be regarded as superior — or even equal — to medicine, which aids the sick with its maternal benevolence, puts our pains to flight, and gives us that which riches and honour are unable to give. . . . Leave aside, O men of the medical arts, those controversies that are prejudicial to the sick; and if you are not able to come to an agreement, consult someone whom you can question without dislike, for every wise man is willing to seek counsel and he is regarded as the most zealous whose frequent questions prove that he is the most wise. At the very beginning of your career in this art you are consecrated by oaths like those of the priests: you promise solemnly to your instructors to hate iniquity and love honesty. . . . Remember that to sin against the health of a person constitutes homicide. When I honour you with the title of *Comes Archiatrorum* so that you will be esteemed among the masters of the art of healing and everyone will ask your opinion, I warn you to demonstrate that you are a just arbiter in this notable art. . . . To the expert archiater may the pulse reveal our internal disorders, may the urines reveal them to his eyes. Enter freely into our palace, with full confidence, and may it be permitted to you to prescribe diets, to say things that one would not dare to hear said, and to prescribe even painful treatment in the interest of our health." This formula shows clearly that there existed at this time a well-organized lay medicine, with a required course of study, and examinations given by the instructors, before whom candidates had to take oaths. Even the fact that these oaths were said to be " like those of the priests " shows that medicine was completely detached from priesthood and that the King of the Ostrogoths had completely accepted Roman medical legislation. The Gothic laws strictly prohibited production of abortions, forbade the activities of the haruspices and sorcerers, imposed severe penalties on those who placed spells on men and animals, regarding them as followers of the

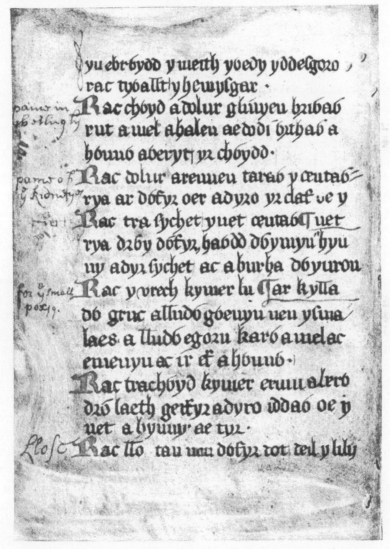

104. *Maddygom Myddfay. A Gaelic manuscript of the thirteenth century containing the prescriptions of the physicians of Myddfay.* (WELLCOME MUSEUM.)

devil, and also condemned those who demanded advice about a sickness from the sorcerers. In the Lombard law known as the Edict of Rotari (Lombard diplomatic code, in Troia: *History of Italy in Middle Ages*), a fine of silver was fixed for blows and injuries to servants, whether of officials or peasants, and payment to the physician is included in the sum. In the law of the Visigoths on the responsibility of the physician (Tit. I, Bk. XI) it is said that no physician, except in the case of emergency, has the right to bleed a young girl unless the father or mother, brother, or some other close relative is present, and that no physician has the right to enter prisons without being accompanied by a custodian, in order that no prisoner could demand or obtain a mortal poison. The law fixes the price of the principal operations and of medical instruction, and decrees that, except in case of homicide, the physician may not be kept in prison before being examined.

After the conquest of Rome, which had been reduced to the state of a village, the successor of Theodoric, his grandson Atalaric, continued the salaries of the public instructors and the maintenance of the schools. The Merovingian and Carolingian kings had their archiaters and the cities had their public physicians. In the Capitularies of 805 and 807 Charlemagne records that he who wishes to dedicate himself to medicine shall be trained in it from his infancy. Thus the laws reveal how the foreign invaders soon accepted the Roman standards and traditions in medicine as in other fields.

Such data suffice to show that the northern conquerors of the Empire well understood the importance of medical practice in the Roman manner. Thus while it was Germanism that furnished the external structure of the social life of the time, the spiritual force of Rome was never entirely extinguished and still lived through the centuries. This same spiritual force little by little ameliorated the severity of the laws of the Lombards, who became Christians and were attracted into the orbit of Rome. This same ancient civilization which took on new life in Christianity, in law, art, and philosophy, also was revivified in medicine. But even as philosophy was clothed at first with mysticism and then with a Neo-Platonism coming from the schools of Alexandria, Antioch, and Cappadocia, medicine, which originated in the same sources, naturally lived a literary life in the shadow of the cloisters in a period when the barbarians were bringing about the dissolution of the corrupt Empire. The long-existing controversy as to whether lay or ecclesiastic medicine predominated in southern Europe need not detain us, as there are abundant indisputable proofs that there were both medical practitioners bearing the same titles and enjoying the same rights as at the time of the Empire, and also ecclesiastics who studied and practised medicine. But if the former were essentially the successors of the ancient Greco-Latin physicians, at least as to form and tradition if not in their steadily weakening studies, the latter conceived medicine as a mystic form of assistance given to the soul rather than to the body, and as a work of charity in which the priest was none other than the interpreter of the divine will and of the divine power to heal which was always an essential attribute of the Saviour. In the sixth century, at the moment when

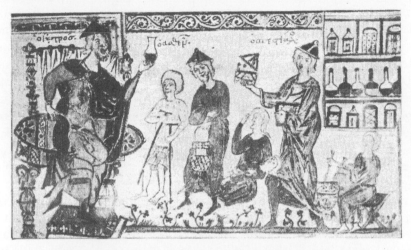

105. *Miniature from the* Antidotarium *of Nicola Mirozzo, a Greek manuscript of the fourteenth century.*   (BIBLIOTHÈQUE NATIONALE, PARIS.)

the long and fierce contests of the Ostrogoths and Byzantium broke out and war, pestilence, and famine ravaged the country worse than ever before, scholarly study in all its forms and manifestations was exclusively reserved to the clerics, because the Church of Rome alone was sufficiently powerful to offer a sure asylum to scholars. Literary medicine took refuge in the churches and cloisters; and the medical learning of the period, as was also the case with philosophy, had its protection and development almost exclusively in the monasteries.

But there is still another reason for the medicine of the period being monastic: following the traditions of the Orient, and the still more ancient Grecian institutions, it was around the monasteries that the hospitals were built. In these times of bloody conflicts no one could find the peace and calm necessary for the care of the sick outside of the religious orders, which had been able to acquire the respect of men of all factions. Religion covered the work of charity with its venerated cloak and thus founded secure asylums where tormented souls could find repose, and where bodies martyrized by ferocious battles or horrible epidemics could find tender care and needed quiet. It is natural that those men who had been driven by the sight of human miseries and fratricidal struggles to embrace the monastic rule of sacrifice and renunciation should be the first and most zealous in treating leprosy and the plague and in succouring the wounded. It is thus that a monastic medicine arose which later flourished, thanks to such orders of chivalry as the Templars and the Knights of St. John. Monastic medicine flourished at Montecassino, where St. Benedict founded the hospice of his order, and Cassiodorus, when he retired from the triumphs of public life to the monastery, brought to it as a distinguished philosopher and physician in the Hippocratic sense his knowledge of ancient literature. Cassiodorus (490–585?), who had carried with him a collection of ancient manuscripts to the monastery founded by him near Squillace (538), was one of the most interesting figures of this period. He recommended to his monks the study of the nature of simples and the composition of medicaments, at the same time placing all their hopes in the Lord. This great scholar, who had been the minister of Theodoric and the predecessor of Charlemagne in the institution of public schools, recommended study of the great herbal of Dioscorides, the books of Hippocrates and Galen in their Latin translations, and other medical books such as those of Aurelianus Cælius. Thus Cassiodorus, who, like St. Augustine and Boethius, took his inspiration from the greatest philosophers of antiquity, reaffirmed the bonds that united Christian philosophy with Greco-Latin thought. Montecassino became, if not an actual medical school, at least an important centre of scholarship in which medicine held a very great part and an invaluable depository of classical manuscripts, both originals and copies. From this ancient monastery the doctrine and practice of St. Benedict extended to numerous other monasteries which rapidly were created at that period. Active centres were established in England at Oxford, Cambridge, and Winchester; in France the prototype was at Tours; while in Germany, Fulda and St. Gall were the best known. Thus little by little hospitals took their place beside the monasteries and interest in medical study spread widely through the monastic order.

Montecassino acquired great fame throughout the West and the teaching of medicine was spread by the Benedictines to the monasteries scattered over Europe. In the library of the ancient monastery of Montecassino there is a valuable collection of important medical manuscripts which show how the medical tradition was preserved there. To the Benedictines, those indefatigable teachers, is due the initiative in the foundation of the cathedral schools of Charlemagne, in which medicine was taught from their beginnings. These schools were to be found throughout his empire, in Paris,

Fulda, Lyon, Metz, Italy, and so on. The course of studies was founded on the so-called trivium and quadrivium: to the trivium belonged arithmetic, grammar and music; to the quadrivium, astronomy, geometry, rhetoric, and dialectic. In 805 Charlemagne ordained that medicine, under the name of physics, should also be introduced into the program. Alcuin (735–804)

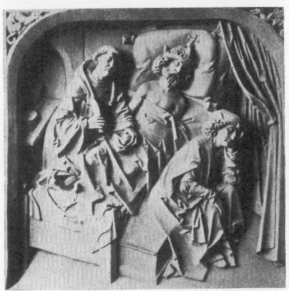

106. *St. Benedict of Norcia performs a lithotomy on the Emperor, and holds in his hand the stone removed from the bladder.*
(*Bas-relief in* BAMBERG CATHEDRAL.)

was the founder of the famous school of Tours, which is properly regarded as the mother of the French monastic schools. Here the work of translating the ancient texts was carried out with the greatest care and among them medical texts unquestionably had considerable importance.

It is probably at this period that the first organized medical instruction began in the monasteries, many traces of which can be found. In the gardens of the cloisters medicinal herbs were planted: thus we know the list of simples planted in the garden of the monastery of St. Gall in 820. We know also that in this monastery there was room for six sick people, a pharmacy, and a special lodging for the physician.

Among these monastery schools in which medicine was taught, the school of Montecassino acquired great renown toward the end of the ninth century. We know that the Abbot Desiderius, born in 1027 and made Pope in 1086 under the name of Victor III, wrote four books on the *Medical Miracles of St. Benedict.* To this monastery the sick came from every part of Europe to undergo cures that recalled those of the ancient temples of Æsculapius. Thus it is told that Henry II of Bavaria (972–1024), suffering from vesical calculus, was cured during "incubation" in the monastery by St. Benedict himself, who appeared to him in a dream, operated upon him, and laid the stone in his hand.

In this period of domination by the northern races few works of importance appeared in medical literature. We know some books that derived from Pliny

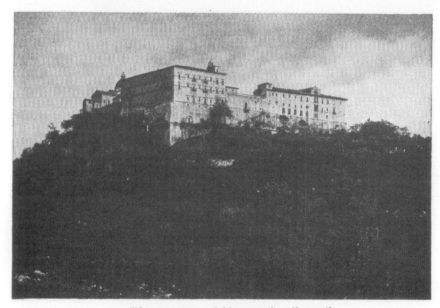

107. *The monastery of Montecassino (in 1938).*

or from the famous herbal of Pseudo-Apuleius, in which is a description of a hundred or more medicinal plants and of their therapeutic virtues. To this period belongs the work of CASSIUS FELIX, written probably about the middle of the fifth century, which contains a short summary of materia medica. Toward the beginning of the sixth century we find medical literature almost exclusively in the hands of the clerics in all the Western countries. The Greek language was more and more forgotten, and rare indeed were even scholars who understood it. Among those who kept the ancient traditions alive in the monasteries, the names of only a few have been preserved from oblivion. One such was ISIDOR OF SEVILLE, the famous Bishop who is known in literature under the name of Isidorus Hispalensis. He was the author of an encyclopædic work entitled *On Origins*, an excellent example of all the books of this kind of the period; in them, beginning with God and the angels, everything in the world is touched upon, even if superficially. In this book there are frequent quotations from ancient medical texts. It served for a long while as a textbook for those who cultivated medicine in the monasteries.

At the height of the troubles produced by the foreign invasions, a centre of scholarly study arose in the most distant part of Western Christianity — in Ireland, where Christianity had been introduced in the fifth century by St. Patrick. In the monasteries founded in the Emerald Isle by mystics and ascetics who were bound by the most rigid discipline, the texts of the great classical writers were studied and knowledge of the Greek tongue was preserved. In the sixth century these monks undertook long journeys to continental Europe, carrying everywhere with them the word of the Gospel and of the Christian sciences. These Irish monks were the founders of many monasteries that attained great renown, such as the monastery of St. Gall, which became a famous centre of medical learning, and of Bobbio near Pavia, which was founded by St. Colombanus, where the love of science equalled that of Montecassino. In England the Benedictines emulated the Irish monks in constantly giving new impulses to learning. Thanks to the pilgrims who visited the various monasteries, the precious medical manuscripts were carried from one to another and were copied, studied, and commented upon by the tranquil inhabitants. Thus there arose a body of medical literature of the monasteries which was extremely important.

It is in this category that should be included the books of the VENERABLE BEDE (672–735), who was the Prior of the monastery of Wearmouth in England, and who compiled a number of treatises of various kinds, among which medicine had a notable place. Also to be mentioned are the authors of the so-called *Hortuli*, books containing descriptions of those simples which were most frequently cultivated in the gardens of the monasteries and from which the medicines were usually prepared. One of the most interesting of these works is that by BENEDETTO CRESPO, Archbishop of Milan, who lived in the first half of the eighth century, whose *editio princeps* was published by Angelo Mai in 1833, following the manuscript in the Vatican library. His *Commentarium medicinale* is an epitome of therapeutics, consisting of a prose introduction and two hundred and forty-one hexameters. The work, written when the author was still a deacon, contains for the most part descriptions of remedies used in popular medicine, with some information drawn from Pliny and Dioscorides. Also worth noting is the *Dietetica*, by ANTHIMUS, physician of Theodoric, and for a time Ambassador to the court of the King of the Franks.

This book, in Latin, was written, according to Pagel, between 511 and 526 and is dedicated to the Prince Thierry, the oldest son of Clovis I. It was published by Roze in 1870. It includes an introduction that explains the need for rational nutrition, also a description of the more common foods, and a series of aphorisms, especially concerning moderation in eating and drinking, methods of preparing medicines, and the care of the sick while travelling. Then follows a list of all the commoner foods, meats, fish, drugs, milk, and so on, with detailed statements as to how they should be prepared and cooked. This is one of the first examples that we possess of those *Advices to a Ruler* which we shall meet more frequently in the literature of the Renaissance. Other medical works in verse are the famous *Lapidarius* of Bishop Marbod of Rennes; the *Physica* of the ABBESS HILDEGARDE; the poem called *De viribus herbarum*, whose author is known under the pseudonym of MACER FLORIDUS. The pharmacological fragment of the Jewish physician SHABBATHAI BEN ABRAHAM (931–982), called Donnolo, born near Otranto, was almost entirely of classical origin. Donnolo enjoyed such a great reputation in his lifetime that high dignitaries of the Church, like the famous Nilo, Abbot of Rossano, came to consult him. Sarton emphasizes the importance of such men in creating a medical focus in southern Italy and thus preparing the way for the prosperity of the school of Salerno.

If we now consider the condition of medical learning and the practice of medicine in Europe in the first centuries of the Middle Ages, we note, on the one hand, the existence of a lay medicine which followed the ancient Roman traditions and held strictly to the teaching of the classics, even though these were none too well comprehended, and, on the other hand, the existence of an ecclesiastical medicine that had its centre in the monasteries. Owing to the influence of the Church and its priests, schools were being founded in France, England, Germany, and Italy; while, thanks especially to the energetic leadership of Charlemagne, the desire for culture gradually spread abroad. Great schools were founded, such as those of York, Winchester, and Canterbury in England; Chartres and Tours in France; Fulda and St. Gall in Germany; and many in Italy, according to the Capitulary of Lothaire (824). The seven liberal arts were taught there, and medicine had its place close beside them. As we have seen, the medical literature was almost entirely ecclesiastical, because the priests were the only ones who knew how to write and to read the ancient texts. This monastic medicine, which spread rapidly throughout western Europe, included among its most illustrious representatives HRABANUS MAURUS, born in Mainz (776–856), a pupil of Alcuin and a monk of the Benedictine monastery of Fulda. He was regarded as the leading educator of Germany. Another was WALAFRID STRABO (died 849), Abbot of the monastery of Reichenau, and author of a didactic medical poem. Monastic medicine had the great merit of having preserved the ancient tradition of learning and of having collected in the small hospitals next to the monasteries the treasury of ancient knowledge, humbly and charitably cherished with ardent devotion at a time when the terrible tempests that raged through Europe were in danger of destroying them entirely.

The decline of monastic medicine, which reached its nadir in the tenth century, was due to several causes. Its very success took monks more and more outside of the monastery and away from their religious duties, so that various Church councils (especially those of Reims, 1131, Innocent II; Tours, 1163, Alexander III; Paris, 1212, Innocent III) restricted medical activities and finally forbade them entirely. The new order of Cistercians, formed from within the Benedictine order, and its most famous representative, St. Bernard, looked more toward agriculture and moral reform than to scholarship, while another important circumstance was the rise of the Dominican and Franciscan orders in the thirteenth century, both of which were avowedly hostile to all scientific activities. Other factors, as we shall see later, were the rise of the cathedral schools, and the growth of large cities and great universities in the thirteenth century.

2. The School of Salerno. First Period

Though not recording any illustrious name or important medical progress, the chronicle of the early centuries of the Middle Ages demonstrates incontestably that even in the most depressing times medical thought continued its advance, no matter how slowly or feebly, and lay medicine exhibited an uninterrupted historical continuity. From these two essential facts, and from all the events that we have just referred to, is derived one of the most significant phenomena in the history of medicine — the formation of the great and memorable school of Salerno. Toward this centre converged successively all the great currents of medical thought, ancient and contemporary: from the Greek schools of lower Italy and Egypt to the monks of western Europe, from the Jews, Arabs, and Orientals to the peoples of northern Europe — an assembly of influences which were absorbed and amalgamated in a secular medical activity to which people of all social classes and religions brought their contributions. The resulting achievement is an admirable example of a characteristic Latin trait: that of utilizing the liveliest jet of each fountain, the soundest germ of every idea, the unspoiled memory of even the apparently dead past, and of giving an eminently practical and lucid trend to every activity. In the smiling bay that the ancient Roman physicians had already regarded as an ideal place for sojourn, in that part of Italy where the contacts between races and civilizations were always the liveliest, where commerce and contact with people from distant parts was a frequent occurrence, there arose the *Civitas Hippocratica*, the seat of the school of Salerno, whose name has remained famous throughout the centuries.

This school, which we first hear spoken of at the beginning of the ninth century, reached its greatest splendour in the twelfth century and

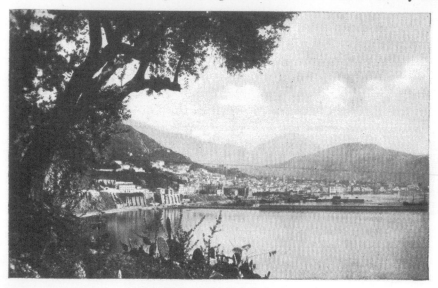

108. *View of Salerno (in 1938).*

preserved its fame to the end of the fourteenth. A distinct tendency to lay medicine early made its appearance there. Its geographical position attracted to the school all the currents of Greek culture which, in spite of wars and invasions, still persisted in lower Italy, chiefly through its uninterrupted commercial contacts with the Levant.

The history of the school of Salerno can be divided into three periods. In the first, it already enjoyed a widespread reputation, which perhaps derived from the time in which a hospital founded by the Benedictines, toward the end of the seventh century, attracted patients from distant parts. Although the information that we have about the early masters is vague, and no historical value can be attached to the legend that the school was founded by four physicians, a Greek, a Latin, a Jew, and a Saracen, nevertheless, this legend deserves to have attributed to it, as Singer has done, the value of a secular tradition. The old Salernitan chronicles that tell about a Master Helinus, who read Hebrew lessons to the Jews, a Master Pontus, who gave instruction to the Greeks, a Master Adela, an Arab who taught in the Arabian tongue, and a Master Salernus, who taught in Latin, thus belong to legend. Be this as it may, we have evidence that already in the year 904 there was a Salernitan physician at the court of the King of France; and that in 984 Alberon, Bishop of Verdun, came to seek the advice of the Salernitan physicians, and that at a later period princes of the Church and secular rulers had recourse to their aid.

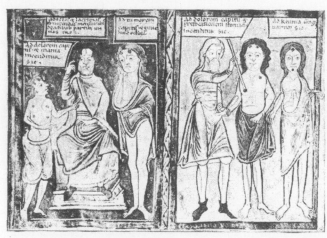

109. *Indication of points for cauterization. Salernitan manuscript of the eleventh century.*   (BRITISH MUSEUM.)

In this first period the instruction at Salerno already possessed a strictly lay character. The ten physicians who composed the *Collegium Hippocraticum* were paid by the students and enjoyed special privileges. The young students of all countries flocked to their lectures. The medical writings of the time seem to be due merely to a desire to prepare manuals for the students. They are almost exclusively summaries or fragments of the old Greek or Latin texts, in which therapy, largely medicinal, without any allusions to magic or astronomy, had the greatest importance.

Our knowledge of the medicine of Salerno at this period is due above all to the intensive studies of the Italian medical historian SALVATORE DE RENZI, whose monumental *Collectio Salernitana* (Naples, 1852–9, five vols.) has thrown an intense light on the history of Salerno and particularly of this first period, which up to that time had remained in obscurity. The investigations of De Renzi were amplified by the studies of Pietro Giacosa (1853–1928), in his *Magistri Salernitani nondum editi* (Turin, 1901), and Pietro Capparoni's book, *Magistri Salernitani nondum cogniti* (London: John Bale, 1923). Daremberg and Sudhoff and the latter's school have also brought important contributions to this subject. Sudhoff has paid especial attention to the Salernitan documents. He has been the most ardent supporter of the lay character of the school and has given interesting explanations of its formative process. The instructive studies of Sigerist and Garuffi should also be mentioned.

Names of many Salernitan physicians of this period have come down to us. The best known is GARIOPONTUS, or GUARINPOTUS, who was the most famous teacher of his time. He lived in the first half of the eleventh century, dying about 1050. Some historians think he was of Greek origin, others that he was a Lombard; while De Renzi believes him to have been a Salernitan. His name is connected with an encyclopædic work which had a great reputation in the eleventh century and even later, called *Passionarius*, drawn largely from the works of Galen, Theodorus Priscianus, Alexander of Tralles, and Paul of Ægina. This work is mostly a compilation made from the Latin translations of the authors just cited; it is divided into five books, with an appendix of three other books which contain a treatise on fevers. From the linguistic point of view, the work of Gariopontus is of special value because it contains the basis of modern medical terminology. In Latinizing the Greek words this Greek author borrowed many words from the living language of the people. Although the *Passionarius* is not an original work but merely a compilation, it cannot be denied merit of an unusual scholastic and linguistic character. A work evidently intended to be studied by pupils, it gives us a clear picture of the most quoted authors of the period and shows that the dominant force in the teaching at Salerno was the Greco-Latin tradition without Arabian influence, which is entirely lacking in this work. On the other hand, the use of words borrowed from the common tongue shows us that the instruction was intended for the laity, for whom a vulgarization of the most important words was necessary. There is not the slightest allusion in the text to mystic or priestly therapeutics. Hippocrates is quoted with the title *omnium peritissimus* (the most expert of all). It is for these reasons that the *Passionarius* deserves an important place in the history of Salernitan medicine, even though its author cuts but a vague figure in history. The first edition is that of Lyon, printed by Antoine Blanchard in 1526.

To the same period belongs another famous physician, Pietro Clerico, or PETRONCELLUS, whose *Practica* (*c.* 1035) was first published by De Renzi. According to De Renzi and other historians, it seems that Petroncellus was a contemporary of Gariopontus and perhaps even his pupil. His book, which is a compilation like the *Passionarius*, contains several chapters which are simple transcriptions from the Greek; many Latinized Greek words occur in it and there are no quotations from Latin authors. A note-worthy item is the frequent recommendation to take cold baths, which are prescribed for a number of diseases.

We cite also among the authors of this first period ALPHANUS I (11th cent.), doubtless the same person who later became Archbishop of Salerno, but not to be confused with another Archbishop of Salerno of the same name. He composed a Latin translation of Nemesius' book on the nature of man and wrote a short treatise on the four humours. A personality who has aroused a lively interest among medical historians for a long time is the woman physician TROTULA, about whose very existence the most varied opinions have been expressed. De Renzi states that she lived at Salerno about the time of the last Lombard prince, before the arrival of Constantinus Africanus. It is certain that very near her own time she is quoted under the name of *sapiens matrona* and *mulier sapientissima*. Odoricus Vitalis speaks of her in his ecclesiastical history, written in the first half of the twelfth century. More recent historians, such as Sudhoff and Singer, however, do not accept that her existence has been proved. A discussion of the question would carry us beyond the limits of this work; it is sufficient to note that the existence of this expert medical woman and of other women who practised medicine is affirmed in the most ancient Salernitan tradition. The book that bears her name, *De passionibus mulierum*, seems to have been, as De Renzi supposes, a later compilation, possibly dating from the thirteenth century. Neuburger regards it as a thirteenth-century elaboration of Trotula's work, whereas some accept it as the work of the woman Trotula herself. The treatment of the material reveals considerable practical experience: especially worthy of attention are the rules about the choice of a wet nurse, who should be neither too far from nor too near her last childbirth; a special diet is prescribed, with abstinence from highly salted foods or an excess of pepper and severe prohibition of garlic and onion. We shall not discuss here the question raised by De Renzi and several other authors as to whether Trotula was really a woman physician or merely a midwife and the wife of the famous physician, JOHANNES PLATEARIUS, or even a generic name for midwives. It is sufficient to note that of the works that pass under her name none may be regarded as original, and that even that part which contains a collection of cosmetic prescriptions was certainly written at a later period. This is not inconsistent with the fact that the book was regarded in Italy as a textbook up to the sixteenth century and quoted by the best authors. It was printed by Aldus in Venice in 1547. It is interesting that this Salernitan female doctor had a certain popularity in old English literature under the name of *Dame Trot* — the *Madame*

Trotte of the thirteenth-century medical trouvère Rutebœuf (*Le Dex de l'Erberie*).

Certain other works that belong to this period should be cited, such as *Speculum hominis,* written about the middle of the eleventh century, a didactic text in verse that treats of man and his diseases in the manner of Isidor of Seville.

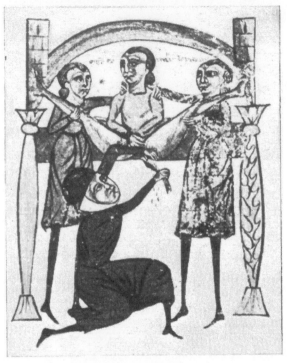

110. *Operation for the stone in the MS. of Roland of Parma.*
(*Codex of the* CASANATENSE LIBRARY.)

Among the other writings of the period is the celebrated *Antidotarium,* the foundation stone of early Salernitan medicine. It was a kind of formulary, made up from the daily practice of the hospitals, and was regarded as a canonical book of standards to be followed by the Salernitan physicians in regard to prescriptions for the patients, similar to the formulas that some hospitals of today draw up for the use of their interns.

The most ancient form of the Salernitan formulary has been lost; that which we possess in the manuscripts of the thirteenth and fourteenth centuries is a later edition bearing the name of the *Antidotarium Nicolai Salernitani,* perhaps prepared in the eleventh century, which underwent a new revision by a French physician in the beginning of the fifteenth century. It then appeared under the title of *Antidotarium Nicolai Præpositi* — probably through confusion, as Sudhoff suggests, with the name of the French physician *Nicole Prévost of Tours*. This Salernitan formulary contains, in addition to the prescriptions known to classical antiquity, a series of medicines borrowed from the Arabian writers and thus constitutes a valuable codification of all the known materia medica. It is highly interesting to compare this, as Sigerist has done, with the formularies of the Middle Ages. The Salernitan formulary is the parent of all those that follow; as the classical text for pharmacists, it had many editions and translations.

Besides these works which belonged to the first period of the school of Salerno, we know a number of others of lesser importance written by such men as RAGENTIFRIDUS, a name certainly of Lombard origin, PETRUS, and GRUNIVALDUS, cited by De Renzi.

3. *The Golden Period of the Salernitan School. Arabian Currents*

The second period of the school of Salerno — that of its greatest splendour — is characterized by the influence of Arabian medicine, which reached it about the end of the eleventh century. It is mostly though not entirely due to one of the great intermediaries of Arabian civilization in the West. CONSTANTINUS AFRICANUS, so called because he was born in Carthage, exercised the same profound influence on medicine that Marsilius Ficinus (1433–99) exerted on literature and humanism. From his earliest youth Constantinus devoted himself to the study of medicine and, according to the chronicle of Petrus Diaconus, made long journeys to Syria, India, Ethiopia, and Egypt. His wide knowledge of Oriental languages and his passion for literary studies took him to Salerno, where he became, according to a history that is largely legendary, the secretary of Robert Guiscard, Duke of Salerno. He soon became one of the most esteemed physicians and famous professors of that school. He remained there several years, then became a Benedictine monk of the monastery of Montecassino, where Desiderius, or Gauferius, the Lombard, was Abbot. The rest of Constantine's life was devoted to intense study until he died there in 1087. We find in him the type with which we shall become better acquainted in the humanism of the fifteenth century, an intensely scholarly man who knows Oriental languages thoroughly and exhibits a marvellous activity in translating the ancient texts, with, however, more facility than exactness.

Like others, Constantine translated everything that came to his hand without distinguishing the rare and precious from mere accumulations of fantastic and extravagant statements. In his translations he often brought together texts from different periods and of greatly different values, sometimes even forgetting the name of the author that he was translating, so that he has been made to pass as the author of the work of others.

The first edition of the works of Constantine appeared in Basel in 1537 in seven volumes. Almost all of the texts of this and later editions are translations from the Arabic. Constantine even translated from the Arabic the *Aphorisms* of Hippocrates and the *Articella* together with Galen's commentaries on the *Aphorisms*. Steinschneider has devoted to Constantine a most interesting study; still earlier Puccinotti published from a manuscript in the Bibliotheca Ambrosiana of Milan a short treatise on anatomy which, though bearing Constantine's name, seems to be of doubtful authenticity. Although the medical value of the work of Constantine is slight, he was greatly admired well into the Middle Ages as the *Magister Orientis et Occidentis*. He is important for having opened the way to a new trend of the school of Salerno by exposing it to the Arabian writers. We must recognize here that the Arabian domination in Sicily lasted almost two centuries and that these writers left great and noble traces of their culture. This current, coming uninterruptedly from Sicily to Naples, established a strong contact between Arabian medicine and the medicine of Salerno. At the very moment when the power of Islam was crumbling, it penetrated into Italy and began to exert its influence in the domain of medical literature, just as it did later in mathematics, astronomy, and art. This is reminiscent of a similar course of events in the history of Greek culture, which commenced to dominate Italy shortly after the fall of the political power of the Hellenes. It is noteworthy that in spite of the penetration of Arabian influences into Italy, the ancient Italian tradition that was based on Greek medicine was not lost, though it appeared dressed in new garments. This applies to the Salernitan physicians of the most glorious period of that school: the family of the PLATEARII, to whom we owe a number of scholastic texts, COPHO, who wrote a book on the anatomy of the pig, which was regarded as the work of Galen up to the end of the sixteenth century, ARCHBISHOP MATTHEW, who wrote a book of advice on the behaviour of the physician; in all these we find indubitable traces of the Hippocratic doctrine without Arabian influences.

The lay character of the school was maintained even though ecclesiastics were always present either as pupils or as teachers. This is proved by the fact that women were admitted to the lectures and to study. Docu-

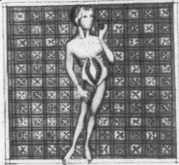

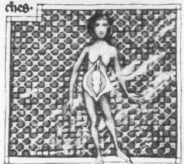

III. A page of Henri de Mondeville's Chirurgia, *from the section on abdominal surgery.*
(From a thirteenth-century manuscript, BIBLIOTHÈQUE NATIONALE, PARIS.*)*

ments also clearly show that the professors were permitted to marry. At the same time we soon find even in the constitution of the school of Salerno the influence of the great Arabian schools of the Orient and Mohammedan Spain. In this kind of school, the teachers formed a close body, so that even their teachings came from the corporation itself and not from an individual; learning was concentrated in the hospitals and in the laboratories; the dig-

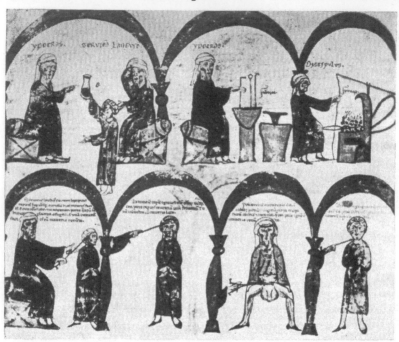

112. *A page of Roland's* Surgery. (*Codex of the* CASANATENSE LIBRARY.) *From left to right, above: Hippocrates prepares to examine the urine, then selects his instruments; finally, a scholar preparing the iron for cauterization. Below: cauterization applied to various surgical conditions.*

nity that the schools conferred on the physicians made them appear essentially as teachers, taking the same pride in their title as did those of ecclesiastical rank; finally the widespread reputation that the physicians enjoyed brought patients to them from all parts of Europe; these are the manifestations that connect the school of Salerno with the tradition of the great Arabian schools. Yet we should not believe on this account that these schools constituted the only model, inasmuch as the Greek and Alexandrian academies also served as prototypes.

The literary fame of the school — and this is also characteristic — is not due to treatises full of philosophic disquisitions or repetitions of scholastic discussions, but above all to that famous poem which under the name of *Flos medicinæ* or *Regimen sanitatis Salernitanum* constitutes, one might say, the backbone of all practical medical literature up to the time of the Renaissance. This poem, which includes within itself all the essential didactic characteristics of the school of Salerno, was committed to memory by thousands of physicians, for whom each of these verses had the quality of Holy Writ. It does not, to be sure, constitute a text of medical treatment that conforms to our present ideas of science; but the seductive quality of the verse had the virtue of spreading these useful, simple, and true maxims throughout the entire civilized world, popularizing with good common sense a sane criticism which evidences a Hippocratic quality that is the greatest glory of the school.

It has been calculated that there are almost three hundred editions of this poem. It has been translated into many languages: eleven times into French, ten into German, several into English, and frequently into Italian. Versions have varied considerably, and additions have been numerous. The school speaks in it as a corporation, and the poem is dedicated to a King of England about whose identity there has been much discussion. Some think that it was written for the benefit of Robert, Duke of Normandy, the oldest son of William the Conqueror, which would place it at the end of the eleventh century. He is known to have spent a winter at Salerno near the end of the century on his way to the Holy Land with his cousin Roger, the reigning Duke of Apulia, and to have visited there again in 1099 on his return. Recently some authors, and among them Sudhoff, who devoted intensive study to the school of Salerno, have supposed that the poem was written much later (probably about the middle of the thirteenth century) than in the flourishing period of the school. Sir Alexander Croake (1830), however, believed that it was written in the earlier period, both because no other king of England has any connection with Salerno and because it had early imitations at Paris and Montpellier, and is referred to by Gilles de Corbeil in the twelfth century. But however true the evidence for its later appearance may be, it cannot rob this famous poem of the great influence that it is known to have had on mediæval medical literature or of its reputation as the incarnation of the essential principles of a school which used dietary regulations and simple drugs as the basis of its treatment.

We quote from this valuable book some of its best-known and most popular verses, according to the 1553 edition of Arnold of Villanova's version. In this edition the poem consists of 362 stanzas; the numerous later additions account for the contradictions that are to be found in other versions. In his *Collectio Salernitana*, De Renzi catalogues all the known editions, among which there is one that contains 3,520 verses. According to him, the earliest edition of the Latin text was printed in Pisa in 1484; Klebs, in *Incunabula scientifica et medica* (1938), assigns the *editio princeps* to Cologne, 1480.

Anglorum Regi scribit schola tota
    Salerni
Si vis incolumem, si vis te reddere
    sanum
Curas tolle graves, irasci crede pro-
    phanum.
Parce mero, cœnato parum: non sit
    tibi vanum
Surgere post epulas, somnum fuge
    meridianum
Non mictum retine, nec comprime
    fortiter anum.
Hæc bene si serves, tu longo tempore
    vives
Si tibi deficiant medici, medici tibi
    fiant
Hæc tria: Mens hilaris, requies, mo-
    derata dieta.

The Salerne Schoole doth by these
    lines impart
All health to Englands King, and
    doth aduise
From care his head to keepe, from
    wrath his heart,
Drinke not much wine, sup light,
    and soone arise,
When meate is gone, long sitting
    breedeth smart:
And after-noone still waking keepe
    your eyes.
When mou'd you find your selfe
    to Natures Needs,
Forbeare them not, for that much
    danger breeds,
Use three Physicians still; first Doc-
    tor Quiet,
Next Doctor Merry-man, and Doc-
    tor Dyet.

Lumina mane manus surgens gelida
    lavet unda
Hac illac modicum pergat, modicum
    sua membra
Extendat, crines pectet, dentes fri-
    cet, ista
Confortant cerebrum, confortant
    cætera membra.

Rise earely in the morne, and
    straight remember,
With water cold to wash your hands
    and eyes,
In gentle fashion retching euery
    member,
And to refresh your braine when as
    you rise,
In heat, in cold, in Iuly and De-
    cember.
Both comb your head, and rub your
    teeth likewise:
If bled you haue, keep coole, if
    bath'd, keepe warme:
If din'd, to stand or walke will do
    no harme.

Sit brevis aut nullus tibi somnus
    meridianus

Some men there are that thinke a
    little nap breeds no ill bloud:

Febris, pigrities, capitis dolor atque catarrhus
Hæc tibi proveniunt ex somno meridiano.

But if you shall herein exceed too farre,
It hurts your health, it cannot be with stood:
Long sleepe at after-noones by stirring fumes,
Breeds Slouth, and Agues, Aking heads and Rheumes:

Quale, quid et quando, quantum, quoties, ubi, dando
Ista notare cibo debet medicus bene doctus.
Ex magna cœna stomacho fit maxima pœna
Ut sis nocte levis, sit tibi cœna brevis
Pone gulæ metas, ut tibi longior ætas.

To keepe good dyet, you should neuer feed
Untill you finde your stomacke cleane and void
Of former eaten meate, for they do breed
Repletion, and will cause you soone be cloid,
None other rule but appetite should need,
When from your mouth a moysture cleare doth void.

Ova recentia, vina rubentia, pinguia iura
Cum similia pura, naturæ sunt valitura.

Egges newly laid, are nutritiue to eate,
And rosted Reare are easie to digest.
Fresh Gascoigne wine is good to drinke with meat,
Broth strengthens nature aboue all the rest.

Lucidus et mundus sit rite habitabilis ær
Infectus neque sit nec olens fœtore cloacæ.

Though all ill sauours do not breed infection,
Yet sure infection commeth most by smelling,

Temporibus veris, modice prandere iuberis
Sed calor æstatis dapibus nocet immoderatis

In Spring your dinner must not much exceed,
In Summers heate but little meate shall need:

Autumni caveas fructus, ne sint tibi
 luctus,
De mensa sume quantum vis tempore
 brumæ.

In Autumne ware you eate not too
 much fruite:
With Winters cold full meates do
 fittest suite.

Lotio post mensam, tibi confert
 munera bina
Mundificat palmas et lumina reddit
 acuta
Si fore vis sanus, ablue sæpe manus.

If in your drinke you mingle Rew
 with Sage,
All poyson is expeld by power of
 those,
And if you would withall Lusts heat
 asswage,
Adde to them two the gentle flowre
 of Rose:
Would not be sea-sicke when seas
 do rage,
Sage-water drinke with wine before
 he goes.
Of washing of your hands much
 good doth rise,
Tis wholesome, cleanely, and re-
 lieues your eyes.

Est caro porcina sine vino peior
 ovina
Si tribuis vina, tunc est cibus et medicina.
Inter prandendum, sit sæpe pa-
 rumque bibendum.

Porke without wine is not so good
 to eate,
As Sheepe with wine, it medicine is
 and meate,
Tho Intrailes of a beast be not the
 best,
Yet are some intrailes better than the
 rest.

Lac ethicis sanum caprinum, post
 chamælinum
Ac nutritivum plus omnibus est
 asininum
Plus nutritivum vaccinum sit et
 ovinum.

'Tis good a Goat or Camels milke to
 drinke,
Cowes-milke and Sheepes doe well,
 but yet an Asses
Is best of all, and all the others passes.

Post pisces nux sit, post carnes caseus
 adsit

To close your stomack well, this
 order sutes,

Unica nux prodest, nocet altera, ter-
tia mors est.

Cheese after flesh, Nuts after fish or
fruits,
Yet some haue said, (beleeue them
as you will)
One Nut doth good, two hurt, the
third doth kill.

Cur moriatur homo, cui salvia cres-
cit in horto?
Contra vim mortis non est medica-
men in hortis,
Salvia confortat nervos, manuumque
tremorem
Tollit et eius ope febris acuta fugit.
Salvia salvatrix, naturæ conciliatrix.

But who can write thy worth (O
soueraigne Sage!).
Some aske how man can die, where
thou dost grow,
Oh that there were a medicine curing age,
Death comes at last, though death
comes ne're so slow:
Sage strengths the sinewes, seuere
heat doth swage,
The Palsy helpes, and rids of mickle
woe.

Motus, longa fames, vomitus, per-
cussio, casus,
Ebrietas, frigus, tinnitum causant in
aure.

These are the things that breed it
[our hearing] most offence,
To sleepe on stomacke full and
drinking hard,
Blowes, fals, and noyse, and fasting
violence,
Great heate and sodaine cooling
afterwards;
All these, as is by sundry proofes
appearing,
Breed tingling in our eares, and hurt
our hearing:

Balnea, vina, Venus, ventus, piper,
allia, fumus
Porri cum cepis, faba, lens fle-
tusque, sinapis

Now shall you see what hurtfull is
for sight:
Wine, women, Bathes, by art to
nature wrought,
Leekes, Onyons, Garlicke, Mustard-
seed, fire and light,

Sol, coitusque, ignis, labor, ictus, acumina, pulvis
Ista nocent oculis, sed vigilare magis.

Smoake, bruises, dust, Pepper to powder brought,
Beanes, Lentiles, strains, Wind, Tears, & Phœbus bright,
And all sharpe things our eye-sight do molest:
Yet watching hurts them more then all the rest.

Sanguine subtracto, sex horis est vigilandum,
Ne somni fumus lædat sensibile corpus,
Ne nervum lædas, non sit tibi plaga profunda,
Sanguine purgatus, ne carpas protinus escas.

Make your incision large and not to deepe
That bloud have speedy issue with the fume
So that from sinewes you all hurt do keepe
Nor may you (as I tougt before) presume
In sixe houres at all to sleepe
Lest some slight bruise in sleep cause an apostume.

Ver, autumnus, hiems, æstas dominantur in anno
Tempore vernali calidus fit aer humidusque
Et nullum tempus melior fit phlebothomiæ
Usus tunc homini Veneris confert moderatus
Corporis et motus, ventrisque solutio, sudor,
Balnea, purgentur tunc corpora cum medicinis
Æstas more calet sicca, nascatur in illa
Tunc quoque praecipue choleram rubeam dominari.
Humida, frigida fercula dentur, sit Venus extra

The spring is moist, of temper good and warme,
Then best it is to bathe, to sweate, and purge,
Then may one ope a veine in either arme,
If boyling bloud or feare of agues vrge:
Then Venus recreation doth no harme,
Yet may too much thereof turne to a scourge.
In Summers heat (when choller hath dominion)
Coole meates and moist are best in some opinion:
The Fall is like the Spring, but endeth colder,

Balnea non prosunt, sint raræ
   phlebothomiæ
Utilis est requies, sit cum modera-
   mine potus.

— Arnold of Villanova, 1553 edition

With Wines and Spice the Winter
   may be bolder.

— Text of Sir John Harington, first published 1607, from *The School of Salernum*
(New York: Paul B. Hoeber; 1920)

One of the classic books of the school of Salerno which permits us to have an idea of the pathology and treatment taught there is the *De ægritudinum curatione*. It is one of those numerous anonymous texts of a period in which writings of several authors were accumulated in a compilation; it is probably of the twelfth century, and gives strong evidence of Arabian influence. It constituted the principal standard work of the Salernitan physicians and the chief textual source of instruction. In the first part of the book, the doctrine of fevers is discussed; in the second, the treatment of all diseases from the crown of the head to the sole of the foot. The second most important part gives the teaching of the seven physicians who were the chief masters of the school: Johannes PLATEARIUS, COPHO, PETRONIUS, AFFLACCIUS, BARTOLOMEUS, FERRARIUS, and TROTULA.

The doctrine of fevers is based on the clinical picture. They are divided into quotidian or ephemeral, and hectic or putrid, the latter being either intermittent or continuous. The treatment is above all dietetic or emollient. The pathology of nervous affections is primitive: mental disorders are regarded as coming from an abscess of the anterior cerebral ventricles. Somnolence or lethargy should be attributed to an abscess of the posterior ventricles.

The treatment of the psychoses consisted in diet, purgatives, blood-letting, and various drugs, but the psychological element is emphasized — for example, by treatment with pleasant words and calming music.

The part that treats of the affections of the respiratory tract is especially interesting because of some observations on the prognosis of consumption. Thus it is maintained that bloody sputum at the beginning of the disease is a good sign. Among the causes of consumption one finds hemoptysis, just as in the older texts; but the treatment recommended emphasizes the necessity of prescribing a generous diet for the patient and a tranquil existence. The differential diagnosis between ascites and tympany is noteworthy: in the first case, percussion gives the sound of a filled bottle; and in the second case, the sound of a drum.

The statements about surgical conditions are primitive and deal almost entirely with a therapy of external applications. The chapter on disorders of the genitalia, on the other hand, is treated in an advanced manner. There are long lists of aphrodisiacs and abortifacients, of drugs that prevent conception, and of many cosmetic medicaments.

Two of the most celebrated physicians who acquired fame in the school of Salerno and were its pupils, were the Jewish Benvenutus Grassus or Grapheus (eleventh, twelfth, or thirteenth century?), and Isaac Judæus.

Benvenutus GRASSUS, who was born in Jerusalem and was a pupil of Nicholæus Præpositus, was the most famous non-Mohammedan oculist of mediæval times. He taught at Salerno and at Montpellier, and wrote a *Practica oculorum* or *Ars probatissima oculorum*, the most popular Latin textbook on the diseases of the eye, as is shown by the number of examples that have been preserved in Latin, English, French, and Provençal (22 manuscripts and 18 printed editions). It has been published by Albertotti and studied intensively by Scalinci (1932). An edition in English was published by Casey Wood in 1929 (Stanford University Press, California). It also has the distinction of being the first printed book on ophthalmology (Ferrara, 1474). Grassus makes frequent references to anatomical studies made by him on the structure of the eye, and his book constitutes a notable advance over the work of the Arabian authors. For five hundred years it was regarded as the classical text on ophthalmology.

Salernitan uroscopy found its classic master in ISAAC JUDÆUS, whose writings constitute the standard for this field. The urine was carefully examined as to colour, density, and content; the different kinds of clouds and precipitates that form on standing were observed, and aided in the deduction of most important and far-reaching conclusions. Though this method had no true diagnostic value and was pushed to fantastic extremes, it held its position for centuries, until eventually laughed out of court by the realistic and better-educated Renaissance.

Pierre GILLES DE CORBEIL (Petrus Ægidius Corboliensis, fl. *c.* 1200) was a celebrated French physician who was a pupil of the school of Salerno and Montpellier and later went to Paris, where he was archiater to Philip Augustus and probably taught in the university. Neuburger has called him the transalpine herald of the glory of the school of Salerno. He was the author of a didascalic poem which enjoyed great contemporary reputation; in it the whole Salernitan doctrine was amplified and paraphrased in Latin hexameters. The description of the different kinds of pulse, methods of examining the patient, of studying the urine, advice about the behaviour of the physician, and invectives against the pharmacists are presented in facile and elegant form. The book on the urine, which is the first in the poem, was regarded up to the end of the sixteenth century as the classical text on uroscopy; it was derived from the famous *Regulæ urinarum* of the Salernitan writer MAGISTER MAURUS (d. 1214). This has been published by De Renzi (*Collectio Salernitana*, III). The poem by Gilles was published by Choulant in Leipzig, 1826, and in a French translation by Vieillard, Paris, 1903.

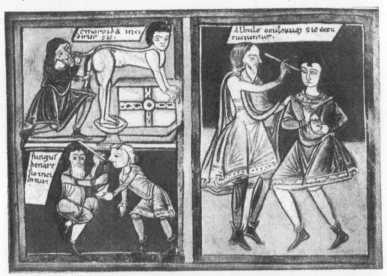

113. *Salernitan surgery. Operations for hemorrhoids, nasal polyp, and cataract.* (*From an eleventh-century manuscript in the* BRITISH MUSEUM.)

The study of anatomy by the dissection of animals was undoubtedly practised at Salerno — one of the chief merits of the Salernitan school. Up to that time anatomy had been taught simply *sicut asserit Galenus* ("thus does Galen declare"). At Salerno the dissection of animals, and particularly of pigs, was carried out systematically. A number of anatomical texts, published in the *Collectio Salernitana* by De Renzi and others, show us that both professors and pupils of Salerno, no matter how attached they were to the teachings of Galen, were beginning to realize the importance of an independent study of anatomy.

The oldest *Anatomia Salernitana*, which, as we have seen, is attributed to Copho, bears no trace of the Greco-Arabic nomenclature introduced by Constantinus Africanus. The *Anatomia* of Magister Maurus, which has been shown by Sudhoff to date from the middle of the twelfth century, and of which four manuscripts are known, already includes such

Arabic terms as *siphac* for the peritoneum, *zirbus* for the omentum, etc.
This shows the slow penetration of Arabian influence at Salerno, a tendency which is confirmed also by later texts. It is interesting to note that
while the texts that we have mentioned thus far were evidently intended
for the practical teaching of anatomy with dissection of the cadavers of
animals, in the later texts there is no mention of anatomical dissections, but

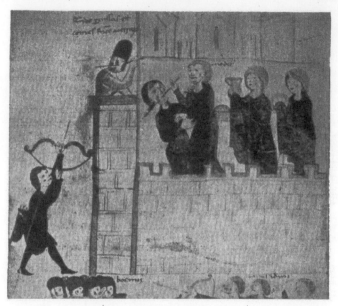

114. *Richard of Acerra is wounded at the siege of Naples and
treated by a physician and two nurses.*
(*From* Carmen de rebus siculis *of Peter of Eboli, twelfth century.*)

only references to the writings of Galen. The *Anatomia* of an anonymous
master, collected by a pupil, concerns itself but little with morphological
data, but rather with physiology and pathology. This fourth Salernitan
anatomy was published by Sudhoff (*Arch. f. Gesch. d. Med.*, 1928), who
believed that it should be ascribed to the Calabrian physician and teacher
URSUS.

Surgery was always practised in southern Italy, frequently by empiricists, as at Norcia and other places; but it is at Salerno that we meet
the first Italian work on surgery worthy of the name. It bears the title,
from the words with which the first chapter opens, of *Post mundi fabricam*
and contains the lectures of one of the greatest of the Salernitan surgeons,
Roger of Salerno (ROGERIUS FRUGARDI), about whose life we possess only
scanty and vague information. This book, which for three centuries was

regarded as a classic, was published in a number of editions with various additions and changes. It is sometimes confused with the work of Roland of Parma, because a master of Parma belonging to the school of Bologna made a new version of it toward the middle of the thirteenth century.

Another text attributed to Salerno is the *Book of the Four Masters* (who were ARCHIMATTHÆUS, PETRONCELLUS or PETRONIUS, PLATEARIUS, and FERRARIUS) on the surgery of Roger of Salerno. As a matter of fact, it probably was inspired by the school of Salerno, and, as Sudhoff has shown, was written at a much later period. In the present state of our knowledge of the history of the period, then, one may accept that Roger of Salerno was the greatest surgeon of the school of Salerno and that all the Salernitan surgeries which appeared under various names were merely elaborations of his lectures.

Though based partly on earlier authorities, such as Constantinus Africanus, Roger's surgery (*Coll. Salern.*, II) contains a considerable amount of the personal experiences of Roger and his contemporaries. It gives an excellent description of herniotomy and recommends the use of mercury salts for chronic and parasitic skin diseases. It is said also to include a remarkable reference to the use of seaweed (iodine) in the treatment of goitre. It treats at length of wounds of the head and brain, even giving the differential diagnosis of injuries of the skull and indications for trephining. For depressed fractures, it is recommended to make a number of holes with the trephine and then slowly raise the fractured bone without damaging the meninges. The chapter on dislocations gives a number of precise indications for reduction. There are many interesting statements in the chapter on lesions of the intestine and peritoneum. If the intestine has protruded and has stayed thus long enough to have become cold, it is recommended to open the abdomen of an animal and to superimpose it on the wounded part until it has been warmed and become somewhat soft. Then with a clean sponge soaked in hot water the intestine is lightly cleansed and replaced in the abdomen, leaving the wound open as long as the intestine is seen to be damaged, after which a drain is inserted and the wound dressed every day.

Surgical treatment of cancer of the rectum and the cervix is regarded as possible, but not advised on account of the poor results obtained. The operations for hernia, hydrocele, and lithotomy are described in the same way as by the classical authors. An interesting item is the description of the examination necessary for the diagnosis of stone in the bladder, and the differential diagnosis between stone and hypertrophy of the prostate.

The *Chirurgia* of Roland of Parma (ROLAND CAPELLUTI) is an elaboration of Roger's work, but somewhat more than a mere commentary, and showing more extensive Arabian influence. It was published in a reproduction of the Latin

Codex 1382 of the *Biblioteca Casanatense* by Giovanni Carbonelli, with an Italian translation and notes (Rome, 1927). This Codex has beautiful illustrations and is one of the most interesting documents of Salernitan surgery. In one place Roland tells of having operated upon and cured a youth of Bologna, a portion of whose lung protruded from between his ribs. Theodoric of Cervia, on the other hand, stated in a manuscript that is preserved in the library of St. Mark's in Venice that this operation was done by Hugh of Lucca, while Roland merely acted as his assistant.

4. *Evolution of Mediæval Medicine. Decadence of the School of Salerno*

The practice of medicine in the early centuries of the Middle Ages was particularly reserved for the ecclesiastics, up to the period in which the school of Salerno became predominantly lay in character. It is in these early times that the foundation of the monastic infirmaries took place, to which St. Benedict devoted a chapter of his rule. Infirmaries were designed exclusively for the monks; and it is only much later that hospitals for the lay sick arose near the infirmaries. The medical attendance in the infirmaries was provided by a physician and an *infirmarius*. About the tenth century these monasteries became more and more rich and powerful, often possessed wide lands, busied themselves with agriculture, and constructed roads and bridges in their domains. Then the monks came to exercise their medical activities even outside of the monasteries, and one often finds them called to the bedside of illustrious patients. In 1130 the Council of Clermont, and in 1139 the Council of the Lateran, forbade monks and regular clerics to practise medicine; in 1219 it was strictly forbidden to every ecclesiastic to go out of the monastery. " *ad physicam legesve mondanas legendas* " (" to read in physic or in civil law "). Finally, Honorius III forbade even the secular ecclesiastics to practise medicine. This brought the practice of medicine more and more into the hands of the laity, and toward the beginning of the thirteenth century, when the first universities were being founded, medicine became almost entirely a lay activity. The school of Salerno marks, as we have seen, the beginning and the flourishing of lay learning, after having been exposed in its beginnings to the influence of monastic medicine. To the ancient monastic medical schools of the Middle Ages, whose activities were limited to the study of a few classical texts and the growth of simples whose medical properties were carefully studied, we should attribute nevertheless the merit of having, in these vexatious times, preserved the traditions of ancient medicine in the tranquil refuge of the cloisters, and of having preached by example the law of charity to the sick and assistance to the weak.

In the course of the twelfth and thirteenth centuries the reputation of the school of Salerno, which was regarded as the centre of medical learning, spread throughout the civilized world. It was to it alone that Frederick II gave the right of conferring on physicians the licence to practise medicine, stating that the study of anatomy on the cadaver should be an important part of the instruction (1240). No one could practise medicine without the approval of the Salernitan Collegium, and, after having completed the five-year course of study, the physician still had for at least one year to practise under the supervision of an experienced physician.

In the legislation of public hygiene in the province of Naples and in Sicily, Frederick II followed the recommendations of the school of Salerno; and in 1267 Charles of Anjou reaffirmed its importance when he reorganized the system of teaching. This begins the third period of the school of Salerno — the period of its decadence. Although it still enjoyed a universal renown, as is shown by the decree of Ladislaus of Hungary (1413) which gave special privileges to its teachers, nevertheless the school was approaching its end. In 1811, when a Napoleonic decree finally suppressed it, it had for a long time existed in name only.

If we regard in its ensemble the work of the school of Salerno, the Civitas Hippocratica, which enjoyed such a great renown up to 1300, we must conclude that it had the tremendous value of presenting the first example of a lay school in which men of all religions and nations worked together toward a common end. There hospitality was extended to Arabs and to Jews, who brought their special contribution of learning and of work; there probably for the first time the official title of *Magister* was introduced, and soon after, the custom of a solemn form of promotion was begun. It is at Salerno that one sees for the first time in Italy a systematic organization of medical study, which, when the young universities began to flourish throughout Europe, took on a new and definitive form during the Renaissance.

Thus the chapter in the history of medicine that concerns this ancient and celebrated school is certainly among those which should interest the scholar most of all. It is the school of Salerno that preserved the concept of Hippocratic pathology and put the practice of medicine back into the hands of the laity independent of dogmatic doctrines. It is at Salerno that was concentrated the activity of those scholars who, with a calm, critical sense, yet fervid enthusiasm, interpreted the ancient texts for the instruction of their students. And, finally, it is at Salerno that that class of lay physicians was created which was to play the most important role in the medicine of the Renaissance; because it was by them that the struggle against scholastic medicine was begun and the new medicine prepared. We find in this ancient school, where, as in the schools of ancient Greece, surgery played an important part, a true *Civitas Hippocratica*, worthy through centuries of this ancient and glorious name. On the shores of the Bay of Pæstum, as at Cos in ancient Greece, masters and pupils came together, concerned especially with the welfare of the patient, in constant contact with human suffering, and far removed from empty speculative discussions and from superstitions and astrology. It is there that a clinical type of instruction developed which may be truly regarded as animating the path-breaking and fertile activities of the universities of the Renaissance.

CHAPTER XV

MEDICINE IN THE LATER

MIDDLE AGES

THE UNIVERSITIES AND HUMANISM. THE PRE-
CURSORS OF THE RENAISSANCE

1. Cultural Currents in the Beginning of the Thirteenth Century

Toward the beginning of the thirteenth century various currents exerted their influence on the evolution of medical thought in Italy. We
have seen the important role played by the school of Salerno in the development of a lay medicine. From it this tendency spread throughout
western Europe, for even though it felt the effect of Arabian medicine in
certain literary forms, it remained essentially Hippocratic in its fundamental concepts. It is the currents from Salerno that fertilized and activated the French school at Montpellier, which is closely attached to Salerno
and its traditions, even though experiencing more directly the influence
of the neighbouring schools in Arab Spain. Soon other schools of western
Europe, together with various isolated centres of medical culture in Sicily
and lower Italy, felt the vitalizing spirit.

Already in 1140 Roger, King of Sicily, had enforced the law prohibiting
from the practice of medicine anyone who had not shown in his State
examination that he had fulfilled the necessary course of studies, " in
order that the King's subjects should not incur dangers through the in-

experience of their physicians." Frederick II, also, recognized the importance of the school of Salerno and promulgated stringent laws (1224) for
the study and practice of medicine. After a preliminary three-year course,
the prospective physician had to take a five-year medical course, followed
by a year with an experienced practitioner, pass a formal examination, and
present testimonials satisfactory to the Imperial authority. The cultural
current which spread from southern Italy and Sicily through the peninsula
had an importance in the history of science which has perhaps not been
properly recognized. Sicily, which from the most distant times had seen
people of different races in constant contact, experienced a marvellous
expansion under the dominion of the Norman rulers and brought together
in an admirable civil organization merchants, artists, and Arabic, Byzantine,
Greek, and Jewish physicians. The court of Palermo became one of the
most flourishing cultural centres of the period. When the Angevin dynasty
followed the Normans, and Charles I of Anjou became King of Naples
and Sicily, this desire to know the classics and to collect a constantly increasing number of precious manuscripts became ever more fervid in
those regions in which, as we have seen, the classical Greek traditions had
never been completely destroyed.

Together with this current of an eminently lay character, another, no
less important, exercised its effect on the development of civilization, science, and art, and consequently on the evolution of medicine. This is the
current of scholastic thought, which, under the stimulus of the Church —
which both strengthened its political power and steadily extended its domination over things of the intellect — monopolized all scholastic activity
and even dominated all thought. Aristotelian philosophy was drawn into
the orbit of Christianity and became the centre about which revolved
the doctrine of Thomas Aquinas, who became the spiritual leader of this
tendency.

The history of medicine of the period continually suggests the presence
of these two great currents, sometimes coming together and sometimes
separating. We should note the influence that the political changes that
occurred in Italy had on the evolution of medical thought, which was
often battered by the different tendencies and was almost always sterilized
by vain discussions. These were the times in which medicine harvested
little or nothing from ancient traditions and new experiences. One almost
has the impression that the silhouette of the physician of the fourteenth
century, familiar to us from the miniatures of the time, entirely preoccupied
with a sumptuous costume, examination of urine, and the day and hour
best suited for blood-letting, is the best symbol that one can find of the

very poor state of medicine at this period. However, if one considers more closely the events and personages of the time, one perceives that in spite of an ignorance of the most elementary facts of anatomy and physiology, and in spite of the apparent vanity of the interminable empty discussions that prevailed, it is precisely at this period that the renaissance of medicine was being prepared. Just as the early painters of the fourteenth century, though ignorant of anatomy and of the laws of perspective, were the precursors of the great masters of the Renaissance, like those humble Sicilian and Tuscan writers of the *dolce stil nuovo,* so the physicians of those times, though derided by Petrarch, the prophet of humanism and of the Renaissance, were the simple but invaluable intermediaries, the unknown and indispensable precursors of the glorious days to come.

2. The Universities. Arabism and Scholasticism

The contest between the various opposing forces was most manifest in the universities which arose in the twelfth and quickly reached their greatest development in the thirteenth century. These, perhaps equally with the magnificent cathedrals, constitute the greatest glory of the Middle Ages. Their creation, one of the most important contributions to civilized culture of all time, though brought about in various ways, was made possible largely by the growth of the mediæval cities, and the accumulation of wealth and power in or near them. The Peace of Constance (1183), which freed the great Italian cities, was another important factor in favouring their development.

The oldest universities probably took their origin from the ancient Latin schools that had survived the decadence of the Empire; but they had no real organization until toward the end of the thirteenth century. The constitution of the first universities reveals their origin. It would be a mistake to assume that from the very beginning there existed schools that all had the same character. In the earliest concept, the word *universitas* indicated only the corporation of the scholars who took the courses of instruction, a corporation to which the communities and rulers who tried to aid the schools in many ways granted the most important privileges. There were schools where medicine alone was taught. Such was the case at Montpellier, which was one of the most ancient, even though the date of its foundation cannot be fixed with certainty. In most of the schools, which were indicated by the term *studium generale,* law, theology, and philosophy were also taught.

The constitution of the various universities and their legal basis differed according to their origins. There were universities supported by the communities, as, for instance, the University of Bologna, which was governed by an autonomous and democratic organization; the rector of the university was elected by the students. In the universities the rights of foreign students were safeguarded with especial care; they enjoyed many privileges and were divided, according to their origin, into various Nations. Together with the corporations of students, there were created later the corporations of teachers or masters, which bore the name *Collegium Doctorum* and enjoyed the *Jus Promovendi* — that is, the right to confer the title giving the licence to practise medicine. The division into different faculties was made at a later time and in different ways. In a number of the more important Italian universities, such as Padua, the medical students belonged to the Faculty of Arts.

Another type of university was that founded at Naples by Frederick II in 1224 and copied by Alfonso VIII and his successors in Spain. These were true State universities, governed by the ruler or his representatives and subject to the regulations that he issued.

A third type of university is that of Paris and the English universities, which were directly under the rule of the ecclesiastical authorities. In all universities, however, the pope and his representatives had the power of supervision; in the earlier periods the masters were almost entirely clerics, and theological instruction dominated the university spirit. No *studium* could be instituted without the express permission of the pontiff, who had always the right to intervene in matters of teaching. The examiners were generally named by the bishop or the legate of the pope; the licence was given in the name of the pope and in church by a high ecclesiastical dignitary, a procedure which gave to this solemnity the character of a religious ceremony.

It was only later when Jews and other non-Catholics entered the universities that this custom fell into disuse and the ceremony often took place in the house of the president of the college. At the beginning of university teaching, in spite of the title of *Studium Generale*, not much importance was given to the subject of medicine; neither did the universities have identical regulations even as regards the type of instruction. In Bologna it was only in 1295 that the medical students obtained the right to elect an independent rector of their own. At Paris the university masters soon formed a corporation and had common rights and duties. The three higher faculties had an elected dean at their head, the Faculty of Liberal Arts having a rector elected by four procurators, themselves named by the four Nations (French, Norman, Picard, and English). A German Nation was added later. Citizens of other countries could be admitted into one or other of these so-called Nations. The faculties and Nations, however, were subordinated to the supreme authority of the chancellor of Notre-Dame, the church in which the university was cradled.

From the year 1200 up to the end of the Middle Ages about eighty universities (the *Studia Generalia*) were founded in Europe, of which there were about 20 in Italy, 19 in France, 14 in the German countries, 5 in Britain, 4 in Spain, 2 in Portugal, and so on.[1] The two chief types were those of Paris and Bologna. Not all the universities gave regular teaching in medicine: of the 19 French universities, for a long time only Montpellier and Paris had regular instruction by medical faculty. The University of Montpellier was the more important in medicine for several centuries, perhaps because the medical school there was practically independent. [At Paris and other universities the *trivium* (grammar, rhetoric, dialectics) and the *quadrivium* (arithmetic, geometry, astronomy, music) constituted the seven liberal arts, taught independently of philosophy, law, and theology. Medicine was often taught as a branch of philosophy (*physica*). The favourite medical textbooks were the *Canon* of Avicenna, Galen's *Ars parva*, the *Isagoge* of Johannitius, the *Liber medicinalis* of Rhazes, and the works of Hippocrates, especially the *Aphorisms, Dietetics,* and *Prognostics*. Even these existed in fragmentary and incorrect translations, as for some time practically no works in the original Greek were available. In succeeding centuries more of the classical medical writers became available, such as Soranus, Paul of Ægina, Aëtius, Alexander of Tralles, Dioscorides, and so on. Toward the end of the period *Consilia* (or *Consortia in Practica*) became popular; they had the practical value of containing descriptions of actual cases rather than mere vague disquisitions. *Ed.*]

In the early times of the universities, as Martinotti has shown in his study of the teaching of anatomy at Bologna, the lectures were given in very humble places or even worse, if it is true that at Paris lectures were sometimes held in houses where prostitutes also were living, as has been affirmed by the chroniclers of the period. It was only much later that the faculties, at first scattered throughout the city, came together near that small but famous street of the Fouarre (or Feurre), called in the Latin documents *Vicus Straminis*, and mentioned by Dante under the name of *Vico degli Strami* (the street of the straw). In summer straw was piled on the floor and in winter hay, on which the teacher and the pupils sat; the teacher had one more bundle of straw so as to be raised above his auditors. Even in 1376 we find the regulation that students should sit on the ground and not on benches, in order that they should not become too proud. In 1271 the entire medical faculty of Paris was composed of six Regents and a Dean. These were the ones who promulgated the first statutes and adopted the square cap and silver medallion.

The origin of this, one of the most famous of all universities, cannot be accurately stated; while some like to believe that Charlemagne was its real founder, others give the chief credit to Peter Abélard (1079–1142). When in 1200 Philip Augustus conferred special privileges on students and teachers, it is apparent that some regular teaching was already in existence. Medical

[1] A list of the world's universities, in the approximately chronological order of their foundation, is given in an Appendix to this volume.

teaching went on there at least from 1210, when Gilles de Corbeil left Salerno to become physician to Philip Augustus. Though the requirements for graduation were often changed, they always were strict according to the standards of the time, and the examinations lasted many hours. The rule that the candidate, in case of failure, had to swear that he would not take revenge on the faculty throws light on the turbulent character of the university students at that time. On graduation with a Baccalaureate degree (a term used from the earliest times and about the origin of which there is much confusion), many of the students stayed on at the university to assist in the teaching. The next higher degree was the Licentiate, attained after taking four special courses and being consecrated by the chancellor of the university following elaborate preliminaries known as the *Paranymphe*. Those who acquired the Doctorate, after an examination called the Vespery, became *ipso facto* members of the faculty.

In many universities, especially outside of Italy, the lectures were held in the houses of the professors. The students paid for the teaching and the use of the benches, while the teachers gave their pupils hospitality and lived with them. From this custom grew the colleges that became widespread, especially in England. Thus Oxford and Cambridge, even in the fourteenth century, had special houses for students (hostels), governed by a responsible principal who furnished the students with food and lodging and books for study. The colleges, many richly endowed, are still the important units in these institutions.

In Bologna the students lived in *ospizi*, paying annually a price that was fixed each year by four *mediatores*, two of whom were chosen from among the students by the rector and the other two by the city. The houses lived in by the students and their families were regarded as under special protection; the proprietor could not expel the students before the end of the term, and if some crime was committed within the house for which its destruction was ordered (a frequent penalty at that time), the execution of the sentence was deferred until the end of the year. If the house was burned down or destroyed without any fault of the students, the city was held responsible for furnishing them with a suitable lodging up to the end of their contracts. The students could live in the hostels with their families and enjoyed exemption from many taxes. All the professors of law and medicine enjoyed the same rights and had the same duties.

Bologna especially, which took great care that the Studium was not disturbed or suppressed but preserved *ut thesaurus preciosissimus*, established in its statutes from 1284 that the students should enjoy all the rights of citizens in addition to a number of exemptions and privileges. The great number of foreign students in the Italian universities is shown by the fact that in the registers of matriculation of the *inclita nazione Alemanna*, even in 1289, one finds the cream of German nobility and intelligence. In most of the Italian universities the autonomous character of the university was preserved to the end of the fourteenth century. It is only at that time that the city began to take a part in the nomination of the lecturers and to give them fixed salaries; but even throughout the fifteenth century the lectures were given in the lecturers' houses or in houses chosen by them.

Soon extremely different tendencies became manifest in the various universities, in accord with the masters who taught there and the liberties that they enjoyed. On the one hand were the largest and most celebrated universities, which obtained from cities and princes great privileges and took on more and more the character of closed corporations constituting a small State within the State, on which the arm of the Church exerted its power. Here science became progressively crystallized in the rigid forms of scholasticism; neither clinical observation nor attempts at experimental investigation could have the slightest effect on this solid edifice. On the other hand were the universities in which lay tendencies predominated, where an obvious tendency away from dogmatism could be detected. This is the period when the schools of the great translators began the task of interpreting the Arabian texts of Avicenna, Rhazes, and Averroes. It is the period when the Greco-Arabian medicine was slowly absorbed by the people of western Europe. Thus medicine, though for a time engulfed in the slough of scholasticism, was preparing itself to progress toward research and observation — the first clear sign of the mingling of the currents from the Orient with the Western world in poetry, science, and art. As it was girding for the great enterprise of the Crusades, the Occident received from such centres as Toledo the forgotten writings of Aristotle and the *Almagest* of Ptolemy. Frederick II gave an enormous stimulus to the activity of the translators; he sent to the doctors of philosophy at Bologna the Latin translation of the works of Aristotle and his commentators, which he had had specially made, " as to the older masters who knew how to bring the new waters from the old wells to eager lips, and who wisely combated dogmas in renewing the ancient works in their teaching." Charles of Anjou followed the same course: he sent scholars to the Orient to seek out ancient medical texts, and had them translated by a Jewish physician of the school of Salerno, Farag ben Salem, who, for instance, put into Latin the colossal work of Rhazes.

Thus developed the first episode of the great contest that lasted for centuries. From the Orient came that last breath of life which delivered the first attack on the edifice of *a priori* science, and it is through medical books that it arrived. Medical science, which always necessarily had to be logical, especially in its contact with the observation of nature, was the advance guard of this movement; thus it is through the translations of Hippocrates and the other Greeks and the commentaries of Averroes that the first breath of humanism came to the West.

Padua soon acquired the reputation of being an Averroist and almost heretical university, chiefly because a leader in its faculty was PIETRO

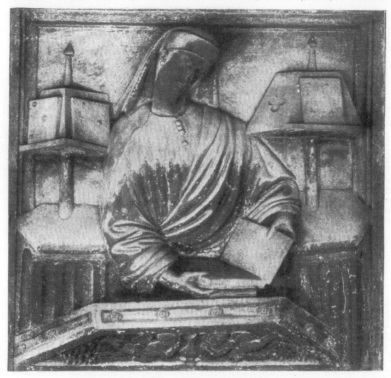

115. *Pietro d'Abano lecturing.*
Bas-relief on the front of the Palazzo della Ragione, Padua.

D'ABANO (Petrus Aponensis) (1250–1316), one of the most illustrious teachers and one of the most persecuted by the Inquisition. Endowed with a highly critical mind, he was placed by his vast scientific and literary knowledge at the head of all the science of his time. He conceived the idea of resolving by the authority of dogma and syllogisms the contradictions that were to be found between Arabian medicine and speculative philosophy. He wished to prepare a complete treatise on theoretical and practical medicine which would harmonize conflicting tendencies, and in which scholars could be instructed both in that natural philosophy which according to the author was the basis of science, as well as in diseases and their remedies. Averroist in thought and dialectician in form, he composed his

Conciliator controversiarum, quæ inter philosophos et medicos versantur (a book which brought the author fame and his name of "Conciliator") according to the methods of ancient dialectics, and resolved differences by almost always submitting empirical data to the syllogism. Nevertheless, beneath all these philosophic discussions one can detect the observational power of a man of genius. Pietro's real master in medicine was Avicenna; like Avicenna, he accepted four phases of disease: the onset, the increase, the fastigium, and the decline. His simple and natural therapeutic measures revealed a physician hostile to all complicated and charlatan-like measures. Cold water is praised as a good remedy in many cases. In his study of the soul, d'Abano generally follows the ideas of Averroes, but does not hesitate to contradict his assertions if need be. Sometimes also he combats both Aristotle and Averroes; without question he shows himself capable of differing from the dominant authorities and disputing the authority of the ancients.

Pietro d'Abano was, as Sante Ferrari has shown, one of the first and most strenuous defenders of Italian Averroism, which was in some ways opposed to Catholic teleological philosophy. Averroes' theory of a union of the soul with the intellect in this life was corrupted by his followers into a theory of a common soul for all mankind, which perforce aroused the opposition of the Church.

One must not forget that Averroism above all means Arabism, and that consequently none of those who had been influenced by Arabian thought could be hostile to the great commentator and to Maimonides, who prepared the way for him. Pietro, however much he was reputed to be hostile to magic practices, had the name of a great astrologer and a powerful magus, and in the literature of the time there are many miracles said to have been accomplished by him with the aid of the devil.

Pietro d'Abano's teachings and books, some of which were regarded as authoritative texts up to the end of the sixteenth century, certainly exerted a profound and widespread influence. The renown of the philosopher who had gone to Constantinople to study Greek and could read Aristotle and Galen in the original, the glory of the scholar who taught medicine at Paris and was regarded there as a great master, all this spread his fame throughout the Western world. His reputation probably was also augmented by the persecutions of the Dominicans, who accused him of heresy because of fifty-five passages in his writings which were contrary to Roman Catholic dogma. When he was called to Padua in 1306 to become Professor of Philosophy at the university, his name was already on the tongue of everyone who devoted himself to philosophy. Already a famous student of medicine, he soon became a much sought-after practitioner, consulted by such dignitaries as the Marquis Azzo d'Este and Pope Honorius IV. The crowd of students that flocked to his lectures was so great that Gentile da Foligno, arriving at the hall where the master was teaching, fell on his knees and cried out: " Hail, O Holy Temple! "

The fame of the scholar and the zeal of the teacher could not leave indifferent those who saw in him a destroyer of mediæval scholasticism as well as a heretic. Accused for the second time by the Inquisition in 1315, one year before his death, when he was already seriously ill, Pietro died while the trial was being prepared; but his death failed to stop it. In 1316 he was condemned to the stake and the sentence was ordered to be carried out on his dead body; but tradition states that loyal hands so concealed his remains that the judgment could be executed only in effigy.

Pietro is known to have exerted a considerable influence on Dante, who perhaps even followed his courses and probably had also attended the lectures of Sigierus in Paris. The thoughts of this greatest of Italian poets and philosophers about the Averroist problem, which necessarily concerned the scholars of that day, were probably much influenced by such contacts. On the 15th of June 1300 Dante was elected Prior of the city of Florence for the guild of the physicians and pharmacists, a nomination, to be sure, which was doubtless due entirely to politics. None the less, one must remember that his poetry contains frequent allusions to diseases, with descriptions that indicate considerable medical knowledge. Even if it cannot be proved, as some have maintained, that he was a physician, it is evident that he was in contact with the physicians of his time and even may have studied medicine at Bologna and at Padua. In all the old representations of Dante that we possess, he is shown with the red robe and the miniver on the cap, a costume which, if not exclusively reserved for physicians, was the one that was usually worn by them.

Among other famous masters in the history of the University of Padua was GENTILE DA FOLIGNO (d. 1348), especially remembered for his *Consilia,* in which are accounts of a number of actual cases studied not without a sense of objectivity. Public dissections of human cadavers were beginning about this time, and it is known that he made one such at Padua in 1341. Among other Paduans were the famous DE SANTA SOFIA family, especially Marsilio and his nephew Galeazzo, Giacomo DEI DONDI (1298–1359) and his son Giovanni; Giacomo DELLA TORRE (Jacobus Forliviensis); Matteo SILVATICO, author of a famous *Pandectæ;* Francesco di PIEDIMONTE, whose *Supplementum Mesuæ* is a good example of the mingling of the Salernitan and Arabian currents; Nicolò FALCUCCI (d. c. 1412), author of a huge *Sermones medicinales* (published in several parts about 1484), summarizing all of mediæval medicine; and Giovanni ARCOLANI (died 1484), whose *Practica* is especially noteworthy in the history of dentistry, having descriptions of gold fillings, dental instruments, and the general surgery of the mouth. These physicians may be regarded as leaders in the attempts to escape from scholasticism and to form objective judgments rather than long dialectic disquisitions. Haeser states that the books studied at Tübingen in the fourteenth century were the first and fourth canons of Avicenna, the ninth book of Rhazes (commentaries of Jacopo da Forli and Arcolani), the *Ars Parva* of Galen (commentary of Torrigiani), and the Aphorisms of Hippocrates.

3. Bologna, Montpellier, and Oxford

The University of Bologna occupies a very important position in the history of medicine. In its early stages it was the seat of a rigid scholasticism, producing the most able commentators and vigorous dialecticians. First among the Bolognese physicians who gained great contemporary renown was Master Taddeo ALDEROTTI (1223, Florence–c. 1300), immortalized in the verses of Dante. He was regarded by his contemporaries as the most illustrious physician of all Italy and it is probable that Dante, who studied at Bologna, attended his lectures.

Taddeo was professor at Bologna from the year 1260. He was the first and most conscientious translator of the Aristotelian maxims and may be regarded as the real founder of the dialectical method in medicine. Taddeo, " the Hippocratist," as Dante called him, commented on Hippocrates, as the jurists did on Justinian, in the style of a period when formalism was beginning to invade medicine, clothing it in brilliant forms but robbing it of all vitality. Author of commentaries that are classic in their knowledge and critical judgment, he revealed himself as faithful to the Greco-Arabian traditions of the school of Salerno. As a practitioner he was much sought after, and he accumulated great wealth. He is known to have charged three thousand crowns in one case, and before undertaking the treatment of Pope Honorius IV, who died under his care, he declared that he would not move for less than a hundred ducats a day — both very large sums when one considers the purchasing power of money at that time.

To Taddeo is owed a new form of medical literature, the so-called *Consilia* — that is, a collection of clinical cases. These were very successful and certainly in this period of scholastic discussions represent an important concession to the need for practical observations. This literary form had, as we shall see, considerable vogue up to the end of the seventeenth century. For his friend Corso Donati he composed a book *Della conservazione della salute*, in which there are some wise hygienic regulations, for instance concerning the care of the mouth and teeth, and frequent daily exercise. It was published for the first time by Puccinotti in his *History of Medicine* (Vol. II, pp. 44 ff.).

We quote a page from this book, which is one of the most ancient medical texts written in the vernacular.

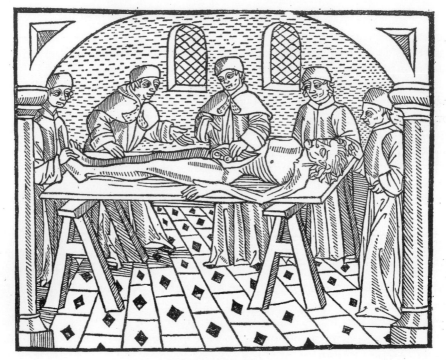

116. *Anatomical dissection.*
(*From the book of Bartolomeus Anglicus:* Les Propriétés des choses, *Lyon, 1493.*)

"When you get up each morning, stretch your limbs; nature is comforted thereby, the natural heat is stimulated, and the limbs strengthened. Then comb your hair, as the combing removes uncleanliness and comforts the brain. Wash your hands and face also with cold water to give your skin a good colour and to stimulate the natural heat. Wash and clean your nose and your chest by expectorating, and also clean your teeth, because the stomach and the chest are aided thereby and your speech becomes clearer. Clean your teeth and your gums with the bark of some odoriferous tree. From time to time fumigate your brain with precious spices; in hot weather use cold things like sandalwood; when it is cold, use hot things like cinnamon, cloves, myrrh, the wood of aloes, and similar articles. This thorough fumigation will open your nostrils and your brain, will keep your hair from degenerating and becoming white, and will keep the face plump. Adorn your body with fine clothing as the spirit is rejoiced thereby; and chew fennel, anise, cloves, because this strengthens the stomach, gives a good appetite, and sweetens the breath; again, use the following things to suppress the vapours and melancholy: daisies, new amber rose, clove pinks, and similar articles. After that, exercise your body as you are accustomed, though in moderation, because fatigue has many virtues; it stimulates the natural heat and burns up superfluities before eating.

"When you come to mealtime it is most essential to encourage your stomach to get rid of the superfluous because that excites the appetite and comforts the stomach. Begin, then, by eating foods that your nature is accustomed to, because you will digest them better; beef is more suitable than chicken to certain stomachs, the same food that is good for one being bad for another, because some have loose movements and others are constipated." (*Cod. Laurenziano*, No. 148 *bis*, entitled " *Zibaldone Andreini*," f. 44 recto.)

The fame of Bologna is indissolubly connected with the first awakenings of modern surgery in the work of Hugh of Lucca, and of his son, Theodoric, both of whom detached themselves from the Salernitan tradition and become bold and successful pioneers.

UGO BORGOGNONI of Lucca (d. 1252) belonged to a well-known family of Lucca which gave many illustrious names to medicine. He was the physician of the Bolognese in Syria and in Egypt during the Crusades and was a courageous and expert surgeon. To him is owed, among other things, a simplification of the treatment of lesions of the extremities and of fractures. Hugh is quoted by his son, but none of his works are in existence today.

Friar THEODORIC OF LUCCA (1205–98), his son, wrongly called a Catalan by some, was Bishop of Cervia after having been Bishop of Bitonto. He belonged to the Order of the Dominicans; his tomb can still be seen in the Church of St. Dominic in Bologna. He was the first to use simple drugs for the treatment of wounds. He maintained that the formation of pus was not necessary and that all the complicated substances that were applied to wounds hindered their healing. The provocation of pus, as Roger and Rolando had taught, was the greatest possible error, " *in stoliditate sua permittuntur errare*."

Going back to the advice of Aristotle, the Borgognoni recommended the application of wine as the best method of healing wounds. Another notable fact is that in one of the books of Theodoric is found for the first time an indication of the use of a kind of narcosis obtained by substances tending to produce sleepfulness during the operation. Sponges were drenched with a narcotic such as opium, jusquiamus, mandragora, that had been dried and kept for the future. Before using, they were put in hot water for an hour and then applied to the nose of the patient, who was instructed to breathe deeply. The operation was not begun until he had gone to sleep. These soporiferous sponges perhaps came into use much earlier; there are some indications of them in the Salernitan surgical works and the receipt books of the early Middle Ages. A receipt of this sort is to be found in the *Antidotarium* of Nicholas of Salerno (Jenson, Venice, 1471, j. 32 verso), but Sigerist found the same prescription in a Bamberg *Antidotarium* of the ninth century, and Sudhoff did likewise in a Montecassino Codex. The sleeping potion, recommended by Dioscorides, apparently never fell into complete disuse, as numerous authors testified. Who is not familiar with the Friar's gift to Juliet?

> Take thou this phial, being then in bed,
> And this distilled liquor drink thou off;
> When presently through all thy veins shall run
> A cold and drowsy humour . . .
> And in this borrow'd likeness of shrunk death
> Thou shalt continue two-and-forty hours,
> And then awake as from a pleasant sleep.
>
> (*Romeo and Juliet*, IV, i)

Interesting also is Theodoric's passage in which the use of mercury is advised in various skin diseases and an abundant salivation after treatment is noted. A six-day treatment with mercurial ointments is prescribed, employing a method that was practised up to our own time. Though reviled by Guy de Chauliac as a plagiarist, Theodoric thus stands out as one of the greatest surgeons of history, and though the practical use of anæsthesia and antisepsis had to wait for some six centuries, he and a slightly later proponent of the same measures, Henri de Mondeville, are nevertheless entitled to the highest praise.[1]

Another great surgeon, perhaps the most renowned of the school of Bologna, was WILLIAM OF SALICETO (Guglielmo Saliceti) (1210–77), of Piacenza. He had the great merit of reintroducing into surgery the use of the knife, which had been almost entirely abolished by the Arabs, who used practically nothing but the cautery. William was also one of the first to try to bring medicine and surgery closer together. He did much to advance the surgery of his country: he sutured nerves that had been severed, he differentiated the spirting arterial blood from venous hemorrhage, emphasized the *sonitus ossis fracti* in the diagnosis of fractures, and in his book on medicine (Ch. 140) gave a notable description of dropsy due to

---

[1] For further details about the Borgognoni, see Giordano's *Scritti e Discorsi* (Milan, 1930).

Bright's disease [1] (*durities in renibus*). His *Cyrurgia*, published at Piacenza in 1476, though much shorter than his work on internal medicine, is much more famous. According to Sudhoff, his Book IV contains the first treatise on regional or surgical anatomy.

The introduction of the new surgery into France was specially due to Guido LANFRANCHI (d. 1315) of Milan, who was exiled by the Visconti in 1290. He went to Lyon, where he wrote his *Chirurgia Parva*. When he reached Paris in 1295, he was unable, as a married man, to teach at the

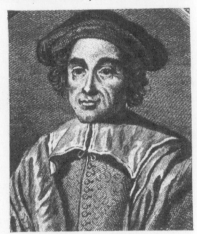

university and was associated with the Collège de St. Côme, which had been organized by Jean Pitard some time before 1260. The *Chirurgia Magna* of Lanfranc, written in 1296 (printed in French at Lyon, 1490), became one of the recognized texts at Paris. Using the cautery rather than the knife, he was cautious with such operations as trephining, removal of cataracts, lithotomy, and treatment of hernia. He was received by the French surgeons with great honour and became the head of the French school of surgery. Daremberg in his great *History of Medicine*, recognizes that France followed Italy in its surgery; in fact, the

117. *Lanfranc, Professor of Surgery at the University of Paris.*

tradition of the great Italian surgeons at Paris was maintained up to the end of the Renaissance. In Lanfranc's book we find some especially remarkable descriptions which show that, far from being a traditional scholastic, he was a profound observer and a skilful operator. The observations on fracture of the skull and the symptoms produced, the indications for trephining, the bandages recommended for hernias, the clear indications for lithotomy are especially noteworthy chapters in his book. One especially interesting item for the history of the surgery of the period is the observation that he made deploring that blood-letting and the other operations of minor surgery should be left to the barbers. He also maintained that "no one can be a good physician if he is ignorant of surgical operations, and no one can perform operations if he does not know medicine." Lanfranc can properly be included among those great surgeons of the thirteenth century who fostered the art throughout Europe, even though some of their best practices were soon to be forgotten.

---

[1] See Haeser's history of Bright's disease, in *Isis*, III, 371 (1848).

Henri de MONDEVILLE (1260–1320), a pupil of William of Saliceto, when he moved to Paris became a protégé of Jean Pitard, and also was a founder of the Collège de St. Côme. He was surgeon to Philip the Fair and Louis X. It is said that he wrote his surgery, uncompleted through ill health, at the suggestion of his friend Bernard of Gordon. Though he relied chiefly on Avicenna, his surgical practice was in advance of his times. He used ligation instead of cautery and belonged to that exalted group previously mentioned who taught that suppuration was a hindrance rather than a necessary factor in the healing of wounds.

The school of Montpellier (*Mons Pessulanus*), next to the school of Salerno the earliest medical school in western Europe, was probably first frequented by Jewish students from Spain, who long endured acrid struggles with the Christian physicians who came thither from Salerno. Though the actual date of the beginning of medical instruction at Montpellier is uncertain, it is known that William IV in 1180 issued a decree that anyone " whoever or of whatever origin he might be should have the right to give medical instruction without being called to account by anyone." By 1220, however, it had become necessary to appeal to the Papal Legate to make regulations for the conduct of the school. It was ordained that no one should teach who had not been properly examined and received a licence from the Bishop of Maguelone, who, with three senior masters, should elect a chancellor. One of the latter's most important duties was to preserve discipline in the unruly students of the time. Much was demanded of them: they had to attend medical lectures for at least five years, and then practise medicine for several months, before being graduated. After three years an examination was given, with each of the masters setting a question, leading to the Baccalaureate degree. After two more years the Master's degree was obtained. The Doctor's degree followed the Triduanes, at which an argument was held for at least an hour on three successive days. It is estimated that it cost the student several thousand dollars to maintain himself while these studies were being carried out. Together with the chancellor, who administered the school, there was a dean, usually the senior master, and two procurators elected from among the masters, who superintended the university, received fees, and so on. In the early days every master and even bachelors were permitted to teach; in 1496 four chairs were established with the requirement of lecturing for the whole year for a stipend of a hundred livres. The dissection of human bodies, only one or two a year and usually of executed criminals, was carried on after 1340. Montpellier reached its greatest height in the thirteenth and fourteenth centuries; among its celebrated pupils and masters were

Gilbertus Anglicus, the Majorcan Raymond Lull, the Catalan Arnold of Villanova, Bernard of Gordon, Petrus Hispanus, Henri de Mondeville, John of Gaddesden, John of Arderne, Guy de Chauliac (its chief glory), and in the fifteenth century the Portuguese Valescus de Taranta. When the popes left Avignon, and the country was decimated by religious wars, the school of Montpellier began to decline, coincidentally with the rise of the University of Paris and of universities in other countries. It enjoyed a brief Renaissance while Rabelais lived there, and even in later times was visited by many great men such as Sydenham, Vieussens, Sylvius, and others.

Although studies are thought to have been conducted at OxFORD, the oldest of English universities, since the ninth century, it did not attain the status of a *studium generale* until at least the twelfth century. According to Rashdall (*Medieval England,* 1924), this occurred rather suddenly when the Anglo-French struggles forced the return of many English students from the University of Paris. Not only were they constrained by an English ordinance to return " as they loved their revenues," but also they were urged thereto by the reprisals that followed a particularly bad students' riot that occurred in Paris in 1228. It is natural, then, that Oxford should have been modelled chiefly after the University of Paris. The number of students at Oxford has been reported as varying from 1,500 to 60,000; in the reign of Henry III it is said to have had nearly 30,000 students. Oxford was more renowned for the classics than as a medical centre. The University of Cambridge, recognized by royal charter in 1217, was fostered by a considerable emigration from Oxford after an unusually severe " town and gown " quarrel. The course of studies included the *Tegni* of Galen or the Aphorisms of Hippocrates on the theoretical side, and either one book of the *Regimen* of Hippocrates or the *Liber Febrium* of Isaac Hebræus or the *Antidotarium* of Nicholas of Salerno. The usual course took about eight years, though bachelors of arts could finish in a much shorter time. The first lecturer on medicine at Oxford whose name we know was Nicholas Tingewick, a Fellow of Balliol at the time of Edward I. Though the universities were not well disposed toward surgery, some surgeons, even barber-surgeons, bore the title of Master, probably having completed their medical course at one of the universities, and university graduates taught at the Barbers' Hall. The licence to practise was granted either by the universities or by the bishops.

4. Anatomical Teaching

BOLOGNA, continuing faithful to scholastic medicine, saw the triumphs of Guglielmo CORVI, known under the name of *Aggregator Brixiensis;* of Torrigiano dei TORRIGIANI, whose commentary on the *Ars Parva* of Galen was regarded as a classic for almost two centuries; of DINO DEL GARBO, commentator on Avicenna, and TOMMASO DEL GARBO, of whom we shall speak later. About now a new current becomes perceptible, especially in the fields of anatomy and surgery. Up to this time anatomy had been taught in the schools exclusively on the text of Galen, which was regarded as a canon about which there could be no dispute. Anatomical dissections were extremely rare, never practised on animals, and never by a physician, but by a surgeon or attendant. Traditions of the Alexandrian school, the Hippocratic doctrines, and the ordinances of Frederick II were either neglected or forgotten. It was at the University of Bologna that the new trend became manifest — an event that sheds everlasting glory on this institution. It appears that anatomical dissections had been practised at Bologna from the beginning of the thirteenth century. Ciasca states that the first autopsy at Bologna was made in 1281, the first female autopsy being performed in 1312 by Mundinus. There is a still earlier reference in Salimbene of Parma's *Chronicon* where he speaks of the dissection of poultry and of a person dying of plague at Cremona in 1286.

BARTOLOMEO DA VARIGNANA, who was first the pupil, then the adversary of Alderotti and was exiled by the Guelph party, seems to have had an important part in this development. From a document dated February 1302, it appears that, a certain Azzolino having died suddenly at Bologna under suspicion of poisoning, an examination of the body was ordered, the dissection being performed by Bartolomeo with another physician and three surgeons. The account of this autopsy, which rejected the theory of poison, shows that Bartolomeo must have already had some considerable practice in dissection. Records of dissections, chiefly on the bodies of executed criminals, taking place in other cities follow in close sequence: Padua, about 1341; Venice and Florence, about 1368–88; Montpellier, about 1366; Paris and Vienna, in 1404; Tübingen, in 1485. Dissections in Padua were sufficiently important to cause an anatomical theatre to be built about 1446,[1] while in Paris four dissections annually were required at this time.

---

[1] The confusion about the date of the first anatomical theatre at Padua appears to be due, according to Töply (Puschmann, II, 201), to a misinterpretation by G. Cervetto of Benedetti, who speaks in a lecture of August 1, 1503 of a "temporary theatre" on the

These dissections, done either in public or in private, to give instruction in anatomy, usually lasted several days and especially in hot weather must have appealed unpleasantly to the senses as well as to the intelligence. It is difficult now to separate them from autopsies done to establish the cause of death. These latter were usually performed, as in the case of Azzolino, where poisoning was suspected, or as matters of State record in the case of exalted persons. Some were necessitated for religious purposes: Galloway, for instance (*Historical Sketches of Old Charing*, London, 1914), points out that Edward I had parts of Queen Eleanor's body deposited in three different tombs erected in her honour.

In William of Saliceto's fourth treatise, written to teach surgeons the anatomy of the body, there are certain statements that do not appear to come entirely from former times, indicating that he had some personal knowledge of dissection.

A famous pupil of William of Saliceto was HENRI DE MONDEVILLE (1260–1320), who brought the new teaching of anatomy to the school of Montpellier, carrying with him anatomical drawings copied by him at Bologna (anatomical texts published by Pagel in 1889; surgical texts by Pagel in 1890–2, and translated into French by Nicaise in 1893). Like his master, he stressed the knowledge of anatomy as part of the surgeon's equipment.

But the first outstanding anatomist worthy of the name was MUNDINUS (Mondino de' Luzzi, 1270?–1326). He was the son of a Bolognese pharmacist, Nerino, who belonged to the Florentine family de Lutiis (Latinized). He was registered at the College of Medicine (1290) and the College of Philosophy; and became public lecturer at the university from 1314 to 1324. He enjoyed a great reputation not only as an anatomist but also as an authoritative statesman, taking part in the government of the city and as Ambassador of Bologna to John, the son of Robert, King of Naples. On his death in Bologna in 1326, he was buried in the parochial church of San Vitale d'Agricola in a granite tomb with a bas-relief by Boso of Parma representing a master in his chair lecturing to his pupils. His uncle Leuzzo, who was also lecturer in medicine, was buried in the same tomb.

The first dissections were practised by Mondino in January 1315, as is stated in his book that speaks of the anatomy of the uterus. The number of cadavers dissected by Mondino cannot be stated, but it was certainly much larger than the two or three that have been suggested by some. Guy

model of those at Rome and Verona. Pietro Tosoni (*Della anatomia degli antichi e della scuola anat. padovana*, Padua, 1844), on the other hand, mentions an anatomical theatre there in 1446 and ceremonious dissections held in March 1465.

de Chauliac, for instance, who was a student at Bologna, states that the anatomical dissections were made by Mondino *multoties*. Although he held strictly in his anatomical teaching to the teleological concepts of Galen, he has the incontestable merit of having been the first to introduce the systematic teaching of anatomy into the program of medical studies. It is from the time of Mondino that the practice began of dissecting different parts of the body one after the other with a careful preparation of each part.

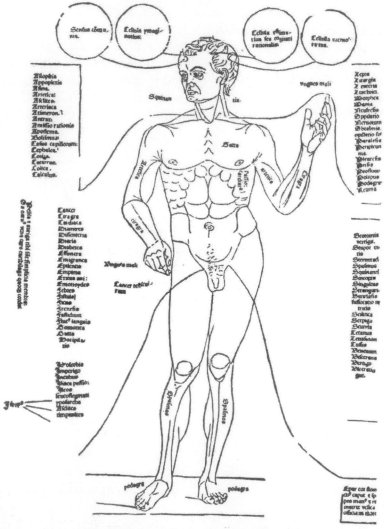

118. *Human anatomy according to Mundinus.*
(*From Ketham's* Fasciculus medicinæ, *Venice, 1493.*)

The *Anathomia* of Mondino was the most used anatomical text up to the end of the sixteenth century, probably partly at least because it contained the most important technical indications in brief and concise form. There are forty or more editions of his work, the oldest of which was printed in Padua in 1478 (reproduced by Wickersheimer, Paris, 1926). The anatomical descriptions are amplified with discussions and scholastic explanations intended to allay any doubts that might arise in the reader's mind. It is possible, as Pagel supposes, that Mondino did not customarily perform the dissections himself, but had the dissected parts demonstrated to students by the dissector, as can be seen from various contemporary illustrations. From the precise technical instructions that he gives, however, he must have either performed the dissections or followed very closely the work of his assistants.

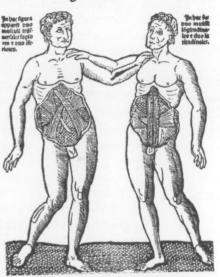

119. *The muscles of the abdomen.* (*From the* Conciliator *of Pietro* d'Abano, Venice, 1496.)

The *Anathomia*, written about 1316, though more of a dissecting manual than a formal treatise, may be regarded as the first anatomical text worthy of the name. The nomenclature is drawn partly from the Arabian and partly from uncertain sources. The instructions seem often superficial and almost always hurried, owing to the fact that the work had to be done rapidly, especially the dissection of the viscera. It is clear that Mondino had made a close study of the Arabian writers, from whom he takes such terms as *mirach* for the abdominal wall, *siphach* for the peritoneum, *zirbus* for the omentum, and many others. However, his text also shows that he had carefully studied the cadaver and had profited by his personal observations.

Dissection, according to Mondino, begins with the opening of the abdomen by means of a vertical cut running *a scuto oris stomachi directe usque ad ossa pectinis*, to which is added a horizontal cut above the umbilicus. The intestinal musculature is fairly well described; the anatomy of the stomach is preceded by a long discussion of its position and function. The wall of the stomach is composed of an internal coat, the seat of sensation, and an external or fleshy coat that serves for digestion. For the examination of the spleen the dissector should remove the false ribs. The liver, according to Mondino, lies higher in the cadaver than in the living body. The *vena chili* (*vena cava*) is described with especial accuracy. The description of the male genitalia is given in much detail. The anatomy of the female genital organs is based entirely on the anatomy of animals, though Mondino doubtless had more than once dissected female cadavers. A new and interesting statement is that the uterus enlarges in menstruation as well as in pregnancy. Noteworthy also are his observations on hernia and its treatment, and on the anatomy of the bladder.

The anatomical descriptions of Mondino reflect the tradition of Galen, on which he also relied for his physiology. The liver has five lobes (as in many animals); the stomach is described as spherical. The yellow bile is secreted by the gall bladder, while the black bile has its origin in the spleen and reaches the stomach by imaginary canals. The pancreatic duct is described with much more accuracy than the pancreas itself. In the heart three ventricles are described. In the right ventricle one sees two orifices — one directed toward the liver, which is larger because the heart draws through it the blood from the liver, and the other the opening of the *vena arterialis* toward the lung. The left ventricle has two orifices: the " *adhorti*," opening with three valves, and the opening of the *arteria venalis* with two valves, through which passes a smoke-like vapour from the lung. The third chamber is described as consisting of various small cavities in the septum, where the blood crossing to the left ventricle may be subtilized.

Examination of the lungs shows the course of the *vena arterialis* (pulmonary artery) and of the *arteria venalis* (pulmonary vein). In the description of the pleura we find a long discussion on the need for distinguishing between true pleurisy, false pleurisy, and pneumonia.

The cranial cavity was apparently opened rarely and with little technical skill, as the directions are extremely vague and inexact. Neuburger points out that in his discussion of the ear Mondino allows that one could study the temporal bone better if it were first boiled, but it would be sinful to do so ("*sed propter peccatum dimittere consuevi*").

The students were taught in the following manner: The lecturer, holding in his hand the classic text which necessarily formed the basis of instruction, read the most important passages, accompanying them with his learned comments. The prosector performed the desired incisions on the cadaver, and the demonstrator indicated with his baton the parts that the prosector had brought to light. Galen was the anatomical authority from whom there was no appeal, but as he was often read in the translations from the Arabic, there were frequent errors and difficulty in interpretation; and the differences between commentators were frequent, as Berengario da Carpi has observed. When the master observed that it was not possible to bring the actual facts into accord with the statements of Galen, it was his pleasure to state that the text of Galen had been changed by the Arabs, or the translators, or the copiers.

Mondino's book soon became a classic text; he was venerated soon after his death as a divine master and anyone who was found differing from his book was regarded as monstrous. For three centuries the lecturers on anatomy were required to use his book in their teaching, as may be seen in the statutes of many medical schools.

5. Medical Teaching

The rapid development of medical teaching in the Italian universities was followed by a similar change in the medical schools of western Europe and especially in France, Spain, Portugal, and England. Among the most ancient of these, as we have seen, were those of Paris and Montpellier, while in some smaller cities like Narbonne and Arles, near the Spanish border, there were Jewish schools where medicine was taught. Raschì (1040, Troyes–1105), the famous commentator on the Talmud, is one such Jewish scholar whose influence on scientific thought was very great in France and much of Europe. The first exact information that we have about the school of Montpellier speaks of oñe ADALBERT OF MAYENCE, who studied medicine there in 1137; the existence of the school in 1153 is shown by a letter of St. Bernard. In 1180 William, Lord of Montpellier, decreed that there should be no limit to the admittance of students, and no matter what his nation or his religion, anyone could be accepted.

The literature of the school of Montpellier is very like that of Salerno. Much the same texts were used in the two schools, one of the best known of which was the *De viribus herbarum,* a poem of two thousand Latin hexameters, attributed to Macer Floridus but probably written by the French physician ODO DE MEUDON (*c.* 1130). Others were the *Lapidarius* of the BISHOP MARBOD (d. 1123), which extols the curative virtues of sixty precious stones, and the *Physica* of ST. HILDEGARDE, written in the first half of the twelfth century.

The great surgeons of Bologna were followed by those of the school of Paris — especially Lanfranc, Henri de Mondeville, and Guy de Chauliac.

GUY DE CHAULIAC (*c.* 1300–67, near Lyon) was the most famous surgeon of the Middle Ages. He studied first at Montpellier, then at Bologna, where he heard the anatomical lectures of Bertuccio, whose teaching from the cadaver he has described. According to Nicaise, he received his title of Magister in 1325. At the time of the great plague he was physician to Pope Clement VI and later to his successors at Avignon, where he came in frequent conflict with Petrarch. His best-known book was his *Chirurgia,* a scholastic work of great importance, which held the same classic position for surgery until the time of Paré that Mondino's treatise held for the field of anatomy. There have been many editions of this work, the first of which was published in French in Paris in 1478 with the title *La Pratique en chirurgie du Maistre Guidon de Chauliac*. The Latin text, *Chirurgia magna*, was first printed in Venice in 1498; a modern edition has been published by Nicaise (Paris, 1890).

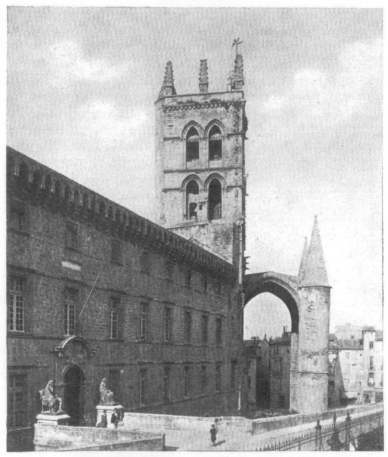

120. Entrance to the Medical School of Montpellier. The building dates from 1364. To the right, the old Cathedral.

The book begins with a *Capitulum singulare*, which contains a historical sketch and a discussion of the importance of surgery. As Streeter has pointed out, this was shown by Symphorien Champier (*Guidon en françoys*, Lyon, 1503) to be the only noteworthy work on medical history since the time of Celsus. It describes various surgical operations, instruments, and the proper contents of a surgical case (*theca vulneraria*). This should contain six instru-

ments: scissors, speculum, razor, scalpel, needle, and lancet. Among the necessary qualifications for the surgeon, Guy places first that of being a man of letters;
second, that of being expert; third, intelligent; fourth, a man of good habits.
Concerning the first of these he adds: " It is necessary that he especially know
anatomy, because without anatomy one can do nothing in surgery." The descriptions of operations performed and demonstrated by Guy contain interesting features, especially when he tries to bring his practical experience into
agreement with the pronouncements of Galen. Though Guy made important contributions to surgery, such as his early removal of cancer with the
knife, treatment of fractures with slings and extension by weights, and operations for hernia and cataract, he was in general a reactionary. Though more
idealistic than his predecessor Henri de Mondeville, he was highly critical of
the latter's writings, while his failure to follow Henri's and Theodoric's simple
methods of treating wounds and his persistence in the meddlesome surgery
of cautery, salves, and plasters, through his great authority retarded surgery
by centuries. Nevertheless, he recognized Nature as the chief workman, whom
the surgeon assists by removing foreign bodies, bringing together separated
parts, and in other ways; he described five methods of controlling hemorrhage:
suture, tamponade, compression, ligature, cautery. To Guy is due the school
of French surgery that prepared the way for Ambroise Paré, generally recognized as the first representative of modern surgery.

In the other countries of Europe at this time surgery still continued in
a primitive state. Worthy of mention, however, is JOHN OF ARDERNE
(1307–90?), an Englishman who studied at Montpellier, practised in
France, and later returned to England, where he was active up to the end
of the fourteenth century. Practising first at Newark, he came to London
in 1370, where he was probably admitted to the fraternity of surgeons.
Working chiefly among the higher classes, he was a sound, practical surgeon, using the best practices of his day. He followed the recent teaching
that wounds should be treated simply and suppuration avoided. According to D'Arcy Power, he invented " the operation for the cure of fistula,
which, after falling into disuse for nearly 500 years, is now universally
employed." His various treatises on the practice of medicine and surgery,
hemorrhoids, fistula, and so on, were written in Latin in his own hand;
English translations were published at various times, and the treatise on
fistula printed in abridged form in 1588. D'Arcy Power's publication
(1922) of Arderne's *De arte phisicali et de cirurgia* gives an English translation, together with photographs of the manuscript, which was written
about 1412.

Jan YPERMAN (born at Ypres in the latter half of the thirteenth century,
died about 1350) was a pupil of Lanfranc at Paris, then returned to his

native land, where he became its leading surgeon, enjoying a wide reputation. He is the author of two surgical works in Latin that were much read by his contemporaries. In these surgical works he showed himself a worthy pupil of his master, collecting many personal observations as well as citations from others, especially Lanfranc, whose teachings about trephining and ligation he largely followed. Neuburger has pointed out that he recognized that some cases of scrofula may get well even without the royal touch. Modern editions of his works have been published by Broeckx (Antwerp, 1863 and 1867) and by van Leersum (Leiden, 1912).

Toward the end of the thirteenth century the best-known physician was the Catalan, ARNALDUS DE VILLANOVA (1235, near Valencia–1315?, Genoa), one of the most distinguished representatives of the school of Montpellier, which from its start had the reputation of being a practical school in which physicians were taught by different methods from those of mere scholastic dogmatism. Arnold is one of the most interesting figures of the Middle Ages; he appears to have studied at both Paris and Montpellier, and perhaps also at Naples or Salerno. He certainly travelled far for his education and had contacts with the most famous physicians of his time. Even in his lifetime he enjoyed a great reputation: princes often called him in consultation. He lived some time at Barcelona, after which he became a professor at Montpellier. He also acted for Spain in various diplomatic matters. For reasons that are still obscure he came in conflict with the Inquisition, which declared one of his books to be heretical. He sought the protection of Boniface VIII, whom he had treated for renal calculus and who also was suspected of heresy after his death on account of this very intimacy with Arnold. Clement V later brought him back into the Church.

He was a voluminous writer, more than sixty of his treatises having been published. The first edition of his collected works was published in Lyon in 1504. Of them the best known is a *Regimen sanitatis*, which, according to some modern criticism, should be attributed to the Milanese Mangino. His commentary is the most famous of all commentaries on the Salernitan poem, and was published in many editions. He also wrote much on materia medica, alchemy, and astrology. Riesman regards his *Parabolæ medicationis* as his most profound work, and his Breviarium as the most influential with his contemporaries.

Neuburger correctly observes that all the medical currents of his time are represented in Arnold's works: Hippocrates and Galen, the Arabs, and the school of Salerno; but one is impressed with his love of truth and his wide experience beyond all scholastic doctrines. He was one of the small band who did not hesitate to contradict even the authority of Galen and Avicenna. Diepgen has published a series of interesting studies on his work (*Arch. f. Gesch. d. Med.*, 1909–10, Vol. III, 115, 188, and 369).

The school of Paris was profoundly influenced by the work of Albert von Bollstaedt (Sanctus ALBERTUS MAGNUS) (1193–1280), born at Laningen in Swabia. He received his doctor's degree at Padua and entered the Order of Dominicans. He was an ardent naturalist and an encyclopædic writer, who is regarded as probably the most learned man of all the Middle Ages. Known as the *Doctor Universalis*, he was regarded as the miracle of

his century; St. Thomas Aquinas, his pupil, called him the "Divine Master." At the College of St. Jacques or on the Place Maubert (abbreviated from Magnus Albertus), when Albertus was in Paris (1222–48), one could see gathered about him the most illustrious scholars of his day — Thomas Aquinas, Roger Bacon, Thomas of Cantimpré, Vincent of Beauvais, Petrus Hispanus, and Michael Scot, one of the founders of Latin Averroism.

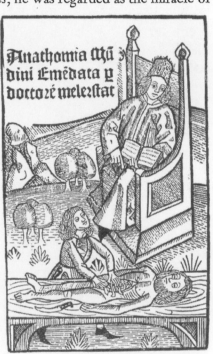

121. *Mundinus lecturing.*
(*Leipzig edition, 1493.*)

His numerous encyclopædic writings are almost all philosophical and theological, but they also treat of the natural sciences and medicine, wherein his interpretations were chiefly influenced by Aristotle and Maimonides. Zoologist, botanist, chemist, and physician, Albertus gave his energy above all to the interpretation of the great Stagyrite, who became for him an absolute authority with whose opinion no other could disagree. The book of Albertus called *Summa naturalium*, which treats of the therapeutic virtues of plants, also served as a text for the history of medicine up to the end of the sixteenth century. The fame of Albertus was so great that many apocrypha were attributed to him. The best known of these was the *Liber aggregationis*, dealing with the magic properties of plants and the *Secreta mulierum*, largely superstitious and astrological. These were the chief reasons for his being frequently quoted as a magician, so that *Ars Albertina* became synonymous with magic, and books are still sold under this title, like the pseudo-Aristotelian *Compleat Masterpiece.*

In the literature of the period encyclopædic works occupied a most important place, which was retained up to the beginning of the sixteenth century. The famous *Thesaurus pauperum*, attributed to PETRUS HISPANUS, who later became Pope under the name of John XXI, dates from

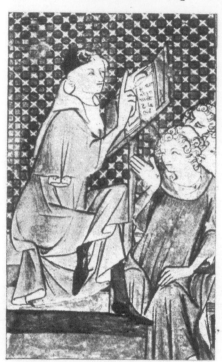

this period. Peter (*c.* 1210, Portugal–1276, Viterbo), the only physician to have reached the papal chair, also wrote a *Liber de oculo*, which was used by Guy de Chauliac and by Michelangelo, whose notes from it still exist in his own hand in the Vatican library. He also wrote a commentary on the book of Isaac Judæus *On Special Diets.* Though a believer in astrology, he made a sincere attempt to avoid superstition and the use of such remedies as the powders of sympathy. Appointed archiater to Gregory X, he rapidly advanced until he followed Adrian V as Pope in 1276. Taking the name of John XXI, he died within eight months beneath the fallen ceiling of his palace at Viterbo. Though thought by some, on account of his great knowledge, to have sold himself to the devil — hence his tragic death — he is mentioned by Dante as the only contemporary Pope whom he meets in Paradise (*Paradiso*, Canto XII, 135).

122. *Henri de Mondeville lecturing to his pupils.*
(*From a 1314 manuscript of his* Chirurgia, BIBLIOTHÈQUE NATIONALE, PARIS.)

A book on materia medica that had a wide reputation was the *Synonyma medicinæ seu clavis sanationis* of SIMON JANUENSIS (Simon of Genoa), physician to Pope Nicholas IV toward the end of the thirteenth century. No less famous was the *Pandectæ medicinæ*, written in the early fourteenth century by Matthæus SYLVATICUS of Mantua (published Naples, 1474).

This was the period in which ROGER BACON (1214–92), the great Franciscan, flourished in England. Called the *Doctor mirabilis*, he was an excellent dialectician who was faithful to the Oxford traditions in his pursuit of physics and chemistry, and in his opposition to dogmatic scholasticism. He taught at Paris about 1240, and one may see in his works how well he understood the dangers to science from the infiltration of scholasticism and appreciated the superiority of observation over reasoning as a basis of knowledge. His *Opus majus*, together with his *Opus minus* and *Opus tertium*, was prohibited by the religious authorities and he was condemned to prison in 1278, where he stayed fourteen years, almost till his death. As soon as he was liberated he published his last work, a *Compendium theologiæ*. This opposition did not cause him to deviate from his unconventional ideas and studies, but it was successful in hindering the spread of his observations through the world of learning.

Though some modern critics do not attribute great importance to the works of Roger Bacon, his true value still remains in doubt on account of the care with which he felt compelled to write his thoughts in obscure language. In the Voynich manuscript, which may be in Bacon's own hand, W. R. Newbold claimed to have found an elaborate cipher which betrayed a knowledge of human anatomy and natural history that was far in advance of his time. According to Newbold, Bacon probably should be credited with the invention of the telescope, the microscope, spectacles, and gunpowder, and he seems to have foreseen flying-machines and mechanical transportation. He may have discovered spermatozoa, seminiferous tubules, and various human cells, announcement of which would have had extremely dangerous consequences for their discoverer. The following from his *Optical Science* touching on these points was written shortly before he was imprisoned: "If a man looks at letters or other small objects through the medium of a crystal or of glass or of some other transparent body placed above the letters, and it is the smaller part of the sphere whose convexity is toward the eye, and the eye is in the air, he will see the letters much better and they will appear larger to him. . . . Therefore this instrument is useful to the aged and to those with weak eyes. . . . The wonders of refracted vision are still greater; for it is easily shown by the rules stated above that very large objects can be made to appear very small, and the reverse, and very distant objects will seem very close at hand, and conversely " (Burke's translation of *Opus majus*, Bk. IV). That Bacon made these discoveries is of course still unsubstantiated; while it is clear that in any case he exerted but little influence on his successors: editions of his works before the seventeenth century are rare, while incunabula are entirely lacking. However, in spite of the ecclesiastical discipline to which he had to submit and the consequent repression of his influence, he stands out as perhaps the first great experimental philosopher. A Platonist who owed much to his English master, Robert Grosseteste, he objected strongly to the Aristotle-loving Albertus and Thomas Aquinas. Some of the titles of his medical works have a modern ring, *On the Retardation of Old Age, Diet for the Aged, Baths for the Aged, On the Preservation of Youth.* Sarton regards the first named as his earliest, poorest, and best-known medical writing. His *De erroribus medicorum,* on the other hand, is a mature criticism, which also expresses his appreciation of the value of experimentation. He was loath to admit his own errors, and in all his writings showed a tendency to original ideas that were independent of mystic speculation. While he recognized the authority of Aristotle, he denied that even the great Stagyrite should be followed blindly. The first edition of his *Opus majus* appeared in London in 1733 (Samuel Jebb); it was translated into English by R. B. Burke (2 vols., 1928). Strange to say, a complete edition of Bacon's work has never been published, more than half of his writings still remaining unpublished, though his seventh centenary, in 1914, occasioned many articles about this great Franciscan scholar.

English medicine of this period, though it was definitely behind that of the Continent, had advanced far beyond the stage of Saxon leechcraft. The Saxon leeches, about whom little is really known, passed on their craft from father to son and often were thought to be possessed of special powers. They practised their craft only as a side issue to their livelihood. As elsewhere, charms and spells were as much in use as the simple herbs and regarded as more potent. With the Norman Conquest came highly educated ecclesiastics, who treated rich and poor in the convents or at court, in addition to their clerical duties. Surgery was mostly military surgery, except for the minor surgery of the barbers. But few names are preserved. We know of two of William the Conqueror's military surgeons, Nigel and Gilbert Maminot, but possess no writings by them. Packer speaks among others of Thomas Weseham, Sargent Surgeon to Henry III, and Fulco of Oxford, who is described as both surgeon and physician. Three university-trained surgeons, the Masters Roger, John, and Peter, are known to have practised at Oxford and Southworth in the early fourteenth century. Of English physicians, one of the best known was GILBERTUS ANGLICUS (d. 1250), who wrote a *Compendium medicinæ,* known also as the *Lilium* or *Laurea* or *Rosa anglicana* (published Lyon, 1510). It is a good mixture of Salernitan and Arabic medicine and contains some interesting descriptions of diseases, such as leprosy, measles, and smallpox, of which Gilbert is said to have been the first to have recognized the contagious nature. He was Chancellor of Montpellier in 1250. BERNARD OF GORDON is usually said to be of Scotch origin, though the cognomen is more probably due to his ascribed birthplace, Gordon en Rouergue, in France. In 1303 he wrote a well-known manual called *Lilium medicinæ* (first printed, Naples, 1480). The great fame that it enjoyed is shown by its frequent reproduction in manuscript form and its passage through seven incunabula editions. Though typically dogmatic and scholastic in form, it is notable for its early description of a truss for inguinal hernia and for possibly the earliest reference to spectacles (*oculus berellinus,* a term that is often taken to indicate spectacles, though perhaps meaning a simple magnifying glass). Bernard recognizes a number of contagious diseases, such as consumption,

scabies, anthrax, trachoma, leprosy, and bubonic plague(?). JOHN OF GADDES-
DEN (1230–1361) was author of a book called *Rosa anglica* (first printed, Pavia,
1492), not to be confused with Gilbert's just-mentioned book. John, a pre-
bendary of St. Paul's and Fellow of Merton College, was physician to Edward II, and is said to have been the original of Chaucer's Doctor of Physic.
RICHARD OF WENDOVER (*Ricardus Anglicus*, d. 1252), physician to Pope Gregory IX and later a practitioner in Paris, and finally in London, was the author
of a *Micrologus* or brief medical encyclopædia. His *Anatomia*, based largely
on Avicenna's *Canon*, is noteworthy as one of the few anatomical works of his
time. It often appears as *De anatomia vivorum*, included in many editions of
Galen's works. JOHANNES DE MIRFELD (d. 1407), a clerk of the Priory of St.
Bartholomew, Smithfield, was the author of a *Breviarium Bartholomei*, a medical
work, and a *Florarium Bartholomei*, a theological treatise that contained one
medical chapter. These were both named after the priory in which he worked
and are chiefly of value as exhibiting the state of English medical knowledge of
the time.

6. Plague in the Fourteenth Century. Other Epidemic Diseases. Sanitary Legislation

Thus at a time when Dante and Boccaccio and Giotto and their schools
were making their glorious contributions to Italian literature and art, Italian
medicine of the fourteenth century was beginning to lead the countries
of western Europe out of the bogs of scholasticism toward a clearer vision
of objective reality. It is at this period that occurred a series of events that
had the most serious consequences for the development of civilization in
Europe. We refer to the epidemics that devastated the world in a manner
that had never before been equalled and have never since been approached.
Chief among these was the pandemic of bubonic plague, known as the
Black Death; but also scourges of leprosy, scurvy, and influenza (many
introduced into Europe by the Crusaders), ergotism, the dancing mania,
and the sweating sickness devastated Europe. Though they were naturally
ascribed at the time to such human or supernatural causes as poisons,
droughts, storms, the stars, and so on, we need hunt no further today than
for such prosaic but important factors as the squalor and dirty habits of the
mediæval cities and the demoralization and mixing of populations caused by
the frequent wars. Especially dramatic was the Black Death, which devastated the whole Continent and reduced flourishing cities almost to a desert
state. The arrest of economic and social life that it determined also had its
effect on the evolution of medicine, imposing the necessity of new lines of

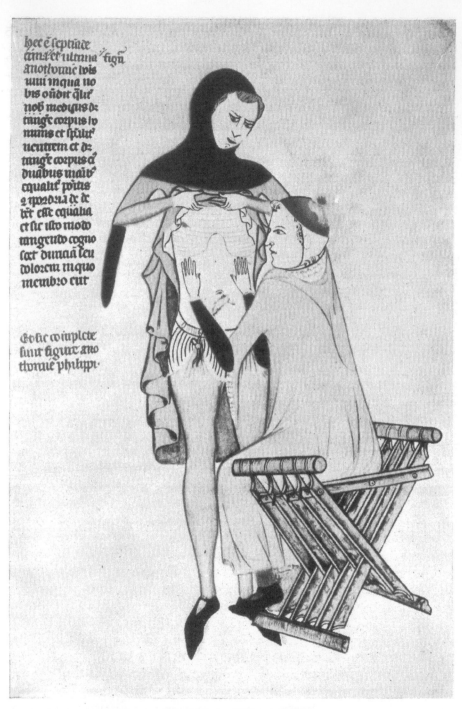

123. *Physician examining a patient.*
(*From the* Anatomy *of Guido da Vigevano, physician to Philip VI, King of France.*
Manuscript in the CONDÉ MUSEUM, CHANTILLY.)

study and above all of urgent provisions for defence. This is the plague so vividly described by Boccaccio, which was often manifested in its pulmonary form. Most of the patients died on the third or fourth day of the disease. The pestilence began in the interior of Asia about the year 1333, to spread toward India and other countries that were on the routes of commerce. The most important of these crossed the Crimea and the Black Sea to Constantinople and entered Egypt by Mesopotamia and Arabia. By the end of 1346 and the beginning of 1347 central Asia, Egypt, and almost all of southern Europe were invaded by this scourge, which fell with frightful violence on the maritime lands of Sicily, Italy, and southern France. Finally, spreading through Holland and France to England, Germany, and Poland in 1349, it reached Russia in 1351-2. By 1353 the epidemic had disappeared from Europe as a pandemic, though it returned periodically in less overwhelming form. In 1357 it appeared in Brabant and along the river Danube; in 1359 Florence was again devastated and in 1360 Avignon. According to the habit of epidemics, less violent recrudescences appeared in 1362 and 1364. These terrible plagues gave rise to a large body of medical and lay literature, consisting of advice about the plague, and to a series of legislative measures, which for the first time in history promulgated defensive laws against infectious diseases.

The first Italian description of the plague is owed to the Franciscan monk Michele Piazza, who in his history of Sicily (*Michælis Platiensis historia Sicula ab anno 1337 ad annum 1361*) described how in the early days of October 1347 thirteen Venetian galleys that took refuge in the harbour of Messina brought the plague to that city. The symptoms of the disease are graphically described: " Because of an infection of the breath passed around among them as they talked, one so infected another that all were seen as if racked with pain, and, in a measure, severely shaken; as a result of the pain, the shaking, and the infection of the breath, pustules appeared on the thigh or arm in the manner of *lenticulæ*, which thus infected and penetrated the body, wherefore they violently spat forth blood; after spitting for three days incessantly without any cure for the dreaded disease, they departed from life; and not only did whoever talked to them die, but indeed whoever bought, touched, or seized anything belonging to them."

Among the early historians of the plague is the Piacenza chronicler Gabriele de Mussi, whose manuscript, now in the Breslau library, was first published by Henschel in 1842. Mussi, who lived in the Orient from 1344 to 1346, had the opportunity of observing the origin of the pandemic in the Crimea and later at Jaffa. The accounts by John Cantacuzene and Nicephorus, Byzantine historiographers, of the plague in Constantinople in 1347 are almost contemporaneous. The description by Boccaccio is the most celebrated of all the his-

tories of the first epidemic (see Major's *Classic Descriptions of Disease*, second
edition, p. 91).

Coluccio Salutati gives much information in his letters about the plague in
Florence and the measures that he took to protect himself, " *quod regimina*

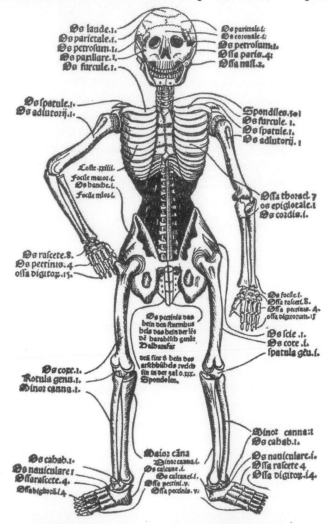

124. *The human skeleton.*   (*From the* Hortus sanitatis, *third edition, 1499.*)

vitæ receperim et pilam aromaticam manu gestem" (" in that I adopted regi-
mens of living and carry around an aromatic pill in my hand "). He also in-
veighs against the citizens who fled from the city on account of the disease
(*Epistolæ*, Novati, Rome, 1891, pp. 96 and 115). The question as to whether
or not the plague-stricken city should be abandoned was frequently discussed

by humanists (cf. the letters of Zabarella, cod. Marc. lat. XIV, 827, cc. 183–94). Florence is said to have lost in the visitation of 1348, described by Villani, more than one hundred thousand persons. Venice and London each lost more than one hundred thousand, and a number of cities, such as Paris and Avignon, more than fifty thousand. According to Richard Fitzralph, Chancellor of Oxford, the students there were reduced from thirty thousand to less than six thousand. The plague even reached Greenland, where, according to Sir Charles Oman, the whole history of North America was altered by the destruction of a community which was already in touch with the American continent.

The spread of the contagion and its principal symptoms, as described by the physicians and chronicles of the period, have been subjects of much study and to it there is little to add. The narrations of Boccaccio and Villani remain classics, not only for the picturesque eloquence with which the desolation of the devasted cities is described, but also for the accurate account of the sanitary measures that were put in force. These certainly contributed considerably to diminishing the violence of the later epidemics. Among the economic results that are bound to follow such profound disruptions were seen the spread of corruption, the rapid increase of crime together with unemployment, and the sudden appearance of a widespread anti-Semitic movement, especially in Germany. And, finally, the appearance of the Flagellants. All of these phenomena, which spread rapidly in the wake of the epidemics, are characteristic of any great scourges that upset humanity, and thus belong to political and social rather than to medical history.

A rich literature on the plague and means of combating it quickly arose in most of the countries of Europe. Sudhoff has devoted a whole series of studies to this literature and has collected the chief writings on the subject that were published between 1348 and 1500 (about two hundred). Among the most important of such works is the *Consilia contra pestilentiam* of Gentile da Foligno, who himself died of the plague in 1348. His advice to the cities of Genoa and Perugia includes precepts about food and drink, purgation, blood-letting, and various medicines to be used. Disinfection was also recommended. Another noteworthy production was the *Medicina practica* by Dionysius Colle (printed at Pesaro, 1617, and referred to by Haeser, Vol. III, p. 169). Haeser also gives the account (1350) by SIMON COVINUS, a Belgian living at the time in France (III, 174). In most of these writings the phenomena of the disease are described and recommendations for treatment given, such as fumigation with pine and larch resin.

In the famous surgical treatise of Guy de Chauliac there is the following description of the plague at Avignon in 1348, where Guy was engaged in the service of the Pope: "It appeared in Avignon in 1348. . . . The disease began in January and lasted seven months. It presented itself in two forms. The first lasted two months with continued fever and the spitting of blood. Death occurred usually in three days. The second lasted for the remainder of the time, also with a continuous fever and abscesses and carbuncles on the external parts, chiefly in the groins and the axillæ. The patients died in five days. So contagious was the disease, especially that with blood-spitting, that no one could approach or even see a patient without taking the disease. The father did not visit the son nor the son the father. Charity was dead and hope abandoned. . . . For self-preservation there was nothing better than to flee the region before becoming infected and to purge oneself with pills of aloes, to diminish the blood by phlebotomy and to improve the air by fire and to comfort the heart with senna and things of good odour and to sooth the humours with Armenian bole and to resist putrefaction by means of acid things. For the cure bleedings, evacuations, and electuaries and cordials were used. The external swellings were softened with figs and cooked onions, peeled and mixed with yeast and butter, then opened and treated like ulcers. Carbuncles were cupped, scarified, and cauterized. As for me, in order to avoid infamy I did not dare absent myself, but with continuous fear preserved myself so that I was able to apply the above-mentioned remedies. Nevertheless toward the end of the epidemic I fell ill with a continuous fever and a swelling in the groin and was ill for six weeks. I was in such danger that my companions believed that I would die, but the abscess became ripe and was treated as I have said and I escaped by the grace of God " (*Chirurgia*, II, Ch. 5). Similar recommendations by Tomaso del Garbo (d. Florence, 1360), a friend of Petrarch, were made, for purgatives, blood-letting, theriacum, and so forth. He gives a number of warnings for those attending the patients, recommending the avoidance of heavy foods and crowded places, and the use of wine rather than water. The advice of Gentile da Foligno was equally popular, appearing in a book called *The Soul of Avicenna*, which was often reproduced in manuscript and print. The *Consilia* of Giovanni Dondi dall' OROLOGIO (1380), who taught at Padua and Pavia, and Franceschino da COLIGNANA (1382) were also well known. Toward the end of the century Pietro da TOSSIGNANO, the famous master of Padua, wrote a letter to Giovanni Galeazzo Visconti in which is found for the first time a series of six remedies against the plague, which were to be changed every day. He forbade marriage during the epidemic and advised strongly against *conversationes politicæ*, probably because he wished the patient to stay in a good humour! Peter affirms that he saw cases of infection by direct contact; there was a widespread conviction in general that contagion could also be spread by clothes. His treatise was published with ample notes and a biography by G. Mazzini (1926).

An important tract was published by the medical faculty of Paris in 1348 called *Compendium de epidemia per Collegium Facultatis Medicorum Parisiis Ordinatum* (printed by Rébouis, 1888). As prophylactic and dietetic measures, the faculty recommended the fumigation with incense and camomile flowers of houses and even of public squares and other crowded places. Poultry and fatty meats should not be eaten, but only dry meat without any condiments. Sleep should not be prolonged after dawn. Fruits should be eaten dry or fresh, but

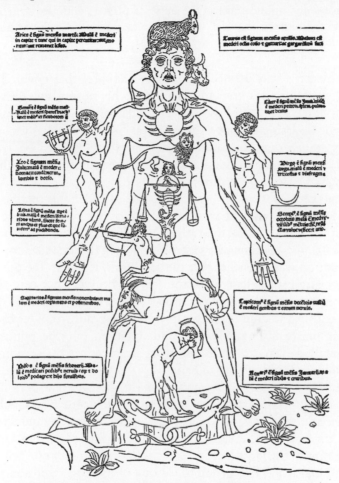

125. *Human figure showing the astrological signs for blood-letting.*
(*From the* Fasciculus medicinæ, *Venice, 1495.*)

olive oil could act fatally. Baths, according to the faculty, could be very dangerous, and sexual intercourse have fatal results. A similar statement was published by the faculty of Montpellier in 1349. Physicians used many precautions to avoid spread of the disease. It was recommended to wash the rooms of the patients frequently with rosewater and vinegar, and to expose vinegar in vases so that the vapours could mix with the exhalations.

Engaging for its descriptions of infallible remedies for the plague is the charlatanesque *Contra pestem*[1] of *Johannes Mercurius* of Correggio. More than a score of remedies are confidently recommended: from theriacum (1 oz. in 3 oz. of *aqua sancta*, t.i.d.) to many herbs — chiefly bitter, such as rue, gentian, dittany — and applications to the bubo of plasters and gems, such as emeralds. These culminated in the " stone of miracles itself," which, however, is discreetly left undescribed.

The physician was dressed in a curious apparel that covered him entirely; he wore long gloves and held before his nose a sponge soaked in vinegar in which had been dissolved a powder of cloves and cinnamon. It was thought desirable to move slowly so as not to inhale any more air in the sick-chamber than was necessary. The room was to be frequently ventilated, and doors and windows opened frequently during the course of the day and at least once during the night.

Various theories were proposed as to the cause of this terrific scourge. Among the most prominent was that it was owing to the conjunction of Saturn, Jupiter, and Mars on the 24th of March 1345 — which naturally suggested catastrophe at a time when astrology was in the ascendancy. Another natural reaction was the belief that the scourge was due to the poisoning of wells, especially by the lepers and the Jews, who were persecuted in large numbers on this account. Any confirmation that was needed for this belief was supplied by the confessions wrung from the unfortunates by torture. Trials thus uniformly resulted in condemnation, but the popular wrath often forestalled even the semblance of legal procedure by burning individuals or groups in buildings out of hand.

Nevertheless the contagious nature of the disease appears to have been definitely recognized. Most of the writers of the plague tracts include such recommendations as *fuge cito, vade longe, rede tarde* (flee quickly, go far, come back slowly). The various books and letters about how to protect oneself belong to the large literature of the *Regimina sanitatis*, which began in the third century. This group has as one of its most interesting manifestations the pseudo-Aristotelian letter dedicated to Alexander the Great and translated into Latin about the middle of the twelfth century by Avendeath, who dedicated it to a Queen of Spain, Tharasia, the daughter of Alfonso VI. This letter, which was regarded up to the end of the thirteenth century as a model of this kind of literature, is related, as Sudhoff has shown,

---

[1] This exists in an apparently unique copy of a publication of about 1500, now in the Library of the College of Physicians of Philadelphia, which has recently been studied by W. B. McDaniel, 2nd. A translation and comments appear in the mimeographed " Fugitive Leaves " of the college for 1935–6.

to the pseudo-epigraphic literature of late Hellenism. After the Black Death one often finds that the *Regimen sanitatis* was transformed to deal chiefly with the plague and means of combating it. Such knowledge soon developed a realization of the necessity of a social protection that was contrary to the theurgic and scholastic principles, which sought in Divinity the supernatural agents and origins of all good and evil and recommended resignation and prayer as the only remedies. At the beginning of the pandemic the municipality of Milan was able by strenuous methods to keep the plague from its doors for several months. When it reappeared toward the end of the fourteenth century, Venice was the first (1374) to forbid entrance into the city of travellers or merchants who were infected or even under suspicion. Other Italian towns followed this example. As early as 1348 the Doge Dandolo had appointed a commission to supervise such precautions as the special removal of corpses, the depth of the graves, prohibition of exposing the dead on the streets, a guard against visiting ships, and so on. The patients were isolated in special places outside of the city, and all who had knowledge of a case were required to declare it. It was on the eastern shore of the Adriatic, in the Republic of Ragusa, that control of sailors was first established (1377). A place distant from the city and harbour was designated for disembarkment, and all those who were suspected of being affected by the plague were required to spend thirty days in the fresh air and sun before being admitted. Anyone who had come in contact with the visitors also had to be isolated. Soon, when it appeared that thirty days was not sufficient, the delay was extended to forty days — a *quarantenaria*, from which our modern word "quarantine" was derived. The selection of forty days was only in part due to observation of the disease: this period was known as the philosophical month by the alchemists, while the numerous forty-day episodes in the Bible probably helped to give the period a certain theological basis. In 1383 Marseille established a special quarantine station. Venice and other maritime cities also codified the public measures to be taken against the plague: the suspected houses were aired and fumigated, furniture was exposed to sunlight, the clothing and linen of those affected were burned, and eventually the roads and water supplies were put under control. Thus from the force of circumstances a sanitary legislation was constructed similar to the more ancient but forgotten measures against the lepers (Council of Lands, 503). Venice, having survived the dangers of its swampy site· and lack of potable water, had shown itself aware of sanitary measures, as, for example, in the collection of rain water in cisterns and submitting it to efficient filtration. It is not surprising, then, that Venice was the first to institute a *magistrato delle acque* and in 1438, as we have seen, created its *provveditori della salute della terra*, to whom were added three delegates from the people for each quarter. In 1385 the Republic created a special *magistrato della sanità* with large powers and resources.

Tournai, in Belgium, offers an early example of ordinances for removal of corpses to a distance from the city and forbidding the assemblage of more than two persons at funerals. At the same time less rational regulations were carried out, such as the prohibition of cursing in order to avoid divine wrath; while the regulations against tolling of bells, the wearing of mourning, and labour over the week-ends might be regarded as having a good psychological and physiological basis. The two saints especially invoked by the faithful were St. Sebastian of the many arrows, who was thought to have stopped the plague in parts of Italy after an altar had been dedicated to him in Rome, and St. Roch (b. Montpellier, thirteenth century). St. Roch, having been himself attacked by the plague and miraculously cured of his bubo, devoted himself to the care of the sick, but later died of a second attack at Montpellier. His bones were venerated as relics and a fraternity founded whose object was the care of the poor and the sick, but especially of the plague-stricken.

Thus we see that the later Middle Ages had acquired some good practical ideas on sanitary defence and by force of circumstances had recognized the need for considerable sanitary legislation. While plague necessarily played the most important part in this development, other epidemics that had devastated Europe between the eleventh and the fourteenth centuries must also be considered.

Leprosy, which had been known to the Hebrews, Greeks, and Romans, began to appear in Europe early in the Middle Ages (sixth to seventh centuries). Its wide spread, however, is probably to be attributed to the movements of large numbers brought about by the Crusades. It reached its height in the thirteenth century, at which time there were more than two thousand leprosaria in France alone (*maladreries* or ladreries), and several hundred in England and Scotland. As many more were considered in detail by Virchow in his exhaustive study of leper houses in Germany — that is, houses or colonies in which the lepers were isolated. The disease most frequently appeared in the well-known nodose form, but the mutilating types were also not absent. Without question, just as in Biblical times, other diseases such as psoriasis and probably syphilis were frequently confused with it, a fact which aggravates the problem considerably for medical historians. As many of the lepers as possible were isolated in separate houses, from which they could emerge only when dressed in special apparel: a black robe with two white hands crossed on the chest and a large hat with a white ribbon. When the leper approached a passer-by he had to give warning with a sort of castanets (in some countries with a horn or bell), and when he wished to buy anything, he had to make use of a long rod. This tragic figure, an outcast from society, and condemned to a symbolic death after official examination (*Lepraschau* in German), formed a frequent topic for the chronicles and romances of the period. The rapid disappearance of leprosy in Europe in the fourteenth century is as mysterious in its way as is the sudden rise of syphilis soon afterwards. The many hospitals that it had occasioned, however, proved most useful in meeting the ravages of syphilis and other epidemics.

Among the severe epidemics that devastated Europe during these centuries was the disease known as *ignis sacer* or St. Anthony's fire (a term first used by Mézeray for the epidemic of 1090). It is not clear whether this was due to the widespread use of diseased rye (ergotism), or whether other infectious skin diseases such as erysipelas were included. St. Anthony, the protector of those afflicted by this disease, is often represented with a fire beside him, in the act of protecting and blessing the sick. First mentioned in the annals of the convent of Zanten (*c.* 857), the disease occurred in at least six epidemics up to 1129, which were described in the chronicles of the time. In most descriptions, the limbs became cold and then burning, with the development of blisters and gangrene. Frequently limbs were lost, but the mutilated patient survived; if the viscera were attacked, the results were fatal. Scurvy reached epidemic proportions at the time of the First Crusade, but remained for centuries the terror of sailors who undertook long voyages, when it caused a frightful mortality. As we know now, this was due entirely to the lack of vitamin C in their necessarily unbalanced diet.

Influenza appeared over centuries in epidemics of more or less severity in periods that bore surprising relations to thirty-year intervals. It was especially attributed to supernatural influences, even the name referring to *influentia cœli* or *influenza del diavolo*. It appeared in both respiratory and gastro-intestinal forms, and possibly in the paralytic and lethargic forms now known as lethargic encephalitis. By many it is thought to have constituted the sweating sickness that was so prevalent in England. The *plica polonica*, named from the masses of matted hair, was another epidemic that appeared after the Mongol invasion of 1287.

Amid all these disturbances and terrible catastrophes that convulsed the social and economic life of the times, psychic epidemics occurred that are not to be wondered at. Under this heading come the manifestations of the

Flagellants who appeared about the middle of the thirteenth century. Bands of semi-naked men and women wandered about the country whipping each other severely. Another form of collective psychosis is that known as the Children's Crusade. In 1312 more than thirty thousand children proceeded to the conquest of the Holy Sepulchre. Thousands died on the way, none reached their goal, and only a small remnant of these unfortunates returned to their homes.

7. The Fifteenth Century and Humanism. Medico-Hygienic Literature. The Herbals

Fifteenth-century medicine exhibits a notable progress, especially in the literature on personal hygiene, impelled thereto by the cruel necessities of the plague. Of great scientific importance was the slow but sure progress of anatomical teaching during this century. Coincident with the development of Humanism, dissections, which were made with more and more frequency, prepared the revival of anatomy as a movment in which the physician played the greatest part. The love of the natural sciences, and especially of botany, is one of the characteristics of Humanism; this tendency was reflected in medicine, to be accentuated toward the end of the century in the renewed study of Pliny and Dioscorides, and the publication of the first printed books with illustrations.

The medical literature of the fifteenth century in the universities consisted for the most part of compilations and commentaries on Greek and Arabian texts, of a few *consilia*, and a number of hygienic writings, those *regimina* of which we have already spoken. This literature arose from the desire of rulers to have at hand the advice of a trusted physician, even though he was far away at the time. All these writings resemble, with few variations, early models such as are found in the Arabian literature or in Arnold of Villanova's treatise. Most of the best-known physicians of the time were authors of such books of advice.

Especially noteworthy among these is the work of Master ALDOBRANDINO of Siena (d. *c.* 1287), written in French under the title *Le Régime du corps* and published by Landouzy and Pépin in a magnificent critical edition based on the manuscripts in the Bibliothèque Nationale and the Bibliothèque de l'Arsenal. This book is an interesting landmark both of the history of medicine and perhaps still more — as the first to be written in French — of the history of the French language. Aldobrandino drew largely from Arabian medicine, reproducing entire pages of the *Canon* of Avicenna, the whole chapter on the hygiene of the stomach by Constantinus Africanus, the dietetics of Isaac Hebræus, and in many parts following Rhazes. Hippocrates and Aristotle, Diogenes and Galen are often quoted by him, but are not the sources of his text. Landouzy and Pépin, endeavouring to find why a physician of Siena should write in French, supposed that he was led thereto by the brilliancy of the French culture of the period and the influence that it exerted on foreigners. It is also known that on his death, at Troyes, he left his goods to the neighbouring mon-

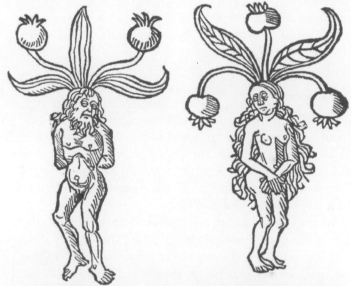

alraun man cclvñ C   alraun fraw cclvñī c

126. *The male and female mandragora.*   (*From a German herbal of 1485.*)

astery. Leaving aside the fact that the earliest manuscripts of this text are in the Walloon tongue, it seems to us that the reason is probably to be found in the fact that the book is dedicated to the Countess of Provence, mother of the Queens of France, England, and Germany and of the Countess of Anjou. This Princess, going to France to visit her daughters, had demanded from the famous physician who accompanied her as attaché to the court of Beatrice a collection of hygienic recommendations for her daughters.

The work of another Sienese physician is one of the earliest to be written in the common tongue. But while Aldobrandino's book is chiefly celebrated as a linguistic monument, the author of the *Trattato utilissimo circa la conservatione della sanitade* is one of the most justly celebrated Italian physicians of the fifteenth century. Ugo BENZI (*c.* 1370–1439), commonly called Hugh of Siena, or Ugone de Benciis, received the doctor's degree at the University of Siena and became Professor of Medicine there in 1395, then at Bologna and at Parma

(1402–16). He was also physician of the Papal Legate with an annual salary of five hundred lire. In 1417 he became lecturer at Siena, and though details about his life are somewhat vague, he certainly taught at Pavia from 1412 to 1427. He was physician at Perugia, as is shown by a passage in his book, and he appears to have given lectures at the Sorbonne. Returning to Italy, he was called by Nicholas III to Ferrara, where he took part in the celebrated Council of 1437. His *Trattato*, dedicated to Nicholas III d'Este, who had been cured by him of a severe skin disease, was first printed at Milan in 1481 by Pietro da Corneno. It was reprinted in 1507, and again in 1618 at Turin with the title *Le Regole della sanità e natura dei cibi con annotazioni di Lodovico Bertalli*, with a new edition shortly after (1620).

Among other authors of the time we note Antonio CERNISONE, professor at Padua from 1414 to 1441, who advocated foot-baths and the use of turpentine for sciatica; Bartolomeo da MONTAGNANA (d. 1460), professor at Padua from 1422 to 1441, who is said to have dissected at least fourteen bodies and was one of the best-known surgeons of his time; Gianmatteo FERRARI di Grado, a devoted Arabist; Antonio GUARNERIO of Pavia; and Michele SAVONAROLA, grandfather of the famous Dominican Gerolamo Savonarola, a physician to Lionel d'Este.

Except for the commentaries on the classic texts, which sometimes contained rich material from personal observations, this period is characterized by a medical literature aimed more at the laity than at physicians, a literature that we speak of today as being on personal hygiene. Attached to this is that medico-botanical literature which had its greatest development in this period.

An interesting chapter in fifteenth-century medical literature and in the history of medical book illustration is furnished by the HERBAL, or, as it is variously known, *Hortus* or *Hortulus*, *Herbarius*, *Hortus sanitatis*, *Gart der Gesundheit*. These books have their origin in the compilations made in the monasteries for the instruction of the monks on medicinal plants. Toward the end of the fifteenth century they began to be printed not only as scientific books but also as popular books to indicate to the laity the curative virtues of plants. Today these books are all rare and command high prices. The *Macer floridus*, published at Naples in 1477 (if this therapeutic poem can properly be called a herbal), is the earliest to have been printed, appearing without illustrations. The earliest printed herbal with illustrations is the *Herbarius* of Pseudo-Apuleius of the fifth century, first published in Rome (J. P. de Lignamine, 1481) and recently published by F. W. T. Hunger in a magnificent folio with facsimile of a ninth-century manuscript at Montecassino (Brill, Leiden, 1936). In 1484 Peter Schoeffer, Gutenberg's pupil, published the first of the *Herbarius* series, which was frequently reprinted in Germany, France, Holland, and Italy. The next year Schoeffer again made publishing history with his *Gart der Gesundheit*, the smaller Ortus. Klebs, who has devoted to this literature an extensive study (*L'Art ancien*, Lugano, 1925), states that this book had the same importance

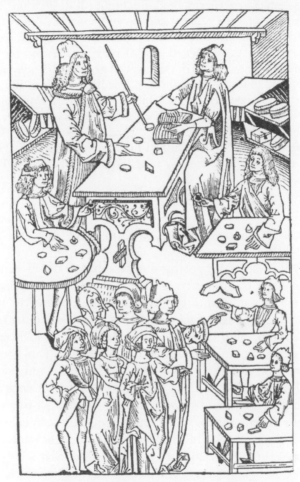

127. *A lapidary shop in which were sold medicinal stones.*
(*From the* Hortus sanitatis, *1491*.)

for the natural sciences that Vesalius' anatomy had for medicine, while Choulant declared it " the most important medical work in natural history with illustrations." The Latin edition was made in Mainz, 1491; the first French edition by Metlinger at Besançon, in 1486 according to Klebs (1490, according to others), with the title of *Arbolayre*. This was the herbal that had the greatest influence of all on the English publications of the type. It was later published as *Le Grant*

Herbier, twice as an incunabulum. These herbals were frequently reprinted and many works of the same type drew their inspiration from them. Among such were Dondi's *Aggregator*, Vincent of Beauvais's *Speculum naturale*, and also the works of Platearius and other Salernitan authors. The edition of the *Herbarius* of Pseudo-Apuleius, earlier quoted, has beautiful illustrations, though perhaps less interesting than the *Hortus sanitatis* of Schoeffer.

All these herbals belong to pre-Renaissance literature, and are extremely valuable documents for the observations that they contain and the picture that they give of the medical ideas of the time. The great herbals describe not only the medicinal plants but also animal drugs, medicinal stones, the examination of urine, and so on, and constitute veritable encyclopædias of popular medicine. In addition to Klebs's important studies, valuable information is to be found in the bibliographical work of L. Choulant (Leipzig, 1841–58), of F. Payne (London, 1901), of Schreiber, who published in 1925 a facsimile of the *Hortus* of 1495, of Sudhoff (1908), and finally, in the classic work of the Prince d'Essling (Florence, 1907–14).

8. *Progress of Anatomy and Surgery in the Fifteenth Century*

If anatomy made no noteworthy progress during the fifteenth century, in its fidelity to the traditions of Galen, nevertheless, it was the time in which dissections became more frequent and thus opened the way for the remarkable revival of anatomy of the Renaissance. Gianmatteo FERRARI (d. 1472) of Grado, who received his doctor's degree at Milan in 1436, taught at Padua, and was physician to the Duchess of Milan, was the author of a commentary on the ninth book of Almansor (first published in Paris, 1471, reproduced by Klebs, 1924). He gives good descriptions of the anatomy of the various organs and seems to have been the first to give the name of ovary to that female organ which had previously been called the feminine testicle. Toward the end of the fifteenth century the study of anatomy on the cadaver was officially authorized by a bull of Sixtus IV (1471–84), who had studied at Bologna and Padua. This was later confirmed by Clement VII (1513–24). This concession of the highest authority of the Church greatly facilitated anatomical progress.

Alessandro ACHILLINI (1463–1512) of Bologna is noteworthy for the frankness, which seemed especially audacious in those times, with which he dared to correct certain errors of Galen (*In Mundini anatomiam annotationes*, Bononiae, 1524). He studied the anatomy of the bladder, the cæcum, and the bile ducts, described the suspensory ligament of the liver, and was the first, according to De Renzi, to recognize the function of the first pair of cerebral nerves. He is also credited with discovery of the fourth cranial nerve and of the hammer and stapes in the middle ear (Sprengel), though the latter discovery was disputed by Morgagni.

Gabriele ZERBI (1468–1505), of Verona, was a Professor of Anatomy

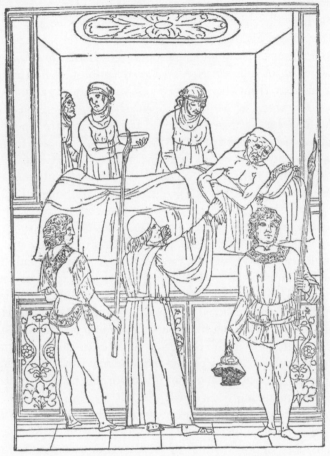

128. *Visit to a plague-stricken patient. Note that the physician holds to his nose an impregnated sponge, while the two servants burn perfumes.* (*From the* Fasciculus medicinæ, *Venice, 1500.*)

at Padua who wrote a treatise (1502) which, among other things, first considered the anatomy of the infant, and described the muscles of the stomach and the outlet of the lachrymal ducts.

Alessandro BENEDETTI (1460–1525), his successor at Padua at the turn of the century, published an *Anatomia* divided into five books and 138 chapters. He maintained the necessity of anatomical dissections independent of the custom then in vogue of supplying the school with cadavers of executed criminals only. In his book, describing a dissection, he speaks of an anatomical theatre at Padua in which from 1490 he gave public demonstrations.

Antonio BENIVIENI (c. 1440–1502), a successful Florentine practitioner who was said by Puccinotti to be the teacher of Benedetti, holds an important place in the history of pathology; in fact, he has been called by De Renzi the father of pathologic anatomy. His book *De abditis nonnullis ac mirandis morborum et sanationum causis* (published posthumously by his brother in 1507 from the Giunta Press) is justly regarded as the first precursor of the work of Morgagni. The *De abditis causis* is important: here for the first time in many centuries are post-mortem studies directed toward finding the internal causes of disease. In the 111 short chapters are notes on twenty autopsies, called incisions and not dissections. They cover cases of intestinal perforation, chronic dysentery, gall-stones, syphilis (which was then raging in Europe), obstructive carcinoma of the bladder, gangrene, tuberculosis(?) of the hip, joint twins, " callus among and obstructing the mesenteric veins," and so on. In the words of Allbutt, Benivieni " opened the bodies of the dead as deliberately and clear-sightedly as any pathologist in the spacious times of Baillie, Bright, and Addison "; nevertheless his importance is rather as a pioneer than for what he actually accomplished. A Galenist, and necessarily a humoralist in theory, he was often wrong in his deductions: post-mortem clots in the heart were of course polyps to him, while a fibrinous pericarditis became for him a part " loaded with hair." Nevertheless this small book may be accepted as the beginning of a small stream of post-mortem observation which in time became the mighty current that was an all-important factor in the development of modern medicine.

Noteworthy for its advanced point of view rather than for any effect produced on a physiologically unenlightened age was the *Dialogue on Statics* (1450) of Nicholas KREBS of Cues (Cardinal CUSANUS, 1401–64). This enlightened churchman and mathematician anticipated the iatrophysical school by advocating estimations of the weight of the blood and urine in clinical disease, and the use of the clepsydra or water clock to determine pulse and respiratory rates in health and disease.

Among the surgeons of the period, especially noteworthy is Pietro D'ARGELATA (d. 1423), the most distinguished pupil of Guy de Chauliac; he taught at Bologna and was the author of a popular *Cirurgia* (printed in Venice, 1480). He treated wounds with dry powders, using sutures and drainage tubes, and was skilled in operating for the stone, the fistula, the hernia, and in dentistry. Leonardo BERTAPAGLIA (d. 1460), professor at Padua, published a *Recollecta super quartum Avicennæ*, a book full of astrology and Arabian polypharmacy. As early as 1330 Master BARNABA DA REGGIO had composed a book on the eye, *De conservanda sanitate oculorum* (published by Albertotti in 1896), which showed a certain amount of originality. The plastic surgery of the BRANCAS was continued through

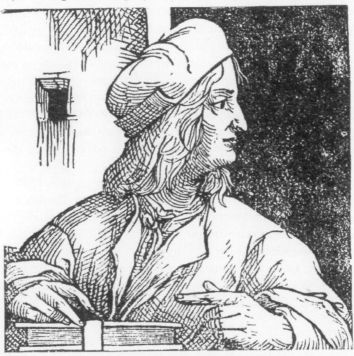

129. Portrait of Alessandro Achillini.

the fifteenth century, to be greatly developed later by Tagliacozzi. Obstetrics and gynæcology, though in their infancy, found certain exponents such as Savonarola, who perhaps was the first to study contracted pelves and their importance at the time of delivery. Benivieni also recommended version in presentation of the feet.

In Germany also, surgery began to be independently studied and described. One of the earliest writers was Heinrich von PFOLSPEUNDT, whose *Bündth-Artzeney* was chiefly concerned with wounds of war, though he appears to have learned some facial plastic surgery from the Italians. The work remained in manuscript from 1460 to 1868, when it was published by Haeser and Middeldorpf. The most important of these German works was the *Buch der Wund-Artzney* (Strassburg, 1497) of Hieronymus

BRUNSCHWIG. Though Pfolspeundt makes some vague allusions to gunshot wounds, Brunschwig is the first to deal explicitly with them in medical literature. He gives many descriptions of operations and technical procedures, while the book is notable as one of the earliest to contain medical illustrations. Thus it is an invaluable document for the history of surgery, and is also important for the history of costumes in the fifteenth century. It depicts so well the surgical instruments, the surgeon at work in the pharmacy, and at the bedside of the patient, preparing for delivery, and handling severe fractures and wounds of all kinds, that it has been reproduced in facsimile by Klein (1911) and by Sigerist (1923). A similar book is Hans von GERSDORFF's *Feldtbuch der Wundartzney* (Strassburg, 1517), based on an experience of forty years and chiefly in various military campaigns. His section on bullet wounds is noteworthy. Wounds were treated with warm (not hot) oil and covered with cotton soaked in oil. Amputation stumps were closed with a flap rather than cauterized, the whole being covered with a moist animal bladder.

One of the earliest books on diseases of children appeared at this time: the *De infantium ægritudinibus et remediis* by Paolo BAGELLARDI. The first edition appeared in Padua in 1472; it was reprinted in 1487 and 1538, and in modern times was published by Sudhoff in *Janus* (1909) and with full commentaries by Simonini (1922). In 1473 appeared Bartholomaeus METLINGER's *Regiment der jungen Kinder* (Augsburg), and shortly after a booklet (Louvain, 1488) by Cornelius Roelans of Mechelen (see Sudhoff, *Janus*, 1909, XIV, 467).

9. Pharmacology in the Fifteenth Century

A widely known practitioner, one SALADINO DI ASCOLI (fl. *c.* 1450), who was physician to the Prince of Tarentum, was driven, in his own words, " by the misdeeds of pharmacists whose ignorance and lack of skill often brought scorn and infamy on the most famous doctors," to write a *Compendium aromatariorum*. In it he treats not only of the kind of examination to which pharmacists should be subjected, but also of all the medicaments described in the famous *Antidotarium* of Nicholas of Salerno, which still constituted the official text of pharmacology. Saladino writes on the weights and the dosage of the drugs, on the way in which the remedy should be prepared, the plants, flowers, roots, and the way of preserving simples and compounds, and finally gives details for organizing and conducting a pharmacy.

Two books that are almost contemporaries of Saladino's are those of SANTE ARDUINO, of Pesaro, and CIRIACO DEGLI AUGUSTI, physician to the Duke of Savoy, who in his *Lumen apothecariorum* (1492) collected all that was known about pharmacology at this time. Paolo SUARDO, of Bergamo, wrote a *Thesaurus aromatariorum*, dedicated to the physicians of Milan; while in Florence there was published toward the end of the century the *Ricettario dei dottori dell'arte*. JACOPO DA FORLÌ or della Torre, who taught at Padua and had such a reputation as a philosopher that he was called by his pupil Savonarola the "Divine Genius," also left certain praiseworthy treatises on materia medica. In this century the study of botany was held in honour, without doubt on account of the return to nature and the observation of plants that Humanism emphasized. Among the most read Humanists who closely followed Pliny was the Latinist Giorgio VALLA, a promoter of a more scientific form of language, who exerted considerable influence on the medical literature of the fifteenth century. Another was Hermolaus BARBARUS, who in his *Castigationes Plinianæ* attempted to purify the text of Pliny that had been corrupted by the copyists and the Arabian translators. He also wrote a commentary on Dioscorides. He was one of the leaders of Humanism. Crowned as a poet at the age of fourteen by Frederick III, he became a doctor at Padua in 1477, made a careful translation of Aristotle, held public office, taught Greek in public, and gathered about him the most illustrious scientists of the end of the century. In 1486 he was Venetian Ambassador to the Emperor Frederick, and in 1489 was Ambassador to Innocent VIII, who created him Cardinal and Patriarch of Aquileia. He died in 1493 before the age of forty, leaving behind him a surprising amount of erudite work that showed a wide knowledge of Greek and of ancient literature.

An eminent position in medical literature must be given to Nicolò da Lonigo, called LEONICENUS (1428–1524). He devoted his early studies to Pliny, whom he criticized severely, as in his famous letter to Politian in which he pointed out the errors committed by the great Roman encyclopædist. Polemics with Barbarus and others resulted, but to Leonicenus remains the credit of having attacked the authority of the greatest naturalist of antiquity, who up to that time had been regarded as impregnable. Leonicenus wrote many translations and commentaries, but his greater value, as Haller and Sprengel have recognized, was that of being the best critic of his period. He refuted not only Pliny and the naturalists but also Serapion and Avicenna, whose distorted translations he confronted with the original classical texts. He did not hesitate to say that they did not know how to read Greek. His principal work is *Plinii et aliorum autorum, qui de sim-*

plicibus medicaminibus scripserunt, errores notati, published in 1492 in
Ferrara, where he spent most of his life. His best-known work is the
Libellus de epidemia quam vulgo morbum gallicum vocant (Venice, 1497).
This is one of the earliest medical texts to give the clinical picture of the

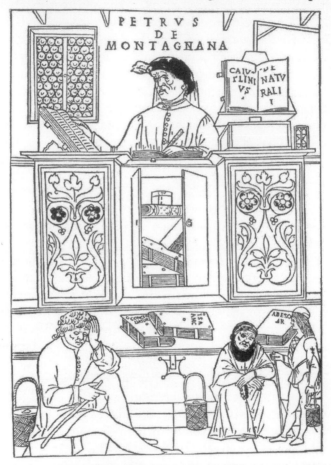

130. *Pietro da Montagnana lecturing at Padua. Note Pliny's* Natural History *on
the lectern and the books of Isaac Judæus and Avenzoar. Below: 3 patients waiting for their urine to be examined.*
(*From the* Fasciculus medicinæ, *Venice, 1500.*)

great pandemic of syphilis; he also speaks of autopsies on syphilitics. The
book has been published in facsimile by Sudhoff in Vol. III of the *Monu-
menta medica* (Milan, 1924). To Leonicenus is also due the credit of
having created at Ferrara a flourishing school to which came pupils from
every part, among them Paracelsus. He is justly regarded as the greatest

clinician of his period, with an outstanding Humanistic culture, acute intellect, and able judgment.

There were many writers on materia medica in this period, such as
Marco GATTINARA, Filippo BEROALDO, Lorenzo MAJOLO of Asti, who was
the teacher of Pico della Mirandola. Thus the study of botany appears to us
as one of the first and most important signs of the approaching renaissance
of medicine, not only on account of the real progress that this discipline
contributed to treatment, but also and especially because these studies
instigated a spirit of observation of natural phenomena and a critical attitude toward the ancients which was most important in preparing the way
to the renaissance in all domains of science. In Germany the little *Artznei-
buch* (Nürnberg, 1477) of ORTOLFF von Bayrlandt attained a popularity
that demanded seven incunabula editions. A popular early work on gynæcology, *Wie sich die schwangern Frawen halten sollen*, is also attributed to
him.

10. The Study and Practice of Medicine at the End of the Middle Ages

During the second half of the fifteenth century, with the first manifestations of Humanism and a return to the study of the classics, one sees more
and more accentuated the tendency of the universities toward a lay type
of medicine. University instruction was well organized, and although there
is still but little question of practical instruction, the first attacks on astrology and magic were taking place and the teaching of anatomy was regularly
given.

By the end of the century the anatomical instruction was not very different
from what it had been at the time of Mondino. Dissections were not practised
even in the larger universities more than once a year; often only every second
or third year. According to the statutes of the University of Bologna in 1405,
only the third-year medical students had the right of attending an anatomical
dissection, and among them only twenty could attend dissection of the male
cadaver, thirty that of the female. Dissections were almost always made at
Christmas time or during Lent; they lasted several days and assumed the proportions of an important public occasion, to which the civil and ecclesiastical
authorities were invited as well as the medical students and faculties of other
institutions. Actually, the teaching was predominantly theoretical.

The medical course usually required four or five years, but sometimes
longer. The bachelor's degree was given after two years of study, the licence
after another two years. The general texts were still those of Galen, Hippocrates, Avicenna, and Averroes, and less frequently the *Isagoge* of Johannitius and

Rhazes' ninth book to Almansor. The examination for the licentiate before
the faculty consisted in comments on one of Hippocrates' Aphorisms, in the
description of certain diseases, and in the long public discussion in connection
with the texts that had been studied. In some universities, before the candidate
could receive his licence, he had to swear that he would not become a surgeon

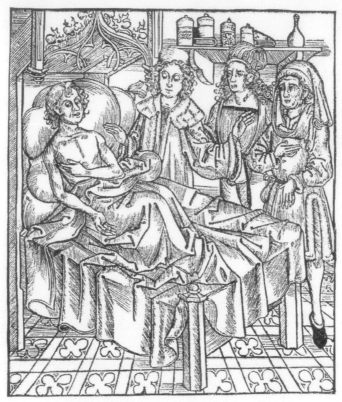

131. *Physicians visiting a plague-stricken patient.*
(*From Brunschwig's* Chirurgia, *1500.*)

and would not operate *cum ferro et igne*. The doctorate was conferred with
special ceremonies and required the payment of heavy fees. The ceremony
generally took place in church with the ringing of bells and the participation
of the entire faculty; toward the beginning of the next century the right to
create doctors was maintained not only by the Pope and the Emperor but
by others to whom this right had been conceded by the Emperor. The libraries
of the universities were for a long time insignificant: in 1395 the faculty of
Paris owned only nine books, of which the *Continens* of Rhazes was held in
the greatest esteem, so much so that when the King borrowed the book in 1371
to have a copy made, he had to leave with the university a large deposit. The

students at Bologna were forbidden under threat of severe punishment to carry books outside of the city. The invention of printing perforce had a very important part in the development of medical culture.

Toward the end of the fifteenth century a great number of books of importance for the history of medicine were printed in rapid succession; and it

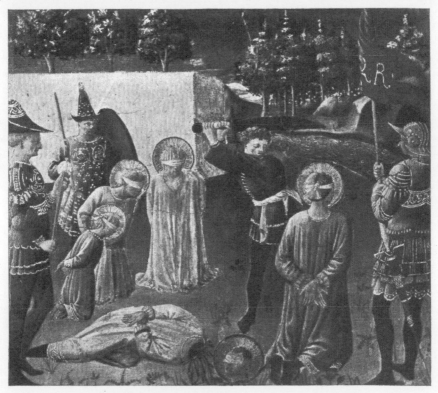

132. *The martyrdom of St. Cosmas and St. Damian.*
(*From a painting by Fra Angelico*, UFFIZI GALLERY, FLORENCE.)

was the diffusion of these publications that made physicians familiar with anatomical figures. This, in turn, gave a new impulse to study and investigation. The illustrated texts were intended in part for physicians and in part for the laity. The oldest illustrations are the reproduction of the Five Figures that are found in the fourteenth-century manuscripts or even earlier. These five (or six) figures represent the skeletal system, the muscles, veins, arteries, and nerves; sometimes a sixth figure is added representing the pregnant female. These figures, found widespread throughout the world, are supposed to have originated in Arabic and Persian manuscripts; they were greatly diffused by the art of printing. Sudhoff has shown that they were not due to direct observation, but were merely copies of ancient designs.

The first medical text with original figures is the *Fasciculus medicinæ* compiled by the German physician JOHANNES DE KETHAM from various separate treatises on such topics as uroscopy, pregnancy, blood-letting, regimen in epidemics, and various surgical procedures. It is especially notable as having been the first printed illustrated medical work, some woodcuts in one of the early editions being in colours. It was printed first in Venice in 1491, and in a number of other editions in the next half-century. The later editions all contained the *Anatomia* of Mondino. Modern reproductions, with translation by Singer, have recently been published (Lier, Florence, 1924 and 1925). A representation of the abdominal muscles is found in the *Conciliator* of Peter of Abano (1496). Other anatomical illustrations are to be found in the *Margarita philosophica* (1503–4) of Gregor REISCH and in the *Antropologium* (1501) of Magnus HUNDT, professor at the University of Leipzig.[1] These pictures were mostly devoted to conventional illustrations of the blood-letting man with the body marked for the best sites for venesection; the zodiac man, with the figures of the zodiac connected with the various viscera; or the planet man, where the planets replaced the signs of the zodiac; the wound man, to show where the arteries should be ligated after wounds of various kinds that are graphically indicated on the body; and the pregnant woman, with the pre-Vesalian *fœtus in utero*. These figures have been traced by Sudhoff to manuscripts of much earlier periods, and to far-distant countries, especially India and Persia.

Of the ancient medical classics there are only a few which appeared in incunabula form; thus the *Ars parva* of Galen was printed first, in the miscellaneous collection called *Articella*, about 1476, and again at Venice five times before 1501. The first Greek edition of Dioscorides — a splendid typographic production — saw the light in the Aldine Press in 1499. The first Latin edition of the collected works of Galen was printed in Venice by Philip Pinzio in 1490. Aristotle's *Physica* appeared in five editions before 1501, his *De Animalibus* in four.

The earliest Roman medical writer to appear in print was Cornelius Celsus in the magnificent edition by Nicolò da Firenze (1478); this was reprinted at Milan in 1481 and Venice in 1493 and 1497. The elder Pliny appeared early: his *editio princeps* came from the press of Giovanni da Spira, of Venice, in

---

[1] Garrison gives a list of eleven so-called " graphic incunabula " of anatomy, the illustrated books on anatomy of the pre-Vesalian period: (1) 33 editions of Mondino; (2) Ketham's *Fasciculus medicinæ*; (3) the skeleton of Richard Helain (1493); (4) the *Conciliator* of Peter of Abano (1496); (5) the *Philosophiæ naturalis compendium* of Johannes Peyligk, which appeared in eight editions between 1499 and 1518; (6) Hundt's *Antropologium* (Leipzig, 1501); (7) Reisch's *Margarita philosophica*; (8) various fugitive sheets on anatomy (see Leroy Crummer's studies, *Ann. Med. Hist.*, 1923, V, 188, and 1925, VII, 1); (9) The *Spiegel der Artzney* of Lorenz Fries (1518); (10) Berengario's commentary on Mondino (1521) and his *Isagogæ breves* (various editions between 1522 and 1535); (11) Dryander's *Anatomiæ pars prior* (Marburg, 1537).

1469. There were eighteen incunabula editions, with the first edition in Italian appearing in 1476. We may deduce, then, that Pliny and Celsus were the most widely read medical writers at this time.

The editions of the *Regimen Salernitanum* were very numerous. It was printed about thirty times before 1501 and the *Antidotarium* of Nicolaus twelve times. Arabian writers to appear most often in early print were: Serapion (first edition, Venice, 1479); Isaac Hebræus (Padua, 1487); Mesue, who had nineteen incunabula editions (Venice, 1471); Avicenna, whose first Latin edition appeared in Milan in 1473, with ten Latin incunabula editions from Venice.

It is interesting to note, in view of these numerous early editions of Celsus, Galen, and the Arabs, that the first editions of the collected works of Hippocrates were not printed until 1525 in Latin, and 1526 in Greek. Systems for aiding the memory, cultivated in classical times by Simonides, Archigenes, and Galen, were included in the domain of medicine at this time. Three such Italian works (printed in many incunabula editions) were those of the physicians Matheolus Perusinus and Johannes M. A. Carrariensis, and the well-known Humanist Jacobus Publicius.

These brief notes suffice to show that medical literature was preparing at the end of the fifteenth century to return to the study of the classics and that in anatomy the elements were ripening to produce a powerful revival.

If now we wish to consider the condition of medicine at the end of this period and to summarize the state of the theoretical knowledge of the time, we see that it had advanced but little beyond the medicine of Galen. Anatomy had made a beginning with the attempts of Mondino and his followers to establish a place for itself in university instruction, but anatomical knowledge was extremely primitive in the profession, which still adhered to the text of Galen. Very few physicians had been present at a dissection even once, and even then stood at a distance from the table. In physiology, knowledge was also elementary; a few facts about the sense organs were beginning to see the light. The theories of Galen about the functions of the heart were still accepted, and in general the humoral theory still reigned supreme. The doctrines of Galen, also, were still in force for the digestive tract; while knowledge of the anatomy and physiology of the genital tract was so scanty that one might say that almost all the progress made in this field by Soranus and his pupils had been forgotten.

Pathology, still based on the theories of the humours and diatheses, made distinction between fevers and acute diseases according to their symptoms. A few rare physicians perhaps based their diagnoses on positive observations and logical deductions; but in general the practitioner drew his conclusions from inspection of the blood, giving special importance to the colour, density, odour, and foam of the fluid; of the sputum, which it was felt permitted a sure diagnosis on the basis of its odour and colour; and above all on the examination of the urine. Various systems of uroscopy gave detailed descriptions of variation in colour, odour, formation of sediment, and so on, together with instructions how to make an exact diagnosis in the greatest variety of diseases. From the layers of sediment that were to be seen in the collecting vessel, the urine was divided into four parts, each of which corresponded to a region of the body. Thus the turbidity of the upper layer indicated a disease of the head, of the lower layer disease of the genital organs or the bladder.

On such foundations therapy could correspond to the disease picture only in an empirical manner. As a matter of fact, being based on the classical principle of *contraria contrariis*, blood-letting was the usual treatment, being applicable in all cases thought to be due to plethora.

The dominant idea was that the blood-letting should deflect the morbific material and make it pass from one organ to another. It was regarded as a revulsive when one drew blood from the side of the body opposite that where the disease was situated; or as derivative, on the other hand, when it was drawn on the same side, in order to diminish the plethora or relieve the patient's pain. The directions for phlebotomy and its technique were extremely minute, determined almost always by astrological considerations, whereby it was permitted only on favourable days and at favourable hours. The question as to whether one should bleed from one vein rather than another, the number of bleedings and the amount of blood withdrawn depending on the age and temperament of the patient, the season of the year, and the locality — these were all the subjects of long and often heated discussions, based on innumerable citations of medical writings. There was much divergence of opinion among the different schools and physicians. Less frequently practised than blood-letting was the application of cups or leeches; other forms of treatment throughout the Middle Ages were the application of blisters, cautery and scarifications, already recommended by the Romans, enemas, and the use of such revulsive remedies as mustard and cantharides. The use of *fontanelle* (issues) and setons is mentioned by the Salernitan physicians. The seton was used by making two parallel incisions in the skin, usually on the neck, and introducing a thread or a small strip of linen to prevent healing; this was drawn further through the channel from time to time to renew the counter-irritation. The *fontanelle*, a small scarification, was kept open by the introduction of a bean or pea or some similar foreign body. These revulsives were chiefly in vogue throughout the fifteenth century, but were widely used up to the eighteenth century and still may be found in backward regions or in veterinary practice. Another revulsive, the *moxa*, we have already met in Oriental medicine.

Among the most popular forms of treatment was the bath, used in various forms, including the steam bath. It was especially in vogue in the Germanic countries, where the public bath (*Badestube*) consisted of huge tubs or vats in which the patients stood or sat. For the steam baths, they were covered to the neck with a cloth, the steam being introduced from below.

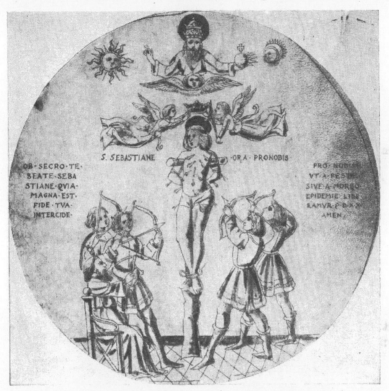

133. *A fugitive sheet against the plague, with the figure of St. Sebastian and an invocation. Lombard master of the fifteenth century.*

Mixed bathing in a state of nature was commonly indulged in, as may be seen in the frequent illustrations by Dürer and the lesser masters of Renaissance art. The practice was often made an occasion for feasting and drinking, while more serious procedures such as the addition of various medicaments or the practice of cupping or blood-letting were also undertaken. The evils that this system produced, however, eventually became apparent. The relaxation in morals that followed in time brought about regulations suppressing mixed bathing, while the increased knowledge of contagion operated toward the elimination of the common bath tank.

Diet played an extremely important part in mediæval therapy, the

physician giving it his closest attention and prescribing the most minute
details even in cases of light illness. A special diet was prescribed before
and after blood-letting; the method of preparing food and drink was closely
outlined and voluminous texts were dedicated exclusively to the explanation
of the proper kind and amount of food for the patients in various diseases.

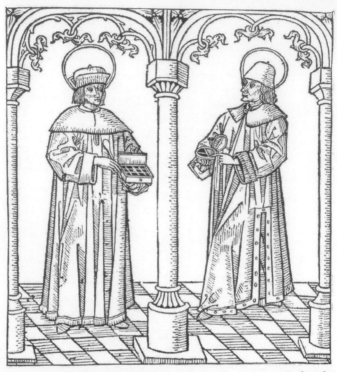

134. *The medical saints Cosmas and Damian in the costume of the physician
(left) and the pharmacist (right) of the period. Spanish print of the late fifteenth century.*

The Hippocratic tisane, broths, milk, which is sometimes indicated as a
sovereign remedy for consumption, and eggs — these were the basic elements of the diet.

The drugs used in treatment were drawn from all sources, but especially from plants, to which was attributed, often correctly, the roles of
digestives, laxatives, emetics, diuretics, diaphoretics, styptics, and so on.
Polypharmacy was at its height, very complicated prescriptions being written that often contained twenty or thirty ingredients. Therapeutic value
was attributed to precious stones, to some of which, like the sapphire, the
emerald, and pearls, were ascribed marvellous virtues.

The prescription that had the greatest vogue throughout this period was the *theriacum* or *triacum* (the origin of our modern word " treacle "), said by ancient historians to have been invented by Andromachus, the physician of Nero, but according to others by Mithridates. The *mithridaticum*, a similar and equally complicated prescription, was more generally attributed to the latter. It is said that the recipe for this compound was cut in

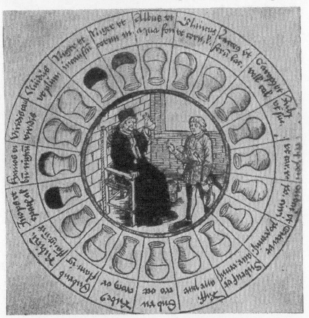

135. *Table for the examination of urine.*
(*From the* Fasciculus medicinæ, *Venice, 1497.*)

bronze in the temple of Æsculapius at Epidaurus. This portentous medicine, about which a whole library has been written, was composed of a great number of drugs that varied according to the time and place. Its fundamental basis was the flesh of vipers, regarded as an excellent remedy against every kind of poison. According to Benedicenti, who has devoted a chapter of his book to this subject, the *theriacum* of Andromachus consisted of fifty-seven substances; its preparation was very difficult and required such special skill that at Venice in the fifteenth century it was prepared in the presence of the *Priori e Consiglieri* of the physicians and pharmacists. At Bologna it was prepared before the public in the court of the arch-gymnasium. From Corradi's studies of the statutes of the pharmacists of Pisa and Florence, it appears that the *theriacum* had to be prepared publicly " by the pharmacists together with the physicians and all the authorities of the said arts," and it could not be sold without the approval of the consuls. Theriacum had a number of imitators, among which was the *orvietan* that was much later placed on the market. This was in great demand throughout Europe, and Venice carried on an extremely valuable commerce in it, of which it was very jealous.

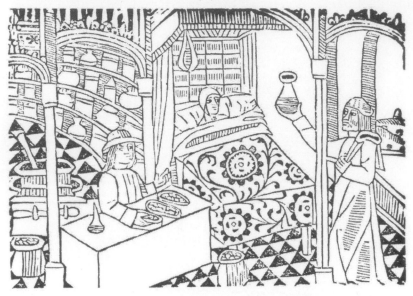

136. *The physician's visit (right) and the shop of the pharmacist (left).*
(*Woodcut from the Spanish edition of Bartolomeus Anglicus;* De las propriedades de las cosas, *Tolosa, 1494.*)

All the factors that we have seen contributing to popular medicine from the most ancient times still continued to exert their influence on treatment as well as on concepts of disease. Mysticism continued to play an important role. In this, suggestion had its part, whether unconsciously or perhaps voluntarily by the more intelligent physicians. Symbolical procedures, analogous to those of primitive peoples, were used even by physicians who otherwise practised their art intelligently. All the amulets used by antiquity are prescribed by such physicians as Arnold of Villanova and Alderotti. To this mystic medicine is allied the miraculous pharmacopœia of the Middle Ages, which often prescribed disgusting animal excretions and such strange drugs as the horns of deer, dragon's blood, the spermatic fluid of frogs, the bile of vipers and snails, and so on. It should be noted, however, that some of these, such as hartshorn, had active qualities, while "dragon's blood" was the name for the red resin of *Calamus draco,* a climbing palm.

The religious sentiment of the period was another important factor in treatment as well as in the concept of disease. This is only to be expected from a time when there was absolute belief in the power of demons and sorcerers, and when such phenomena as impotence and loss of memory were regarded as due to hostile spells. For the treatment of such disorders, naturally, exorcism became an important therapeutic practice; and the priest was substituted for the physician, who was powerless to cure these diseases due to malignant spirits.

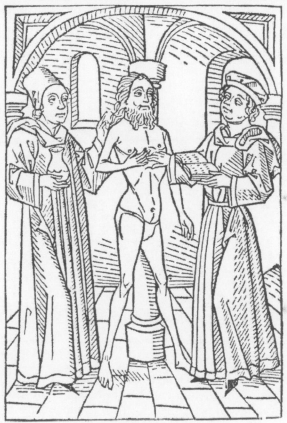

137. *The examination of the patient.*
(*Frontispiece of the* Regimen sanitatis, *Augusta, 1482.*)

The cult of relics became widespread, and certain prayers were ordered to be repeated to cure various symptoms and diseases. Thus Arnold of Villanova gives many prayers to such and such a saint as the best means of relieving this or that disease. Similar procedures are still in use, and their efficiency still in dispute.

Belief in the cure of scrofula by the royal touch had its origin in the Middle Ages and was continued for many centuries. Scrofula was early known in England as the king's evil; and we find in the chronicles of Edward the Confessor records of cures obtained by the imposition of the royal hands on the diseased part. About the same time the same power was claimed for the hands of the Most Christian King of France. Actually the tradition and the use of this healing power as a divine or royal attribute goes back to much earlier times. The figure of Æsculapius found in the Temple at Athens, for instance, is in the act of placing his hands on the patient (Sudhoff, *Arch. Gesch. Med.*, 1926, No. 3). Pliny tells of Pyrrhus curing diseases of the spleen, Tacitus of Ves-

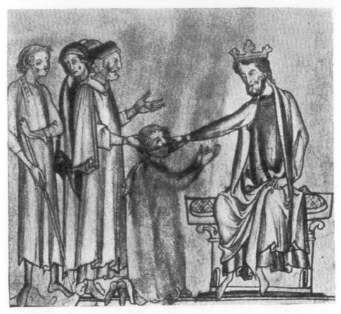

138. *Edward the Confessor curing the scrofulous. English miniature of the thir-teenth century.*   (UNIVERSITY OF CAMBRIDGE.)

pasian curing the blind, and of Hadrian curing dropsy by the Imperial touch. Similar is the Christian tradition of cure by the laying on of hands.

Edward the Confessor, who died in 1056, undoubtedly treated a great number of patients for scrofula in this way. Gilbertus Anglicus says in his *Compendium medicinæ* that scrofula was called "*morbus regius quia reges hunc morbum curant.*" In the household accounts (1277-8) of Edward I we find the records of 73 persons touched by the King on the 4th of April, 192 the next week, and 288 on Easter 1277. After Richard II there was no mention of the practice in the English chronicles until 1462, when Henry VI appears to have revived it and distributed gold angels as touchpieces. In France, accord-ing to Tillemond's description in his *Life of Saint Louis* (1849, Vol. VII, p. 360), the cure was performed as follows: "After having prepared for the ceremony by fasts and prayers, and having taken the Holy Sacrament, and worshipped for three days at the Tomb of St. Marcolph at Corbigny, the King received the patients who were arranged before him. He placed his fingers on the diseased part, making the sign of the cross and pronouncing the words: 'The King touches thee and God heals thee.' He then blessed the patient, who was given food and money for his journey home." The healing touch was thought to come to the kings after they had been consecrated with the holy oil. The number of patients touched by the kings of France was enormous: Philip of Valois is said to have touched fifteen hundred persons at one sitting. John

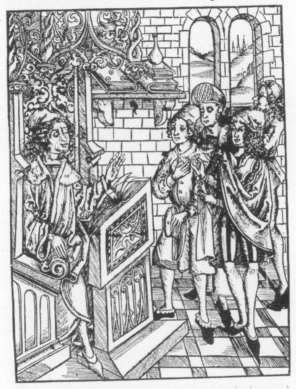

139. *Medical teaching. (From the* Hortus sanitatis, *1499.)*

of Gaddesden (1280–1361) in his *Rosa anglica*, after having recommended various diets and drugs for scrofula, adds: "If this does not suffice, go to the King that he may touch and bless you; because this disease is called the royal disease and the touch of the Most Serene King of the English is valuable for it." It is only when this treatment failed that the patient was advised to have recourse to the surgeon.

Interesting details of the ceremony are given by William Clowes, physician to Queen Elizabeth, and also by one Tooker, her chaplain, who goes at length into the priority of the kings of England over the kings of France. The French affirmed that it was Clovis who had first used the healing power after his baptism and coronation, A.D. 496; while the English maintained that the kings of France had only inherited this power from their relatives the kings of England. Richard Wiseman, the famous surgeon of the time of Charles II, gives a classic account of the king's evil, while Shakespeare refers to the royal touch and the golden angel in *Macbeth* (IV, iii). Samuel Johnson was touched by Queen Anne, but apparently without much help to the great lexicographer. In England the practice fell into disuse shortly after his time. In France the practice continued into the nineteenth century. Louis XVI at the time of his

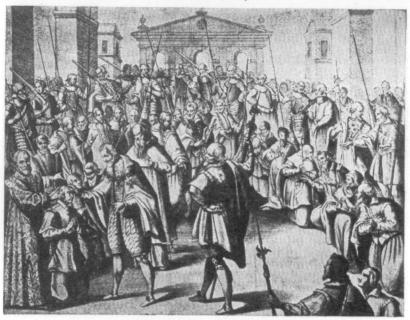

140. *Henry IV, King of France, curing the scrofulous.*
(*Frontispiece of A. Laurens's* De mirabili strumas sanandi vi, *1609.*)

coronation in 1775 touched 2,400 patients; and Charles X in 1824, touched 121 patients who had been presented before him by the two famous physicians Alibert and Dupuytren.

The knowledge of surgery in the later centuries of the Middle Ages was considerably influenced by Greek and Byzantine traditions, as well as by the writings of the Arabs and the school of Salerno. Surgical treatment was almost entirely limited to wounds, fractures, dislocations, amputations and the opening of abscesses and fistulas. The objective nature of surgical treatment and the ability to see results directed surgical concepts into a healthy development that was less hampered than was medicine by the theorizing of scholasticism. Surgery, however, was practically limited to certain simple operative procedures, which themselves often were done with considerable technical skill, while difficult and complicated operations existed almost exclusively in the literature and were rarely put into practice. The operation for inguinal hernia, though frequently practised, appears not to have produced favourable results. Lithotomy, practised in the traditional Greco-Latin manner with the patient in the position still generally used today, was accompanied by great loss of blood and often was followed by

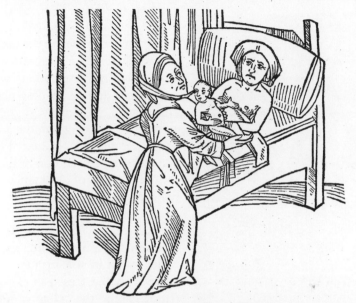

141. *The midwife attending childbirth.*
(*From Lichtenberger's* Prognosticatio, *Heidelberg, 1488.*)

a fatal infection. Suturing of wounds was known, but was rarely put into practice. Obstetrics was almost entirely in the hands of midwives; intervention by the surgeon, as far as we can determine from the written record, was based on very insufficient knowledge; mediæval obstetrics had fallen far behind the time of Soranus and Paul of Ægina. Embryotomy was often practised because the obstetrician rarely knew how to perform version. Often, according to an ancient Hippocratic practice, the woman about to give birth was shaken violently, which was thought to facilitate delivery. Delivery was accomplished in special chairs, of which numerous specimens have been preserved and are still in use in certain countries. Cæsarian section existed at this time only in the literature and, forgotten from classical times, was brought back into practice, as we shall see, only at a much later period.

The operation for cataract was in especial favour with the Arabian physicians, from whom it was borrowed by the West, together with puncture and couching of the lens.

It is to this period that we owe the highly important invention of spectacles. Long discussions have risen as to whether it came by accident or as the result of long study. It is generally accepted that the ancients knew that objects appeared larger when looked at through glass spheres. Ac-

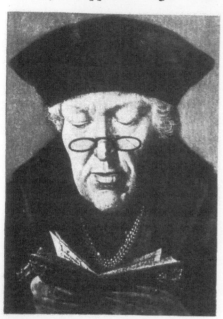

cording to Pliny, Nero used an emerald for this purpose. Alhazan noted the distortion as well as the magnification of objects by a glass sphere, while Roger Bacon's descriptions were apparently of appliances designed to aid failing sight. Gilbertus Anglicus' reference to *oculus berellinus* has already been commented upon. The evidence raised by certain authors that the invention of spectacles should be credited to SALVINO DEGLI ARMATI (d. Florence, 1317) seems insufficient to Albertotti. It is certain, on the other hand, that spectacles were in use in 1352, as may be seen in the fresco of Thomas of Modena in the chapter-house at Treviso representing Hugh of Provence with spectacles on his nose. In a miniature in the convent of St. Mark at Florence the Apostle St. Matthew is represented before a table,

142. *Portrait of Thomas More, Chancellor of Henry VIII, by the Elder Holbein, showing spectacles of the period.*
(AIX-LES-BAINS MUSEUM.)

reading with a pair of spectacles. Finally, in the chapter on Venetian art illustrated by Monticoli and Cecchetti and dating from that period penalties are given for glassworkers who made spectacles from glass instead of from crystal. Thus it seems possible that the invention of spectacles is of Venetian origin and that they were already being made there on a large scale in the fourteenth century. The problem is complicated by the confusion that exists between true spectacles and instruments that may well have been mere simple lenses or eye-shields.

11. The Practice of Medicine, Surgery, and Pharmacy

The practice of the healing arts in the late centuries of the Middle Ages developed rapidly along the lines of the Salernitan traditions and from that time on was entirely in the hands of the laity. Already about the beginning of the fourteenth century the first fruits of the new order were to be observed in Italy, where, on the one hand, the free development of study began in the universities, and, on the other hand, physicians began to be organized into a body that was jealous of its rights, which were protected by the

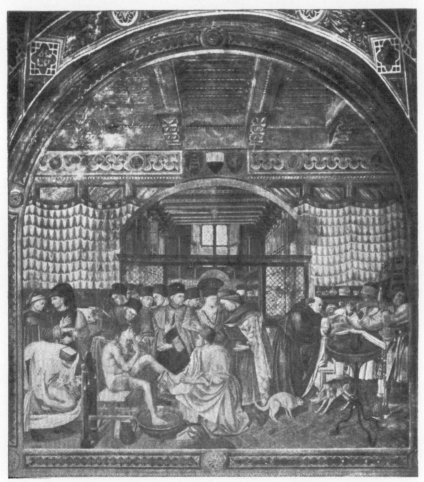

143. *The treatment of the sick. Fresco by Domenico di Bartolo in the infirmary of the Pellegrinaio in the Hospital of Santa Maria della Scala, Siena.*

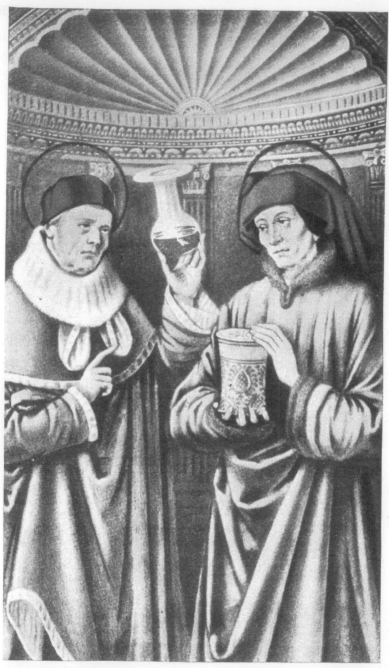

144. *Saints Cosmas and Damian, from the prayer book of Anne of Brittany.*
(Fifteenth-century manuscript, BIBLIOTHÈQUE NATIONALE, PARIS.)

law. It is at this time that the " guilds " were formed, with strict regulations guaranteeing that no one could practise the profession without possessing the requisite knowledge and having made the required studies. At the same time a number of factors contributed to the recognition of the need for hospitals where pilgrims, soldiers, strangers, artisans, and others could be treated. Important factors in this development were the effects of the Crusades with the large movements of soldiers and the constantly in-

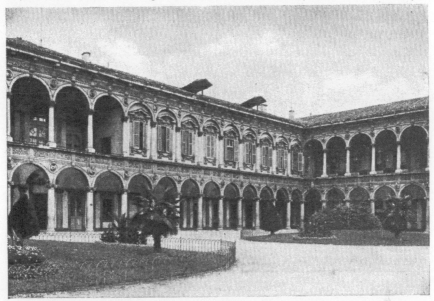

145. *The courtyard of the Spedale Maggiore of Milan, said to have been designed by Bramante.*

creasing traffic with the Levant, both of which brought about a tendency toward adoption of measures that would safeguard the public health. Examples thereto had not been lacking in the former civilizations, the Roman, the Byzantine, and the Saracen. Thus throughout Europe began the slow development of institutions which in some cities reached an exemplary standard.

Toward the end of the fifteenth century hospitals were already well organized, and especially in the larger Italian cities magnificent edifices with notable sculptures were erected to receive the sick. The Hospital of the Ceppo at Pistoja is ornamented with the marvellous bas-reliefs of Giovanni della Robbia (1469–1529), the chefs-d'œuvre of this artist and an important iconographic contribution to the history of medicine. The hospital of Siena, with the valuable frescoes of Dominico di Bartolo, the

Hospital of Milan, magnificent in Lombard art, the Hospital of Santa Maria Nuova at Florence (1288), and many others too numerous to mention, speak eloquently of a period when charitable sentiment was active and Italian cities were quite aware of the importance of an establishment consecrated to the care of the sick.

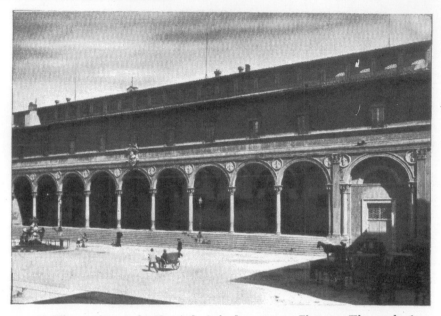

146. *The portico of the Hospital of the Innocents at Florence. The work of Brunelleschi, with medallions by Della Robbia.*

An evidence of the generous scale on which Italian cities maintained the hospitals is the gift of more than twenty-five thousand florins in the single year of 1348 to the Hospital of Santa Maria Nuova, as Villani has pointed out. The money was well spent, as the hospital " gave its alms freely and found itself abundantly provided with many patients, men and women." While the act that founded the hospital speaks of places for 17 patients, the documents published by Corsini show that toward the middle of the fourteenth century there was room for 220 patients. The inventory published by Chiapelli and Corsini in 1923 is extremely interesting also for the great wealth of manuscripts and *objets d'art* that it lists.

At the same time, we see the appearance of laws, doubtless inspired by the legislation of Frederick II, which regulate the sale of foods, forbid the sale of poisons, and give instructions for the burial of the dead.

In spite of the strict laws of Frederick II, the practice of medicine was abused by persons who had no right thereto and had not made the necessary studies, as is shown by the famous verses attributed to the school of Salerno, but certainly of much later date:

Fingit se medicus, quivis idiota, pro-
    fanus
Iudæus, monachus, histrio, rasor, anus
Sicuti alchemista medicus fit aut sa-
    ponista,
Aut balneator, falsarius aut oculista
Hic dum lucra quærit, virtus in arte
    perit.

The role of physician may be assumed
    by any ignoramus or heretical
Jew, monk, actor, barber, or old
    woman,
Just as the physician may become an
    alchemist, or cosmetician,
Bath-attendant, forger, or eye quack.
As soon as lucre is sought, the merit in
    the art departs.

The practice of medicine was by now entirely in the hands of the laity: Honorius III had forbidden the clergy to practise. Each city was much interested in the success of its university; in the year 1300 Bologna, for in-

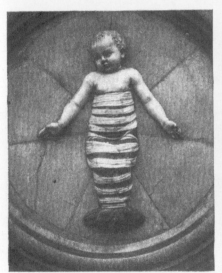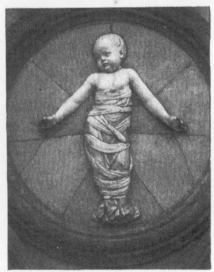

147, 148. Della Robbia medallions on the Hospital of the Innocents, Florence.

stance, spent a good half of its municipal receipts, not less than twenty thousand florins, to support its university. There was the greatest rivalry between the best-known universities to procure the most famous lecturers with cash offers or to retain them by means of contracts, oaths and threats.

The physician who had obtained the university licentiate and had the title of Master — the title of Doctor being first reserved for the professors

— was free to exercise his art wherever it seemed best. As one may see in contemporary pictures, the physician went to the pharmacy to order the drugs by pointing them out with his baton; and it is only much later in the Renaissance that the custom of writing prescriptions grew up. Particular honours were reserved for the physicians of rulers, who, as we have seen, were specially concerned with issuing hygienic and dietetic advice, often

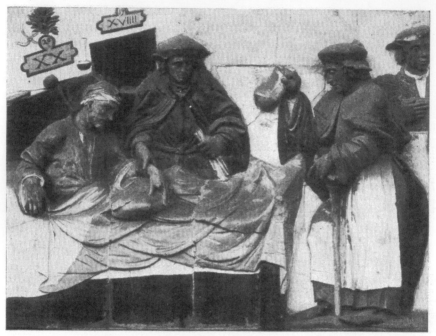

149. *Visit to the sick.*
Frieze by Della Robbia in the Hospital of the Ceppo, Pistoia.

based on astrology. They sometimes had the responsibility of supervising the food or of testing its effects to remove any danger of poisoning. The larger cities often had municipal physicians who were responsible for the care of the indigent sick and the supervision of the sanitary laws. Physicians, like notaries, masters, and magistrates, were engaged by the city in a special contract; and often grave contests arose between cities or rulers in the endeavour to procure some illustrious physician.

The financial reward of physicians during the Middle Ages was often considerable, partly because the number of physicians in practice was relatively small. We know that the most successful physicians of wide reputation amassed considerable fortunes, and demanded remuneration that even today would seem very high. But from chronicles, wills, and public acts we may infer that even practitioners who did not enjoy a great renown made a good living from their occupation, could live honourably, often bought house and land, and sometimes became possessors of valuable works of art. Even at this time patients sought to be treated free of charge and to avoid paying honoraria to the physician, as is shown by the many recommendations that authors gave to their colleagues about watching over their own interests. The following verses, attributed to the school of Salerno though probably written much later, show a good knowledge of the psychology of the patient.

Non didici gratis, nec musa sagax Hippocratis	Don't give your services gratis; let not the wise muse of Hippocrates
Ægris in stratis serviet, absque datis.	Serve the sick in bed without reward.
Empta solet care multum medicina juvare;	For medicine bought dearly benefits much;
Si quæ detur gratis, nil affert utilitatis.	If something is given for nothing, no good results.
Res dare pro rebus pro verbis verba solemus:	We are accustomed to give things for things; words for words.
Pro vanis verbis montanis utimur herbis	For profitless words we give back mountain herbs,
Pro caris rebus, pigmentis et speciebus,	For high rewards we give unguents and spices,
Est medicinalis Medicis data regula talis,	A medical rule is given to the physician thuswis
Ut dicatur: da! da! dum profert languidus ha! ha!	That he should say: give, give, until the patient cries ah! ah!
Dum dolet infirmus Medicus sit pignore firmus;	While the patient is suffering let the physician be firm in his demand;
Instanter quærat nummos, vel pignus habere;	Let him ask for immediate payment or get security;
Fidum nam antiquum conservat pignus amicum,	For the faithful pledge preserves the ancient friend,
Nam si post quæris, quærens inimicus haberis.	But if you seek it later, you will be held as an enemy.

The Italian novelists of the fourteenth century often speak of physicians, describe their clothes, and tell of the jokes that were played upon them. A passage from Boccaccio's *Decameron* (the ninth story of the eighth day) is illustrative of some of the medical customs and costumes of the time. " A certain Master Simone da Villa, richer in inherited goods than in learning, returned hither, no great while since, a Doctor of Medicine, according to his own account, clad all in scarlet and with a great miniver hood, and took a house in the street which we call nowadays the Via del Cocomero." Shortly after we read that friend Bruno, " so he might not appear ungrateful for the hospitality shown him, had painted Master Simone a picture of the lenten season in his salon, also an Agnus Dei at the entrance of his chamber and a chamber-pot over the street door, so those who had occasion for his advice might know how to distinguish him from the others."

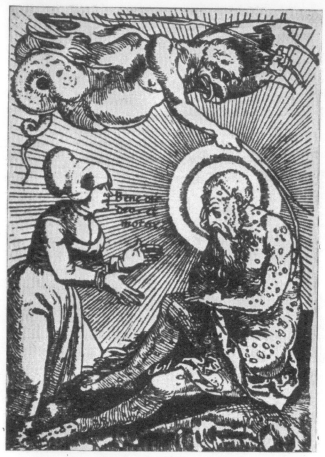

150. *The Leper, by Hans Wechtlin.*

Many more such tales could be quoted to show how the medical men of the period laid great weight on appearances and on their costumes, even though people often ridiculed them for their ignorance. As a matter of fact, they were persons of importance and had the right to go through the streets in luxurious costumes with belts of silver thread and wearing pearls and precious stones. Even the wives of physicians could evade the strict laws about costume and adorn themselves with clothing that was forbidden to other women. Petrarch waxes highly indignant about the luxury of physicians, as may be seen in one

of his letters to Boccaccio: " Add to that an indecent display of usurped clothing, purple mixed with other colours, sparkling rings, golden spurs; and tell
me that I, no matter how normal, would not remain lowered before so much
splendour." Perrens, who bases his information on Boccaccio and Sacchetti,
thus describes the costume of the Florentine physician: " Miniver fur on new
clothing, a mantel of miniver on the shoulders, a velvet bonnet, embroidered
gloves, a valet and a horse — these are the signs by which the physician is recog-

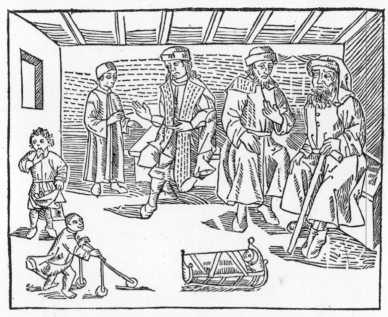

151. *Patients awaiting the doctor at the hospital.*
(*From Bartolomeus Anglicus'* De la propriété des choses, *Lyon, 1500.*)

nized." One might add to this characteristic costume the red robe (*lucco*) in
which Dante is often represented.

We quote here the famous letter of Petrarch to Pope Clement VI which
started his quarrel with Guy de Chauliac, the physician of the Pope: " I know
that your bedside is beleaguered by doctors, and naturally this fills me with
fear. Their opinions are always conflicting, and he who has nothing new to
say suffers the shame of limping behind the others. As Pliny said, in order to
make a name for themselves through some novelty, they traffic with our lives.
With them — not as with other trades — it is sufficient to be called a physician
to be believed to the last word, and yet a physician's lie harbours more danger
than any other. Only sweet hope causes us not to think of the situation. They
learn their art at our expense, and even our death brings them experience:
the physician alone has the right to kill with impunity. Oh, Most Gentle Father,
look upon their band as an army of enemies. Remember the warning epitaph

which that unfortunate man had inscribed on his tombstone: 'I died of too
many physicians.' Entirely appropriate to our time is the prophecy of the
ancient Cato: 'When the Greeks have flooded us with their literature, and
especially their physicians, they will ruin everything for us.' As we fear to

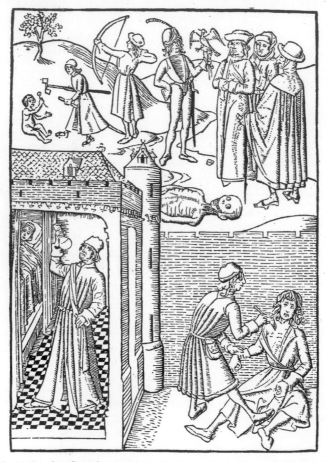

152. *A visit by the physician and a surgical operation; above, the inspection of a
cadaver. (From the 1485 edition [Harlem] of Bartolomeus Anglicus.)*

live without physicians, although countless nations have lived, better perhaps
and healthier, without them — Pliny says the Romans themselves lived so for
more than six hundred years at the time of their greatest epoch — then find
yourself a single one of their band who is worthy, not on account of the grace
of his expressions, but because of his knowledge and his integrity. For in the
act of forgetting their profession, they are eager to step out of their sphere;
they set their feet upon the blooming acres of poesy and the wide fields of
rhetoric, as though it were not their province to heal but to convince." (Pe-

trarch's *Letters*, Vol. II, Bk. 5, Letter XIX, Le Monnier, 1864 translation in V. Robinson's *Story of Medicine*.)

The Pope, in spite of the recommendations of Petrarch, had the letter read to Guy de Chauliac, thus giving rise to the famous quarrel and the satires of Petrarch against physicians.

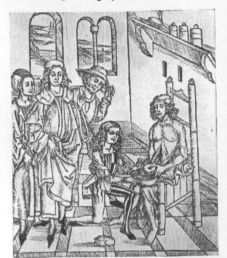 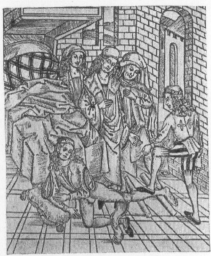

153. *Treatment of a perforating wound of the abdomen and a dislocation.*
(*From Brunschwig's* Chirurgia, *Strassburg, 1494.*)

Thus we find well-organized medical schools at the end of the fifteenth century and laws governing the practice of medicine, with severe penalties for those who practised without the necessary licence. Ethical rules were observed. It was forbidden to a physician to make a grave or even qualified prognosis about his patient's disease without consultation with a colleague. A fine was inflicted on any physician who spoke evil of another in public. The practice of medicine was entirely in the hands of the laity. It is at this time that we first find a body of professional laws so adequate and well thought out that even up to our own times it has not been necessary to make any considerable changes.

The medical physicians, masters or doctors in medicine as they were later called (though in reality this title only belonged to the university lecturers), usually did not deign to practise surgery, which was regarded as an inferior art and unworthy of scholars. The physician, however, often gave written surgical advice, as, for instance, did Dino del Garbo and Gentile da Foligno; but he abstained from all practice of surgery, which was left to the surgeons proper and to the barbers.

The surgeon at this period did not possess university rank. While the physicians were regarded as academicians and gave their services to the popes and princes and occupied university chairs, the surgeons were of a lower order who rarely knew Latin. They often went from one country to another, practising the operations for the stone, hernia, and cataract, which were grave and difficult operations that required a high degree of skill and profound knowledge

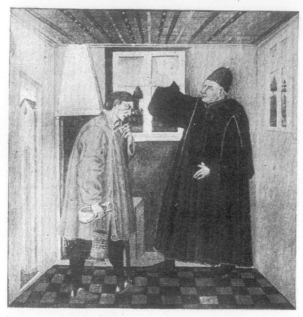

154. *The doctor and the patient.*
(*Miniature from the Hebraic Codex of Avicenna in the* UNIVERSITY OF BOLOGNA.)

of their art. From the surgeon's rooms where the young men were taught who wished to dedicate themselves to the art, there issued forth men ignorant of scholastic disquisitions but often very expert. The contrast between physicians and surgeons was so great that in the fourteenth century the student of medicine in Paris, for instance, had to swear that he would not do any surgical operations. Blood-letting was forbidden to physicians, who thought it unworthy of them, although the best writers of the time, such as Alderotti, Pietro d'Abano, and Gentile da Foligno wrote at length on the appropriate diseases and the proper time and place in which to practise it.

The barber, who in German countries was generally connected with baths and thus had the name *Bader*, and who also let blood, sold unguents, pulled teeth, applied cups, and gave enemas, was a highly important figure in mediæval medicine; in fact, almost up to the eighteenth century. Often he was confused with the surgeon and generally had the right to practise surgery. The barbers began to acquire importance about 1100, when the monks, who required their services for the tonsure, also had recourse to them for blood-letting, which monks were obliged to undergo regularly by ecclesiastical law. The barber of the monastery was called *Rasor et Minutor* (barber and blood remover) because to let blood in the Latin of the time was called *minuere sanguinem*. No one could avoid the periodic blood-letting unless he was seriously ill. The extensive practice of surgery by the barbers is revealed by an observation of Bruno di Longoburgo in his *Chirurgia Magna*. He complains of the fact that physicians regarded it as undignified to practise surgery, and especially blood-letting, but left them both in the hands of the barbers: " *Ac operationes scarificationis et flebotomiæ noluerunt medici propter indecentiam exercere; sed illas barberiorum in manibus reliquerunt.*" Lanfranc, who certainly was in a position to know the condition of the surgery of his time, also observed that blood-letting was relinquished to the barbers on account of medical pride, though it formerly was the task of the physician and later of the surgeons proper. The Collège de St. Côme of Paris, founded about 1210, made a clear distinction between the surgeons of the long robe and the barbers, or the surgeons of the short robe, for whom successive royal decrees prohibited the practice of surgery without their having undergone a special examination. In 1365 there were forty barber-surgeons in Paris. The Statutes of the *Communauté des Barbiers* date from 1361 and were confirmed by an ordinance of 1383, according to which " the king's first barber and valet controls the trade of the barbers of the city of Paris " and was also " head of the barbers and surgeons of the kingdom." The ordinance of Charles V in 1372 shows that already the barbers were concerned with the treatment of various surgical diseases, " boils, lumps, and open wounds, if the wounds are not fatal." The Faculty of Medicine in its rivalry with the Collège de St. Côme established a course for the barbers (1505), but as the lectures were given in Latin until the beginning of the sixteenth century they probably were not of much help.

In England, the London barbers began as a religious guild, but later dropped the religious element and were recognized by the charter of Edward IV in 1462. In 1540 the Barber Company joined the surgeons with a charter granted them by Henry VIII, as may be seen in the magnificent painting by the younger Holbein that still hangs in Barbers' Hall. The picture of Thomas Vicary, the first Master, receiving the charter, surrounded by his companion barber-surgeons, affords an excellent example of the surgical costumes of the period. The union of the barbers and surgeons lasted until 1745; four years after the dissolution of the Surgeons' Company the present Royal College of Surgeons was founded (1800). That conditions were différent in Italy may be seen from the *Statuti dell' arte dei medici e speziali* of Florence. In the Statute of 1349, Chapter 23 reads: " that all and every one of those who practise the said art should subscribe to the said art under oath and submit themselves to the consuls of the said art "; it further states: " So that no doubt may arise about those who are pharmacists and druggists, we declare that all and every one of those who practise medicine or surgery, set bones, and take care of the mouth in the city and province of Florence, whether they prescribe in writing or without writing. . . ." In an appendix of December 1374, in the writing of the Judge Nicolò di Cambione, and bearing the signature of the notary Tino di ser Ottaviano, it states: " all barbers and every one of them of those who practise the trade of barbers should be called, regarded as, and accepted as physicians, should take the oath, and should submit to the said art and to the consuls of the said art." Thus the distinction between physicians and surgeons was certainly less accentuated in Italy than elsewhere, possibly because of the able surgeons who taught anatomy in the Italian universities at that time. From contemporary chronicles it does not appear that the controversies between physicians and surgeons ever were so violent in Italy as in other countries.

Toward the end of the thirteenth century the first public pharmacies were established in Italy. The statute of the Guild of Physicians and Pharmacists of Venice dates from 1258, and the statute of the Florentine pharmacists from 1300. The pharmacy, which followed the Arabian model, began its development in the richer monasteries and then in the courts of rulers; finally it appeared as private property. The pharmacist of the fourteenth century was often an astrologer or an alchemist to whom the people attributed magic powers, and he created in his pharmacy a sort of scientific circle. The shop, with its high shelves on which were arranged the pots and jars full of medical drugs, odoriferous extracts, candles, old books, and hundreds of strange and rare objects, exhaled a special atmosphere of mystery and a certain air of the supernatural.

In Ciasca's book on the Florentine physicians and pharmacists from the twelfth to the fifteenth century, there are many interesting facts about the privileged position of the pharmacists and about the price of drugs, methods of purchase, and the monopolies on spices, and so on. In mediæval Latin the pharmacist is called *stationarius;* though this word has disappeared from modern Italian, it is probably the origin of the English word " stationery," to indicate the shop where books, paper, and writing-material are sold, which in Italy was done in the pharmacy. The pharmacy had its special sign, like the inns. Some of them were quite famous, such as the " Golden Pine Cone," mentioned by Vasari, where the Florentine painter Perin del Vaga was apprenticed. The great wooden counter was placed opposite the entrance, the walls were covered with oaken panels, and often there was a niche in the centre for a statue of Æsculapius or Hygeia. The pharmacist was enthroned behind the counter. The physician and the notables of the city gathered about him; in Italy the pharmacy was the first place for scientific, literary, and political meetings. The pharmacist, belonging, like the physician, to one of the more important guilds, often received in his shop patients who were waiting for the physician, a custom which was maintained in certain parts of Italy almost up to our day. It is not strange, then, that in old Italian illustrations the physician should often be shown in a pharmacy, about to prescribe medicine or

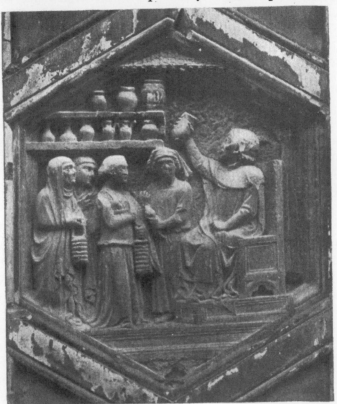

155. *The guilds of the physicians and the pharmacists. Bas-relief on Giotto's Campanile of the Cathedral of Florence.*

raising in his right hand the flask of urine toward the light for the uroscopy. This typical scene appears in the celebrated bas-relief of Andrea Pisano on the Campanile of the Cathedral of Florence. It was for a long time wrongly interpreted as the art of the potter, because pots are prominent in it, but for the reasons given it undoubtedly represents medicine and pharmacy, as Schlosser and Hollaender have observed. Both the costume and the high chair of a master of the university show that the seated figure is that of a physician. When this representation is compared with others of the same period, such as that of the *Taccuinum sanitatis* of the Cerruti family in the State Museum of Vienna, the similarity of the two is apparent, the bas-relief obviously representing the interior of a pharmacy with the physician examining the urine and surrounded by patients and their servants. The characteristic form of the jars suffices to show that they were destined to contain medicaments. The engraving in Brunschwig's *Cirurgia* (1497) evidently reproduces a similar scene: the physician chooses the medicine by pointing to it with his staff. It is also found in a miniature of a manuscript of Avicenna at Bologna that has been reproduced by Giacosa: here the physician is seen examining urine which has been brought to him in a vessel carried in a wooden or wicker basket, of cylindrical form and provided with a handle. Thus the pharmacy constituted the centre where much of the physician's activity was carried on up to the time of its transfer to the hospital. From the point of view of the history of art the study of pharmacy is of considerable importance, because it is to pharmacy that one of the most flourishing Italian arts owes its greatest development. The first awakening of the ceramic art in Italy came from the Orient along with the commerce in drugs. Already by the end of the fifteenth century there had arisen a remarkable trade in these magnificent pharmacy jars, which are much sought after today for their beauty of form and decorations.

Such is the state of the healing art in Europe toward the end of the fifteenth century. Much valuable preparatory work had been done, although teaching strictly followed the classical texts and a conservative tradition swayed medicine rather than the spirit of observation. With scholarship in the hands of the laity, universities now opened their doors to the new doctrines which tended to free medicine from its ancient bonds. The return to the classical texts, advocated vigorously by the Humanists, brought the Western world into intimate relation with Hellenism. If, on the one hand, the use of the classics in their original form might seem to strengthen their authority and to make any study or criticism that varied from them more vulnerable, on the other hand these classical texts stimulated the admiration of scholars, who found in them healthy reasoning, acute observation, and that freedom of investigation and criticism which seemed in the intervening centuries to have been forgotten. Western Europe began to understand that, much more than the maxims of the classics, it was the spirit that dictated these maxims that was to be appreciated. It is essentially from this Humanism that arose a free and fertile spirit of criticism that flourished in medicine as in art, together with the desire to see new things and to think with one's own mind instead of bowing meekly before the dogmatic assertions of scholasticism. Humanism, of which Petrarch was a chief prophet, is defined by J. A. Symonds as " a just perception of the dignity of man as a rational, volitional and sentient being, born upon this earth with a right to use it and enjoy it." It is in this spirit that the principal factor in the renaissance of medicine is to be found — a revival that was prepared by the later Middle Ages with those early studies on the cadaver and the beginnings of clinical observation which are characteristic of Humanism. Art also gave a halo of nobility and beauty to medicine. The pictures of the great painters that adorned the hospitals or recorded the miracles of the saints, especially Cosmas and Damian, or reproduced interesting medical scenes, such as those of Pollaiuolo, Ghirlandaio, and others, the clear engravings of anatomical figures, the pure architectural lines of the hospitals — all these opened the path of medicine toward the Renaissance.

Toward the end of the fifteenth century the newly invented art of printing permitted the rapid diffusion of medical texts, which up to that time could be only rarely and inaccurately reproduced, often by ignorant copyists. The power that printing conferred in making classical texts and the commentaries of recent authors accessible to a wider and wider circle of scholars made acquaintance with them possible to those who lived far from the great libraries and universities. The desire for instruction and the thirst for fame, innate qualities of the men of the early Renaissance, are the most important of the factors that prepared the great innovations in the domain of medicine.

CHAPTER XVI

THE RENAISSANCE

THE REVIVAL OF ANATOMY AND PHYSIOLOGY. BIOLOGICAL AND CLINICAL TRENDS

1. Factors Contributing to the Renaissance of Medicine

THE SITUATION in Europe at the end of the fifteenth century, and the principal factors that led to the renaissance of art and science, have already been touched upon. This remarkable period of transition from mediæval to modern civilization has been well defined as " the entrance of European nations upon a fresh stage of vital energy in general " (Symonds). It is connected with such a number of major events within a single half-century that it constitutes one of the most striking changes in our civilization. But it would be both impossible to fix accurately and also a mistake to assign a certain historical date to the beginning of the Renaissance; for already in the fourteenth century tendencies and points of view characteristic of the new era had become apparent; while, on the other hand, vigorous dogmatic and scholastic influences persisted well into the period that is usually called the Renaissance. If the Renaissance can no longer be regarded, as was done for a long while, as a period of history in which the critical spirit suddenly became fully autonomous and the arts, science, and literature sprang up magnificently in an arid and almost desert soil, it is not to be denied that at this time there took place simultaneously events which were decisive in the history of human thought. This period produced the double phenomenon of a return to the classic past (prepared in the fifteenth century by the renewed realization of human dignity freed from the bonds of dogmatic scholasticism); and also of the revival of the individuality, manifested by a renewed appreciation of the human body and its beauty, a striving for glory that is reminiscent of classic Greece, by a desire for freedom of thought and expression that could not be withstood. This was the very moment when the system of Copernicus was shaking one of the basic tenets of mediæval scholasticism, when civil wars were affirming the right of the people to a free government based on the model of the ancient republics, when the discovery of America was opening apparently infinite horizons to commerce, navigation, and exploration, and when the loss of Constantinople to the Turks drove toward the west the ideas, books, and men who were well versed in the ancient Greek traditions.

When Luther proclaimed his rebellion against the authority of the Roman Church and thus started the religious wars that lasted for centuries, there was also initiated the historical period in which thought assumed its true critical functions, science invoked the aid of personal experience, and art began one of the most marvellous developments yet known. Among a tumult of·new sentiments, new sensations, and new ideas there arose the concept according to which man is the centre of human thought, and the classic tradition of human beauty returned in its full strength. This Greek concept, which had been shattered by early Christians and almost forgotten, was revived by the discovery of classic statues, which were admired almost to the point of adoration by the crowd, and by the study of the ancient poets, whose verses after centuries of neglect once more delighted the souls of men in the new Western dawn that followed the night of suffering, wars, pestilences, and famine.

The Christian viewpoint, which made disease a consequence of sin, gave way to the Hellenic idea, according to which disease is a lack of harmony which nature should cure — an idea emanating from a hedonistic concept of life. The principle that caused death to be regarded with horror or with a resigned indifference was overwhelmed by the return of the desire to live and enjoy life. The attitude that banned dissection of cadavers as showing a lack of respect for the human body, " the temple of the soul," gave place to a thought that was at the same time both new and ancient: namely, that only by the actual study of the human body itself could one know perfect beauty, that no one could be an artist who had not studied the human body at first hand, and that no one would be worthy of depicting the human body without having devoted a fervent and intensive study to his subject. Just as in the earliest times medicine was born of terror and was strengthened by faith, and later Hippocratic medicine found its basis in philosophy; just as finally in the Middle Ages, while preserving a measure of vitality in popular tradition, it had become the slave of theology and scholasticism; so in the renaissance of human thought medicine followed a path parallel to that of art and literature. This place was prepared for it by the study of anatomy, stimulated by a new concept of art and by the free conscience of the individual critic; the new desire for life also was a stimulus to investigate the deepest mysteries, such as the problem of death, which had to be solved if one wanted to explain the problem of life.

This Renaissance naturally took different forms in different countries. In Germany and the North, even as Luther strove to abolish classical beauty and ancient culture, so Paracelsus brought about a violent revolution against the authority of the ancients. In Italy the conflicts were less violent: in cultural fields the Renaissance pivoted on men like Machiavelli and Guicciardini, profound historians and politicians of their age, whose writings reflect its characteristic shortcomings as well as its virtues. In medicine it was the new anatomy that led the rebellion against scholasticism and gave a huge impulse to the development of the arts and sciences.

2. The Renaissance of Anatomy

In this preparation for the renaissance of medicine, it is highly significant that one of the greatest precursors of the movement should have embodied in his marvellous personality all the characteristics of the Renaissance — we refer to LEONARDO DA VINCI. This genius, the greatest artist of his day, painter and sculptor, not only was a great scientist, architect, geologist, physicist, and mechanical engineer but also left ineradicable traces in the field of biology. His was " the grandest effort ever made by any man to explore and interpret the universe." His manuscripts have revealed numerous inventions for the rediscovery of which the world had to wait often for centuries. It is characteristic of the time that one endowed with such an ingenious mind, with such a concise and clear vision of all nature, with such gifts of invention and criticism, should have been the one to initiate the new era of anatomical and physiological study and have been a leader in the acquisition of the new knowledge that developed from them.

Leonardo began his anatomical studies without concerning himself in the least with Mondino or Galen and consequently paying not the slightest attention to scholastic tradition. He viewed anatomy with those piercing eyes which could see beyond mortal limits, and dedicated himself to the study of the human body with the enthusiasm and tireless energy that he brought to all his work from youth to old age. Herein lies the secret of Leonardo's grandeur — this, and his independence of authority in anatomy

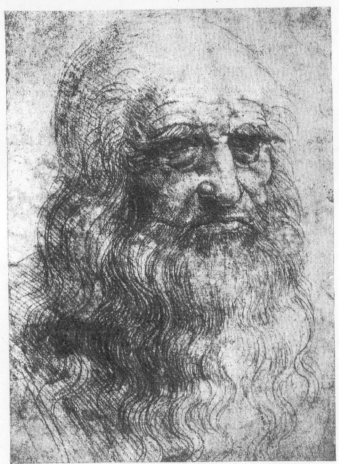

156. *Leonardo da Vinci, self-portrait.*   (ROYAL LIBRARY OF TURIN.)

as in art. Before Francis Bacon and before Galileo, this magnificent man re-lied on his own intellect and experience to affirm with that proud certainty that is characteristic of all his work as investigator and observer: " I disclose to men the origin of the first or perhaps the second cause of their existence."

Leonardo was the friend of Marco Antonio DELLA TORRE, who, accord-ing to Vasari, " was among the first to cast a real light on anatomy, which up to that time had existed in the deepest shadows of ignorance; and in this

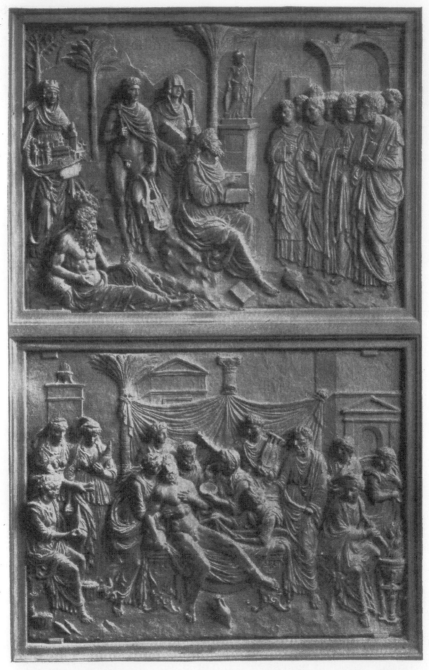

157. *Funereal monument of the Della Torre. Bas-relief by Andrea Riccio. Above, the physician lecturing; below, visit to the patient. Note Apollo in the background.* (LOUVRE MUSEUM.)

he was marvellously served by the genius, work, and hand of Leonardo, who made a book of drawings in red crayon, outlined with the pen, of bodies from which he had removed the skin with his own hand and which he sketched with the greatest care. In the book Leonardo drew the entire osseous system, to which were joined all the nerves (tendons) in order and the muscular coverings." Marco Antonio della Torre (1478–1511), of Verona, is connected with work of another great Italian artist: the great monument by Andrea Riccio to Marco Antonio and his father, Girolamo, who was also a worthy physician. The bronze bas-reliefs from the monument in the Church of San Fermo in Verona may be seen in the Louvre at Paris; the portrait medallions of the two physicians are still in their original position.

Leonardo performed careful dissections; according to the memoirs of the Cardinal of Aragon, he dissected thirty males and females of various ages, of which ten were for the study of the veins alone. In Leonardo's ambitious program, his treatise on anatomy was to consist of one hundred and twenty books, from the birth of man to his death, from the head to the soles of the feet, and was to include physiology and comparative anatomy. This indefatigable searcher for technical perfection in all of his activities had a remarkable anatomical technique: he appears to have used injections into the veins, liquid wax in cavities, and gross serial sections. But the most admirable part of his work are his drawings of the things he observed; these were made with a perfection and fidelity that have never been surpassed.

Most of the manuscripts of Leonardo's biological work are to be found in the library of Windsor Castle. Sixty notebooks containing about five hundred designs were published in Paris in 1898, under the title of *Fogli A*, and in 1901 at Turin as *Fogli B*, published by Sabachnikoff with translation and notes by Piumati. The second and earlier-composed part of the Windsor manuscripts, consisting of one hundred and twenty-nine leaves, and about ten hundred and fifty drawings, was published by Vangensten, Fonahn and Hopstock (1911–1916, Christiania, 6 vols.). *Notes et Desseins* of Leonardo was also published in twelve volumes by Rouveyre (Paris, 1901), but there are doubtless many other notes and drawings that have not yet seen the light.

Leonardo was concerned with all parts of anatomy; he studied the embryos of animals before observing the human fetus in the uterus. He was the first to give an accurate representation of the uterus, which up to that time had been shown as an inverted vessel with rigid walls. He represented the human uterus as unilocular, instead of identifying it with the two-horned uteri of other mammals, as was customary. The membranes of the fetus are accurately de-

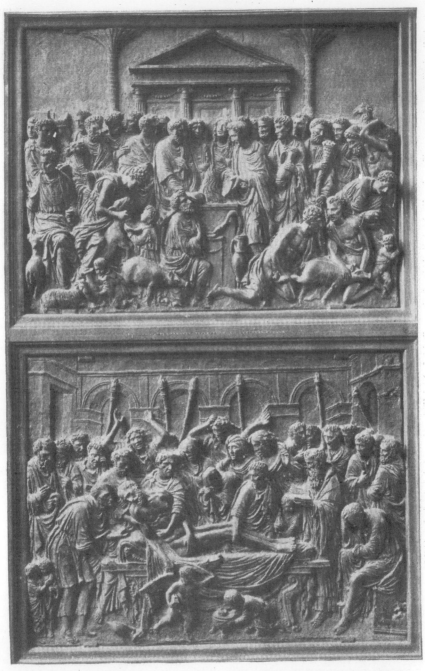

158. *Funereal monument of the Della Torre. Bas-relief by Andrea Riccio.*
Above, the sacrifice to Æsculapius and the serpent; below, death of the patient.
(LOUVRE MUSEUM.)

scribed: "The infant within the womb has three envelopes which surround it; of which the first is called *amnius*, the second, *alantoydea*, and the third, *secundina*. The womb is connected with this third membrane by means of the cotyledons, and all are brought together at the umbilicus, which is composed of veins" (Q. 9 — f. 8 V.). Thus the amnius corresponds to the amnion, the secundina to the chorion, and although he does not describe the placenta, his

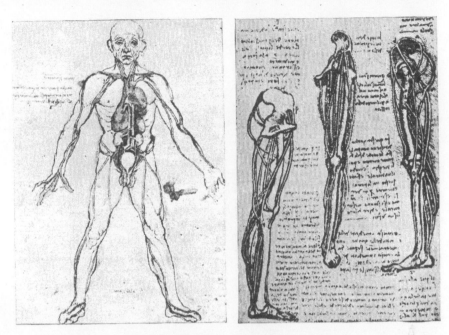

159. *The circulation of the blood, by Leonardo.*
160. *Anatomy of the lower extremity, by Leonardo. The bones are joined by cords to indicate the lines of muscular traction. (Quaderno V, folio 4r.)*

drawings show how the chorion is joined to the internal surface of the uterus and the projecting cotyledons of the chorion are embraced by the uterine endometrium.

He studied muscles and bones carefully, as is well shown by his drawings. He made sections of the brain and was concerned with the cerebral nerves. He had a clear idea of respiration, and studied all aspects of the circulation, a problem which interested him especially, perhaps on account of its relations with mechanics and hydraulics, subjects that he had studied in his youth. He made frequent studies of the function of the valves; he injected wax into the beef heart to examine the shape of the various chambers. Although there is no proof that he solved the great problem of the circulation, it is clear that he upset many of the false statements of his predecessors, and he indicated the correct lines of progress in the study of the cadaver and in rational experimentation.

To Leonardo belongs the credit of having first delineated the space in the upper maxilla that he called " the cavity of the bone which sustains the cheek

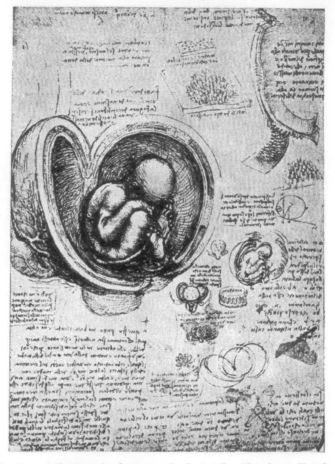

161. *Position of the fetus in the uterus, by Leonardo.* (*Quaderno V, folio 8v.*)

or the armament of it," now known as the antrum of Highmore. He was the first to describe the moderator band (*catena*) of the right ventricle of the heart, which Wright thought should be called " the band of Leonardo." His copious notes interspersed through the sketches are all in mirror writing, for reasons that have not been explained.

Although Leonardo thus showed the intuition and accomplishments of genius in the field of anatomy, and although historically he should be regarded as the first to have considered human anatomy objectively and free from Galenic tradition, nevertheless it must be admitted that his work did not have the immediate recognition that it deserved. His manuscripts, known only to a few persons and most of these not physicians, virtually fell into an oblivion from which they were rescued only several centuries later. It seems probable that Vesalius had some knowledge of them and that he even followed some in his drawings; but whatever curious coincidences may be suspected, it cannot be maintained that Vesalius owes any of his ideas to Leonardo.

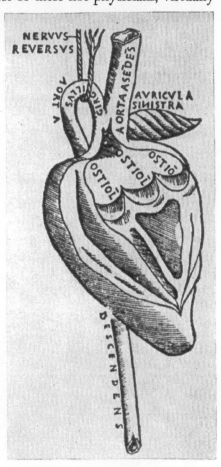

162. *The heart.*
(*From the* Isagogæ, *1523, of Berengario da Carpi.*)

Several other Italian anatomists had entered the new paths just before the time of Vesalius. In addition to della Torre, previously mentioned, there was Jacopo BERENGARIO DA CARPI (1470–1530), one of the greatest physicians of his time, although Cellini, who was under his care, does not speak of him in very favourable terms. He was famous throughout Italy for having been among the first to use mercurial ointment for the treatment of syphilis (but see Section 5). He was a patient investigator and an accurate, even gifted student of anatomy; to him is owed the first description of the sphenoid sinuses, the first careful examination of the tympanum and of the pineal gland. He first described the vermiform appendix and the arytenoid cartilages, described the valves of the heart, and made a detailed study of the brain, in which he distinguished the lateral ventricles and the formation of the choroid plexus. Berengario was professor at Bologna between 1502 and 1522, after which he devoted himself to his considerable and lucrative surgical practice until his death at Ferrara in 1530. He was the first to have embellished his work with fine engravings. His *De fractura calvariæ s. cranii* was published in Bologna in 1518; his *Commentaria . . . super anatomia Mundini*, with drawings from nature, in Bologna in 1521. His *Isagogæ*, in which the anatomy of the heart is well handled, was published in 1522.

Important in the history of anatomy is the book of GIOVANNI BATTISTA CANANO (1515–79), of Ferrara: the *Musculorum humani corporis picturata dissectio* (Ferrara, 1541?), a facsimile of which has been published by Lier (1925), with notes by Cushing and Streeter. It is a valuable production of one of the gifted precursors of Vesalius, revealing depth of observation and boldness of interpretation. Canano, who was a pupil of della Torre at Pavia, had prepared a program for a large treatise of anatomy, of which this part alone was finished. Why did Canano leave his project uncompleted? It is logical to suppose, as Streeter suggests, that when the magnificent work of Vesalius appeared, Canano, realizing the futility of attempting to equal this stupendous achievement, not only interrupted his work but withdrew the first fasciculus from circulation. Canano was the first to describe the valves in the veins, which discovery he communicated to Vesalius, as appears from a statement by the latter; but the discovery was soon forgotten. He died on January 29, 1579, and is buried in the sacristy of St. Dominic in Ferrara.

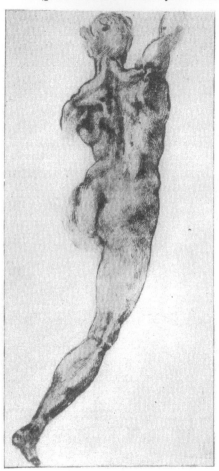

163. *A study in surface anatomy, by Michelangelo.*

Andreas VESALIUS (December 31, 1514–October 2, 1564), a Fleming of German origin from Wesel on the Rhine, occupies one of the foremost places in the history of medicine, not only as the inaugurator of a real science of anatomy, but also as a founder, with Harvey, of modern medical science based on fact rather than tradition. He had a far from tranquil life. Descendant of a family of physicians, son of a pharmacist who seems to have had some connection with the court of

Charles V, he was born at Brussels and studied first at Louvain, Montpellier, and Paris, under Guido Guidi (Vidius) and Jacques Dubois (Sylvius), an able anatomist but intense Galenist. From Paris the young Vesalius returned to Louvain and then proceeded to Padua, where he taught anatomy. It was during this teaching period (1537–46) that he most completely demonstrated his magnificent gifts of observation and description.

At the University of Padua, which was then at the height of its splendour and taught students from all parts of Europe, Vesalius found an op-

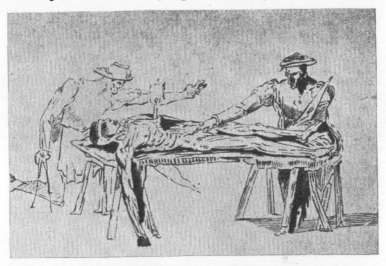

164. *Michelangelo (?) at the dissecting table.*
(*His sketch, now in the* OXFORD MUSEUM.)

portunity for free research and a sympathy for the new thought which made possible the completion of work so audacious that even he, faithful Galenist in principle, did not clearly realize its significance. He undermined the foundations of Galen's anatomical pronouncements, which the entire world regarded as an indisputable canon, and on which the Church itself had conferred the aureole of true dogma. He showed that Galen's statements applied only to animals and that much that concerned the human body was scantily or incorrectly set down. Though teaching from the very chair in which for three centuries the masters had bowed to the authority of the great Pergamene, he found it necessary to start the study of anatomy from its beginning. It seems the height of audacity for a youth of scarcely twenty-nine to undertake this task; the struggle was hard, but, sure of the validity of his ideas and driven by the necessity of sweeping away all the old errors, Vesalius forged ahead.

In 1538 he published the now excessively rare six *Tabulæ Anatomicæ*, and in 1541 he took part in the translation of Galen for the Giunta edition. In 1543 appeared his epoch-making work *De humani corporis fabrica libri septem*, published, practically contemporaneously with the *Epitome* of it, by Andreas Oporinus of Basel. These publications aroused among scholars tempests of hitherto unknown violence. The Galenists, who formed the

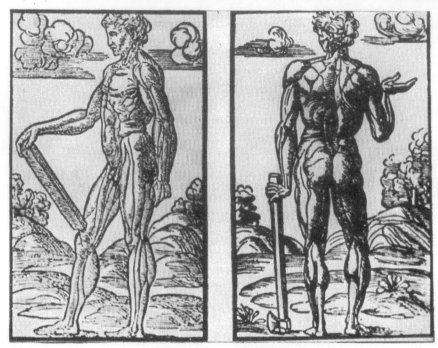

165. *Human figures showing the muscular system.*
(*From Berengario's* Anatomy, *Bologna, 1521.*)

majority of the university physicians, joined to a man in denying absolutely and vehemently the truth of Vesalius' statements. After the publication of the *Fabrica*, Vesalius, who had already made anatomical dissections at Bologna and Pisa, returned to Basel, where he prepared a skeleton which is still to be seen. Then new editions of his great work began to appear: at Lyon without illustrations in 1552; another, with many additions, at Basel, 1555; and another at Venice in 1568. Thus while his fame as an anatomist became greater and greater, on every side the most violent accusations arose. Sylvius, his former teacher, took the field against him, while Realdus Colombus and other anatomists also attacked him. Perhaps irritated by these hostilities, perhaps even fearful of the threatening authority of the Church, Vesalius left Padua to become physician to the court of the Emperor Charles V, and in 1556 to his successor, Philip II, at Madrid. During his years at court he apparently followed the progress of the new anatomy and read with pleasure the works of his successor

Fallopius, but had no opportunity to pursue his own studies further. In 1563, perhaps on account of these difficulties, and perhaps for other reasons, but surely not for the need of expiating the alleged sin of vivisection, he undertook a voyage to Jerusalem. After several days at Venice, where he learned of the death of Fallopius, he departed for the Holy Land. It has been suggested that he had hopes of returning to Padua to fill the vacant chair of anatomy there, but on the return voyage his ship was wrecked at Zante and he was stricken by a severe illness, probably typhoid. He died there alone and far from his family, scarcely fifty years old, without returning to that Italy where, as he had stated, he had passed the most beautiful years of his life. His body recognized by a goldsmith, he was buried in the simple Church of the Virgin at Zante.

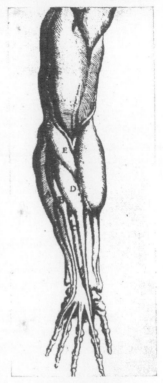

166. *The musculature of the arm.* (*From Canano's* Musculorum . . . dissectio, *Ferrara, 1543* [*1541*].)

Vesalius' achievements in anatomy were truly epochal. His book, with the magnificent engravings by Stephen Calcar, slowly but surely reached that eminent position from which it has never been removed. Still today it stands as a valuable and practical anatomical text as well as one possessing the distinction of being the masterpiece of a hardy pioneer who did not hesitate to affirm the new truths as he saw them without directly attacking Galen. In Osler's opinion it was the greatest medical book ever written, from which modern medicine starts. Published in a magnificent volume with illustrations by a great artist who himself must have studied the cadaver closely, and so well that some think that Calcar's anatomical knowledge was as great as that of Vesalius, this book is a document of the highest rank in the history of science. Yet the man who wrote it was scarcely twenty-nine years old when it was completed, and it might be said that with it his work as an anatomist was finished. Here for the first time the text was greatly aided by the illustrations; Vesalius himself closely supervised the execution of the engravings. He chose the kind of paper to be used, and took pleasure in the beauty of the frontispiece, in which in a symbolic scene full of life and worthy of the spirit of the Renaissance the teaching of anatomy assumes the aspect of a ceremony.

Vesalius, in contradicting the authority of Galen, described for the

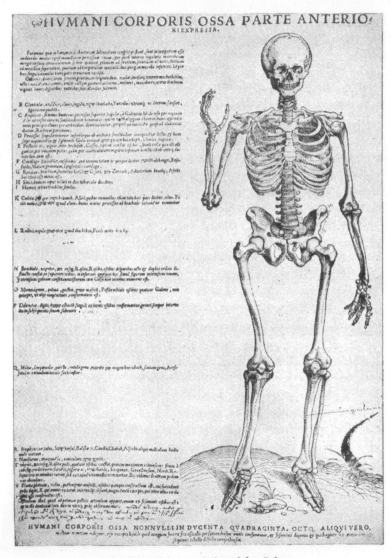

167. *The skeleton, designed by Calcar.*
(*From Vesalius' Anatomical Tables, Venice, 1538.*)

first time the course of the veins and the anatomy of the human heart, and expressly states that he had not seen pores in the ventricular septum. He appears to have accepted Galen's teaching on this point, not because he believed that it was the truth, but because he did not yet have sufficient confidence in himself to be able to affirm the contrary. He finally states:

"I do not see how even the smallest amount of blood could pass from the right ventricle to the left through the septum." The anatomy of the mediastinum and of the mesentery was carefully described; many of Galen's errors about the anatomy of the liver, the bile ducts, the uterus, and the maxillæ are corrected by Vesalius' observations. He refutes Galen's thesis as to the reason for the curvature of the femur and the humerus; he shows the proper structure of the sternum and the number of bones that form the sacrum. He describes correctly the arytenoid cartilages and the articular surfaces of the hand and the knee; he also describes the corpus luteum. His book closes with a chapter on vivisection, in which the author takes issue with the experiments of Galen and shows that with artificial respiration the life of the animal can be maintained after the thorax has been opened. He also notes the variations

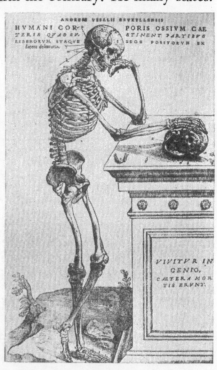

168. *The skeleton in meditation. Note the inscription: "Only through his genius may man survive, everything else will die." (From Vesalius' Fabrica.)*

in the shape of the skulls of different races, such as the brachycephaly of the Germans, and the dolichocephaly of the Flemings.

Not all, to be sure, of the observations and descriptions of Vesalius are correct: for example, he accepts the existence of a seventh ocular muscle, of an internal muscle of the nose; he thinks that the lens is in the centre of the eye, and that the *vena cava* starts in the liver. But in spite of such errors of observation, and although he has no concept of the circulation of the blood, still it should be recognized that he invades all parts of the body with the sureness of a conqueror, and that he brings to his work a valuable spirit of independent observation. This reformer of anatomy, German in origin, Bel-

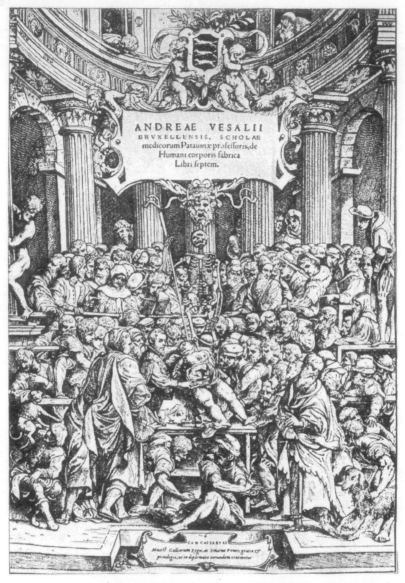

169. *Frontispiece of the first edition of Vesalius'* De humani corporis fabrica.
*Note the attitude of the old man with the beard to the right of the dissecting
table, and the animals near the two lower corners. The dissector is regarded as
a portrait of Vesalius.*

gian by birth, found in an Italian university a soil favourable for his work; it was only in the ferment of renascent Italy that it was possible to conceive and carry out this marvellous revolution.

In addition to the works of Vesalius already mentioned, there are several others listed in the preface of his *Opera omnia*, collected by Boerhaave and Albini (Leiden, 1725). A beautiful volume of *Icones anatomicæ* containing the reprints of the anatomical figures from the original blocks, has been published jointly by the New York Academy of Medicine and the University of Munich (Munich: Lehmann; 1935).

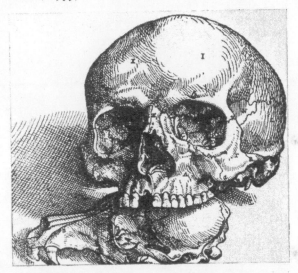

170. *The skull.*   (*From Vesalius'* Fabrica.)

Vesalius' work did not at once have the important success that it deserved; only with difficulty and slowly were the truths established that he had audaciously put forth. But even if the teaching of Galen continued to occupy an important place in the universities for another century, progress in a real study of anatomy continued without a break and demonstrated even more forcibly the need of getting rid of the incorrect classical texts. Thus the first breach was opened in the fortress of Galenism.

Gabriele Fallopio (or Falloppia; Latin: Fallopius) (1523–62) was without doubt the most illustrious of the Italian anatomists of the sixteenth century. He began his studies at Ferrara, where he also taught, and continued them at Pisa and finally at Padua. He was the most courageous of the anatomical pioneers and had the boldness to attack the teachings of Galen even more decisively than Vesalius had done. Daremberg even affirms that Fallopius was a genius while Vesalius was only a scientist. Toeply, in his history of anatomy in Puschmann's *Handbuch,* calls him the equal of Vesalius and stresses the importance of his discoveries. Fallopius, to be sure, did not publish a voluminous work as Vesalius did, nor did he attribute such great importance to illustrations, but he was a most earnest student of anat-

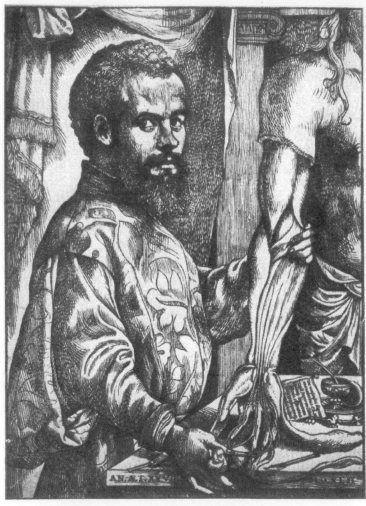

171. *Portrait of Vesalius.*
Woodcut by Stephen Calcar in the first edition of the Fabrica.

omy, *indefessus magnus inventor,* as Haller called him, and in his polemics with Vesalius the impartial critic recognizes that he often was right. Among his meritorious contributions was his description of the ear; he corrected Vesalius about the course of the cerebral arteries, which the latter maintained arose from the sinus; he described the clitoris and the *arteria pro-funda* of the penis, as well as the tubes that bear his name; he gave an ex-cellent account of the ocular muscles and the cerebral nerves. He was the first to describe the *chorda tympani*, the semicircular canals, and the circular folds of the small intestine called the valves of Kerckring; also, as Romiti has observed, the inguinal band known as Poupart's ligament. His contributions to knowledge of the tissues entitles him to be regarded as the precursor of Malpighi and Bichat. The first edition of his most im-portant work, the *Observationes anatomicæ*, was published in Venice in 1561, and was followed by several later editions in and outside of Italy. His *Opera omnia* were published in Venice in 1584; in Frankfurt in 1600, and again in Venice in 1606.

Like Herophilus and Erasistratus, Berengarius and Vesalius, Fallopius was accused of having performed human vivisection. Vesalius, as has been already stated, wroted about animal vivisection (illustrating it with a cut that is suspi-ciously like the illustration in the Giunta Galen); and as these anatomists were all surgeons, their operations on the living might easily be confused with hu-man vivisection. Fioravanti, on the other hand, calmly allows that he had per-formed living dissection on an infidel Saracen — apparently a sufficient justi-fication! The matter is further discussed by Giordano (*Scritti e discorsi*, pp. 1–24).

GEROLAMO FABRIZIO D'ACQUAPENDENTE (*c.* 1533–1619), a pupil of Fallopius, was a great surgeon as well as anatomist and physiologist. He was the first to publish a good description of the valves of the veins; yet he believed that the blood of the veins flowed away from the heart. He was the teacher of Harvey at Padua and doubtless stimulated the latter's interest in the movement of the blood. In view of Harvey's other great book, on embryology, it is significant that Fabricius' best work was on the anatomy and physiology of the fetus and on generation and childbirth. In his time was constructed the present anatomical theatre at Padua, which is the only Renaissance structure of its kind to be still completely preserved. Hirsch lists some twenty-four of his separate publications, most of which were gathered into his *Opera omnia anatomica et physiologica* (Padua, 1625; Leipzig, 1657, 1687; Leiden, 1738).

A number of other anatomists should be given the credit of helping to place the sixteenth-century Italian school of anatomy at the forefront of medical progress. GIULIO CESARE ARANZIO (1530–89), Professor of Anat-omy at Bologna, devoted himself especially to the anatomy of the fetus; he was the discoverer of the *ductus arteriosus* (sometimes called the *ductus*

Botalli [1]), and of the *ductus venosus* of the fetus that runs to the umbilical cord, also of the *corpora Arantii* in the valves of the heart. BARTOLOMEO EUSTACCHIO (1520–74), who was a Galenist in his teaching at Rome, later became an enthusiastic adherent of the new school. He discovered the tube that bears his name, also the thoracic duct, and the adrenal glands (*glandulæ renibus incumbentes*), and advanced the study of com-

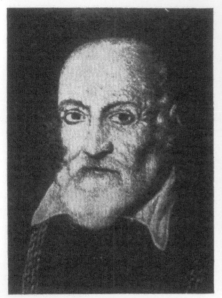

172. *Fabrizio d' Acquapendente.*
An oil painting of the seventeenth
century in the ANATOMICAL INSTI-
TUTE OF PADUA.

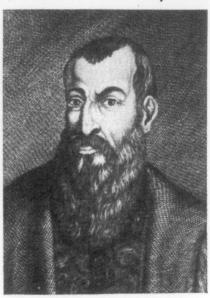

173. *Gian Filippo Ingrassia.*
From the frontispiece of the com-
mentary on De ossibus *of Galen*
(*Palermo, 1603*).

parative anatomy and of the finer structure of the teeth. His *Tabulæ anatomicæ* were left unpublished at his death and remained in various private hands for many years. They were finally published in 1714 by the great clinician Lancisi, with his own notes. Eustacchio's commentaries on his drawings have never yet been found. The plates are exceedingly well and accurately executed and have the distinction of being the first medical illustrations on copper. GIAN FILIPPO INGRASSIA (1510–80), a Sicilian who was professor at Naples and from 1563 at Palermo, was a distinguished osteologist. In his commentaries on Galen he pointed out that the latter had often described the bones of monkeys as well as human

---

[1] Medical history has a bad score in the case of Botallo: his name is linked with the ductus arteriosus, apparently because he called the *foramen ovale* a *ductus;* he is often said to have been born in 1530, the year he was graduated, and to have been the pupil of Lanfranc, who lived some three centuries earlier (Puschmann, II, 235).

beings. His work on the anatomy of the cranium was important, especially that on the mastoid cells, the stapes, which he discovered, and his denial of the existence of the inframaxillary bone. His name is also connected with the discovery of the seminal vesicles. He was a good epidemiologist, and wrote on the plague of Palermo in 1575 and 1576, against which he led the attack. In his book *De tumoribus præter naturam* (Naples, 1533), he was the first to describe scarlatina (*rossalia* or *rossania*), clearly distinguishing it from measles, and was probably the first to recognize chickenpox as a separate disease.

Costanzo Varolio (Bologna, 1543–Rome, 1575) is remembered for his studies on the anatomy of the brain, and his description of the pons that bears his name. His chief work, *De nervis opticis* (containing descriptions of the *crura cerebri*, the pons, the optic commissures, and so on), was published at Padua in 1573. To Arcangelo Piccolomini (1525–86) Capparoni has devoted a careful and laudatory study; Sprengel, however, in his study of the sixteenth-century anatomists (Vol. III of his history), regards him as of only mediocre ability. Giambattista Carcano (1536–1606), of Milan, pupil of Fallopius and Professor of Anatomy at Pavia, in a book on the course of the great vessels of the heart in the fetus (1593), was the first to describe the *foramen ovale* and the *ductus arteriosus*.[1] He was also the first to give an adequate description of the eye muscles and the lachrymal gland.

The Italian school of anatomy had many famous pupils from other parts. The custom of seeking instruction in various countries was well developed, and it was but natural that many should come to Italy at a time when it was playing such a leading role. Among such were Volcher Coiter, Plater (Platter), Bauhin, and Valverde. Volcher Coiter (Gröningen, 1534–90?) studied under Fallopio, Eustacchio, Aranzio in Italy and under Rondelet at Montpellier. He was especially noted for his studies of osteology and the formation of bones in the fetus and of exudates of the brain and spinal cord (meningitis). His experiments on decapitated animals are still remembered. He was a thorough believer in the importance of pathologic anatomy and was successfully insistent with the civil authorities on the need for autopsies in the study of disease. Felix Plater (1536–1614), of Basel, after studying in various countries, returned to his home city to serve as Professor of Medicine for some forty years. He was the earliest supporter of Vesalius north of the Alps; he also founded a Botanical Garden and Anatomical Theatre, with chairs in both subjects. Pieter Paaw (1564–

---

[1] Consult Sprengel for a good discussion of these vexed questions, and Antonio Scarpa (1813) for Carcano's special merits.

1617), of Amsterdam, studied at Leiden, Paris, and Rostock, and at Padua under Fabricius. Professor at Leiden (1589), he secured the construction of an anatomical theatre there and wrote a number of anatomical works which exploited the new anatomy in the Low Countries. JUAN VALVERDE

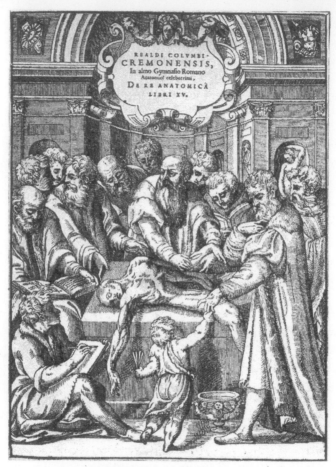

174. *Frontispiece of the* De re anatomica *of Realdus Columbus (Venice, 1559). Compare the figure of the old man with the beard with the same figure in the frontispiece of the work of Vesalius (Fig. 169).*

de Amusco (fl. mid sixteenth century), a pupil of Colombo, was the outstanding Spanish anatomist to replace the authority of Galen by the newer Vesalian anatomy. His *Historia de la composición del cuerpo humano* was published in Spanish in 1556, in Italian at Rome in 1560, in Latin at Venice 1589, and so on. It was one of the most widely read anatomical works of the Renaissance.

Throughout the Renaissance the leadership in anatomy remained with Italy. It was easy to obtain material for dissection there, as Vesalius states, because the judges condemned criminals to the kind of death best adapted for subsequent dissection, and sometimes modified the form of capital punishment so that the cadaver would better serve the anatomist's purpose. When Vesalius was teaching at Pisa, where he gave seven-week courses in anatomy, Cosimo de' Medici had the body of a monk, who had just died in Florence, brought in a boat along the Arno so that the skeleton could

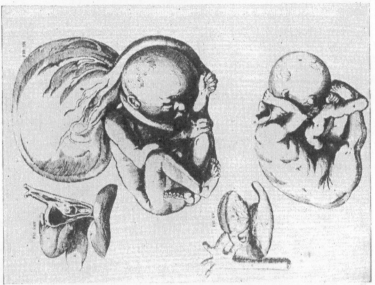

175. *Anatomical drawings from the* De formato fœtu (*Venice, 1604*), *of Fabricius of Aquapendente.*

be prepared. Anatomists in other countries complained that it was not possible to obtain bodies or even a skull, while Fallopius says that he had a large quantity of bones at his disposal, and Realdus Colombus affirms that he had examined a thousand cadavers. At any rate, Haller's estimate of the Italian school of anatomy appears to be justified: " This school taught all of Europe for a century and a half, so that there were very.few dissectors who did not come out of it."

3. *The Beginnings of Physiology — The Discovery of the Circulation of the Blood*

It was the progress in anatomy that determined the earliest advances in physiology worthy of the name. After the anatomy of the bones, joints, cartilages, and muscles had been learned, their functions were investigated with different concepts from the teleological ones which had hitherto dominated. Fabricius of Acquapendente was one of the anatomists who brought valuable contributions to the physiology of movement. His study of the musculature of the extremities and of the various phases of walking, jumping, and so on, and of the effort exerted in overcoming resistance, an-

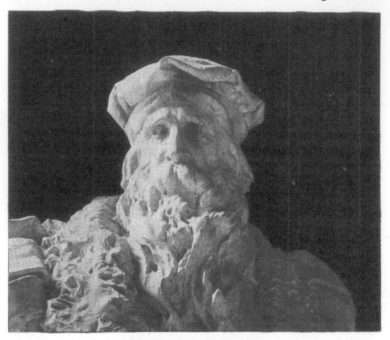

176. *Bartolomeo Eustacchio.*
Marble bust by Ercole Rosa at San Severino Marche.

ticipate, as De Renzi has noted, the more famous studies of Borelli. In the physiology of sight, also, Fabricius made valuable contributions; he is the first to speak of the mobility of the pupil, which he says was revealed to him by Fra Paolo Sarpi (one of the most interesting Renaissance personalities, and important also in medicine, where he figures in the study of the circulation). Fabricius wrote at length about the functions of respiration and speech. It is said that one day in 1588 all the scholars of the German " Nation " deserted the lecture when it seemed to them that in the explanation of the muscles of the tongue he had derided their pronunciation of Italian. Among the anatomists who contributed to the study of the physiology of hearing, Fallopius and Eustachius were especially prominent.

The most interesting chapter in Renaissance physiology is without any doubt that which is concerned with the circulation of the blood. This subject constitutes the fulcrum of all physiological knowledge; in fact, one cannot speak of true progress in physiology until the secret of the circulation was revealed — a secret that had challenged attention since classical times without having resulted in much progress. It might even be said that up to the time of Leonardo and Vesalius, who may have guessed at the truth, the functions of the heart were given the same explanations as in the classical texts.

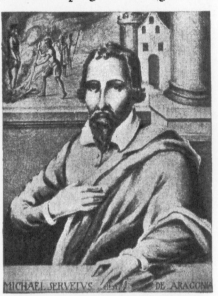

Up to this time it was believed that the liver was the centre of the circulation of the blood, so that in the priestly medicine of ancient times the greatest importance was given to the liver. It was thought that in the liver the blood mixed with the chyle which had been brought there by the "meseraic" veins and from there spread throughout the body. According to the classical idea the left ventricle of the heart contained air, or blood mixed with air, which left the right side of the heart through pores which, though invisible, were assumed to exist in the ventricular septum (see fig. 83, p. 218).

177. Michael Servetus. In the left upper corner is shown his death at the stake.

The air, passing through the arteries, carried the vital spirit throughout the body, reaching the heart from the lungs by means of the *arteria venalis*. Only the veins carried blood. The first step necessary in clearing away false ideas was to recognize the error of the presence of invisible pores in the septum. Leonardo and Berengario had doubts of their existence and Vesalius had at least a vision of the truth. The valves of the heart were well described by Berengario, who indicated clearly that the tricuspid valves served to hinder the passage of the blood from the ventricle to the auricle, and that the semilunar valves closed the pulmonary artery and opposed the passage of blood from the aorta into the ventricle. Thus an anatomical basis was beginning to be laid.

Who was really the first to have a clear idea of the circulation of the blood? Who was it who created the basis for the new physiology in destroying the old but solid concepts of Galen? With but few exceptions historians outside of Italy are in agreement in giving this credit to Harvey, who, as we shall see later, without question deserves the highest credit. He is the one who collected in clear and definite form ideas which until then had been stated but not confirmed by experiment, and who erected an edifice of original and definite achievement based on his own ideas as well as those of others. But if credit is to be properly apportioned between those who first evolved a concept and those who did the effective work, then the part that Harvey's precursors played in this discovery must be recognized. Michael Servetus (1511–53), of Villanueva, near Lerida in Spain, a theologian and anti-Arabist physician, in 1553 stated in his *Chris-*

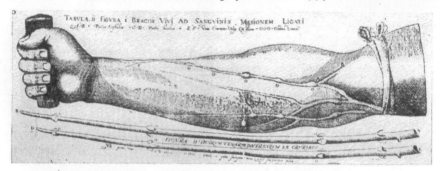

178. *The valves of the veins. From* De venarum ostiolis *(Padua, 1603), of Fabricius. Compare this figure with Harvey's illustration of the same subject.*

tianismi restitutio the hypothesis of the pulmonary circulation, a concept that appears in the original draft of 1546. He states that the blood enters the lungs by way of the pulmonary artery in greater quantities than is necessary for the nutrition of the lung, and that after being mixed with the pneuma in the lung (which could not happen in the atria of the heart on account of the restricted space) it returns to the heart by the pulmonary veins.

Servetus had a tragic career on account of his theological doctrines, and especially because of his attack on the dogma of the Trinity. He studied at Lyon with Symphorien Champier, one of the leading French Humanists, and then at Paris with Dubois and Fernel, and succeeded Vesalius as prosector to Günther of Andernach. He practised at Avignon and other places in France until he was accused by the Calvinists of heresy, arrested at Geneva, and burned at the stake on October 27, 1553. Two copies of his *Restitutio* were burned with him, and many others were burned in other places. Only three copies are known still to exist (at Vienna, at Paris, and an incomplete copy at Edinburgh), though the work has been reproduced in the original Latin and in German. To Servetus belongs the undeniable credit of having been the first to state that the ventricular septum was not perforated as had been previously maintained, and to describe the lesser or pulmonary circulation. His discovery, however, attracted but little attention, probably because it was a short, incidental statement in a theological work.

REALDO COLOMBO of Cremona (1510– ?), successor of Vesalius in the chair of anatomy at Padua, shortly afterwards (March 4, 1558), published his book *De re anatomica*, in all probability without knowing about Servetus' work; it was written, according to his own statement, before the *Restitutio* appeared. In it the concept of the circulation is clearly stated. An indication that Colombo was not acquainted with Servetus' work is found in the fact that the Spaniard Valverde, in his treatise on anatomy in 1556, repeats the views of Colombo that he had already stated publicly. Colombo deals with this vexed question in the description of the cardiac ventricles, wherein he refers to the septum, through which general opinion attributed a pathway for the blood from the right to the left ventricle. "But they," he adds, "follow a false path, because the blood goes through the *vena arteriosa* to the lungs and there is attenuated; then, mixed with air, it goes through the *arteria venosa* to the left heart, just as everyone may observe, but which no one has observed up to this day and no one has stated in his writings."

One of the most essential points in the problem, the non-existence of the supposed passage through the septum, together with the whole concept of the lesser circulation, was thus well known and described by Colombo, to whom belongs the further merit of having definitely stated that the *arteria venosa* carried blood and not air, as had been supposed, and that there were no such things as the assumed particles which according to the ancient anatomists were formed in the heart and were transported from it. In Book VI, speaking of the four great vessels of the heart, he notes that two were constructed so as to bring the blood to the heart, which happens during diastole, and two others to carry blood from the heart during systole.

Then he continues: "When the heart dilates it receives the blood of the *vena cava* into the right ventricle, and at the same time the left ventricle receives the blood mixed with air by means of the *arteria venosa*, and for this purpose the membranes (valves) are lowered and permit ingress; then while the heart contracts those are closed, so that the blood cannot flow out in the same way; at the same moment the valves of the large artery, as well as those of the *vena arteriosa*, open and let the aerated blood pass, which is spread throughout the body, at the same time the natural (venous) blood is carried to the lung."

Harvey knew of the work of Colombo and quoted from it without attributing to it its full importance. Furthermore, Colombo's discovery was generally known, as is shown by the fact, cited by Richet, that Primrose in his acrid controversy with Harvey reproved him (1639) for merely repeating but not testing the statements of Colombo.

Thus it appears that Colombo had visualized the larger circulation in its general lines; and although he continued the error of attributing to the veins the function of carrying the nutritive blood through the body and of still allocating to the liver the central position attributed to it in classic times, still it should be recognized that an important step toward the great discovery was made by the gifted Cremonese anatomist, whose views on the movements and contractions of the heart were supported by experiments on living animals. The work of Colombo, which is not sufficiently appreciated by some historians, made a great stir throughout Italy. It began in the field of physiology the demolition of Galenism, which from then on appeared inevitable to acute observers.

GUIDO GUIDI (Vidius), who was an eminent anatomist as well as surgeon, confirmed the observations of Colombo with his own work, stating that the septum did not have pores and that therefore not even a drop of blood could pass directly from the right heart to the left.

Aranzio was another who strove to resolve the problem as to how the blood could go from the *vena cava* to the left ventricle if not through the pores in the septum. He also had a vision of the lesser circulation, but was arrested by the spectre of the role of the liver, which was regarded as a *noli me tangere* of physiology. It is evident that the problem could not be solved until the liver was shown not to have a central role in the movements of the blood or to play an essential part in the circulation.

ANDREA CESALPINO (1519?–1603), of Arezzo, was Professor of Medicine at Pisa and later Director of the Botanical Garden there. Finally he was called to Rome by Clement VIII and was given the chair of medicine at the Sapienza. Aristotelian in his viewpoints, he was keenly devoted to biology, botany, mineralogy, and zoology; he was creator of a philosophic system which was well received and brought him the name of " the Pope of Philosophers."

Cesalpino held to the concept of the microcosm in the macrocosm; and accepted a single principle as responsible for all cosmic phenomena, and an analogous principle in man by which the functions of organic and psychic life were governed, a principle that he called *anima* in the sense of the philosophers. But differing from them — and this establishes his eminence also in philosophy —

Cesalpino did not hold that there were different vital principles for the various functions; he believed in a unique principle which he therefore called the anima, one and indivisible, which ruled all the functions of the body. The seat of this principle, according to Cesalpino, was the heart. The animating force materialized its power through heat, and the heat, according to the philosopher, had its principle precisely in the heart, because by means of the blood the heat was

spread throughout the body. Thus, affirms Cesalpino, Galen is clearly in error in holding it possible to divide the spirit into various forms, attributing the nutritive factor to the liver, and the sensitive to the brain. By means of the blood, heat and with it life are diffused to all parts of the body. From all these parts it returns to the heart as its beginning. The anima therefore is identified with the blood, and its centre is in the heart; the arteries and the veins, which are designed to transport it, are but the continuation of the heart, as he shows with an able anatomical description of the great vessels and the valves.

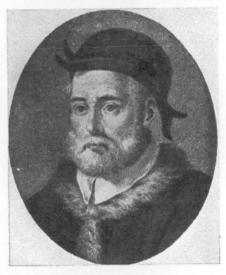

179. Andrea Cesalpino.
(BOTANICAL INSTITUTE OF THE UNIVERSITY OF PISA.)

The concept of the circulation, then, is clearly indicated in its general outline by Cesalpino. We quote a passage in which this appears (*Quæst. medic.*, 1593, Bk. II, Ch. 17): " The orifices of the heart are made by nature in such a way that the blood enters the right ventricle of the heart by the *vena cava*, from which the exit from the heart opens into the lungs. From the lungs there is another entrance into the left ventricle, from which, in its turn, opens the orifice of the aorta. Certain membranes placed at the openings of the vessels prevent the blood from returning, so that the movement is constant from the *vena cava* through the heart and through the lungs to the aorta."

The most important error that Cesalpino attacks in his argument, then, is the Galenical concept regarding the liver as the centre of the movements of the blood. This he was not content to undermine with philosophic arguments, but he also attacked it with anatomical evidence showing that the *vena cava* is of larger size near the heart than near the liver, which would not be the case if, as Galen supposed, the veins started in the liver. The pulmonary circulation is clearly viewed in his concept. The lung, into which the hot blood of the right ventricle comes by way of the *vena ar-*

teriosa, transmits it by means of anastomosis into the *arteria venosa*, which enters the left ventricle of the heart. He knows that the blood that reaches the lungs from the heart is distributed into fine branches and comes in contact with the air that penetrates the finest air passages; also that the air

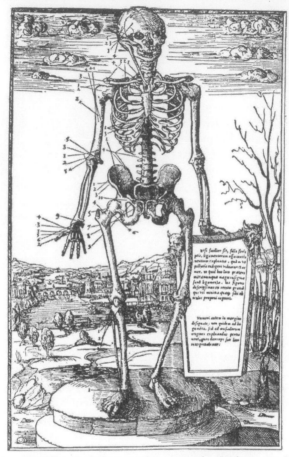

180. *Skeleton, from* De dissectione partium corporis *(Paris, 1545), by Carolus Stephanus* (ESTIENNE).

tempers the heat of the blood — not by direct contact, as Galen erroneously maintained, but only by its proximity to the vessels.

Thus another of the fundamental errors of Galen's doctrines was destroyed. No one who reads Cesalpino impartially can deny the eminent part that he played in the discovery of the circulation of the blood, even if he did not demonstrate the mechanics of the greater circulation; neither is it correct to state, as some historians have suggested, that he merely proposed various nebulous suppositions. This is not the place to quote all the pertinent statements from his work, which, in any case, have been fully discussed by De Renzi, Ceradini, Bilancioni, and others. It is true that the work of Cesalpino was little known and not appreciated by his contemporaries, even though this great man was called by Cuvier the first creator of mineralogic methods and by Linnæus the first systematist in bot-

any. It cannot be definitely stated whether the reason is to be found, as De Renzi observes, in the fact that Fabricius of Aquapendente, who was faithful to the ancient concepts, was absolute ruler of Italian medicine at the time, or whether it should be ascribed to other circumstances difficult to reconstruct. Certainly today, after four centuries, studying the actual words of the Aretine, the author believes, regardless of the views of others, that he was the first to point the way. The priority of the discovery, then, cannot be in doubt. The several editions of Cesalpino's works before Harvey's arrival at Padua suffice to show the error in the frequently repeated statement that the discoveries of Cesalpino were unknown in Italy. Thus Cesalpino deserves an eminent position in the renaissance of medicine, even though he may have been somewhat neg-

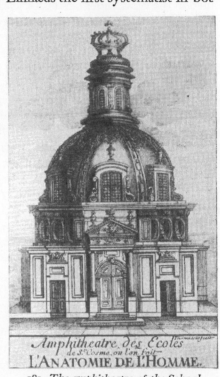

181. *The amphitheatre of the School of St. Cosmas at Paris, where anatomical dissections were made.*

lected by his contemporaries and his successors. In the history of scientific thought, success is not the factor that should influence the critical judgment of the impartial historian. Among the opinions of European writers who have recognized the merits of Cesalpino that of Flourens should be noted: "The concept of the general circulation could not have been better conceived or better and more concisely defined." Charles Richet also states: "Perhaps as great as Michael Servetus and as Harvey is Andreas Cesalpino, who discovered the general circulation. It is he who was the first to use the word 'circulation,' in 1559. Cesalpino observed what happened in the veins when one ligated the arm, he saw that the veins filled below and not

above the ligature . . . and demonstrated the circulation in its entirety "
(*Æsculape*, 1926, XVI, 49).

[It has been pointed out by some critics that Cesalpino still believed that
some of the blood went from the right ventricle to the left by way of invisible
pores in the septum; that he apparently believed in the ebb and flow of nutrient
blood in the veins, though in his *De plantis* (1583, Bk. 1, Ch. 2, p. 3), to be sure,
he speaks of veins carrying nourishment to the heart; and that his use of the
word " circulation " might well have been in the sense of the French gendarme's
" *circulez*," merely as an order to keep moving. Unfortunately his latest word
on the subject (*Praxis universalis*, 1606) shows his uncertainty: " the blood flows
and is distributed from the heart through aorta and pulmonary artery, and also
through the *vena cava* and pulmonary vein." Much hinges on the interpretation
of the word " discovery," as is frequently the case in the often fruitless discussions of priority. Granted that more than one pioneer had made significant
observations and statements that contributed materially to the problem of the
circulation, it appears to most students that Harvey is entitled to be named as
the discoverer of the circulation, because of his masterly synthesis of the observations of others with his own observations, experiments, and reasoning into
an impregnable doctrine based on fact. Though the views of Cesalpino and his
predecessors were known for thirty years before Harvey's work, they had no
practical effect on the current of medical thought. Harvey's book, on the other
hand, after overcoming a violent but natural reaction, became the very centre of
all medical concepts dealing with the circulation; even more — with Vesalius'
Fabrica it constituted the turning-point into the stream of modern medicine.
Ed.]

The description of the valves in the veins, discovered by Canano in
1541 but quite overlooked, is owed to Fabricius of Aquapendente (1574).
In 1603, the year in which Harvey left Italy, Fabricius published his work
De venarum ostiolis, with a description of the valves, so that his pupil
Harvey must have been influenced by these anatomical researches in his
demonstration of the true function of the valves. We shall see in the chapter on the seventeenth century the part that the great Englishman played
in this discovery.[1]

In the field of PATHOLOGICAL ANATOMY, the sixteenth century can be regarded as a period of preparation. The number of dissections, carefully
carried out, and their use in medical teaching, were the chief factors in
developing this discipline. All the great anatomists of the sixteenth century

---

[1] [In his *Anatomia del cavallo, infermità e suoi rimedii* (1598), Carlo Ruini taught that
the left ventricle sent blood and vital spirits to all parts of the body but the lung. This, however, was not original with him and is hardly a sufficient reason for the tablet that was set
up in the Veterinary School in Bologna honouring him as the discoverer of the circulation. Ed.]

concerned themselves with pathological anatomy. It is stated that Vesalius performed a number of pathological examinations and even had the intention of publishing his results. He speaks occasionally of pathological changes in his *Fabrica*. In the same way Ingrassia, Realdo Colombo, and Aranzio made pathological as well as anatomical observations, as did AMATUS LUSITANUS (1511–61), a Portuguese who, after studying medicine at Salamanca, was driven by the persecutions of the Jews to Antwerp

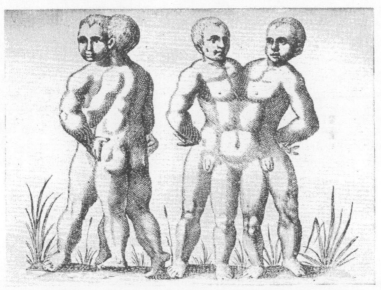

182. *Illustrations of monsters from* De monstris *of Liceto, 1534 edition.*

and later became professor of Medicine at Ferrara. He is chiefly known for his *Curationum medicinalium centuriæ septem* (Venice, 1563), which includes many able observations on symptomatology, diagnosis, and treatment. FELIX PLATER (1536–1614), Professor of Anatomy at Basel, is said by Chiari to have dissected more than three hundred bodies in fifty years. He made numerous original pathological observations (for example, "stone beneath the tongue," giantism, enlarged thymus, intestinal parasites, cystic liver and kidney). His *Praxis medica* (1602–8) gave what amounts to the first modern attempt at the classification of disease, especially mental disease. Rembertus DODOENS (Dodonæus) (1517–85), physician to the Emperors Maximilian II and Rudolph II, made various pathological observations in pneumonia, concretions of the lungs, tumours of the stomach, and so on. He is best known today as a botanist. His *Cruydboeck* (Antwerp, 1553) was assembled with other of his writings in a huge *Stirpium historiæ* (Antwerp, 1583), which was a model for Gerard's *Herball*. Johann Schenck von Grafenberg (1530–98), a practising physician of Strassburg and Freiburg, has left us a valuable *Observationum medicarum rararum . . . volumen* (1597), which combined his own extensive experiences with many concise pathological reports from practically all important works since classical times, all classified and indexed in an orderly manner. Among others may be cited his reference to Avenzoar's *verruca ventriculi* (gastric cancer?), Bauhinus' example of cerebral hemorrhage, and Garnerus' case of splenomegaly. Schenck was an ardent upholder of the value of post-mortem examinations. Charles Estienne (Carolus Stephanus) (*c.* 1500–64) was a member of the famous family of book-publishers. Among his publications in various fields of learning, anatomy held an important place: his *De dissectione partium corporis humani* (Paris, 1545) is a magnificent folio that contains illustrations of diseased as well as normal anatomy. The work of Ambroise Paré, the great surgeon, should also be noticed here on account of the number of pathologic descriptions and illustrations that it contains. The books of Caspar Bauhin (1560–1624) and of Fortunio Liceto (1577–1657), appearing in the early part of the seventeenth century, contain numerous descriptions and illustrations of animal and human monsters, many of which, however, are either exaggerated or entirely imaginary.

At Padua pathological anatomy was already being taught in the sixteenth century, as can be seen in documents of the German "Nation" of that university, where the Professors Oddi and Bottoni had decided to perform autopsies on women who died at the hospital, to show students the origins and sites of diseases.

4. Concepts of Disease

Against the still dominant system of Galen a revolt was thus preparing which was undermining the basis of this hitherto undisputed authority. We have seen that Cesalpino had attacked the very centre of the Galenic system and that others were contributing to its downfall. In Italy the first to rebel against Galen's authority were Giovanni Manardi (1462–1536), pupil of Leoniceno; Luigi Mondella of Brescia, professor at Padua; A. Musa Brasavola of Ferrara, and Girolamo Fracastoro, of whom we shall speak later. Giovanni Battista da Monte (Montanus) (1498–1552) is especially important historically for having restored after many centuries the teaching of clinical medicine at the bedside of the patient. It is from this development at Padua, continued by his successors Bottoni and Oddi, that Johann HEURNIUS (1543–1601) carried the custom to Leiden, where bedside instruction was definitely established by Otto HEURNIUS, his son, and Ewald SCHREVELIUS. Here, under the stimulating and authoritative guidance of Boerhaave, this all-important method of clinical instruction was firmly established. Americans like to follow its spread from Leiden to Edinburgh and then to the American colonies, so that the sound eighteenth-century bedside instruction, later lost for a while, can be directly traced to Boerhaave and Montanus.

Jean FERNEL (1497–1558), of Amiens, Professor of Medicine at Paris, not only was influential in breaking down the authority of Galen in France, but also contributed much to medical progress in his writings. His *Universa medicina* (1554), a standard work throughout Europe, includes in its three parts physiology, pathology, and therapeutics – a classification that is far in advance of anything proposed up to that time. E. R. Long speaks of his *Pathologiæ Libri VII* as "the first medical work to be called a text of pathology," even though its author still holds to the ancient teaching of the humours. His description of the "iliac passion," with postmortem examination (1567), is the earliest clear record of what we now know as appendicitis. He was also one of the first to suggest the syphilitic origin of many aneurysms.

Among the German writers of the period, Johann LANGE (1485–1565), of Löwenberg in Silesia, insisted on the need for direct study of the classics. In France, Pierre BRISSOT (1478–1522) upheld the banner of Hippocratism against the Arabists. He was one of their most pugnacious opponents on a problem which was being solved in indifferent ways, and which, at that time, seemed of the greatest importance. The question revolved on the point at which phlebotomy should be performed in pleurisy and pneumonia. The Arabians had maintained that at the beginning of the disease bleeding should be practised to a small extent at a site distant from the diseased area; they believed that bleeding near the diseased part was weakening. Hippocrates, on the other hand, believed in taking large amounts of blood from near the diseased part. Brissot, whose dissertation was published at Paris three years after his death, returning to this view, became a reformer of the first rank. These events will not surprise those conversant with the history of great revolutions and reforms, which often start from disagreements whose insignificance is properly evaluated at a later period when the subject of the quarrels is no longer of moment. Brissot succeeded in getting the support of the University of Paris for his views, but his adversaries retaliated with a decree from Parliament for-

bidding the use of his method. Brissot retired to Portugal, where he continued the agitation, thus exposing himself to further persecution. Charles V
was asked to condemn him, his enemies maintaining that his method was just
as damnable as the Lutheran heresy. All medicine was divided into two
camps: among Brissot's adversaries were the famous Günther of Andernach,
Trincavella, Antonio Donato d'Altamura, Thomas Erastus, the enemy of

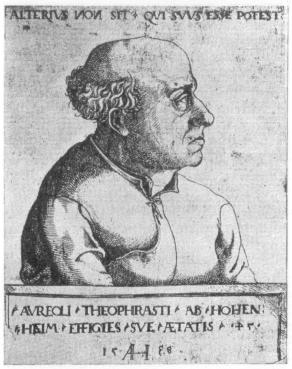

183. *Paracelsus. Copper engraving by A. Hirschvogel.* (VIENNA STATE LIBRARY.)

Paracelsus, and many others. Among his supporters were Manardi, Jerome
Cardan, Emilio Campolongo, Vesalius, Guido Guidi, and others. Botallo
was one of the warmest partisans of frequent and free bleeding. The whole
problem was discussed from one end of Europe to the other, the significant feature being whether or not the authority of the Arabians was to
be upheld. This controversy, which lasted several decades, at least had
the good effect of hastening the return to Hippocratism. The change from
Aristotle, as rigidified by scholasticism, to the higher sphere of Platonist
concepts went parallel in philosophy with the progress from Galenic concepts to the free investigations of the Hippocratic method.

The most violent reform in Renaissance medicine centred on Philippus

Aureolus Theophrastus Bombastus PARACELSUS von Hohenheim (1493–1541).[1] Though very differently evaluated by different times and writers, he played, without any doubt, a very important role in the history of medicine, which owed new life and direction to his revolutionary spirit. Paracelsus was born at Einsiedeln in Switzerland, the son of a physician; after studying at Basel he travelled widely in Italy and Germany. He studied at various universities, especially concerning himself with minerals and metals and the pursuit of alchemy. His questing spirit could not remain oblivious of the astrological superstitions which at that time dominated even the wisest scholars throughout Europe.

Paracelsus frequented the University at Ferrara, where he heard the lectures of Leonicenus, who, imbued with the Neo-Platonism of Marsilio Ficino, was one of the first who had dared to attack the authority of Galen. He began his career away from the close atmosphere of the schools, following nature and life as he found them. He regarded men and things with the bold opinions of youth, a rebel from all authority, and was keen to shake off the yoke of dogmatism, beneath which even the most able and illustrious had bowed. Endowed with a high estimate of his own value, he placed no limit on his destructive criticism, and did not stop even before the truth of classical knowledge.

He came to Basel at the invitation of the famous printer Froben, his great friend, taught there in 1527 and 1528, and was appointed town physician and professor at the university. He is said to have expressed his antagonism to traditional medicine by publicly burning the works of Avicenna, Galen, and others. He taught pharmacology and medicine, discoursing on the Aphorisms of Hippocrates and on surgical diseases in Germany, in ways that greatly antagonized his colleagues. His opinions, which attacked the very foundations of ancient medicine, added to the violence and impetuosity of his personality and produced such enmities that his stay at the university became impossible.

" Very few physicians," he wrote at this time, " have exact knowledge of diseases and their causes: but my books are not written like those of other physicians, copying Hippocrates and Galen; I have composed them on the basis of experience, which is the greatest master of everything, and with indefatigable labor. If any of you feel the desire of penetrating into the divine secrets of medicine and feel like acquiring the whole medical

---

[1] The owner of this peculiar name started life without the second and fifth items. The " Aureolus " appears to have been owing to his golden hair, the " Paracelsus " to his penchant for the prefix " para " (cf. the cryptic titles of several of his works). It has been taken by some to signify that he ranked himself above Celsus. The derivation of our common noun " bombast " is easily traced to its possessor's temperamental behaviour.

art in a short time, come to me at Basel and you will find much more than I can promise with my words." Against such statements the professors and the faculty immediately took determined stand, all the more because Paracelsus refused to take part in the solemn ceremonies and in the dissertational disputations. They excluded him from the university halls, but he continued to give his lectures, both in German and in Latin. His adversaries, professors and students, inveighed against him more and more; finally the entire city became hostile to him and he had to leave Basel secretly without protectors. For almost ten years he continued to wander about Germany, persecuted by his enemies, without even finding a printer who would publish his manuscripts or a university which would permit their publication. He died, probably of cancer, according to Sudhoff, at the age of forty-eight at Salzburg, where his monument is still to be seen.

Paracelsus was fortunate enough to have some enthusiastic admirers who even during his life placed him on a pedestal as the liberator of Germany from foreign influences. But he was still more fortunate, four centuries after his death, in acquiring in Karl Sudhoff a most enthusiastic student of his personality, investigator of his writings, and indefatigable commentator on his work. As a result we have a better estimate of Paracelsus than of any of the great physicians who preceded him. Like all great innovators, he was the butt of the most infamous accusations of those who regarded him as a dangerous heretic, worthy of the stake. He was enthusiastically praised, on the other hand, by those who saw in him the Luther of medicine and, struck by the truth of his statements, followed him throughout, even when his verbal violence led him into iconoclastic extremes. Such violence was perhaps necessary in a country where the classical traditions were so profoundly rooted. Perhaps his iconoclasm was needed to destroy the adventitious structures that deformed the essential edifice of Hippocratic theory.

Paracelsus saw clearly the need for beginning over again in medicine and for proceeding on the basis of experience and reason (*experimentum ac ratio*). He returned to the bedside of the sick; he became a clinician in the true sense of the word, utilizing the observations that he made during his travels and the histories that he got from the workmen, peasants, and merchants with whom he fortunately had much more contact than with the masters and philosophers. His practical soul saw things simply and clearly and always was suspicious of the grandiloquence of the university scholars. Hostile to the academies and faithful to the people from whom he drew his strength, Paracelsus is without doubt one of the most interesting figures of the Renaissance, if not the most representative, as is sometimes maintained. He cannot be regarded as truly representative because he possessed, one might say, almost a double personality. Continual internal dissension, and mixture of concise ideas and concepts with uncertain oscillations between the study of nature and magic, between mathematical observations and abstruse lucubrations, prevent us from forming the same definite opinion about him as is possible of such other pioneers as Galileo and Luther, who were consistent in their ideas. On the other hand, in practice he exhibits the true temperament of the practitioner, learning from his daily

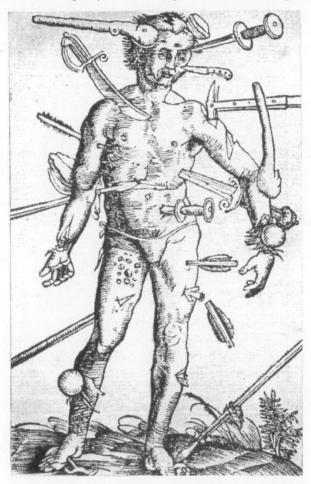

184. The "wound man," indicating the various injuries from different weapons.
(From the Grosse Wundartzney, 1536, of Paracelsus.)

contact with the patient much more than from books, and living in a state of un-certainty, where the successes of today are replaced by the discouragements of tomorrow. His tendency to mysticism is characteristically Teutonic; he reflects in his person the essential qualities of the race from which he came — in his type of intellect, his passionate, even violent activities, his tendency to ab-struse and metaphysical meditations, from which he emerges only by a romantic return to nature. One of the secrets of his success was undoubtedly his appeal to the common people in lecturing and writing in their own language. Up to and well after that time in Germany, as elsewhere, scholars universally used Latin. It was his habit to gather his pupils about the bedside of patients rather than in the universities; if he frequently changed his abode, it was because his restless indomitable spirit could not abide the restraint of authority.

Many of Paracelsus' works were published soon after his death. They were all written in a style that was difficult to comprehend; the most worthy of study is the *Paramirum*, which contains interesting concepts characteristic of his youthful enthusiasm. According to Paracelsus, nature constitutes the macrocosm, the highest development of which is man, who, formed by the same materials and subject to the same laws, repeats in himself all the phenomena of nature and is subject to all the cosmic and telluric influences which regulate the universe. Microcosm and macrocosm are in constant and reciprocal relations; processes develop in the body that correspond to metallic sublimation, combustion, and reduction to ashes. Thus Paracelsus also calls the macrocosm the " exterior man." Salt, sulphur, and mercury are the components of all metals, and also of all living matter. These apparently were to be taken symbolically, however: salt, the solid, indestructible by fire; mercury, the fluid, vaporized but unchanged by fire; suphur, both changed and destroyed by fire. These elements were contained in the *Mysterium Magnum*, whence were developed the four elements: air, water, earth, and fire. Each of these contained an *archæus* — that is, an active principle that possessed an innate force over dead matter. From the union of these organic elements, life is derived, the essential element that constitutes the " quintessence." This brief résumé shows that his concept of nature was clear neither in its aims nor in its exposition; but obviously it had a symbolic significance in the mind of its author. In actual fact, it represented the need for creating a new system to be opposed to the system of Galen. The weakness of Paracelsus' system lies in the support that he sought for this symbolic mysticism in magic, astrology, and alchemy.

When he enters the field of practical medicine, however, we find him becoming again the physician and philosopher who — in his own quotation from Hippocrates — is divine; here we find the courageous and vital sentiments that constitute his chief claim to fame: " The physician should not be a masquerader, nor an impostor, nor an executioner, nor a frivolous person. He should be above all a good and true man."

The doctrines which brought Paracelsus the greatest popularity among the philosophers of his time now possess merely a historical value. Such, for instance, was his theory of disease as due to the five *entia:* the stars, foods and poisons, diathesis, the mind, and divine purpose. His more valuable achievements are various original observations, many of which are to be found in the *Paragranum* (first published in 1530), where he maintains that medical studies should be based on nature and its physical laws, the comprehension of vital phenomena, and the preparation of remedies,

especially by chemistry; but important above all was *virtus* — that is, the spirit of sacrifice whereby the physician gives his all to his patients.

In the second edition of the *Paramirum* — written between 1530 and 1531 — his principles are further elaborated. In Book 2, which treats of " tartaric " conditions, he deals with those diseases that give rise to pathological secretions, concrements, calcifications, and other deposits; and he states that gout, rheumatism, arthritis, and, in general, almost all those diseases loosely grouped under the term " exudative " diathesis, belong to a clearly defined pathological group. In his *De generatione stultorum* he linked cretinism with endemic goitre with remarkable prescience.

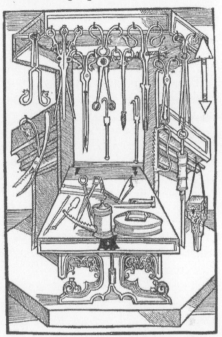

185. *Surgical instruments.*
(*From the* Grosse Wundartzney *of Paracelsus.*)

Paracelsus was the first to promote the use of chemical substances in treatment; he recommended new forms of medicinal preparations such as extracts and tinctures, as more efficaceous than the electuaries and syrups which had been in vogue up to that time. He sustained the " doctrine of signatures," which for a long time enjoyed great popularity in the treatment of disease. This is based on the idea that drugs often appeared in the form or colour of the diseased organs for which they were useful in treatment; thus *pulmonaria* was indicated for diseases of the lung; gold, connected by alchemy with the heart, was indicated for cardiac diseases; the spotted skin of the lizard was indicated as a remedy for malignant tumours (secondary nodules?), and so on at great length. The essential task of the physician consisted in finding the specific remedy for each disease.

In the field of neurology Paracelsus made important observations on epilepsy, and he related paralysis and speech disturbances to injuries of the head. His comments on the origin of invisible diseases are still worth reading. His acute observations on the *Bergsucht* (fibroid phthisis) of miners constitute one of the earliest studies of an occupational disease. His observations on syphilitic ulcerations (which he must have had plenty of chance to see at that time) and their treatment, his surgical studies, particularly of the treatment of wounds, reveal a marvellous activity, especially when the circumstances of his restless existence are considered.

His concept of medicine is eminently chemical; for him chemical and vital laws dominate all manifestations of the organism, so that, as Sudhoff has pointed out, he should be regarded as a chemicopathologist and vitalist.

Paracelsus is known to have composed more than three hundred separate works, written in German, though many later were translated into Latin, dealing with various diseases, different phases of surgery, alchemy, polemics, impostors, and so on. His works were recently translated into modern German, with commentaries, by B. Aschner (1926–32). A very complete definitive edition of Paracelsus' medical works was completed by Sudhoff between 1922 and 1933 as Part 1 of a complete study. (It is uncertain whether Part 2, covering the philosophical and metaphysical works, will be published.)

Paracelsus' doctrines gathered many pupils about him; but unfortunately many of them were driven chiefly by a desire for lucre and only utilized those parts of his teachings that furthered a charlatanism cloaked in glittering formulas.

The best-known Paracelsists in Germany were Adam von BODENSTEIN, Michael SCHÜTZ, Michael DÖRING (d. 1644) of Giessen, Günther von ANDERNACH; in England, Robert FLUDD (1574–1637), of pulse timing and early vaccinating fame. Several of these were able men who were receptive at least to the therapeutic teachings of Paracelsus. Peter Soerensen (SEVERINUS) (1540–1602) published a letter in defence of Paracelsus (Florence, 1570) and later exploited his views in a book, *Idea medicinæ philosophicæ*, that had a great success. He extended his master's ideas about invisible agents of disease in the concept of *pathologia animata*.

The enemies of Paracelsus conducted against him a violent campaign full of abuse and grave accusations, especially in Germany and in Basel. In France many medical men rallied to his defence; especially JACQUES GOHORY, professor at Paris, who in 1567 published a summary of the philosophy and medicine of Paracelsus. Other supporters were ISRAEL HARVET, PIERRE DE LA POTERIE (POTERIUS), and Joseph du Chesne (QUERCETANUS), whose introduction of Paracelsian antimony into France was opposed by that spirit of constant denial, Jean Riolan.

The Paracelsian development was but one of various manifestations of the Renaissance in medicine, which now began to show signs of division into some of its specialties. Toward the end of the sixteenth century appeared a book by GIACOMO TRONCONI which was one of the earliest treatises on pediatrics (Florence, 1593). A healthy sign of the times was the appearance of pediatric works written in the vernacular: in England, the *Boke on Children* of THOMAS PHAYRE (d. 1560) appeared in 1545, though Roesslin's

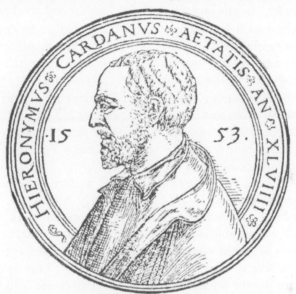

186. *Gerolamo Cardano.*

Rosengarten had previously been translated into English; in Spain, LOBERA DE AVILA's *Libro del regimiento de la salud . . . y de las enfermedades de los niños* was published in Valladolid in 1551; and in France, Simon de VALLAMBERT's *De la manière de gouverner les enfants dès leur naissance* was the first to appear on the subject in French (Poictiers, 1565).

In the field of psychiatry the Renaissance marked a new era: G. B. DA MONTE, for instance, especially concerned himself with melancholics, for whom he prescribed frequent baths, blood-letting, and so on. GEROLAMO MERCURIALE, who was the author of several famous works, *De morbis puerorum* (Venice, 1583), a treatise on medical gymnastics, *De arte gymnastica* (1573) (first printed Venice, 1569, under the title *Artis gymnasticæ apud antiquos libri VI*), and *De morbis cutaneis* (Venice, 1572), maintained that the frequency of melancholia was due to the life of pleasure and unrestrained luxury to which people were giving way in ever greater numbers. He traced its origin to a disturbance of the imaginative faculties. He distinguished three kinds of mania: sanguineous, for which he recommended blood-letting; bilious, for which he prescribed cholagogues; and melancholic, where frequent purgations and cautery were indicated. The first to attempt a classification of the psychoses was the Swiss Felix PLATER (1546–1614), who has already been noticed in the previous section. While recognizing the diabolic origin of melancholia, he distinguished four types of mental diseases: *mentis imbecillitas* (state of mental weakness); *mentis consternatio* (in which mental activity is suspended, as in epilepsy, catalepsy, and apoplexy); *mentis alienatio* (true alienation, mania, hydrophobia, and phrenitis); and, finally, *mentis defatigatio* (hyperexcited states). He fought against the use of forced restraint in the treatment of the insane.

PROSPERO ALPINO (1553–1617) studied melancholia long and objectively. He practised for many years as physician at Cairo and has left an excellent historical work on the medicine of the ancient Egyptians, as well as various epidemiological studies. Jerome CARDAN (1501–76), of Pavia, a man of brilliant intellect, was one of the pioneers in psychiatry. In his book *De utilitate ex adversis capienda* (1561), written after the beheading of his son, Giovanni Battista, who had poisoned his own wife, he gives a description of immorality as corresponding to a moral mania, maintaining that " immorality is nothing more than a disease of the spirit, and malignant stupidity, which does not reach the point of total insanity because even the immoral are able to control their will-power to a certain extent." He distinguished among the wicked the *vecordes* or perverse, and those whom he called *perfidi*, who do wrong only through vehemence of their passions, as in righteous indignation or amorous transport or extreme misery, without attaining to the point of wickedness (cf. E. Rivari: *Rivista di storia delle scienze mediche e naturali;* 1922). An accurate observer, he distinguished exanthematic typhus from other contagious diseases, and left important works on pathologic anatomy and teratology. He also wrote on astrology, physics, and mathematics and had a wide reputation as a practitioner, with princes and popes as his clients. He finished his life in misery, opposed by his contemporaries; but the excellence of his various achievements is witness of his great intellect.

5. Contagious Diseases. Syphilis. Sweating Sickness. Exanthematic Typhus. Sanitary Legislation

The Renaissance brought highly important changes in the kinds of epidemic disease that afflicted the peoples of Europe. Plague especially was greatly diminished, and from this time on remained chiefly endemic in Oriental countries with occasional epidemics still appearing in the Western countries. It was the same with leprosy, which was manifest only in much smaller numbers and in occasional epidemic foci. Collective mental disorders, such as St. Vitus's dance, which scourged the Middle Ages, practically disappeared. One might say that with the new life of the Renaissance, and probably connected with the effect of the hygienic and prophylactic measures that had been adopted in Europe, the general conditions of public health were greatly improved. On the other hand, the sixteenth century saw the spread of other diseases which up to that time had been absent in the West or hardly recognized; SMALLPOX, MEASLES, and CHICKEN-POX became prominent. In 1510 INFLUENZA spread throughout Europe in severe epidemic form. It reappeared in 1557, and again in 1580 and 1593 in pandemic form that resembled its ravages at the time of the World War. The tendency to a return in approximate periods of thirty years, or once in a generation, has been emphasized by various historians. Exanthematic typhus was another disease which was recognized and studied in its symptoms and course. Just before the turn of the century also SYPHILIS made its appearance in such severe and epidemic form that it mowed down thousands of victims.

The discussion as to whether syphilis was brought to Europe from Spain after the discovery of America, or whether it had already existed there in less striking form, has given rise to a long and heated controversy which is still active and by no means settled. In recent times the European origin of the pandemic has been upheld by Sudhoff and his school, Vorberg, Singer, and in this country by Butler and Holcomb. Their views are chiefly based on the two arguments that syphilis can be shown to have existed in Europe before the return of Columbus and his sailors, and that the arguments in favour of its spread by the latter are unsound. On the other hand, the exponents of the theory of the American origin of European syphilis (among whom are Ivan Bloch, Barduzzi, Jeanselme, and in America, Pusey) find support in various contemporary accounts and in the dubious nature of the evidence of pre-Columbian syphilis in Europe, with reliance necessarily limited to bone lesions, and even these not absolutely diagnostic. It is certainly strange that more pre-Columbian bones that have been accepted as syphilitic have not been found in Europe. On the other hand, evidence of syphilitic lesions in North and South American bones before the arrival of Columbus has been recently accumulated to an imposing degree (H. U. Williams, J. R. Sharpsteen, Krumbhaar, etc.).

It is not opportune here to pursue the matter further. In order to receive adequate treatment, it would demand a lengthy exposition and detailed critique of historical documents. In our opinion, the truth is to be found in a middle ground; that is, one should accept that syphilis was probably noted in Europe before the return of Columbus and that the doubtful allusions of early writers really apply to syphilis; but that it was only after 1493, because of the great movements of troops throughout Europe, and especially the invasion of Italy by the French army that the disease was so widely distributed. Perhaps also it was brought back from the New World in more virulent form. If there is little doubt that syphilis or something very close to it existed in the New World before the arrival of Columbus, it seems best to assume, for the moment at least, that syphilis had existed on both continents for undetermined periods, even though the reason for its sudden increase in Europe has not been satisfactorily explained. The historian should note the first Spanish writers to mention the disease. The first statement that syphilis was brought to Europe from the West is to be found in the writings of a Spanish physician, Ruy Díaz de l'Isla (between 1504 and 1506). He states that on the return voyage from Hispaniola a malady attacked one of the Pinzon brothers, the pilot of Columbus, covering the skin with frightful and bizarre eruptions. The author also states that he himself treated sailors attacked by this disease at Barcelona. Another writer who is frequently quoted on the American origin of syphilis is Oviedo, a non-medical Spanish writer, who was in Barcelona in 1493 and in touch with Columbus and his companions. He was Governor of the West Indies in 1515, and in 1525 he sent to Charles V a report on the subject which contains such obvious impossibilities that it should carry but little weight as historical evidence. Another Spanish author who wrote on syphilis was the priest Francisco Delicado, who himself was severely attacked by the disease. After twenty-three years of extreme suffering, he was cured in Rome by guaiac. Out of " pity for others " he wrote a book entitled *Il modo de adoperar il legno de India occidentale* . . . (Venice, 1529), which is chiefly remarkable for its mention of what he regarded as this disease as present in Europe in 1488. Delicado was also the author of a book entitled *La Lozana andalusa*, purporting to be the diary of a Spanish courtesan living in Rome in the early part of the sixteenth century. It gives extremely interesting details about the life of the period, and also a curious account of the various measures practised by courtesans at that time, and of the medicaments they used for cosmetic purposes.

Whatever its origin, syphilis undoubtedly spread through Europe with frightful rapidity in the early sixteenth century, especially in the upper classes. [The histories of the period leave no doubt that it was disseminated in epidemic form; many cases apparently were not transmitted by sexual intercourse. *Ed.*] Thought to have first broken out when the army of Charles VIII invaded Italy (though Sudhoff even doubts that this particular disease was syphilis), the disease was called by the French the " Neapolitan disease." The Italians, however, were more successful in establishing their terminology, as it was generally known as " *morbus Gallicus* " throughout Europe.

The earliest descriptions of the disease emphasize the external lesions, especially on the genital organs, which, after three or four days, were accompanied by a change in the general appearance of the patient and of his humours.

It was generally thought that the chancre appeared several days after the infection. It was observed that the second stage of the disease was manifested by skin lesions and pains in the joints. These were at first regarded as the most important and characteristic signs of syphilis. The secondary stages were

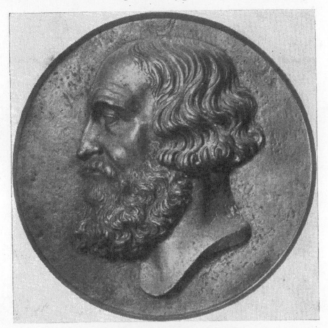

187. *Gerolamo Fracastoro. Medallion by Giovanni Cavino.*
(PADUA CIVIC MUSEUM.)

thought to begin from thirty days to four months after the infection, as Fracastoro held. The pains never appeared at the same time as the skin lesions; there was even a certain antagonism suspected, whereby the one disappeared when the other became manifest. The pustules which appeared over all the body were carefully described: their shape, colour, size, and so on. These were the *pustulæ malæ*, which gave rise to some of the names by which the disease was then known. The destructive lesions which appeared in the throat, lips, and eyes were extremely serious, even occasionally causing the death of the patient. In the tertiary stage affections of the bones and large swellings were observed, with much destruction of the tissues. Writers spoke of frequent sudden death from the disease. There were various conjectures as to its cause, which was ascribed by the Church to divine punishment for the lax morals of the time.

Some physicians tried to relate syphilis to other better-known afflictions;

but almost all thought that they were dealing with a new and hitherto unknown disease. The astrologers spoke of the influence of the stars, such as the conjunction of Saturn and Mars, an opinion that was especially prevalent in Italy. However, the contagious nature of the disease was soon recognized and even a *con-*

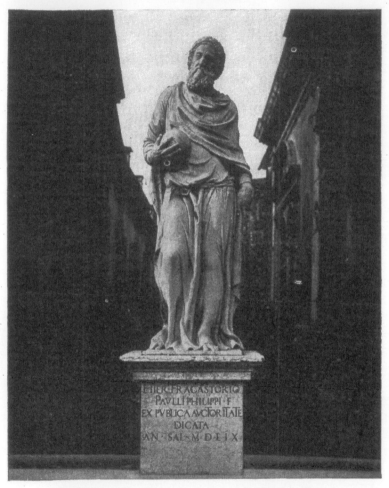

188. *Statue of Fracastoro in the Piazza dei Signori, Verona.*

tagium vivum considered. ULRICH VON HUTTEN, one of the early writers on the subject, made the supposition that it was perhaps a question of small winged worms (*vermiculi alati*). Some thought that syphilis was due to a mixture of existing diseases, such as Paracelsus' combination of leprosy with *cambucca*. ULSENIUS, in 1496, stated that it was due exclusively to contagion, as did Fracastoro's *De contagiosis morbis* (Bk. II, Ch. 2).

GEROLAMO FRACASTORO (1478–1553) was born in Verona of a patrician family that already included well known physicians, such as Aventino Fracastoro, in the early part of the fourteenth century. Gerolamo completed his medical studies at Padua together with Copernicus, who was matriculated with the Faculty of Medicine there in 1501. He was a pupil of Achillini, and the Aristotelian Pietro Pomponazzi (1462–1525). In 1502 he was made Professor of Logic at Padua, and then went to Verona with M. A. della Torre and Andrea Riccio. He was a close student of classical literature, but also a tireless investigator of the scientific truths to be found in the laws of nature.

In 1545 he was called by Pope Paul III to the high office of Physician of the Council of Trent. When a number of cases of plague broke out there in 1547, Fracastoro advised the transfer of the Council to Bologna, where he remained with it for some time, in contact with the most illustrious princes of the Church. He then returned to the quiet leisure of his villa at Incaffi, carrying on his studies and a correspondence with the greatest litterateurs of his time, and especially with G. B. Rannusio and Jacopo Sannazzaro two well-known writers of this time. His death there, August 6, 1553, was widely lamented throughout Italy and a monument was erected to him in Verona.

Geographer and astronomer, eminent poet and musician, mathematician and biologist, he is an excellent example of the universal interests possessed by the Renaissance leaders. But if he is best known today by his poem on syphilis, it is his *De contagione et contagiosis morbis* (Venice, 1546) that best exhibits his profound scientific vision and places him among the great biologists of his time. Fracastoro, whom Charles and Dorothy Singer have called the father of modern pathology, was the most scientific student of the epidemic diseases of his time — typhus, plague, syphilis — and of their origins and spread. Unhandicapped by superstition and tradition, he distinguished three forms of contagion: (1) by simple contact, as in scabies, phthisis, leprosy; (2) by indirect contact, by means of what he calls *fomites* (that is, vehicles of infection, such as clothing and bedclothes) which can carry the seeds of contagion (*seminaria prima*) without being corrupted; and (3) by transmission from a distance, without direct or indirect contact, which may happen in plague, Egyptian ophthalmia, and smallpox. To explain how contagion may take effect at a distance, he imagined that the *seminaria* spread themselves by selecting the humours for which they have an affinity (Bk. 1, Ch. 7), and by attraction, being drawn into the vessels. They then could be absorbed by the breath and adhere to the humours, which carry them to the heart. Fracastoro contemplated various affinities

in infection. " There are diseases of plants which do not contaminate animals, and vice versa animal diseases which do not attack plants; there are
other diseases limited to man or to certain animals, as cattle, horses and
so on. Certain diseases have a special affinity for certain individuals or certain organs." Again, when he considers whether infection is a kind of

189. The first page of first edition of Fracastoro's poem, Syphilis sive morbus
gallicus *(Verona, 1530).*

putrefaction (Ch. 9): " Sometimes putrefaction consists of a simple dissolution . . . but at other times it is a question of a new formation that
has a particular form." He concludes: " If we consider the contagions inductively, we shall see that the contagion of a putrefaction goes from one
body to another whether adjacent or distant "; and again in Chapter 12:
" These seeds have the faculty of multiplying and propagating rapidly."
Such statements, perhaps inspired in Fracastoro by the atom theory of
Lucretius, show a good understanding of the specific nature of contagions,

so that he is worthy of being accepted as one of the great precursors of the modern theory of infection and of being included among the greatest scientists of the Renaissance. Among the writers on syphilis, also, Fracastoro occupies an eminent position. To him is owed the name of the disease, which is derived from his poem *Syphilis sive morbus Gallicus* (Verona, 1530), which quickly became very popular and was published in many editions and languages. This poem is worth reading from the literary as well as the medico-historical point of view.

It recounts the adventures of the rich and beautiful young shepherd Syphilus who had insulted Apollo. The god avenged himself by the infliction of a terrible disease, the manifestations of which are described in polished verses: The limbs are stripped of their flesh, exposing the bare bones, the mouth loses its teeth, the breath is fetid, the voice is reduced to a feeble whisper, mercury and guaiac wisely administered will eventually restore the patient to health. The discovery of the latter, which was called the Holy Wood, and the portrayal of the unfortunate condition of Italy at that time, are two sections that are especially well written. The poem, composed in 1521 on the model of Vergil's Georgics, opens as follows: "What varied fortunes and what germinations have produced a fierce and rare disease, never before seen for centuries, which ravaged all of Europe and the flourishing cities of Asia and Libya, and invaded Italy in that unfortunate war whence from the Gauls it has its name — all this I shall tell in this my song. And here I shall tell of the new treatments, by whom discovered, and how human wisdom has proudly fought this grave calamity, and what was the divine aid and the rewards. And I shall seek the secret causes in the profound mystery of the air and the stellar spaces."

Fracastoro doubts that syphilis was brought from America by Columbus's sailors for one good reason — that it appeared simultaneously in countries far apart — and for one poor reason — because astronomers had predicted its coming some years before. In his book on contagious diseases (Bk. 2, Ch. 11) he gives the following description: "This contagion did not leave *fomites* behind, or only when some especially favourable opportunity occurred, nor did it propagate itself to a distant object. It did not manifest itself at once, but remained latent for a certain time, sometimes for a month, sometimes for two months, and often even for four months. . . . At last, in the majority of cases, small ulcers began to appear on the sexual organs . . . and would not depart. . . . Next, the skin broke out with incrusted pustules, in some cases beginning with the scalp. . . . Next, these ulcerated pustules ate away the skin, as do those ulcers which are called phagedenic; and they sometimes infected not only the fleshy parts but even the very bones as well. In cases where the malady was firmly established in the upper parts of the body, the patients suffered from pernicious catarrh which eroded the palate or the uvula, or the pharynx and tonsils. In some cases

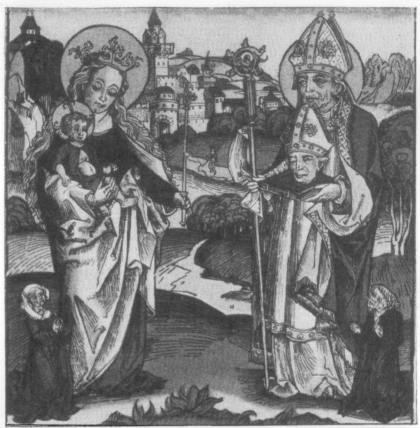

Aller heyligister vater vñ grofmechtiger nothelfer Dyonisi:ein ercz
bischoff vñ loblicher martrer.O du himelischer lerer:der von fräck-
reich apostel:vñ teutzscher landt gewaltiger regierer.Wehuet mich vor der
erschreklichen krancheit mala franzos genant: von welcher du ein grosse
schar des christenlichen volks in franckreich erleledigt hast:So dy kosten
das wasser des lebédigen prunnen der onder deine aller heiligisten korper
entsprang:Wehuet mich vor diser gewerlichen kranckheit:O aller genedi
gister vater Dyonisi:biß ich mein sunde mit dem ich got meinen herren be
laidigt hab: pussen mug:vñ nach dysem lebé erlangen:dy freud der ewigé
saligkeit:das verleich mir xps iesus der dich in dé aller vinstersten kercker
verschlossen trostlichen haym gesuechet:vñ mit seiné aller heiligisten leich
nam ond pluet dich speiset sprach:dy lieb vñ guttikait dy du hast zu mir al
leczeit:dar omb wer wirt bitten der wirt gewert:Welcher sey gebenedeit in
ewigkait Amen.

190. *Invocation by St. Dionysius against the "French malady" (Nürnberg, c. 1496).
Note the two patients, kneeling at the corners.*

the lips or nose or eyes were eaten away, or in others the whole of the sexual organs. Moreover, many patients suffered from the great deformity of gummata . . . violent pains attacked the muscles. . . . Meanwhile there was lassitude of all the organs; the body became emaciated. . . . Sometimes these symptoms were accompanied by slight fever, but rarely. . . . I use the past tense in describing these symptoms, because, though the contagion is still flourishing today, it seems to have changed its character since those earliest periods of its

appearance. I mean that, within the last twenty years or so, fewer pustules began to appear, but more gummata, whereas the contrary had been the case in the earlier years" (translation of W. C. Wright).

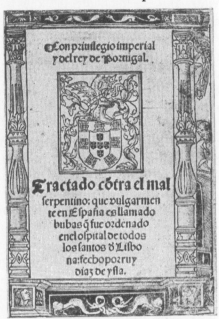

191. *Frontispiece of Díaz de l'Isla's treatise on syphilis (Sevilla, 1539).*

Many contemporary authors wrote about syphilis and its treatment, as is easily understandable in view of the widespread character and severity of the disease. Sudhoff collected in facsimile eight of the earliest works (1495 and 1496) that mention the disease (Leipzig, 1912). In various publications he considered the evidence of pre-Columbian literature bearing on the subject and demolished much of the flimsy evidence that connected its sudden spread with the return of Columbus's sailors. In summing up he says that before that time its existence in Europe is indicated by various prescriptions in use by mediæval physicians that would be efficient against syphilis, and by the existence of a number of names of skin infections — probably including syphilis together with leprosy, psoriasis, and other diseases. In 1496 Joseph GRÜNPECK wrote a *Tractatus de pestilentiali scorba* and in 1503 a *Libellus de mentulagra*, which contains detailed observations about the disease, from which the author himself suffered. Johannes WIDMANN (1440–1524) wrote one of the best of the fifteenth-century syphilis tracts, *De pustulis quæ vulgato nomine dicuntur mal de Franzos* (Strassburg, 1497). In 1497 the Humanist Leonicenus wrote a *Libellus de epidemia* on the same subject, and in 1498 Francisco Lopez de VILLALOBOS his *Sumario de la medicina con un tratado sobre las pestiferas bubas* (Salamanca). Fallopius established the unity of the disease manifestations and refuted the hypotheses of others that based its occurrence on a disorder of the cardinal humours; Botallus courageously attacked the doctrine which made the liver the seat of the evil and therefore prescribed abundant purges. Fallopius, recognizing individual differences in susceptibility, stated that for ten people who were exposed to the infection there would be scarcely four who would become infected; thus his great authority contributed to alleviate the terror that the disease inspired in Italy. The Paduan NICOLÒ MASSA (d. 1569) was one of the best known syphilologists of his time, to whom many patients came for treatment from all parts of Europe. He described cases in which contagion was carried by the linen, and is thought to have been the first to describe gummata (*materiæ albæ viscosæ*) in his book *De morbo gallico* (Venice, 1532).

The treatment of syphilis at first consisted in the use of purgatives or antitoxic drugs, such as theriacum and mithridaticum. Soon treatment entered a more efficient phase with the widespread use of mercury. Already used for various skin diseases, this anti-syphilitic specific was naturally used in a condition where pustules were the most striking signs. The first results of mercurial treatment were most auspicious. But it was much abused by empiricists and charlatans, who affirmed that they were the only ones who possessed this secret and who sold it at high prices. Charlatanism and superstition were rampant; even healthy individuals were told that they had the disease so that large sums might be extorted from them for treatment. At first the treatment of syphilis remained almost entirely in the hands of surgeons; it was a current phrase at the time that they had finally resolved the great problem of alchemy and had transmuted mercury into gold. In the simpler prescriptions mercury was combined with pork fat for inunction; later aromatic substances were added, then sulphur and myrrh and incense. Mercurial salivation was soon observed and even fatal cases; but the mercurial treatment continued to spread. Berengario da Carpi treated Benvenuto Cellini with mercury for high fees, as Cellini notes in his Memoirs, and still earlier mercurial treatments appear in a letter of Giorgio Sommariva, a patrician of Verona, to the physician Bartolomeo Niger de Ruico, of Treviso, which was printed by Cristoforo da Cremona at Venice in 1496.

A second form of treatment was introduced with guaiac, the Holy Wood, which was used by the natives of the American continent and early brought to Europe by the Spaniards. Its use, in the form of infusions which were taken for a month after prolonged fastings, was said to be followed by marvellous successes.

The remedy was especially popular in Germany where Ulrich von Hutten recommended it enthusiastically. In his *De guaiaci medicina et morbo Gallico* (1519) he described how he himself had been cured by the Holy Wood of a severe attack of syphilis that had racked him for a number of years. Paracelsus was one of the first to combat the use of guaiac, which he declared to be of little

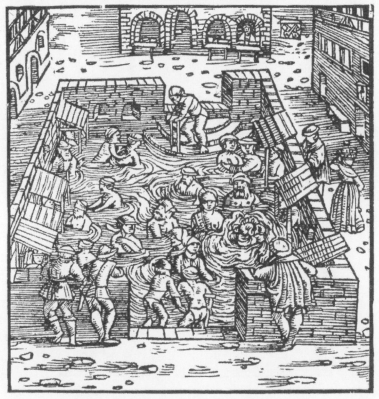

192. *A bath establishment of the sixteenth century.*
(*From the book of Johann Stumpff, Zurich, 1548*).

value. In spite of this and the opposition of other high authorities, however, guaiac treatment was widespread in Europe up to the end of the sixteenth century.

Thanks to the ample opportunities for physicians to observe the disease and effects of treatment, and thanks to the rapid diffusion of knowledge about public health afforded by printing, the Renaissance quickly acquired a full picture of the course of syphilis and of various desirable therapeutic procedures. One might say that by 1520 any intelligent physician was in possession of current knowledge about the disease, the danger of contagion, and its various manifestations and the treatment to be recommended. Fournier brought this out well in the imaginary letter from Jean de Vigo to nineteenth-century syphilographers that composes the preface of his translation of Vigo's chapter on syphilis in Book 5 of his *Surgery* (1514).

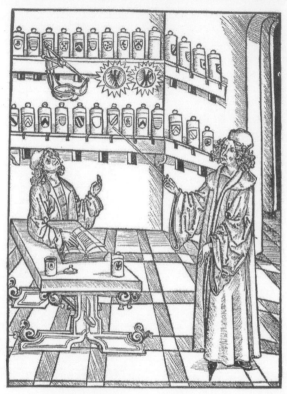

193. *The physician in the pharmacy shop.* (*From Brunschwig's* Chirurgia, *1497.*)

Corradi's *Storia della malattie veneree* gives many interesting facts about syphilis in Italy. He collected fifty ancient documents about syphilis, many of which had hitherto been unpublished. The oldest is by Ser Tommaso di Silvestro of Orvieto, dated 1498, which contains a good account of a case of syphilis. He dwells on the great diffusion of prostitution and the official steps to supervise it; also on the development of sodomy, which, according to the Venetian chronicler Marino Sanudo, spread through Italy in the fifteenth century. In Venice prostitution was most highly developed; the census of 1509 gives no less than 11,654 *femene da partido* among the 300,000 inhabitants. In Rome at the end of the fifteenth century, according to Infessura, there were more than 6,800 public prostitutes, without counting those who remained hidden. When Pius V tried to exile the courtesans from Rome, the entire city rebelled and the

Pope had to give way. In a book by the Count of Oxford on the laws and memorials of prostitution in Venice, a " catalogue of the most important and honoured courtesans in Venice " is reproduced, giving not only their addresses but also their fees. The courtesans were distinguished from the prostitutes and not included in the prohibition against their mingling with the nobles and the bourgeois. With the rapid spread of the disease it was to be expected that governments would seek for measures of control. Already in 1496 prostitutes were expelled from Bologna, Ferrara, and other places, because it had been found " that the women had a secret kind of pox which others called the leprosy of St. Job." In 1552 Venice ordained that all those " ulcerated and afflicted with the French disease should go for treatment to the places designated for them " — that is, the Hospital of the Incurables. The officials of this hospital had to keep an exact list of the patients, male and female, with their first names, day of entry, and discharge. The Confraternity of Ferrara in 1505 was licensed by Alphonso I to seek contributions for a hospital for syphilitics (*Spedale dei Franciosati*). A document that is especially interesting for the study of public hygiene is the statute of Faenza of 1507 in which it states that: " women desiring to devote themselves to prostitution should present themselves at the office called the Guard so that it may be known if they come from a suspect locality and if they have a healthy body; and no one of them should be permitted to serve who had the French disease." This occurred at a time when the Diet of Worms knew no better way of combating the new disease than by exhortations not to blaspheme. Gaspare Torella, physician of the Borgias and bishop, made a special demand on Pope Alexander VI to institute a regular examination of the prostitutes and to obtain the aid of the secular authorities to transport them to a hospital to be submitted to the necessary treatment. In 1496, also, the barbers were forbidden to admit syphilitics to their shops or to make use of instruments that they had employed.

Soon special hospitals were opened for syphilitics. At Bamberg, in 1497, syphilitics were forbidden all contacts with healthy individuals and could not enter the inns or even the churches. In the same year the Parliament issued an edict according to which all syphilitics who had no fixed residence had to leave Paris within four hours by two gates that were expressly named, and the others had to show that they were taking medical treatment. The poor had to go to a special hospital for appropriate treatment.

At the same time the Church began energetically to combat the spread of the disease, preaching chastity as the single prophylactic measure necessary.

The continued use of energetic treatment and the wide diffusion of knowledge of the disease undoubtedly had their influence in bringing syphilis slowly into the group of infectious diseases without its ever having assumed the same pandemic dimensions of leprosy and plague.

The epidemic of syphilis of the sixteenth century might be regarded as the crucial test of the new medicine. It clearly shows the new spirit that guided physicians, who no longer addressed themselves to ancient texts in the face of imminent peril, but forced themselves to construct the noso-logical picture of the disease and its treatment according to personal ob-servations and tests.

One of the diseases that was most prominent in the Renaissance is that known as the *sudor anglicus*, or SWEATING SICKNESS, which appeared in the first quarter of the century, without having given any evidence of its ex-istence up to that time in the history of medicine. It first appeared in England in a severe epidemic in 1485, shortly before the battle of Bosworth Field, and again in 1507, 1528, 1551, and 1578 in a violent epidemic which decimated the population of England.

The universities of Oxford and Cambridge lost many of their teachers and pupils, and, according to a chronicler of the period, thousands died in the two cities. Ireland and Scotland were not attacked. In 1529 a fourth severe epidemic arose in England, beginning in London in the month of May, but this time it spread to Denmark, Sweden, Germany, Poland, Russia, and the Low Countries.

The disease became manifest in a most acute form and with a high fever; death sometimes occurred a few hours after the first signs of fever and almost all cases were fatal. Hamburg lost more than a thousand persons in several days, after which the disease spread rapidly through Germany, reaching Bavaria and Austria in the autumn. In the single city of Aix more than a thousand persons died in the first five days, and there were hundreds of deaths in Strassburg. A severe epidemic broke out in London in April 1551, with a high mortality, but it did not spread beyond England, where it died out in September. It was first described by John Caius in 1552 (" A boke, or counseill against the disease com-monly called the sweate, or sweatynge sicknesse," London: Grafton). This first original description of a specific disease as observed by the writer has recently been reprinted in facsimile from the copy in the New York Academy of Medicine.

The principal phenomena were high fever with chills, formications in the hands and feet, pains in the nails and extremities, and cramps in the feet. Next, severe pains over the heart were experienced, with a sensation of anguish, difficulty in breathing, often cyanosis of the face and a rapid, irregular pulse. Some authors state that this irregularity even continued after convalescence and sometimes for a number of years or even permanently. In the severe cases there were clonic contractions of the muscles, nausea and vomiting, and grave cerebral phenomena: hallucinations, delirium, and especially a profound stupor which was emphasized by all writers as constant — *invincibilis somnus subethicus*. The height of the disease lasted from a minimum of several hours to a maximum of twenty-four; recovery followed profuse sweats. Patients appeared to have completely recovered after eight to fifteen days, though relapses were frequent and often repeated three or four times. The treatment consisted especially in diaphoretic measures. The estimates that can be made from the descriptions of contemporary authors suggest that the epidemic may have been similar to influenza, which it certainly resembled in the rapidity of its spread and the number of people attacked. On the other hand, epidemics of influenza are on record at different periods, and Hirsch in his *Handbuch* regards it as a separate disease. After 1578 no further epidemics of the sweating sickness were encountered either in England or in Europe. It was more than a hundred years later (1718) that another epidemic appeared with sweating as a prominent feature — the *suette des Picards* (miliary fever).

Among sixteenth-century diseases that were observed for the first time, or rather that were first studied with any recognizable precision, was exanthematic or petechial TYPHUS, so called on account of its characteristic spotted rash.

According to De Renzi, the first information that we have on this subject comes from a chronicler of the convent of La Cava near Salerno, who states that in the month of August 1083 he saw in this convent a " very severe " and malignant fever with petechia and parotitis. In a Parmense notebook of 1477, published by Muratori, there is a high mortality record at Milan in this year, following an epidemic of a severe acute fever that attacked many people. This appears also to have been typhus; likewise the Italian *peste marranica*, of 1492 and 1493, which was said to have been spread by the Jews who had been expelled from Spain. Cardano also gave an early account of the disease (1536) under the name *morbus pulicaris*. To Fracastoro belongs the merit of having first accurately described the disease. In his classic *De contagione* . . . (1546) is a clear account of typhus, which up to that time had been confused with plague and other diseases, with a description of *lenticulæ, vel puncticulæ aut pesticulæ*. In 1505 and 1528 there had been a severe epidemic of typhus in Italy, coming from Cyprus and its adjacent islands. Fracastoro was the first to emphasize the character and importance of the rash and to connect the influence of war and famine with the spread of the epidemic. His grasp of the epidemic diseases, and especially of typhus, even though with Galen he thought that they were due to air infection, contributed significantly to a new impulse in the doctrine of contagious diseases. Ingrassia and Prospero Alpino were also warm supporters of the theory of contagion. The epidemics that occurred in the first half of the century were described by other authors such as Massa, Luigi Mondella, and Giovanni Colle. In Spain the disease, which was called *tabardillo*, or " little cloak," was well described by LUIZ DE MERCADO (1541–1606), FRANCISCO VALLES (1524–92), and others. In Mexico it was described by FRANCISCO BRAVO in his *Opera Medica* (Mexico, 1570), the earliest medical publication of the American continent.

In France typhus seems to have been more frequent toward the end of the sixteenth century; in Germany it was described in the last ten years of the century under the name *febris puncticularis*. *Morbus Hungaricus*, which overran the camps of Europe (1501–66), was probably this same disease. In Cobert's *Observationes castrenses* (1606) a connection between it and lice was surmised. In England typhus broke out in characteristic form in civil prisoners in the famous Black Assizes of Cambridge (1522), Oxford (1577), and Exeter (1586) (Holinshed's *Chronicles*, II, 1547). The accounts of the disease evidently raised the difficulty of arranging it in the Galenical system of hitherto known fevers. The explanations in the classical texts were unsatisfactory for the physicians of the period; they were soon able to recognize that phlebotomy, which had been hitherto recommended for all sorts of fevers, proved useless.

It should be noted that Fracastoro's ideas of contagion were definitely opposed to Galenical concepts and had returned to the Hippocratic method of observation of the patient at the bedside, together with consideration of atmospheric conditions and any other phenomena that might possibly explain the disease. Though his concepts did not become immediately established, he nevertheless should be regarded as the first and greatest reformer of ideas about the nature and treatment of the contagious diseases.

The contagiosity of various diseases was clearly indicated by Fracastoro in his epoch-making book.

" The principle of infection which resides in solid bodies is apparently of a different nature from that which is contained in liquid or soft matter; so that as soon as it has passed from the infected spot into a solid body, it can persist there for a long time without the least alteration; so that one may be astonished by the objects infected by consumptives or plague-stricken patients, such as bed, clothing, pieces of wood, and similar matter; we have often seen the poison persist for two or even three years even though no molecule emanating from the putrified matter would seem able to keep such a power for so long a time " (Bk. I, Ch. 4).

The recommendations of Fracastoro about the treatment of consumption are of interest. He is especially concerned with this disease, and he is certainly the first physician to express the idea of destroying the germs of the disease in the lung. If an early case is being treated, he recommends aiming entirely at the germs: " If it were possible to destroy them by the use of caustics, there would be no better remedy; but because such agents cannot be employed without danger to the organ, it is necessary to treat them through adjacent organs. Some ancient authors have recommended inhalations of *sandarac* (orpiment) into the lung. . . . You can also use various roots in the form of decoctions, such as iris, scordium, Cretan dittany, theriacum, and similar remedies."

" If the disease has already passed the initial stages and has started the catarrh in motion, then one can try to attack both the germs and the substance involved. But you should always remember that the most important thing is to combat the germs and oppose the contagium. The best remedy is turpentine and the resins in general, such as larch, pine, myrrh, and styrax. They can be administered singly or mixed with the afore-mentioned remedies. It is desirable to avoid styptics and astringents which impede expectoration; on the other hand, emollient drugs should be added, such as honey or sugar. Decoctions are highly to be recommended as they penetrate most deeply; they are to be taken with a little sugar in fresh water; the root of squinium is warmly recommended as it is very drying and induces sweat " (Bk. III, Ch. 8).

Cap. viii. de duobus lateribus.

HAEC Duo latera, quorum subsidia tanto-pere forceps inhiat, huiusmodi ordine confi ciuntur. Calescat igitur Chalibs igne follibus in-suflato. Calefactusq; in formam tetusæ latitudinis, quorum talis est.

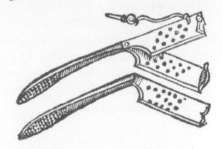

From the above we must recognize that while therapeutics had not made great advances in the four previous centuries, if the prescriptions of Fra-castoro had received the recognition

194. *Instruments, from* De lapide renum (*Venice, 1535*) *of Mariano Santo of Barletta.*

that they deserved, many mistakes and much suffering would have been avoided. Following Fracastoro, the concept of the contagiosity of phthisis began to be spread throughout Europe. For instance, Settala, the Milanese physician quoted by Manzoni in the description of the plague of Milan, says that the contagium of consumption must be endowed with a fat and viscous nature, which, according to the ideas of the time, was necessary for the explanation of its spread.

Various epidemic diseases remained prominent or were first recognized in the sixteenth century. The long voyages of the great explorers produced ideal conditions for the development of SCURVY, which on Vasco de Gama's voyage of 1498 killed fifty-five of his sailors. In Jacques Cartier's exploration of Canada in 1535 his sailors were ravaged by a violent form of scurvy, though to them it was a mysterious and unknown disease. Its connection with dietary deficiency was not established for another two centuries, when James LIND's *Treatise on the Scurvy* (1753) demonstrated the curative effects of lemon juice. Lind's *Essay on the Health of Seamen* . . . (1757), an important milestone in the history of naval hygiene, further emphasized this form of treatment, though it was many years before it became established — in the Royal Navy. In 1573 Volcher COITER (Koyter) first described CEREBRO-SPINAL MENINGITIS, though the epidemicity of the disease was not recognized till the nineteenth century. Guillaume de BAILLOU (Ballonius) (1538–1616) was one of the most influential in leading the University of Paris from Galenism into the new paths of learning. He was especially concerned with epidemic disease and was the first to describe an epidemic of WHOOPING COUGH in 1578 under the name of " quinta " or " quintana " (*Epidem. et ephemer.*, Lib. II, p. 237, published posthumously, 1640). This disease was later called " *coqueluche* " or " little hat," a term which unfortunately was also used for other diseases. Baillou also described (ibid., Bk. 1, p. 55) as RUBIOLA a disease, occurring in 1574, with the characteristics of scarlatina, thus anticipating Sydenham's better-known description. Baillou's *Liber de rheumatismo*, according to Major (2nd ed., p. 220), is the first to describe an affection under the name of " rheumatism," recognizing both acute and chronic forms. The term, used, to be sure, in a humoral sense, goes back at least to Galen, but not to Celsus or Hippocrates.

6. Surgery, Obstetrics, and Ophthalmology

During the Renaissance, surgery began to attain a higher position in medicine than in previous periods. The art, which had been almost entirely in the hands of the barbers, came to be regarded as worthy of the higher-trained physicians who began to practise it. Thus we see a revival, first in Italy and next in France, of its former dignity in the hands of such worthy representatives as William of Saliceto, Lanfranc, Henri de Mondeville, and Guy de Chauliac.

Among the better-known Italian surgeons were GIOVANNI DA VIGO (Rapallo, 1460–1525), surgeon to Pope Julius II, whose chief work, *Practica copiosa in arte chirurgica* (Rome, 1514), passed through more than forty editions and was translated into French, Italian, Spanish, German, and English. In 1517 he published a compendium of the larger work which was also highly successful. It was divided into nine books, of which the first deals with the anatomical knowledge necessary for a surgeon, while the others consider other surgical conditions and their treatment. Noteworthy in Vigo's work is the indication as to how the great vessels should be ligated, *intromittendo acum sub vena desuper filum stringendo* (by inserting the needle beneath the vein and tightening the thread from above). This procedure had been practically abandoned since the time of Celsus. Believing that wounds were poisoned, he advocated their treatment by cautery, and by a plaster containing ground-up frogs, worms, and vipers. He describes a trephine that he invented and a number of new instruments.

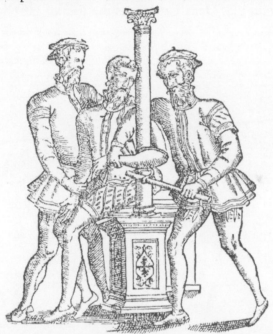

195. *Reduction of a dislocation of the elbow.* (*From Paré's* Chirurgia, *1573.*)

Vigo believed that major operations should be left by the physicians to the surgeon.

His pupil MARIANO SANTO of Barletta (b. *c.* 1490) was especially famous for his operation for lithotomy, which was known as the *metodo Mariano* or *apparatus magnus.* He wrote a successful *Compendium in chirurgia* (1514). The lateral incision that he recommends in his *De lapide ex vesica per incisionem extrahendo* (Rome, 1522) was especially popular with the French lithotomists, such as Colot and his followers. MICHEL-ANGELO BIONDO (1497–1565), a Venetian who practised in Naples, was an early proponent of the treatment of wounds and contusions with applications of cold water. To him also are owed such therapeutic recommendations as the avoidance of the use of irritating drugs on wounds, which he observed had the effect of retarding healing. Fallopius, who has already been mentioned as a great anatomist, was also a well-known surgeon; he ligated vessels and sought for healing of wounds with simple medicaments. GIOVANNI ANDREA DELLA CROCE, of Venice, was the author of several popular works on surgery, two of which were printed in Venice in 1573 and had numerous later editions. He gives good descriptions of the surgical instruments in use at that time and of those introduced by him. Burg correctly observes that Della Croce was the first to introduce synonyms

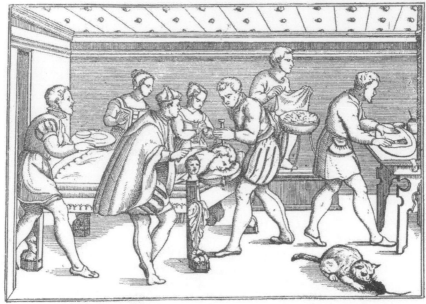

196. *Trephining the skull.* (*From the* Chirurgia *of Andrea Della Croce, 1573.*)

for the Greek, Arabian, and Latin names of diseases. He paid especial attention to gunshot wounds, the indications for trephining, and the different types of instruments needed for this procedure.

GUIDO GUIDI (Vidius) (d. 1569) was a Florentine who became the royal physician and professor at the Collège de France, thus arousing the antagonism of the university faculty, who wanted the position for Dubois. Guidi was recalled to Italy in 1547 by Cosimo I, who made him Professor of Philosophy and Medicine at Pisa. His *Chirurgia e Græco in Latinum conversa* was printed in 1544 by Pierre Gautier at the home of his friend Cellini. It contains a number of fine illustrations that have an extra interest as they appear to have been done by Primaticcio. Inspired by classical illustrations, they show how the Renaissance imitated the instruments and operations of the ancient Romans. Guidi's work was translated into French

(Lyon, 1565; Paris, 1634). His name is preserved in anatomy by the Vidian nerve and Vidian canal that he first described.

FABRICIUS OF AQUAPENDENTE (1533–1619) was famous both as surgeon and anatomist. He was made Professor of Surgery at Padua in 1665, and of Anatomy in 1671. After teaching for many years and receiving many honours, he was given the right to choose his successor, his choice falling on Julius Casserio, who had been his attendant in the Hall of Anatomy. His services were sought by the most illustrious, so that at his death he left his niece a fortune of more than two hundred thousand ducats. Acquainted with the classical works, especially those of Celsus and Paul of Ægina, he was a prudent surgeon who avoided dangerous operations and guarded carefully against the loss of blood. He ligated arteries (*Pentateuchos*, Bk. VI, Ch. 2, Frankfurt, 1592) and described techniques for tracheotomy, thoracentesis, and urethral surgery. His book contains illustrations of orthopedic apparatus for wry neck, spinal curvatures, and so on. He was no doubt the leading Renaissance surgeon in Italy. Eminent among Renaissance Italian surgeons was GASPARE TAGLIACOZZI

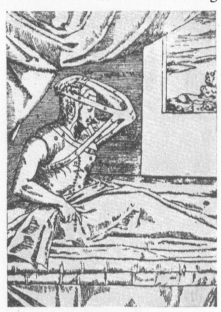

197. *Rhinoplasty.*
(*From the* Chirurgia curtorum per insitionem [*Venice, 1597*] *of Tagliacozzi.*)

(1545–99), who is especially linked with the history of plastic surgery. He was the first to practise rhinoplasty on a basis of solid anatomical knowledge. He was also successful in the plastic surgery on the ear and lips. His system consisted in loosening strips of skin from the arm, which were transplanted to the nose while still connected with the arm. The arm was held rigidly bound in contact with the nose until the transplant had taken root in its new surroundings. But rhinoplasty was strenuously opposed by most surgeons, such as Paré and Fallopius, and was prohibited by the Church. It was not brought back into use until 1822, by Dieffenbach.

Rhinoplasty, which, as we have seen, was known to the ancient Hindus, had been practised in the fifteenth century by surgeons belonging to the Branca family in Sicily, to which it had probably been introduced by Arabian surgeons.

In Calabria it became the secret of the family of Vianeo di Maida and of the Boiano family of Tropea. It was sometimes called *Magia tropœsiarium*. The names *Norcini* and *Preciani* were given to the surgeons of Norcia (near Perugia) and in the suburb of Preci who practised the operations for the stone and for cataract for many generations. The earliest of these surgeons known to us were the fifteenth-century SCACCHI DELLE PRECI, who was physician to the King of France; and later BENEDETTO DA NORCIA, who was professor at Perugia and phy-

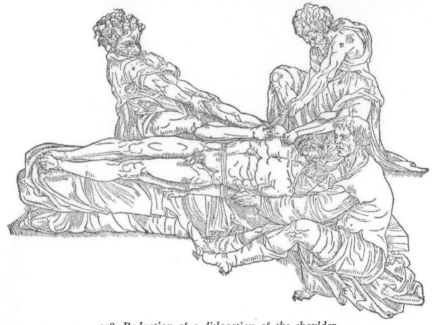

198. *Reduction of a dislocation of the shoulder.*
(*From the* Chirurgia [*Paris, 1544*] *of Guido Guidi.*)

sician to Sixtus IV and Francesco Sforza, Duke of Milan. Fabricius speaks of ORAZIO DA NORCIA as a skilful operator for hernia and describes his method. Records exist of twenty-seven of these families of surgeons who practised lithotomy and the surgery of the eye up to the eighteenth century; eventually other empirical surgeons were included in the term *Norcini* who were not related to the ancient families and did not come from Norcia.

One of the greatest figures of the Renaissance, and unquestionably its greatest surgeon, was AMBROISE PARÉ, who was born about 1510 at Bourg-Hersent near Laval in Mayenne. He began his study in a barber shop and it was during his service at the Hôtel Dieu, where he started at nineteen as companion-surgeon for three or four years, that he acquired much of his practical knowledge. The campaigns in Italy from 1536 to 1545 afforded him a vast experience in military surgery. In his *Méthode de traicter les playes* (Paris, 1545, 1552, etc.) he recommended the ligation of the artery at the site of the hemorrhage, first practised by Damvillers. He knew no Latin and therefore wrote in French. In 1554 he became a member of the

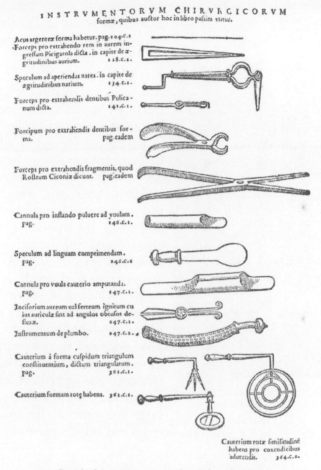

199. *Surgical instruments of the sixteenth century.*
(*From the* Commentaria [*Venice, 1542*] *of Herculanus.*)

College of St. Cosmas, in spite of the opposition of the professors of the Sorbonne, who could not conceive of a member of the college not knowing Latin. He was surgeon to Henry II, Francis II, and Charles IX, who was said to have protected him during the Massacre of St. Bartholomew by hiding him in his bedchamber, and also to Henry III. In 1573 he published his *Deux Livres de chirurgie* (Paris, Wechel), the first part of which includes obstetrics, and the second monsters and wounds of the nerves; in 1582 appeared his discourse (Paris, Buon) on mummies and unicorns, in which he asserted their uselessness as remedies, though they were much sought after and prescribed by the Parisian professors. For such reasons he was in frequent conflict with the conservative elements, and it was only much later that his authority and honour as a surgeon were indisputably established.

200. *The dentist. Engraving by Lucas van Leyden, 1523.*

Paré is responsible for the abolition of the method employed by the Arabians, and of those who followed them, of applying the cautery and boiling oil to wounds. During a battle in which the supply of oil gave out he began to use simple bandages and was surprised to find the next morning that those who were treated in this way were in much better condition than the others. He at once championed the new method, and generally introduced into operative surgery simpler methods of procedure. Control of hemorrhage by ligation of arteries had been frequently recommended, but it was Paré who first practised it systematically and brought it into general use. He reintroduced the operation for hare-lip, which had been practically forgotten since the time of the Arabians; he popularized the *trepan à couronne* and various other improvements in the treatment of fractures.

We reproduce the passage that describes his discovery that revolutionized the treatment of wounds: " In the year of our Lord 1536, Francis the French King . . . sent a puissant Army beyond the Alpes. . . . I was in the King's Army the Chirurgion of Monsieur of Montejan, Generall of the foote. The Imperialists had taken the straits of Suze, the Castle of Villane, and all the other passages; so that the King's army was not able to drive them from their fortifications but by fight. In this conflict there were many wounded on both sides with all sorts of weapons but cheefely with bullets. I will tell the truth, I was not very expert at that time in matters of Chirurgery; neither was I used to dresse wounds made by gunshot. Now I had read in *Iohn de Vigo* that wounds made by Gunshot were venenate or poisoned, and that by reason of the Gunpouder; Wherefore for their cure, it was expedient to burne or cauterize them with oyle of Elders scalding hot, with a little Treacle mixed therewith.

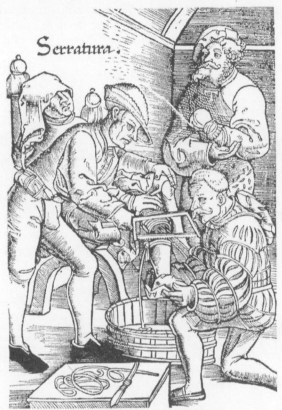

201. *Amputation of the leg.*
(*From the* Feldtbuch der Wundartzney [*Strassburg, 1517*],
by Hans von Gersdorf.)

"But for that I gave no great credit neither to the author, nor remedy, because I knew that caustickes could not be powred into wounds, without excessive paine; I, before I would runne a hazard, determined to see whether the Chirurgions, who went with me in the army, used any other manner of dressing to these wounds. I observed and saw that all of them used that Method of dressing which *Vigo* prescribes; and that they filled as full as they could, the wounds made by Gunshot with Tents and pledgets dipped in the scalding Oyle, at the first dressings; which encouraged me to doe the like to those, who came to be dressed of me.

"It chanced on a time, that by reason of the multitude that were hurt, I wanted this Oyle. Now because there were some few left to be dressed, I was forced, that I might seeme to want nothing, and that I might not leave them undrest, to apply a digestive made of the yolke of an egg, oyle of Roses, and Turpentine. I could not sleep all that night, for I was troubled in minde, and the dressing of the precedent day, (which I judged unfit) troubled my thoughts; and I feared that the next day I should finde them dead, or at the point of death by the poyson of the wound, whom I had not dressed with the scalding oyle.

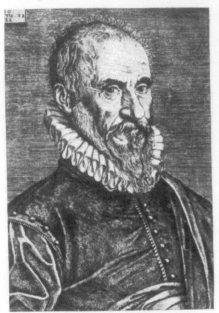

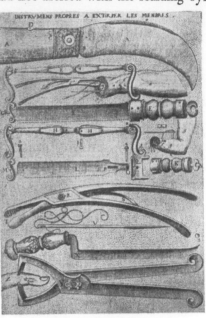

202. *Ambroise Paré.*
Sixteenth-century French engraving.

203. *Some of Paré's surgical instru-*
ments.

Therefore I rose early in the morning, I visited my patients, and beyond expectation, I found such as I had dressed with a digestive onely, free from vehemencie of paine to have had good rest, and that their wounds were not inflamed, nor tumifyed; but on the contrary the others that were burnt with the scalding oyle were feaverish, tormented with much paine, and the parts about their wounds were swolne. When I had many times tryed this in divers others I thought this much, that neither I nor any other should ever cauterize any wounded with Gun-shot . . ." (translation in D. W. Singer's *Selections from the Works of Ambroise Paré*, London, 1924).

The figure of this man of genius, indefatigable worker, honest to the highest degree, endowed with but little culture but with a magnificent spirit of observation, is one of the most vital in the great pageant of medical history. This Huguenot, who by his industry, intelligence, courage, and technical ability raised himself to become the adviser and friend of several kings of France, successfully maintained a violent strife against scholasticism and dogmatism and against the medical authorities who did not wish to recognize this offspring of the people. An audacious pioneer, he personifies all the tendencies of the new period, intolerant of the bonds of scholastic tradition. He was not only a great surgeon but a physician who had a profound faith in the healing force of nature. To him is owed the famous remark, made when he was being congratulated on the cure of a difficult case: " *Je le pansay, Dieu le guarit* (I treated him, but God cured him)." Between his first little book (1545), which bears on its title-page the name of the author with the modest title of *maistre Barbier, Chirurgien*, and the *Œuvres de M. Ambroise Paré, conseiller, et premier chirurgien du Roy*, a magnificent folio of 945 pages, which came out in 1575 (Buon, Paris), appeared numerous works that illustrate his originality, wisdom, and profound honesty. A complete bibliography of Paré's work by Janet Doe has recently appeared (University of Chicago Press, 1937).

Paré's best-known pupils were ADRIEN and JACQUES AMBOISE, BARTHÉLEMY CABROL, and PIERRE FRANCO, the celebrated Huguenot surgeon and lithotomist of Provence, the first to perform suprapubic cystotomy. Of Franco's two rare treatises on surgery, the *Petit Traité* (1556) was reprinted in the *Deutsches Archiv für Geschichte der Medizin* (1881, 1882) and in the *Revue de Chirurgie* (1884); the *Grand Traité* (1561), one of the most complete in Renaissance times, was republished by Nicaise (Paris, 1895).

Among his contemporaries who recommended the milder treatment of gunshot wounds, and perhaps independently of Paré, was Leonardo BOTALLO (b. 1530), who also was physician to Charles IX and Henry III and lived most of his life in Paris. In his greatest book, *De curandis vulneribus sclopetorum* (Lyon, 1560), he combated the theory of the poisonous nature of gunshot wounds, but was a fervent advocate of frequent and copious blood-letting. Among his best-known pupils were BARTOLOMEO MAGGI (1516–52), Professor of Anatomy and Surgery at Bologna and physician to Julius III, who in a posthumous work (1552) also recommended the simple treatment of gunshot wounds without hindrance to the normal secretions. This book was probably written independently of Paré.

Among the German surgeons of this period one of the best known was FELIX WÜRTZ (1518?–74) of Zurich, a friend of Paracelsus, who followed him in the simple treatment of wounds. His *Practica der Wundartzney*, however, limits itself to the treatment of wounds, fractures, and dislocations, without dealing with operative surgery and exhibiting little anatomical knowledge. He deserves credit, however, for having been the first in Germany to combat the treatment of wounds with cautery, unguents, and plasters. His book was published in Basel in 1563 and had fifteen editions in a little more than a century. The work of another German surgeon, the *Practica copiosa* (1559) of CASPAR STROMAYR, which

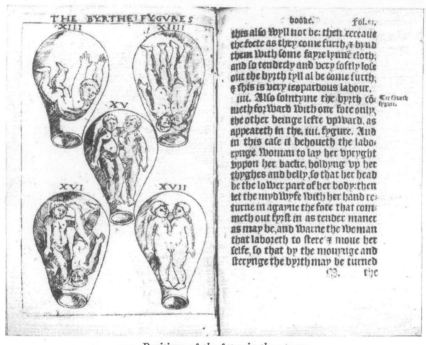

204. *Positions of the fetus in the uterus.*
(*From* The Byrth of Mankynde *by Roesslin, translated by R. Jonas, London, 1540.*)

has recently been printed from the original manuscript by Walther von Brunn (Berlin, 1925), with its fine coloured drawings, gives an excellent survey of the state of surgery at the time. Perhaps the best known of these German surgeons was Wilhelm Fabry, of Hilden near Düsseldorf (FABRICIUS HILDANUS) (1560–1624), who is often referred to as the father of German surgery. He studied in Italy and France, and practised surgery in Bern. The best known of his numerous surgical writings is the *Observationes medico-chirurgicæ* (Basel, 1606). He is said to have been the first to recommend amputation above a gangrenous part (*De gangraena et sphacelo*, Cologne, 1593), and to amputate the thigh, controlling hemorrhage with a tourniquet. He adhered, however, to the cautery and the weapon-salve, which was often applied to the weapon instead of the wound! The *Armamentarium chirurgicum* (Ulm, 1653) of JOHANN SCULTETUS contains excellent illustrations of the surgical instruments in use at that time as well as good descriptions of most of the operations then in common use.

In the British Isles, WILLIAM CLOWES (1540–1604) was an experi-enced military surgeon who was phy-sician to Queen Elizabeth. Norman Moore regards his work as the " very best surgical writings of the Eliza-bethan age." PETER LOWE (*c.* 1550–1612), a Scot, studied in the Paris col-lege of surgery and spent many years in France and Flanders in military surgery, attached to the King of France. Later in life he returned to Glasgow, where he wrote *The Whole Course of Chirurgerie* (London, 1596, and many subsequent editions). A second edition of this work con-tained *The Booke of the Presages of the Divine Hippocrates*, which is noteworthy as the first English at-tempt to reproduce the works of the great Greek physician. He was a founder of the Faculty of Physicians and Surgeons at Glasgow (1599) and

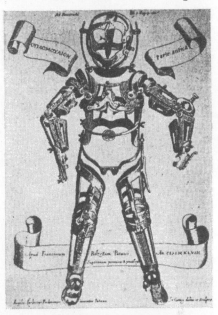

205. *Prosthetic aids.*
(*From the* Chirurgia [*Paris, 1613*] *of Fabricius of Acquapendente.*)

long the outstanding surgeon in the west of Scotland. THOMAS GALE (1507–86) was another who advocated in England, in his excellent *Treatise of Wounds from Gonneshot* (London, 1563), the non-irritating treatment of wounds.

Of various Spanish surgeons whose names have come down to us FRANCISCO DÍAZ is especially to be remembered as author of one of the first works on the urinary tract (1588), so that Lejeune calls him the founder of urology.

OBSTETRICS developed a noteworthy literature during the Renaissance. In 1513 appeared EUCHARIUS ROESSLIN's *Der Swangern Frawen und He-bammen Rosengarten*. The author was a practising physician at Worms and then at Frankfurt. His text is little more than a compilation of Greek and Latin works, so that it would have little importance except for the twenty woodcuts and for the vernacular language, used here for the first time in obstetrics. In spite of the inadequate text and primitive nature of the illustrations, the book had an enormous success and was translated into many languages in numerous editions up to the eighteenth century. It was translated into English by Richard Jonas as *The Byrth of Mankynde* (London, 1540). Walther Ryff, who published a poor plagiarism of Roesslin's book, should not be confused with the Swiss surgeon JACOB RUEFF

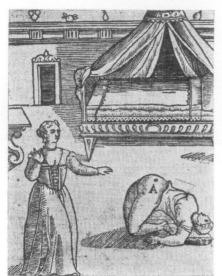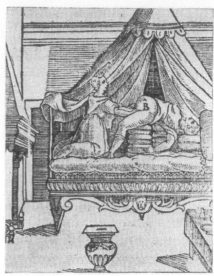

206. *Preparation for childbirth.*
(*From* La comare, *1595, of Scipione Mercurio.*)

(1500–58), who published a *Trostbüchle* (Zurich, 1554) that is a sound work on contemporary obstetrics and pictures interesting instruments such as a speculum and long-toothed forceps used to extract the dead fetus.

Anatomical and surgical progress had a distinct influence on obstetrics; and almost all of the great men of the time, such as Vesalius, Fallopio, Realdo Colombo, and Fabrizio, dealt with the various deformities of the pelvis and the mechanism of childbirth. Of great importance is the work of the French surgeons, and especially of Paré, who should be regarded as one of the founders of modern obstetrics. His book, *De la génération de l'homme* (Paris, 1573, in his *Deux Livres*) is a good combination of Hippocratic principles with his own observations and modifications, especially in his energetic recommendation of podalic version. Paré, who says that he learned this procedure from de Héry and Lambert, two barber surgeons of Paris, advocates a different position of the patient from that of lithotomy, extracting first one foot and then the other with simultaneous pressure on the abdomen. According to Fasbender, Paré deserves the credit for having been the first to describe this method and put it into successful practice.

Among Paré's pupils were Jacques GUILLEMEAU (1550–1613), an

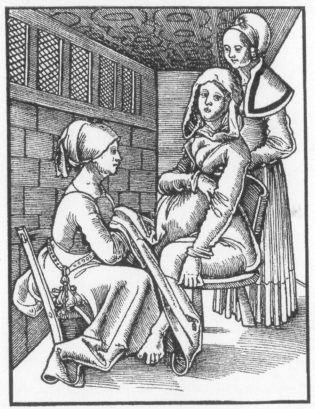

207. *Delivery on the birth stool.*
(*From* Der Swangern Frawen Rosengarten [*Hagenau, 1531*] *of Roesslin.*)
The woodcut is by Conrad Merkel, the friend of Dürer.

oculist surgeon and obstetrician whose best-known book was on *L'Heureux Accouchement des femmes* (Paris, 1609). He followed his master in recommending podalic version, and the avoidance of Cæsarian section in the living, which, however, he recommended on the pregnant woman who had just died. The best-known Italian was SCIPIONE MERCURIO, whose *La comare o raccoglitrice* (1595) was one of the most celebrated medical books of the whole Renaissance and was republished in an incredible number of editions well into the eighteenth century. Mercurio, a pupil of Aranzio, appears to have practised obstetrics in France; he is one of the first to maintain that contracted pelvis is an indication for Cæsarean section.

The outstanding Renaissance description of Cæsarean section occurs in the *Traité nouveau de l'hysterotomotokie* (Paris, 1581) of FRANÇOIS ROUSSET (b. 1535). On the basis of fifteen successful cases he maintained that it was not so dangerous an operation as was commonly believed at the time.

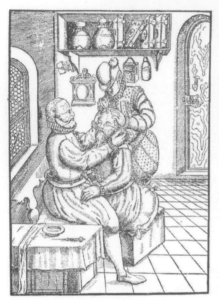 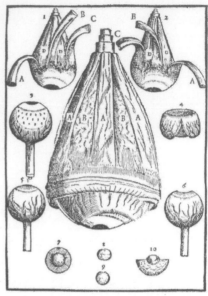

208. *Operation on the eye.*   209. *Anatomy of the eye.*
(*From the* Ophthalmodouleia [*Dresden, 1583*] *of Georg Bartisch.*)

The first Renaissance book on the surgery of the EYE was written by GEORG BARTISCH (1535–1607), a skilful and fortunate peripatetic operator who was the oculist of August of Saxony. The *Ophthalmodouleia* (service of the eyes) first appeared at Dresden in 1583 and attained a phenomenal success, both on account of the number of its anatomical illustrations and of the numerous procedures described, which give a good idea of the state of this specialty at the time. Bartisch, for instance, distinguishes five kinds of cataract and describes the method for their extraction. He gives conscientious directions for the necessary pre-operative measures on the part of both patient (fasting, etc.) and operator (abstention from drink and venery, etc.). He is said to have been the first to describe excision of the eye in living man, and it is of interest that he devoted chapters to the care of the mouth, skin, and so on in relation to diseases of the eye.

7. Pharmacology

Enthusiasm for the study of nature, which is one of the characteristics of the Renaissance, brought about a more careful study of plants and their qualities and consequently a notable revival in therapeutics. The therapy derived from the Arabians had become too heavy a burden; the enormous number of drugs, the difficulties in preparation, the infinite number of heterogeneous items mixed in one prescription (sometimes containing forty or more different substances), all this had contributed to a state of affairs which made the rational application of drugs quite illusory.

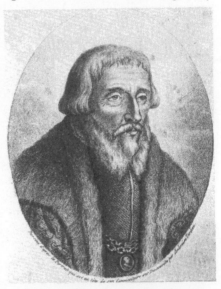

Among the Italians who sought to liberate pharmacology from Arabian traditions, an important figure was Pietro Andrea MATTIOLI (1501–77), of Siena. Having studied at Padua, Siena, Perugia, and Rome, he went to Trent, where he became the friend of the Prince-Bishop Bernardus Clesius. In 1540 he was called to Gorizia to fight a severe epidemic, where his fame spread so rapidly that in 1554 he was called to be the physician of Ferdinand I, and later of Maximilian II. In 1562 he returned to Trent, where he died of plague

210. *P. A. Mattioli. A seventeenth-century engraving.*

in 1577. Mattioli was one of the most venerated physicians of his time. In his *Commentary on Dioscorides* (Venice, 1554), which can be regarded as an encyclopædia of Renaissance pharmacology, he collected the results of his long-continued observations and careful studies. He examined and described hundreds of plants, while the illustrations of his book are far superior to anything previously published in Italy in this field, so that it is not to be wondered at that it was the classic text for almost two centuries.

Among the early botanical gardens were those created at Padua by Francesco BONAFEDE (1545) and at Pisa by Luca GHINI, who was followed as lecturer on simples by his pupil Anguillara.

One of the most interesting naturalists and biologists in Renaissance medicine was the Bolognese Ulysses ALDOVRANDI (1522–1605), who founded the Botanical Garden (1567) of the Museum of Natural History at Bologna. He wrote a *Storia naturale* in thirteen volumes, only four of which were published before his death. Giovanni MANARDI (1462–1536), of Ferrara, physician to Alphonso d'Este and Ariosto, was among the first, according to Haller, to switch from the impure texts of the Arabians to the original Greek. His *Epistolæ medicinales* was published in many editions; at Lyon in 1536 with a preface by Rabelais. The *Erbario novo* (Venice, 1584) of the Umbrian Castore DURANTE (d. 1590) went through many editions. Antonio Musa BRASAVOLA (b. 1500), a pupil of Leonicenus, reintroduced into medicine many new plants, such as black hellebore, and was also one of the first to use guaiac and *radix chinæ* in Italy. The Venetian Prospero ALPINO (1553–1617) spent three years in the Orient studying the local customs, drugs, and diseases, which resulted in several botanical works, among which his *De plantis exoticis* included descriptions of more than fifty hitherto unknown plants. He is credited with the introduction of coffee and moxa from the Orient. We also meet Alpino in connection with medical history in his *De medicina Ægyptiorum* (Venice, 1591), and also in his book on prognosis, *De præsagienda vita et morte ægrotantium* (Venice, 1601).

A famous German physician and pharmacologist was LEONARD FUCHS (1501–66), Professor first of Philosophy and then of Medicine at Ingolstadt, physician of the Margrave Georg of Brandenburg, then professor at Tübingen for thirty-one years. A fervid Hippocratist and writer of numerous works, he is best known for his *De historia stirpium* (Basel, 1542). The beautiful engravings in this magnificent botanical work give it a bibliographical as well as a scientific value. It went through a number of editions, including smaller reprints for popular consumption. Another popular work was the *Kreuterbuch* (Frankfurt, 1555) of Adam LONICERUS (1499–1595). North of the Alps herbals and bestiaries (with descriptions of real and fanciful animals of all kinds) were much in vogue. Far superior to the popular Horti of the fifteenth century, for instance, was the *Herbarum vivæ icones* (Strassburg, 1530–6) of Otho BRUNFELS (1464–1534), which contains 135 excellent original woodcuts of plants. The brilliant Valerius CORDUS (1515–44), of Erfurt, in his short twenty-nine years left permanent traces in science, with his discovery of sulphuric ether (1540), his description of some five hundred new plant species, his commentary on Dioscorides (published posthumously by Gesner, Strassburg, 1561), and his publication of the first adequate pharmacopœia, the *Dispensatorium* of 1535 (Nürnberg). This set the fashion for similar works, often published by cities such as Basel, Antwerp, Augsburg (see T. Schirch, *Janus*, 1905, X, 281 ff.).

A striking figure, typically Renaissance in his universality, was the Swiss Conrad Gesner (1515–65), whose attainments in botany, zoology, medicine and surgery, philology and general scholarship brought him the name of the " German Pliny." In spite of years of poverty and physical ailments, he produced important works on many subjects, from the century bird to the Lord's prayer, typified in his *Bibliotheca universalis* (20 vols., Zurich, 1545–9), the best general bibliography before Haller.

In materia medica, as we have seen, Paracelsus was a leader in popularizing mineral drugs such as mercury, while guaiac and sarsaparilla were brought into widespread use in the epidemic of syphilis (see Ulrich von Hutten). Pharmacy shops acquired greater importance during the Renaissance and contributed noteworthy works of art in their pharmacy jars. The most celebrated potters of Faenza and Urbino and Pesaro competed in the production of artistic jars, especially for the pharmacies of the princes and the convents, which constitute valuable documents of the ceramic art of the Renaissance.

8. The Study and Practice of Renaissance Medicine

During the Renaissance medical science, and later the practice of medicine, were entirely in the hands of the laity. The improved economic position of western Europe, the spread of hygienic concepts through the better-organized states, and the introduction of many public health measures — all these brought about great improvement in the practice and social position of the physician. Physicians belonged to the wealthier classes and lived in easy circumstances. They generally received their education in the universities, those of Italy being at the height of their fame in the sixteenth century. During the Renaissance Padua reached its climax, receiving many foreign students who were organized into various " nations " (German, English, Polish, Hungarian, and so on), which exerted a considerable influence on academic life.

The Senate of the Venetian Republic appreciated the political importance of the university and gave it many privileges; it opened its doors to all religions and refused to admit the restrictions of the Church universities on the form of study and the doctor's degree. Students were well received in Padua and throughout the Republic. Protestants as well as Hebrews enjoyed full liberty; in vain did the Jesuits attempt to found a university of their own at Padua in 1591. When Pius IV in his bull *In sacrosancta*

(1565) ruled that the degree could be given only to those of the Catholic faith, the Venetian Senate, in accordance with the ecclesiastical policy of the Republic and affirming its absolute sovereignty also in cultural affairs, named a Procurator who had the power to grant the degree without regard to the faith of the candidate. Those who could not attain academic grades because they were not Catholics generally had recourse to the counts palatine, to whom the emperors had given the privilege of conferring

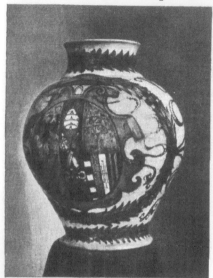
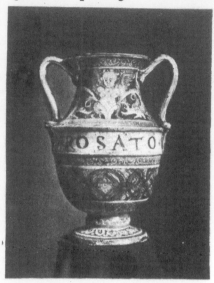

211. *Tuscan pharmacy jar with the coat of arms of the Duke of Urbino, 1500.*　　212. *Sienese pharmacy jar with two handles, early sixteenth century.*

(COLLECTION OF A. CASTIGLIONI.)

academic degrees. These doctors, who customarily were examined by the professors of the university, were called *Doctores bullati* as opposed to *Doctores academici promoti*. In 1589 such a diploma was given to the Jewish physician Salomone Lotio by the Count Sigismondo Capodilista, the same Count Palatine who in 1602 conferred the degree on William Harvey. It was in 1616 that as a result of a quarrel with the Church and by the advice of Fra Paolo Sarpi the Venetian Senate considered the foundation of a *Collegio Veneto*, in which the degrees were conferred *auctoritate veneta*. These are the first diplomas that can be properly regarded as diplomas of the State.

Many famous Europeans studied in Italy during the Renaissance, such as Copernicus and the Hungarian Josephus STRUTHIUS (1510–78), physician of Sigismund August, King of Poland. He made an important contribution to clinical medicine with his *Ars sphigmica* (1555), which contains noteworthy diagnostic and clinical information on the action of the heart and blood vessels. Ferrara was so well thought of by the Portuguese Amatus Lusitanus that he advised his compatriots to study there. Germans, Flemish, French, Catalans, and English attended the Italian universities in great numbers — Caius (Dr. Keys) and William Harvey, for instance. Bologna at-

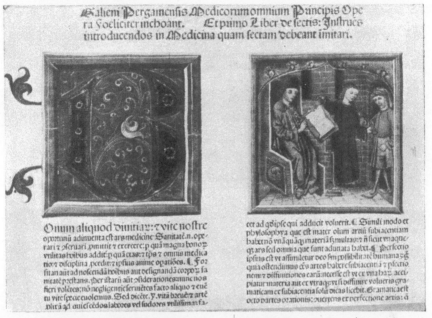

213. *The first page of the editio princeps of Galen's* Opera *(Venice, 1541).*

tracted students through the great reputation of its anatomists and surgeons; Rome, the intellectual and artistic centre of the world at that time, attracted the sons of high officials and noble families in other countries to hear the lectures of the famous doctors of the Sapienza, as the university was called. The story of the *Collegium Mediolanensium Medicorum* was told (Milan, 1607) by G. B. SILVATICUS (*c.* 1550–1621), who was also one of the first to write a treatise on malingering (*De iis qui morbum simulant deprehendendis*, 1595).

The constitution of the Italian universities placed great power in the hands of the students, who elected the rectors and other officials of the university and even supervised the course of studies, at a time when the rest of Europe was being desolated by the religious wars. The recompense of university professors varied in the different countries. In the German universities, according to Baas, they were poorly paid, while the Italians probably received the highest pay. The professors at Heidelberg had an annual salary of fifty to sixty florins, while Vesalius at Pisa received eight hundred florins. For the two chairs created in the Paris Faculty in 1505 the stipend consisted of twelve livres annually. There was considerable rivalry between the various universities to procure the most famous teachers, so that it was unusual to find a professor of the sixteenth century staying for a long time in the same university.

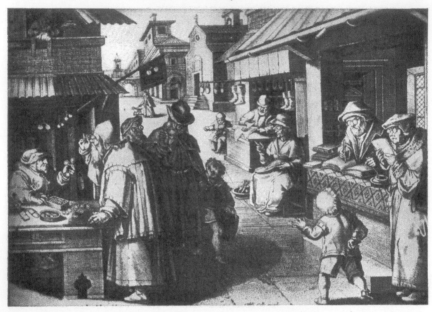

214. *The vendor of spectacles. French print.*

Sixteenth-century medical teaching was still, superficially at least, of the classic type; and although the texts of Galen and Avicenna and the rest were rigorously prescribed, and although the anatomy of Galen continued to be the chief anatomical text long after the time of Mondino, it is nevertheless true that the new orientations made headway in spite of the conservative spirit of the professors. Public dissections were practised carefully and in greater numbers than heretofore. The ancient custom of reading from a text of anatomy, while often a clumsy assistant mishandled the organs, was going out of fashion, although still preserved in Paris by Jacobus Sylvius. More teachers of anatomy did their dissections in person; anatomical theatres began to be constructed toward the end of the sixteenth century. Vesalius taught in a temporary theatre at Bologna and Padua, as he states in the first edition of the *Fabrica,* but the first permanent anatomical theatre was apparently constructed later at Bologna, and the second at Padua by Fabricius. Up to the end of the century anatomy was taught together with surgery. It was only in 1570 that a special chair was created for each subject, and they were combined in most schools well into the eighteenth century.

Thus anatomy began to take its place in university instruction. Soon dissection of the cadaver was prescribed as an essential and regular part of the instruction. The teaching of pathology began also in this century, as is shown by a document of 1587 in the University of Padua.

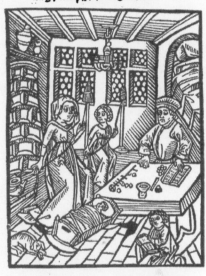

Ein regiment der jungen kinder
Wie man sy halten vnd erziehen sol von
irer gepurt biß sy zu iren tagen kōmen.

215. *Frontispiece of Metlinger's early work on pediatrics (1473).*

After the university professorships the posts most sought after by physicians were in the courts of princes or the great cities. The physicians sometimes worked by contract under advantageous conditions; they were required to prepare medical *consilia* and regulations in case of epidemics. The pay of physicians was high, as we have seen in the case of Fabricius, Massa, and Berengario. The medical household of Louis XII, King of France, consisted of a physician receiving eight hundred livres annually, five ordinary physicians at five hundred livres, five surgeons at one hundred and eighty livres, two barbers, an apothecary, and an astrologer. The chief physician of Henry II received twelve hundred livres; while Fernel is said to have received ten thousand *écus* at each of the ten accouchements of Catherine de' Medici. Throughout Europe special laws regulated the course that physicians should follow in the preparation of medicines and in their prices. Regular visits were made to the pharmacies to supervise the quality of the medicines. In various countries an actual tariff of medical charges was in use. Surgery began to be practised by doctors of medicine and even by university professors.

The quarrels between the surgeons and the physicians of the faculty, especially at Paris, constitute almost a special chapter in the history of the practice of medicine of the time. The surgeons enjoyed a great reputation, even though they had no academic culture. The King of France himself had twelve surgeons attached to his person, but the most important were those who accompanied the armies, being engaged for each campaign. In Germany it was only in 1548 that surgery was declared to be an honourable profession and that doctors of medicine retained their dignity in practising it. However, for a long time inferior types continued to go from village to village practising minor surgery together with other trades and throwing discredit on the profession. Nevertheless, the better type of surgeon, especially in Italy and France, was beginning to bring about a worthy revival in surgical practice.

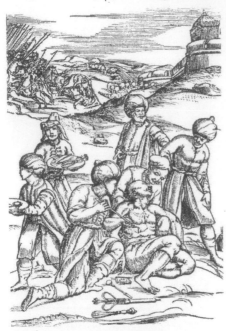

216. *Cauterization of wounds on the battlefield.*
(*From the* Officina chirurgica [*Venice, 1596*] *of Andrea Della Croce.*)

MILITARY MEDICINE had occupied the special attention of states and military leaders from the end of the fifteenth century. True military hospitals had been founded at the siege of Alora (1484) and at Baza (1489), as may be seen in the letter of Peter Martyr to the Archbishop of Milan; they were greatly developed during the Renaissance. The great progress of surgery in France is really due to a military surgeon, Ambroise Paré. The greater use of firearms, which at first were thought to make poisoned wounds, considerably developed the activities of the military surgeons.

The physician of the Renaissance took on a very different character from that of his mediæval predecessor. Even though most practitioners still consulted astrology and based their diagnosis on uroscopy and their treatment on blood-letting; and even though empiricists, charlatans, barbers, and farriers flourished over Europe, and even were sought after by rulers, it is no less true that the best physicians acquired great reputations and were held in high esteem. It was during the Renaissance that the physician became a scholar. He often devoted himself to the observation of nature after freeing himself from metaphysics and dialectic. The great physicians had a profound knowledge of classical literature and were often Humanists and men of letters; many were collectors of works of art and were prominent in politics. The iconography and literature of the Renaissance portray them for us in sumptuous garments but with a composed and grave expression, in the act of dissecting or of studying the ancient texts. The pictures of the physicians with the urine glass in hand become rarer. In Renaissance society the medical man occupied an important position. As Wickersheimer states: " The physicians did not give way to the gentlemen; Legrand is the friend of Brantôme and Marc Miron is both physician to Henry III and his companion." A physician had sufficient influence on Charles VIII to make him decide to undertake an expedition to Italy. Physicians were often the boon companions of enlightened princes such as

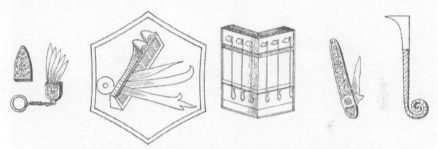

217. *Sixteenth-century instruments for blood-letting. The second figure from the left is the emblem of the Manfredi, Dukes of Faenza, who used the symbol for blood-letting in their coat of arms.*

Cosimo de' Medici and artists such as Leonardo and Michelangelo. It was for physicians that the most valuable editions of books were printed and beautiful illustrations of anatomical works made by famous engravers.

The history of Renaissance medicine is inextricably bound to the glorious Renaissance of art. Anatomical progress certainly was due in part at least to the new spirit which animated the artists of the period. The greatest painters and sculptors felt the need of returning to the study of nature, of examining the position of the muscles in the *écorchés* and the structure of the bones in prepared skeletons. Thus artists and anatomists had a similar goal; we have seen how Leonardo was the collaborator of Della Torre; we know that Michelangelo was the pupil of Realdo Colombo, and that Paolo Veronese was probably the designer of the frontispiece of Realdo's famous book. The anatomical plates of Vesalius were drawn by Calcar, the pupil of Titian, and the tradition persists that some of the drawings were by Titian himself. The anatomical plates of Eustachius were designed by a Venetian painter, De Musis. Raphael himself was a close student of anatomy, as is shown by his numerous drawings. The German painters were no less concerned with such studies, as is shown by the drawings of Dürer, Holbein, and Cranach. One of the most interesting of

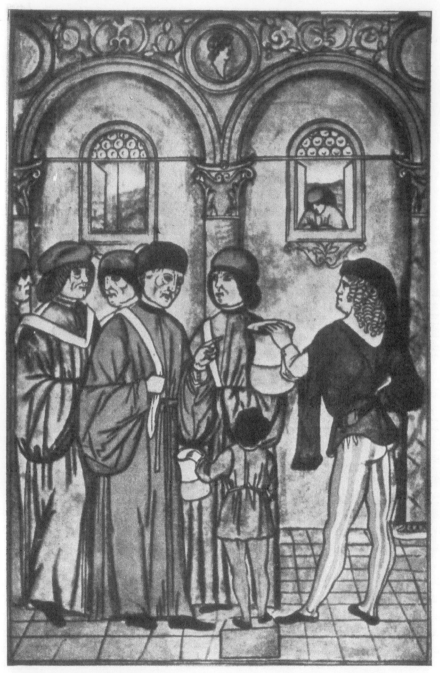

218. *Medical consultation.* (*From Ketham's* Fasciculus medicinæ, *Venice, 1512.*)

Dürer's drawings is one that he sent to his physician, pointing out a painful area on his body. As we may see, he is obviously referring to a painful spleen, probably due to an attack of malaria that he contracted during his sojourn at Venice. But in addition to these anatomical pictures the Renaissance painters were attracted by many other medical scenes. The plague was often the subject of their paintings, as in the celebrated design of

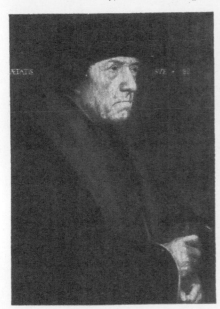

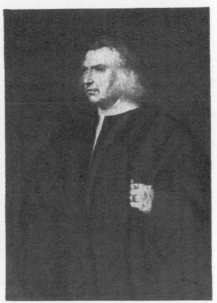

219. *Portrait of John Chambers,*
physician to Henry VIII, by the
younger Holbein.
(LICHTENSTEIN GALLERY, VIENNA.)

220. *Portrait of the physician*
Parma, attributed to Titian.
(STATE MUSEUM, VIENNA.)

Raphael. Francesco Carotto, of Verona, represented St. Roch showing his inguinal bubo; the same subject can be seen in the pictures of Tintoretto (at Venice), Andrea del Sarto (in the Pitti Museum), and Guido Reni (at Dresden). It is of historical significance that leprosy, which was often reproduced in the fourteenth and fifteenth centuries, when it was common in Europe, disappeared almost entirely from the illustrations of the Renaissance. The first representations of syphilis date from the last years of the fifteenth century; among them one of the most famous is Dürer's picture of a syphilitic that he made in Nürnberg in 1496.

Portraits of illustrious physicians became more and more frequent, another indication of the social importance of physicians at this time. Outstanding among these are the alleged portrait of Vesalius and that of the artist's physician, Parma, both attributed to Titian (Vienna State Museum). One of the masterpieces of Renaissance portraiture is the superb picture of John Chambers, physician to Henry VIII, by Hans Holbein the younger, in the Lichtenstein Gallery in Vienna. The portrait of Paracelsus

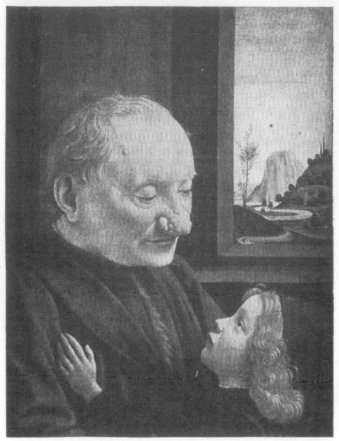

221. *The man with rhinophyma. Ghirlandaio.*   (LOUVRE MUSEUM, PARIS.)

in the Bern Museum, attributed to Holbein, is also of artistic and historical interest.

The figure of the physician as given by the writers of the period is very different from that of preceding centuries. We have seen how the physicians of the fourteenth and fifteenth centuries were often described in a contemptuous way as ignorant persons of scanty culture; the writers of the Renaissance speak of physicians with greater respect as, often, famous persons esteemed by princes and connoisseurs of literature and art. The physicians mentioned by Benvenuto Cellini in his autobiography give us a vivid picture of the conditions in which medicine was practised. In a fine satire published with a commentary by Capparoni, Ariosto borrows the words of a vendor of medicinal herbs to proclaim their virtues. Many of the writers of the period allude to physicians and to medical treatment.

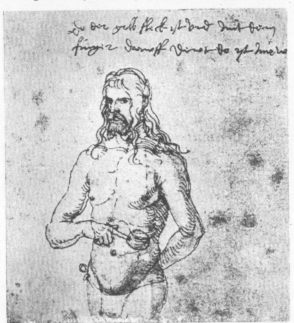

222. *Albrecht Dürer. His sketch sent to his physician to show a painful area (acute splenic tumour?).*

Among the French writers who are most concerned with medical matters is the vital figure of François RABELAIS (1483–1553), the famous cleric and satirist who studied medicine at Montpellier and lectured on Hippocrates and on Galen at that university. In 1532 he studied at Lyon, where he published his immortal satires, *Gargantua* and *Pantagruel;* but at the same time he was writing his commentaries on Hippocrates and Galen and editing a fine edition of the *Epistolæ* of Manardi. Rabelais was physician to the hospital of Lyon, and often visited Italy on important missions, thus becoming familiar with Italian art and literature. Finally, after many quarrels with the Church, he became curate of Meudon, where he died in solitude. He ridicules the charlatanesque forms of treatment and the numerous medical superstitions as well as the antiquated methods of teaching from faulty texts, cherishing the Greek ideals of developing all aspects of man.

The statement that he was the first to lecture at Montpellier with the Greek text before him is probably incorrect.

During the sixteenth century, with the establishment of the independence of scholarship from the control of the authorities, astrology, which had been strenuously upheld by physicians, commenced to lose ground. The belief in witches, however, and the power that they could exercise

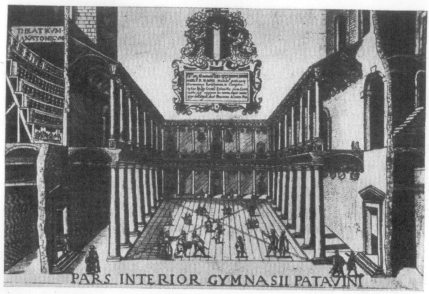

223. *The atrium of the University of Padua. In the upper left-hand corner is seen the anatomical theatre of Fabricius.*

was at its height, though it had less of a hold in Italy than in the northern countries. Ever since the publication of Jacobus Sprenger's *Malleus maleficarum* (*c.* 1485), indicating that the Church and the Inquisition recognized witches as their enemies, persecution had become widespread. In 1562 witchcraft was made a capital offence in England (not repealed until 1735), and progressive spirits such as Sir Thomas Browne, Johan Lange, Paré, and Fernel believed in the powers of witchcraft. The Salem trials of 1692 are well known to Americans; while in Austria even in the eighteenth century de Haen supported the error. Against the view that witches were accomplices or victims of the devil, to be condemned to the stake, appeared the memorable and courageous work of the physician JOHANN WEYER (1555–88), known under the Latin name of Wierus. In 1563 Weyer published his work *De præstigiis dæmonum*, in which he maintained that witches were merely poor people who had lost control of their emotions and whose minds had become distorted. He believed that the confessions extorted from witches as the result of torture were horrible mistakes; he denied the transformation of men into animals and that witches flew through the air on broomsticks. Incubi and succubi, according to Weyer, were merely manifestations of apprehension and anguish; philtres, magic, and witchcraft sometimes could lead to insanity but never to the attain-

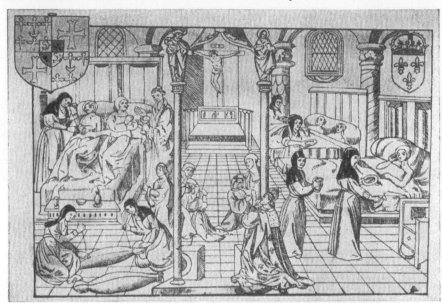

224. *A sick-room in the Hôtel Dieu, Paris.*
(*From a woodcut in the Cabinet of Prints of the* BIBLIOTHÈQUE NATIONALE, PARIS.)

ment of the desired magic ends. The diabolic arts and their bugbears should not frighten anyone. Weyer examined such cases one by one and showed that in each it was a question of sickness or rascality; and he called the judges butchers who condemned these miserable wretches. Weyer's book had remarkable success, especially considering the strength of his opponents, and passed through several editions even during his lifetime. Gregory Zilboorg in his recent book *The Medical Man and the Witch during the Renaissance* (Johns Hopkins Press, 1935) states that Weyer might well be called the founder of modern psychiatry. Another courageous opponent of superstition was REGINALD SCOT (1538–99), who in his *Discoverie of Witchcraft* (London, 1584) supported the ideas of Weyer. Little by little other physicians were won over to the more enlightened point of view, though the last executions for witchcraft in Germany and Switzerland were in 1775 and 1782 respectively. In general, the Renaissance saw considerable progress in the opposition of physicians to ancient superstitions.

A summary of the advance made by medicine during the Renaissance reveals enormous progress: medical thought evolved rapidly, and, together with the replacement of rigid Aristotelian systems by Neo-Platonism, scholarship advanced with quick and certain step to objectivity of observation

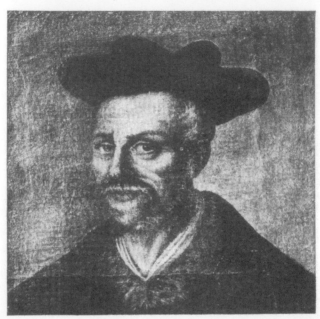

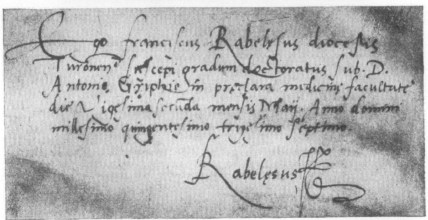

225. *François Rabelais. Portrait, early seventeenth century. Below, Rabelais's autograph accepting his degree from the Medical Faculty of Montpellier, May 22, 1537.*

and experiment. Thus it returned to the Hippocratic concept at the same time that anatomy, thanks to such great men as Leonardo, Vesalius, Fallopius, and Cesalpino, acquired a basic, firm position in science. The observation of Nature, which is one of the most important gifts of Humanism to the Renaissance, found its widest application in the study of anatomy,

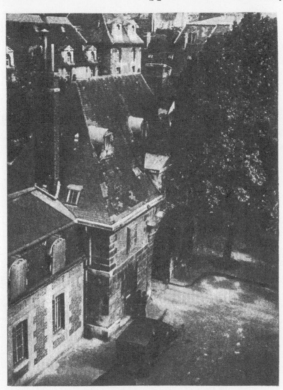

226. *The Hospital of St. Louis at Paris, built by Henry IV at the end of the sixteenth century for plague patients. The original façade is preserved.*

physiology, and chemistry. The study of the human organism, its behaviour, and its diseases from now on has an integral part in the program of medicine, which abandoned the study of the text to return to the study of the patient, a concept interpreted in its most representative and violent form by Paracelsus.

At the same time surgery, under the enlightened leadership of Paré, made noteworthy progress in close connection with the anatomical discoveries. The gifted statements of Fracastoro opened the way to new concepts in the field of epidemic diseases. The study of syphilis constitutes the best possible demonstration that medicine had attained a position to handle the most difficult and complex problems efficiently. The establishment of the experimental method by the scientific work of Galileo, the formulation of natural laws at the moment when Descartes announced his view that the body is nothing but an automatically operating machine — all these gave a new impulse to the naturalistic concept of the universe.

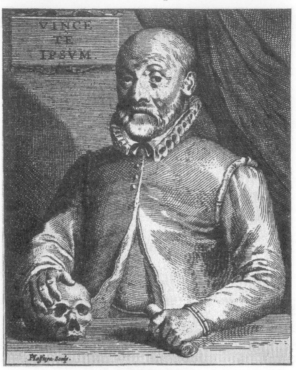

227. *Johann Weyer.*

The publication of medical texts during the Renaissance flourished; the most famous printers of Europe competed in the publication of magnificent editions of classical medical works. In addition to the *Fabrica,* Étienne's *Anatomy,* and the great herbals, the *Opera Omnia* of Galen was published by the Giunta Press in Greek in 1525, and in Latin 1541–2. The first Latin edition of Hippocrates was published at Rome in 1525.

Thus in this marvellous period of the Renaissance, which marks the return to the ancient concepts of Hellenism, in philosophy as in art, in medicine as in literature, vivid sparks emerged from the forge in which the new forces of the world were being tempered. At this period when even discussions of religious dogmas were carried on, the outmoded concepts of Galenism finally fell beneath the attacks of investigators, almost simultaneously with the ancient ideas about our planetary system. Disencumbered from the rigid structure of scholasticism, the horizon revealed the striking profile of the new science, founded on the free, critical, and individualistic philosophy of Hippocratism and nourished by the new investigations and gifted observations of the men of the Renaissance, guided no less by ancient traditions than by the firm desire to engrave deeply their own record in the pages of history.

CHAPTER XVII

THE SEVENTEENTH CENTURY

*DAWN OF SCIENTIFIC LIBERTY. BIOLOGICAL
AND EXPERIMENTAL TRENDS IN MEDICINE*

1. Evolution of Philosophical and Medical Thought in the Seventeenth Century. Great Discoveries. Academies

THE EVOLUTION of medical thought in the seventeenth century strikingly reflects the tendencies of the period, as exhibited in political and social events and the spiritual revolution of the time. It was a tempestuous period, when new ideas flourished and political revolutions against foreign domination were accompanied by revolt against restraint on research; a time also that marked a grave economic crisis for Italy, because the discoveries of Columbus and other great explorers necessarily diminished the maritime importance of Italian ports by opening up new commercial routes. The power of Venice and Genoa was beginning to lessen, Lombardy was ravaged by the French, Germans, and Spaniards. The little Italian duchies were torn by princely rivalry and by the armies of mercenaries. All these struggles found their bloody epilogue in the War of the Spanish Succession. In Germany, also, desolated by the sanguinary religious contests, the Thirty Years' War destroyed the most flourishing cities, interrupted commerce, ruined industries, and in certain regions almost blotted out a population that had been reduced to misery and decimated by all these misfortunes. It is a period, on the other hand, in which Holland and England reached the

[504]

height of their maritime power, and it is in these two countries that science found its best supporters and medicine had its most flourishing development. The glory of the Elizabethan age and the period following, with the literature of Shakespeare and Milton and the science of Newton, Francis Bacon, William Gilbert, and a host of others too numerous to mention, is a

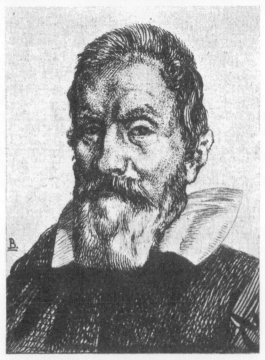

228. *Galileo. After the portrait by Ottavio Leoni, 1686.*

good example of that mysterious combination of circumstances which occasionally brings a people, like the Greeks in the age of Pericles, to produce giants in many fields of human activity, all in a few generations. The period was one of great individualism in medicine as in other activities, with many individual discoveries, a state of affairs which almost necessarily was accompanied by a decreased emphasis on such collective activities as the hospital care of the sick.

Italy, which in the two preceding centuries had done so much to prepare the way for profitable investigation and free, penetrating criticism, suffered from the effects of severe struggles in the field of science as well as of politics. The revolutionary movement which the Reformation had let loose against the Papacy in the name of a renewed faith and freedom of conscience opened the way to the spread of democratic ideas in overturn-ing the political structure of the Middle Ages. A corresponding movement was carried on in Italy by certain men who, without leaving the Church, nevertheless attacked the political principles and essential tenets of Catholi-cism. This is not the place to consider whether the Counter-Reformation in Italy was useful for the Latin world as Croce believes, or, as some modern writers have maintained, that it marked a period of intellectual arrest.

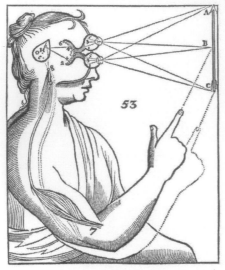

229. *Vision.*
(*From Descartes's* De homine, *1664.*)

There is no question, however, that its effects were manifest on the philo-sophic thought of the period. The names and sufferings of Giordano Bruno, Campanella, and Galileo are witnesses to the strivings toward freedom of thought and to the dawn of scientific liberty which penetrated the peninsula two centuries before its political and economic freedom.

The political and economic con-ditions in Italy, by obstructing that immediate and fertile co-operation which is possible only when research progresses unhampered and the ex-change of ideas is free and rapid, only too often caused the seed to fall on sterile ground. However, this period, when poetry was seeking Arcadia and art turning toward the baroque, was not a period of decadence, but one of preparation and transition. Practical medicine, to be sure, made no great progress beyond that of the Renais-sance. Most physicians still held, as we shall see, to sterile formulas and vain discussions and relied on the authority of the classical texts without appre-ciating the lessons of their great thinkers and scholars; but the voices of those who were attacking the ancient edifice and bringing to light the fundamental truths were being raised ever more loudly. The voice of con-science was being awakened, the voice of the individual was heard — voices that a blind authority could silence but not extinguish. In this period, much more important historically than was formerly accepted when it was thought in Italy to be a decadent period in art, letters, and sciences, medi-cine followed the direction given it by the great naturalists and anatomists of the Renaissance in a spirit of ever developing liberty. Medicine was pre-paring itself to penetrate more and more deeply into the innermost secrets of life; it was stimulated to these studies on the one hand by the philosophic movement, and on the other by the experimental orientation of science in direct relation to it.

It was during this century that Latin philosophy manifested a violent opposition to mediæval doctrines, an opposition that was hit hard by the penalties of counter-reform. For it, anyone who tried to change science

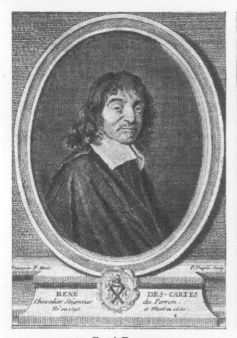

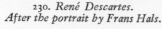

230. René Descartes.
After the portrait by Frans Hals.

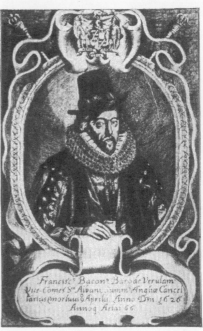

231. Francis Bacon,
Baron Verulam

was an enemy of religion, even when the desire to change the method of study was stronger than the idea of attacking established dogma, as in the case of the two philosophers and poets Giordano Bruno and Campanella.

There is an essential connection between the philosophy of Bruno and that of René DESCARTES (Cartesius) (1596–1650), whose name has great importance for the history of medicine, not only on account of his personal contributions as physiologist and pathologist, but also on account of the effect that the Cartesian philosophy exerted on the evolution of medicine. St. Augustine, developing the idea of Plato, had already maintained that our intelligence knew nothing as certainly as that which confronts it at the moment, and that nothing is more present in our thought than the thought itself. Descartes made this idea the basis of his philosophy. He maintained that knowledge of our own thoughts is the only absolutely certain fact. "*Cogito, ergo sum* (I think, therefore I exist)." The affirmation of this principle weakens the evidence of the senses as compared with reasoning. At a time when the establishment of the Copernican doctrine proved the superiority of mathematical concepts and exact calculations over

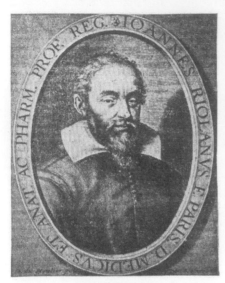 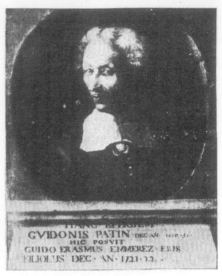

232a. *Jean Riolan.*   232b. *Guy Patin.*
Both were professors at the University of Paris, and ardent defenders of Galenism.

sensation, it was logical to place the source of consciousness in the reasoning power.

Descartes's profound intellect not only had a vast knowledge of the mathematical and natural sciences, but also of anatomy and physiology, so that his book *De homine* (1662) has been accepted as the first physiological text. His work established the idea of an infinite and perfect being, the concept of God and of the corporeal world outside of our own being. Besides Divinity and the corporeal world — matter which occupies all space and is infinitely divisible — he recognized the thinking substance, the spirit. The smallest particles of matter are in motion and produce by their movements natural phenomena that we observe. These movements, in Descartes's almost prophetic concept, were not in a straight line but in an undulating motion. The human body is a machine created by God, and in it dwells the soul, which synthesizes the thinking substance. But the only true essence is Divinity; the body and the spirit are merely the forms in which the Divinity manifests itself.

From these considerations of Descartes and his belief that all the activities of the organism are forms of motion and that this motion can be submitted to precise physical and mathematical examination was born the concept of iatrophysical medicine. His observations of chemical phenomena that took place in the organism, however, were sufficient to justify the veneration that the iatrochemical school had for the great French philosopher whom they considered as their master.

At this time when new ideas frequently arose from the violent shock of minds and events, there was an ever increasing appreciation of the correlation between human problems and the possibilities of human knowledge. The philosophies of Campanella, Sarpi, and Galileo took this specially into account. Among the medical philosophers of the time and a pioneer in optics was Giambattista della Porta (1540–1615), the inventor of the camera obscura (1563) and the opera glass (1590). Having discovered the principle of the former as a boy of fifteen, according to his own account, he became convinced that vision was due, not to rays leaving the eye, but to something that entered the eye. The Accademia dei Segreti that he founded about 1560 furnished him with observations for his work on *Magia Naturalis* (1589). Fortunius Licetus of Rapallo (1577–1657) developed the Aristotelian doctrine of the activity of the senses, dominated, however, by the power of the spirit. Licetus, one of the less effective opponents of Harvey's doctrine, was a prolific writer who enjoyed a popularity even in northern Europe that is hard to explain today. The fact that it was in the ranks of medicine that philosophy found some of its most outstanding representatives is a good indication of the close connection that existed between philosophic and medical studies at this time.

If it was these philosophic tendencies that determined the orientation of medicine, the effect of the great pioneers who opened the ways of experimental science was even more remarkable. The great animating spirit was that of GALILEO GALILEI (1564–1642), whose gigantic individuality dominated all this historical period. Thanks to his investigations, astronomical studies revealed new worlds unknown to Biblical scholars. In the realms of physics, mathematics, and chemistry a febrile activity developed which rapidly produced marvellous results; while in zoology and botany new investigations produced greater and greater knowledge of the laws of nature. All those who adopted the method of scientifically controlled observation followed his lead. Galileo is the first to pose the basis for the experimental method. He affirms the need for examining facts in the light of criticism and for reproducing known phenomena experimentally in order to ascertain their causes and, above all, their explanation. The greatness of Galileo's method consists in the fact that he was not content, like Bacon, to discover the reasons for a fact and the motives that determined it, but he wished to search out the exact mathematical laws that regulated phenomena. " Nature is written in mathematical symbols," declared the great genius of Arcetri. Thus continuing the vision of Leonardo da Vinci, who had made a start along the same road, Galileo established that, uncontrolled by reasoning, the perception of the senses is just as much a source of error as is poor reasoning deprived of confirmation. The importance of this line of thought in the field of medicine is easily understood.

Francis BACON, Lord Verulam (1561–1626), impressed by the shortcomings of mediæval philosophy, endeavoured to formulate the underlying theory of the new type of study. " To extend more widely the limits of the power and greatness of man," he planned his celebrated inductive method: all recorded facts, new observations, and experimental results were to be collected and tabulated, so that the connections between phenomena and their resultant general laws would become manifest. Bacon, however, is less important historically than Galileo and Descartes as an animator of experimental science. His writings appear to have had but little influence on the scientists of his day, except Robert Boyle, so that one finds hardly any references to him, for instance, in the medical literature of the first half of the seventeenth century. It was only later, and in the eighteenth century, that Bacon's inductive science deeply influenced scientific thought. Bacon was not himself a great discoverer of scientific fact, though he was well aware of the special need of his age for proved facts rather than theories.

Important as were the contributions of great thinkers like Descartes and Bacon, it is open to question how much they directly influenced their medical contemporaries. The new spirit was already in the air. Vesalius had already revolutionized anatomy, and Paré had modernized surgery; Harvey's physiological studies were under way and Paracelsus had launched medical reform. The philosophers were characteristic figures and leading exponents of their age rather than important pioneers and guides of medicine. Many were the discoveries in this century which demonstrated the excellence of the principles both that nature should be studied directly and unhesitatingly and that legends and superstitions had to be ignored and dogmas swept aside in order to inspire the new spirit of investigation with the living breath of objective criticism. In physics, Isaac Newton discovered the law of gravitation; in mathematics, Johann Kepler established the laws of the movements of the planets; Pascal determined barometric pressure and elucidated the theory of probabilities; Robert Boyle scientifically attacked numerous physical and chemical problems; Evangelista Torricelli's studies of liquids in a vacuum led to his invention of the barometer; the Jesuit Francesco Maria Grimaldi preceded Newton in the discovery of the refraction of light; von Guericke, of Magdeburg, invented the air pump; J. B. van Helmont opened new methods of chemical research; Napier invented logarithms; and Newton created the differential calculus.

In this infinite desire for knowledge, this thirst for penetrating into the innermost secrets of Nature, one sees arising the desire to amplify the powers of the organs of sense, to increase the possibilities of seeing, studying, investigating. It is this period that gave to science one of the most valuable of all its instruments of investigation: the microscope. The studies that we have mentioned and the spirit that animated them crystallized the need for more perfect instruments to investigate the mysteries of nature in the fields of the infinitely great and the infinitely small. This we owe also to Galileo, the inventor of the telescope and the first scientific user of the microscope. Govi has shown that already in 1610 Galileo had adapted the telescope to extremely small objects, and that he had constructed an instrument for the examination of the organs of very small animals. In 1614 he spoke about it to several friends, and Détarde, who visited him at Florence, states that he had seen, thanks to this instrument, flies that were as big as sheep, and had observed that they were covered with hair and provided with angular joints. In the *Saggiatore* Galileo speaks of this instrument, to which the name "microscope" was given by a member of the Accademia dei Lincei, Demisciano or Fabre. Thus this discovery, later perfected by excellent technicians, reduced philosophic speculations to concrete facts, controlled and demonstrated experimentally. While the early history of the microscope is enveloped in considerable obscurity, it is usually accepted that the first compound microscope was probably constructed by Zacharias JANSEN, a spectacle-maker of Middelburg, about 1590. Hooke's compound microscope, a half-century later, is much better known; but none of these probably had a resolving power equal to the biconvex single lens that Leeuwenhoek made for himself, literally hundreds of times. It is easy to understand that in all the enthusiasm for exact study, the pursuit of the sciences played an important role.

It is about this time that the study of botany took on a truly scientific character. Marcello Malpighi is the creator of the modern anatomy of plants in a work that he presented to the Royal Society of London in 1675. In zoology we recall the names of Marco Aurelio Severino, of Calabria; Antonio Maria Valsalva, who studied the sensory organs of animals; Antonio Pacchioni, who made detailed investigations on the meninges of animals; Antonio Vallisnieri, who was particularly concerned with the anatomy of worms; Malpighi, whose studies on the anatomy of the silkworm were highly praised by Cuvier and Haller. Malpighi also discovered the respiratory organs of insects and their vascular circulation, the structure of the optic nerve of fishes, and made many other important discoveries. Gian Alfonso Borelli, the leader of the Iatro-physicists, was a profound student of the physiology of animals, and Francesco Redi, an eminent physician, anatomist, physiologist, and littérateur, was the first to repudiate, as we shall see, the spontaneous generation of insects. Francesco STELLUTI (1577–1651) was one of the first microscopists to study the eyes, antennæ, and heads of bees, publishing excellent illustrations in the Italian translation of Persius (1630). Robert HOOKE (1635–1703), in his *Micrographia* (London, 1665), gave a brief description of the cellular nature of plant tissue, as seen by him in razor cuts of cork, where the word " cell " was used for the first time. The study was further developed by Nehemiah GREW (1641–1712) in his *Anatomie of Plantes* (1682), which contained much more adequate illustrations of the cellular nature of plants. Jan SWAMMERDAM (1637–80) published in 1669 his *Historia insectorum*, dealing with the metamorphoses of insects, the effect on animals of the deprivation of blood, and similar subjects. His *Bijbel der Natuure* was not published until long after his death, by Boerhaave in 1737. This contains what was probably the earliest observation of animal erythrocytes, a discovery that was made independently by Malpighi and Leeuwenhoek. Thus in various biological fields in all the countries of Europe studies were fermenting which led the way to better knowledge of the functions of organs, tissues, and cells, and of the forms and manifestations of life.

One of the most important factors in the evolution of scientific thought in this century was the creation of various scientific academies. Culture was spreading rapidly and in ever wider circles, as Giacosa has observed in his study of Redi. The upper classes of the day had a lively interest in all forms of intellectual activity: scientific investigations, as well as works of art and literature. Purely scientific gatherings were extended to include types of men whom today one would regard as not competent for or interested in such discussions. It was in the wide diffusion of this love of scientific research, and perhaps also the desire for literary or medical *conversazioni*, that arose the desire to form societies where scholars and those who wished to pass as scholars could gather and communicate the results of their work. In each little town of Italy these academies sprang up. The most ancient, the Accademia dei Lincei (Academy of the Lynx-eyed, from its device of a lynx, as a symbol of sharpness of vision), founded at Rome in 1603 by Prince Cesi, can properly be regarded as the first of all these scientific bodies. One of the earliest scientific societies was the Societas Ermeneutica, founded at Rostock in 1622, which, however, lasted only a short time. In 1652 there was founded in Germany the Collegium Naturæ Curiosorum, essentially a gathering of physicians, which in 1677 became the Academia Cæsarea Leopoldina-Carolina. Shortly after it began publication of a *Miscellanea curiosa sive ephemerides medico-physicorum germanorum*, which took high rank among the scientific publications of the seventeenth century. In 1648, under Ferdinand II, Grand Duke of Tuscany, the foundations were laid for the famous Accademia del Cimento (Academy of Experiment), which was definitely organized by the Prince-Cardinal Leopold of Tuscany in 1657. The Cardinal himself, who enthusiastically conducted physical experiments, was a member of the Academy, which met in the palace of the Grand Duke. This Academy was the beacon of the scientific ardour that enlightened Italy at this time. Its members included such gifted spirits as Borelli, the brothers Del Buono, Viviani, Redi, and Magalotti, the secretary. The Academy, which was generously supported by Leopold, would undoubtedly have exerted a decisive influence on scientific development in Italy if it had not been dissolved by the Prince in 1667. In Bologna, a small " *Coro Anatomico* " was organized by Bartolomeo Massari, with nine members, including Malpighi. In 1645 an " Invisible College " had been founded in London, including Boyle, Wren and other advanced spirits; this later joined with a Philosophical Society at Oxford, and in 1662 received its charter from Charles II as the famous Royal Society of London. Two years later it began to publish its *Philosophical Transactions*, which has continued to the present time as one of the best-known scientific journals in the world. It attained such a high standard that communications were made to it from many of the leading scientists of Europe, such as Malpighi and Leeuwenhoek. The French Académie des Sciences, following the foundation of the Académie Française by Richelieu in 1635, was founded by Colbert in 1665 and began publishing its transactions in 1699.

These academies, which were rapidly augmented by many others, such as those of Brescia, Bologna, Dublin, and Berlin, became the centres of scientific activity. Perhaps for the first time in history experimental work profited from the intelligent and cordial collaboration of men working in various fields of knowledge. In the history of science the academies completed the work of the universities in the Renaissance period and prepared the way for the laboratories of modern schools. Finally, it is important to note that it is to the academies that we owe the publication of the reports of their meetings, and these in turn gave rise to the first scientific journals. The earliest of these was the *Journal des Sçavants* (Paris, 1665). We shall speak later in more detail of this literary movement, which was an important factor in the development of medical science in the last half of the seventeenth century.

Thus we see that the principal characteristic of this century should be sought in a decisive orientation of medicine toward the natural sciences and experimental research, an orientation, as we have tried to show, that was also determined by the philosophic trends of the time. In a period when the philosophy of Descartes posed the problem of dualism and the investigations of Galileo demonstrated the necessity of probing the depths of natural phenomena and raised a corner of the mysterious veil of Nature, it is easy to trace the route that medicine was to follow. Science became experimental; medicine followed philosophy because philosophy itself turned to Nature, to keep step with the natural sciences, chemistry, and physics, fields in which physicians intuitively realized that the secrets of life were to be most directly sought. Objective criticism and collaboration became indispensable from the very character of these studies. The earlier philosophers could by themselves in the silence of their studies create the basis of philosophic systems without being concerned with what was being produced about them, but the investigator of this century, desiring to explore physics and botany and chemistry, could not remain by himself. He had to seek the aid of his companions in research; he had to give such aid himself. From this necessity arose the academies and the scientific journals. For the same reasons a new type of university came into existence, destined no longer to be merely a meeting-place for students where each professor, even though from a foreign country, gave lectures on his own account; but rather a work-place of intellectual labour founded on a vast collaboration which rapidly became international.

It is in this century that one can begin to speak of a real international science. There had been a medicine of Babylon, Egypt, India, the Jews, Greece, and Rome, each in its turn having its effect on other civilized peoples, but only through a simple penetration of ideas without any collaboration between physicians or scientists of different countries. During the Renaissance science had been chiefly Neo-Latin; it was chiefly in the Latin universities that there was a highly organized scientific instruction. But in the seventeenth century in all civilized countries this collaboration of scientists became a decisive as well as a characteristic feature. The relations between countries became intensified. The results of discoveries were quickly spread abroad; the work of Boyle was known in Italy almost as soon as in England; Malpighi became no less popular in London than in Bologna; Harvey announced his discoveries almost simultaneously in Flanders, England, and Germany, and they were discussed immediately afterwards on a vast scale and throughout civilized Europe. Having considered the characteristic factors in the evolution of medical thought in the seventeenth century, let us now examine the great discoveries, the most significant lines of progress, and the most representative men of the period.

2. Anatomy and Physiology

Anatomy and physiology underwent a marvellous development in this century. The problem of the circulation of the blood, perhaps already visualized by Leonardo, had been partly solved by Servetus' announcement of the pulmonary circulation, Realdo Colombo's denial of the pores in the septum, and the discovery of the valves in the veins by Canano and Fabricius. The concept was still further advanced by the contributions of Cesalpino. But it was the genius of William Harvey (1578–1657) that completed the solution of the problem, with a true vision of its importance and masterly comprehension of its details, a rare technical skill in experimental demonstration, and a marvellous clarity in the exposition of his results. He was able to comprehend the problem in its broadest phases, definitely outline the main factors of the circulation, and demonstrate the truth of his hypothesis with a logically arranged and successfully prosecuted series of experiments. William HARVEY was born on April 2, 1578, at Folkestone, England. After graduating from Canterbury Grammar School, he entered Caius College, Cambridge, in 1593, where he received a B.A. degree four years later. Wishing to study on the Continent, he naturally turned to Padua, where he was the pupil of Casserius and Fabricius, who was, as we have seen, himself closely connected with the study of the circulation. Receiving his M.D. degree in Padua in 1602, Harvey returned to London, became physician to St. Bartholomew's Hospital, and later Professor of Anatomy and Surgery and physician to James I and Charles I. Having followed the fortunes of the King in the Civil War, he returned to London, where he devoted as much time as possible to his studies. Though he was made President of the Royal College of Physicians, he was not especially successful in practice, perhaps on account of the suspicions engendered by his physiological studies. After the publication of his immortal work on the circulation, his scientific activities were for many years concerned with the complex study of generation. His conclusions were eventually published in

1651 through the efforts of his friend Sir George Ent, under the title *Exercitationes de generatione animalium*. This work played by no means so important a role in the complicated study of embryology as did his discovery of the circulation in its field. However, nothing had equalled it in this field since the time of Aristotle. In fact, without the use of the micro-

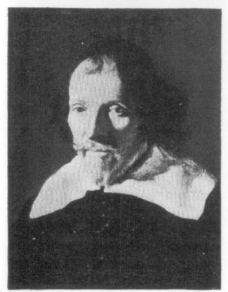

233. *William Harvey.*
(*From the portrait in* CAIUS COLLEGE,.
CAMBRIDGE.)

scope it is obvious that the subject could not have been greatly advanced at that time. Harvey recognized the importance of pathologic anatomy and was concerned with it. It was he who was ordered to do the autopsy on Old Parr, who died at the age of 152 (report published in 1669), and he gave one of the earliest descriptions of spontaneous rupture of the heart. Many of his manuscripts were lost when his lodgings at Whitehall were stripped by the Roundheads, and probably still others when the old building of the College of Physicians was destroyed in the Fire of London. Shortly before his death from gout, with a terminal " palsy giving him an easy passport," he transferred his property to the Royal College of

Physicians to provide for a librarian and an annual oration, which is still given by the most eminent members of the profession in Great Britain.

The experiments of Harvey, establishing the mechanics of the circulation, lasted almost twenty years. His crabbed manuscript notes, in a curious mixture of English and hog Latin, for his Lumleian Lectures in 1616 have fortunately been preserved at the British Museum. From these we know that his theory was already sufficiently well formulated for him to say: " It is proved by the structure of the heart that the blood is perpetually transferred through the lungs into the aorta, as by two clacks of a water bellows to raise water. It is proved by the ligature that there is a transit of blood from the arteries to the veins; whereby it is demonstrated that the perpetual movement of the blood in a circle is brought about by the beat of the heart. Is this for the sake of nutrition, or the better preservation of the blood and members by infusion of heat, the blood in turn being cooled by heating the members and heated by the heart? " Not for another twelve years, however, did he publish in Frankfurt (1628) his famous book *Exercitatio anatomica de motu cordis et sanguinis in animalibus*, which definitely upset the erroneous views of Galen that still formed the basis of instruction in the schools of the period. In seventeen chapters, condensing the results of his years of experimentation, Harvey established beyond any doubt the phenomena of the circulation. He demonstrated that

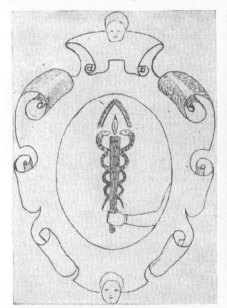

234. *Harvey's* stemma *in the atrium of the* UNIVERSITY OF PADUA.

235. *The frontispiece of Harvey's* De motu cordis (*Frankfurt, 1628*).

the heart contracts during systole, and that the blood is forced from the right heart by way of the pulmonary artery through the lung and from the left heart into the general circulation; and that during diastole the blood flows from the great veins into the auricles and then passes into the ventricles.

Harvey's great merit, which makes him one of the greatest figures in the history of science, is that of having proved the various steps of the problem by a series of inductively arranged physical demonstrations. He demonstrated the return of the blood to the heart by way of the veins and also that it was a mathematical necessity. Garrison observes that it is the first time in the history of medicine that mathematical proof and exact calculations were used in biological research. Harvey states that the heart is a pump, functioning by muscular force. Observing, as in Fabricius' experiment, that a vein swells below a ligature — that is, away from the heart — he was the first to interpret this phenomenon properly and to show that the statements of Galen were erroneous. His series of experiments on the exposed hearts of living animals demonstrated the occurrence of systole and diastole, the heart-beat occurring during systole and the pulse wave in the arteries distinctly later. He was the first to note the movement of the auricles of the heart and to perceive that this motion was transmitted to the ventricles, and he correctly states that this part of the heart is the *ultimum moriens*. To establish the pulmonary circulation, Harvey was not content with experiments on animals, but also utilized the mathematical evidence of the comparison of the capacity of the veins and the pulmonary arteries

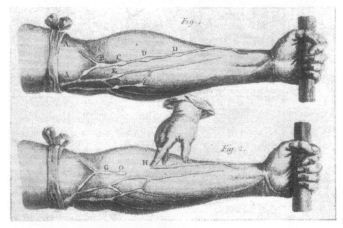

236. *Harvey's demonstration of the direction of the blood flow in the veins. Compare this with Fabricius' illustration of the same topic (Fig. 178).*

with that of other vessels. Mechanics led him to the conclusion that the beat of the pulse in the arteries came from the impact of the column of the blood against their elastic walls.

In regard to the direction of the current in the veins, Harvey utilized the existence of the valves and their position in the great veins above as well as below the heart to deduce correctly that they served, not merely to counteract the effect of gravity in the veins, as his predecessors had thought, but to prevent a reflux from the heart. Calculation of the volume of blood in the body in comparison to the time and number of pulsations was also used by him in filling out a definite and complete picture of the circulation. As the capillaries were not known to Harvey, he suggested an imaginary anastomosis between arteries and veins in order to make the complete circle possible.

We give here from his *De motu cordis* the historic words in which Harvey summarized his concept of the circulation: " And now I may be allowed to give in brief my view of the circulation of the blood, and to propose it for general adoption. Since all things, both argument and ocular demonstration, show that the blood passes through the lungs and heart by the action of the [auricles and [1]] ventricles, and is sent for distribution to all parts of the body, where it makes its way into the veins and pores of the flesh, and then flows by the veins from the circumference on every side to the centre, from the lesser to the greater veins, and is by them finally discharged into the vena cava and right auricle of the heart, and this in such a quantity or in such a flux and reflux thither by the arteries, hither by the veins, as cannot possibly be supplied by the ingesta, and is much greater than can be required for mere purposes of nutrition; it is absolutely necessary to conclude that the blood in the animal body is impelled in a circle, and is in a state of ceaseless motion; that this is the act or function which the heart performs by means of its pulse; and that it is the sole and only end of the motion and contraction of the heart " (Ch. 14, translation by R. Willis, Sydenham Society Publications).

There was still one link of the chain lacking for the complete demonstration: the proof of the existence of blood capillaries. This was furnished by Malpighi, who in 1661, with the aid of the microscope, discovered their existence and substituted them for Harvey's imaginary anastomosis.

Harvey's announcement of the discovery of the circulation excited violent opposition. Many writers took pains to demonstrate the inconsistency of his statements, among whom was James PRIMROSE, the son of a Scottish emigrant to France. His book against Harvey, said to have been written in fourteen days, was to serve as a good example of a Galenist attacking the new doctrine by fair means or foul. Other opponents were Gassendi, Caspar Hoffmann, and Giovanni della Torre, who emphasized the scandal caused by this man who was trying to demolish so many " succulent dogmas " and magnificent theses. The most cultured and most violent of Harvey's adversaries was Jean RIOLAN (1577–1657), who, in Baas's phrase, proved that eternal opposition could procure a certain kind of immortality. Riolan maintained that if dissections no longer agreed with the descriptions of Galen, it should be attributed to the fact that Nature had changed since Galen's time, but that one should not admit that Galen had been wrong. Riolan is one of the few whom Harvey dignified with a written reply; in 1649 he addressed two Anatomical Disquisitions to him that were chiefly concerned with combating the various objections that had been raised to his theory. GUY PATIN (1601–72), an eminent member of the Faculty of Paris, declared Harvey's theory " paradoxical, useless, false, impossible, absurd, and harmful." This statement is characteristic of Patin, one of the most interesting figures in the French medicine of the century. He carried on violent quarrels in the name of the faculty with all innovators,

---

[1] These two words do not occur in the original text.

against the physicians of Montpellier, against Renaudot, van Helmont, and many others. His letters, republished by Pic in 1911, give a vivid and bold picture of the condition of physicians and of the Paris Faculty at that time.

But against these opponents who attempted to cover Harvey with contumely, more eminent and authoritative voices arose in his support. The Dane Niels STENSEN (1638–86), the Frenchman Raymond de VIEUSSENS (1641–1715), the Germans Werner ROLFINK (1599–1677), professor at Jena, and Hermann CONRING (1606–81), the Dutchmen Franciscus SYLVIUS and Jan de Wale (WALÆUS) (1604–49), and the latter's pupil, the Dane Thomas BARTHOLINUS (1616–80), and Harvey's countryman Richard LOWER (1631–91), and his friend Sir George ENT, all warmly upheld Harvey's theory and proved its correctness by further studies on the anatomy and function of the heart and great vessels.

Technical improvements, to some of which we have already referred, helped materially in the intensification and productivity of research. The gross injection of vessels, which had already been suggested by Leonardo and was practised by Eustachius with coloured fluids, became a much used method. In 1668 de Graaf, for instance, injected the spermatic vessels with mercury. Especially important were the low melting-point materials used by Swammerdam. He first used suet (*Proceedings of the Royal Society*, 1672) and later changed to the more efficient wax (1677), training Ruysch in their uses. Similar methods were employed by Domenico MARCHETTI (1626–88), of Padua, and Steven BLANKAART, of Middelburg (1650–1702).

Knowledge of the circulation of the body fluids received support from the discovery of the chyliferous vessels (lymphatics) by Gaspare ASELLI, of Cremona (1581–1625). His book, *De lactibus sive lacteis venis*, was published in 1627, just before the *De motu* of Harvey, who had not appreciated Aselli's discovery and perhaps was not aware of it. Lacteals were already known to the ancient Greeks, and Fallopius seems to have seen them when he speaks of veins coursing over the intestines full of a yellow matter and going to the liver and the lung. It seems that Eustachius had also seen them, as he describes a similar appearance and speaks of a whitish canal going from the clavicular area to lower parts. But these were merely sporadic observations; the observers of these vessels had no comprehension of their function or importance.

Aselli, while he was doing an autopsy on a dog on July 23, 1622, to show some friends the recurrent laryngeal nerves, also wished to observe the movements of the diaphragm. Opening the abdomen and holding back the stomach and intestines, of a sudden he noticed whitish cords spread over all the mesentery and intestine in numerous branches. At first Aselli thought he was dealing with nerve filaments, but then he saw that the intestinal nerves were entirely different and distinct. Undecided as to their nature, he cut across one of the largest of these cords and saw a white cream-like liquid exude. Turning to his colleague, Alexander Tadino, and to the Senator Settala, President of the Council of Health, he cried out: " Eureka! " This observation, which Aselli hastened to repeat carefully, led him to describe the new vessels under the name of *venæ albæ et lacteæ.* He described the valvules at the point of departure of the intestinal vessels and the course of the lymphatics, and, before the publication of Harvey's book, wrote these remarkable words about the circulation: " Perhaps it would not be absurd to suppose that the blood brought to the lung by the *vena arteriosa* (pulmonary artery), mingled with the air attenuated by the lung and returned to the left ventricle through the *arteria venosa* (pulmonary vein). Perhaps it is not necessary to imagine the passages that Galen supposed to exist in the interventricular septum, which could not have any use."

In 1647 Jean PECQUET (1622–74), of Dieppe, discovered the thoracic duct of the dog, and the canal that joins it with the superior *vena cava* (*canalis Pecqueti*); his experiments (*Experimenta nova anatomica*, Paris, 1651) confirmed Harvey's theories and the earlier studies of Aselli. Olaf RUDBECK (1630–1702), of Sweden, a student at the University of Padua, on January 27, 1651 discovered the lymphatic vessels of the intestine, distinguishing them from the lacteals (*Nova exerc. anat.*, Westerås, 1653). Bartholinus re-examined the relations between the lacteals and the lymphatics and gave the first adequate description of the lymphatic system as a whole.

This is not the place to describe the acrid discussion that arose between Rudbeck and Bartholinus as to the priority of this discovery. It will suffice to state that the discoveries of both these illustrious scientists definitely mark an important event in the history of medicine, in permanently eradicating the central position of the liver in the economy of the organism. Bartholinus wrote the last page of this episode with an epitaph on the liver, " whose empire is dead." It was not rehabilitated by Della Torre's hymn *Pro sanguifico hepate* (1666), which Daremberg quotes in his discussion of this whole episode.

Giovanni Guglielmo RIVA (1627–77), of Asti, was Professor of Anatomy at Rome, teacher of Lancisi, and surgeon to Louis XIV and Clement X. This distinguished anatomist and surgeon created an important anatomical museum, which unfortunately has been lost, and left a series of unpublished anatomical plates, including a graphic presentation of the entire lymphatic system. He also started a society for the discussion of pathological observations, to which he made notable communications — among other things, on the then little-known subject of aortic aneurysm.

The story of the circulation of the blood can be closed with the gifted work of one of Italy's most distinguished scientists, Marcello MALPIGHI (1628–94), of Crevalcore near Bologna, who was one of the leading anatomists and histologists of history. It is not without significance that the subject of his doctoral thesis was the superiority of the Hippocratic doctrine.

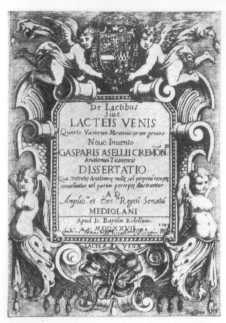

237. *Frontispiece of Aselli's* De lacteis venis (*Milan, 1627*).

Pupil of Borelli, one of the boldest pioneers in experimental medicine, Malpighi was already a professor at the University of Pisa at the age of twenty-eight. A few years later, having returned to Bologna, he began the publication of his numerous discoveries, but he encountered such hostility from the physicians of Bologna, faithful conservators and obstinate champions of the theories of Galen, that it seemed impossible for him to remain there. He accepted the invitation of the Senate of the University of Messina, where he taught for four years, not without finding there also the same opposition from the Galenists. Once more returning to Bologna, he was much comforted by his election in 1669 to the Royal Society of London.

Malpighi's life is a good example of the hostility that had to be borne by those who dared to combat the ancient ideas. Such was the force of dogmatism and the inveterate respect for classical opinions that anatomical demonstration and microscopic proof were insufficient to convince these enemies of all progress. His fiercest enemies were Paolo Mini, Professor of Anatomy, and Giovanni Sbaraglia, lecturer on medicine and anatomy at Pisa, who insisted that the truth must lie with Galen and the ancients, and publicly criticized and derided the observations and discoveries of Malpighi. The struggle became so violent that in 1689 he was assaulted by two of his masked colleagues of the university, as is told by him in a letter that was published by Medici (*Compendio storico della scuola anatomica bolognese*, 1857). Malpighi spent his later years in Rome under the patronage of Innocent XII, who made him his physician and had a high appreciation of his worth.

Malpighi is the founder of knowledge of the anatomy of the tissues. He was one of the first biological scientists to make use of the microscope, which opened up a vast field to his extraordinary genius for research. A worthy botanist, he established the foundations for future botanical research in his great work *Anatomia plantarum*, which was published by the Royal Society of London, in two volumes (1675–9). His studies on animals, and especially on the silkworm, were no less profound. From these he passed to the study of the lungs (*De pulmonibus*, 1661), in which he was the first to demonstrate the vesicular structure, and

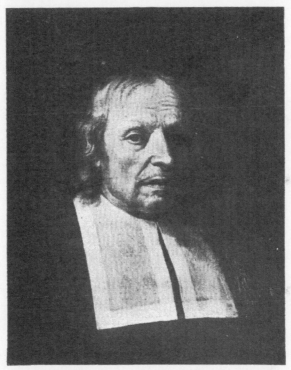

238. *Marcello Malpighi. Painting by C. Cignani.*
(COLLECTION OF PROF. PUTTI, BOLOGNA.)

to the development of the ovum (*De formatione pulli*, 1673). In 1661 he made the important discovery of the existence of capillaries in the lungs and in the mesentery of the frog. In 1665 he described in the blood the corpuscles which we now recognize as the erythrocytes. His histological studies were extended to many species, from the eagle to the butterfly, from the glowworm to the earthworm, from fishes to parasites. He made a profound study of the structure of the lymph nodes and the spleen (*De viscerum structura*, London, 1659), distinguishing in the spleen the corpuscles which bear his name, and the glomeruli in the kidney. More than anyone else he was the creator of microscopic anatomy, a tireless investigator, unshakable in his defence of the truth, penetrating in his observations, scientifically honest in his conclusions, and a genius in his productions. He was the founder of the new anatomical school of Bologna, and as teacher of Valsalva led the direct line to Morgagni, Scarpa, and Panizza.

We quote Malpighi's description of the capillaries: "I saw the blood, showered down in tiny streams through the arteries, after the fashion of a flood, and I might have believed that the blood itself escaped into an empty space and was gathered up again by a gaping vessel, but an objection to the view was afforded by the movement of the blood being tortuous and scattered in different directions and by its being united again in a determinate part. My doubt was changed to a certainty by the dried lung of a frog which to a marked extent had preserved the redness of the blood in very minute tracts, which were afterwards found to be vessels, where by the help of a glass I saw not scattered points but vessels joined together in a ring-like fashion. And such is the wandering about of these vessels as they proceed on this side from the vein and on the other from the artery that the vessels no longer maintain a straight direction, but there appears a network made up of the continuations of the two vessels. . . . Hence it was clear to the senses that the blood flowed along sinuous vessels and was not poured into spaces, but was always contained within tubules, and that its dispersion is due to the multiple winding of the vessels" (translation in V. Robinson's *Story of Medicine*).

One of the most illustrious anatomists of the period was Francis GLISSON (1597–1677), pupil of Harvey, and later professor at Cambridge, whose studies on the liver are perpetuated in the "capsule of Glisson" (*De hepate*, London, 1654). He also was a noteworthy early contributor to the knowledge of rickets. Thomas WHARTON (1614–73), on the basis of his discovery of the duct of the submaxillary gland, Wharton's duct, announced that all glands had their secretory ducts (*Adenographia*, London, 1656). This led Niels STENSEN (Steno) (1638–86) to a more detailed study of the anatomy of glands and his discovery of the parotid and lachrymal ducts (see his *Observationes anatomicæ*, Leiden, 1662). Stensen travelled widely through Europe and especially in Italy, where he was converted to Catholicism and nominated as Bishop of Titiopolis. He lived many years at the court of Tuscany, where he was a close friend of the Duke Cosmo III. Among the many individual discoveries that followed in rapid order about this time should be mentioned Nathaniel HIGHMORE's antrum (*Corporis humani disquisitio anatomica*, The Hague, 1651); Thomas WILLIS's circle of cerebral vessels (*Cerebri anatome*, London, 1664); R. LOWER's tubercle and other structures of the heart (*Tractatus de corde*, London, 1669); Clopton HAVERS's canals in the bone (*Osteologia nova*, London, 1691); J. C. BRUNNER's duodenal glands (*Glandulae duodeni*, Frankfurt, 1687); H. MEIBOM's glands of the conjunctivæ (*De vasis palpebrarum*, Helmstädt, 1666); A. NUCK's salivary ducts (*De ductu salivali*, Leiden, 1685); J. C. PEYER's patches in the intestine (*De glandulis intestinorum*, Schaffhausen, 1677); T. KERCKRING's *valvulæ conniventes* (*Spicilegium anatomicum*, Amsterdam, 1670).

Among eminent Italian anatomists was Lorenzo Bellini (1643–1704), of Florence, pupil of Redi and Borelli, who occupied the chair of medicine at Pisa at the early age of twenty-one. He was a tireless investigator and keen observer, noted for the elegance and clarity of his literary style. His study of the structure of the kidney, published at the age of nineteen (*De structura renum*, 1662), demonstrated among other things that the striations on the cut surface were minute tubules and not cords, as had been supposed. His descriptions of the organs of taste are also worthy of note.

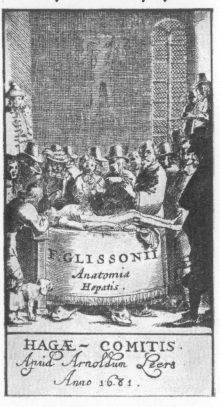

Antonio Maria Valsalva (1666–1723), pupil of Malpighi and teacher of Morgagni, was especially noted for his studies on the anatomy and physiology of the ear: the functions of the ear-drum, ossicles, and semicircular canal. To this end he practised hundreds of dissections; his book, *De aure humana* (1704), constituted a standard on the subject for more than a century.

Valsalva was the first to subdivide the ear into its external, middle, and internal portions, a division that was quickly accepted by all anatomists. He also described the sebaceous glands of

239. *Frontispiece of Glisson's* Anatomia hepatis (*1681*).

the skin of the lobe of the ear, which he related to those in other parts of the body, and the preauricular lymph node, connecting it through its structure and relations with the lymphatics and the parotid ducts.

The muscles of the external ear, as Politzer, the Viennese otologist, who was a great admirer of Valsalva, observes, had escaped previous students on account of the difficulty in bringing them out in anatomical preparations. Valsalva also described the superior bundle of the anterior ligament of the ear and the spine of the helix. He accurately outlined the external auditory canal, and, better than his predecessor Duverney, described the incisuras, of which the most anterior bears the name of " the great incisura of Valsalva." His observations on the middle and internal ear were no less important. He described and named the

Eustachian tube. He carefully studied the function of the labyrinth, searched carefully for the supposed *foramen Livini*, studied the form and capacity of the tympanic cavity, examined the auditory apparatus of the fetus, in fact was concerned with all the anatomical, physiological, and pathological problems of the ear. He is chiefly recalled to medical students today by the eponymic sinuses behind the semilunar valves of the aorta. They are described on pages 129–31 of his *Opera* (Venice, 1740).

Throughout his writings Valsalva manifested a devoted attachment to Malpighi, whose stimulus as a friend and colleague determined his methods

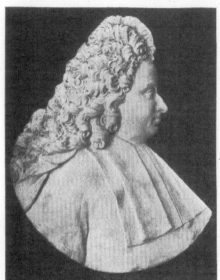

of study and investigation. According to his pupil Morgagni, who left a biographical monument to his master, Valsalva was an excellent physician and surgeon as well as anatomist. Suffering from ill health toward the end of his life, he worked unceasingly and enthusiastically, and if, as Politzer has remarked, practical otology did not receive from him all the benefits that might have been expected from his profound anatomical and pathological knowledge, one finds in his work nevertheless a beginning of a rational treatment that opened new ways and perspectives. Valsalva was also one of the first to introduce a humane treatment of the insane, who up to that time were

240. *Antonio Maria Valsalva.*
Bas-relief in the Library of Imola.

still treated, according to the phrase of Celsus, "by hunger, chains, and torments."

Another distinguished Italian anatomist of the seventeenth century was Giulio Casseri (1552–1616), one of Harvey's teachers at Padua. In 1604 he became lecturer on anatomy at Padua and in 1627 (Venice) published a *Tabulæ anatomicæ*, which contained excellent illustrations of the anatomy of the organs of speech and hearing.

Antonio Pacchioni, of Reggio Emilia, friend and pupil of Malpighi, with whom he collaborated in the publication of the anatomical plates of Eustachius, was particularly concerned with the anatomy and function of the dura mater. According to him, it was to be regarded as a muscular tissue whose contractions served to push the nervous fluid toward the periphery. He described in the dura mater the small bodies that bear his name and the incisura of the *tentorium cerebelli.*

Another disciple of Fabricius who contributed to anatomy was Adrian SPIGELIUS (van den Spiegel) (1567–1625), whose name is connected with the caudate lobe of the liver and the *linea alba,* on the midline aponeurosis of the abdominal muscles. Born at Brussels, Spigelius studied at Padua,

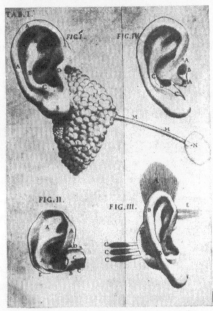

241. *The ear.*
(*From Valsalva's* De aure humana,
1704.)

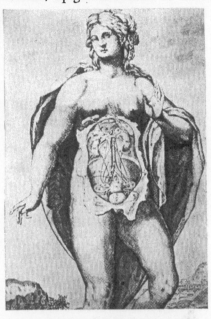

242. *The abdominal organs.*
(*From the anatomy of Giulio
Casseri, Venice, 1627.*)

where he was inscribed in the registry of the " German Nation." He received his doctorate in 1605, and, with Fabricius, treated Fra Paolo Sarpi, who had been severely wounded by an assassin. He taught anatomy at Padua from 1618 to 1624. In Favaro's biography we learn that, like many contemporary anatomists, he was also a good surgeon and often practised trephining of the skull.

Among other well-known foreign anatomists who studied at Padua was Johann VESLINGIUS (Wesling) (1598–1649), of Minden in Westphalia, whose *Syntagma anatomicum* (Padua, 1641) was translated into many languages and for more than fifty years was the anatomy text most generally employed in the universities. Choulant regards it also as an important landmark in the history of anatomical illustration. Johann Georg WIRSUNG (1600–43), a Bavarian, was Wesling's prosector and the discoverer of the pancreatic duct (recorded on a unique copperplate, 1642). He was killed by a shot from an arquebus in a private quarrel with a Belgian.

Anatomical illustration was promoted in the seventeenth century by the use of copper engravings, which surpassed even the splendid woodcuts of the Renaissance. After Casseri's *Tabulæ* follow the *Anatomia* (1685) of Govert BIDLOO (1649–1713) and of Bernardo GENGA (1691). The *Thesauri Anatomici X* (1701–16) of Frederik Ruysch (1638–1731) profited by his knowledge of coloured injections and by the special charm of the quaint illustrations. Ruysch's anatomical preparations, and especially the so-called "mummies," acquired a great contemporary reputation. His laboratory

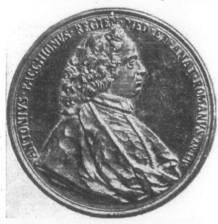

243. *Antonio Pacchioni.*
Bronze medal by Hamerani.

was visited by Peter the Great, who bought some of them to be used in anatomical instruction in St. Petersburg. Ruysch was also an able microscopist, who studied especially the structure of various organs such as the kidney and the testicles, and the anatomy of the placenta. The engravings in the *Anatomy of Human Bodies* (Oxford, 1698) of William COWPER (1666–1709) were largely plagiarized from Bidloo, a discreditable procedure even in those days, which was promptly excoriated by Bidloo in a published communication

to the Royal Society. The urethral glands named after Cowper were described in his *Glandularum quarundam nuper detectarum . . . descriptio* (London, 1702). They had previously been described by Méry in 1684. The *Catoptron microcosmicum* of Johann Remmelin (born 1583, Ulm), with its superimposed visceral plates, is perhaps the best known of this type of anatomical illustration, which also figured in the fugitive sheets of this and earlier periods (see Leroy Crummer, in *Annals of Medical History*, 1923, V, 189).

To Antoni van LEEUWENHOEK (1632–1723), of Delft, belongs the high merit of having been the first to use the microscope systematically and of having brought the construction of the simple microscope in his own hands to a high degree of perfection. One of Leeuwenhoek's microscopes that is still preserved at Utrecht has been shown to have extraordinarily good resolving power and a magnification of almost two hundred diameters. Self-taught and never having attended a university, ignorant of Latin and

Greek and of the classical texts, he became one of the greatest and most expert microscopists, thanks to the sagacity of his observations and the perfection of his technique. He was constantly constructing new microscopes, always of the simple variety (a single biconvex lens), but varying in construction, depending on the type of material to be examined. Leeuwenhoek

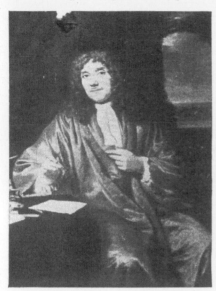 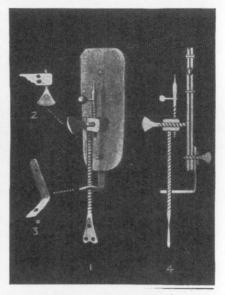

244. *Antoni van Leeuwenhoek. (From the 1695 edition of his* Works.)
245. *Leeuwenhoek's microscope. (From Dobell's* A. van Leeuwenhoek and His Little Animals, *London, 1932.) 1 shows the instrument seen from behind; 4 is a lateral view. The biconvex lens is mounted between two metal plates prepared with appropriate seating for the lens. In this instrument the object to be examined is placed on the metal point, which can be moved by the means of a screw. Another screw serves for the lateral movement of the optical part of the instrument. 2 and 3 show details of the construction. The eye is placed close to the lens. Other instruments were designed to examine liquids or spreads on glass plates.*

regarded microscopic examination as the means to an end rather than an end itself. His contemporaries have stated that he often stayed for hours at a time examining the most varied objects microscopically: liquids, organic tissues, " little insects," without any predetermined program or any preconceived ideas, occupied only with seeing and understanding.

Leeuwenhoek discovered and made fairly accurate estimates on the size of the red blood corpuscles in both vertebrates and invertebrates; he studied the walls of the vessels that controlled the movement of the blood in the capillaries, and even attempted to estimate the blood velocity. He was the first to describe the anatomical structure of the teeth and to study the blood vessels. He examined the structure of muscles, observing their fibres and their increased size in contraction. He was the first to discover the laminated structure of the lens of the eye and to explain accommodation, and he also contributed to the knowledge of the anatomy of the nerves and of the skin. He was the first to describe the spermatozoa and protozoa and to demonstrate micro-organismsion the teeth, giving what constitutes the first illustration of various kinds of bacteria (September 17, 1683). Most (375) of his observations were communicated to the Royal Society, his work finally being collected in his *Ontledingen en Ontdekkingen* (Leiden, 1685), his *Brieven* (4 vols., 1685–1718), and in his *Opera omnia* (Leiden, 1722).

He lived quietly at Delft, a placid burgher attending to the small details of a modest existence, but always enthusiastically pursuing his microscopic studies. His letters, many of which are published in Dobell's biography, are illustrative of his patient and diligent work. Though neither the inventor nor the first user of the microscope, as some historians have stated, he undoubtedly deserves the credit of having been one of the earliest and most successful microscopists, whose personal characteristics place him high among the contributors to this field.

Diacinto CESTONI (1637–1718), of Leghorn, a pharmacist to Cosimo III, was the first to describe the acarus as the etiologic agent in scabies, in a letter to Redi, written together with his friend the physician Giovanni Cosimo BONOMO (1687). Though scabies had been recognized as contagious since Biblical times and was one of the eight diseases generally accepted as contagious in the Renaissance, its definite cause had never been previously observed. This discovery constitutes the first proof of an organism of microscopic size being the cause of a definite disease. Though their discovery was translated into Latin and English, it was soon forgotten, resurrected by Wichmann in 1786, forgotten again, eventually to be established with experimental as well as clinical proof by RENUCCI, pupil of Alibert, in the Hôpital St. Louis at Paris.

An early microscopist of note was Father Athanasius KIRCHER (1602–80), born at Geysa in Germany, later professor at Würzburg, until he abandoned Germany for Italy during the Thirty Years' War. He became Professor of Mathematics at the College of Rome, and on his death left a valuable archæological museum. Though a mystic and often given to confused and fantastic ideas, he accomplished historically important work in the natural sciences, especially his studies which led him to believe that invisible animals were present in putrefied tissue and that the contagion of plague was due to similar minute bodies (*Scrutinium physico-medicum*, Rome, 1658).

Holland was especially distinguished for its anatomists in this century.

This was, as we have seen, the period in which Holland was asserting its political liberty and reaching the height of its commercial expansion and financial prosperity. The portraits of these illustrious anatomists have been transmitted to us in many paintings by Dutch artists, who also led the world at that time. Group portraiture was much in vogue. In that country, where

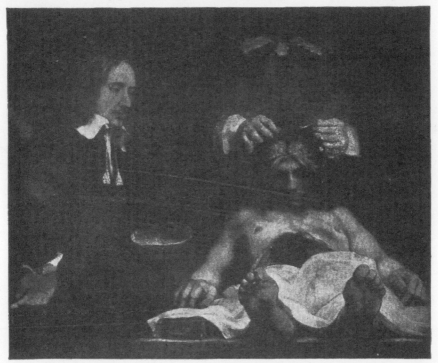

246. The Lesson in Anatomy of Dr. Johan Deyman, *by Rembrandt.*
(*A fragment in the* AMSTERDAM MUSEUM.)

a cultured, free, and powerful bourgeoisie held in skilful hands the conduct of the State, and proud and flourishing cities led the commerce and economics of half the world, physicians enjoyed a high social rank. The people showed a particular interest in science and especially in anatomy. Possession of an anatomical theatre was regarded by a city as being as much of an asset as an art museum would be to a city of today.

Pieter PAAW had founded the first Dutch anatomical theatre at Leiden in 1597; De Ghein's painting (engraved by A. Stog) shows him in it surrounded by his friends and pupils. Nicholas TULP (1593–1674), Professor of Anatomy at Amsterdam, with his pupils forms the subject of that marvellous painting by Rembrandt *The Lesson in Anatomy*, which is one of the great artist's masterpieces and one of the most valuable paintings of all time. Sebastian Egbert DE VRIJ is portrayed in two celebrated pictures, one by A. Pietersz (Amsterdam, 1603), the other by Thomas de Keyser (Amsterdam, 1619). The names of all the surgeons who surrounded the Professor of Anatomy are known; so that it appears that such lessons were not followed only by students but also by physicians, often by high officials or

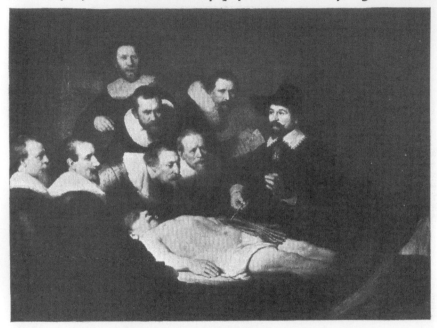

247. *The Lesson in Anatomy of Dr. Tulp, by Rembrandt.*
(THE HAGUE MUSEUM.)

rich citizens who wished to attend the distinguished performance. Another of these interesting historical documents is the painting by Juriaen Pool (1666–1745), the nephew of Ruysch, representing Boekelman, the President of the Society of Surgeons, showing to his colleague, Six, a heart with injected arteries.

Regnier DE GRAAF (1641–73) was a Dutch anatomist and physiologist who was celebrated for his work on digestion as well as on the anatomy of the genital organs, *vasa deferentia*, and the tubules of the testicle (*De virorum organis generationi inservientibus*, Leiden, 1668). He discovered the ovarian follicle (1672), to which Haller gave the name " Graafian." In his *De natura et usu succi pancreatici* (Leiden, 1664) de Graaf demonstrated the function of this organ after collecting the pancreatic juice in an experimental fistula. He also studied the nature of the bile collected in the same way from a biliary fistula. Philip VERHEYEN (1647–1710) was the author of a treatise on anatomy (1693, and a larger edition in 1710) which contained interesting microscopic studies. He maintained that the blood plasma was the really important part of the blood in the nutrition of the body. Frederik DEKKERS, of Leiden (1648–1720), enjoyed a wide reputation as physician and surgeon, but concerns us more as an early contributor to clinical pathology with his discovery of albumin in the urine (1694), which could be detected by boiling it with acetic acid.

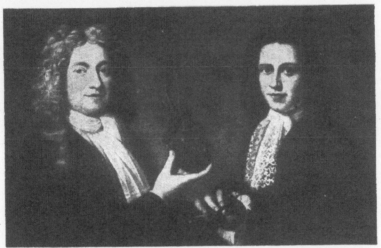

248. *Boekelman, the President of the Company of Surgeons, shows his colleague, Six, a heart in which the arteries have been injected — by Juriaen Pool.*

In France the study of anatomy was promoted especially by Claude PERRAULT (1613–88), Joseph Guichard DUVERNEY (1648–1730), who wrote an early treatise on otology (1683), Pierre VERNEY (1678–1730), and Raymond de VIEUSSENS (1641–1730), professor at Montpellier, who contributed especially to the anatomy of the nervous system (*Neurologia universalis*, 1685), the ear, and the heart. He was the first to give an adequate description of the structure of the left ventricle, the coronary sinus, and the distribution of the coronary vessels. He observed pericardial adhesions and effusions, described and depicted aortic insufficiency long before Corrigan, and mitral stenosis before Morgagni and Corvisart (*Traité . . . du cœur*, Toulouse, 1715).

In pathology, Theophilus BONETUS (1628–89), of Geneva, collected in his *Sepulchretum sive anatomica practica* (Geneva, 1679) a large and extraordinary amount of pathological material, describing some three thousand cases.

Although his book contains many inaccuracies, partly due to the relatively few cases that were observed by him directly, and although the cases are classified clinically in anatomical order rather than pathologically, nevertheless his work constitutes an invaluable document in the history of pathology, and Haller was justified in accepting this book as worth a whole pathological library. However, the *Sepulchretum* was chiefly a storehouse of miscellaneous observations; the synthesis of such observations into a systematic whole had to await the masterly hand of Morgagni. Aided by an excellent index, the reader today can find many cases that are still interesting clinico-pathologically. For instance, Observation 46 of the first section gives little doubt that a cyst of the pituitary gland is being described, perhaps for the first time. Particularly important is Bonetus' contribution to pulmonary tuberculosis, of which he includes more than one hundred and fifty cases. Though vague and obscure about the etiology of tuberculosis, he groups consumption and tabes of glands and bones in the same chapter and gives a clear description of miliary tuberculosis (Case 17 quoted from Heurnius): "the whole parenchyma of the lung was seeded with minute tubercles." Among the circulatory diseases he includes Lower's case of tricuspid endocarditis, also his experimental production of œdema, and ruptured aortic aneurysm. He describes cases of syphilis and tumours of bones, dropsy from obstruction of veins by abdominal tumours, nephritis chiefly from ascending infection, and gives many other interesting clinico-pathological correlations. The case described by Jean Jacques Manget, who republished Bonetus' book in 1700 with the addition of personal observations, is of particular interest. In a young man who had died of consumption, minute granulations (*grandines*) were found scattered through the lungs, liver, kidney, intestine, and mesentery glands. Manget was the first to compare these granulations to millet seeds (*magnitudine seminum milii*). He clearly observed the cheesy degeneration of tubercles, which he said he had also found in cattle, pigs, and poultry. He believed that it was these tubercles that formed the cavities and that it was the cavities that produced consumption; but these very interesting observations passed almost unobserved.

The concept of consumption owed a stimulus to the classical *Phthisiologia* (1689) of Richard MORTON (1637–89), of London. A careful observer and skilled physician, Morton described tubercles, which he regarded as formed by the obstruction of certain glandular parts of the lung. He noted that the tubercles were "sometimes bad, gangrenous and very dangerous," at other times "more benign, which one often observes in hard, cold swellings that develop chronically but change into plaster-like material presenting the consistency of honey." He also described the tuberculous glands which form about the trachea and the roots of the bronchi and considered their importance as probable causes of pulmonary tuberculosis; but these observations remained as dead letters for the clinicians of the period, who completely ignored them.

The post-mortem studies of Johann Jacob WEPFER (1620–95), of Schaffhausen, first clearly revealed the causative relation of cerebral hemorrhage to apoplexy (*Observationes anatomiæ ex cadaveribus eorum quos sustulit apoplexia*, Schaffhausen, 1658). The striking signs of apoplexy had concerned the ancients since the time when Nabal became as a stone for ten days before he died (I Samuel xxv, 37). The classical writers had

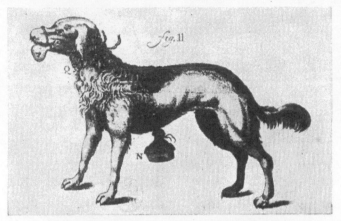

249. *Experimental pancreatic fistula.* (*From De Graaf's* De succo pancreatico, *1664.*)

observed its phenomena and estimated its prognosis, but had confused the condition with various other sudden deaths and offered quite fanciful explanations of its cause. Wepfer's discovery, which was not one of chance, thus constitutes an important landmark in pathological anatomy. He was a famous physician who recognized the great value of autopsies and went to great trouble to procure them. When he died of " asthma," his body was examined " as customary "; and an extensive sclerosis and calcification of the aorta were found.

3. *Iatrophysical (Iatromechanical, Iatromathematical), Iatrochemical Schools. Beginnings of Experimental Research*

At the moment when anatomy was entering into its most flourishing period, physiology and pathology developed a movement toward the experimental method based on the mathematical and philosophical trends that have been earlier described — the great schools of the iatrophysicists and iatrochemists. They represent the first efforts to impose the control of exact calculation and objective observation on medical research. Though their efforts teemed with errors in calculation and conclusions, these schools thus represent an important step in medical progress. Sanctorius' metabolic studies of patients on his famous scale, Borelli's use of mechanical laws to explain vital phenomena, van Helmont's attempts to reduce the doctrines

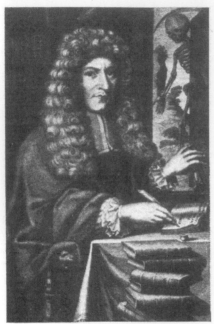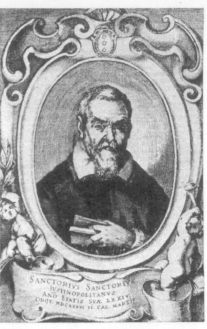

250. *Theophilus Bonetus.*
(*Portrait from his* Sepulchretum,
Geneva, 1700.)

251. *Santorio Santorio. Engraving
by Piccini.*
(*From the 1600 edition of his*
Opera omnia.)

of Paracelsus and Sylvius to formula as a scientific basis for the humoral theory — all these are examples of a trend that was less important in its immediate results than as an introduction of quantitative, objective methods in experimental medicine.

Santorio SANTORIO (Sanctorius) (1561–1636), of Capodistria, professor at Padua and leading representative of the IATROPHYSICAL SCHOOL, with his quantitative experiments opened a new line in medicine, the importance of which he appears to have realized. Before Sanctorius only qualitative changes had been the object of medical study. With his innovations, and particularly his studies of " the insensible perspiration," as he called it, the first investigation of metabolism in pathology and physiology brought to research a quantitative basis controlled by instruments of precision.

The ancients had already supposed the existence of an evaporation, and Galen had spoken of a *diapnoe* — that is, a respiration through the skin of the whole body in the form of a light vapour. Sanctorius understood the importance of evaluating this respiration by exact measurements. His invention, which at that period was something new and unheard of, as he states, consisted in the use of the balance as the instrument of control. He placed his work-table and his bed and all that he needed for existence on a specially constructed balance and thus was able to investigate the alterations in his body weight produced by solid and liquid secretions in various normal and pathological conditions. His experiments, which he continued with admirable patience and pertinacity for more than thirty years, were described in a series of aphorisms in his *De statica medicina* (Venice, 1614). The success of the book was phenomenal; it was translated into all European languages and went through many editions. But more important even than the practical results is the value of this book in making proved experiments the basis of all his observations and conclusions, thus constituting one of the most courageous affirmations of experimental medicine. He had numerous followers; among them Dodart, Gorter, Lining, and Bryan. His investigations stimulated his followers up to the time of Lavoisier and Séguin, whose more precise measurements superseded those of Sanctorius.

One can of course oppose many objections to his "insensible perspiration" and its importance. One must admit, however, the value of the physiological concept of this physician, mechanist, and mathematician, for whom every disturbance in the humours could cause disease and for whom this disturbance was largely produced by an excretion of these substances through the skin.

Further evidence of the innovating quantitative spirit of this great Italian is afforded by other instruments invented or successfully applied by him: he used a thermometer to measure the temperature of the body, being perhaps the first to do so; he invented a hygrometer and a pulsimeter to register the movements of the pulse, and a kind of water bed, together with various surgical and other instruments. (See Castiglioni on Sanctorius, 1920; English translation, *Medical Life*, 1931.)

Another leader of the iatrophysical school was Gian Alfonso BORELLI (1608–79), of Naples, a pupil of Galileo and a teacher of Malpighi. In an efficient laboratory in his own house at Pisa, he applied the laws of mechanics and statics to all physical phenomena. According to Borelli the human organism should be regarded as a machine which functions according to determined laws: the circulation, respiration, and bodily movements are mechanical facts. The soul is the effective cause of animal movements; for, as he says, no one will deny that animate beings live because of their soul and that once they are dead — that is, once the action of the soul is finished — all movement also is stopped. Again, according to Borelli, the immediate instruments by means of which the soul brings about movement are muscles, which receive the motive force by way of the nerves. The anatomy and physiology of the muscles found a diligent investigator in

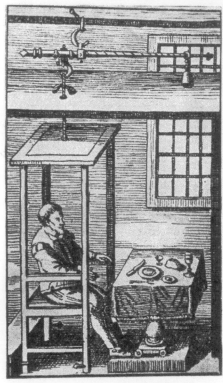

Borelli. He distinguished muscles of various forms and structures. He maintained that one could distinguish between the individual action of the fibres and a voluntary action. Borelli's book *De motu animalium* (1679) includes many mathematical calculations on the motor force of single muscles.

Borelli's explanations of the mechanical basis of the respiration and the circulation of the blood produced some very interesting observations, such as the importance of the intercostal muscles and of the diaphragm in respiration. But all his theories on the separation of the blood from the urine in the kidney, and of the bile in the liver, all his hypotheses of the circulation of a nervous fluid (*succus nerveus*) analogous to that of the blood, his entire theory of painful movements coming from a twitching of the nerves, and of febrile heat coming from fermentation of the nerve juice — all these definitely belong to the realm of empty hypothesis. In one case,

252. *Santorio on his balance.*
(*From* De statica medicina, *Venice,* 1614.)

however, his work had a lasting influence: his neurogenic theory of the heartbeat, which until modern times held the field against the myogenic theory with varying success, attributed the heart action to the action of the nerve juice on the heart through its various nerves. Borelli belongs to that class of scientists who when they are following a system which they have found confirmed in certain ways apply it inflexibly in other domains and modify the fact so as not to have to consider the problem of changing or modifying the system. However, he occupies a creditable position in physiology as a leader in the mechanical orientation of medicine which gave rise to a medical school of thought to which modern medicine owes much: the principle of regarding the living organism as subject to immutable and inescapable physical laws.

A pupil of Malpighi, Giorgio BAGLIVI (Ragusa, 1668–1706), whom we shall meet later in the section on clinical medicine, represents the extremes to which the iatrophysical school later proceeded. He divided the body machine into many smaller machines, comparing the teeth to scissors, the stomach to a flask, the heart and blood vessels to a system of water-works, the thorax to bellows, and so on. Baglivi was the first to distinguish smooth from striped muscle (1700).

Together with this mechanistic tendency, there developed an important movement toward a chemical explanation of vital phenomena — the IATROCHEMICAL SCHOOL. Jean Baptiste VAN HELMONT, of Brussels (1577–1644), a Capuchin friar and able chemist, can be regarded as the precursor of this school. He was a pioneer in the chemistry of gases, having invented the name "gas" (derived from the Greek *chaos*, as used by Paracelsus in the general sense of air). He was the first to discover carbonic-acid gas and made notable con-

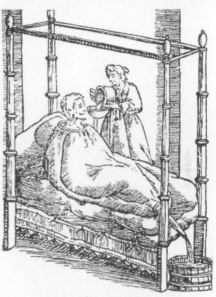

253. *The continuous bath invented by Santorio.*

tributions to pharmacology. His attempts to add to knowledge of renal function by weighing twenty-four-hour specimens of urine show at least an appreciation of quantitative methods, though they appear to have produced no practical results. His iatrochemical theories, however, which were derived from the system of Paracelsus, have none but a historical value.

Van Helmont was one of the most interesting medical figures of the seventeenth century. Agitated by passionate controversies and fierce persecution, even to the point of being denounced to the Inquisition by his rivals, he swayed between science and mysticism. As is shown by his own statement, he had apocalyptic visions in the Capuchin convent of Louvain which led him to the fervid analysis of Dioscorides and Hippocrates. His life reflects the history of his century, oscillating between anguished doubts and returns to the faith, between spiritual revolts and acts of contrition. In 1599 van Helmont became a physician; whereupon, falling seriously ill during a long voyage, he called in two physicians whose bedside discussions he later recalled with fierce irony. Losing all faith in medicine, he continued his travels, but later returned to the path of Paracelsus, whom he surpassed in the profundity of his observations and his scientific knowledge. Though exalted by some historians, his work on close examination does not deserve the high merit sometimes attributed to it. His theories neither explain nor dimly grasp the secrets of vital phenomena. His explanations of different *archæi*, of which the supreme *archæus* governs fecundity, not only explained nothing but did not even seem clear in the mind of their author. In the field of physiology van Helmont was not a convinced supporter of Harvey, according to Daremberg. For the physiology of the gastro-intestinal tract he relied on the authority of Hippocrates and created six ferments for his six types of digestion. He regarded nature as derived from divine power, which is represented in man by a vital body force, *archæus insitus*, and an *archæus influus*, the divine force which regulates physical and mental phenomena in man. Every modification of the *archæus* produced by the *idea morbosa* results in disease, every alteration of the regulating germ has as a secondary consequence the alteration of matter.

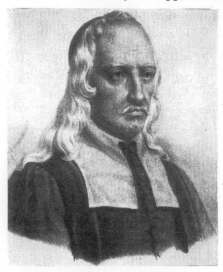

254. *Giovanni Alfonso Borelli.*
From a contemporary print.

Disease, according to the new concept of van Helmont, is an actual entity existing as an invisible principle endowed with various properties. This is not an opposition of two forces or a diathesis resulting from the struggle of contraries or an imbalance of the humours; disease is regarded as due to the operation of *idea* and of "seeds" in which the *idea* were included, aided by the intervention of the *archæus*. The products of disease are seminal generations, so that they depend on the seeds that are reproduced. This will serve as a brief illustration of the concept of van Helmont, who stated that he was inspired by God, to whom he often had recourse for his inspiration. These extraordinary lucubrations from an erudite and experienced scientist, who had violently attacked the ancient traditions, merely substituted for them an even more baseless system. It seems, then, that to him should only be attributed the merit, but a very significant one, of having given a new impulse along the chemical path indicated by Paracelsus. His physiological speculations, which were long the objects of admiring study, can be dismissed as nothing but non-constructive baroque hypotheses. His principal work, the *Ortus medicinæ, id est initia physicæ inaudita*, was published by the Elzeviers of Amsterdam four years after his death.

The real founder of the iatrochemical school was the Dutch scientist FRANÇOIS DE LA BOE, or du Bois, Latinized SYLVIUS (1614–72). Having studied at Dutch and German universities and being graduated at Basel, he became professor at the University of Leiden, where his attractive personality, handsome appearance, and outstanding lectures drew students from all parts of Europe. Founding his system on the newer knowledge of anatomy, physiology, and clinical medicine — the circulation, the lymphatics, glandular action — Sylvius was an important factor in constructing a more rational system of the practice of medicine. His humoral physiology stressed the triumvirate of the saliva, the pancreatic juice, and the bile, all bodily forces being subjected to the chemical processes of fermentation and effervescence. The saliva promoted digestion in the stomach, the pancreatic juice and the bile determined the direction of the ingested food into the blood and fæces. The blood was the centre where the most important processes of normal and pathological life were produced. As Daremberg has observed, Sylvius constructed a chemical picture in a purely Galenical frame. All diseases are explained and treated chemically, and the indications for treatment are based on a supposed chemical relation between the disease and the drug. Sylvius was a determined supporter of Harvey's doctrine. An able investigator, his name is connected in anatomy with the aqueduct and the fossa that bear his name; in physiology, he envisaged the concept of acidosis and explored the functions of the ductless glands and of the thermal and tactile senses. Not only was Sylvius the first to describe tubercles but he clearly related them to consumption and observed their progress into cavities. However, he remained faithful to classical medicine in regarding them as the result of hemorrhage, peripneumonia, and empyema. He wrote: "I found more than once larger and smaller tubercles in the lung, which on section were shown to contain pus. I believe that these tubercles become purulent and are changed into cavities, which are lined with a thin membrane. In these tubercles I hold that not infrequently phthisis has its origin." His therapeutic ideas are illustrated by the following: " If all the blood is black, that indicates that acid predominates, while if it is red, the bile predominates. In the former case it is necessary to diminish the acid in the body and the blood; in the latter to diminish the bile and weaken its strength." Sylvius recommended sudorifics, absorbents, and emetics and condemned blood-letting.

In England the head of the iatrochemical school was Thomas WILLIS (1621–75), of Oxford. Willis was an acute clinical observer: he was the first to notice the sweetish taste of diabetic urine (1670), to describe the disease now known as myasthenia gravis (1671), to describe and name puerperal fever, and to note that certain deaf people appeared to hear better in the presence of noise (*paracusis Willisii*). In addition, his *Cerebri anatome* (1664) was the best account of the nervous system that had yet been written, giving the first description of the eleventh or spinal accessory nerve (nerve of Willis) and of the communicating arteries at the base of the brain, known as the "circle of Willis." Another English iatrochemist was John MAYOW (1645–79), who was one of the most important precursors of Lavoisier in the physiology of the respiration. His experiments showing that venous blood was made red by the addition of his nitro-aerial spirit, obtained from nitre, came close to the later-established oxygenation of the blood in the lungs. William CROONE (1633–84) held similar views and also wrote enlightened monographs on embryology, *De ovo* (*Philosophical Transactions*), *De ratione motus musculorum* (Amsterdam, 1676). He is better remembered today by the Croonian lectures of the Royal Society that were endowed by his widow. Opposed to the iatrochemical school of thought were Robert BOYLE of the Chemical Society, and Henry STUBBES in clinical medicine, while John FREIND (1675–1728), the medical historian, opposed the iatrochemical views on ferments. In Holland, the chief representative of the iatrochemists was Cornelius BONTEKOE (1647–87), whose book (German translation, *Die Lehre vom Alcali und Acido durch Wirckung der Fermentation und Effervescentz,* 1721), asserted that thickening of the blood was the cause of all disease. Tea-drinking, by thinning the blood, was therefore a panacea; but here Bontekoe has been accused of partiality, being in the pay of the newly prominent group of Dutch tea-merchants. In Germany, iatrochemistry had as a precursor Daniel SENNERT (1572–1637), whose corpuscular theory attempted a compromise between the chemical doctrines of Paracelsus and those of Aristotle and Galen, though, like most of his contemporaries, he was a firm believer in witches and pacts with the devil. Among German iatrochemists were Michael ETTMÜLLER (1644–83), Wolfgang WEDEL (1645–1721), Christian SCHELLHAMMER (died 1716), and Baron Ignatius von BEINTEMA, the physician of the Emperor. Opposed to them, however, were the more eminent J. C. BRUNNER, J. N. PECHLIN, CONRING, Johann BOHN, and eventually Friedrich HOFFMANN. In France, there were many supporters of the theory: the younger Riolan, Guy Patin, Nicolas de Blégny, who founded an Iatrochemical Academy in Paris, Vieussens, Astruc, and lesser lights. In Italy, iatrochemistry found few supporters, and these inconspicuous.

PHYSIOLOGY, profiting by the anatomical discoveries of the age, leaned more on exact calculations and control experiments and less on philosophic speculation. In embryology particularly was progress to be noted, practically for the first time since the classical Greeks. As we have seen, Harvey in his *Exercitationes de generatione animalium* showed that the embryo developed from the egg by the process of " epigenesis " (that is, not pre-formed in the ovum, but growing by a successive appearance and develop-ment of the various structures). De Graaf and Malpighi contributed significantly to knowledge of the ovum and the ovarian follicle, and Swammerdam to generation in the lower animals. In 1677 the Dutch pupil of Leeuwenhoek, Johann HAM, of Arnhem (1650–1723), discov-ered the spermatozoon (*animalcula seminis*). A. Vallisnieri taught in *The History of Generation of Man and Animals* the fundamental doc-trine of the various stages of genera-tion. He showed the significance of the egg, and its passage through the Fallopian tube, the construction of hydatids, and their fundamental dif-ference from the ovaries. In the con-test which arose between the so-called " Oviparists " and the " Animalcul-ists," following Ham's discovery, Antonio VALLISNIERI (1662–1730), professor at Padua, made decisive contributions in favour of the impor-tance of the ovum. Other important

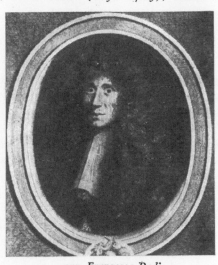

255. *Francesco Redi.*
(*From his* Opere, *Venice, 1712.*)

studies were made by Domenico SANTORINI (1681–1737), whose name is preserved in the pancreatic duct that bears his name and who first described the corpus luteum.

Francesco REDI (1626–68), of Arezzo, is without any doubt one of the most interesting figures in Italian medicine. De Renzi is correct in calling him the Father of Helminthology, while his studies on the poison of vipers (1664) and on the generation of lower animals place him in the first rank of biological investigators. His *Osservazioni intorno agli animali viventi che si trovano negli animali viventi* (1684) is one of the earliest and best works on parasitology. He was the first to demonstrate the repro-ductive organs of ascaris and described more than one hundred species of parasites. He was never tired of studying chrysalids, snakes, pigeons, fish, tortoises, insects, in the various stages of their existence. A facile writer, spirited in polemic, he developed his arguments with subtle logic and clar-ity of interpretation. He is regarded as one of the best Italian poets of this century, but as Giacosa has stated, even without his *Bacco in Toscana*, his

Poemetti and *Sonetti*, his scientific writings would have revealed the artist in their precision, clarity, and elegance of style. A man of extraordinary good sense, reserved in statement and calm in judgment, he avoided all grandiloquence and pedantry. His *Consulti* reveal an honest thinker and capable physician who is concerned above all with aiding his patients, protecting them from charlatans and the abuse of drugs, and leading them toward a temperate life and wise dietary.

A passage from his *Esperienze intorno alla generazione degli insetti* (1668) shows how well the scientific writers of that day were able to express their thoughts in clear diction understandable by the laity: " From many observations that I have made, I am inclined to believe that since the first plants and first animals were produced in the first days of the world by the command of the sovereign and omnipotent Pastor, the earth has never of itself produced any herb, or tree, or animal, perfect or imperfect, and that everything that has been born in the past and everything that we see born in it or from it comes entirely from the real and veritable seed and plant of the animals, which preserve their species by means of this seed. . . . In closed bottles, I have never seen even a worm produced after many months had passed since the bodies (of animals) had been introduced. One day I killed a large number of worms that were produced in some beef flesh and put some in a closed vessel and others in an open vessel. In the first, nothing more was produced, though in the second, worms appeared which changed into eggs, then into ordinary flies; and the same phenomenon was repeated with a large number of these flies killed and placed in similar vessels, some open and others shut, for nothing was ever seen to be produced in the closed vessel."

Among those who founded physiological doctrines that flourished in this century was Francis Glisson, whom we have already mentioned in connection with the capsule of the liver. Glisson, who in a certain sense approaches the theories of Borelli, supposed that there existed in every living body the faculty of being stimulated by external influences of activity and movement, to which faculty he gave the name of " irritability."

Thus in his work on the anatomy of the liver Glisson asked himself what are the causes that make the bile ducts secrete a larger amount of bile under certain circumstances, answering that this happens when the vessels are in a state of irritation: " Every part that suffers from an incommodity seeks to disembarrass itself. That might be called an irritation, and the parts capable of perceiving the damage and reacting against it can be said to be capable of irritation."

In later works, *Tractatus de naturæ substantia energetica* (London, 1672), and *De ventriculo et intestinis* (Amsterdam, 1677) he maintained that " irritability " was the prime cause not only of muscular movement but also of life itself. Materialistic and mechanistic, Glisson's theory takes origin from psychology and metaphysics as regards his idea of sensibility, and is connected with physiology by this new concept of irritability. According to Glisson, the powers of movement and life in general are properties of the organs. Irritability is the property of the muscle fibre in perceiving irritation and reacting to it. When the irritation stops, contraction stops also and the muscular fibre relaxes. Matter is energetic; crude matter is endowed with movement and, up to a certain point, with intelligence. In the various fibres there are different kinds of movements, depending on whether they come from the brain, as is the case in animal movement, or from an agent that has no well-defined site, but is carried from the heart by way of the blood (natural movement).

Glisson's hypotheses are the interesting attempts of an able thinker to explain important physiological phenomena. His views on nervous irritability, which were much praised by Haller, who had his own view on the importance of this property, constitute an important step in physiology. In practical medicine Glisson wrote what should be regarded as the original account of infantile rickets (*De rachitide*, 1650); according to the English historian Norman Moore, Daniel Whistler's slightly earlier account (*De morbo puerili anglorum*, 1645) is of minor importance and probably based on what he had learned from Glisson.

An important Italian physiologist was the Florentine Lorenzo BELLINI (1643–1704), pupil of Borelli and Redi, who was the author of a book on the anatomy and physiology of the organs of taste (*Gustus organum . . .* 1665), and of a larger work on the arterial pulse, together with some considerations on the origin of fever (*De urinis et pulsibus*, 1683). He also studied phlebotomy, investigating the utility of this procedure in clinical medicine.

Italy was still regarded as the leader in physiology, as is shown by Junken's statement of about 1700: " Let him who seeks skilful physicians go to Italy because it is only there that one can find men who are trying to unveil the secrets of nature and to explain on the basis of mechanical principles the hidden cause of diseases."

4. Clinical Medicine

The most characteristic tendency in the evolution of medical thought in the seventeenth century was the orientation toward the exact sciences. This trend to research and to experimental studies, however, brought with it the danger of again separating the physician from the bedside of the patient. Some of the great anatomists and physiologists of this period, some of the great investigators, discoverers, and founders of new schools, actually practised medicine little if at all, so that one might have had the impression that the chief function of the physician was to devote himself to anatomical study or to mathematical calculations rather than to the study of the patient. The frequent appearance of new theories and hypotheses tended to turn the attention of the physician from practical medicine, or at least to separate the investigating physician from the clinicians, who were pleased to call themselves Hippocratists. It also introduced the danger of erecting systems and schools maintaining that practical medicine had no other basis than experimentation.

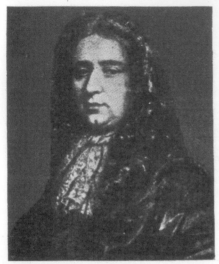

256. *Thomas Sydenham.*

It was an English physician, Thomas SYDENHAM (1624–89), who had the great merit of recognizing the need for returning to common sense and practical methods, faithful to the true principles of Hippocrates, where the supreme goal of medicine was the care of the patient. It was Sydenham who brought medicine back to clinical observation and personal experience. While iatrochemists and iatrophysicists conducted their violent polemics, Sydenham returned to Hippocrates, affirming the need for living close to the patient and for not constructing the house, as he said, before the foundations were established. Born at Winford-Eagle, in Dorsetshire, Sydenham studied at Oxford and perhaps also at Montpellier, but interrupted his studies to enlist with the Parliamentarians in the Civil War which had just broken out. Chancing to take up the study of medicine, he received his doctorate in medicine at Cambridge, and began in London a practice which soon became very large. He believed that the cause of all diseases should be sought for in nature and that their cure was due to nature.

In his reaction against the ultra-literary developments of medicine, especially in Italy, he doubtless went too far in ridding himself of all literary baggage. To a friend who asked what was the best book for a young physician to use as a practical guide, he advised the reading of *Don Quixote*. He regarded disease as an entity independent of the individual invaded and maintained that the body tried to rid itself of all morbid material through the blood. He recognized in fever a process which aimed to purify the blood of the disease, distinguishing acute diseases in which the febrile process developed rapidly, and chronic diseases in which it took place slowly and with difficulty. He returned to the Constitution concept, believing that Nature possessed a secret instinct that directed it. He suggested the existence of an Animal Constitution, predisposing to certain diseases at certain seasons (such as pneumonia at the beginning and end of winter), and an Epidemic Constitution coming from various meteorologic factors. Following the example of Hippocrates and his book on Epidemics, he carefully studied the epidemics that occurred in London at the time.

His therapy is fundamentally Hippocratic. He followed the antiphlogistic method, chiefly using diet, purgatives, and bleeding. Among specific drugs, he was among the first to recognize the curative powers of cinchona bark, which had just been brought to Europe from Peru, and of opium, in the form of Sydenham's Drops, which he regarded as an excellent remedy for the heart. With such a therapeutic arsenal, in which simples played a prominent part, he left the chief role to the healing powers of nature.

The title of " the English Hippocrates," given to him by his contemporaries, and the lasting veneration of subsequent English physicians, were eminently deserved by this man who, without following any system or allying himself with any school, put the Hippocratic concept of good sense and clinical observation back in its former position of honour. His epidemiological observations also were in line with the straight Hippocratic tradition, while his chief aim seems to have been to bring medicine back to simple and practical lines. His extraordinary success in practical medicine is not surprising in view of his intelligent and close attention to the symptoms and course of the individual disease, instead of the long dissertations to the patient, couched in abstruse terms, which were still the fashion. He left excellent clinical descriptions of many diseases: smallpox, malaria, consumption, rheumatic polyarthritis (*Observationes medicæ*, vi, Ch. 5), scarlatina, which he named and differentiated from measles (1675), the acute febrile form of St. Vitus's dance, which is still known as Sydenham's chorea (1686), and hysteria (from *hysteron*, the uterus), which he recognized as occurring in males as well as females. Best known is his classic *Tractatus de podagra* (1683), which contains such a vivid account of an acute attack of gout that it should be read by every medical student. His *Opera universa* (1685), reprinted a score of times in the next century, was frequently translated into English and several other languages. His *Processus integri* (1695), was the favourite therapeutic vade mecum in England until the nineteenth century.

It seems logical that this reaction against the baroque in medical literature should have taken place in a country where the healthy criterion of common sense and moderation in criticism has always predominated. Thus Sydenham appears, not as a violent revolutionary, but as an able, common-sense practitioner who understood that the great need of medicine was the careful bedside observation of clinical phenomena, and that the chief aim of the physician should be to make himself useful to the patient. Of all the returns to Hippocrates that are to be found in the important periods of medical history, Sydenham's is without any doubt one of the most significant. It is noteworthy that this return to the Hellenic idea in medicine occurred at a period when the Greek ideal of political liberty was revived in England by Cromwell and the spirit of the Greek drama was being equalled by Shakespeare.

Boerhaave, who, as we shall see, led clinical teaching in the next century, derived in a direct line from the school of Sydenham.

Italy in this period also possessed a noteworthy pioneer in clinical medicine, Giorgio Baglivi, the iatrophysicist, who, however, is shown in his book *De praxi medica* (1696) to have been a profound observer and eminently practical clinician. Students flocked to Rome to hear his lectures, his practice was extending rapidly, and he was at the height of his fame when he died at the early age of thirty-nine. He can be regarded as the master of Italian clinicians. His teaching can be condensed in his simple phrase: " Let the young know that they will never find a more interesting, more instructive book than the patient himself." In another place he says: " Idle talk is of no use; one should only study in the light of reason and experience and indefatigably investigate the truth. . . . Let those who read my book think that experience alone has guided me, that vain hypotheses and grandiloquent systems serve no purpose. To study medicine, it is necessary to compare disease with disease, moment with moment, and man with man, and to abandon for ever these interminable discussions and logomachies, for which I find no other explanation than the anger of an outraged and avenging God who has inflicted them on man."

Among the physicians who followed the return to Hippocrates was Bernardino RAMAZZINI, a renowned student of disease and medical practitioner of whom we shall speak later in regard to his outstanding work as the founder of a new discipline in medicine, the study of occupational disease. Glisson, Bonomo, Vieussens, Willis, Freind, Bartholinus, and B. de Moor (1649–1724), to whom Neuburger (1898) attributes original ideas on hysteria, all followed the new trends. The Leiden anatomist Ysbrand van DIEMERBROECK (1609–74) is remembered not only for his studies of the plague (1644), but especially for his *Anatome corporis humani* (1672), which enjoyed considerable popularity throughout Europe. In 1642 was published the *De medicina Indorum* of Jacob BONTIUS (1598–1631), a book notable not only as an early work on tropical medicine but also for its first description of beriberi. He seems to have been well aware of the curative virtues of lemons in certain diseases. Other celebrated books on tropical medicine were those by Willem PISO (1611–78): *De Indiæ utriusque re naturali et medica* (Amsterdam, 1658), and *Historia naturalis Brasiliæ* (1648), which contained the first description of yaws. Publications in special branches of medicine were increasing in number, though of course written by general practitioners, often the most important contributions to medicine being included as a part of a more general work. Thus in the

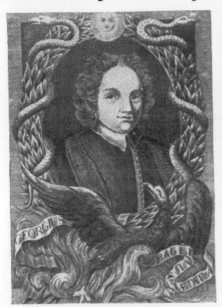

257. *Giorgio Baglivi.*
(*Frontispiece of the Lyon edition of his* Works, *1704.*)

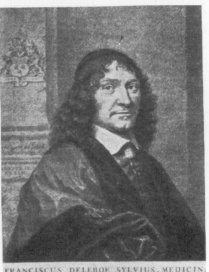

258. *Franciscus Sylvius (De La Boe).*
(*From a contemporary engraving.*)

field of pediatrics Sennert's *De mulierum et infantium morbis* occurs as Bk. IV of his *Practica medicinæ* (Wittenberg, 1632); and the description of whooping cough (quinta) by Guillaume de BAILLOU (1536–1616) is to be found in his posthumous *Epidemicorum . . . libri duo* (1640).

Whistler's and Glisson's descriptions of rickets have already been referred to; also Plater's account of sudden thymic death in infants, a condition the actual existence of which still remains in doubt. Sydenham, Willis, and others made valuable contributions to the knowledge of children's diseases. The first book on the subject in Dutch was the *Ziekten der Kinderen* (Amsterdam, 1684) by Stephen Blankaart. In England the best known is the *De morbis acutis infantum* (London, 1689) by Walter Harris (1647–1732), which " attained a reputation far beyond its merits and was quoted and requoted for at least a hundred years " (Still).

In a quite different field England was beginning her long and valuable contribution to the progress of medicine through the study of VITAL STATISTICS, the Political Arithmetick of the day. Though the census was not yet in existence, a number of London parishes had joined in publishing Bills of Mortality. These were analysed by John GRAUNT (1620–74), a London haberdasher, for the total number of deaths and their distribution in different districts, the various diseases and their incidence, and similar items. His friend Sir William PETTY (1623–87) continued this pioneer work in *Essays in Political Arithmetick* (1683–7), which was carried still further by Gregory KING (1648–1712), whose *Natural and Political Observations* (1696) extended the study of demography to include economic problems of housing, family income, and so on. Edmund HALLEY (1656–1742), the astronomer, also published the mortality tables of Breslau (*Philosophical Transactions*, 1693) with applications to the calculation of life annuities. These studies, especially Halley's, gradually found their counterparts in other countries, especially Holland.

5. Surgery

The progress of surgery during the seventeenth century was neither so marked nor so important as might be supposed from the advances made in anatomy and pathology. But knowledge of anatomical discoveries diffused slowly and it was only much later that their full effect on medical progress became visible. Also the surgeons of the period lacked the scientific preparation that was even then available. Although the situation was improving daily, the abyss that separated them from physicians was still considerable.

Among the precursors of modern surgery is one whose name has largely been overlooked — Cesare MAGATI (1579–1647), of Scandiano. In his book *De rara medicatione vulnerum* (1616) he proposed a rational treatment of wounds, which, in spite of the example set by Paré, were still being treated with unguents of various kinds. He maintained that frequent exposure of wounds to the air was deplorable, and that the introduction of sounds and lint produced dangerous putrefaction. He denied the need for cleaning and anointing and prescribed bandaging with simple linen, to be renewed only after five or six days. These precepts, like those of Paré, were soon forgotten, however, and the old errors were continued into the eighteenth century.

Marco Aurelio SEVERINO (1580–1656), a well-known anatomist, was also a famous surgeon, who repeatedly practised tracheotomy during the Naples epidemic of diphtheria — a procedure that had already been recommended by Guidi, Fabricius, and Sanctorius. The last had even constructed a special sort of trocar to facilitate the operation. Severino's works, *De efficaci medicina* (Frankfurt, 1646), *Trimembris Chirurgia* (Frankfurt,

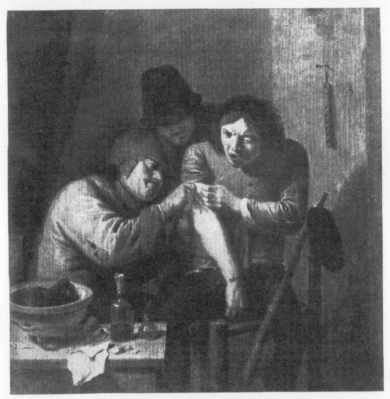

259. A surgical operation. Painted by Adrian Brouwer.

1663), and *De recondita abscessuum natura* (Naples, 1632), are noteworthy. The last named work, which included descriptions of neoplasms, granulomatas, buboes, and other lesions, as well as abscesses, is an important landmark in the history of surgical pathology. One of the earliest experimental surgeons of these times was Giuseppe ZAMBECCARI, of Florence, a pupil of Redi, who was the first known to have performed an experimental splenectomy. He successfully accomplished the experimental removal, wholly or in part, of various other abdominal organs (see Neuburger, *Medicinisch-Chirurgisches Centralblatt*, 1896, XXI, 368).

The history of BLOOD TRANSFUSION begins in this century, even though vague references to it can be found in older writers. The first definite description of blood transfusion was made by Giovanni COLLE (1558–1630), of Belluno, Professor of Medicine at Padua, and physician to Cosimo II of Florence, in the seventh chapter of his *Methodus facile procu-*

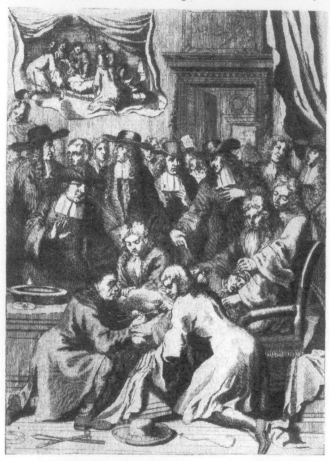

260. *Jacques de Beaulieu (Frère Jacques) cutting for the stone. Early eighteenth-century engraving.*

randi tuta et nova medicamenta (1628). Francesco FOLLI (1623?–85), of Poppi, in his *Stadera medici* (1680), advised transfusion by insertion of a silver tube in the artery of the donor and a bone cannula in the vein of the recipient, uniting the two by means of a tube especially made from an animal blood vessel. In 1665 the Cornishman Richard LOWER (1631–91) performed blood transfusion between animals (*Philosophical Transactions of 1666*, London, 1700, III, 226); and in the next year Jean Baptiste DENIS, physician of Louis XIV and professor of the Faculty of Paris, transfused blood from a lamb to a patient, with the help of the surgeon Emeret. The patient, who had been greatly weakened by a tremendous phlebotomy, improved for a while, but then died (from hemolysis by incompatible blood?). In spite of later successful attempts by other surgeons such as Riva (1668) and Manfredi (c. 1670), the above and similar results led the Paris Faculty of Medicine to secure the interdiction of blood transfusion, first by an Act of Parliament and later by a Papal bull, so that it fell into disuse for more than a century.

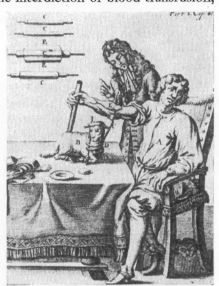

The most illustrious French surgeon of this century was Pierre DIONIS (b. Paris; d. 1718). He was surgeon to the royal house of France, and to him is owed the first idea of the foundation of the Royal Academy of Surgery. His *Cours d'opérations de chirurgie* (1707) was the best-known work on the subject during this century. The operation for lithotomy was so much in vogue that many operators were known as lithotomists. Such was the COLLOT family of whom the most famous, Laurent Collot, was lithotomist to Henry II, Francis II, and Charles IX. The last of the family, François (d. 1707), wrote a treatise on the subject. Jacques de BEAULIEU (1651–1714), a simple labourer, was one of the most celebrated lithotomists in France. Becoming a Franciscan, under the name Frère Jacques, he continued his surgical work and appears to have been one of the first to use the lateral incision. Other well-known lithotomists were Jean MÉRY (1645–1722), Barthélemy SAVIARD (1656–1702), and Georges MARÉCHAL (1658–1736), surgeon to Louis XIV.

261. Blood transfusion from animal to man.
(From Purmann's book on military surgery, 1721.)

Among German surgeons of the period were Fabricius Hildanus and Scultetus, who have already been considered in the previous chapter. M. G. PURMANN (1649–1711) was a skilful and courageous military surgeon who appears to have been an able writer, though a believer in sympathetic powders and in the weapon-salve for healing by absent treatment. In his numerous writings he describes a large number of surgical operations, including the transfusion of blood and forty cases of trephining of the skull.

Military surgery had a special development in Prussia in the hands of the Great Elector (1620–88), who introduced a good sanitary organization in his armies, fixing the pay and standing of his physicians and surgeons.

In England the outstanding surgeon was Richard Wiseman (1625–86), body surgeon to James I, Sydenham's contemporary, and a Royalist in the Civil War, who held in English surgery a position similar to Sydenham's in medicine. He was a skilful amputator, relieved strictures by external urethrotomy, and was the first to describe *tumor albus,* the white swelling of the joints due to tuberculosis. James Yonge's (1646–1721) *Triumphant Car of Antimony* (in Latin, 1679) is reminiscent of a similar title by Basil Valentine; it is full of original surgical ideas and observations, such as the use of flaps in amputations. Stephen Bradwell's *Helps in Suddain Accidents* (1633) is said by Garrison to be the earliest book on first aid to the injured.

Instruction of deaf mutes made considerable headway in this century. The principles of Pedro Ponce de León (1520–84), set down by J. P. Bonet (*Reduccion de las letras . . .* Madrid, 1620), were carried by Sir Kenelm Digby from Madrid to England, and by others to Italy. Giovanni Bonifacio's *L'Arte dei cenni* (Art of Signs) (Vicenza, 1616), and various British publications (by John Bulwer, John Wallis, W. Holder, and G. Dalgarno) and the *Surdus loquens* (1692) by J. C. Amman (1669–1724) are evidences of the speed with which this useful method made headway.

Veterinary medicine began to take form in this century; we have already noticed Carlo Ruini's work on the anatomy of the horse in connection with the discovery of the circulation. In Germany, Martin Böhme's *Artzeney . . .* (1618) was the standard for nearly a century, while in England Andrew Snape's *Anatomy of an Horse* (London, 1686) held a similar position. Noteworthy too was Jacques de Solleysel's observation that glanders was a transmissible disease in horses (1664).

6. Obstetrics and Gynæcology

In the history of obstetrics in the seventeenth century an important event was the introduction of obstetrical forceps, the use of which had already been suggested by Pierre Franco in 1561. Franco had pictured a speculum with three valves to be used for the extraction of the head. In 1647 a member of the Chamberlen family, probably Pierre, constructed a practical forceps in a fenestrated form with a curved head, not very different from the modern forms. The secret of the forceps was jealously preserved in his family, and the instrument was shown to no one. Several members of the family practised successfully with its aid in London, gaining considerable sums of money. Hugh Chamberlen tried to sell the forceps in Paris for a high price, but an unfortunate fatal result, with laceration of the uterus in a patient of Mauriceau, forced him to return to England without a sale. He eventually sold the secret in Holland to Roger Roonhuysen, and to various other physicians, but it was almost fifty years before it came into common use.

The story of the various attempts to construct obstetrical forceps, their varieties, the attempts to discover the secret of the Chamberlens, and their exploitation of the invention constitutes an interesting chapter in the history of obstetrics (see Fasbender, Fischer, and others). Jean PALFYN (b. Courtrai, 1650–1730) invented a popular forceps of two uncrossed valves, which was modified by Heister, Levret, and others.

One of the great masters of obstetrics was François MAURICEAU (1637–1709), whose celebrated treatise *Des maladies des femmes grosses*

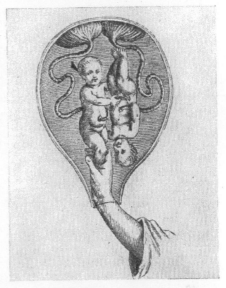

262. *Delivery of twins.*
(*From Viardel's* Observations, *1671.*)

et de celles qui sont accouchées (1668) went through many editions and was translated into English, German, Dutch, and Italian. Two collections of clinical records of his also experienced great popularity. Mauriceau, who was an ordinary surgeon and not a doctor of medicine, was a skilful practitioner and an acute observer, publishing his observations in an admirably concise and clear form.

Mauriceau was the first to study the conformation of the female pelvis, showing that in a woman with a large pelvis birth could take place without separation of the bones. He studied the movements of the fetus in different positions, the circulation in the pregnant uterus, and the formation of milk. He advised the bimanual extraction of the head, and was the first to describe the complication of strangulation of the newborn by the umbilical cord. He strongly condemned cephalic version, and introduced a number of technical improvements. His treatment of hemorrhage was excellent, and he gave careful rules for the treatment of *placenta previa*. He condemned Cæsarian section, which he regarded as fatal. Contrary to the opinion of his predecessors, he recognized the puerperal flow as a secretion analogous to the suppuration of a wound.

Important among Mauriceau's contemporaries was Cosmé VIARDEL, whose *Observations sur la pratique des accouchemens* . . . (1671) contains much of value, together with many odd statements that indicate the incomplete status of the subject at that time. Another contemporary and

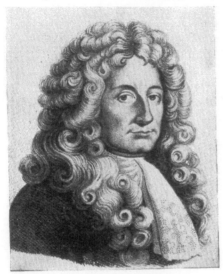

263. *François Mauriceau.*
From an original engraving.

supporter of Mauriceau, Paul PORTAL (d. 1703), of Montpellier, favoured podalic version, but treated facial presentations expectantly. He is credited with the discovery of the condition known as *placenta previa*. Philippe PEU (d. 1717 at an advanced age), an enemy of Mauriceau, published a *Pratique des accouchemens* (1694) based on four thousand deliveries, giving directions for delivery and version in case of foot presentation, following the ideas of Benivieni. Guillaume Mauquest DE LA MOTTE (1655–1737), a skilful and successful operator who studied the contracted pelvis, closes this list of the great French obstetricians of the century.

Among the Dutch physicians, the best-known were Ruysch, the anatomist, a pioneer in the study of the mechanics of childbirth, and Henrik van DEVENTER (1651–1724), who wrote on the same subject.

About this time surgeons were beginning to be admitted to normal deliveries. Previously only midwives, who had complete charge of the pregnant woman, could attend. Maternity institutes were first founded in France under expert surgeons; and this is the explanation of the rapid and marked development of obstetrics that we have just noted in France. But it should also be recognized that some of the midwives were skilful and capable of making valuable observations.

Thus in the history of the obstetrics of the century importance attaches to the work of Louise BOURGEOIS, or Boursier (1563–1636). She was a pupil of Ambroise Paré and the most famous of midwives, and was attached to the person of Queen Marie de Medicis. Reputed for her caution and great skill, she was much sought after by the French aristocracy after the fortunate delivery of the future Louis XIII. He was born in a state of asphyxia, but is said to have been saved by the midwife, who forced into his mouth a few drops of wine. She attended the birth of six royal princes, but was fiercely attacked by her enemies, particularly after the death of the Queen's daughter-in-law, Marie de Bourbon Montpensier, who died of a puerperal peritonitis for which la Boursier was held responsible. When one reads the report of the physicians today, the accusation seems to have but little foundation. However that may be, she made a number of valuable observations, especially as to detachment of the placenta. The most important of her works, dedicated to the Queen, was her *Observations diverses sur la stérilité, perte de fruicts, fécondité, accouchements, maladies des femmes et nouveaux naiz* (1609).

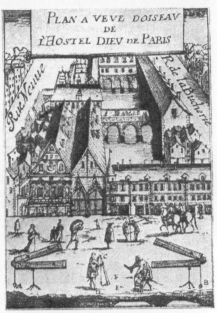

264. *Bird's-eye view of the Hôtel-Dieu of Paris, at the end of the seventeenth century.*

7. Legal Medicine

Legal medicine was a new medical discipline that naturally followed the anatomical and surgical progress of the period. Occasionally autopsies for legal purposes, to be sure, had been reported in earlier centuries, but it was only at the beginning of the seventeenth century that the special problems of the subject began to be envisaged and systematically pursued, especially in Italy. One of its earliest pioneers was Battista CODRONCHI, of Imola, who studied various aspects of the subject, such as the effect of poisons (*De morbis veneficis*, Venice, 1595). Fortunato FEDELE (1550–1630) was a better-known investigator of the subject (*De relationes medicorum*, Palermo, 1602), who in turn was surpassed by Paolo ZACCHIA (1584–1659), whose *Quæstiones medico-legales* (Rome, 1621–35) is a landmark in the early history of the subject.

Few physicians enjoyed more universal respect from their contemporaries than did Zacchia, whose vast knowledge led Pope Innocent X to confide to him the most delicate missions for the public health of the Papal States. The writings of his contemporaries reveal his authoritative position in the legal profession as well as among physicians. His book, which contains an extraordinary amount of legal information, was regarded as a classic text throughout Europe. Haller spoke of it with high praise, and Portal a century and a half later demanded that it should be publicly placed on view in all the universities of France. Platner praised its profound erudition. Up to the beginning of the nineteenth century no book on the subject failed to show the impress of this man of real genius. In the last of the ten books there are eighty-five cases (*Consilia*) with the replies and decision of the courts. All the problems that were posed were solved in the light of medical and legal authority, with citation of the most important legislative decisions of all times. Thus whoever wishes to study this discipline finds in Zacchia's book a veritable treasure of important documents. Another noteworthy production in this field is the *Medicus politicus* (1614) of Roderigo da CASTRO, a Lisbon Jew who established himself at Hamburg in 1598 and fulfilled the functions of a medico-legal expert for many years.

Germany was quick in following Italy's lead with the work of B. Saevus, J. F. Pfeiffer, G. Welsch, and especially of P. Ammann and Johann Bohn (1640–1718). Bohn's book on the examination of mortal wounds, *De renuntiatione vulnerum* . . . (Leipzig, 1689), was the first to treat this subject scientifically; he insisted that all the cavities of the body should be opened in medico-legal autopsies, and gave exact directions for the autopsy procedure.

An important step in legal medicine was the proper recognition of infanticide, which was greatly helped by Swammerdam's discovery that the lungs of an infant will float in water when it has once breathed (*Tractatus de Respiratione*, Leiden, 1667). This was shortly after, in 1682, applied in a legal case by J. SCHREYER.

8. *Pharmacology*

It is easy to understand that at a time when chemistry was much in favour, pharmacology should have made such notable progress that it is only in this century that scientific therapeutics founded on experiments may be said to have started. It was at this time that the wider use began of mercury, arsenic, and other metals in a rational manner justified by experiments. The use of opium became more extensive and better controlled; Sydenham was one of its advocates, and it was regarded as a sort of panacea by many. Antimony, though vigorously combated by the faculties, enjoyed considerable popularity among physicians and patients.

One of the most important events in the history of therapeutics was the introduction into Europe of cinchona bark by the Jesuits in 1632, and later, in 1640, by Juan DEL VEGA, physician of the Count Chinchon, Viceroy of Peru. The wife of the Viceroy, who in 1638 suffered from a tertian fever, was quickly cured by this miraculous remedy. Markham does not accept the general view that the virtues of the bark were known to the Indians at the time of the Incas. According to him, when the Countess returned to Spain with her husband at the end of his Viceregal term, she carried a supply of the wonderful bark with her, so that it was long known as the Countess's powder (*pulvis comitissæ*).[1] De Vega returned to Spain with a quantity of cinchona, which he sold at Seville at the high price of a hundred reals per pound. The spread of cinchona bark through Europe was extremely rapid, though it aroused acrid polemics. One might say that all Europe was divided into two camps, for or against its virtues. Strange to say, a religious factor entered into the controversy, as cinchona was brought from America in large quantities by the Jesuits, who were greatly enriched thereby, a circumstance which stirred up furious attacks from their enemies. However, cinchona soon achieved a definite place in the materia medica of the century. In England it was popularized by Sydenham and Morton. It was introduced into France by the Englishman Talbot, who with it cured the King and the Dukes of Burgundy and Anjou. It was given either as a powder or steeped in wine or in pills.

This was one of the most significant events in completing the downfall of Galenism. Up to this time the Galenists had maintained the absolute necessity of treating the sick with purgatives. They even thought that that was the reason for the success of mercury in the treatment of syphilis, maintaining that salivation was nothing more than the elimination of the *materies morbi*. However, no hypothesis of this kind could possibly explain the effect of the cinchona bark. Nevertheless, the faithful supporters of Galenism conducted a violent campaign against the introduction of this new remedy on the ground of its being irrational. One cannot but admire the insight of Ramazzini, who affirmed that the revolution brought about by cinchona in the history of medicine could only be compared with the effect of the introduction of gunpowder in the art of war.

Another new and important drug was the root of ipecacuanha, the

[1] At the London celebration of the three-hundredth anniversary of the introduction of cinchona bark into Europe, the Peruvian Minister, Alfred Gonzales-Prada, pointed out that documents discovered since the publication of C. R. Markham's *Memoir of Lady Ana de Osorio, Countess of Chinchon* (London, 1874) show that Doña Ana died in Spain before her husband became Viceroy of Peru, so that it must have been his second wife, Doña Francisca Henriquez de Rivera (d. 1641) who was cured by the Jesuits' bark.

therapeutic virtue of which had been known by the natives of Brazil. The French physician LE GRAS brought it to Europe in 1672; but its wide use was chiefly due to a Dutch physician, Hadrian HELVETIUS (1661–1727), who with it cured the Dauphin from an attack of dysentery. From it Helvetius acquired a large fortune. Already in 1685 Baglivi was advocating ipecac as an excellent remedy against dysentery.

Digitalis leaves were introduced into medicine during this century as a remedy for scrofula, and the root of colombo was recommended by Redi. The introduction of antimony has a peculiar history; the *Triumphant Chariot of Antimony* (1604) by the mythical fifteenth-century monk BASIL VALENTINE (Johann Thölde) popularized the use of antimony in many fevers. Lazare RIVIÈRE (Riverius) (1589–1655), who introduced the teaching of chemistry at Montpellier, upheld the benefits of antimony, about which violent controversies arose. Fallen out of fashion, its vogue was re-established when after its use Louis XIV recovered from an attack of continued fever (typhoid?). Many secret remedies, purgative pills, mineral waters, and powders of all sorts constituted an important part of the therapeutic arsenal of the century. During the century various food products were first introduced into Europe from newly discovered colonies: the potato, tea, coffee, cocoa, and tobacco. This has a certain importance in medicine, as various diseases were also attributed to them. A nervous constitution was attributed to the use of coffee and tea, and scrofula to the excessive use of potatoes. Severe laws were promulgated against the use of tobacco, especially in England; but no legislation was able to halt the increasing use of these products throughout Europe.

9. *Epidemics. Progress in Hygiene*

The epidemics of this century were among the most severe in history. Scurvy raged throughout northern Europe, in Scandinavia and on the shores of the Baltic; but also in the interior of Germany, so that the doctrine of a Scorbutic Constitution was invoked.

Malaria was epidemic in Italy, especially in the province of Naples. G. B. Cavallari stated in his book of 1602 that it had killed no less than forty thousand people. In the second half of the century new epidemics appeared, especially in England, in 1657 and 1664. In his book *De febribus* (1662), Willis stated that in 1657 almost all England was reduced to the state of one large hospital. The fever appears to have been of an irregular intermittent type, like that observed in Pisa by Borelli in 1661.

Epidemics of typhus occurred in France, Germany, and the Low Countries, especially during the Thirty Years' War, and in Italy from 1628 to 1632, and again toward the end of the century with great violence throughout northern Europe.

Bubonic plague, which was never long absent from Europe, returned in this century with the greatest violence since the Black Death. In a ter-

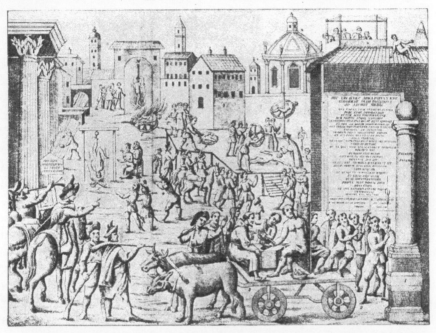

265. The column of infamy and the torture of the anointers, Milan, 1630.

rible epidemic in Lyon (1628–9) almost half the population died. Its occurrence in epidemic form in Italy (1629–31) is described by Manzoni in his *Promessi sposi*. He not only reveals the terrible consequences of the epidemic, but recounts the means employed by the physicians, the authorities, and the clergy to oppose its spread. He laments the ignorance of its cause, which still prevailed even among the cultivated classes, who were still dominated by astrological concepts. Milan, in 1630, lost 86,000 persons, and no less than 500,000 died in the Venetian Republic. Haeser regards this affliction as an important factor in the decline of Venice. Corradi, basing his estimates on accurate documents, states that between 1630 and 1631 there were 1,000,000 victims of plague in northern Italy alone.

It spread rapidly through Holland and Germany. From 1654 to 1656 it decimated the peoples of eastern Europe, then returned to Italy, to devastate particularly the Neapolitan provinces and some of the cities of northern Italy – Genoa was said to have lost 65,000 in one year. In London in 1665 the violence of the epidemic was the greatest since the Black Death. The catastrophe was made even more terrible by the Great Fire, which, during three days, destroyed a great part of the city. However, the evacuation that the fire necessitated, and the number of rats that it must have killed, seem to have had a beneficial effect in limiting further ravages. In 1679 the plague killed about 100,000 people in Vienna and was equally devastating at Prague.

Smallpox appeared with a special violence in this century in eastern Europe, and in England (1666–75), where it was described by Sydenham. It was common also along the Atlantic coast of the American colonies, especially in New England, Pennsylvania, and Charleston. Scarlatina, which, as Corradi has shown, was already known in the Middle Ages and described by Ingrassia (1550) under the name of *rossania*, but was then confused with measles, was carefully studied and described by Sydenham, and by Morton in 1671. These authors also made careful observations of the epidemic of dysentery.

In this century appeared the first adequate descriptions of diphtheria, a disease to which ancient authors had referred, especially in the Talmud (*askara*, from the Greek *eschara*). Aretæus and Ætius speak of a pestilential disease with ulcerations in the throat and white and grey eschars. Early descriptions of the disease are found in Spanish around the turn of the century, under the name *enfermedad del garrotillo* (after the running noose that was used in Spain to strangle criminals). From Spain diphtheria reached Naples, where it was described by F. Nola (1620) and others. Already in 1610 Severino had practised tracheotomy in Naples.

During this century, cursed with epidemics, medical hygiene profited by various studies and observations that paved the way for the great developments of modern hygiene.

Giovanni Maria LANCISI (1654–1720) was one of the outstanding Italian clinicians of the century, as well as a great epidemiologist. His *De subitaneis mortibus* (Rome, 1707), written to explain the number of sudden deaths in Rome in 1706, included acute cardiac dilatation as one of the causes, described vegetations on the valves, and classified various cardiac diseases. His work on aneurysm, *De motu cordis et aneurysmatibus* (Naples, 1728), considered the various causes and types of aneurysms and emphasized the frequency of cardiac aneurysms. As a hygienist he studied the quality of the airs and waters of Rome, seeking in the exhalations of the Pontine Marshes the causes of the diseases current at the time.

During an epidemic of influenza Lancisi proposed a series of hygienic measures. His book *De noxiis paludum effluviis* (1717) offers profound observations on the evil effects of stagnant water, which, if they had been appreciated, would have saved Italy inestimable loss of life and fortune. Lancisi maintained the need of draining pools and swamps as the only means of making healthy those places where pernicious fevers reigned. He regarded it as the duty of the government to oppose forest destruction, because trees with tall trunks improve the quality

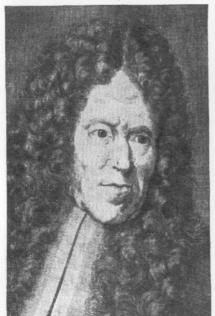

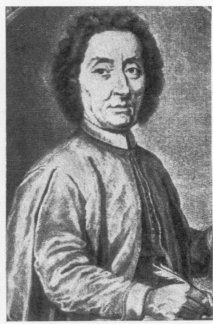

266. *Bernardino Ramazzini.*
(*From a contemporary engraving.*)

267. *Giovanni Maria Lancisi.*
From a contemporary engraving.

of the air. Lancisi maintained that cinchona bark was a specific for the cure of swamp fever (malaria). His efforts to improve the health of Italy were continued by those of other scientists, such as Giambattista Doni, who studied the sanitation of the Ager Romanus.

The first principles of MILITARY HYGIENE are to be found in the work of the Florentine Orazio Monti, entitled *Trattato della consuetudine, con il modo di governare gli eserciti ed i naviganti.* . . . This was followed by the *De militum in castris sanitate tuenda* (Vienna, 1685) of A. Porzio, who on his campaigns made interesting observations on the avoidance of epidemics in armies, and on the bad results of allowing soldiers who were suffering from contagious diseases to mingle in barracks with companions who were allowed to circulate through the city

Bernardino RAMAZZINI, of Carpi, near Modena, was professor at Modena (1682–1700) and at Padua until his death in 1714. Called by Koelsch the father of industrial hygiene, he was the author of the famous *De morbis artificum* (Modena, 1700; 2nd, larger edition, Padua, 1713), which is the first systematic treatise on OCCUPATIONAL DISEASE. Before him Paracelsus had been concerned with diseases of miners in the Tyrol, and an unknown

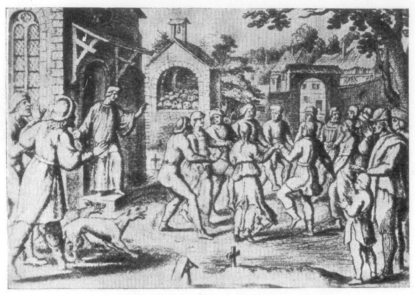

268. *An epidemic of St. Vitus's dance in a cemetery.*
(*Copper engraving from J. Gottfried's* Chronicle, *Frankfurt, 1632.*)

author had written about diseases in desert regions (edited by C. Singer, Oxford, 1915), but these were but detached sporadic observations. Ramazzini collected all that had been written before him on the subject and set himself to investigate the diseases of artisans, their causes, and the relations that existed between the disease and the occupation. In a series of masterly observations, still worthy of being read with interest and profit, he recognized the harmful effects of metals used in this or that technique, noting the damage produced by mercury in surgeons using mercurial inunctions, in chemists and pharmacists who prepared the remedies, and in gilders. He described various disorders that attack painters (Ch. 8) due to lead poisoning, though he apparently did not recognize the connection. He speaks authoritatively of the diseases of tinners, and of coloured-glass workers who handle antimony. The diseases of painters and of all other tradesmen form the subject of special study. Few classical works equal Ramazzini's book in the pleasure they give today. Wisely conceived, logically carried out, it reveals the work of a cultivated writer and courteous polemicist, as well as a profound scholar. In epidemiology also Ramazzini was an observer of the first rank, so that he may be regarded, with Baglivi, as one of the most illustrious Italian clinicians of his time.

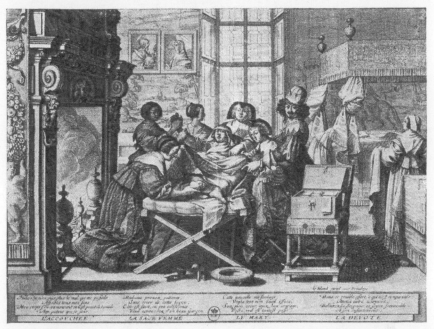

269. *Childbirth, by Abraham Bosse.* (BIBLIOTHÈQUE NATIONALE, PARIS.)

Ramazzini was not only the founder and greatest exponent of a new medical discipline, the study of occupational disease, but he was also an excellent general clinician. His philosophy of medicine and his teaching were clear and logical, directed toward the examination of disease pictures and their symptoms in pathological changes, so that he might proceed objectively toward the proper treatment. In therapy, therefore, he also stands out among his contemporaries. He attempted no form of treatment that was not fully justified; an ardent supporter in the use of cinchona bark in the intermittent fevers, where he regarded it as a specific, he opposed the tendency of the time to prescribe it for all febrile states without discrimination. He recognized the value of single medicaments, and preferred to use simple remedies because, as he said: " In unsuitable combinations the quality of drugs changes and one should not combine different remedies where one does not exactly know their compatibility." In a period when phlebotomy was much in favour, and when, in his words, " it seems as if the phlebotomist grasped the Delphic sword in his hand to exterminate the innocent victims rather than to destroy the disease," he strenuously combated this abuse. For him the duty of the physician was to " exhaust himself in infinite examinations, in continual experiments, to try to resolve the greatest as well as the most insignificant medical problems."

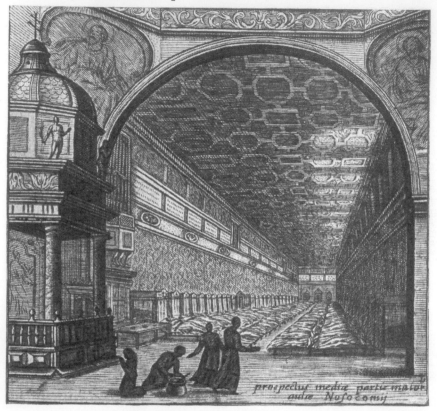

270. *A ward in the Santo Spirito Hospital of Rome, seventeenth century.*

Toward the end of the seventeenth century significant steps were made in the domain of social and SANITARY LEGISLATION. Already in 1656, when the plague broke out in Rome, Monsignor GASTALDI, special Papal commissary of health, adopted the following interesting sanitary measures: Sanitary guards were placed at the gates of the city and at the frontiers. A certification of health was required from all travellers, the streets and sewers were cleaned, aqueducts regularly inspected, places designated for the disinfection of clothing, all popular gatherings forbidden. Gastaldi's work, *De avertenda et profliganda peste* (1684), contains two hundred and forty-five sanitary edicts issued during the campaign against the plague — an important historical document. In July 1699 the General Health Council of the Republic of Lucca publicly stated that " in the future there shall not be danger or prejudice to the health of the human body from the clothing that remains after the death of persons sick of consumption and other similar diseases." At the same time it was decided to ask the College of Physicians that " these gentlemen should make known the persons, no matter of what sex or condition, that they have treated in the past six months for the diseases mentioned in the following decree, so that all the precautions may be taken that seem opportune." Shortly after, the report of the College of Physicians was returned to the Health Council with the names of consumptives, or those suspected of having consumption, who lived in Lucca. The authorities took the necessary measures for disinfection and gave permits to physicians to perform autopsies on those dying from consumption, in order to study the nature of the disease. The time was not yet ripe, however. These measures were soon revoked on account of the hostility of the citizens and the difficulties that arose in their execution.

The first attempts at military hygiene took place in this century in the German armies. It was even tried to regulate prostitution, a plague which had reached frightful proportions.

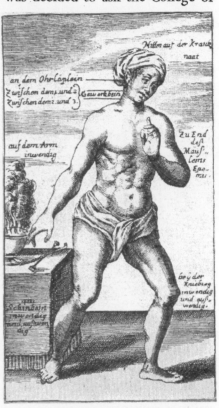

271. *Directions for the application of fontanelles.*
(*From the German edition of the* Chirurgie *of Tiberius Marcus, Nürnberg, 1676.*)

Friedrich Schiller narrates that at the siege of Nürnberg (1632) there were no less than fifteen thousand prostitutes in the camp of Wallenstein. Contemporary historians said that in 1648 the Imperial armies were followed by prostitutes who were more than twice as numerous as the soldiers in the army. This horde of women (*Weibertross*), often accompanied by their illegitimate children, constituted an enormous danger for the armies. The regulation of the authorities did little to ameliorate the situation, which remained much the same up to the middle of the eighteenth century.

10. Medical Teaching and the Social Position of Physicians

The importance of the Italian universities, for reasons that we have given, diminished in this century; no longer did they receive large crowds of students from all parts of Europe. Padua, Bologna, and Rome still preserved their prestige, thanks to their eminent professors, but gradually the northern universities acquired greater importance. In France, Holland, England, and Denmark the medical schools took an active part in scientific progress, though the German universities were retarded by the religious wars. But the teaching of the classics still dominated the great schools of Europe. Hippocrates, Galen, and Avicenna held the place of honour; chemistry and physics played an important part. Clinical teaching, in the modern sense of the word, which had been inaugurated by Montanus in Italy and Heurnius in Holland, was employed by Baglivi in Rome, and by Franciscus Sylvius in the twelve beds of his little infirmary at Leiden. An interesting change in university teaching that took place during this century was that the corporations of students in the universities gradually lost their power over the choice of professors and the kind of teaching, while the professors of the faculty were well and solidly organized and assumed more and more control. It is during this century also that one finds the first systematic attempts at combined theoretical and practical teaching and at lectures at the bedside of the patient.

The teaching of anatomy was obligatory in all universities, though it was usually left to the surgeon, as the physician still regarded it as unworthy of his social position. It was only toward the end of the century that this tradition gave way and the anatomist was accepted as a respected member of the college of professors.

Surgery continued to be regarded as an art inferior to medicine, especially in France, where conflicts were constantly arising in the bosom of the Paris Faculty. In this respect Italy was an honourable exception: although there were still surgeons and barbers who occupied themselves exclusively with bleedings, minor operations, clysters, and such things, the physician also performed surgical operations which he regarded as in conformity with the dignity of his art. In the northern countries, on the other hand, the division was still distinct, so that almost all the surgeons of this century were products of the barbers' guild and usually lacked the proper scientific foundations. This of course did not prevent some of the barber surgeons from acquiring an honourable position in the history of surgery through their great technical skill, which permitted them to undertake the boldest operations.

In this century also the teaching of obstetrics to physicians and midwives began to be organized. The old theoretical instruction was still dominant; thus admission to the delivery rooms of the Hôtel-Dieu in Paris was strictly forbidden to physicians; but the spirit of progress was in the air

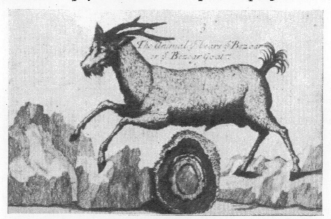

272. *Bezoar Stone and Bezoar Goat. From Pomet's* Histoire des drogues.

and we find toward the end of the century many physicians who had good practical knowledge and skilled obstetrical technique. Midwives were officially taught in Paris in a three months' course, but generally their knowledge was extremely slight and their reputation poor.

During the seventeenth century there was a great improvement in the social position of physicians. They began to enjoy more consideration and occupy a more respected position in society.

Practitioners, however, were for the most part men of little culture who were content to write prescriptions and accompany them with long discourses. The type of physician immortalized by Le Sage and Molière, although surely exaggerated, may be taken as characteristic of the average physician of the time. Dr. Sangrado, of *Gil Blas*, whom " all Valladolid regarded as a Hippocrates, had a grave air and his expressions had a particular accent of nobility. His reasonings were geometrical and his opinions very individual." Hear him at the bedside: " Others in my place without doubt would order saline, urinous, volatile, or mercurial remedies; but purgatives and sudorifics are pernicious drugs invented by charlatans." No sooner said than he called the surgeon to remove six ounces of blood from the unfortunate patient and ordained that he drink three pints of hot water.

Molière speaks through the mouth of the doctors Diafoirus, father and son, in the *Malade imaginaire:* " But above all what pleases me and him, and wherein he follows my example, is that he follows blindly the opinions of our ancestors, and that he has never tried to understand or listen to the theories and experiences of the pretended discoverers of our century concerning the circulation of the blood and other opinions on the same foolishness." In the burlesque ceremony

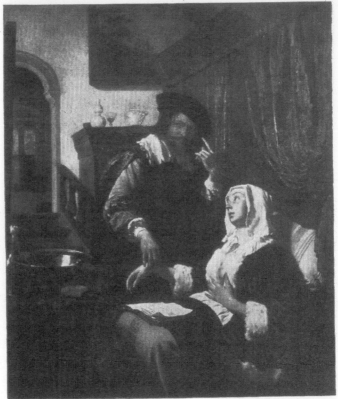

273. The Physician's Visit, *by Frans van Mieris.*   (VIENNA STATE MUSEUM.)

in that play an assemblage composed of eight syringe-bearers, six apothecaries, two doctors, eight dancing surgeons, and two singers proceeds to the examination of the candidate. The bachelor responds to the questions proposed by the doctors with the approval of the Dean. The treatment is the same for all patients: clysters, phlebotomy, purgation: " *Clysterium donare — Postea seignare — Ensuita purgare.*" In especially grave cases it is necessary to " *Reseignare, repurgare et reclysterisare.*" The chorus gives its enthusiastic approval with these responses: " *Bene, bene, bene respondere — dignus, dignus est intrare in nostro docto corpore.*" After the new doctor has taken the oath always to agree with the oldest colleague and only to use remedies approved by the Faculty, they confer the doctoral bonnet on him which gives him the power: " *Medi-*

candi, Purgandi, Seignandi, Perçandi, Taillandi, et Occidandi, Impune per totam terram."

It would of course be wrong to evaluate the physicians of the time on the basis of caricatures by dramatic writers. But perusal of the prescriptions and most of the medical treatises of the period indicates that the satirists were justi-

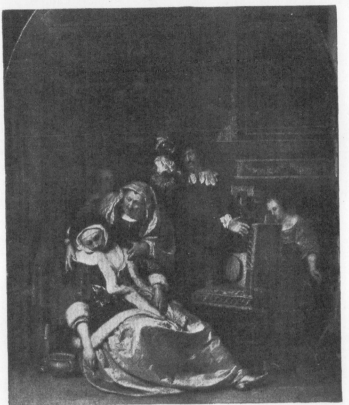

274. The Sick Lady, *by Frans van Mieris.*   (MUNICH PINACOTHEK.)

fied in their attacks on the empty grandiloquence of the physicians of the seventeenth century.

It was a period when there was a number of scientific physicians but not yet a scientific medicine. In the schools, where the ancient doctrines were deeply rooted, the many innovations were poorly tolerated. As a result, most physicians of the time followed the policy of the ostrich in hiding its head under the sand as the storm approaches and swore allegiance to Galen so as to avoid problems for which they did not feel themselves prepared. The penetration of new ideas and the diffusion of new discoveries met a violent resistance even in this century. It seems as if the scholastic doctrines outdid themselves in a last effort to defend the traditional positions.

Medical literature assumed an important position at this time, not only for the scientific knowledge that it diffused, but also as regards medical teaching and the attitude of the physician to the patient and to the pharmacist.

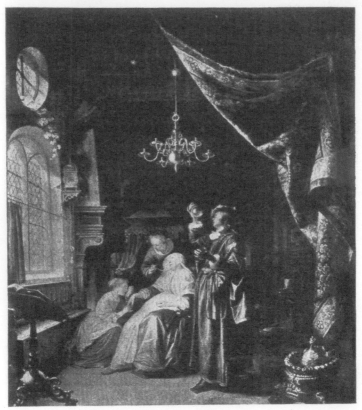

275. The Woman with Dropsy, *by Gerard Dou.*   (LOUVRE MUSEUM.)

Lancisi, in his *De recta medicorum studiorum ratione instituenda* (1715), proposed a reorganization of medical studies, emphasizing for physicians the need for extensive culture and especially for long courses of training. He was the first to maintain that physicians should familiarize themselves with the use of the thermometer and the microscope and become acquainted with pathology. Other authors also, such as Paolo Zacchia, wrote on the dignity of the medical profession and the duties of the physician toward the State.

The grave dissensions between physicians, the vogue of charlatans and superstitions, and the persistence of the Galenic tradition gave rise to a number of writings against physicians and against medicine, such as *Le Confusioni dei medici* (1633) of Antonio CARERA, writing under the pseudonym of Raffele Carrara. Another popular and much quoted book was *Il Mondo ingannato da falsi medici* (1716) by Giuseppe GAZZOLA, physician of the Emperor Leopold.

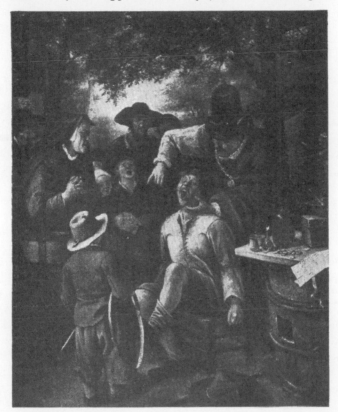

276. The Dentist, *by Jan Steen.*   (THE HAGUE MUSEUM.)

We quote the following: " Without at all understanding philosophy, mathematics, chemistry, or anatomy, without having studied diagnosis, symptomatology, dietetics, or physiology, anyone can become a physician. . . . It suffices for him to know by heart four aphorisms of Hippocrates, a dozen passages from Galen, and several other small quotations from a classical author, together with the names of various diseases, all of which could be included in one page of writing. . . . One often sees how effrontery, manners of the servile courtier, affectations, boldness, and false religion cause certain persons to be accepted as excellent." Attacks like this were frequent in the seventeenth century and provoked answers from eminent physicians.

The growth of medical journalism, due in part to the publications of the newly founded scientific societies, was a natural sequel of the private News Letters, such as the Fuggers', and of the development of newspapers in quick succession in Italy, the Low Countries, Germany, England, and France. The movement toward the formation of scientific journals, which in Italy were called literary, was led by the *Journal des sçavans* (first published, Paris, 1665, by Jean Cusson), which was founded and directed by Daniel de Selle under the pseudonym M. de Hedouville. The journal appeared every Sunday in duodecimo fasciculi, and included frequent medical articles and reports. Only a few months later followed the publication of the celebrated *Philosophical Transactions* of the Royal Society of London. The earliest Italian journal to include scientific material was the *Giornale dei letterati* (1668), founded by F. Nazari, Professor of Philosophy at the Sapienza in Rome, in imitation of the *Journal des sçavans*.

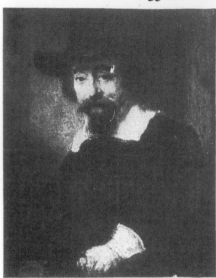

277. *Portrait of Doctor Ephraim Bonus, by Rembrandt.*
(SIX GALLERY, AMSTERDAM.)

More directly concerned with medicine was the *Giornale Veneto dei letterati*, founded by Dr. Pietro Moretti at Venice in 1671; for instance, the number of April 20, 1672 included Observations made at the Medical Theatre of Venice on the Foetus outside of the Uterus. The first medical journal properly so called was the *Journal des Nouvelles découvertes sur toutes les parties de la médecine*, published at Paris in 1679 by Nicolas DE BLÉGNY (1652–1722), a former beadle of the Medical Faculty who had risen to an important position at court. De Blégny also had some historical importance as the inventor of the truss for inguinal hernia (1676), and for his work on the then youthful subject of legal medicine, especially in its relations to surgery (Lyon, 1684). The journal was successful, and when its editor was imprisoned for various intrigues, it continued to appear for some time at Amsterdam, and in a Latin translation at Geneva and a German translation at Hamburg. These first attempts at journalism, however, did not find successors until the beginning of the eighteenth century.

To be mentioned here is the name of a great French physician who founded the first political journal, *La Gazette de France* (1631). Its founder, publisher, and editor was Theophraste RENAUDOT (1584–1653), physician to the King and commissary general of the poor of the Kingdom. He created wisely administered charity institutions where free medical treatment was given to the poor. He was also the founder of the first pawnshops (*monts de piété*) in France, and a friend of Richelieu, who held him in great esteem. Guy Patin, who called him " The Gazetteer," covered him with insults, and the Paris Faculty, always ultra-

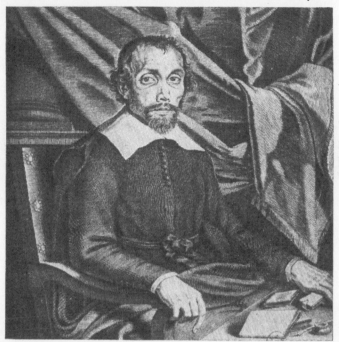

278. *Theophraste Renaudot, physician and journalist. Engraving of 1631.*

conservative, carried on a fierce struggle against him which ended only with his death. France has dedicated to this great physician and journalist a beautiful monument.

Medical subjects figured prominently in the work of the great artists, as we have already seen in the section on Anatomy. Physicians and patients were particularly popular subjects with the Dutch painters, such as Rembrandt, Frans van Mieris, Gerard Dou, Jan Steen, David Teniers, and Peter Breughel. Their skilful paintings on the greatest variety of medical subjects — the lame, the halt, and the blind, idiots, malingerers, lepers, syphilitics, and especially chlorotics, suffering from the " love sickness " — are full of interest for the history of medicine. The Spanish painters also recorded many medical conditions in their masterly canvasses. Velasquez's dwarfs and hydrocephalics and achondroplastics, Ribera's paralytics, and Murillo's idiots can still be seen in the museums of Europe as well as in their proper Spanish background.

Progress was much slower in the practice than in the science of medicine. The discoveries of the famous anatomists and physiologists were but little read and understood by the majority of the profession — a phenomenon that would be hard to understand for one who was not acquainted

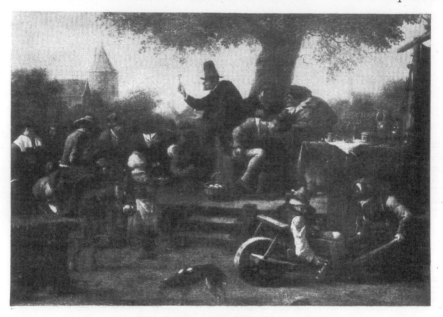

279. The Dentist at the Fair, *by Jan Steen.*

with the evolutionary processes of medical thought throughout history. We see the most illustrious clinicians and the most ignorant charlatans each surrounded by many pupils and faithful followers, often occupying eminent positions side by side. We see the most marvellous discoveries proclaimed from the chairs of one university, while in another the most obsolete principles and metaphysical doctrines are being obstinately repeated. We see a small number of courageous men armed only with their convictions and passion for the truth combating the ignorant, superstitious, and often deceitful, who used governmental authority, the tradition of ancient texts, and the stupidity of the credulous as a rampart to obstruct every attempt at research and every effort to illuminate the darkness. Often the individual succumbed but the idea remained victorious. Once having penetrated into the investigative field, which had hitherto been closed to it, medicine advanced first with faltering steps, then with increasing security. The diffusion of medical culture became more and more extended, the exchange of knowledge became international, the small number of courageous men became in time a larger group and finally a formidable crowd, against which the arts of the enemy could not prevail. Thus at the end of this century, when the co-operation of medicine and the natural sciences was being emphasized, we already see outlines of the essential features of the great structure of experimental medical science. Already various specialties began to be detached from the main trunk. Surgery became an art comparable in dignity to medicine. Anatomy, removed from the hands of the barber surgeons, became an exact science on which physicians leaned with respect. Hygiene, sanitation, and legal medicine codified their principles; obstetrics, ophthalmology, and dentistry became disciplines organized on scientific foundations. Finally, beside the universities, academies arose which were the cradles of the future scientific societies, just as the first literary journals that were founded in this century became the precursors of scientific journals.

Here we have an extensive preparation for modern medicine. The need was being felt of replacing the inadequate systems of medicine by others which would incorporate all the scientific discoveries and investigations of the century and would be better able to explain the pathological and biological problems of the future.

CHAPTER XVIII

THE EIGHTEENTH CENTURY

FROM SPECULATIVE SYSTEMS TO PATHO-LOGICAL AND CLINICAL CONCEPTS

1. General Considerations

THE EIGHTEENTH century was a period in the history of civilization, and especially in that of medicine, which occupies a distinct if not a detached position in the historical evolution of medical thought. Whereas the seventeenth century was dominated by political and social movements and by an orientation toward free investigation, the eighteenth represents a logical evolution of facts and ideas in their most ample and complex manifestations. It ended with a great political reaction against dominant institutions, a reaction determined by a spirit of revolutionary idealism which tended more and more to the liberation of peoples and of individual consciences. This idealism found its spiritual origin in a decisive orientation toward the natural and exact sciences and in the dominance of inductive philosophy.

The great cities were becoming ever richer and more flourishing, the corporations more affluent and powerful, the bourgeoisie more aware of its importance. The same evolutionary processes which brought about the American and the French Revolutions also exerted important influences on scientific development. Enlightened princes, like Joseph II of Austria, Catherine II of Russia, Frederick the Great of Prussia, were turning in no uncertain way toward intellectual liberalism, giving an enormous impetus to scientific culture.

[578]

During this century, when religious controversies were less violent but nevertheless attacked scholastic dogmatism in its very essence, the need for new concepts and classifications was being affirmed in all branches of political and intellectual life, to replace those that it was felt should be destroyed. The architects of these new doctrines, in politics, literature, political economy, and medicine, were those systematists who endeavoured to bring the most important problems of life in accord with the results of experimental study and the discoveries of science. On these foundations they attempted to state the laws underlying the new concepts, in which new factors, often created by metaphysical speculation, but thought to be derived from positive research, should replace values that were regarded as definitely negligible. The first part of the eighteenth century, then, was a time when the influence of philosophers predominated, when it seemed that every problem could be solved by appropriate reasoning. It was the philosophers, such as Montesquieu and Rousseau, who determined new social and political forms, and they exerted on medicine an equally remarkable influence. Of this sort was Gottfried Wilhelm LEIBNITZ (1646–1716), scientist, mathematician, and statesman, above all a synthetic and systematic intellect, a man who could be regarded as the first representative of that school of German philosophy which at the beginning of the century took on, one might say, the guidance of European civilization. His system of philosophy, which was published about the beginning of the century by his pupil Christian VON WOLFF (1679–1754), was based on the existence of infinitely small and indivisible units, the so-called "monads," alive and thinking, essential parts of all bodies and all beings, of which they constitute the soul. The clarity of the representations of the monads corresponds to the level of the individual's intelligence. The monads of man have the clearest representations and thus man is capable of the greatest intelligence. The single atoms or automats come from a central monad, which is none other than God, and are united with each other and with God by a pre-established harmony. Thus everything that happens is for the best, according to the philosophy of Leibnitz. (To a follower of Leibnitz who had attacked Voltaire in print, the latter replied: "When you have shown why so many men cut their throats in the best of all possible worlds, I shall be exceedingly obliged to you. I await your arguments, your verses, and your abuse; and assure you from the bottom of my heart that neither of us knows anything about the matter.") The influence of the philosophy of Leibnitz on medicine is due to the frequent contact that he and his disciples had with the greatest physicians of his time and to the diffusion of his philosophical ideas, especially in Germany.

Emmanuel KANT (1724–1804) maintained that the origins of science should be sought in the human intellect and founded a critical system in which the results of human knowledge are fixed. He thus launched a concept which, in the hands of his followers, Fichte, Schelling, and especially Hegel, led to the conclusion that philosophy is the queen of all the sciences, and that it is for her to utter the latest word even in the problems of the natural sciences. It is easy to imagine the effect of this *a priori* argument on the evolution of German medical thought. But in other countries also, and especially in the work of the French Encyclopædists, the philosophers exerted a more or less direct influence on the evolution of scientific thought.

Much more important was the influence of progress in the exact sciences. The chemistry of this century, for instance, with the discovery of oxygen and a number of other gases (carbon dioxide by Black, 1757; hydrogen by Cavendish, 1766; nitrogen by Rutherford, 1772), finally overthrew the phlogiston fallacy and laid a sound basis for knowledge of the physiology of respiration.

During the eighteenth century the electrical discoveries of Luigi GALVANI (1737–98) and of Alessandro VOLTA (1745–1827) opened new horizons of physical laws and gave to medicine new investigative possibilities in physiology and pathology and new perspectives in therapeutics. The studies of LINNÆUS (1707–78), the gifted Swedish botanist and physician, resulted in the first modern system of botany, in which for the first time the classification of plants was made on the basis of the characteristics of the stamen and pistils. Linnæus excelled in his descriptions and was the first to introduce the binomial nomenclature for living beings and to classify man as *Homo sapiens* in the order of the primates. His classical work, the *Systema naturæ*, first published in 1735, went through twelve editions during his lifetime.

The Abbé Felice FONTANA (1720–1805), of Pomarolo (Rovereto), a distinguished naturalist and physiologist, founded the Florentine Museum of Natural History and enriched it with more than fifteen hundred well-constructed wax preparations. His studies on the venom of vipers (1767) are especially noteworthy as initiating a long line of investigations on this subject, which still continue. He was the first, as Castaldi has noted, to describe the cell as a uniform body endowed with a spot in the centre, thus foreshadowing the cell nucleus (1781). Credit for the first description of the cell nucleus is usually given to R. Brown (*Transactions*, Linnean Society of London, 1833, XVI, 685). Fontana was also the first (1781) to describe the tubules of the kidney and the nerve sheaths that bear the name of Henle. He is eponymically connected with the *sinus venosus* of the sclera and the space at the angle of the iris.

Modern embryology may be said to have been launched by Caspar Friedrich WOLFF (1733–94), of Berlin, with his doctoral thesis on *Theoria generationis* (1759; enlarged German version, 1764). In 1764 Wolff became a member of the Academy of Sciences of St. Petersburg, where he wrote his important *De formatione intestinorum*, a work which was largely overlooked until it was reprinted in German by Meckel (1812). Wolff supported Harvey's theory of epigenesis, as opposed to the preformation view, and recognized the development of the body from small sacs, even foreshadowing von Baer's recognition of the embryonal layers. He maintained that all parts of plants are nothing but transformed leaves. In anatomy his name is preserved in the Wolffian ducts. The studies of Goethe (1749–1832) on comparative anatomy (the intermaxillary bone) and on the physiology of plants, those of Buffon (1707–78), in which can be seen ideas pointing toward the Darwinian theory of evolution, and those of Lazzaro Spallanzani (1729–99) on spontaneous generation – these all manifest the tendency throughout Europe toward a systematic arrangement of newly acquired knowledge.

Among other factors aiding in the development of medical thought during the century was the increasing interest of the various social classes in scientific problems. The academies that we have spoken of were changing from gatherings of leisurely dilettanti to assemblages of scholars who devoted themselves to earnest scientific investigations. The intelligentsia, even the " socialites " of the day, crowded to scientific discussions and demonstrations as never before. The scientific journals, which were steadily multiplying, spread throughout Europe the news of the numerous discoveries. The renewed study of the best ancient authors contributed to the return to true Hippocratic principles, a return which has been so frequently observed in the important periods of medical history. On the other hand, mysticism, which spread especially through Germany and France toward the end of the century but gained some ground throughout Europe, created a new and mysterious pseudo-scientific atmosphere which prepared the way for impostors and adventurers.

To summarize the principal characteristics of the century, we see on the one hand a tendency to construct systems in the effort to explain the most important physiological and pathological phenomena; and on the other hand, under the stimulus of the discoveries made in the exact sciences, a persistent tendency to experiment, to search and re-search, and thus to give more weight to the forces of nature, accepting man as a part of the cosmos rather than as the more important figure that he had assumed in scholastic and metaphysical medicine. It is thus a period of trial and error and also of fundamental construction, so that there is some basis for the attitude of the historians who regard this century as of prime importance for modern medicine. It was during this century, as a matter of fact, that the foundations of scientific thought, methods, and accomplishments

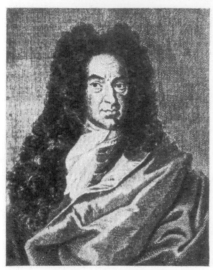 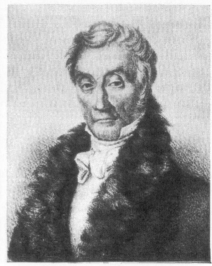

280. *Georg Ernst Stahl.*   281. *Giovanni Rasori.*

were being laid which remained intact even after the destruction of the various systems of that day. And it was the advances of this period which established in a definite way that no one can try to explain the human organism, healthy or diseased, while ignoring, as in the past, anatomy, physiology, and the complex phenomena of physics and chemistry. Thus even the systems dominated by philosophy require study by the medical historian: the steps by which the work of the past was blotted out or resumed, or made the basis of progress, or even led to false conclusions when medicine abandoned concrete investigation to hurl itself into the adventure of transcendental hypotheses. In history, the study of errors is no less instructive than the study of successes.

2. Medical Systems

The medical systems of the eighteenth century naturally reflect the influence of all the tendencies toward reform arising from the Aristotelian doctrine of the preceding centuries. The mechanistic and chemical tendencies which dominated medicine at that time found an imposing adversary in the person of Georg Ernst STAHL (1660–1734).

G. E. Stahl, born at Ansbach, and from 1694 Professor of Pathology, Dietetics, Physiology, Botany, and Pharmacology at Halle, was a rigid personality, blunt in his expressions, a fervent believer, and profoundly convinced of the absolute truth of his views, which he would not permit even to be discussed. A fertile writer, he was the author of no fewer than three hundred publications, of which the most important was his *Theoria medica vera* (Halle, 1707). He carried on many controversies, even with those who had been his best friends, such as Hoffmann. In 1716 he left Halle, which, thanks to him and Hoffmann, had become the centre of the philosophic movement in Germany, to go to Berlin, where he was given the position of court physician, dedicating himself otherwise entirely to his investigations.

Stahl's system of Animism represents an attempt to deny the dualism of Descartes, who separated the life of the immaterial soul from that of the body. Stahl maintained that the supreme principle of life, the *anima*, should be identified not with the intelligence but rather with Nature. According to him, the anima represents the unity of the entire organism, protecting it against the deterioration toward which it tends, and against the putrefaction which occurs when the anima abandons the body. The anima provokes in the organism the movements on which life depends. These are not always the same or co-ordinated, but it is only by them that the anima can be recognized, so that one cannot speak abstractly of an activity of the anima, but only of the *anima agens*. When the movements that represent normal life are altered by the body or its organs, disease supervenes. Thus disease is nothing else than the tendency of the anima (or of nature) to re-establish the normal order of tonic movements as quickly and efficiently as possible.

The activity of nature is produced through the circulatory system. The increase of temperature and the rate of the pulse, which for Stahl is much more characteristic, a symptom to which he was not the first to attribute importance, represent a more rapid succession of movements which are nature's attempts to bring the organism back to a normal state. It is therefore more correct to call Stahl a dynamist rather than a vitalist, as many have done. Stahl's erroneous phlogiston theory of combustion, however, retarded chemistry for the best part of the century. Even though Mayow had shown that some substances gain in weight when burned (by oxidation), Stahl maintained that burning matter was dephlogisticated —

that is, lost the hypothetical phlogiston — an error that was eventually corrected by Lavoisier's discovery of oxygen and its role in respiration.

In practice, Stahl's doctrine led him to many erroneous conclusions. Starting with the essential humoral concept that all disease phenomena arise in the blood, he maintained that most diseases come from a stasis in the blood vessels and that the anima remedies this by spontaneous hemorrhages. Stahl thus attributed great importance to hemorrhoids, and thought that stopping "the hemorrhoidal flux" gave rise to chronic diseases and especially to hypochondriasis and melancholia. He denied the utility of quinine and opium, preferring purgatives instead. He disdained anatomy and physiology and maintained that the best theorists were the worst practitioners. However, in spite of the many errors in his system, he is entitled to the merit of having conceived a vitalist or dynamic theory, whichever one chooses to call it, the truths of which are still apparent.

If, on the one hand, Stahl can be regarded as a pioneer in the biological trend of medicine, on the other hand Friedrich HOFFMANN (1660–1742) appears as the creator of an influential system of medicine reposing on mechanistic foundations. A disciple of G. W. Wedel (1645–1721), a prominent iatrochemist, and from 1694 professor at the University of Halle, Hoffmann was an intimate friend of Robert Boyle (1627–91), the great English chemist and physicist, and of Ramazzini and other contemporary Italian scholars. In philosophy he was much influenced by Leibnitz, and maintained that our knowledge, being founded on the senses, is necessarily limited and that ultimate causes are inscrutable. Force is inherent in matter and manifests itself by mechanical movements that can be determined by measurements, numbers, weights. In the living organism also the vital forces are manifested in this way. Life is nothing but movement, and death the cessation of movement. Hoffmann assembled his doctrines in a work entitled *Medicina rationalis systematica* (9 vols., Halle, 1718–40), which he designed especially as an effort to serve the practice of medicine. Reasoning and observation, according to him, should be the basis of medical knowledge, which should be elucidated by physics, chemistry, and anatomy. The living organism is entirely formed of fibres, having a special characteristic *tonus*, with the ability to contract and dilate. The tonus of the fibres is stimulated or regulated through the nervous system by a "nervous ether," so called because it is like the atmospheric ether. This fluid has its seat in the brain, whence it is transported to all organs of the body by a systole and diastole of the meninges. When the tonus is normal, the body is healthy, every modification of the tonus bringing with it a disturbance of health.

The principal cause of disease, according to Hoffmann, is plethora (fullness), which acts indirectly through the stomach and intestines, so that it is to these organs that the physician should devote his closest attention. Fever has its origin in the spinal cord following a contraction of the arteries and veins, and should be regarded as a disease and not as a healing process. Partisan of the healing powers of nature, Hoffmann maintained that farmers got well better and quicker without the medical care that was available to the inhabitants of cities. He proposed fourteen therapeutic measures, most of which come directly from Hippocrates.

Treatment, according to Hoffmann, should be sedative, corroborant, tonic, or evacuant, according to the case and to the necessity of stimulating or quieting the tonus of the fibres. He deserves credit for having recognized — perhaps the first to do so — that the effect of drugs depends not entirely on their pharmacological action but also on the constitution of the patient. If this is ignored or not sufficiently appreciated, all treatment will be vague and uncertain. He introduced into therapeutics a number of drugs — and sold them himself at a handsome profit — such as the famous Hoffmann's Drops and Anodyne, which still appear in some pharmacopœias. To Hoffmann is due also the employment of such drugs as quinine, iron, and ether in chronic diseases. The prominence of "tonics" in modern treatment is testimony to the deep impression made by his doctrines. He was above all a chemist, who had a clear view of disease in many respects, even though one finds strange supernatural explanations of diseases which he called "diabolic," as, for example, impotency, which he thought due to a mystic influence exerted through the ether. However, his chemical and biological knowledge often led him into proper paths in practical medicine. He was the first to introduce mineral waters into therapeutics and explained the effects of the so-called "muriatic" waters as due to the presence of alkali. Also one must not forget his recognition of the importance of the nervous system in disease, which led him to attribute to the nervous system, for the first time in medical history, a role of prime importance in the vital functions of the body.

The honourable position that many historians attribute to him is not undeserved. Although his system contained many errors, and his very facility of expression led him to a prolixity that tires anyone studying his voluminous output, one must recognize nevertheless that he was a profound thinker and tireless investigator.

Hoffmann's neural concept of disease had an important advocate in William CULLEN (1712–90), of Edinburgh, a founder of the medical school at Glasgow (1744). Cullen maintained that the cause of normal tonus of the solid parts is found in the energy emanating from the nervous system. Contractions or relaxations are produced when the tonus is increased or diminished by external stimuli. A thoughtful observer, Cullen supposed that gout, which was then extremely common in Great Britain, came from an atony of the digestive system which caused vicarious conges-tion in the joints. Medicines acted through the stomach, according to him, reflexly or by sympathy. Some, such as wine, quinine, camphor, should be regarded as tonics of the nervous system. Treatment with laxatives and purgatives, which was then in great vogue, should be regarded as without foundation and dangerous. Cullen was a believer in the Hippocratic doc-trine of critical days. His theory represents some progress beyond that of Hoffmann; and, without accepting the estimate by some historians of Cul-len as the father of the neural concept of disease, we must admit that his doctrines contain principles that later became important in modern con-cepts of the pathology of the nervous system. His ideas still persist in more subtle form in such modern expressions as " nervous energy " and in the whole gamut of the neuroses. A promoter of the Glasgow medical school, he was unrivalled as a lecturer, and one of the first to give clinical lectures in the vernacular. Cullen's principal work, *First Lines of the Practice of Physick* (4 vols., London, 1777), soon became the chief textbook of its kind throughout Europe, and especially in Germany, whose universities had many connections with the English universities. Like his *Treatise of the Materia Medica* (1789), it was translated into the leading languages of Europe. But soon it was the turn of another systematist to receive the approbation of widespread medical and scientific circles.

John BROWN (1735–88), a pupil of Cullen's, was the creator of an ex-traordinarily popular system in its day — Brunonism — which affirmed that life is essentially not a normal spontaneous state but one maintained by con-tinuous stimuli. The normal excitability of organs and the proper dosage of the stimuli thus constitute the state of health. Every deviation from this normal state, and therefore every disproportion between stimulus and ex-citability, results in a morbid state, which is sthenic if the excitation is too strong, or asthenic if it is too weak. Diagnosis depended chiefly on the pulse and the temperature, as with Stahl, but also on various other items of the general state of the body. In therapeutics Brown obviously prescribed sedatives in the case of too much excitation, and stimulants in the state of depression.

Another medical system that issued from the ideas which we have men-tioned is Vitalism, or the doctrine of the vital force. This system, which has certain analogies with that of Cullen, but which also reflects the physio-logical studies of Haller and the animism of Stahl, found its maximum de-velopment in the French schools of Montpellier and Paris. Its most cele-brated representative was Théophile DE BORDEU (1722–76). Author of a number of physiological treatises and a book on the history of medicine

(1764), Bordeu maintained that the lymphatic glands as well as the solid parts of the musculo-nervous system had a characteristic vital activity. He asserted therefore that secretion is a phenomenon that is neither purely physical nor chemical. The *vita propria* resided in every part of the body and, dependent on the laws of nature, regulated function by means of sensibility and motility. Bordeu's belief that the blood contained extracts from all parts of the body — special humours made in the laboratories of the organs — is an interesting forecast of our present theory of internal secretion, but nothing more than a forecast (see Neuburger, *Janus*, 1903, VIII, 26). Among his pupils was Joseph BARTHEZ (1734–1806), who introduced the term " vital principle " and maintained the point of view that every abnormality of function of normal life constituted disease. Another pupil was Philippe PINEL (1745–1826), who, under the influence of the philosopher Condillac, attempted the analysis of the various elements that underlie normal and pathological processes. His popular *Nosographie philosophique* (2 vols., 1789) is an attempt to align medicine with the natural sciences, assigning diseases to various classes, orders, and genera. The chief importance of this division is as an early attempt to show that certain tissues were subject to certain diseases, from which grew the highly important studies of Bichat. We shall also meet Pinel later in this chapter in connection with the humane treatment of the insane. In this French school, different from other theoretical systems of medicine of the time, there was a basis of good sense and a calm moderation of reasoning that is characteristic of French medico-philosophic speculation, a saving feature that protected scientists and physicians from the metaphysical exaggerations of various systems that were popular in this period.

In Germany vitalism had as its chief representatives J. F. BLUMENBACH (1752–1840), the founder of scientific anthropology, and J. C. REIL (1759–1813), of Halle and Berlin, clinician and anatomist whose name persists eponymically in the " island of Reil " of the cerebrum. Reil was the first editor of the *Archiv für Physiologie* (Halle, 1795), the first physiological journal, which later merged into the greater *Müller's Archiv*.

The tendency to romanticism that predominated in Germany at the end of the century and the orientation to mystic phantasy, led to the birth of other systems that require notice on account of their importance to the history of the medicine of the period, and also because they left significant traces in modern medicine. In this century, for instance, was born the concept of animal magnetism, or mesmerism, which was called after its founder, Franz Anton MESMER (1734–1815), who studied medicine in Vienna. In his doctoral dissertation he had supported the concept of the influence of the planets on physiological and pathological phenomena. Mesmer's idea thus resembles that of the mediæval astrologers; but he added to it "magnetic therapy," derived from the imposition of hands on the patient, a method that he asserted had given him astonishing cures.

Mesmerism is related to the primitive practices of magic medicine and is based on suggestion, the track of which, as we have seen, can be followed uninterruptedly through the whole history of medicine. The most interesting example perhaps is the cure of the scrofulous by the royal touch, as we have seen in Chapter xvi. In England especially, throughout the seventeenth century, charlatans flourished who claimed to cure all sorts of diseases, especially the rheumatic diseases, by the imposition of hands. The most celebrated was the Irishman Valentine GREATRAKES, who included some of the most illustrious men of his time among his clients.

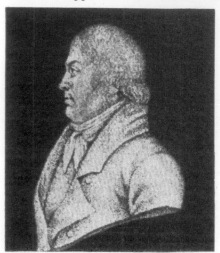

282. *Franz Mesmer.*

Mesmer, whether consciously or unconsciously, adopted this ancient idea of curing by the imposition of hands. To give it a scientific basis he created a complete doctrine according to which every living body possesses a magnetic fluid which circulates and gives out a special force that animates both the living and the inorganic world and produces connections between living beings. Recalling Molière's sarcastic phrase, where "a principle gives sleep because it contains the sleep principle," here the sleep principle merely had to be changed to the "magnetic virtue."

Mesmer's theories, but still more the reports of his cures and of his power of preventing pain and curing disease by producing a state of somnambulism or clairvoyancy, procured an enormous celebrity for the man and his system. Although the medical faculties and scientific societies rapidly and energetically denied the truth of his assertions on the basis of many experiments, patients flocked to him enthusiastically throughout Europe. His doctrine is set forth in his *Mémoire sur la découverte du magnétisme animal* (1779).

Mesmerism was especially popular in France. Mesmer came to Paris in 1768, boasting of miraculous cures and obtaining fabulous sums from his enthusiastic admirers, though he refused to present his results to the Medical Society. He was given the protection of Marie Antoinette, and the King offered him ten thousand francs to found a Magnetic Institute, and a grant of twenty thousand francs for his personal use. He included among his clients Lafayette and many of the most eminent littérateurs, politicians, and aristocrats of the time. He received his patients in a magnificent apartment in the middle of which was a large

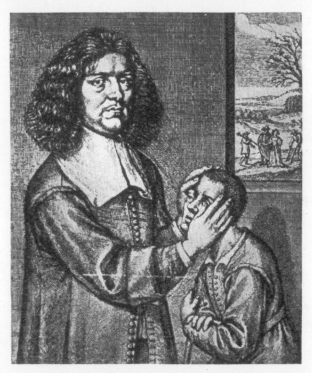

283. Valentine Greatrakes laying on hands.
From a seventeenth-century English print.

tub of a weak solution of sulphuric acid. From the tub emerged iron bars for the patients to grasp and cords to conduct the magnetic currents. The patients, placed in a circle around the magic tub, held the contacts in their hands or joined hands to form a circle. With many artifices, such as theatrical costumes, perfumes, and dramatic illuminations, Mesmer gave his treatment by touching the patient on different spots and bringing him into a hypnoidal state, in which he suggested cure. Driven from Paris by the fierce opposition of the physicians, he retired to Spa, but returned to Paris in 1784 and was acclaimed with enthusiasm by the court and all classes of people. The Academy of Medicine, however, again reported unfavourably on his activities. The French Revolution forced Mesmer to abandon France, with the loss of all his wealth. He retired to Frauenfeld in Switzerland, where he practiced until 1813, dying at Meersburg in 1815.

Mesmer was followed by a number of philosophers, physicians, and mystics. In a general way, he attracted all those whose tendency to the supernatural, the occult and mysterious responded to his method — a tendency that was one of the characteristics of the end of the century. Among others who belonged to his school were Eschenmayer, and the physician poet J. Kerner (1786-1862), who even subscribed to the doctrine of demons and magic practices. But intelligent scientists, such as Hufeland and Heim, took it up seriously, so that one might say that during the last decades of the eighteenth and in the early nineteenth century, contemporary with the development of romanticism, magnetic and occult medicine flourished in central Europe. The notorious London "Temple of Health" (1780) of James GRAHAM was an unworthy English variant of the Mesmer craze. The errors to which collective suggestion can drive even intelligent scientists is shown by the example of a German physician, D. G. KIESER (1779-1862), who believed in a solar brain which was active during the day, and a "telluric ganglion," a sort of lower psychic centre which regulated spiritual functions during the night.

As has been so often the case in medical history, however, this irregular and fantastic doctrine contained a modicum of truth which is still being sifted from the mass of chaff. Not only was mesmerism a dramatic example of the power of suggestion, which eventually has become fairly well evaluated and is intelligently used by the modern physician, but also it brought forward hypnotism, a true psychic phenomenon that has found definite allocation in mental pathology and therapy.

With mesmerism, magnetizers of all kinds appeared. A few among them apparently sought in good faith to give a scientific sanction to the new theory with the aid of " natural philosophy," which was beginning to make its appearance at that time, especially in Germany. Others, mostly impostors and charlatans, of whom the most celebrated was Giuseppe Balsamo, Count CAGLIOSTRO, were activated by the great opportunity offered to crafty and unscrupulous persons to exploit the credulous, the suffering, and the ingenuous; in other words, almost everyone. They even spoke seriously of spiritual or magnetic fertilization between the magnetizer and the magnetized, and there resulted much grotesque discussion, spiritualist séances, fantastic experiments, " polarity of sensations," and so on. America's contribution was the famous metallic tractors of Elisha PERKINS, a respected practitioner of Norwich, Connecticut. These were two metal rods, selling for five guineas a pair, which he claimed could extract disease when drawn downward over the part affected. First America then England was taken by storm, especially after the publication of his son Benjamin's *The Influence of Metallic Tractors*, etc. (1798). The fraud was castigated by Christopher Caustic (T. G. Fessenden) in his *Terrible Tractoration* (1803) and fell into disrepute after J. H. Haygarth of Bath had showed that dummies made of wood were no less potent (1799).

About the same time there arose another system which has perhaps not been given sufficient importance by historians: namely, homeopathy. Christian Friedrich Samuel HAHNEMANN (1755–1843), thinking that he had observed that cinchona bark produced febrile exacerbations, proclaimed the principle of *similia similibus:* that many diseases are cured by the administration of drugs which produce a condition similar to the disease. Thus hot compresses were prescribed for burns, opium to cure somnolence, and so on. According to Hahnemann, treatment should be directed entirely against the symptoms and not against the disease, about the nature of which it is useless to argue. The name " homeopathy " comes from the principle of like treating like, as opposed to so-called " allopathy," *contraria contrariis*, where, for instance, sedatives are given in excited states and stimulants in depressed states.

According to Hahnemann, drugs were thought to act by modifying the vital force so as to cause the disappearance of symptoms by increasing the energy of the vital force. Hahnemann was an empiric who thought that a successful result should be the index for treatment, and that this was the entire aim of medicine. Another fundamental doctrine of homeopathy was the belief that the effects of a drug became more powerful the smaller the doses in which it was given — the Theory of Potencies. For liquids, Hahnemann recommended the thirtieth potency; that is, an original tincture is prepared of which two drops are diluted with ninety-eight drops of alcohol; one drop of this solution is further diluted in ninety-nine drops of alcohol, and so on, for thirty times. With solid drugs the procedure is the same, mixing the original material with sugar of milk.

Hahnemann's disease concepts were no less strange. Chronic diseases were divided into three categories: those due to syphilis; those derived from *sykosis* (a morbid form that was thought to be cured by the juice of arbor vitæ in a potency of decillions); and, finally, those that come from scabies (*psora*), the commonest cause of chronic disease. In 1810 Hahnemann published his *Organon der rationellen Heilkunde*. In spite of the campaign of opposition conducted by the leading physicians of the time, he acquired a great reputation and found numerous followers. Homeopathic clinics, societies and journals were rapidly founded in many parts of Europe and America. Schools of homeopathic medicine came into existence, a few of which still survive. His disciples evolved new schools, such as isopathy, founded by Constantine HERING, of New York, according to which the disease should be treated by the very products of that disease; thus persons suffering from tapeworm were given tapeworm heads by mouth; those suffering from gonorrhœa were treated with gonorrhœal pus, and so on. Long and heated discussions were held on the merits of these systems, of which homeopathy still manages to survive, especially in America. [Here, too, as in the case of mesmerism, an irregular system based on false, even absurd, principles had an unwarranted vogue, yet contained a germ of truth that had a beneficial influence on the main current of medical treatment. The minute, homeopathic doses at least did no harm at a time when polypharmacy and " shot-gun " prescriptions held sway in the ranks of the medical élite. Just as Paré found that wounds would heal better without boiling oil, so physicians learned that diseases often did better when exposed to fewer remedies or to none at all, except to those few that had been proved efficacious. Today this type of " therapeutic nihilism " has justified itself, and the number of drugs that have so proved themselves is now satisfactorily on the increase. *Ed.*]

All these systems found fewer followers in Italy. The most popular was the Brunonian theory, which, probably on account of its simplicity, made rapid headway in the universities and academies of the peninsula. Brown's *Elements of Medicine* (1788) was translated in 1792 by Giovanni Rasori (1766–1837), of Parma, a young and enthusiastic admirer of the theories of Brown, whom he compared to Bacon and Newton. Numerous articles appeared on the subject in the medical journals, but most of the Italian physicians of the time declared themselves against it. Among its partisans were the professors Borda of Pavia, Brera of Padua, Tommasini of Bologna, Emiliani, Mocini, and many others. Against them were ranged F. Vaccà-Berlinghieri (1732–1812), who maintained that morbid and vital stimuli were essentially different, and Domenico Cotugno (1736–1833), who stated that " medicine does not have masters; it has but one teacher, Nature."

Rasori, professor at Pavia, was the chief exponent of the Brunonian system in Italy. Relying on experiments, the absence of which he lamented in Brown's writings, he founded the Theory of Counter-stimuli, substances which diminished excitability by an effect contrary to that produced by stimuli. His book (1799) attacking Hippocratism, ancient and modern, provoked a veritable tempest in university circles. Rasori was an extraordinary personality who was prominent among the revolutionaries and French partisans of the time. At Pavia the violence of his polemics drove him from the city. Returning to Milan, he abandoned Brown's system and substituted " the diatheses of stimulation and of counter-stimulation " for Brown's *sthenia* and *asthenia*. From one point of view at least, Rasori's doctrine was meritorious, in that it prescribed the careful study of the effect of drugs and prohibited the use of more than one drug at a time, so as not to prevent the proper study of its effect. He regarded blood-letting as a sure means of diagnosis, in the sense that subsequent improvement indicated the diagnosis of a diathesis of stimulation; and aggravation of the condition, a diathesis of counter-stimulation. Rasori and his pupils prescribed enormous doses: for a case of syphilis, 134 grams of extract of aconite in eight days; for a case of pleurisy, 4 to 5 grams of antimony tartrate in four days with a blood-letting of 4,230 grams, and so on. Antimony and phlebotomy consti- tuted the basis of his therapy, which had, as one might imagine, catastrophic results. When the French returned to Milan after Marengo, Rasori was made chief physician of the military hospital and professor of the clinic. He began the publication of a journal entitled *Annali di medicina*, published his translation of Erasmus Darwin's *Zoonomia*, and acquired new fame and many new enemies. It was said that the theories of Brown and Rasori claimed more victims than the French Revolution, and much was written to show the dangers of this form of treatment. In 1812 Rasori was deposed from his chair and in 1814 he was con- demned to two years in prison by the Austrians for participation in the con- spiracy of the Carbonari.

The last of the great Italian systematists was Giacomo TOMMASINI (1768–1846), Professor of Physiology and Pathology at Parma (1794), and of Clinical Medicine at Bologna (1816). At first a partisan and even champion of Rasori, he later parted from him in his *Della nuova dottrina medica italiana* (Bologna, 1817), believing that irritation is always local and not the result of a diathesis, and distinguishing between general and local diseases.

3. Anatomy

Though the formation of theoretical systems was, as we have seen, characteristic of the eighteenth century, the valuable progress made was along the lines of observation and experimentation in the natural sciences, a trend which had made an auspicious start in the previous century. The necessities of historical exposition have required us to follow these two tendencies separately, but it should be recognized that there were actually many contacts between the great systematists and the great observers of the period. We have seen that the former found many followers throughout Europe; we are about to see that the latter had a much wider and deeper influence on medical thought. The distinction between these two groups should not be understood as a rigid division determined by entirely different objectives. It merely indicated the two great routes along which eight- eenth-century medicine proceeded: on the one hand toward mysticism and theory, directed by philosophic speculation; on the other toward positivism and a materialism in which observation and experiment predominated.

General anatomy had become well established as a teaching discipline in most European countries in the eighteenth century, though important discoveries were less frequent than in the preceding century. The centre of anatomical study shifted from Holland to Paris and to Edinburgh, where the dynasty of the three Monros held sway for more than a century. This was started by Alexander Monro primus (1697–1767), the son of John

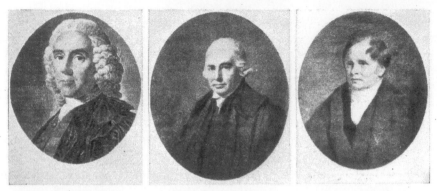

284. *The Three Alexander Monros, Professors of Anatomy at Edinburgh, 1720–1846. (The portrait of Alexander Monro primus is from a contemporary engraving, that of secundus after a portrait by Raeburn, that of tertius from an original portrait in the* EDINBURGH ROYAL COLLEGE OF SURGEONS.)

Monro, a Scottish army surgeon. Alexander, familiar with the superior condition of medicine on the Continent began a course of lectures in 1720, which was continued for nearly forty years, being followed in 1758 by those of his son, Alexander Monro secundus (1733–1817), who had been trained to follow his father in anatomical teaching. The foramen of Monro, connecting the third with the lateral ventricles, was described in his *Treatise on the Brain, the Eye and the Ear* (1797), the last of his four chief works, all published after his fiftieth year. A greater and more successful teacher than his father, he in turn was followed by his son, Alexander Monro tertius (1773–1859), in whose hands the standard of the teaching eventually degenerated. Monro tertius is said to have used his grandfather's lecture notes verbatim, even including such remarks as: " When I was a student at Leiden in 1719."

Anatomy was still mostly in the hands of the surgeons, of whom William CHESELDEN (1688–1752), of St. Thomas's Hospital, London, is a good example. His *Anatomy of the Human Body* (1713) and *Osteography* (1733) were deservedly popular, though the latter aroused the ire of a

London Scot, JOHN DOUGLAS (d. 1759), to the point of publishing an *Animadversion* (1735) thereto. JAMES DOUGLAS (1675–1742), an older brother, wrote on comparative myology (London, 1707) and is remembered by the " pouch of Douglas " (*Description of the Peritoneum*, London, 1730). In France the anatomical trend was represented by Joseph LIEUTAUD (1703–80), whose name is also remembered in connection with Lieutaud's triangle in the bladder.

Probably the most influential anatomist of the century was the Dane Jakob Benignus WINSLOW (1669–1760), who, turned toward anatomy by his teacher Duverney, and having become a Catholic, remained in Paris, where he numbered Haller among his many pupils. His textbook (1732) was a favourite for a full half-century. Best remembered among his numerous observations is that of the peritoneal foramen that bears his name.

The outstanding descriptive anatomist of his time was Bernhard Siegfried ALBINUS (b. Frankfurt, 1697–1770), of Leiden, the eldest of three eminent sons of a well-known father. A pupil of Bidloo, Rau, and Boerhaave, he brought out with the last named an excellent edition of Vesalius' works, and published praiseworthy atlases on the bones (1726) and muscles (1734), and a splendid *Tabulæ sceleti et musculorum corporis humani* (1747), all beautifully illustrated by Wandelaar.

In Germany, three generations of MECKELS ably advanced the subject. The grandfather, Johann Friedrich (1714–74), gave the first description of the spheno-palatine (Meckel's) and the submaxillary ganglia, in his inaugural dissertation, *De quinto pari nervorum* (1748). The dissertation of his son, Philipp Friedrich Theodor (Berlin, 1756–Halle, 1803), *De labyrinthi auris contentis*, also made history, though he later turned to surgery and to obstetrics at the court of the Czar. The grandson, Johann Friedrich (1781–1833), the greatest of the three, was one of the leading figures in the German medicine of the time. He wrote valuable treatises on normal (1815) and pathological anatomy (1812–18) and on malformations (1817–26). His several works on comparative anatomy (Halle, 1806; Leipzig, 1808–12; *Archiv für Physiologie*, 1808; Halle, 1821–30, etc.), for which he has been called the German Cuvier, made Germany the centre for this discipline in the early nineteenth century. His studies of normal and pathological development revealed the comparatively late differentiation of sex and the tendency of higher forms to pass through stages of development each similar to the end stages of lower forms. " Meckel's diverticulum " is named after him. To Abraham VATER (1684–1751), of Wittenberg, is owed the description of the ampulla of the common bile duct (*Dissertatio Anatomica*, 1720), one of many anatomical discoveries too numerous to describe here (see Garrison, 4th ed., pp. 332 ff.). Somewhat later, S. T. von Sömmerring (1755–1830) was an able, industrious contributor to anatomical progress. His numerous investigations were well set forth in remarkably accurate illustrations, made by himself and his pupil Christoph Koeck. Descriptive anatomy has been said to have reached its greatest height with Sömmerring.

The most famous English anatomist of the eighteenth century was WILLIAM HUNTER (1718–83), of Long Calderwood, Scotland. A pupil, then an assistant of Smellie in London, in 1746 he became Professor of Anatomy of the Society of Navy Surgeons, and in 1750 received the medical degree from the University of Glasgow. After a journey to the Continent, where he made the acquaintance of Albinus, he turned to gynæcology and obstetrics, but in 1768 became Professor of Anatomy at the newly established Royal Academy of Arts, of which he was later President. His lectures on anatomy, surgery, and obstetrics were continued in the famous anatomical theatre and museum on Great Windmill Street, built in 1768. His greatest work, *The Anatomy of the Human Gravid Uterus*, published by the celebrated Baskerville Press of Birmingham as their only medical publication (1774), contains twenty-four masterpieces of anatomical illustration. This atlas was reprinted by the Sydenham Society in the next century. Hunter, though jealous and needlessly controversial, "worked till he dropped and lectured when he was dying" (Stephen Paget). The great sums of money that he accumulated were devoted entirely to medical purposes; he left more than one hundred thousand pounds sterling for the anatomical museum at Glasgow.

His even more famous younger brother, JOHN HUNTER (1728–93), was one of the greatest figures in English medical history. His anatomical museum, containing thousands of preparations, forms the basis of the marvellous collection at the Royal College of Surgeons of London. He was the founder of pathological anatomy in England, and raised English surgery from the position of a technical trade to its proper rank in medicine, to be pursued in the same scientific manner as medicine itself and its various specialties. Above all is he important in the history of medicine for his lifelong insistence on investigation and experimentation, so that Garrison places him as a biologist with Haller and Johannes Müller, and with Paré and Lister as one of the three greatest surgeons of all time. His chief publications were *The Natural History of the Human Teeth* (1771); *On the Venereal Disease* (1786); *Observations on Certain Parts of the Animal Oeconomy* (1787); and *On the Nature of the Blood, Inflammation and Gun Shot Wounds* (1794, published posthumously by his brother-in-law,

Everard Home). His bibliography contains also a large number of articles on the greatest variety of subjects.

Hunter was a rare type of great natural intelligence and penetrative observation, who, arriving in London without the slightest scientific preparation, entered rapidly upon a successful practical and scientific career. Tireless in his anatomical and pathological studies, desiring above all to observe with his own eyes, the sworn enemy of the mazes of academic and scholastic medicine, an

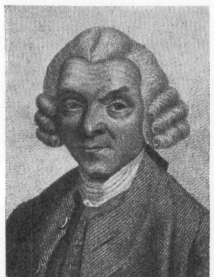

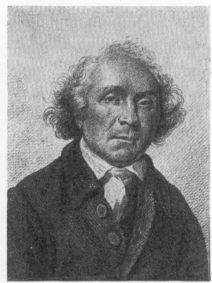

285. William Hunter.   *286. John Hunter.*

unremitting investigator, but sometimes hazardous in his hypotheses, John Hunter represents the typical Scot, endowed with a dominating, vigorous common sense, an iron will, and a marvellous energy. His method is illustrated by his reply to Jenner, regarding the latter's ideas on hibernation in hedgehogs: "Don't think, try." To the many branches of experimental and surgical pathology, Hunter successfully applied his passionate love for research. To him is owed the differentiation of the hard and soft chancre and valuable observations on the collateral circulation. He studied hibernation with the cessation of digestion which occurs during that period, and the repair of ruptured tendons following an accident to his own person. He pursued many novel lines of study and his very lack of previous education prevented him from wasting time on the many confused hypotheses of the day. Among his errors was his controversy with Spallanzani on the nature of digestion and his identification of gonorrhœa with syphilis, following his inoculation of himself and his delay in treatment in order to study the development of the disease. His death occurred in a dramatic manner at a board meeting in St. George's Hospital. Subject to attacks of angina, he recognized that " my life is in the hands of any rascal who chooses to annoy and tease me." Opposition about the appointment of his successor at the hospital roused his ire and brought on a fatal attack. Cheselden and the Hunters will be met again in the section on surgery.

An eminent pupil of Hunter was his brusque successor, John ABERNETHY (1764–1831), who attained wide fame as a skilful surgeon and performed various major operations successfully for the first time. William HEWSON (1739–74), a pupil of both Hunters, worked out the lymphatics in various lower animals (1769) – an important step in the development of knowledge of absorption by the body. His *Experimental Inquiry into the Properties of the Blood* (1771) illuminated the phenomena of blood coagulation and the behaviour of the colourless corpuscles (leucocytes). His untimely death, from a dissection wound at the age of thirty-five, sent his family to Philadelphia, where they still continue in medicine in an unbroken line of male descent. William C. CRUIKSHANK (1745–1800), who succeeded Hewson as William Hunter's assistant and after the latter's death took over the Great Windmill Street school, combined a large and generously conducted practice with various scientific investigations, especially the continuation of the Hunters' study of the lymphatic system.

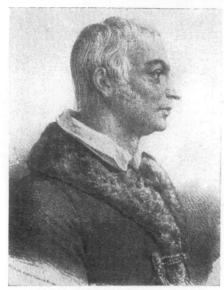

287. *Paolo Mascagni, by Antonio Verrico.*

In the young American colonies, for a long time first-hand knowledge of anatomy was exceedingly difficult to obtain. Dissections were almost non-existent and only a few autopsies for medico-legal purposes are on record. The first anatomical lectures (1730?) were given by the Philadelphian Thomas CADWALADER (1708–79) on his return from medical study in Europe. Cadwalader held a leading position in the medicine of the colonies and also wrote two notable articles. His *Essay on the West-India Dry-Gripes* (published by Benjamin Franklin, 1745) is an account of chronic lead poisoning from rum distilled in lead pipes, while his description of *An Extraordinary Case in Physick* (published in the same work) is the first known description of *mollities ossium*. In 1752 Thomas Wood of New York advertised a course in anatomy (though it is not known if it ever was given); and for several years William Hunter (1730?–77), of Newport, gave highly successful anatomical lectures. The most important anatomical event for the colonies, however, was the gift by the Quaker physician John Fothergill of "curious anatomical casts and drawings" (the latter beautifully executed in 1755 by J. van Riemsdyck after dissec-

tions by Jenty) to the young William Shippen (1736–1808) for use in teaching at the Quaker Pennsylvania Hospital. This was an important step toward the founding (1765) by Shippen and John Morgan (1735–89) of the School of Medicine of the University of Pennsylvania, the first medical school in the American colonies. Systematic anatomical teaching was started in New York by Samuel Clossy in 1763 (continued from 1768 on in the medical department of King's College, now the College of Physicians and Surgeons, and in Baltimore about the same time by C. F. Wiesenthal). In Boston the first public lecture was given by John Jeffries (of English ballooning fame) shortly before the Revolution; and when Harvard College formed a Medical

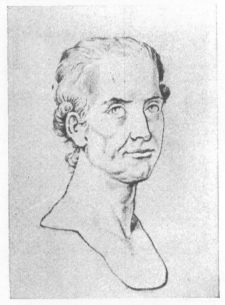

288. *Domenico Cotugno.*
(*Frontispiece of his* Opuscula omnia, *Naples, 1826.*)

School in 1782, John Warren became its first Professor of Anatomy and Surgery. In 1779 Thomas Jefferson had brought about the creation of a Professorship of Anatomy, Medicine, and Chemistry at William and Mary College. Though doubtless inconspicuous in contemporary medicine abroad, these steps are important both locally and as illustrating the development of medicine in a country where development occurred late in medical history.

Among the chief Italian anatomists of the century was G. B. Bianchi (1681–1761), who contributed to the anatomy of the liver, the lachrymal ducts, and the genital organs. G. D. Santorini (1681–1737) published valuable anatomical observations on the musculature of the face, larynx, and penis, and on the accessory duct of the pancreas that bears his name. His anatomical illustrations, published in 1765 after his death, by Girard, were regarded by Daremberg as one of the masterpieces of the century, belonging to that magnificent series of anatomical works that are characteristic of the period.

Leopoldo CALDANI (1725–1813), who succeeded Morgagni in the chair of anatomy at Padua, was a great admirer of Haller and his theories, endeavouring to correlate them with the doctrines of his master. He was

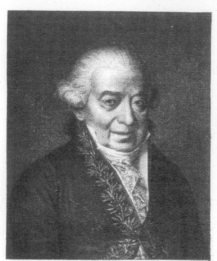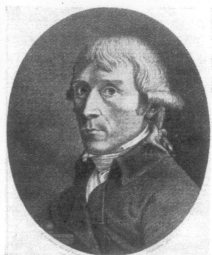

289. *Leopoldo Marcantonio Caldani, by Natale Schiavoni.*
290. *Antonio Scarpa, by G. Cattaneo.*

especially concerned with comparative anatomy and physiology, acquiring valuable knowledge through animal experimentation. A lecture upholding Haller's doctrines of irritability (1760) gave rise to such opposition that Caldani was forced to leave Bologna. He accepted the chair of medicine at Padua, and in 1771 the chair of anatomy there. His anatomical plates, published after his death by his nephew, Floriano (Venice, 1813), illustrate his studies on the structure of bones and the anatomy of the ganglia and the nervous plexuses.

In 1787 Paolo MASCAGNI (1752–1815), who became Professor of Anatomy at Siena, published his great work on the lymphatics, with beautiful copper engravings. It was long accepted as a classical work and passed through many editions. It includes a notable passage on the diapedesis of the blood corpuscles through the blood vessels in areas of inflammation. Many of his anatomical plates were published in 1819 by Francesco Anton-marchi, Napoleon's physician at St. Helena, and still other plates by Farnese in 1821 and Berlinghieri in 1823–32.

Antonio SCARPA (1752–1832), pupil of Morgagni, at the age of twenty became Professor of Anatomy at Modena, where he organized a model department. In 1783 he was called to the chair of anatomy at Pavia, where he reconstructed the Anatomical Institute, and from 1787 to 1812 was also Professor of Clinical Surgery. He was succeeded in the chair of anatomy in 1803 by his pupil Panizza. His first study, on the *Round Window of the Ear*, was published at the age of twenty; he gave the first description of the naso-palatine nerve and of Scarpa's triangle of the thigh, of the cremasteric fascia (known as Scarpa's fascia), and of the secondary membrane of the tympanum (known as Scarpa's membrane). He made valuable observations on the nerves of the heart (*Tabulæ Nevrologicæ*, 1794) and on the intimate structure of bones, their development, and the bony callus, and recognized changes in the intima of arteries in arteriosclerosis. His works, *Anatomicæ annotationes* (1779), *Anatomicæ disquisitiones de auditu et olfactu* (1789), *Sui piedi torti congeniti* (1803), *Sull'aneurisma* (1804), laid a deserved basis for his wide fame. His *Osservazioni sulle principali malattìe degli occhi* (1801) was the classic text of ophthalmology for several decades in the last century and passed through several editions in Italian, German, English, French, and Dutch. With Spallanzani, Volta, and Frank, Scarpa formed a group which brought Pavia to the height of its fame as one of the greatest European universities.

Domenico COTUGNO (1736–1822), of Naples, was not only a scholarly scientist and penetrating observer, but also a fervid Italian patriot. A remarkable hygienist, he was a pioneer in the prophylaxis of tuberculosis. He discovered the cerebro-spinal fluid, which has since assumed a highly important role in pathology, and also was the first to have established experimentally the abnormal presence of albumin in the urine. Gradenigo (*Atti R. Acc. di Torino*, 1919) attributes to Cotugno the priority for the concept of hearing that a century later was established by Helmholtz. Cotugno also wrote a masterly description of ischialgia (Naples, 1764), recommending the use of blisters and cauterizations.

3a. Pathological Anatomy. G. B. Morgagni

In this century pathological anatomy made its greatest advances thus far in the achievements of Giovanni Battista MORGAGNI (1682–1771), of Forlí. Morgagni was not only one of the most fertile observers in the history of medicine but also a profound and tireless investigator. He was a master in the best sense of the word in the limpid clarity of his thought, the masterly form of its exposition, and the pertinacity with which he applied his life to the studies that resulted in his immortal *De sedibus et causis morborum per anatomen indagatis* (1761), the high-water mark of clinico-pathological description.

His ability was demonstrated at an early age; he was scarcely fourteen when he composed essays and poetry and publicly discussed philosophical essays. At

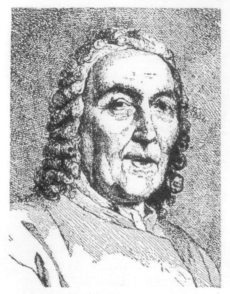

sixteen he became a pupil of Valsalva at Bologna, from whom he received the stimulus for his life work in pathology. Receiving his degree in 1701, in 1706, when he had just been made President of the Academia Inquietorum, he published his first medical work, *Adversaria anatomica prima*, which, *inter alia*, contained valuable observations on the anatomy of the larynx. At twenty-five he was nominated lecturer at the University and prosector in the Anatomical Theatre of Bologna, and four years later was called to teach theoretical medicine at Padua. In 1715 he was given the chair of anatomy at Padua, and was one of the greatest to hold this distinguished position. During this period he published his second work, *Adversaria anatomica altera*, which dealt especially with adipose tissue, the musculature of the di-

291. *Giovanni Battista Morgagni, by Angelica Kauffmann.*

gestive tract, the structure of the lungs and biliary tract. His other anatomical works gained the esteem of his Italian colleagues and of such eminent foreigners as Boerhaave, Winslow, and Ruysch. Last and greatest of his works was his *De sedibus*, which presented his entire experience in the field of pathological anatomy. In addition to writing his medical works he was a student of the classics and wrote on Cornelius Celsus; he was a skilful archæologist, describing the antiquities of Forlí in the *Lettere Emiliane*. He also compiled biographies of Guglielmini and Valsalva.

He continued teaching to the last year of his life, in which he held lectures regularly in spite of the excessive cold of that winter. When John Morgan of Philadelphia visited him at Padua in 1764, Morgan recorded in his journal that the octogenarian was as hale as a man of fifty and still worked without spectacles. The legend is unfortunately incorrect that Morgagni, in the copy of *De sedibus* (now in the College of Physicians of Philadelphia) that he gave Morgan, inscribed himself as a cousin — doubtless suggested by the similarity of the two names. Already in 1727 Heister dedicated his *Compendium anatomicum* to the young Morgagni, calling him leader in the anatomical art. In 1769 the *Natio*

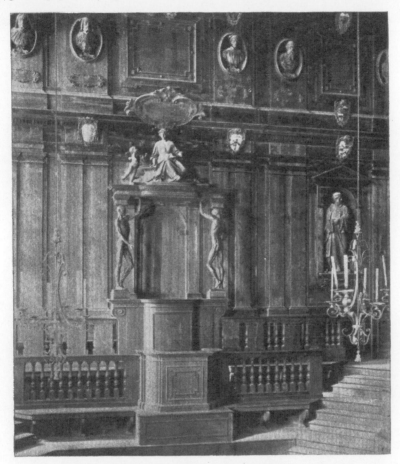

292. *The anatomical theatre of the University of Bologna. The carved figures are by E. Lelli, eighteenth century.*

Germanica of the Paduan Athenæum proclaimed him publicly in the magnificent anatomical theatre of the university as *anatomicorum totius Europæ princeps*. Admirers, perhaps tinged with envy, often called him in Italy " His Anatomical Majesty." Forlí jealously preserves his memory; in 1931 his monument was unveiled in the piazza that bears his name. The volume published on this occasion bears evidence of the high esteem in which he was held and contains a voluminous catalogue of Morgagniana. *De sedibus* was frequently reprinted, and has been translated into French, and into English by B. Alexander (London, 1769). His bibliography appears in Fiorentini's *Saggio di bibliografia sintetica* (Bologna, 1930).

In Morgagni's classic work we see an anatomist and pathologist combining his special knowledge of the autopsy room with the bedside obser-

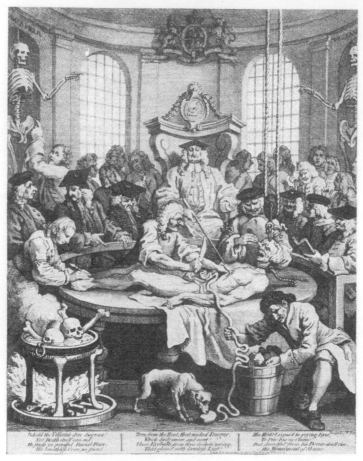

293. *Hogarth's* Reward of Cruelty, *caricaturing the dissecting methods of the time.*

vations of the clinician. He brought medicine to its true fountain-head – the pathology that the Hippocratists had foreseen without penetrating into its mysteries. Pathologic anatomy, which had not existed as a science up to that time, had in a single stroke assumed its vital position in medical science.

It must of course not be forgotten that there were pathologists before Morgagni who had made notable contributions to pathological anatomy. From the time of Benivieni to the *Sepulchretum* (1679) of Bonetus and steadily thereafter, many valuable pathological observations had prepared the way for this great work. But just as Harvey's glory is in no way dimmed by the notable work of his predecessors, so Morgagni's by its very size, intelligence of observation, and critical judgment, is entitled to its pre-eminent position in establishing pathological anatomy on a scientific basis in modern medicine. Morgagni's masterly analysis of the enormous amount of material that he had gathered over many years, and his systematic and logical construction of phenomena, succeeded in bringing out, as never before, the connection between the changes in the diseased organ and the manifestations of the disease. He noted the anatomical differences between the normal and the pathological organ and demonstrated that for every anatomical change there was a corresponding change in function. It is for these reasons that Morgagni can be regarded not only as the founder of pathologic anatomy but also as a great contributor to clinical medicine.

If we analyse Morgagni's *De sedibus*, which was written in the form of letters, we at once find a fundamental principle stated by the author in the dedication of the first book. He tells us that autopsies are only useful when made by an experienced physician who has a profound knowledge of normal anatomy (which he regards as the torch of pathological anatomy), and when they are accompanied by a detailed, accurate history of the disease. When these conditions are lacking, pathological anatomy is necessarily sterile, because one cannot properly correlate anatomical lesions with the clinical symptoms. It is evident that the best post-mortem descriptions are useless unless accompanied by knowledge of the functional changes that the lesions produced during life.

An essential difference between the pathology of Morgagni and that of his predecessors is that it is founded on a system of logical reasoning and is not a mere collection of isolated individual observations. With a clear vision not only of his own investigations, but still more of the proper method of investigation — which to us constitutes his great merit — Morgagni appreciates that the most important step in medicine is the objective search for the origin of the disease, even though, as he recognizes, it may give rise to frequent errors, such as mistaking post-mortem changes for actual lesions, or of attributing a causal relationship to phenomena that have nothing to do with the cause. How avoid these errors, or at least how reduce them to a minimum? With sure intuition Morgagni establishes the method that the study should follow: The dissection should be made with the greatest care, and no detail of any organ should escape the observer. He should always bear in mind the possible cause of the disease, the clinical phenomena observed, and the lesions previously discovered in patients attacked by the same disease. The pathologist should appreciate the frequency or rarity of the lesions observed. By objective observation the pathologist should endeavour to reconstruct the nature of the disease in question.

Thus Morgagni follows the Hippocratic line of thought and conducts it into a region that Hippocrates had not penetrated: the search for the origins of disease and the visible changes that it produces in the dead body. Morgagni's erudition was equalled by his modesty. He published his great work only after many years of study, and even then was stimulated thereto by a young physician for whom he wished to summarize his experiences, declaring that his work should be regarded only as a continuation of the work of Bonetus.

Morgagni's masterpiece, *De sedibus*, written at the ripe age of seventy-nine, contains some seven hundred cases with adequate clinical histories and reports of autopsies performed by himself or his assistants, covering practically every phase of gross pathological anatomy. The five books deal with: Diseases of the Head, Thorax, Abdomen, Surgical Diseases, and those involving the whole body, and Addenda.

The difficulty of considering Morgagni's discoveries in detail is obvious. We may, however, refer to the masterly description of the state of the heart in angina pectoris, in myocardial degeneration, and in vegetative endocarditis (one of these following gonorrhœa). He recognized the post-mortem nature of those clots in the heart chambers which until his time had generally been regarded as polyps — that is, ante-mortem pathological phenomena. He detected the slow pulse and epileptiform seizures later known as Adams-Stokes disease. He made original observations on pulmonary tuberculosis; his descriptions of a tubercle in the process of liquefaction can still be studied today with profit. Especially noteworthy are his observations on tumours of the pylorus, and on blenorrhagia and its difference from urethral ulcer, which had been accepted as due to the blenorrhagia. He was the first to describe the cuneiform cartilages of Wrisberg (1739–1808), which Sappey and Fraenkel proposed to call the " cartilages of Morgagni." He is also eponymically connected with those small vesicles in the genital tract known as the " hydatids of Morgagni."

Morgagni knew that apoplexy came from changes in the blood vessels and not from a lesion in the cerebrum itself. He was the first to connect syphilis with lesions of the cerebral vessels, though he made no direct statement to that effect. He was of course familiar with syphilis of the skin and its destructive effect on bones, and described gummata of the liver and brain, the latter apparently for the first time. He appreciated that in pneumonia the lung had " the substance of liver " (i.e., hepatization); that cerebral abscess was the result, not the cause, of a discharging ear. He described cirrhosis of the liver and what we now call acute yellow atrophy, also various calculi, and numerous tumours, including one in the adrenal body. He observed that hemiplegia was manifested on the opposite side from the cerebral lesion and threw doubt on the hemiplegia said to be caused by damage to the cerebellum. At a distance of two centuries his work appears so convincing that the attacks directed on him by Broussais and others now merely cause a smile. One can hardly give higher praise to his work than to recognize that one can still reconstruct exact diagnoses of the cases that he has included in his immortal pages.

Characteristic of Morgagni was his study of Valsalva, who had assembled a vast amount of data for his work on the human ear. Morgagni, with a profound devotion to his master, utilized this material for a study which demonstrated not only the admiration and gratitude that the pupil had for the master, but also assured Valsalva his important position in the history of medicine. After fifteen years of collection and study Morgagni published his magnificent work *De vita et scriptis Antonii Mariæ Valsalvæ* (1740), followed by twenty letters on anatomy, almost all referring to Valsalva's works. In these two large volumes Morgagni also gives the results of his personal studies.

We quote one of the most interesting of Morgagni's descriptions, an early observation of the permanently slow pulse of heart block:

" This man was a merchant, at Padua, of sixty-four years of age, of a square stature, and of a fat habit of body; but not to excess. He, having been formerly subject to rheumatism, and contractions of the nerves, had been cur'd by medical remedies: so that notwithstanding he was taken up with many and various businesses continually, he was nevertheless, in good health, to that very age which I just now spoke of; when, of a sudden, some circumstances happen'd, from whence he was seiz'd with very violent affections of the mind, with terror, fear, anger, and sadness. A few days after these commotions, a kind of vertigo coming on, he fell down. And, on the day following, he began to be troubled with convulsive motions, together with an attack similar to an epilepsy. . . . The pulse was, at that time, strong indeed, but hard and rare. . . . The rareness of the pulse in particular, was found by me to be so great, that the number of pulsations was less, by about two third parts, than it ought to be. . . . And this rareness, which was perpetual, and had been so for many months, was perceiv'd to be even more considerable, as often as ever the attacks were at hand. . . . And his death happen'd, at length, on the last day but one of September, in the same year 1747; on which day three or four attacks had preceded. . . . On the day following I was present at the dissection of the body, according to desire . . . the heart was very large, by reason of the ventricles being dilated; and not from the parietes being become thicker " (*De sedibus*, Letter 64, Art. 5; from English translation by B. Alexander, London, 1769).

Together with Morgagni's systematic correlation of clinical and pathological observations, pathology was also being pursued in the older manner of miscellaneous pathological observations and uncorrelated descriptions. A prominent eighteenth-century representative of the collector type was Edward SANDIFORT (1742–1814), of Leiden, a pupil of Albinus, who carried the methods of museums and atlases into pathology. His *Observationes anatomicæ-pathologicæ* (1777–81) and *Museum . . . descriptum* (1793–1835) beautifully describe the contents of the Leiden museum, illustrating such specimens as congenital lesions of the heart and other viscera, hernias and intestinal obstructions, bony ankyloses and inflammations, ulcerative endocarditis, and so on.

The most successful teacher of pathology of his day was Jerome David GAUB (1705–80), Boerhaave's successor at Leiden. In his popular *Institutiones pathologiæ medicinalis* (1758) he endeavoured to conciliate humoral and vitalistic pathology. This is an interesting example of a sterile exposition of a modified humoral theory, blind to the growing accumulation of sound pathological anatomical knowledge. First appearing three years before Morgagni's *De sedibus*, it continued unchanged in several editions for another score of years. We search through it in vain for the solid facts that had accumulated in the previous century. Pathology, the theory of the morbid states of man, to be sure, is regarded as treating of disordered function as well as structure, the divisions of general and special pathology are considered, and its causative factors are subdivided into the familiar predisposing and active, remote and proximal causes (we even read of substances resembling hormones and animate causes of disease), but no meat clings to these dry bones. " Chemical analysis " of the body shows that it is composed of wet substance (the most mobile), inflammable (the food of fire), saline (the friend of water), and earthy (resisting fire and water). Disease comes from improper mixtures of these; putridity, for instance, is a kind of corruption that easily ensues if there is a copious supply of wet and inflammable. Deficiency of the natural cohesion of the body matter causes debility, tenuity, or dissolution (hemorrhages, diarrhœa, ptyalism, pustules); excessive cohesion causes undue tenacity, " spissitude " (stagnation, obstruction, infarction, tumours). We hopefully meet " aneurysma," " anastomosis," only to find that these are terms used for diseases of the contents of solid structures, or cavities which admit or emit too much laxity! The five hundred and twelve pages of this archaic uselessness were soon discarded after the author's death.

A new type of pathological exposition was inaugurated by *The Morbid Anatomy of Some of the Most Important Parts of the Human Body* (1793).

In this book Matthew BAILLIE (1761–1823), nephew of the Hunters, from whom he received his start both in scientific medicine and in a lucrative practice, codified his pathological knowledge into the first systematic text on pathological anatomy in any language. Though brief and not covering the entire body, it described in simple, clear language the lesions that the several organs and systems were prone to, much as in the special pathology

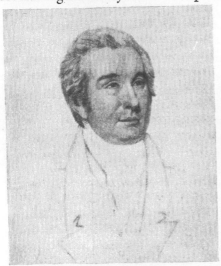

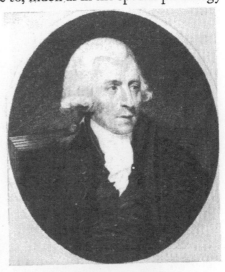

294. *Matthew Baillie.*
From a contemporary unfinished stipple engraving.

295. *William Withering.*
From a contemporary engraving.

sections of modern textbooks. Case reports were not included, though they were added in the German translation; in other words, pathology was now treated for the first time as an independent science. The success of the book was prompt: a second and larger edition appeared in 1797 (here rheumatism of the heart was for the first time mentioned in print), and a supplementary atlas, also the first of its kind, was published from 1799 to 1802. In the atlas the illustrations of an ovarian teratoma and a hydatidiform mole are especially well known. Baillie's book was translated into German, French, and Italian, setting the vogue in those countries for similar works, out of which our modern textbooks of pathology have grown.

4. Physiology. Haller, Spallanzani. English School

A leader in eighteenth-century physiology was Albrecht von HALLER (1708–77), of Bern, one of the most famous men of his period both for the profundity and extent of his knowledge and for his versatility in many fields.

Haller, called "the Great" even in his lifetime, possessing the universal admiration of his contemporaries, was one of those intellectual geniuses who recall the types of the Renaissance. A *Wunderkind*, who as a young child composed

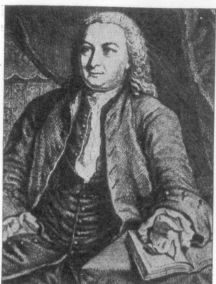

grammars, poems, biographies, and classical translations, this Bernese aristocrat was a poet of uncommon value, illustrious statesman, botanist, philosopher, and physician. He began his studies at the University of Tübingen at the age of fifteen, after which he studied at Leiden as a pupil of Boerhaave. His crowded life took him to Basel, Göttingen for seventeen years at the newly established university, and back to his native Bern, where in 1745 he became a member of the Swiss Council and was active as public health officer, economist, founder of a philological seminary and a State orphan asylum, the head of his Canton. Although carrying an enormous load, Haller never abandoned his scientific labours and left to posterity an incredible amount of work that can barely be touched upon here. His most important

296. *Albrecht von Haller.*
(*Frontispiece of his* Works, *1757.*)

works are his commentaries on the *Institutiones* of Boerhaave (1739–44), his work on physiology called *Primæ lineæ physiologiæ* (1747), and his famous *Elementa physiologiæ corporis humani* (8 vols., 1757–66). In this last-named work he assembled with great industry and critical sense the treasures of all physiological observations made up to that time, and co-ordinated various theories into an organic unit which constitutes the basis for scientific physiology. Though this work alone would have sufficed to occupy a lifetime, Haller also published an *Icones anatomicæ* in eight volumes (1743–56) and colossal bibliographies in twenty volumes on botany (1771–2), anatomy (1774–7), surgery (1774–7), and medicine (1776–8). He corresponded with hundreds of scientists of his period (the Bern Library contains sixty-seven stout volumes of his later correspondence), composed thousands of shorter reports, wrote on the history of medicine, and composed a volume of poems which had an important influence at a critical moment on the development of German poetry. One of the many anecdotes about Haller concerns Voltaire, who had spoken about Haller with the greatest enthusiasm. When one of his assistants remarked that it was strange for him to express such an opinion after the great physiologist had spoken of Voltaire in no favourable terms, " Who knows? " answered Voltaire, smiling; " perhaps we were both wrong." Haller enjoyed an extraordinary reputation during his lifetime; he even appears in the memoirs of Casanova, who was struck by the profundity of his knowledge and his exquisite courtesy.

Haller's most important work is on the physiology of the blood vessels and of the nervous system — especially noteworthy is his doctrine of ir-

ritability. We recall that Glisson had already advanced the concept of irritability, which he regarded as an innate faculty of all organic matter. In a series of experiments Haller showed, on the contrary, that it is a property of muscle fibres, and that sensibility is the property of the nervous system or of muscular tissue through which nerves are passing. Muscles have also the capacity of contracting independently of nervous action, but sensibility is exclusively of nervous origin. This observation of Haller's is the foundation of the myogenic theory of the heart-beat, which, over a century later, finally overcame the neurogenic theory of Borelli.

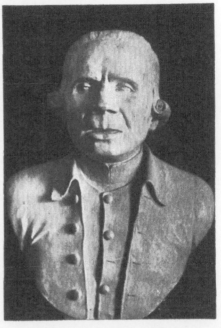

297. *Lazzaro Spallanzani.*
Terracotta bust in the Insane Asylum
of St. Lazzaro in Reggio Emilia.

In hundreds of experiments Haller illuminated the most varied medical problems. In physiology he recognized the role of the bile in the digestion of fats; he was correct in denying the current doctrine of irritability of the dura mater and of motility in the brain; on the other hand, he refused to place the psyche in the central nervous system, and opposed Wolff's correct embryological views. In experimental pathology he studied the fate of septic material when injected into the body, and also the results of interfering with the muscular transmission of the cardiac impulse. His small *Opuscula pathologica* (1768) is one of his less important works, containing but eighty short observations (an early example of a fusiform aneurysm of the aortic arch, the *corpus luteum*, a very early fetus, and so on). In the field of medical history he wrote a *Methodus studii medici* (Amsterdam, 1751), which was one of the best works on the subject since the time of Guy de Chauliac. His scientific theories were not immediately successful. Many adversaries opposed his views, the importance of which, however, has eventually become firmly established.

Knowledge of the physiology of digestion was materially advanced in the eighteenth century, especially by the work of R. de RÉAUMUR (1683–1757), whom Foster regards " as one of the most striking men of science of the eighteenth century and, indeed, in some respects of all time." Though he was better known for his thermometer (1731) and the temperature scale that bears his name, his outstanding work was on *The Digestion of Birds* (1752). By ingenious experiments on a kite, which is able to unload its stomach easily, and later on other animals, he established that the gastric juice could dissolve various but not all kinds of food, and did so by a process that was the opposite of putrefaction, which had hitherto been accepted as the mechanism of gastric digestion.

Another great physiologist, who ranks close to Haller in the extent of his culture and the profundity of his investigations, is Lazzaro SPALLANZANI (1729–99), who perhaps even more than Haller determined new directions for physiology.

Spallanzani was born at Scandiano, and first studied law at the University of Bologna. He was Professor of Logic and Metaphysics, first at Reggio, than at Modena, finally at Pavia, where he became Professor of Natural History and Director of the Museum. Among his most important works was his vigorous attack on the theory of spontaneous generation: *Saggio di osservazioni microscopiche relative al sistema della generazione dei Signori Needham e Buffon* (Modena, 1765); of equal importance were his studies on regeneration of animal tissues, *Prodromo di un' opera da imprimersi sopra le riproduzioni animali* (Modena, 1768), and on the circulation in embryos and in cold-blooded animals (*Dei fenomeni della circolazione osservata nel giro universale dei vasi* (Modena, 1777).

The problem of spontaneous generation (that is, that various animals can develop *de novo* in putrefying matter) was being actively discussed. We have seen that Redi was one of the most stubborn champions of the thesis *Omne vivum ex ovo* and denied the possibility of spontaneous generation. But the enemy camp maintained that the experiments of Redi, Vallisnieri, and others could only be applied to the infusoria. Spallanzani's patient and careful investigations led him to overcome what had hitherto been the stumbling-block in the problem, by showing that fertilization could not occur without direct contact of the spermatazoon with the ovum. For fertilization to be possible, therefore, it was necessary to accept the existence of an ovum in the female genital apparatus. He studied fertilization in frogs and toads: when the male parts were covered with a waxed linen, the ova remained unfertile after mating. He collected the liquid that was in the sac and found that when it was placed in contact with the female ova they were fertilized. He obtained artificial fertilization of mammals by injecting the dog's sperm into the uterus of a bitch. These experiments not only became the foundation of the doctrine of generation, but also constituted the strongest arguments against the theory of spontaneous generation, which had been accepted as dogma for centuries. In the physiology of the circulation Spallanzani was a bold and valuable explorer: he was the first to show that the impulse given to the blood by the heart-beat maintained the circulation throughout the arterial tree down to the smallest capillaries. He recognized that the heart emptied itself of blood during systole. He studied the role of the heart and the blood vessels from the embryo to the adult and noted the velocity of the blood, the arterial dilatation produced by systole, and the circulation of the blood in the lungs. In the physiology of digestion he extended Réaumur's methods and observations, experimenting on himself by the production of vomiting and by swallowing bags and tubes which were recovered *per anum*. He recognized that mastication and Borelli's gastric trituration served as preliminaries toward more rapid digestion, and came very near re-establishing the acid nature of the gastric juice, which had been forgotten since the time of van Helmont. In the physiology of respiration he utilized the discoveries of Lavoisier and of the English school, as controlled by his own objective experiments, to construct an excellent picture of the process. It was Spallanzani who showed that the death of animals from lack of air was not due to arrest of the circulation, as had been believed, but to phenomena in the nervous system determined by lack of oxygen. Spallanzani also revised the idea of Sanctorius and showed in numerous experiments that the perspiration of the skin produced phenomena on the surface of the body that were analogous to respiration in the lungs. He even showed that under special circumstances cutaneous respiration could substitute up to a certain point for pulmonary respiration (posthumously, Geneva, 1803). This tireless investigator, deep thinker, experienced traveller, and brilliant conversationalist is one of the finest scientific figures of the century. Not always sufficiently appreciated, he recently came into his own when he was selected for special honour at the 1935 International Congress of Physiology at Rome. A chapter in de Kruif's *Microbe Hunters* (1932) gives a vivid picture of his life and times.

English physiology contributed in this century to knowledge of the lymphatics (see Hewson and Cruikshank, Sect. 2), of the nervous system (see Robert Whytt, Sect. 5), also of the circulation, through an English clergyman, Stephen HALES (1677–1761). His *Statical Essays* (2 vols., 1731–3) not only threw light on such matters as the hydrostatics of sap movement in plants, but, more important, made the first quantitative estimates of blood pressure. A glass tube inserted in the femoral artery of a horse permitted him to measure directly the height of the column of blood — the first quantitative experiment in what has become an important part of medical as well as physiological study, and the most important step in knowledge of the circulation between Malpighi and Poiseuille. Hales also studied the behaviour of the pulse (with the sphygmoscope) and made good estimates of the capacity of the heart and of blood velocity in mammals.

Chemistry contributed notably to physiology in this century, especially in solving the problem of respiration, which, after being tantalizingly approached by Boyle's discovery and Mayow's " igneous particles " in the preceding century, had been thrown into confusion by Stahl's erroneous phlogiston theory. Boerhaave, for instance, had to be content with " an occult virtue in air that contained the secret food of life." In 1754 Joseph BLACK (1728–99), from his experiments on quicklime, rediscovered van Helmont's *gas sylvestre*, giving it the name " fixed air " (carbon dioxide). Nitrogen was discovered by Rutherford (1772), though not named until later by Chaptal. Joseph PRIESTLEY (1733–1804), though a believer in the phlogiston theory, actually prepared oxygen (1774), which he called " dephlogisticated air." He recognized also its importance in combustion and in the maintenance of animal life, and that it was given off by living plants. The actual discovery of oxygen, however, and of its role in fresh and devitalized air, was due to Antoine Laurence LAVOISIER (1743–94). Lavoisier, who was to lose his life under the guillotine as a victim of the French Revolution, definitely demonstrated the chemical nature of respiration. In the second volume of his memoirs he showed that respiration decomposed the inspired air and that in restricted quarters the air is quickly vitiated by the absorption of oxygen and expiration of carbon dioxide, with diminution in volume but increase in weight. It had to be concluded, then, that some of the air which entered the lungs did not come out in the same state, and that some of the oxygen, or " vital air," as he called it, is taken into the blood. Lavoisier was the first to apply these results hygienically and to maintain the need for a certain amount of air space in places inhabited by one or more persons.

5. Clinical Medicine

Medical writers, especially in Germany, were seeking at this time for philosophical explanations of normal and pathological existence, and attempting to correlate philosophy with medicine, or rather to accommodate medicine to the subjective constructions of philosophy. On the other hand, thanks especially to Morgagni, the fundamental concepts of pathology were stimulating the formation of schools of real clinical medicine, in which teaching was based on the examination of the patient and his diseased organs, rather than on the study of classical texts, metaphysical discussions and dogmatic statements. The master of clinical medicine in this century — and this title cannot be disputed even by those who prefer to regard him as the greatest of the systematists — was Hermann BOERHAAVE (1668–1738), born at Voorhout, a suburb of Leiden.

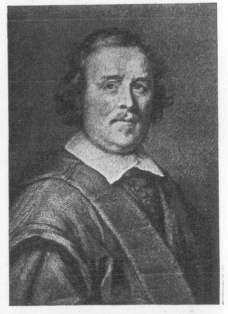

298. *Hermann Boerhaave.*

Boerhaave studied medicine in the famous University of Leiden, and in 1701 obtained the chair of theoretical medicine there. He began his lectures with a discourse, *De commendando studio Hippocratico*, which can be regarded as the program for his entire scientific activity, emphasizing the need for returning to the study of the Hippocratic texts. Boerhaave soon became the most famous clinician in Europe. He was so well known that it was said that he received promptly a letter from China, with the simple address " To Mr. Boerhaave in Europe." Students came to his lectures from all countries, and the most illustrious patients came to seek his advice. His pupil, the great Haller, called him *Communis totius Europæ præceptor* (The Common Teacher of all Europe). He was surrounded by the admiration, or rather the adoration, of his pupils and fellow citizens; and when he died, leaving more than ten million florins, acquired entirely from the practice of his profession, his mortal remains were given truly regal honours. The visitor to Leiden finds many tangible evidences of his presence there — his country house at Oegstgeest, his town house, where he died, on the Rapenburg, his funeral urn in the Church of St. Peter, and his heroic-size statue in front of the Boerhaave laboratories of the university.

Boerhaave was perhaps the most deserving of the title, which he desired above all others, " disciple of Hippocrates." His concept of medicine and of the way that it should be practised is entirely Hippocratic, as is his belief that the principal aim of medicine is to cure the patient, and his axiom that all theoretical discussion should cease at the bedside of the patient. Hippocratic also is the form of his teaching and writing, given in the form of short aphorisms containing valuable observations and rules for treatment. Quite in the spirit of Hippocrates is his calm and objective consideration of the phenomena of health and disease, in the attempt to draw from his observations the simplest and clearest possible conclusions. Thus Boerhaave can be regarded as the master of the systematists, if one understands by systematist, not the physician who adapts himself to preconceived systems and ancient concepts, but one who seeks to arrange the problems of nature in logical sequence, considering man as a part of the cosmos. He deserves at the same time to be regarded as the first of clinicians, bringing back the patient as the centre of medical attention. Up to this time theories had been constructed first and observations adapted to the theories, and the patient treated accordingly. Boerhaave taught the examination of the patient first and later consideration of the disease in the construction of theories. He was an eclectic. He utilized the knowledge and concepts of the iatrochemists as well as the iatrophysicists. He distinguished disease of the solid parts from disease of the humours. These latter he thought might be due to quantitative or qualitative changes, to a superabundance or an insufficiency of the humours, or an alteration in their composition. Disease of the solid parts, on the other hand, he thought to be due to something abnormal in the shape, size, or tension of the tissues, or in the capacity of the vessels. Inflammation, according to Boerhaave, came from a conglomeration of blood determined by the construction of the small arteries and by a change in the constitution of the plasma. Interesting are his ideas on fever, which he thought came from an increase in the action of the heart meeting the resistance of the capillary vessels. Without making any great single discoveries, he promoted the many sides of medicine in which he was active. His *Institutiones medicæ* (1708) was virtually an excellent book of physiology, and, like his *Aphorisms* (1709), went through an incredible number of editions and translations — even into Arabic. As may be seen in his *Opera medica omnia* (Venice, 1766), he wrote important treatises on chemistry (1731), nervous diseases (1761), the eyes (1746), syphilis (1751), and on methods of teaching (1726). The Botanical Garden that he founded for the University of Leiden, and described in 1710, is still to be seen in the heart of the city. He realized the importance of post-mortem examinations and left at least two noteworthy descriptions: one of a large fatty tumour of the mediastinum, and the

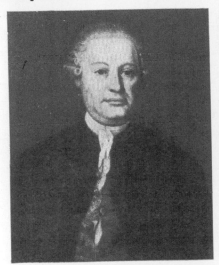
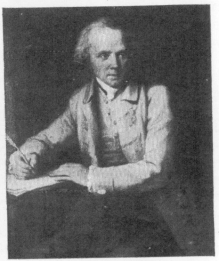

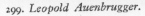
299. *Leopold Auenbrugger.*

300. *S. A. Tissot.*
Portrait by Angelica Kauffmann.

other of Baron Wassenaer's ruptured esophagus. He also gave an early description of heat stroke (insolation).

Through his pupils Boerhaave influenced medicine in far-distant countries — van Swieten was the founder of the old Vienna school; Gaub had an important influence on German medical thought; and through Cullen and Pringle his influence spread through England and Scotland. Especially was it felt in the Edinburgh school, and at a time when students from the American colonies were beginning to flock to Edinburgh for a better education than could be got at home. Thus Americans, too, could trace a direct influence on their clinical medicine and teaching to Boerhaave, and less directly to the Italian Montanus, the founder of bedside teaching, through the pupils who carried his message to Leiden.

The OLD VIENNA SCHOOL was founded, one might say, by Gerard VAN SWIETEN (1700–72), who was called from Leiden to Vienna in 1745 by Maria Theresa to the task of reorganizing medical instruction in this ancient university, and of placing the public health service on a new and better basis. Van Swieten was thus one of the founders of modern clinical medicine. His comments on the *Aphorisms* of Boerhaave, published in five large volumes between 1754 and 1755, constitute one of the most interesting documents of the Hippocratic trend, which found its principal seat in the Viennese school. Vienna, the capital of a rich and powerful Austria, which at that time was dominant from the Near East to Flanders and over a large part of Italy, was the predestined centre for this rapid and vigorous new development in clinical medicine. Open to the influence of the German schools of philosophy, though but little inclined to follow their heavy and mystical systems to extremes, the Viennese school also was in contact with the cultural centres of northern Italy, where experimental studies flourished. Here, as in many other intellectual activities in Austria, its special role is revealed in absorbing and often fusing currents of diverse origin. Following van Swieten to Austria was his compatriot Anton DE HAEN (1704–76), who, though a believer in witchcraft and of a quarrelsome, dictatorial nature, made real contributions to clinical medicine by his use of the thermometer and with his treatise on therapeutics, in fifteen volumes. He is said to have been the first to have performed autopsies routinely before medical students. Anton STOERCK (1731–1803), the pharmacologist, Maximilian STOLL (1742–87), the epidemiologist and writer on medical ethics, M. A. von PLENKIZ (1704–86), who carried on the tradition of a *contagium animatum*, J. J. von PLENCK (1732–1807), a classifier of skin diseases, and above all Auenbrugger and Frank, complete the Viennese group.

Leopold AUENBRUGGER (1722–1809), one of the immortals of medical history, inaugurated the art of physical diagnosis with his discovery of percussion as a diagnostic measure. Observing that the level of fluids in his native wine casks could be ascertained by thumping, he was led to study the same phenomenon in the human thorax, and eventually realized the possibility of " the determination of the internal condition of its cavity by the varying resonance of the sounds thus produced." His results were published in a modest little volume, *Inventum novum* (1761). In spite of its great importance it escaped notice for many years until it was revived by Corvisart, the great physician of Napoleon I, and then was rapidly made known to the entire medical world.

We translate herewith the fundamental statements of this classic booklet:

" I. The thorax of a healthy person sounds, when struck.

" II. The sound thus elicited from the healthy chest resembles the muffled sound of a drum covered with a thick woollen cloth or other envelope. . . .

" IV. The thorax ought to be struck, slowly and gently, with the points of the fingers, brought close together and at the same time extended.

" V. During percussion the shirt is to be drawn tight over the chest, or the hand of the operator is covered with a glove made of unpolished leather. If the naked chest is struck by the naked hand, the contact of the smooth surfaces produces a kind of noise which alters or obscures the natural character of the sound.

" VI. During the application of percussion the patient is first to go on breathing in the natural manner, and then is to hold his breath after a full inspiration. The difference of sound during inspiration and expiration and the retention of the breath is important in fixing our diagnosis. . . .

" XI. If, then, a distinct sound, equal on both sides, and commensurate to the degree of percussion, is not obtained from the sonorous regions above mentioned, a morbid condition of some of the parts within the chest is indicated.

" XII. If a sonorous part of the chest struck with the same intensity yields a sound deeper than natural, that part is diseased where the note is deeper.

" XIII. If a sonorous part of the chest struck with the same intensity yields a sound duller than natural, disease exists in that part. . . . I have opened the bodies of many dead from this disease [consumption] and I have always found the lungs firmly bound to the pleura, and the lobes on that side where the obscure sound has existed callous, indurated, and more or less purulent." (Mostly from John Forbes's translation.)

The ENGLISH schools of clinical medicine in this century produced many whose names are still familiar and who continued the practical traditions of Sydenham and Boerhaave. John HUXHAM (1692–1768), of Devonshire, and a pupil of Boerhaave, was an especially acute observer of the infectious diseases. His *Essay on Fevers* (1739) and his *Dissertation on the Malignant Ulcerous Sore Throat* (London, 1750) are his best-known works; while his eponymic tincture of cinchona, his use of a vegetable diet in scurvy, and his discovery of Devonshire colic are important clinical landmarks. In the first work he recognized the importance of fresh fruit and vegetables in the treatment of scurvy on long sea voyages; but it was not until some years after publication of the *Treatise of the Scurvy* (1753) by James LIND (1716–94) that the British Navy adopted Lind's similar ideas (1795) and quickly eradicated scurvy from its ships. The Devonshire colic was later (1767) shown by Sir George BAKER (1722–1809) to be due to poisoning from the lead that lined the apparatus used in preparing cider. Sir John PRINGLE (1707–82), another pupil of Boerhaave and a pioneer in military medicine in Great Britain, differentiated various forms of dysentery and correlated typhus with hospital and " jayl " fevers. His *Observations on the Diseases of the Army* (1752) was important in securing better sanitation in jails, hospitals, and other institutions as well as in barracks and military camps. In the Preface he describes how the Earl of Stair proposed to the French the demilitarization of the French and

British hospitals — the germ of the Red Cross idea. One of the most successful clinical observers and practitioners of the period was the scholarly William HEBERDEN (1710–1801), whose numerous valuable observations were reported at various times to the Royal College of Physicians and published posthumously — *Commentarii de morborum historia et curatione* (London, 1802). His original description of angina pectoris (1768) — the first reported case being that of the Earl of Clarendon, described in his memoirs by his son (1632) — is a classic which fortunately is now easily available to readers in Major and other modern reprints. He also described the rheumatic nodules on the phalanges called Heberden's nodes, chickenpox (1767), and night blindness (1785) and made acute observations on hitherto unobserved peculiarities of various diseases and on the superstitious fallacies of polypharmacy. Two Quakers reached medical eminence. John FOTHERGILL (1712–80), "a man who devoted his labours and fortune to public good" to become "one of the first physicians of the age," in Lettsom's words, used his great influence to improve the conditions of jails, to install public baths and effect other sanitary measures in collaboration with his friend John Howard. A graduate of Edinburgh, where all five of his professors were pupils of Boerhaave, Fothergill wrote an important *Account of the Putrid Sore Throat* (1748), which contained good clinical descriptions of a severe and highly contagious epidemic, which seemed to include both diphtheria and scarlatinal streptococcic angina. He should be held in grateful memory by Americans, not only for his pacific efforts with his friend Benjamin Franklin in the pre-Revolutionary period, but also for his sympathy and financial encouragement to the colonies. His friend, John Coakley LETTSOM (1744–1815), also a Quaker philanthropist, stands as a familiar figure before us in the engraving of the first meeting of the Medical Society of London, which he founded in 1773. His writings on tea-drinking received the widest notice, but he also wrote an interesting *History of the Origin of Medicine* (1778).

An important therapeutic advance, which came like Jenner's discovery of vaccination through the ability to see important scientific truths in unexpected places, was William WITHERING's (1741–99) discovery of the use of foxglove (digitalis) in cases of dropsy, especially when of cardiac origin. Finding that remarkable ability to help the dropsical was possessed by a family of Shropshire farmers, he traced their success to the use of a mixture containing foxglove, and thereupon not only established the proper method of administering the remedy, but also demonstrated the important fact that dropsy, which had been accepted as a primary disease, could be due to cardiac weakness. His *Account of the Fox-Glove* (1785) is his masterpiece, deservedly an English classic. An eminent clinician of Bath was Caleb H. PARRY (1755–1822), whose name has missed being attached to exophthalmic goitre, a disease especially rich in eponyms — Flaiani, Graves, Basedow; yet the first of his eight cases, the description of which appeared posthumously in his *Unpublished Medical Writings* (1825), was observed by him in 1786, before any published accounts. In pediatrics an important step was made by George ARMSTRONG (fl. 1767), who in 1769 opened the first " Dispensary for the Infant Poor " (described in his *General Account*, 1772); he also was the first to describe infantile pyloric stenosis (1771).

Progressive medicine in AMERICA, still in its infancy in the eighteenth century, owed much to those coming from Europe and to those who had had the advantage of a European education, especially at Edinburgh. Others had to depend solely on the apprentice system for their education. A few personalities emerge. The role of Morgan and other Edinburgh graduates in promoting American medical education will be considered later. Another Scot, Peter MIDDLETON (d. 1781) of New York, who with John Bard performed a much cited early autopsy on a criminal, was influential in founding the King's College Medical School; yet another Scot, Alexander GARDEN (1728–91), after whom the gardenia is named, was a distinguished practitioner in Charleston for thirty years. The all-pervading Benjamin FRANKLIN left his mark on American medicine, not only directly by his invention of bifocal spectacles, his gospel of fresh air, and his modern views on " catching cold," but also indirectly in founding the Pennsylvania Hospital, and through his great influence on younger men. He was undoubtedly a considerable factor in making Philadelphia the cradle of American medicine. The brothers Thomas (1712–84) and Phineas (1717–73) BOND were distinguished physicians, the former especially to be remembered for his part in the formation of the Pennsylvania Hospital, where he took the important step of giving the first clinical instruction in America (1766) controlled by observations in the dead-house. John (1716–99) and Samuel (1742–1821) BARD, father and son, were among the most eminent physicians in New York; the former is chiefly remembered for his contribution to the proper handling of ship fever and yellow fever; the latter for his part in founding the King's College Medical School and his book on diphtheria, *Angina suffocativa* (1771), though his favourite occupation was midwifery. Hezekiah BEARDSLEY's (1748–90) original account of a " scirrhus " in the pylorus of an infant (1788) is noteworthy both for its superiority to Armstrong's account in the previous decade, and also as one of the very first American contributions to nosography.

Best known of all was Benjamin Rush (1745–1813), the "American Sydenham," as Lettsom called him; "the greatest historical figure in American medicine," according to Welch. Rush, to be sure, has many items on the debit as well as the credit side of his balance. His expressed views on the cause of yellow fever seem fantastic today, yet he gave one of the best descriptions of the Philadelphia epidemic of 1793 and observed that mosquitoes were especially prominent in times of epidemics. He wrote the

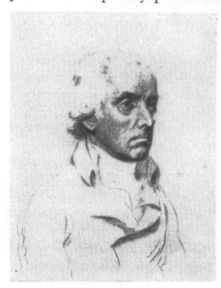

301. *Benjamin Rush.*
Original drawing by Hames.

only systematic American treatise on insanity, according to C. K. Mills, before our own time; yet he advocated a barbarous "tranquilising chair" just when Pinel "struck the chains from the mentally afflicted." His chief reliance in treatment was on the lancet and on calomel, which he called his Samson (according to his detractors, because it had slain its thousands); yet he observed and wrote ably on cholera infantum, on the harmful effects of drinking cold water when overheated, on military and camp hygiene, and on the evil effects of alcoholism. He independently described dengue in 1780, one year after the original description by D. Bylon, and was probably the first to record that general disease (arthritis, epilepsy) could be relieved by the extraction of decayed teeth. A signer of the Declaration of Independence, yet a member of the Conway Cabal, he was undoubtedly the most influential and one of the ablest American physicians of his period.

In Germany the leading clinicians of the period were undoubtedly Stahl and Hoffmann, who have already been mentioned. Others of note were P. G. Werlhof (1699–1767), whose name is preserved in his original description of *purpura hæmorrhagica* (1735), appearing in his *Opera omnia* (1775). C. W. Hufeland (1762–1836), friend of the poets Goethe, Schiller, and Herder, was a valuable influence in combating the extravagant systems of the day and in promoting Jenner's vaccination in Germany. His famous *Journal der praktischen Arzneikunde* (1795–1836) is still remembered as "Hufeland's *Journal*." Two Swiss physicians attained a distinguished position: the Genevan Theodore TRONCHIN (1709–81), pupil of Boerhaave and physician to Voltaire, an enthusiastic supporter of smallpox inoculation and an early describer of lead poisoning (*De colica Pictonum* [Poitou colic],[1] Geneva, 1757); and S. A. TISSOT (1728–97), of Lausanne, who wrote especially on nervous diseases. He is best known, however, for his famous work on onanism, and his popular book on hygiene, *Avis au peuple sur la santé* (1760).

The ITALIAN clinicians who chiefly represented the return to Hippocratism in this century were the previously mentioned Lancisi, and Torti, Borsieri, Sarcone, and Testa. Francesco TORTI (1658–1741) wrote notably on malaria (Modena, 1709) and was one of the first to use cinchona bark in Italy. He introduced the term *mal aria* (bad air) for the disease, which was long thought to be due to poisonous exhalations from swamps. G. B. BORSIERI (1725–85), pupil of Morgagni, was Professor of Clinical Medicine at Pavia; his chief work was an *Institutiones medicinæ practicæ* (4 vols., Milan, 1781–8), which was translated from the Latin into Italian, German, and English. One of the most interesting Italian figures of the period was Domenico CIRILLO (1739–99), of Naples, a man of great intellect, an eloquent orator and fervent patriot. A friend of Pringle and Hunter, and member of the Royal Society of London, he was an eminent botanist and student of medicine and was a real pioneer in the new medical trends. A founder of the shortlived Parthenopean Republic, he was condemned to death on its fall and was executed in spite of the active protests of Lord Nelson and Lady Hamilton.

The first studies on pellagra appeared in this century: it was first described by Gaspar CASAL (1679–1759), a Spanish physician whose description, written in 1735, was not published until 1762. F. THIÉRY in the meantime had published (1755) his book on the same disease, which was called *mal de la rosa*. Francesco FRAPOLLI (d. 1773) wrote an excellent description of the disease in his book published in Milan in 1771, and was the first to give it the name " pellagra," which he derived from *pellarella*, a term used in the registers of the Milan Hospital since the end of the sixteenth century to indicate a cutaneous disorder of the same nature. Publications on the subject increased in number, the most important of which was that

---

[1] This should not be confused with *colica pictorum* (painter's colic), though by coincidence both were due to lead poisoning. The Poitou colic, due to drinking water that had passed through lead pipes, was known long before Tronchin. Citois (Citesius), in his *De novo et populari apud pictones dolore colico bilioso diatriba* (Poitiers, 1616; partly translated in Major, 2nd ed.), had described the condition; and lead poisoning appears to have been known to Nikander and Paul of Ægina.

(1786) of Gaetano STRAMBIO (1753–1831), director of the Milan Hospice for pellagrins. He showed that the disease had long been known by the Milanese under the name *mal rosso*, and that it was not a true skin disease but a general disease whose origin should be sought in spoiled bread or polenta. The role played in its production by lack of vitamins was of course not discovered until the present century.

Among the FRENCH clinicians of the period Jean SENAC (1705–70) is to be especially mentioned. His book on diseases of the heart (*Traité de la structure du cœur*, etc., 2 vols., 1749) is a classic for its precise observations of symptoms and lesions; asthma, orthopnea, blood-spitting, œdema of the legs, are all noted as important signs of cardiac disease. Another eminent clinician was F. R. QUESNAY (1694–1774), Professor of Surgery and surgeon to Louis XV, one of the greatest economists of his time (the founder of the physiocratic system), and author of a well-known book on the continued fevers (1753).

6. Surgery

During this century surgery definitely emerged from its inferior position with respect to medicine. In this the FRENCH surgeons took the lead. One of the most important was F. G. DE LA PEYRONIE (1678–1747), who in 1743 procured a definite separation of the surgeons from the barbers. A skilful operator, especially on hernia and wounds of the intestine, he was one of the founders of the Royal Academy of Surgery (1731). J. B. Baseilhac (1703–81), better known as FRÈRE CÔME, was the inventor of the *lithotome caché*, which he and his nephew used on several thousand cases in spite of great opposition. He also practised the *haut appareil* (suprapubic extraction of vesical calculi). Jean ASTRUC (1685–1766) was a noted writer on syphilis and obstetrics, and was the first to describe blenorrhagic ophthalmia. His *De morbis venereis* is a valuable source of information on the history of venereal disease. J. L. PETIT (1674–1760), the inventor of the screw tourniquet and of numerous successful surgical procedures, including mastoidectomy, was the most eminent surgeon of the first half of the century and the greatest contributor to his subject in France since the time of Paré. His literary chef-d'œuvre was *L'Art de guérir les maladies des os* (Paris, 1705). Pierre DESAULT (1744–95) was one of the best-known surgeons of his time. He was professor in the School of Practical Surgery and surgeon-in-chief of the Hôtel-Dieu, where he founded the first surgical clinic. His bandage for the fractured clavicle is well known to medical students. F. R. CHOPART (1743–95), with a reputation also as a physiologist and pathologist, was a pioneer in the surgery of the urinary tract. His method of amputating the foot (1792) still is known by his name.

First among ITALIAN surgeons of the period was A. SCARPA (1752–1832), whose anatomical achievements have already been noted. He also made important studies on the cure of aneurysm and treatment of inguinal hernia and cataract. An outstanding surgeon and anatomist was Giuseppe FLAIANI (1741–1808), who was the first to publish a description of ex-ophthalmic goitre (1802), which therefore is sometimes known as "Flaiani's disease." Founder of the anatomical museum of the Hospital of the Holy Spirit in Sassia, he was also a skilful surgeon and lithotomist, who had a most extensive practice.

In the history of military surgery an important part was played by G. A. BRAMBILLA (1728–1800), of Pavia, who was given by the Emperor Joseph II the task of reorganizing the teaching of military medicine.

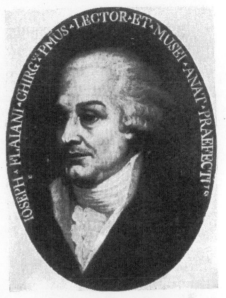

302. *Giuseppe Flaiani.*
Portrait by Pompeo Batoni.

His influence with the Emperor enriched the University of Pavia in its anatomical and natural-history collections. He also founded the university library and obtained the nomination of Scarpa as Professor of Anatomy at the university. In Vienna he instituted the Josephinum, an academy of military medicine and surgery (1785), where regular instruction was given for military surgeons. He also wrote a *Storia delle scoperte fisico-medico-anatomico-chirurgiche fatte dagli uomini illustri italiani* (1777) and a number of surgical studies. He was one of a number of Italian physicians who successfully practised medicine in Vienna about the turn of the century.

M. TROIA (1747–1828), of Naples, was a skilful operator who wrote especially on the surgery of the bladder and of the bones. Studying the regeneration of bone, he described in 1814 the perforating connective-tissue fibres usually known as Sharpey's fibres (Castaldi).

In GERMANY the separation of surgeons and barbers came much later, though surgeons worthy of the name were already to be found. Such was

Lorenz HEISTER (1683–1758), whose *Chirurgie* (1718) was one of the first systematic treatises on the subject and is especially interesting for its illustrations. Heister, who, like most surgeons of the time, was an excellent anatomist, had an important influence in raising the standards of surgical teaching in Germany. One of the best known of the German surgeons of the period was A. G. RICHTER (1742–1812), professor at Göttingen, where his teaching made the clinic one of the most famous in Europe. He was a pioneer in the surgical treatment of hernia (1777–9); he wrote a well-

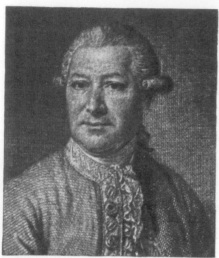

known textbook (Göttingen, 1782–1804) and was editor of the first surgical journal: *Chirurgische Bibliothek* (15 vols., 1771–97). His contemporary, K. K. von SIEBOLD (1736–1807), was founder of the surgical school of Würzburg and the first of a distinguished family of scientists, which is traced through four generations in Hirsch (2nd ed., Vol. V, p. 258). Military surgery in Germany was raised by the Hohenzollerns from a lowly trade pursued by barbers and executioners to a worthy branch of the medical profession. A Collegium Medicum Chirurgicum was expanded (1724) from the Berlin Theatrum

303. *Giovanni Alessandro Brambilla.*

Anatomicum (founded 1713), and the Charité Hospital created in an endeavour to prepare surgeons for the army. In 1785 the college was devoted entirely to this task.

The chief representative of ENGLISH surgery in the first half of the century was the St. Thomas's Hospital surgeon William CHESELDEN (1688–1752). At a time when operative speed was a prime consideration, he was known to have extracted a bladder stone in less than one minute. His *Anatomy of the Human Body*, which also contained many surgical observations, was extremely popular, eleven editions appearing between 1713 and 1778. His *Treatise on the High Operation for the Stone* (1723) and his later advocacy of the lateral operation are indications of the importance of this condition in the surgery of the period. Prominent in English surgery were the two Hunters, whom we have already met among the anatomists. William HUNTER, like his brother, John, great in surgery as in anatomy, was the first to describe arteriovenous aneurysm (1762) and retroversion of the uterus (1770). He did not hesitate to tap ovarian cysts, but was averse to the use of forceps in difficult labour. John, whose interests covered the entire field of nature, " chased that damn'd guinea " with best results in practical surgery. He explored the treatment of club foot and of ruptured tendons, after having ruptured his own Achilles' tendon. Having experimented on the collateral circulation of stags' antlers in the

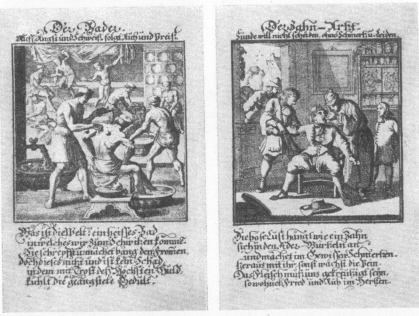

304. *The barber surgeon.* 305. *The dentist.*
Eighteenth-century German engravings after Caspar Luyken of Amsterdam.

royal park at Windsor, he was led to the important step of treating peripheral aneurysms with a single proximal ligature instead of by amputation (this had previously been done empirically by the French surgeons Guillemeau and Anel). In fact, all his surgical writings exhibit his unsurpassed skill in the application of inductive reasoning and patient research. In Mather's words, he " found surgery a mere mechanical art . . . he left it a beautiful science." Percivall POTT (1714–88), of St. Bartholomew's Hospital, London, the most successful English surgeon of the latter half of the century, is responsible for many able surgical descriptions, of which two come down to us still connected with his name. " Pott's fracture " indicates the common and characteristic break of one or both bones above the ankle, which he described in 1769 (*Some Few General Remarks on Fractures*). The statement is probably incorrect, however, that the compound fracture of the leg that he suffered in a fall from his horse in 1769 was of this variety. His other best-known achievement was his description of the curvature of the spine, frequently with paralysis, called " Pott's disease " (1779), which in 1782 he recognized as being related to phthisis. This connection, however, had been known by Hippocrates, who said: " They [the humpbacked] have also as a rule hard and unripened tubercles in the lungs, for the origin of the curvature and contraction is in most cases due to such gatherings." (*On Joints*, Sect. 41). The condition was more completely described by J. P. David in 1779, the same year as that of Pott's publication.

Toward the end of the century AMERICAN surgery was taking its first steps toward its brilliant course in the next century. Philip Wright Post (1763–1828), his courses in anatomy in New York being interrupted by the " Doctors' Mob " in 1792, was appointed Professor of Surgery at Columbia College Medical School. In 1796 he successfully repeated his master's, John Hunter's, ligation of the femoral artery for popliteal aneurysm; he ligated the common carotid (1813) and followed Dorsey in ligating the external iliac (1814). He was the first to ligate the subclavian artery above the clavicle for brachial aneurysm (1817). James LLOYD (1728–1810), a pupil of Cheselden, William Hunter, and Smellie, was the most prominent surgeon in Boston, where he introduced lithotomy, the use of ligatures in the control of hemorrhage, and Cheselden's flap method for amputated limbs. John JONES (1729–91), of New York, who studied under Cadwalader, Pott, William Hunter, Petit, and Le Dran, was the first Professor of Surgery at King's College. His *Plain Concise and Practical Remarks on the Treatment of Wounds and Fractures* was the chief text on military surgery used during the Revolution. Moving to Philadelphia in 1780, he became surgeon to the Pennsylvania Hospital and was one of the founders of the College of Physicians there. He attended Washington and Franklin, of whose last illness he left an interesting account.

7. Obstetrics and Gynæcology

The eighteenth century was extremely important in the history of obstetrics and gynæcology. Knowledge of the anatomy and physiology of the genital tract was greatly promoted by the work of Mascagni, Santorini, Haller, Sandifort, and Spallanzani. The old controversy between the ovists and the animalculists as to the nature of generation had been decided in favour of the former, but the ovists had already divided into two camps.

One, following Haller, accepted the theory of palingenesis, or preformation, according to which all the organs were already preformed in the egg; while the others adhered to the theory of epigenesis — that is, the gradual and continuous new formation of organs.

The FRENCH were the greatest masters at this time in the field of obstetrics. Physicians and students came to the French schools from all parts of the world; and although the professors limited themselves almost exclusively to theoretical teaching and practice on mannequins, having access to but little clinical material, nevertheless the most important progress in obstetrics is due to the French surgeons. Eminent among them was Nicolas Puzos (1686–1753), who was the first to recognize the importance of bimanual examination of the uterus and of protection of the perineum during delivery. André Levret (1730–80) was one of the most illustrious obstetricians of all times, known for his studies of extra-uterine pregnancy and placenta previa and his delivery procedures for the different presentations. He also introduced a number of instruments, some of which in more or less modified form are still employed. He is responsible for the greater use of the forceps which the master barber Jean Palfyn (1650–1730), of Courtrai in Flanders, had presented to the Paris Academy in 1724. J. L. Baudelocque (1746–1810), pupil of Solayres (1737–72), a founder of the theory of the normal birth mechanism, was one of the most illustrious figures in the history of French medicine and obstetrics. To him is owed the systematic pre-partum measurement of the pelvis and the establishment of its importance in prognosis and treatment. He studied the different positions of the fetus *in utero*, and the best methods of delivery to be adopted in each case. His obstetrical teaching had an international reputation, and his book *Principes des accouchements* (1775) went through many large editions and translations. Other notable figures were J. R. Sigault, the first to practise symphyseotomy (1777), and J. Lebas (1717–97), of Montpellier, who introduced a transverse incision for Cæsarean section.

Prominent in the history of English obstetrics was William Hunter, whom we have already met in the sections on anatomy and surgery. An experienced practitioner in the specialty, he made important studies on the retroversion of the gravid uterus; his most famous work, as mentioned before, is the *Anatomy of the Human Gravid Uterus*, published by Baskerville in 1774. But the greatest figure in English obstetrics was William Smellie (1697–1763), who, after twenty years of village practice, came to London to devote himself to the teaching and practice of obstetrics. According to Fischer, in ten years he gave two hundred and eighty courses of lectures, which were attended by thousands of pupils. To him are owed the first attempts to measure the fetal cranium *in utero,* and also important studies on the mechanism of delivery and the methods to be pursued in cases of placenta previa and retroversion of the uterus. His influence was especially felt in the use of the obstetrical forceps, which toward the end of the century became widespread among obstetricians, especially in England. His *Midwifery* (1752) was reprinted by the Sydenham Society (1876–8). Among other prominent English obstetricians were Benjamin

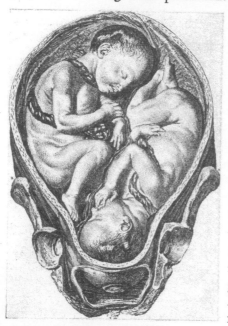

306. *Twin pregnancy.*
(*From Smellie's* A Set of Anatomical Tables, *London, 1761.*)

PUGH of Chelmsford, who in 1740 used curved forceps before Levret; and two pupils of Smellie, R. W. JOHNSON, and the Irishman William DEASE, who upheld the minimum use of instruments in childbirth. His view that attempts to expel the placenta should be approached with caution gave rise to the procedure that became known as "the Dublin method." An important precursor of Holmes and Semmelweis was Charles WHITE (1728–1813), of Manchester, whose insistence on surgical cleanliness (*On the Management of Pregnant and Lying-In Women,* 1773) greatly improved conditions in the Manchester Hospital. If adopted more generally, they would have largely prevented the horrible conditions in the maternity wards of the succeeding century. While it is doubtful if White recognized that puerperal fever could be transmitted by the doctor and nurse, he unquestionably appreciated the advantages of cleanliness and isolation for the woman in childbirth and the need for segregation of cases of puerperal fever as they arose. White was the leading surgeon of his time in the north of England and was instrumental, at the early age of twenty-four, in the foundation of the celebrated Manchester Infirmary (1752), and later of the Lying-In Charity (1790).

In ITALY the first chair of obstetrics was founded in Florence in 1760. Morgagni had written in detail on such obstetrical subjects as repeated abortions, the mobile symphysis, and so on. Among Italian obstetricians were Giuseppe VESPA (1727–1804), and Paolo ASSALINI (1759–1840), who described various new instruments in his book *Nuovi strumenti di ostetricia* (1811). Francesco ASDRUBALI (1756–1832) published two works, *Elementi di ostetricia* (2 vols., 1795–7) and a comprehensive *Trattato generale dell'ostetricia* (5 vols., 1812), that were among the best European works on the subject.

In the GERMANIC countries obstetrics also made notable progress. It began to be taught in the universities in 1737, and toward the middle of the century the first schools for midwives were placed under university authority. Outstanding among German obstetricians was J. G. ROEDERER (1726–63), who made notable anatomical and physiological studies on the fetal circulation, the position of the fetus, and the mechanism of delivery. His principal work was *Elementa artis obstetriciæ* (1753). Also to be mentioned are G. W. STEIN (1731–1803), of Marburg, the champion of Levret's ideas in Germany, and F. B. OSIANDER (1759–1822), of Göttingen, an extreme representative of the interventionist tendency, which has made such progress in recent years. Only fifty-four per cent of the deliveries in his clinic occurred spontaneously, the use of the forceps being almost routine. L. J. BOER (1751–1835), Professor of Theoretical and Practical Obstetrics at the University of Vienna, on the other hand, was an energetic upholder of the doctrine of the natural development of pregnancy, instead of regarding it as a troublesome process often requiring intervention.

8. *Ophthalmology*

Progress in the knowledge of the anatomy and physiology of the eye in the eighteenth century had a considerable influence on the scientific development of ophthalmology. In this period fall the achievements of François and Étienne POURFOUR DU PETIT, father and son, on cataract (1730 and 1746); and of Thomas Young on the mechanism of optics (1801); of Haller on the lamina cribrosa and the choroid coat (1749); of Carlo MONDINO on the choroidal pigment (1748); of Morgagni on the muscles of accommodation; of Fontana on the movements of the iris (1775); and of LA HIRE (1706) and others on the anatomy of the lens. In 1702 Stahl described lachrymal fistula; in 1767 Heberden first described night blindness (nyctalopia); in 1782 Buzzi discovered the *macula lutea*; in 1784 Benjamin Franklin invented bifocal spectacles; in 1794 John DALTON described colour blindness (Daltonism). The earliest Italian treatise on the eye is the compilation of BILLI, of Ancona, largely taken from the French and German (1749). The revolution in the field of optics was determined by Newton's theory of light and colour. The studies of Haller, Mariotte, and others brought a complete revision of the science of the eye, which is especially due to the French.

Antoine MAÎTRE-JEAN (1650?–1730), the founder of French ophthalmology, was one of the first to recognize the true nature of cataract, which had been suspected by Morgagni and the Italian anatomists. In 1706 he presented his views to the Academy of Sciences at Paris and in the same year published an excellent treatise on diseases of the eye. Michel BRISSEAU (1677–1743), of Tournai, independently of Maître-Jean, showed that cataract consists of a hardening and clouding of the lens, and in 1708 " couched," or reclined, the cataractous lens in the living. He also wrote on glaucoma (Paris, 1709). The most noteworthy step in the treatment of cataract, however, is due to Jacques DAVIEL (1716–62), regarded throughout Europe as the best oculist of his time. In 1750 he began his first attempts at the extraction of cataract, an operation that had often been tried but without much success. In the single year 1752 he operated on 206 patients, with successful results in 182. Although his priority has been long and passionately discussed, it must be accepted that to him is due the credit of having invented a practical operation for the extraction of the cataract and established the technique through his teaching and example.

A leader among English students of the eye was the remarkable Thomas YOUNG (1773–1829), the pupil of John Hunter and Baillie. One of the most learned and versatile scientists of his time, he contributed to many non-medical fields, such as his translation of the hieroglyphics on the Rosetta Stone. In ophthalmology his treatise On the Mechanism of the Eye (1801) gave the first description of astigmatism; he also announced a theory of colour vision, which is still known as the Young-Helmholtz theory; he evolved a wave theory of light due to undulations of the ether (1801–3), which, in 1809, he applied to refraction by crystals. Thus he has been called the " Father of Physiological Optics," and by the great Helmholtz, " one of the most clear-sighted men who ever lived." Of quite a different nature was the notorious, self-styled Chevalier, John TAYLOR (1708–67). Though in some ways a clever oculist — for instance, he early described the conical cornea and invented a cataract needle and other optical instruments — he was really a " clever buffoon," who travelled about Europe in startling costume in a gaudily painted carriage, distributing leaflets that boasted of his ability. At any rate, he accumulated thousands of patients and great wealth. A similar charlatan was Sir William READ, who was less successful as a tailor than when he practised ophthalmology and so imposed on Queen Anne that he was knighted for his services. His book on eye diseases was supposed to have been written for him by a hireling.

The establishment of the Vienna school of Ophthalmology (1773) may be regarded as the beginning of modern ophthalmology on the Continent. Joseph BARTH was installed there by the Empress Maria Theresa as the first lecturer on diseases of the eye in Europe, to be followed by J. A. SCHMIDT in 1795, and by Beer in 1812. For the most part, however, the practical surgery of the eye was accomplished in this century by the better general surgeons, such as Heister and Scarpa, or even medical practitioners such as Boerhaave.

9. Psychiatry and Legal Medicine

Psychiatry as a separate branch of medicine can be regarded as beginning toward the end of this century, before which time the care of mental patients had been entirely custodial; they were treated in the most barbarous fashion, kept in chains, and abandoned to the treatment of the ignorant and the cruel. Valsalva had made a beginning in combating this mode of treatment and showed himself a precursor of the now well-established principle of " no restraint." An illustrious Italian physician, Vincenzo CHIARUGI (1759–1820), courageously maintained against great odds the need for a fundamental reform in the treatment of the mentally afflicted. In the model Florentine institute directed by him he demonstrated the usefulness of a humane treatment of the alienated. Leopold I of Tuscany in 1774 had established principles for the proper treatment of the insane in special institutions and had established the Bonifazio Hospital, of which Chiarugi assumed the directorship in 1788. A decree of the ephemeral Kingdom of Etruria shortly afterwards (1802) initiated the teaching of psychiatry from a chair confided to Chiarugi.

Chiarugi, in his book *Della pazzia in genere e in ispecie* (1793), ably presented the diagnosis and prognosis of mental diseases, dividing insanity, which was thought to be due to an imbalance in the activity of the sensorium, into melancholia, mania, and dementia. In melancholia there was but a partial insanity, limited to one or more subjects; in mania, a general insanity that exaggerated audacity of volition; dementia was regarded as a general insanity without emotional manifestations, characterized by deficiency both of intelligence and of the will. His book contains observations on hundreds of cases, many of them controlled by autopsies. He maintained the importance of psychotherapy and of a treatment that was either stimulating or sedative, depending on whether the condition was caused by hyperactivity or atony. The studies of Padovani (Ferrara, 1927) have emphasized the credit that is due in the treatment of the insane to Joseph DAQUIN (born at Chambéry, 1733), who wrote a book on *Philosophie de la folie* (1791) in which he recommended the abolition of chains and confinement in cells and regarded imprisonment as extremely harmful for the insane. This book also contains a valuable bibliography on the subject.

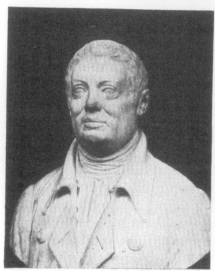

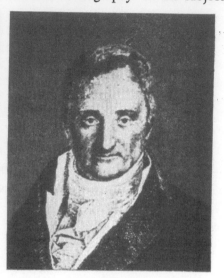

307. *Vincenzo Chiarugi.*
Marble bust in the Insane Asylum of Florence.

308. *Philippe Pinel.*
Portrait at the Salpêtrière, Paris.

The most famous reformer in the treatment of the insane, however, was Philippe PINEL (1745–1826), physician at the Bicêtre Hospital of Paris and shortly after at the Salpêtrière, who devoted himself to psychiatry after having been profoundly impressed by the plight of a friend who had been attacked by a grave mental disorder.

Pinel was the pupil of Barthez, and therefore a vitalist. Following the views of the great philosopher Condillac, he affirmed the necessity of the analytic method in the study of medicine, and thus provided a scientific and philosophical basis for pathological investigations. Pinel taught that it is not possible to understand diseases properly except by analysing the various phenomena and tracing them back to their sources in organic lesions. The organs being composed of different elements, he maintained that it was necessary to examine the functional changes of each of these elements; thus he was the precursor of Bichat, whose great contribution was the establishment of the various tissues rather than the organs as the significant units of study.

His *Traité médico-philosophique sur l'aliénation mentale* (1801) affirmed the origin of mental disease in pathological changes in the brain. In 1796 he obtained permission from the National Assembly to remove the chains from the forty-nine insane patients at the Bicêtre. His pupils,

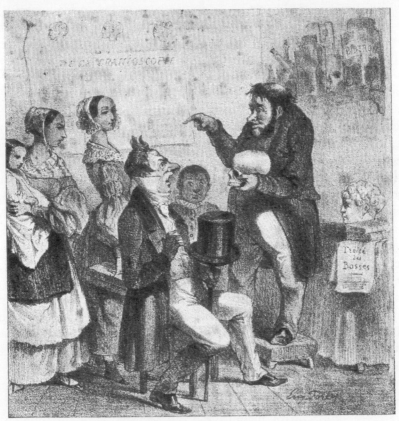

309. *The phrenologist.*
French caricature, late eighteenth century.

especially E. D. ESQUIROL (1772–1840) and A. M. FERRUS (1784–1861), were influential in promoting the principles proposed by their master. In Germany, Reil advanced Pinel's views and proposed the construction of institutions with gardens to hasten the recovery of the insane. The idea was followed up in other countries, in England especially, by John CONOLLY (1796–1866), whose book on the *Treatment of the Insane without Mechanical Restraints* (1856) found the " no restraint " system definitely introduced into psychiatry and operating on more than ten thousand inmates of twenty-four English institutions. It is difficult now to picture the difficulties to which these men were subjected by the authorities and violent reactionaries before they could establish these humane principles. Conolly had been preceded in England by William Tuke's Quaker institution at York (1794), which through three generations of Tukes gave practical demonstration of the efficacy of the humane treatment of the insane.

One of the most interesting medical figures of the end of the century is that of F. J. Gall (1758–1828), of Tiefenbronn in Germany, the founder of the pseudo-science of phrenology. He studied at the University of Vienna as a pupil of van Swieten, concentrating on the anatomy of the brain and on attempts to trace the tracts of white matter to their connections with the grey matter of the cortex. In his lectures at Vienna in 1796, published in the *Neuer Deutscher Mercur* in 1798, Gall maintained that certain areas of the brain are especially connected with certain intellectual functions, and that the strength of these functions in the individual (i.e., the various mental characteristics and emotions) is manifested by variations in the protuberances of the cranium, so that it is possible to diagnose the intellectual and moral qualities of the individual by inspection and palpation of the skull. Gall's doctrine, which found many passionate partisans, was condemned by the Emperor and the ecclesiastical authorities, but continued to be energetically defended by his disciples, especially by J. C. Spurzheim (1776–1832). In 1805 they travelled together through Europe spreading their doctrine, and later Spurzheim went to America, where he found many proselytes. Gall's own skull is preserved in his collection of skulls and models, which after his death went to the Jardin des Plantes in Paris. However fantastic their theory may seem today, it is generally accepted that Gall and Spurzheim were sincere believers in phrenology and had the further merit of launching the doctrine of the localization in parts of the brain of various cerebral processes. Gall also recognized and demonstrated the fibres of the medulla and the decussation of the pyramids, a discovery first made by Domenico Mistichelli, of Fermo, in 1709. Moebius, Froriep, and Neuburger have all emphasized the historical importance of Gall's work.

A somewhat similar theory, the relation of physiognomy to mental attributes, was developed by the Swiss clergyman and physician J. K. Lavater (1741–1801). His theory, which was especially popular in Germany and France, had been preceded by the views of G. B. Dalla Porta, whose *De humana physiognomonia* maintained the possibility of estimating the character of the individual from his facial appearance.

Legal medicine, which, as we have seen in the previous chapter, was largely created by the Italians Fedele and Zacchia, during this period prepared the way for the greater progress of the nineteenth century. Among the more important works on the subject were the *Corpus juris medico-legale* of M. B. VALENTINE (1657–1729), of Giessen, and the studies on hanging by Antoine LOUIS (1723–92), Secretary of the Royal Academy of Surgery. Louis was the collaborator of Joseph Ignace GUILLOTIN (1738–1814), the inventor of the guillotine, the advantages of which were presented to the Academy in 1791. In England *Elements of Medical Jurisprudence* (1788) by Samuel FARR (1741–95) was influential; while in France the treatise of F. E. FODÉRÉ (1764–1835) on *Les Lois éclairées par les sciences physiques* (1798) was accepted as a classic for half a century and brought its author the title of the Nestor of legal medicine in France. Among the Italians prominent in this field were G. V. BONONI (1728–1803), professor at Ferrara and author of a treatise on legal medicine (1780);

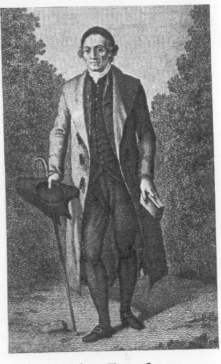

310. *Johann Kaspar Lavater.*

and Giuseppe TORTOSA (1743–1811), of Vicenza, whose treatise on the subject (1801) emphasized the need for more university instruction in this field, which at the moment in Italy was taught only in Pavia.

10. Hygiene and Social Medicine

Physicians had long been forced into a lively interest in the contagious diseases, but it was not until the eighteenth century that systematic and accurate descriptions were made and that scientific societies began to regard control of these diseases as an important part of their program. In the second half of the century hygiene assumed the character of an independent science; about the same time arose the realistic and political concept that the common people were entitled to better economic conditions of existence and that it was the duty of the State to provide them.

The various epidemics were not manifested with the same intensity as in previous centuries; but we can detect in the study of the clinical phenomena and the social results of epidemics the trace of logical lines of thought leading to clear, precise conclusions. We can see the differentiation of clinical syndromes, which toward the end of the century were sufficiently well defined to permit a much improved differential diagnosis of the epidemic diseases. Bubonic plague continued to afflict Europe, especially in the epidemic of 1709, which destroyed more than three hundred thousand lives in Prussia alone. Important but less severe were the epidemics in the Ukraine in 1737, at Messina in 1743, and at Cherso (Istria) in 1783. One of the most violent was the epidemic of Moscow (1789–1811), which was described and energetically fought by Gustaf ORRAEUS (1739–1811), who is said to have been condemned to death by Catherine II, for having insisted on recognizing the severity of the epidemic. Thousands of persons died in a few months.

Epidemics of exanthematic typhus were numerous, if only because of the many wars that afflicted Europe in this century. In 1741 it is calculated that more than thirty thousand French died of the disease at Prague. In the second half of the century typhus raged in Spain and Italy.

Typhoid fever, or abdominal typhus, probably was the most important element in the epidemic described by J. J. ROEDERER (1726–63), the first Professor of Obstetrics at Göttingen, and C. G. WAGLER (1732–78), of Brunswick, in their work *De morbo mucoso* (1760). This condition, which they ascribed to the contamination of well water, they regarded as intimately connected with dysentery and malaria. Typhoid was in all probability the " mesenteric fever " of Baglivi and the *febris nervosa lenta* which Huxham distinguished from the *febris putrida* (typhus?). Its intestinal lesions were also observed by Morgagni, but it was not to be demonstrated as a definite clinical entity until the next century by the French school of Louis. Epidemics of malaria were frequent, especially in France, Germany, and Hungary between 1770 and 1772, and in Holland between 1779 and 1781. Diagnosed as ague or as intermittent fever, it was prevalent in the English-speaking countries; but with different habits of living and the draining of swamps for economic reasons, it gradually diminished in frequency there long before any connection with the mosquito had been established. Dysentery was common in Europe, as in the German epidemic of 1720, and also endemically. Diphtheria, which in the previous century had been observed chiefly in Spain and Italy, was now spreading throughout the world. Influenza raged through most of Europe with more or less severity at more or less regular intervals, and was also common in America. The great pandemic of 1767 appeared in both continents, diffusing more slowly than it does at the present time, when the speed and frequency of travel are greatly increased. The wide diffusion of whooping cough in the eighteenth century is noteworthy; it spread rapidly in severe form toward the end of the century, especially in the northern countries; in Sweden, for instance, forty thousand children died of this disease between 1749 and 1764.

Scarlet fever, first observed in the preceding century, is known to have spread rapidly toward the end of the eighteenth century, even though its differentiation from measles was still uncertain. However, of all the infectious diseases, especially those that attack children, none reached the violence of smallpox, which appeared almost everywhere with high mortality. In the single epidemic of 1719 Paris lost fourteen thousand; in 1770 more than three million persons died of smallpox in India. All the great European states were ravaged by the disease and pock-marks on those that recovered were the rule rather than the exception. It was the very severity of the smallpox epidemics that led to the courageous attempts at preventive treatment that we shall speak of shortly.

Among the exotic diseases that began to reach Europe in this century, especially prominent was yellow fever, which previously had been found almost exclusively in America. Since the first epidemic observed on the western continent — Guadeloupe, 1635 — yellow fever had never been absent there. In the American colonies a good account of the 1741–2 epidemic was written by John Mitchell of Virginia in 1744. Excellent descriptions of the most severe of all the American epidemics — that of 1793 — were written by Matthew Carey and Benjamin Rush in Philadelphia and by John Lining of Charleston, South Carolina. In 1723 yellow fever appeared in epidemic form in Lisbon and endemic foci became manifest in the various maritime cities of Portugal and Spain. Late in the century, when public health conditions in Europe were at a low ebb, various epidemics of yellow fever appeared through western Europe.

Toward the end of the century hygienic provisions, even in the great capitals, were still primitive. It was the rule for excrement to be dumped in the streets, which were unpaved and filthy. In London it was only in 1782 that sidewalks began to be installed. Water closets appeared in Paris at the beginning of the century, but only in few houses, and they were entirely lacking in the rest of continental Europe. Street-cleaning began in Paris in the latter half of the century; the use of baths, which during the Renaissance had been widespread, had become a luxury in the eighteenth century. The first city to institute public baths was Liverpool, toward the end of the century. The private stationary bathtub made its first appearance in America in the next century and is still a rarity in some civilized countries.

Even this brief summary of the hygiene of the period is sufficient to explain the wide diffusion of infectious diseases, a phenomenon which was still further promoted by the migration of the countryfolk into the large cities and the enlargement of urban centres coincident with the beginnings of industrialization. On the other hand, and perhaps because of the situation just described, realization of the need for better hygiene began to take form, or rather to show a revival. We have had occasion to note even in ancient times the installation of real hygienic regulations. While many of these were dietetic, important steps were also taken in the hygiene of water, baths, massage, and so on. We have seen the influence of Fracastorius in the recognition of contagion, which necessarily led to the development of hygienic measures as defences against infectious diseases. We have seen also how the studies of the microscopists led to a better comprehension of contagious diseases and recognition of the need for prophylactic measures.

It is not without interest that Michele Rosa (1731–1812), of Rimini, professor at Modena (1782), believed that contagious diseases could be derived from disease germs, from the physical condition of the air, or from emanations from the ground. He attributed special importance to so-called abnormal physical constitutions (alterations of the atmosphere which modify the organism so as to predispose it to disease). This concept of the physical constitution was developed by various Italians such as F. Asti of Mantua, and C. Allioni, in his study of miliary fever in Piedmont (1758).

To England belongs the credit for having given new impulse to public hygiene and having improved the care of the sick in hospitals, which were in a deplorable condition throughout Europe at this time. It was England that led the hygienic movement in the second half of the century and maintained this honourable post throughout this past century — a circumstance that will not seem strange to those who realize that the development of hygiene always accompanies the economic well-being of a national culture. Toward the end of the century England went through a period of great commercial expansion. Humanitarian institutions flourished and the education of the young far surpassed that of the other countries of Europe. It was the Englishman John Howard (1726–90) who, after having been imprisoned in France and learned at first hand the terrible condition of the French prisons, undertook a pilgrimage through the prisons and hospitals of Europe and dedicated his life and fortune to this study. The material that he collected was published in his *Account of the Principal Lazarettos in Europe* (1789), which, in the numerous translations that were made, influenced many countries. Another Englishman, John HEYS-HAM (1753–1834), founded at Carlisle the first poor-law dispensary (1781) and commenced there the collection of vital statistics which formed the basis of J. Milne's famous " Carlisle Tables " (1816).

It was another English physician, Edward Jenner, who at the close of the century discovered vaccination against smallpox, an event of prime importance not only on its own account but also as the first step in the scientific prophylaxis of disease. The possibility of protection from small-pox by means of " variolization " — that is, the inoculation of human pus from smallpox cases — had been known since far-distant times. The an-cient Chinese had the custom of introducing scabs of the smallpox pustules into the nose of the healthy person in order to protect him from contagion. The Greek physician Emanuel Timoni (Timonius), according to Sudhoff, tells (1713) that Circassian women had the habit of pricking the body with needles bathed in smallpox pus to acquire a benign type of the in-fection. Lady Mary Wortley Montagu, wife of the English Ambassador at Constantinople, practised this method on her own children (1718–21) and brought the news to England, where it had considerable vogue until replaced by Jenner's discovery of vaccination. The doctrine of inocula-tion spread rapidly in the American colonies, as can be seen in the papers by B. Colman, Isaac Greenwood, Cotton Mather, William Cooper, William Douglass, all appearing in 1721 and 1722. Zabdiel Boylston's account (1726) of its use in the Boston epidemic of 1721 is the best known of the early American contributions; while Benjamin Franklin, John Morgan, and Rush all wrote in favour of the procedure. The Swiss Theodore Tronchin, and the Tuscan Angelo Gatti (1730–98), were especially influential in popularizing the method on the Continent. It was Gatti, one of the best Italian physicians of the century, who recommended the use of the pus extracted from artificially produced pustules, and also of the powder ob-tained from crushing the scabs. He wrote *Réflexions sur les préjugés qui s'opposent à l'inoculation* (Brussels, 1764) and *Nouvelles Réflexions* (1767), which were translated into English, German, and Italian. Gatti's method was well received in Paris, but soon he was forced into a long polemic with the Academy. He emerged victorious from this, however, and was given the task of inoculating the pupils of the École Militaire. Inoculation was especially well received in Italy, which is perhaps the reason that vaccina-tion also found less opposition there than in some other European countries. However, in spite of the successes obtained, inoculation was never adopted in a general way, both on account of the danger of infection from the germs of other diseases and because of the scars and sometimes severe, even fatal, attacks of smallpox produced.

Edward JENNER (1749–1823), born at Berkeley in Gloucestershire, is one of the finest figures in the history of medicine. This active and able

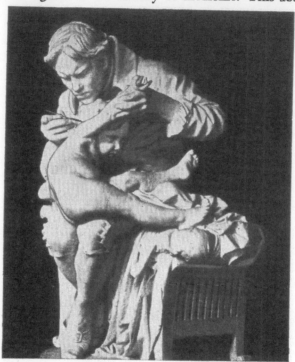

311. *Jenner vaccinating a child.*
Marble group by Giulio Monteverde, Genoa.

yet modest investigator and practitioner, on whom success smiled abundantly in his lifetime, remained throughout life a calm and clear-headed observer who united the best qualities of the good physician. Pupil and friend of John Hunter in London, he returned to the west of England, where he soon acquired a successful practice. As early as 1768 he had been told by a patient that she could not take smallpox because she had had cowpox. He observed the truth of this observation in his own practice among the farmers and their families, and continued to study the problem through many years. Finally convinced of the idea that cowpox (vaccinia) was a sure defence against smallpox, on May 14, 1796 he vaccinated a country boy, James Phipps, with pus from the milkmaid Sarah Nelmes, who was in the active stages of cowpox. The experiment succeeded perfectly: Jenner tried to infect the child with pus from human smallpox, and the infection did not take. He repeated his observations and experiments many times, and in 1798 published his results in a small book entitled *An Inquiry into the Causes and Effects of the Variolæ Vaccinæ* (London, 1798).

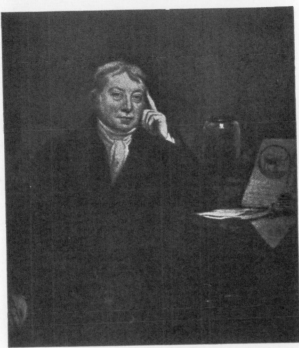

312. *Edward Jenner.*

One cannot imagine the emotion aroused throughout the civilized world by Jenner's publication.. Within a few years the method was known and used everywhere. In 1799 the Swiss physician Jean DE CARRO practised the first vaccinations at Vienna; in Italy, Luigi SACCO (1769–1836) was the first and most enthusiastic apostle of the new method. In Germany, Hufeland and Heim were its chief proponents. In the United States vaccination was first performed by Benjamin WATERHOUSE (1754–1846), who in July 1800 vaccinated, with serum received from London, his own children, who later failed to take smallpox when exposed to it. The vaccine was successfully used by Crawford of Baltimore, Coxe of Philadelphia, Elisha North, and Nathan Smith and, in spite of temporary failures by Jackson of Boston and Miller of New York, was well established in a decade. In England, its use spread rapidly; in 1802 Parliament voted Jenner a national gift of ten thousand pounds; in 1807 a second gift of twenty thousand pounds. Smallpox, which had been hitherto one of the greatest of human plagues, began to diminish rapidly wherever vaccination was enforced, and epidemics became ever more rare. But in spite of the compelling statistics throughout the world to show the efficacy of this prophylactic measure, efforts of the misguided and ignorant still continued to combat its compulsory use, and the number of cases occurring annually

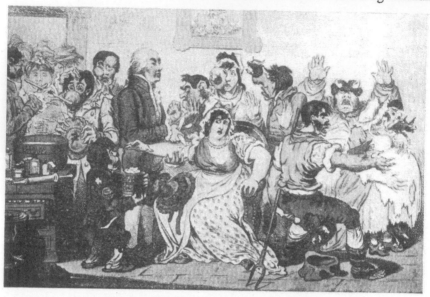

313. A Rowlandson caricature of vaccination.

throughout the world among the unvaccinated is still considerable. In enlightened countries where vaccination has long been in force, cases of smallpox have long been almost a curiosity. Jenner's discovery is an excellent example of the triumphs of scientific observation and of experiment, modestly and accurately set forth in print, and quickly confirmed by the organized profession. His *Inquiry* also includes observations of the effect of inoculation in persons who had previously had cowpox that constitute an interesting precursor of the present doctrine of anaphylaxis.

While Jenner was making these all-important observations, the whole structure of modern systematic hygiene was being outlined by Johann Peter FRANK (1745–1821), who was professor at Pavia for nine years and from 1795 at Vienna. An excellent clinician of the school of van Swieten, Frank was a remarkable organizer, who collected in his *System einer vollständigen medizinischen Polizey* (1779–1819) the most important principles of State hygiene. Carrying out Mirabeau's thought that the health of the public was the responsibility of the State, he maintained that the government not only should take charge when the public health was endangered by grave diseases, but should also be responsible for the public health at all times.

His book also contains chapters on conjugal hygiene, on the protection of women engaged in manual labour, the education of children, and the hygiene of schools.

Frank had an international reputation; tall, good-looking, with distinguished silver hair, he was sought by the greatest persons and monarchs of Europe. Napoleon, while the French were occupying Vienna, tried to get him to Paris, but this was made impossible by the jealousy of Corvisart. He was a man of great intellect, noted for his bons mots, which were often not without sarcasm. When he had eight of his colleagues in consultation at his deathbed,

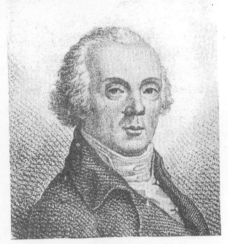

314. *Johann Peter Frank.*

smiling he said: " I call to mind a grenadier of Wagram who was dying of eight gunshot wounds. ' The devil,' he said, ' does it take eight balls to kill a French grenadier? ' "

The theories pronounced by Frank in his gifted book, which should be regarded as a cornerstone of modern hygiene, found support in the work of Benjamin Thomson, COUNT RUMFORD (1753–1814), of Woburn, Massachusetts. Rumford was a successful agitator for better public hygiene and concerned himself particularly with the improvement of the condition of the poor, lowering the cost of living, building inexpensive healthful houses, creating soup kitchens, supplying warm meals for school-children, emphasizing the hygiene of proper clothing, and urging proper inexpensive illumination and heating of the houses of the poor.

Anti-tuberculosis legislation had begun in Italy, as we have seen, toward the end of the seventeenth century. In 1735 the far-sighted Republic of Venice made special provisions for the tuberculous, who could not be admitted to the ordinary hospitals. In 1754 the Grand Duke of Tuscany, following a report of Antonio Cocchi, published an edict forbidding the sale or exportation of anything belonging to consumptives without proper disinfection. In 1782 a similar edict was announced with the sound of trumpets at Naples by the Tribunal of

Public Health, and severe penalties were decreed for those who failed to disinfect the clothing and houses of consumptives — a fine of three hundred ducats and ten years' imprisonment or banishment of the culpable physician for the second offence. In 1783 a special hospital was even considered; but these wise

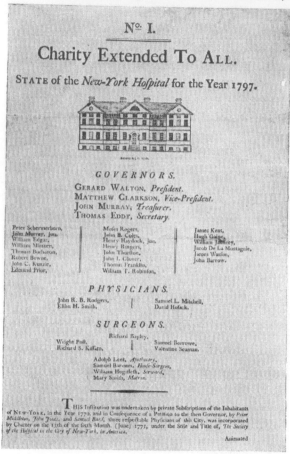

N°. I.

Charity Extended To All.

STATE of the *New-York Hospital* for the Year 1797.

GOVERNORS.

GERARD WALTON, *Prefident.*
MATTHEW CLARKSON, *Vice-Prefident.*
JOHN MURRAY, *Treafurer.*
THOMAS EDDY, *Secretary.*

Peter Schermerhorn,	Mofes Rogers,	James Kent,
John Murray, jun.	John B. Coles,	Hugh Gaine,
William Edgar,	Henry Haydock, jun.	William Janncey,
William Minturn,	Henry Rutgers,	Jacob De La Montagnie,
Thomas Buchanon,	John Thurfton,	James Watfon,
Robert Bowne,	John I. Glover,	John Barrow.
John C. Kunzie,	Thomas Franklin,	
Edmund Prior,	William T. Robinfon,	

PHYSICIANS.

John R. B. Rodgers,	Samuel L. Mitchell,
Elihu H. Smith,	David Hofack.

SURGEONS.

Richard Bayley,

Wright Poft,	Samuel Borrowe,
Richard S. Kiffam,	Valentine Seaman.

Adolph Lent, *Apothecary,*
Samuel Barnum, *Houfe-Surgeon,*
William Hogarth, *Steward,*
Mary Smith, *Matron.*

THIS Inftitution was undertaken by private Subfcriptions of the Inhabitants of NEW-YORK, in the Year 1770, and in Confequence of a Petition to the then Governor, by *Peter Middleton, John Jones,* and *Samuel Bard,* three refpectable Phyficians of this City, was incorporated by Charter on the 13th of the fixth Month, (June) 1771, under the Stile and Title of, *The Society of the Hofpital in the City of New-York, in America.*

Animated

315. *Announcement of the state of the New York Hospital for the year 1797.*

measures were soon abrogated by the opposition of short-sighted individuals of the kind who always are opposed to hygienic laws which demand some sacrifice from the individual in favour of the common interest. These laws, nevertheless, constitute important documents in the history of social hygiene. Further anti-tuberculosis measures were taken by the Republic of Venice in the law of 1772 (published by Pasinetti, Siena, 1926).

Among the precursors of modern hygiene should also be mentioned the great chemist Lavoisier, who, like Pinel, Chiarugi, Howard, and Heys-ham, especially studied the construction of prisons and pointed out the need for abolishing for prisoners the damp, dark, subterranean chambers where fresh air never penetrated. To Lavoisier is also owed a legislative project for protection against contagious disease. He was the first to demand that when a suspect is accepted in an establishment, his clothes should be boiled in a special apparatus and the patient himself carefully bathed.

Although we cannot yet speak of a veritable sanitary legislation in this century, we see progress toward an understanding of the problem and of the role that the State should play in the protection of the public health. The outlines of the sanitary legislation of the next century began to appear together with ideas which later were transferred into practice. Gifted visions of the objectives to be reached and the means to be employed were appearing in print at this time, and practical applications of great value were being made. Thus it can be said that toward the end of the century hygiene was well started on its way toward the solution of the most important problems of public health.

11. Therapeutics and Pharmacology

In the seventeenth century the Hippocratic doctrine of the curative powers of nature dominated therapeutics — a tendency manifested by Sydenham and continued by Boerhaave, who regarded fever as an important factor toward cure and advised the physician not to interfere in the evolution of the disease except by aiding the forces of nature. On the other hand, Friedrich Hoffmann, who did not admit that nature cured except by accident, maintained the necessity of active therapeutic intervention, especially in chronic diseases. Stahl, for his part, thought, like the Hippocratists, that the processes of healing are natural ones and that the effect of fever was to rid the body of harmful substances. He was one of the firmest believers in expectant therapy. The old Vienna school, following the doctrines of Boerhaave, placed this Hippocratic principle at the foundation of its therapeutics, to which Vienna remained faithful up to the middle of the past century. The French school of Bordeu felt the influence of Stahl; Montpellier was vitalistic and thus favoured the healing powers of nature. Pinel demanded of the physician " a profound wisdom and skill in putting to profit the healing powers of nature . . . and a strict differentiation of the diseases that it is dangerous to try to cure from those that demand prompt and intelligent aid." The same tendencies were followed in the teaching of the greatest physiologists and clinicians of Germany and Italy, so that, as Neuburger has shown, the eighteenth century should be regarded as the Hippocratic century par excellence. During this century bizarre medicaments began to disappear from the pharmacopœia and some of the most important that we use today made their appearance. Thus digitalis became established in the treatment of heart disease, and cinchona bark acquired its definite place in the therapeutic arsenal. F. R. TORTI

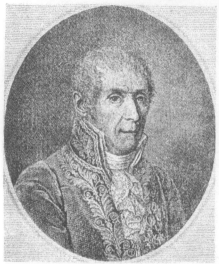

(1658–1741) was one of the most vigorous upholders of the therapeutic effect of quinine in his classic work on intermittent fever, *Therapeutice specialis ad febres periodicas perniciosas*, etc. (Modena, 1709). Warmly received throughout Europe and frequently reprinted, it is this book, according to Pagel, that brought about the final victory of cinchona bark.

Among other drugs introduced into medicine were jusquiamus, colchicum, aqua laurocerasi (by Byles, 1773), tar water for skin diseases (by Bishop Berkeley). Arsenic was prescribed in liquid form by Thomas

316. *Alessandro Volta.*

FOWLER (1736–1801) in the well-known "Fowler's solution." At this period therapeutics showed a tendency to return more and more to natural means of treatment. Cures at spas and treatment with natural mineral waters received once more the favour that they had enjoyed in the Middle Ages and with Paracelsus. Better chemical knowledge permitted a more accurate analysis of these waters and better indications for their use. As we have seen, Hoffmann was an excellent chemist, who analysed a number of different waters, which he prescribed in various diseases.

Hydrotherapy returned to the honourable position that it had held in the time of Hippocrates and in Italy in the hands of Savonarola (1424), Christopher Barzizio (1450), and Settala. Cirillo warmly recommended cold baths, a form of treatment that was popular in England, as may be seen in Sir John Floyer's *Inquiry into the Right Use of the Hot, Cold and Temperate Baths in England* (eight editions between 1697 and 1722). In Germany, Johann Sigmund HAHN (1664–1742) constructed an entire system of treatment of disease based on bathing in and drinking cold water

— *Psychroluposia* (Leiden, 1738). His doctrines were continued by his son, Johann Gottfried.

A new discipline, electrotherapy, was inaugurated with the work of the clinician and anatomist Luigi GALVANI (1737–98) at Bologna, and of

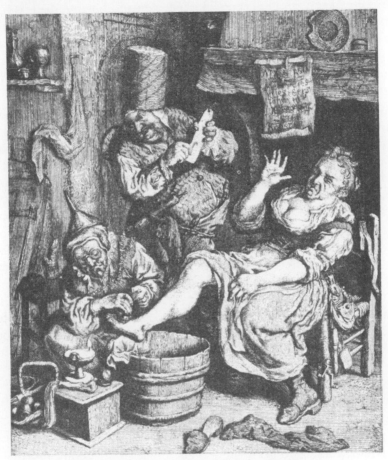

317. *Application of cups. A Dutch print, 1695.*

Alessandro VOLTA (1745–1827), of Como. Volta showed that a muscle could be put in a state of constant tetanic contraction by the application of electricity; and, although not a physician, he tried to apply the electric motor to the cure of disorders of hearing. A close friend of Spallanzani, he made many studies in the natural sciences, and was a pioneer in electrotherapy, a form of treatment that was later widely developed. Christian Gottlieb KRATZENSTEIN (1723–95), of Copenhagen, was one of the first to use electricity in the treatment of paralysis. Its use in the treatment of disease was popularized by Benjamin Franklin, G. F. Rössler, and others, so that static machines were to be found in many hospitals before the end of the century.

In spite of the great advances in chemistry and botany, materia medica did not make the progress that might be expected of it in this century. Perusal of lists of the most frequently used drugs shows that physicians and public still had recourse to many composed of strange ingredients of doubtful utility. Although authoritative scientists condemned the use of such drugs as theriacum, crayfish eye, pearls, and the flesh of vipers, they continued to be in frequent use. Toward the end of the century, however, new and more rational drugs began to be known and their value recognized; at the same time special secret remedies, which often made the fortunes of physicians and pharmacists, appeared in practice. The pharmacy shop of the eighteenth century had considerable social importance, especially in Italy and France. It was there that the scientists and the notables of the towns and cities came together and the problems of chemistry and natural history as well as those of medicine and politics were discussed. The Italian pharmacies, and especially those of Venice, were often splendidly decorated, the furniture and the sculptured woodwork designed by good artists. The large, beautifully coloured pharmacy jars, the bronze mortars, and the allegorical pictures combined to make the pharmacy shop a place worthy of respect and admiration and a centre of mundane life. Artists of the period often recorded their splendour in paintings and engravings.

12. The Study and Practice of Medicine

The eighteenth century was a period of philosophies and systems in its earlier part, leading to grave upheavals in the political and social life of Europe in its latter half. These upheavals in turn had a profound influence on the intellectual currents which brought them about. In this century arose the philosophic and scientific currents which tended toward positivism. From Leibnitz to Comte the path is marked by an ever increasing trend toward the positivistic concept, supported at each step by discoveries that revealed some of the mysteries of nature that had hitherto been accepted as inaccessible. We have already referred to the part played by medicine in this development. Let us now consider the events that determined the progress of science, which was rapid at this time and was fostered by the general spread of culture and the international collaboration of scientists of all countries.

Important contributors to this development were the MEDICAL JOURNALS, which began to acquire importance in this century.

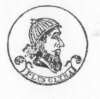

Lately published, by LOCKYER DAVIS.

1. A New Edition of Dr. Heister's General System of Surgery. Containing the Doctrine and Management, of Wounds, Fractures, Luxations, Tumors, and Ulcers, of all Kinds. 2. Of the several Operations performed on all Parts of the Body. 3. Of the several Bandages applied in all Operations and Disorders. To which is prefixed, an Introduction concerning the Nature, Origin, Progress, and Improvements of Surgery. With such other Preliminaries as are necessary to be known by the younger Surgeons. Illustrated with Forty Copper Plates, exhibiting all the Operations, Instruments, Bandages, and Improvements, according to the modern and most approved Practice. Translated from the Author's last Edition, greatly improved. 4to. 1l. 1s.

2. Mr. Chapman's Treatise on the Improvement of Midwifery. Third Edition, 4s.

3. The Medical Works of Dr. Wintringham, collected and published entire, by his Son Sir Clifton Wintringham, M.D. F.R.S. 2 vols. 10s.

4. Cases and Consultations in Physic, by the late eminent John Woodward, M.D. Published by Dr. Templeman, 5s.

5. Dr. Ball's Female Physician. Wherein is summarily described, all that is necessary to be known in the Cure of the several Disorders to which the Fair Sex are liable. Delivered in a Manner so concise, familiar, and intelligible, that every Woman of common Capacity may be able, upon most Occasions, to relieve herself by the Methods and Remedies herein contained. A Work of great Utility to young Physicians, Surgeons, and Apothecaries, 2s.

6. Pharmacopeia Domestica Nova, praecipue in usum eorum, qui vel Ruri vel Partibus Transmarinis Artem Medicam exercent, ut Apothecas, privatas sibimet construant, editio 4ta. Auctore Johanne Ball, M.D. 2s.

7. Mr. Warner's Account of the Testicles, their common Coverings and Costs: the Diseases to which they are liable, with the Method of treating them. 8vo. 2s.

8. Dr. Parsons's Analogy between the Propagation of Animals and that of Vegetables, 4s. 6d.

9. Dr. Birch's Collection of the Yearly Bills of Mortality for 100 Years back. To which are added, several curious Tracts written on this Subject, 9s. in Boards. 4to.

10. Mr. Da Costa's Natural History of Fossils, 12s. 6d. in Boards. 4to.

CASES AND OBSERVATIONS;

BY THE

MEDICAL SOCIETY

OF NEW-HAVEN COUNTY, IN THE

STATE OF CONNECTICUT,

Instituted in the Year 1784.

New-Haven: Printed by J. Meigs, 1788.

318. *The first American medical journal.*

In 1683 Jean Paul de la Roque, who had been one of the editors of *Journal des scavans*, began the publication of the shortlived *Journal de médecine*. From 1695 to 1709 Claude Brunet published *Le Progrès de la médecine* in monthly duodecimo fasciculi. This early attempt, which was stopped by the death of Brunet, had no lasting success and found no imitators. It was only in the latter half of the century that French medical journalism became triumphantly established. The *Journal de médecine, chirurgie*, etc., was begun in 1754 by Bernard, Bertrand, Grasse, and others and continued monthly publication until 1794. It was begun again in 1801 by Corvisart, the celebrated physician of Napoleon. The *Journal de médecine militaire* was published at Paris in seven volumes between 1782 and 1788; the *Journal de chirurgie* lasted but two years (1791–2), a common occurrence for journals of those days.

Germany produced the largest number of eighteenth-century journals, though mostly shortlived. *Der patriotische Medicus* was published in Hamburg from 1724 to 1726. In 1721 the pharmacist R. A. Vogel began the publication at Erfurt of the *Medizinische Bibliothek,* which carried a number of contributions of considerable scientific value. Reil's *Archiv für Physiologie* lasted from

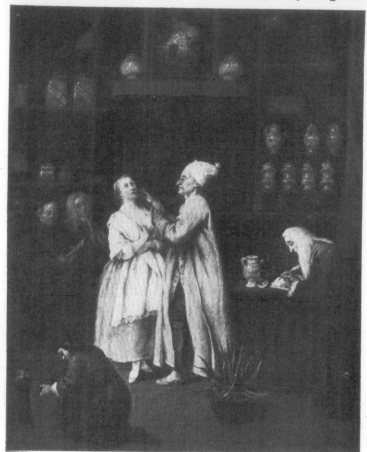

319. *A consultation in the pharmacy, by Pietro Longhi, eighteenth century.*
(ROYAL ACADEMY, VENICE.)

1795 to 1815. Earlier in the century in Germany, as elsewhere, medical articles had appeared in scientific journals, such as the *Acta eruditorum* of Leipzig, begun by Gross and Gleditsch in 1682.

In Italy the first medical journal properly so called was the *Giornale di medicina,* published for Pietro Orteschi by the printer Benedetto Milocco in Venice in 1763. Orteschi, who was a physician of wide culture and an able writer, dedicated the first volume of his journal to Haller, to whom he expressed his regrets that Haller's publication of his *Extracts of European Literature* had been

suspended. Orteschi's journal lasted until 1777 and then reappeared for a single
year in 1781. In 1783 Francesco Aglietti and his colleagues in Venice began the
publication of the *Giornale per servire alla storia ragionata della medicina di
questo secolo* (Journal for the Study of the History of the Medicine of this
Century) at Venice, printed by G. B. Pasquali. In 1773 G. Targioni began at
Florence the publication of *Raccolta di opuscoli medico-pratici*, of which six
volumes were published within ten years. Holland is represented by two eighteenth-century periodicals, the *Weekelijk Discours over de Pest* (Amsterdam,

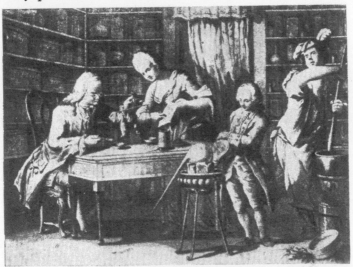

320. *The apothecary. Eighteenth-century Italian engraving.*

1721–2) and *Esculapius* (Amsterdam, 1723). Among eighteenth-century medical journals in England, all shortlived and first appearing toward the end of the
century, we find the *Medical Observations and Inquiries by a Society of Physicians in London* (6 vols., 1757–84); the *London Medical Journal* (11 vols., 1781–
90); *Medical Commentaries* (1780–95), a continuation of the *Medical and Philosophical Commentaries; Medical Communications* (1784–90); *The Medical
Spectator* (1791–3); and *The Medical and Physical Journal* (1799–1814). The
United States contributed two medical journals before 1800: *Cases and Observations by the Medical Society of New-Haven County, Connecticut* (instituted
in 1784) and *The Medical Repository* (1797–1824). An excellent and accurate
list of medical journals in all languages is to be found in the supplementary
volume of the Index Catalogue of the Surgeon Generals Library (First Series,
Washington, 1880–95).

Together with the progress of medical science in the eighteenth century there occurred a profound change in the lot of the medical profession

and in the forms of medical practice. The physician consolidated both his scientific and his material position. The best-known clinicians received pupils and patients from all parts of Europe. Eminent physicians no longer were attached to the courts of princes, but practised their profession independently, acquiring great honour and financial gain. The practice of medicine was especially well organized in England, where the social position of the physician reached such a point that he occupied a high rank

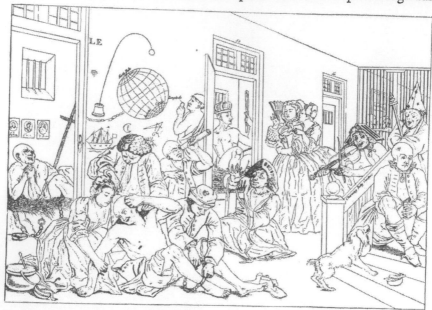

321. *Bedlam Insane Asylum, at the end of the eighteenth century, by Hogarth.*

in society and gained large financial return. Richard Mead made as much as seven thousand pounds in a year, and John Fothergill was able at his death to leave many thousands of pounds to the poor.

The physician no longer made use of alchemy and astrology and horoscopes in the practice of medicine. Physicians no longer were peripatetic or frequently changed their residence as in the preceding century, but established themselves in cities and small towns. The tendency toward literary and philosophic studies was accentuated, and we often see physicians eminent in science acquiring a reputation in literature. Such were Redi, Magalotti, Haller, and the medical poet Giovanni Meli, who was called " the Sicilian Anacreon." In England we find the physician to Queen Anne, John ARBUTHNOT (1667–1735), writing under the pseudonym Martinus Scriblerus. His humorous *History of John Bull* immortalized the nickname by which the English people have since been known. Sir Hans SLOANE (1660–1753) was another who acquired great wealth and a patent of nobility to boot; his memory is preserved in several place-names in London as well as at the British Museum, which was founded on the nucleus of his private museum and library. Sir Samuel GARTH (1661–

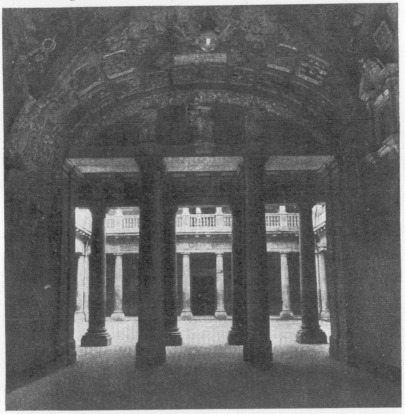

322. *Atrium of the University of Padua, with the coats-of-arms of the students.*

1719), a distinguished practitioner and author of *The Dispensary* (1703), a satirical poem of historical value for its description of the contest between the physicians and the apothecaries, was the only medical member of the celebrated Kit-Kat Club; his portrait by Kneller is familiar to many in mezzotint or in the Houbraken engraving. Redolent of the times is William Macmichael's story of *The Gold-Headed Cane* (1827), an adornment that was then a conspicuous part of the physician's insignia. This particular one passed successively through the hands of Radcliffe, Mead, Askew, William and David Pitcairn, and Matthew Baillie, whose widow presented it to the Royal College of Physicians. Much of the English medical life of the century can be found included in the account of the lives of these eminent men. John RADCLIFFE (1650–1729), founder of an equally famous library, infirmary, and observatory, whose secret of success was to " use all mankind ill "; Richard MEAD (1673–1754), who, in Samuel Johnson's phrase, " lived more in the broad sunshine of life than almost any

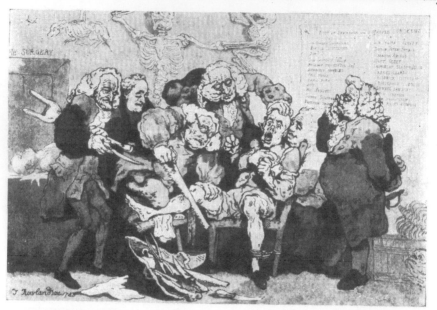

323. *Amputation.*　　　　　　　　　　　*Caricature by Rowlandson.*

man "; William PITCAIRN (1711–91), who is said to have been the first, in his lectures of 1788, to have connected rheumatic fever with heart disease; and Matthew BAILLIE (1761–1823), the Hunters' nephew, whose *Morbid Anatomy* (1793) is the first systematic and independent, though brief, textbook on the subject in any language.

In the eighteenth century family practitioners customarily did not practise surgery or obstetrics. The university degree no longer gave the right to practise beyond the boundaries of the state in which it was issued, except in the case of physicians of the highest reputation.

Medical teaching in the universities progressed systematically. The student was required to have first studied the classics. Anatomical instruction was steadily becoming more widespread, and special institutions of anatomy were being created. The first university clinic was instituted at Vienna by van Swieten in 1754; at Pavia a clinic was started by Borsieri in

1770. The hospitals were for the most part still wretchedly maintained, so that they served but poorly for instruction. In most of the great hospitals, such as the Hôtel-Dieu at Paris, toward the end of the century two or even more patients were habitually placed in one bed. The faculties were small — usually four or five professors, with several subjects assigned to each. Anatomy, surgery, and obstetrics were usually taught by the same professor; clinical medicine, chemistry, botany, and pharmacology

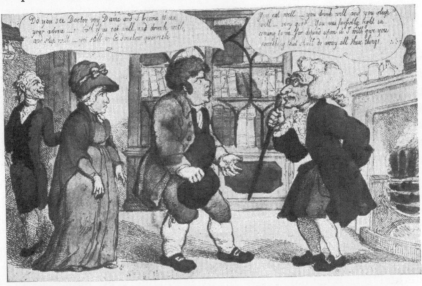

324. *A visit to the doctor.*   *Caricature by Rowlandson.*

by another. Each professor collected fees for his own course, a practice still maintained in some universities, and issued tickets of admission, which were often printed on the back of playing-cards. Examinations differed in the various universities, but were almost entirely theoretical. The Doctor's degree was given after the candidate had delivered a public address and discussed his inaugural thesis. The Italian universities still enjoyed a good reputation, especially Padua, Bologna, Rome, and Pavia. Paris and Montpellier continued in the lead in France, attracting physicians and students from various parts of Europe. In London the old-established hospitals began clinical instruction, which later developed into medical schools (now collected under the fostering wing of London University). Teaching began at Guy's Hospital as early as 1723; at St. Bartholomew's clinical instruction was given by Pitcairn and Abernethy in 1792 if not earlier; and at the London Hospital Medical School in 1785. The Edinburgh Hospital started clinical teaching in 1736, and the Meath Hospital in Dublin in 1756.

In this century surgery finally attained a position equal to that of medicine, the barbers continuing to practise minor surgery and dentistry. The guilds of barber surgeons, especially in England and France, in the early part of the century still possessed great importance; many famous surgeons acquired their skill in the shops of the barbers, but little by little the situation was changing. In France an important event that led to the emancipation of the surgeons from the barber association was C. F. Felix's cure (1686) of the anal fistula of Louis XIV. Such was the popularity of the Roi Soleil that this operation immediately became fashionable and the surgeons correspondingly important. The Collège de St. Côme, through Mareschal, expanded its teaching (1724) in spite of the protests of the Faculty of Medicine, and in 1731 the Royal Academy of Surgery was founded. A final step in the elevation of the surgeon was the decree by Louis XV forbidding the barbers to practise surgery (1743). In England the corporation of surgeons was separated from the barbers in 1745. The barbers' guild, however, still continued and it was not until 1800 that the Royal College of Surgeons received its charter. Surgical teaching in the universities, the social importance of the leading surgeons, and the spread of anatomical studies with the manifest need of such training for surgeons, were all factors in the evolution of the surgeon's social position. In England and in Germany, thanks especially to John Hunter and Heister, surgeons began to occupy university chairs and to be accepted as scientists by their colleagues. However, much of the practice of surgery still remained in the hands of empiricists, charlatans, and peripatetic operators, such as the famous Dr. Eisenbarth. In Germany the treatment of wounds and ulcers, according to the decree of Frederick the Great (1744), was open to the executioners of high justice. Even toward the end of the century the surgeons of the Prussian army were simple barbers, and it was only in 1785, as we have seen, that a military academy was founded at Vienna.

The teaching of obstetrics began, as we have seen, in this century. Proper schools of obstetrics were founded in the universities, and teaching was organized for midwives, from whom a diploma was required. Private schools also flourished, such as that of Grégoire in Paris (1720) and at the Maternité under Baudelocque (1797). Teaching of midwifery started at Vienna in 1748, at Göttingen and Berlin in 1751, and in many other cities of continental Europe before the end of the century. Similar developments took place in Great Britain, chairs of midwifery being established at Edinburgh in 1739 and at Dublin in 1743. The great Rotunda

Hospital at Dublin was founded (1751-7) by Mosse; the British Lying-in Hospital in London in 1749, and Queen Charlotte's in 1752.

The organization of public health services in the cities progressed slowly. In almost all the leading countries a national health service was beginning to be organized, with a central office in the capital headed by

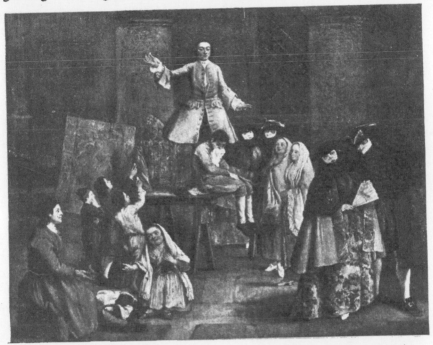

325. *The charlatan, by Pietro Longhi.*   (BRERA ACADEMY, MILAN.)

men of first rank. In the smaller cities and towns the health service was still deficient; but legislation to remedy the situation was already apparent.

It was only toward the end of the century that, thanks to the work of Howard, a definite campaign was made to improve the scandalous condition of the hospitals and prisons of Europe. True reforms were inaugurated in the rational treatment of the sick; asylums for the insane were erected where these unfortunates were treated patiently and kindly, and barbarous methods, such as chains, forced bathing, bastonade, isolation in cells, were abandoned after centuries of abuse.

In North America the institution of the first hospitals, medical schools and societies began in the second half of the century. The Pennsylvania Hospital, founded in 1751 by Benjamin Franklin, Thomas Bond, and others, is the oldest independent hospital of the American colonies; though there

is evidence that the present Philadelphia General Hospital has had a con-
tinuous existence, starting as the Infirmary of the Almshouse, since 1731.
The Bellevue Hospital in New York has a similar history starting in 1735.
In New Orleans a combined hospital and almshouse was opened in 1737.
The New York Hospital, now combined with the Cornell Medical School
in a magnificent Medical Centre in New York City, was chartered in 1771,

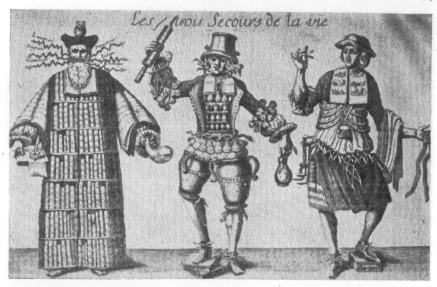

326. *The costumes of the physician (long robe), the pharmacist, and the surgeon
(short robe). French caricature of the late eighteenth century.*

through the efforts of Middleton, Bard, and Jones. Dispensaries were
founded in Philadelphia in 1786 and in New York in 1791. Medical instruction, except for the few who could study abroad, had perforce been
by the apprentice method. The evident advantages of more formal teaching at the hospitals led to the formation of several medical schools before the
close of the century. The earliest was the School of the College of Philadelphia (now the University of Pennsylvania), founded by John Morgan
on the lines of the Edinburgh School, with Morgan, Shippen, Adam Kuhn,
and Rush as the original faculty. The first degrees (M.B.) were conferred
in 1768, the first M.D. in 1771; so that the King's College School (now
the College of Physicians and Surgeons of Columbia University), though
founded in 1767, was the first to give the degree of M.D. in course (1770)
in the present United States.[1] Harvard, the oldest American college, did

[1] The first actual M.D. degree, an honorary one, was given by Yale College in 1723 to
Daniel Turner – his enemies suggesting that the letters stood for *multa donavit*. It is said that

not start a medical school until 1783 and for twenty years many would-be physicians came on horseback to the Quaker City for their medical instruction. The other schools to be founded in the United States in the eighteenth century were Dartmouth College School (by Nathan Smith,

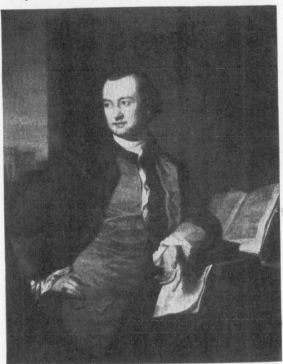

327. *John Morgan, founder of the first medical school in the United States. (After a portrait by Angelica Kauffmann, at the* UNIVERSITY OF PENNSYLVANIA.)

1796) and the now defunct Transylvania University School, in Kentucky (1799).

In spite of the better organization of medical practice and of severe laws aiming to control the abuses that were common, the eighteenth century was a flourishing period for adventurers and charlatans. Vendors of panaceas and secret remedies were common. While the charlatans of the sixteenth and seventeenth centuries were content to sell their remedies to the lower classes in the public squares and to practise minor surgery in the small towns and villages of the provinces, the eighteenth century presents a new type of the elegant adven-

his acceptance included the odd remark that " he appreciated it just as much as if it had been from an institution of higher learning "! Lane (*Annals of Medical History*, 1919, II, 367) points out that Toner was wrong in giving the date as 1720.

turer, surrounded with much scenic apparatus, disdaining the public square and country fairs as the scenes of his exploits. He was no longer content to narrate ancient romances while he described his remedies for a few pennies; he now travelled with a whole troupe of comedians and gave plays as he sold his remedies. He easily penetrated to palaces, and even to royal courts, and knew how to exploit the credulity of the public in a really extraordinary manner. We have already met one of the most celebrated, the self-created Count Cagliostro, vendor of powders, ointments, and waters of youth for the ladies, and inventor of an elixir of long life, by means of which he was able to extract large sums from the wealthy. Showered with gifts from the sick of Europe, he tried his tricks in Paris, where he came in contact with the court and the high aristocracy; but he soon passed to another kind of activity in the occult arts which brought him both fame and trouble. The Count of Saint-Germain, the king of impostors of his time, also invented an elixir which conferred immortality. He claimed to cure all diseases with a medicine that he called the " Universal Archæus."

Fantastic powers were still attributed to supernatural beings such as the blood-sucking vampires and hobgoblins that spread epidemics. J. K. WESTPHAL (d. 1722), member of the Academy of the Curious about Nature, in his *Pathologia demoniaca* (1707), tells many stories of bewitched women. Friedrich Hoffmann accepted as a proved fact that evil spirits entered the body, causing spasms and convulsive diseases. Miraculous cures have always found a favourable soil in France. The Jansenist and thaumaturgist François Paris was accepted as a performer of miracles, and about the year 1730 hundreds of epileptics crowded to his grave in the Cemetery of St. Médard to be cured. Montgeron, Councillor of the Parliament of Paris, described these miracles in a book which he presented to the King of France, who eventually was forced to close the cemetery to the public.

Charlatans and adventurers were no less successful in England. Some of them, such as Jane Stevens and a certain Mrs. Mapp, accumulated considerable fortunes. Stevens's remedy for stone in the bladder was bought by the English

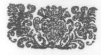

NUOVO METODO

Da offervarfi in avvenire per lo fpurgo delle Stanze, dove fono morte Perfone per cagione di male di 'Etisia, approvato dagl' Illuftriffimi Signori Confervatori di Sanità fotto il giorno 12. Febbrajo 1767.

I deve prima ben fpazzare pulita tutta la ftanza, e dopoi ftuccare con calcina diligentemente tutti li buchi, e fiffure, si delle porte, come delle fineftre, a riferva di un folo ingreffo; fi prenderà poi libbre tre Pecie greca, e libbre tre Zoifo, e meffo cio dentro un tegame in mezzo di detta ftanza, fe gli darà fuoco, con' un poco di ftipa, e dopo fi ferrerà detto ingreffo, ftuccandolo con calcina e con diligenza come fopra acciò non efca il profumo, dopo due giorni fi potrà riaprire, con lavare le muraglia, porte, e fineftre, con una forte lifciva, con paffarvi più volte fopra il tutto il pennello da Imbiancatore, e con l'ifteffa lifciva ancora fi lavarà il pavimento, e dopoi fi faranno dare due mani di Bianco alle muraglia di detta ftanza, come ancora al foffito, avvertendo che vi fia qualche giorno di mezzo da un imbianco all'altro

E quanto al detto fpurgo della ftanza dovrà la fpefa foffrirfi dal Proprietario, o fia Livellario della medefima Cafa, in cui faranno feguite morti per cagione del detto male di Etis a &c.

In fede &c.

NICOLAO RICCI CANC.

IN LUCCA 1784. Preffo FILIPPO MARIA BENEDINI.

328. *Edict of the Health office of Lucca for the disinfection of rooms in which consumptives had died.*

government by Act of Parliament, but on examination was found to be composed of ingredients that had no therapeutic value whatever.

Common also was the mountebank physician who had completed more or less medical study in order to practise his trade in public places. One of the most notable of these was Bonafede Vitali, " Mountebank," as he was proud to call

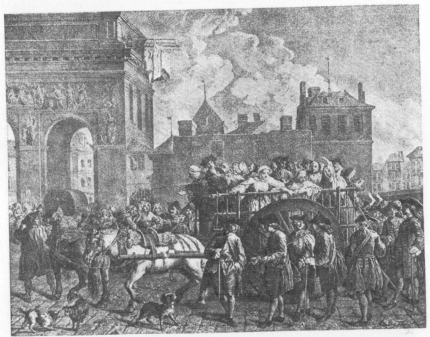

329. Filles de joie *being transported to the hospital. Eighteenth-century print.*

himself, but who was very famous, and was called *the Anonymus*. He had doges and grand dukes, the Pope, Charles XII, and Louis XIV among his patients, who showered him with gifts. Though the superstitious and charlatans have always been with us, they seem to have flourished particularly toward the end of the eighteenth century, when intercommunication was much increased, yet credulity and ignorance were widespread, even among the higher classes of society.

The literature of the period naturally reflected this state of affairs. If it shows us the illustrious scientists and famous physicians on the one hand, it is equally rich in sharp satires, especially by the humorists, exposing the tricks of the charlatans, their false remedies, and their dubious practices. Among those who delighted to expose the medical profession was the dramatist Carlo Goldoni, himself the son of a physician. His *La Finta ammalata (Malingerer)*, like Molière's *Malade imaginaire* of the previous century, exposes the ignorant physician and pharmacist, but also portrays the figure of the honest physician. Other comedies show us patients who prefer the remedies of the cobbler to those of the physician; and physicians, some ready to improvise voluble explanations, while others disinterestedly and conscientiously take care of the sick; such, for instance, is *The Dutch Physician*, representing Boerhaave. Vivid pictures of the physicians of the time are to be found in the novels, plays, and biographies of the period, such as Casanova's autobiography and the letters of Mme de Sévigné.

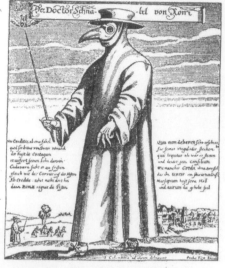

330. *The plague physician. Engraving by A. Colombina.*

Medical caricatures were popular at this time and were often made by great artists: one by Boucher represents a vendor of orvietan (1736); the remarkable pictures of Longhi were often reproduced. Satirical pictures of physicians and medical scenes by the famous Polish painter Daniel Chodowiecki (1726–1801) were much appreciated. The vigorous caricatures of Gillray, Rowlandson, and the Cruikshanks were very popular in England. Engravings of famous physicians, medical scenes, extraordinary cases, and remarkable cures were much in demand. Thus literature and art faithfully reflected the doctrine of the medical life of the century; it would be erroneous, however, to judge this life too severely on the basis of these criteria. These elegantly perfumed and bewigged physicians loved to promenade majestically, wearing their three-cornered hats and flourishing their gold-headed canes, using grandiloquent and often abstruse forms of speech. Beside them, to be sure, were the ignorant and the charlatans, but also serious scholars, keen, profound observers, men cultivated in the sciences as well as in letters. They moved in that curious and interesting eighteenth-century society where adventurers were on a par with ministers, and charlatans gave laws to the realm. Sometimes they favoured the most bizarre and ridiculous forms of treatment; at other times they were revealed as sincere, courageous apostles of humanity and scientific progress. Some of these men exerted a much greater influence on the intellectual and political life of the time than is apparent in the pages of history; to many, science was a stimulating leader. The historian of civilization can never forget the efforts of Pinel, Chiarugi, and the Tukes toward a rational treatment of the insane; or the campaign for improvement of infant mortality under the leadership of Rousseau. Neither can history forget the foundation of the great medical libraries, such as those created

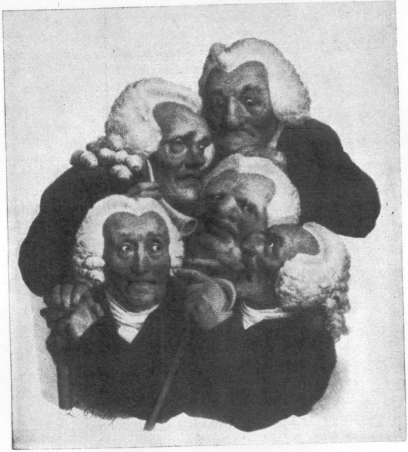

331. *Doctors in consultation, by L. L. Boilly.*

by Lancisi (1711), by the Faculty of Medicine in Paris (greatly enlarged in 1733), by the British Museum, and by J. Radcliffe. Great museums were founded by Aldovrandi (on natural history), the Hunters, Flaiani, Scarpa, and others. Many great scientific societies were formed, such as the Royal Academy of Berlin (1700), the Paris Academy of Surgery (1731), the Medical Societies of Edinburgh (1737) and London (1773). Even the North American colonies had their local medical societies, beginning with

Boston in 1735; and seven states had formed societies before the end of the century. The Massachusetts Medical Society (1781), the Medical and Chirurgical Faculty of Maryland (1784), the College of Physicians of Philadelphia (1787), and a few others still flourish, the last named sharing with the Army Medical Library and the New York Academy of Medicine the distinction of having the best medical libraries in the country.

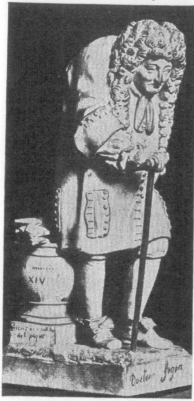

332. *Guy Crescent Fagon, physician of Louis XIV.*
(*Porcelain statuette in the* CARNAVALET MUSEUM, PARIS.)

If, then, the medicine of the century, though delivered from Galenic dogmatism, had not yet found its true gait and was too much dominated by transcendental mysticism, it nevertheless was regarded by some as a golden age of the medical profession, gathering the fruits of the seed sowed by the Renaissance. Scientific medicine was no longer the monopoly of a few isolated scholars, but had become the patrimony of many physicians. Though empiricists and charlatans were only too numerous, in all branches of medicine physicians were appearing whose knowledge reposed on a scientific basis. The increased possibilities of rapid diffusion of scientific discoveries, the vast organization of teaching and research in universities, the differentiation of medicine into various branches of equal dignity, and, finally, the recognition of that fundamental truth that anatomical, physiological, and pathological knowledge constitutes the basis of all medical study — these are the important foundations on which, after the great political upheavals had subsided, humanity was enabled to erect the structure of modern medicine.

CHAPTER XIX

FIRST HALF OF THE NINETEENTH

CENTURY

EXPERIMENTAL AND BIOLOGICAL CONCEPTS.
THE CELL DOCTRINE

~~~~~~

1. General Considerations

MEDICINE in the early part of the nineteenth century has its special characteristics, influenced by the vigorous intellectual, political, and social currents of the time. Medical progress, which had been slowed during the period of the French and American Revolutions and the almost contemporaneous upheavals in the countries of central Europe, gained momentum especially in France after the Napoleonic victories brought to that country a flourishing period in the arts and sciences. The liberty of word and thought that accompanied the French Revolution contributed notably to the evolution of science. The freer atmosphere of politics favoured rebellion against dogmatism, metaphysics, and the many influences that restricted human thought. The new position of the bourgeoisie gave the Third Estate access to the courses in higher learning. With the opening of the doors of the university, free from religious and political control, the privilege of culture as well as of political sovereignty came within the reach of the lower classes. The rapid progress of industries, the development of urban centres, where the growing population insisted on better

[667]

sanitary conditions, and other factors of a similar nature obliged statesmen and physicians alike to concern themselves with the problems of public health that were daily becoming more urgent and important. The remarkable development of the new United States of America, the enormous increase in traffic on land and sea determined by new means of communication, the great increase in the interchange of ideas and scientific discoveries among the different countries of Europe and America, brought an impulse to science that determined its rapid and vast expansion with a steadily accelerating rhythm.

Together with the great increase in material and cultural growth, a deeper sense of human dignity was penetrating even to the lowest social classes; on the other hand, especially in the Latin countries, a realistic tendency was manifested against the idealism of the eighteenth century. This realistic tendency and the pursuit of materialistic aims was a general phenomenon through Europe, eventually leading to a romantic orientation that emphasized a national ideal, in antithesis to the humanitarian ideal of the French Revolution. This orientation, in which the dualism of Kant and, still more important for medical thought, the doctrines of the philosopher F. W. von Schelling played an important part, naturally contributed to overcome metaphysical and transcendental tendencies and to further the progress of the natural sciences. It was in the study of nature, in constant experimental investigation, in the observation of all forms of life, that the scientists of the period now found the necessary basis for their work. It was in objective and controlled observations that they sought the solution of the most complex biological problems, abandoning any reliance on philosophical hypotheses. Medicine felt the result of this new orientation in the most direct manner.

At the same time the progress of chemistry and physics stimulated the development of those studies that depend especially on these sciences, and the new disciplines of physiological and pathological chemistry came into existence. Technical progress was equally important to the evolution of science and medicine, in giving to investigators instruments of greater and greater precision, to chemical laboratories more reliable reagents, and to therapeutics drugs that had been better studied and evaluated in their effects and combinations.

Under the influence of political and social events, and of intellectual currents, which were sometimes causes and sometimes results, the materialistic tendency, which necessarily owes its importance to a development of technique and of the natural sciences, became ever more dominant. Auguste Comte founded the philosophy of Positivism, seeking for the laws that rule phenomena through positive reasoning, solely considering actual facts based on objective and accurate methods.

Close examination of the factors that determined the trend toward positivism, and therefore the development of medicine in the nineteenth century, reveals the importance of the discoveries at the beginning of the century in botany, zoology, chemistry, and physics, which tended to upset idealistic and metaphysical systems and opened up new paths of thought and study. It was biology and the natural sciences that furnished the background of the philosophic thought of the time.

The achievements of Georges CUVIER (1769–1832) in comparative anatomy, in the classification of zoological types, and in the new discipline of vertebrate palæontology, were necessary for the solution of many biological problems.

Schleiden and Schwann's recognition of the cellular nature of living structure and Robert Brown's discovery of the cell nucleus, together with Virchow's doctrine of cellular pathology, laid the necessary foundations for modern biology. Bassi's discovery of the microscopic cause of silkworm disease, Pasteur's demonstration that fermentation was due to living organisms, and later the foundation of the new discipline of bacteriology by Pasteur and Koch revolutionized the whole concept of infectious diseases. Two other doctrines of the greatest importance for medical science were announced toward the middle of the century: first, the law of the Conservation of Energy, discovered by Julius Robert MAYER (1814–78) in 1842 (Liebig's *Annals*), and almost contemporaneously by James Prescott JOULE (1818–89), and applied to all matter by Helmholtz in 1847; and second, the law of Natural Selection, established by Charles Darwin and published in his immortal *On the Origin of Species by Means of Natural Selection* (London, 1859).

CHARLES ROBERT DARWIN (1809–82), grandson of the celebrated physician ERASMUS DARWIN (1751–1802), who also had announced original views on evolution, began the study of medicine in Edinburgh in 1825. Turning to botany and the natural sciences, he joined the H.M.S. *Beagle* on a voyage of exploration that lasted five years, during which time he was constantly gathering material on the differences between species. On his return, in spite of considerable ill health, he devoted himself exclusively to his studies, which after twenty years resulted in the publication of one of the most important of scientific works. It immediately aroused great interest and also opposition and in a few years was translated into most modern languages. Darwin upheld the thesis that different species came into existence by a process of evolution depending on various selective factors, of which natural selection (survival of the fittest) was the most important, thus definitely attacking the idea of immutability of species. In addition to the theory of natural selection, it should not be forgotten that Darwin invoked other phenomena, such as sexual selection, as factors in the development of new species. A score of books elaborating the general theme were written by him during his long, active career. The enormous amount of material that Darwin gathered for his observations, and the masterly deductions and generalizations that he was able to make from them, prove him to have been not only a

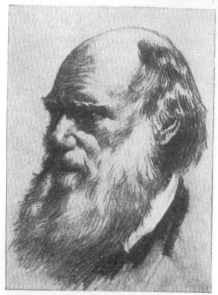

careful, intelligent, and eager scientist but also a man of genius who accomplished one of the most remarkable generalizations in the history of human thought. Among his precursors should be mentioned Étienne Geoffroy Saint-Hilaire (1772–1844), who advanced the hypothesis of successive changes in species (1828), Buffon, Lamarck, and the poet Goethe, who in his *Metamorphoses of Plants* (1790) stated some of the fundamental principles of the theory of descent. Alfred Russel Wallace (1823–1913) had simultaneously with Darwin arrived at similar conclusions, published in 1858, but his broad-minded spirit recognized the priority of Darwin's studies, which began twenty years before the publication of the *Origin of Species*, and the

333. *Charles Darwin.*

two men continued friendly intercourse throughout their lives. Among the best-known followers of Darwin were the biologist Thomas Henry Huxley (1825–95), who was a brilliant exponent of Darwin's evolutionary idea, and the zoologist-anatomist Richard Owen (1804–92), the discoverer of the trichina. Many opponents of Darwinism arose, however, even such eminent scientists as von Baer and Virchow. Ernst Haeckel (1834–1919) was the chief supporter of the theory of evolution in Germany; his *Generelle Morphologie der Organismen* (1866) and his *Anthropogenie* (1874) classified organic animal structures on the evolutionary and hereditary basis. His museum at Jena contains the world's best exhibition illustrating the theory of evolution.

These important advances in the domain of the natural sciences were accompanied or followed by discoveries in physics and chemistry which were of great importance in the development of medical science. In fact, it might even be said that modern medical research is largely founded on physics and chemistry, which continue to contribute more and more to the solution of fundamental problems of normal and pathological physiology.

A number of important therapeutic measures, such as electrotherapy, massage, and orthopedics, are derived directly or indirectly from physics. Enunciation by John Dalton, the discoverer of colour blindness, of the law of multiple proportions in 1802, and of the atomic theory in 1803, were basic events in the science of physics. Volta's discoveries in the fields of electricity and therapeutics, and the discovery of the induction of electric currents by Michael Faraday (1791–1867) have proved to be fundamental for progress in medicine as well as in industry. Hermann von HELMHOLTZ (1821–94), inventor of the ophthalmoscope, is another physicist who was of great importance in the history of medicine for his theories of electrodynamics and galvanic polarization; Heinrich HERTZ (1857–94) in 1885 made the important discovery of the electric waves that have played such an important part in the development of the radio. Equally important discoveries were made in chemistry; in 1828 Friedrich WÖHLER (1800–82) founded organic chemistry with his artificial synthesis of urea, showing that organic compounds were subject to ordinary chemical laws. Thomas GRAHAM (1805–69) was the founder of the enormously important colloid chemistry; Justus von LIEBIG (1803–73), in his fundamental work on *Die Thierchemie oder organische Chemie in ihrer Anwendung auf Agrikultur und Physiologie* (1842), was the first to affirm the necessity of searching in the laws of chemistry for the explanation of the important phenomena of metabolism, thus becoming one of the chief pioneers in physiological chemistry. The studies of A. W. von HOFFMANN on organic nitrogenous substances and on synthetic chemistry were useful in advancing physiological chemistry and led toward the recognition of a number of new drugs useful to the physician.

Such discoveries illustrate the decisive reaction against the metaphysical systems of the previous century and of the natural philosophy of the Germans, which culminated in the philosophical speculations of Oken and other purely theoretical systems such as mesmerism, homeopathy, and Broussais's dogma of the irritability of the intestinal tract as the basis of all disease. The reactive tendencies, which many attribute to the influence of Haller, must also be accepted as having been due at least in part to the Italians, who had never wholly accepted the metaphysical trends; Rokitansky, for instance, saw fit to engrave the title of Morgagni's book on the façade of his institute. Spallanzani, Fontana, and Corti were the first Italian investigators properly to be regarded as the initiators of the new trend. Medical supremacy, however, passed to the French in the first part of the nineteenth century, later to rest with the Germans, at the time of the political and industrial ascendency of Germany.

The progress of science in the early nineteenth century reveals numerous currents and determining factors — a circumstance that makes the history of this epoch unusually interesting and yet difficult to follow. A division into different periods cannot be more than approximate and cannot coincide with exact chronological dates. With this reservation, we regard as the first period in the development of medical thought in this century that which extends from about 1800, with the tendencies that we have just discussed, up to the establishment of the modern pathological concept of disease, about 1850.

It is obvious that with the enormous development of hospitals, clinics, and medical publications, the history of this period can merely be sketched in its main features. We can mention only those concepts, discoveries, and eminent individuals that had a determining importance from the historical point of view, or gave a characteristic note to the evolution of the art and science of medicine.

2. Anatomy

The modern study of anatomy, begun with the epoch-making work of Vesalius, had continued through the eighteenth century to be limited to the gross anatomy of organs, muscles, and bones in their visible form. This knowledge had steadily become more detailed and accurate; had included the comparative anatomy of the lower animals, and the relations of parts to one another — often learned by the student from his own dissection rather than as a demonstration by others. With the new century, however, vitally important progress was made in extending knowledge of the body structure along two lines: first, Bichat's studies of tissues rather than organs, and, second, microscopic anatomy and the establishment of the cell theory.

Histology, or the study of the tissues (ἱστος, a tissue), had in a sense existed since the days of the ancients, and in the seventeenth century some microscopic observations had been made. The systematic study of tissues, however, and emphasis on them as important units of normal and pathological structure, is owed to the gifted Marie François Xavier BICHAT (1771–1802), who from this point of view is entitled to be accepted as at least one of the fathers of histology. Born at Thoisette in the Jura, Bichat studied at the University of Montpellier and at the Hôtel-Dieu in that city with such enthusiasm that he is said to have performed no less than six hundred autopsies before his early death from tuberculosis. Stimulated by the ideas of his master, Pinel, and of Andreas Bonn of Amsterdam, Bichat proceeded, without the aid of the microscope, to found a system of normal and pathological structure based on the tissues rather than on organs as the important biological units. He distinguished twenty-one kinds: nervous, vascular, mucous, serous, connective, and so on, which were regarded as the elementary structures, each having its characteristic vital property in the Stahlian sense, which when sufficiently weakened permitted the exist-

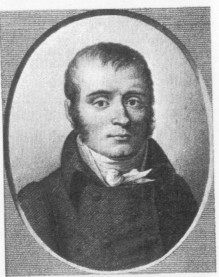

334. *Marie François Xavier Bichat.*

ence of disease. He announced the important concept that disease of a tissue is essentially the same, in whatever organ it may be located. These ideas are developed in his *Traité des membranes* (1800), *Sur la vie et la mort* (1800), and his *Anatomie générale* (4 vols., 1801); he also wrote a *Traité d'anatomie descriptive* (5 vols., 1801–3) and other works that can still be bought from book dealers for relatively small sums. His views on contractility, irritability, and toxicity recall those of Haller and other predecessors; of permanent value are such statements as: "The invariability of the laws that govern physical phenomena allows all the sciences that depend upon them to be submitted to calculation." These doctrines, applied to clinical medicine, gave rise to the great French school, which, in spite of the exaggerations of a few such as Broussais, brought a magnificent contribution to modern medicine.

Without the microscope, anatomical research could not proceed much further. With the introduction of achromatic lenses and improved compound microscopes in the 1820's, however, the study of histology, both normal and pathological, was made possible to an extent and accuracy hitherto undreamed of. While these technical improvements were undoubtedly important factors in promoting progress in microscopic anatomy, it must also be accepted that the time had become favourable, as is so often the case in major scientific developments. The desire to know had to be awakened before the fundamentally important cell doctrine of living structures could be established by Schleiden and Schwann in 1838 and 1839. Much more could have been discovered before their day with the tools at hand, and actually so many significant observations had been made that there is a tendency in some quarters to give the chief credit to others. Pure speculation, too, in the writings of Oken and others, not having at that time sunk to the unwarrantedly discredited position that it occupies in biology today, had contributed in preparing the soil. Furthermore, MILNE-EDWARDS (Paris thesis, 1823) had stated that every animal tissue that he studied was composed of "spherical corpuscles" about 1/300 mm. in diameter; and R. J. DUTROCHET, in particular, had clearly observed (1824) the universal cellular structure of animal and plant tissues and had appreciated that growth consisted in the formation of new cells. He recognized the structural individuality of each cell and, still more surprising, discovered cellular osmosis, coining the term "endosmosis" to signify impulsion within a body by the osmotic force.

Renewed interest in embryology, practically dormant since Harvey's time, was undoubtedly another factor in promoting the cellular concept of living structures. The segmentation of the frog's ovum was described by Prévost and Dumas in 1826; the mammalian ovum was discovered by von Baer the next year; the cell nucleus by R. BROWN in 1832 (published 1833); the nucleolus by VALENTIN (1836); the germinal spot of the animal egg by J. V. COSTE (1807–73) of Paris in 1837. Spermatozoa, known since the seventeenth century, had been shown by Spallanzani to be essential to fertilization (1786). Their cellular origin, however, was not established till 1841 (Kölliker), and their nucleus and cytoplasm were demonstrated by Schweigger-Seidel (1865). The chromosomes were first described much later, by Flemming in the seventies, and named by Waldeyer. In any case, we must recognize that, whatever the reason, these earlier studies were not fertile; whereas shortly after 1839, and due to Schleiden's and Schwann's publications, the concept of the cell theory was firmly established in the biological world, with less opposition than has attended most major scientific discoveries. Much credit for this important step is undoubtedly due to the great Johannes Müller, whose many-sided achievements will be further considered in the next section. He had himself worked with the microscope for several years and in fact in 1838 he published the first volume, the only one published, of his great book on tumours (*Über den feineren Bau und die Formen der krankhaften Geschwülste*), based on the cellular ideas of his pupil Schwann, and recognizing that the cell is by far the most frequent element of morbid growth.

Mathias SCHLEIDEN (1804–81) was an erratic, melancholic character who turned to the natural sciences only in 1831 after he had despondently shot himself in the head for his supposed failure at law. He betook himself to the microscopic study of plant structure so successfully, however, that in 1838 appeared his *Beiträge zur Phytogenese* (*Müller's Archiv*). Though wrong in his concept of cell formation from an unorganized cytoblast, he did recognize the universality of the cell in plant structure, which he correctly regarded as a community of cells, and that plant growth is due to increase in the number of cells. Equally important perhaps was the conversation he is said to have had over the coffee cups with Theodor SCHWANN (1810–82), which led the latter to study the application of Schleiden's theories to animal life, looking for and finding cells in all animal tissues, even in the embryonic stage (*Mikroskopische Untersuchungen über die Uebereinstimmung in der Struktur und dem Wachstum der Thiere und Pflanzen*, 1839). Schwann recognized that cells, in a limited number of forms, were the structural units of animals as well as plants, practically universally present in the tissues; also he regarded non-cellular elements as coming from the cells. Though he, like Schleiden, was wrong in his view of the animal cell as a vesicle, his concept of the cell as an important unit of life in animal as well as vegetable tissue was of prime importance. It was quickly accepted and stimulated active progress in many lines.

While these new paths of the highest importance were being broken in the field of histology, gross anatomy was not idle. In GREAT BRITAIN its leading exponent was Sir Charles BELL (1774–1842), who like many energetic Scotsmen spent more of his life in London than in Scotland. Like his brother, John, an able surgeon who had a private school of anatomy at Edinburgh, Charles conducted a successful general practice, though it did not seem to hinder a large output of scientific studies in anatomy and physiology. (*Medical classics*, October 1936, lists 143 items in his bibliography.) Bell's name is perpetuated in Bell's Law, that the anterior spinal roots are motor; the posterior, sensory (*New Anatomy of the Brain*, London, 1811); Bell's nerve, the exterior respiratory nerve (1821); Bell's palsy (1821), of the facial nerve; and Bell's phenomenon (1823), the changed ocular rotation in facial palsy; and the observation that the trigeminal nerve was both motor and sensory. Atlases, wax models, and " artificial anatomies," like those of Auzouz in Paris and Chovet in Philadelphia, were being replaced by actual dissections, the material for which, however, was still hard to procure. The indiscreet and unfortunate Robert KNOX (1791–1862), Professor of Anatomy at Edinburgh, is better remembered today for his involuntary and innocent connection with "burking" (murder to procure bodies for dissection) than for his really valuable services in teaching the newer type of anatomy. The very number of students attracted to his courses made it the more difficult to provide sufficient anatomical material. At a time when body-snatching and grave-robbing (the "Resurrectionists" and the "Sack-em-up Men") were practically necessitated by the lack of laws to provide dissecting material, Knox bought bodies for dissection from two rascals, Burke and Hare. When they were eventually convicted of murdering a number of unfortunates in order to sell their bodies, Knox's medical career was finished, even though it was admitted that he knew nothing of the crimes that were committed. Similar events occurred elsewhere (see the *History of the London Burkers*, London, 1832), but the practice soon ceased when the sale of bodies for dissection was legalized by Warburton's Anatomy Act of 1832. It was not long before similar acts began to operate in all enlightened countries. The shortlived English anatomist Henry GRAY (1825–61) is known to every English-speaking medical student through his *Anatomy* (1858), which has now reached its twenty-third edition. His promise as an investigator is shown by his prize-winning essays on the optic nerves (1849) and on the spleen (1854), the latter of which contained important facts about its function that lay buried for seventy years.

A leader in AMERICAN anatomy was Caspar WISTAR (1760–1818), Professor of Anatomy at Pennsylvania, highly reputed teacher, and writer of the first American textbook on the subject. W. E. HORNER (1793–1853), a later incumbent of the same chair, is recalled as the discoverer of the tensor tarsi muscles; he also observed that the "rice water" stools of cholera owe their appearance to the masses of desquamated epithelium. It is perhaps noteworthy that this chair, in the 174 years of its existence, has had but eight occupants — Shippen, Wistar, Dorsey (one year), Physick, Horner, Leidy, Piersol, E. R. Clark. Of these undoubtedly the ablest, and the leading anatomist of his time in this country, was Joseph LEIDY (1823–91). Uncanny in his knowledge of comparative osteology, Leidy was also an expert on fossils, worms, and parasites, and was the discoverer of trichina in pork (1846), and the hookworm in cats in the United States (1886). He studied cancer in subcutaneous transplants, independently observed amœboid motion of leucocytes, and was the first to describe parasitic amœbæ. A valuable contributor also to botany, zoology, geology, and mineralogy, he is entitled to high rank among the descriptive naturalists.

In GERMANY, the impulse given to the study of anatomy by the Meckels in the previous century was continued, especially by Jacob HENLE (1809–85), whose broad interests and powerful intellect greatly aided in making Germany a leader in nineteenth-century medical science. He discovered the renal tubules that bear his name (1862), the endothelium and smooth muscle of the blood vessels (1840), and described the structure and development of the larynx, and the relations of various cerebral lobes. One of the first to appreciate the importance of the cell theory, he described and evaluated the different kinds of epithelium in the body and made many important contributions to comparative anatomy and to pathology. His *Allgemeine Anatomie* (1841) already included many microscopic details, used as a basis for knowledge of function, though his *Handbuch der rationellen Pathologie* (1846–53) shows but little influence of the newer trends. On the other hand, his 1840 essay *On Miasms and Contagions* (translated by Rosen and recently reprinted by Sigerist's Institute) is the best pre-Pasteurian statement of the micro-organismal causes of infectious disease. His *Handbuch der systematischen Anatomie* (3 vols., 1866–71) is the best work of its kind that had appeared up to that time. One of the world's leaders in descriptive anatomy was Josef HYRTL (1811–94), of Vienna, whose textbook of human anatomy (1846) was the German equivalent of Gray's, passing through twenty-two editions. His *Handbuch der topographischen Anatomie* (1847), equally the standard for regional anatomy, and his dissecting manual (1860) indicate his bent toward teaching by established methods, in which he was unexcelled, though he also made many contributions to anatomical progress and to the history of his specialty.

One of the most illustrious FRENCH anatomists of the period was Baron Antoine PORTAL (1742–1832), who taught at the Collège de France for sixty-four years, and for fifty-five years at the Jardin du Roi. In 1803 he published a *Cours d'anatomie médicale* in five volumes. Hippolyte CLOQUET (1787–1840) prepared for the Paris Faculty a popular *Traité d'anatomie descriptive* (2 vols., 1816), which was followed by a more celebrated atlas, *Planches d'anatomie descriptive*, republished in several countries. In Russia, Leopold Wenceslas GRUBER (1814–90) founded the anatomical museum at St. Petersburg, where he was Professor of Anatomy. He was a prolific writer, especially on teratology.

Among the ITALIAN anatomists of the first half of the century, pupils of Morgagni and Mascagni, first of all should be mentioned Bartolomeo PANIZZA (1785–1867), Professor of Anatomy at Pavia.

Panizza was the author of a number of studies on the eye (1821), on the lymphatic system of reptiles (1833), venous absorption (1842), and the parotid gland (1843). He enlarged the anatomical museum of Pavia, and founded and directed for twenty-five years the *Gazzetta medica lombarda*. His most important work was on the lymphatics and on the ninth cranial nerve, and the localization of the cortical centre of vision in the occipital lobes. As Grassi observes, this entitles him to be included among the founders of the doctrine of cerebral localization. He was the first to establish in Italy a course on microscopic anatomy.

Luigi ROLANDO (1773–1831) was especially concerned with the structure of the spinal cord (Turin, 1824) and of the brain in man and animals (Sassari, 1809). His name has been given to the fissure of Rolando in the brain and to the gelatinous substances over the posterior horns of the spinal cords, as well as to several other structural units, such as the *tuber cinereum*. Alfonso CORTI (1821–76), who spent many years at Vienna and Würzburg and wrote mostly in French and German, returned to Turin in 1853. His studies on the ear (*Récherches sur l'organ de l'ouie des mammifères*) have recently been reprinted with a full biography by B. Pincherle (Coll. " Valsalva," 1932). He also made important studies on the structure of the retina and on the organ of the internal ear that bears his name (1851).

One of the earliest Italian histologists was Filippo PACINI (1812–83), who in 1835, when still a student, discovered the sensory corpuscles that bear his name. He published studies on the retina (1844) and on the electric organs of fish; in 1854 he described the " cholerigenic vibrios " and the intestinal lesions that they produced.

Mauro RUSCONI (1776–1849), an eminent embryologist and comparative anatomist, published important studies on the anatomy and embryology of fish and reptiles, and on toxins produced by micro-organisms; he was without doubt the best-known Italian scientist of his time. Giambattista AMICI (1786–1863), naturalist, astronomer, and mathematician, aided medical science with his improvements of the achromatic lens (1827) and the invention of the immersion objective (1850). To anatomy he contributed the " bands of Amici " in the muscle fibres; he demonstrated the production of toxins by parasites and made observations on the oidium of grapes.

Following the establishment of the cell doctrine, microscopic anatomy advanced with astonishing rapidity. At Breslau, the Czech, Johannes Evangelista Purkinje (1787–1869), who had won the admiration and aid of Goethe with his thesis on vision (1819), established the first official physiological laboratory (1842). He utilized the microscope to good advantage in exploring the structure of the skin, bones, blood vessels, seminal vesicles, teeth, and so on ("Purkinje cells" in the cerebellum, 1837; "Purkinje fibres" in the heart, 1839). He was the first (1839) to use the term "protoplasm" for embryologic material (applied by von Mohl to cell cyto-

plasm in 1846), and by 1837 had recognized the similar cellular structure of animals and plants. Technically, he was the first to prepare sections with a microtome instead of free hand with the razor, and to make glass slide preparations with balsam. An able pharmacologist and physiologist, he preceded Bárány in producing artificial nystagmus, and recognized the importance of fingerprints (1823) long before Galton. His eminence in all these fields is still to be appreciated. His best work was finished before he moved to Prague in 1850, though, like Ludwig, he continued to advance biology through guidance of his many productive pu-

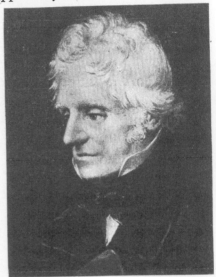

335. Giambattista Amici.

pils. Other histologists who contributed to Germany's leading position in this field were Robert Remak (1815–65), among whose many original observations were the discovery of the non-medullated nerve fibres (1838), "Remak's ganglia" in the heart (1848), and the epithelial nature of carcinoma (1852); and the Swiss, Albrecht von Kölliker (1817–1907), Henle's prosector at Zurich and professor for half a century at Würzburg. Kölliker was a pioneer in applying the cell doctrine to embryology, recognizing the segmentation of the ovum, the development of spermatozoa in the testis, and their role in fertilization. He isolated the smooth muscle fibre, and showed the connection of the medullated nerve fibre to the nerve cell, an important step in the development of the neurone theory. In C. S. Minot's phrase, he "knew more by direct personal observation of the microscopic structure of animals than anyone else who has ever lived." The next great step in knowledge of microscopic structure came with the development of special selective stains in the latter half of the century.

3. Physiology

The first half of the nineteenth century was a decisive period for physiology, when it definitely passed from the domain of metaphysical speculation to that of a natural science based on physics and chemistry. Galvani's discovery that a muscle could be made to contract by an electric current,

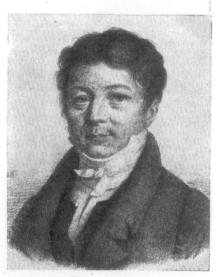

336. *François Magendie.*

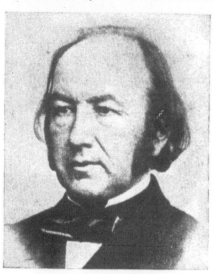

337. *Claude Bernard.*

and Volta's analysis of this current, formed the basis for the whole study of animal electricity that now forms such an important part of neurophysiology.

In the experimental field, the French physiologists led the way. Among their precursors an honourable position must be given to Stefano GALLINI (1756–1836), of the University of Padua. His books on the physics of the human body (1802 and 1818) emphasized the need for basing physiology and pathology on physical laws. But the greatest credit for having established the need for an experimental basis for physiologic as of all other biologic research is due to François MAGENDIE (1783–1855), of Bordeaux. Already in 1809 he published an energetic polemic against vitalism, insisting that one could not speak of a single vital force, but that different organs possessed different functions that could be explained only on the basis of experimental observations. Throughout his life Magendie refused to place any credence in statements that had not been confirmed by experiment.

An investigator of all sorts of isolated phenomena and always ready to experiment in any field of science, he called himself a " rag-picker " who would gather up anything that he found in his path. He was a fervent apostle of animal experimentation. Anyone who studies the work of this destructive critic and revolutionist in physiological method must recognize that he sometimes went too far in setting down without critical analysis experimental results that could not withstand a strict objective examination. However, his work on cardiac function, on digestion, on the importance of the blood in disease, his study of typhus by the intravenous injection of virulent material, his injections of egg albumin into the veins of rabbits, and his pharmacological studies on the localization of the site of drug action (which gave a scientific basis for the introduction into practice of such drugs as strychnine, morphine, and veratrine) constitute his imperishable claims to the gratitude of science. He was the first to show adequately that section of the anterior roots of the spinal cord affected motility but not sensation, and vice versa as to the posterior roots. Thus he completed the work of Bell, who had merely observed that the posterior roots could be cut " without convulsing the muscles " while a mere touch of the anterior roots caused convulsions. The so-called Bell-Magendie law was confirmed by Foderà and Bellingeri, and in 1831 by Johannes Müller. In Magendie's words: " I had under my eye the posterior roots of the lumbar and sacral nerves, and raising them successively with the blades of small scissors, I could cut each, the cord remaining intact. . . . I first thought that the limb corresponding to the cut nerves would be entirely paralysed; it was insensible to pricks and to stronger pressure. It seemed to me to be immobile; but soon, to my surprise, I saw that it moved distinctly although sensation was entirely absent. The second and third experiments gave me exactly the same result; I began to regard it as probable that the posterior roots of the spinal nerve could have different functions from the anterior roots, and that they were especially concerned with sensation."

A prominent pupil of Magendie, J. J. C. LEGALLOIS (1770–1814), showed that bilateral section of the vagus led to broncho-pneumonia (1812), and he was the first to localize the respiratory centre in the medulla (1812). Like Borelli, he believed in the nervous origin of the heart-beat. J. M. P. FLOURENS (1794–1867), Professor of Comparative Anatomy at Paris, was the author of *Recherches expérimentales sur les propriétés et les fonctions du système nerveux* (1824). He was the first to consider the cerebral hemispheres as organs of sensation and of the will, and in a series of able experiments showed that the cerebellum controlled the co-ordination of movements. In 1837 his experiments led him to affirm the existence of a " vital node," the respiratory centre in the medulla; he also gave an excellent picture of the localization of reflexes and of the importance of the spinal cord for movement and sensation. His *History of the Discovery of the Circulation of the Blood* (1857) and his *Essay on Longevity* (1855) are still frequently consulted.

François Achille LONGET (1811–71) published a classical text on *L'Anatomie et la physiologie du système nerveux*, which added to the existing knowledge on the subject his own studies on the functions of the spinal cord and on the inner-vation of the larynx. He was also the author of the first great *Traité de physio-logie* (1850-2). His experimental and clinico-pathological studies (1841) car-ried the Bell-Magendie concept one step further in demonstrating that motor impulses were transmitted in the white matter of the anterior portion of the cord, the sensory stimuli in that of the posterior portion. Another important member of this group of French physiologists was J. L. M. POISEUILLE (1799–1869), who made important contributions to knowledge of the circulation and of the blood pressure and viscosity. He was the first to introduce the mercury manometer for the measurement of blood pressure, and in 1828 constructed a hemodynamometer which Karl Ludwig later improved, as the kymograph, by connecting a movable float with a point that recorded on moving smoked paper (1847). Poiseuille also invented a viscosimeter, and made such progress in the study of the velocity of the blood that he was able to construct mathematical equations that gave quantitative expression to the factors influencing velocity (Poiseuille's Law). An able German pioneer in quantitative studies of the circu-lation was Karl von VIERORDT (1818–84), the most celebrated professor of the University of Tübingen. Patient, modest, industrious, able, and brilliant, he studied human blood pressure twenty-five years before Marey, in 1852, made the first accurate erythrocyte counts, reported the first sphygmograph (published in 1855), and in 1858 invented a hemotachometer, to record the velocity of the blood.

The greatest of French physiologists was Claude BERNARD (1813–78), of Villefranche. This man of genius, who first studied pharmacy, took up literature and play-writing, and then became the favourite pupil of Ma-gendie, can properly be called one of the greatest figures in the history of physiology. Logical and thorough in his system of study, admirable in the rectitude of his scientific thought, marvellous in the clarity of his exposition, he differed from Magendie in not limiting his doctrines and beliefs entirely to the results of his own experiments, as well as in the greatness of his dis-coveries. His well-known aphorism that on entering the laboratory one should divest oneself of the imagination as one does an overcoat included the thought that one should put on the overcoat again on emerging from the laboratory. Few indeed are, like Claude Bernard, sufficiently equipped with both great constructive imagination and experimental ability; the possessor of either, therefore, should be specially cherished by science. Scientists today are becoming more aware of this century's trend to over-emphasize the importance of facts to the discredit of speculative theory; both are necessary in their proper sphere. Claude Bernard was a firm sup-porter of determinism as the fundamental basis of physiological research.

His achievements, which touched almost every branch of physiology, were of permanent value in many fields.

A number of volumes, published between 1854 and 1878, presented his lectures at the Collège de France, where he succeeded Magendie. The *Comptes rendus* of the Académie des Sciences and other bodies include many reports of his studies. Best known of his discoveries was that of the glycogenic function of the liver, which is based on the observation that one finds sugar-issuing from the liver of a dog whether fed on meat or sugar (1848–50). By 1857 the theory of the glycogenic function of the liver was well established; glycogen had been isolated and was known to be consumed by muscular activity. These studies, which gave rise to the concept of animal glycogen and of its metabolic relation to diabetes mellitus, place Bernard as an important pioneer in endocrinology. No less important were his studies on the vasomotor nerves. He observed the results of cutting the sympathetics (1851–2) and realized the importance of the vasomotor nerves for secretion. In the physiology of the digestive tract, by the use of the experimental pancreatic fistula, he discovered the importance of the pancreatic juice for digestion (1849–56), which until that time had been regarded largely as a gastric affair. He showed that the pancreatic juice split the fats of the diet, changed starch into sugar, and broke down proteins further than they had been by the gastric juice. In the domain of pharmacology and toxicology he made important studies on curare and on carbon monoxide and other poisons. Probably the greatest of his biological concepts was his last published work, his doctrine of the constancy of vital phenomena independently of external factors: the " internal environment " or *milieu intérieur* (*Leçons sur les phénomènes de la vie*, Paris, Baillière, 1878, 2 vols.). Relatively neglected for many years, until the recognition of the interrelationship of the glands of internal secretion and of the equilibria of many body processes (Cannon's " homeostasis "), Bernard's concept is now accepted as one of the very basic principles in animal physiology, and has already exerted great influence on modern study.

An incomparable master of his subject, he was entirely worthy of the high recognition that he received from his government and of the universal veneration and enthusiastic admiration that were brought to him from scientists throughout the world. In his admirable book *Introduction à l'étude de la médecine expérimentale* (1865), which should be read by all medical students, he presents his entire program of intellectual and laboratory activity. " One must break the bonds of philosophic and scientific systems as one would break the chains of scientific slavery. Systems tend to enslave the human spirit."

Another member of the classic school of French physiologists was Étienne Jules MAREY (1830–1904), who contributed especially to the knowledge of the circulation through his invention of a practical sphygmograph (1860). Though he was preceded in this field by Vierordt, through the technical efficiency of his instrument it became possible for the first time to make accurate objective studies of the rhythm and form of the pulse waves. Also belonging to the French school was Charles Edward BROWN-SÉQUARD (1818–94), who was born in Mauritius, studied at Paris, taught several years at Harvard, and became the successor at Paris of Claude Bernard on the death of the latter in 1878. This gifted and far-sighted scientist may be regarded as also one of the founders of endocrinology and especially of modern organotherapy (excision of the adrenal glands, 1856–8; use of testicular and other organ extracts, 1889–91). He also recognized the increased reflex response below the level of a resected spinal cord, and observed vasomotor and other sympathetic effects following the application of heat to the cerebral cortex.

In Germany, Schelling's effort to solve the fundamental problems of the natural sciences by philosophical reasoning was followed by pregnant observations and experimental studies of the greatest importance. One of the greatest masters of physiology of the nineteenth century, ranking with Claude Bernard and Karl Ludwig, was Johannes MÜLLER (1801–58), born at Coblenz, whose versatility in many fields of natural history is reminiscent of the great figures of the Renaissance. His remarkable activity as a student and observer, as an able investigator and incomparable stimulator of younger men, has left imperishable traces in the history of human physiology. As Garrison remarks, through his influence on such pupils as Schwann, Henle, Kölliker, Virchow, Dú Bois-Reymond, Helmholtz, and Brücke " we may trace the main currents of modern German medicine."

His *Handbuch der Physiologie des Menschen* (Coblenz, 1833–40) is especially valuable in outlining the road to systematic experimental study and contains many fundamental observations and conclusions on comparative anatomy and pathology, as well as on physiology. An able zoologist, a zealous investigator of the smallest details of the life of inferior organisms, Müller passed by natural transition from his early studies to the subject of human physiology. Through his own endeavours and the work of his pupils, he made many valuable discoveries, of which only the most important can be mentioned here: his explanation of colour sensation on the retina (1826), the law of eccentric projection of sensation from the peripheral sense organs and other nerve terminals (1833), his experiments on phonation and the vocal cords (1835–57), his law of specific nerve energy (1840), which states that every sensory organ responds to the stimulus with its particular sensation (set forth in his *Handbuch*). We have already mentioned the important part that he played in establishing the doctrine of the cell theory and his great book on tumours, of which unfortunately only the first volume was published. As Du Bois-Reymond correctly states in his classic biography, Johannes Müller had all the characteristics of a great reformer and pioneer. His literary activity seems today inexplicable in view of the enormous amount of work and teaching that he also accomplished. Author of a large textbook, he was also for many years the active director of Meckels' *Archiv für Anatomie und Physiologie*, which, popularly known as *Müller's Archiv*, was

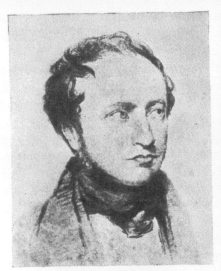 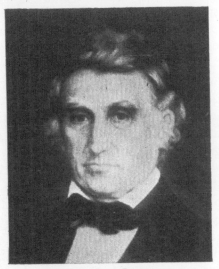

338. *Johannes Müller.*

339. *William Beaumont.*
(*From a photograph at the* COLLEGE OF PHYSICIANS, PHILADELPHIA.)

long the leading journal of its kind. Physiologist, experimental investigator, strict but just critic, he never forgot the need for philosophic speculation, and for a logical co-ordination of the different scientific disciplines. His aphorism: "No one can be a psychologist without being a physiologist" is a good example of this trend of thought.

Among the illustrious scientists who carried on the scientific inheritance of this master were the three brothers WEBER — Ernst Heinrich, Eduard Friedrich, Wilhelm — two of whom were anatomists and physiologists and the other a physicist. Their studies were particularly directed to the application of physics and mathematics to physiology, especially in the mechanics of motion. Most important was the discovery by the first two of the inhibitory action of the vagus nerve (1845), which not only helped understanding of the heart action, but also opened up a new field of neurophysiology. The way toward knowledge of reflex action had been prepared by Descartes's study of eye-blinking, by observations on decapitated cold-blooded animals (Bayle, J. Bohn, Hales), and by the discovery of the motor and sensory nerve roots. This knowledge was further developed by Marshall HALL (1790–1857), of Nottingham and London, in his two communications to the Royal Society: *The Reflex Function of the Medulla Oblongata and Medulla Spinalis* (1833), and *The True Spinal Marrow Excitatory System of Nerves* (1837). Though Hall wrongly assumed a special set of " excito-motor " nerve fibres, he showed the central position of the spinal cord itself in reflex action (which function, like strychnine convulsions, was abolished when the cord was destroyed).

Two notable contributions to the physiology of digestion were made by Americans in this period. John Richardson YOUNG (1782–1804), in his graduating thesis from the University of Pennsylvania (*An Experimental Inquiry into Principles of Nutrition and the Digestive Processes*, 1803), demonstrated that gastric digestion was due to the solvent action of the gastric juice, rather than to trituration, as was generally held at that time, and that its effect was owing in part to its acid nature. The discovery that the acidity of gastric juice is due to hydrochloric acid (1824) was made by William PROUT (1785–1850), an observation shortly after confirmed by Friedrich TIEDEMANN (1781–1861) and Leopold GMELIN (1788–1853). The other important American contribution was made by William BEAUMONT (1785–1853), a United States Army surgeon from Connecticut, who in 1822 fortunately had to treat a certain Alexis St. Martin for a gunshot wound of the stomach. When this healed with a permanent fistula, Beaumont made good use of the opportunity to study the appearance and function of the exposed living stomach over a number of years. He was able to demonstrate the characteristics of gastric motility and the intermittent quality of its secretion; and confirmed the presence in the stomach of hydrochloric acid and of another active substance (which in 1846 was shown by Schwann, in an article in Müller's *Archiv*, to be the enzyme pepsin). Beaumont's *Experiments and Observations on Gastric Juice and the Physiology of Digestion* (Plattsburg, 1833) is one of the landmarks of American medical literature and a prominent milestone on the road to Pavlov's experiments almost a century later.

Modern PHYSIOLOGICAL CHEMISTRY practically began about this time. One of its founders and one of the most illustrious chemists of the century was Justus von LIEBIG (1803–73), Professor of Chemistry at Giessen and later at Munich.

Liebig made a searching study of organic chemistry in its relation to the normal and pathological physiology of the animal organism. Continuing the approach of John DALTON (1766–1844) and of J. B. J. D. BOUSSINGAULT (1802–

87), he carefully examined all matter taken into and excreted from the body, and discovered the excretion of urea, a substance of the highest importance in animal life. In his laboratory (the first of its kind to be established in connection with university teaching, 1826), he investigated numerous organic compounds, discovered hippuric acid and other uric-acid compounds, chloral, and chloroform. "Liebig's extract" is still in use today. His *Annalen* (1832–74) was a leading chemical journal of the time, while his book *Die organische Chemie* (1840) was the first adequate statement on the subject. The most important step in establishing the new organic chemistry was the artificial production of urea (1828) by Friedrich Wöhler (1800–82), thus proving that organic substances could be made synthetically, whereas up to that time it had been thought that they could be created only by living tissue. Other chemists rapidly contributed to the new field. The scientific basis of nutrition was established by Max von Pettenkofer (1818–1901) and Karl Voit (1831–1908), who, with the aid of special apparatus capable of enclosing a large animal, and even man, observed the utilization of food substances (metabolism) during activity and repose and measured oxygen-consumption and heat-production (calorimetry). Pettenkofer was a great believer in the importance of the soil, both in public health and in the spread of specific diseases. His belief that typhoid fever was spread in this way once led him to drink a brew of typhoid bacilli to demonstrate the

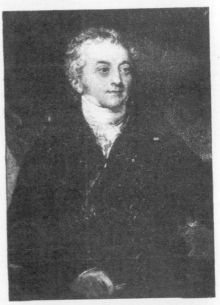

340. *Thomas Young. Engraved from a portrait by Sir Thomas Lawrence.*

falsity of the bacterial theory of the cause of that disease. Fortunately for him, no fever developed, but the bacterial cause of typhoid fever thereby became the harder to establish in Germany. He brought about much-needed improvements in sewage disposal, which at that time was often discharged untreated into streams or the open sea. The English chemist Frankland advanced the study of nutrition with his calculations of the caloric values of the important food substances; and Georg Meissner (1829–1901), a student of Müller's, elucidated the formation of urea and uric acid. Notable progress in the chemistry of the blood was made by one of the masters of modern physiological chemistry, E. F. Hoppe-Seyler (1825–95), especially on the spectroscopy of hemoglobin, the isolation of hemoglobin crystals, and other blood pigments, of which he obtained the chemical formulas in some cases. He was the founder of the *Zeit-*

schrift für physiologische Chemie and author of one of the best texts on physiological chemistry (1877–81).

An event of the greatest importance for physiological chemistry was the distinction made between colloids and crystalloids (1861) by Thomas GRAHAM (1805–69), of Glasgow, and Professor of Chemistry at London University (1837). From his study of the colloidal state (that is, particles in a degree of dispersion larger than the typical molecule or ion but smaller than those of a mechanical suspension) has grown a special discipline, colloid chemistry, which is of especial value in biology, as all living tissues, proteins, fats, carbohydrates, and many other substances, either exist or may occur in this form. Graham followed the classic Greeks in the concept of atoms and in the importance he attributed to motion; to him, for instance, diversity in motion was the only basis for diversity of material. He evolved laws governing the diffusion of gases, and those of osmosis (after Dutrochet) and studied the dialysis of solutions through semi-permeable membranes. A true modern, he paved the way for Willard Gibbs, van't Hoff, Arrhenius, Hamburger, and the numerous exponents of physical chemistry of the present century.

The physics of physiology was greatly advanced by the work of Hermann Ludwig von HELMHOLTZ (1821–94), who introduced the graphic method of studying musculature contractions, and measured the speed of the propagation of the impulse in the motor nerves of frogs — an achievement that Johannes Müller only a few years before had declared to be impossible. Helmholtz was the inventor of the ophthalmoscope (1851), an instrument of the greatest importance for the development of ophthalmology. He wrote a masterly treatise on physiological optics, which supported Young's theory of colour vision, and found the explanation of the changes in the curvature of the lens. Most important of all of his contributions to general science was his monograph *Über die Erhaltung der Kraft* (1847), which gave the general application of the law of the conservation of energy, previously stated by Robert Mayer. This established the first law of thermodynamics: that all kinds of energy can be transformed from one form to another but cannot be destroyed or created. (The second law of thermodynamics, elaborated independently by Clausius and Lord Kelvin, 1850–2, established that energy has a constant tendency to move in the direction of dissipation rather than of concentration.) The macula lutea in the eye, which had been discovered by Mariotte in the seventeenth century, was first shown by Helmholtz to be insensitive to light. In acoustics, he announced the doctrines of tonal sensations as a physiological basis of the theory of music.

While Italy had good physiologists in this period, it is not surprising that the difficult political situation of the time, agitated by wars and revolutions, greatly handicapped their activity. We note Bartolomeo PANIZZA (1785–1867), of Pavia; Filippo LUSSANA (1820–97), who studied the physiology of the brain and was the author of an important textbook; Carlo MATTEUCCI (1811–68), of Forlí, pupil of Müller's and, according to Grassi, the intellectual leader of Du Bois-Reymond.

Following the path in galvanometry of Leopoldo NOBILI (1784–1834), and of Stefano MARIANINI (1790–1866), Matteucci described the phenomenon more generally known as " the current of Du Bois-Reymond." He discovered that if an electrode was placed on the cut section of a frog's muscle and another on the external surface, the galvanometer indicated the presence of an electrical current. In 1841 he showed that the nerve from a frog's muscle in contact with the muscle of another frog caused the contraction of the latter when the nerve was stimulated. Thus he was the first to prove beyond doubt that muscular activity is accompanied by electrical changes. Salvatore TOMMASI (1813–88), author of an important book on electrophysiology (1844), was one of the best-known Italian physiologists of the period. Francesco SELMI (1817–81), professor at Bologna, is remembered for his discovery of ptomaines, which he named.

Two foreign physiologists, one from Germany and one from Holland, contributed notably to Italian physiology. Moritz SCHIFF (1823–96), of Frankfurt, forced to leave Germany after the Revolution of 1848, became the first Professor of Comparative Anatomy at Bern till 1863, when he accepted the chair of physiology at Florence (1863–76). After 1876 he taught at the University of Geneva. His studies of the physiology of the nervous system, with recognition of the vagus as the controlling nerve of the heart; his observations on the functions of the cerebrum and the cerebellum and on the mechanism of peristalsis; and his prolific contributions to physiological literature have been posthumously collected in four volumes (Lausanne, 1894–6). Of greatest significance today is his pioneer work in endocrinology, especially his experimental excision of the thyroid with the prevention of deleterious effects by the use of thyroid grafts or the administration of thyroid extracts. The Dutchman Jakob MOLESCHOTT (1822–93) in 1856 became Professor of Physiology in Zurich, in 1861 at Turin, and in 1879 at Rome. His works were published at Giessen (1857–85) in thirteen volumes. Moleschott was an enthusiastic supporter of Darwin and enthusiastically maintained the superiority of materialism over dogmatism.

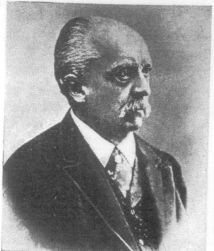

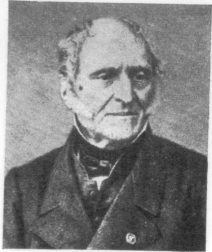

341. *Hermann Ludwig von Helmholtz.*   342. *Jean Baptiste Cruveilhier.*

4. Pathology

In the nineteenth century pathology was based more completely than at any other time on pathologic anatomy. It was during this period that the solid foundation of the new medicine was laid by the discoveries in pathologic anatomy, when the great clinicians no less than the professional pathologists trained themselves thoroughly in this discipline. In France, the anatomist Bichat and the clinician Laënnec were thoroughly aware of the importance of pathology in the science of medicine and each wrote far-sightedly on that subject. J. B. CRUVEILHIER (1791–1874), the first occupant of the newly established chair at the University of Paris (1836), was the leader of French pathology and the first to give an adequate description of disseminated sclerosis and of progressive muscular atrophy. His great atlas, *Anatomie pathologique,* in two folio volumes (Paris, 1829–42), represents the greatest height ever reached in the illustration of gross pathology. His system of general pathology, however, was marred by his belief that " phlebitis dominates all pathology," which sometimes led him far from the narrow path of objective observation. Gabriel ANDRAL (1797–1876), Professor of General Pathology at Paris, was a pioneer in emphasizing the chemical study of the blood in disease. His *Essais d'hématologie pathologique* (1843) was one of the first to be written on this subject. Prominent among the clinicians who made careful studies in pathology was the surgeon Guillaume DUPUYTREN (1777–1835), who left a legacy of 200,000

francs to found the chair of pathological anatomy, first occupied by Cruveilhier. Among physicians, P. C. A. Louis (1787–1872) was noteworthy
for his clinico-pathological studies on tuberculosis and on typhoid fever,
and particularly for his introduction of the statistical method as a means
for the scientific clinical investigation of disease. Another clinician, Pierre
Bretonneau (1778–1862), in 1826 wrote an important monograph on
Diphthérite (his own term), which definitely established this clinical entity
and proved its identity with croup and malignant angina, a matter that
had remained obscure since the days of Aretæus. He also, under the term

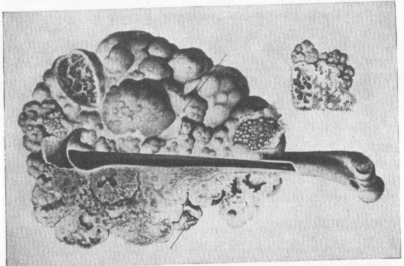

343. *Osteochondroma.*   (*From Cruveilhier's* Anatomie pathologique.)

" dothienentérite," described the intestinal lesions of the condition gradually becoming recognized as typhoid fever. The highly important pathological observations of Corvisart and Laënnec will be considered later under
clinical medicine. One more French achievement in pathology remains
to be noted. In 1819, at the suggestion of Cuvier, the first independent
chair of pathological anatomy was established, at the then French University of Strasbourg, for J. F. Lobstein (1777–1835). Lobstein's *Traité
d'anatomie pathologique* (Paris, 1829), unfortunately never completed, is
interesting both for its historical review of pathology from the time of the
Pharaohs, and for the advance that it records over Gaub's text, which had
dominated instruction in the previous half-century. The book was conceived in the spirit that " it is not the dead organ that medicine wishes to
understand, but the living organ, exercising the functions peculiar to it."
It had the threefold merit of clear pathologic description, comprehension of
the pathogenesis of disease (a term coined by Lobstein), and correlation of

morbid anatomy with symptoms, and it also emphasized the need for animal experimentation.

Among contemporary Italian pathologists were the Bolognese Floriano CALDANI (1776–1836); Eusebio VALLI (1762–1816), a precursor of Pasteur in the field of vaccination, who died from yellow fever contracted at Havana in the course of his investigations; M. V. MALACARNE (1744–1816), of Pavia and Padua; G. B. PALETTA (1747–1832); F. L. FANZAGO (1764–

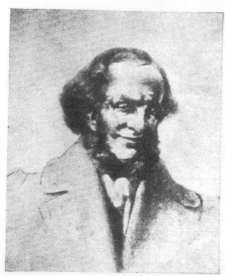

344. *Agostino Bassi.*

1836). Francesco Enrico ACERBI (1785–1827) was a precursor of modern bacteriology, who in his *Dottrina teorico-pratica del morbo petecchiale* (1822) maintained that the cause of contagious disease was a specific organized substance capable of maintaining existence and of reproduction according to the common laws of living beings.

Great credit for opening new paths in micropathology is due to Agostino BASSI (1773–1857), of Lodi, who was the first to show that the silkworm disease, *mal del segno* or *calcino* (muscardine) was caused by a micro-organism. The work of this distinguished man places him among the important pioneers of bacteriology. His studies on the silkworm disease, lasting from 1807 to 1835, established that it was produced by a " living vegetable cryptogamous parasite," and led to his generalization that many diseases of plants, animals, and man are caused by animal or vegetable parasites. He found that *Botrytis paradoxa* was the cause of the disease and recommended various physical and chemical methods of destroying it. He also recognized the importance of the relationship of the number of infective organisms to the incidence of infection, a principle later put forth by Flügge. In 1846 he wrote the following significant lines: " While many if not almost all scientists believed and still believe that contagious materials are of a special kind, they are actually living substances — that is to say, animal or vegetable parasites." This decisive statement, based on countless observations and long years of microscopic study, anticipated by ten years Pasteur's discovery of the micro-organismal causes of disease, as Martinotti (1894) and Grassi have observed. It was a clear vision of a great truth which was amplified and further illuminated by the discoveries that were to follow. His complete works were published in 1925 by the Medico-Chirurgical Society of Pavia. According to Schönlein's statement, it was Bassi's discovery that led him to search for the microscopic cause of favus — the *achorion Schönleinii* (1839). Henle also grasped the importance of Bassi's discovery and doubtless passed on the idea to his pupil Robert Koch.

Luigi PORTA (1800–75) was not only an illustrious surgeon but also a notable figure in surgical pathology. He created the Anatomico-surgical Museum of Pavia, and published more than fifty monographs, including an extensive study on the pathological changes in the arteries after ligature or compression (1845). This work included some six hundred experiments over a period of nine years. He also made important contributions to the study of the thyroid gland (1849) and of sebaceous tumours (1856). Atto TIGRI (1813–75), who came near demonstrating the presence of bacteria in tuberculosis (1850), later confirmed the discovery by his friend Pacini of the cholera vibrio in the intestine, recognizing its comma-like shape. In 1863 Tigri saw the typhoid bacillus in the blood of typhoid patients and he is credited with being the first to describe the reticular tissue in the spleen (1849), calling it *trama microscopica*. The Sicilian Michele FODERÀ (1792–1848), a pupil of Magendie, became a member of the Institut de France at the early age of thirty. Grassi credits him with the discovery in 1822 of the law of absorption (osmosis), which was later clearly demonstrated by Dutrochet.

Pathology in the British Isles was marked in this period especially in the delineation of new disease entities by the able correlation, mostly by clinicians, of clinical signs and symptoms with the gross findings at autopsy. One has but to recall the imperishable achievements of Bright, Hodgkin, and Addison, of Graves, Corrigan, and Stokes, to realize the heights reached by the masterly application of this method. The more usual type of pathological study is represented in England by such studies as those of Joseph HODGSON (1788–1869), *On the Diseases of Arteries and Veins* (1815). This book not only gave the best illustrations of aneurysms of various kinds that had thus far been published, but also contains excellent illustrations of aortic valvular endocarditis (one fungating and perforated, one chronic) and what is said to be the first description of aneurysmal dilatation of the aortic arch. The work so impressed the French, to whom it owed little, that they often spoke of aortic aneurysm as the *maladie d'Hodgson*. Gross pathological illustration was worthily represented. James HOPE (1801–41), a surgeon of St. George's Hospital, London, in 1834 published his *Principles and Illustrations of Morbid Anatomy*, which in spite of the rather crude illustrations went through several editions and was translated into German and Russian. His popular *Treatise on Diseases of the Heart and Great Vessels* (1831) is important for its comments (Preface) on Laënnec and its many original observations (especially the signs of aortic, mitral, and pulmonary stenosis and of aortic regurgitation). He did much to establish the new discoveries of the French school in conservative England and to co-ordinate the new knowledge of heart disease. The *Illustrations of the Elementary Forms of Disease* (1838) of Sir Robert CARSWELL (1793–1857) stands midway in technical and textual excellence between Hope's and Cruveilhier's productions.

In the latter part of this period the Viennese school assumed the leadership of the world's pathology. Karl ROKITANSKY (1804–78) became Professor of Pathological Anatomy at Vienna in 1844, remaining in that capacity until four years before his death. This man of genius, one of the greatest of all gross descriptive pathologists, was able to base his lifelong study of disease on an enormous amount of material; suffice it to recall that in 1866 he had already performed not less than thirty thousand autopsies. Rokitansky was one of the chief founders of the new Vienna school, which appears to have derived more from Morgagni than from the French school, and was recognized by Wunderlich as early as 1841 as the initiator of German leadership in world medicine. Like Morgagni, Rokitansky reported his pathological observations with admirable clarity. The following quotation from his final lecture will indicate his attitude toward the subject: " Pathological anatomy has been presented by me to my students as the essential basis of pathological physiology and the elementary doctrine for medical research. On pathological anatomy clinical knowledge is founded, developed, and perfected. It has been further developed by pathological histology, has shown the way to chemical pathology, and has called experimental pathology into being."

Rokitansky's scientific publications constitute a monumental edifice; their value is very great from the historical point of view, even though later studies negated some of his doctrines. They are models of medical writing for clarity of demonstration and reasoning power. Most important is his *Handbuch der pathologischen Anatomie* (1842–6), which far surpassed any previous texts on the subject. Among his special contributions may be noted his studies on goitre (1849), diseases of the arteries (1852), abnormalities of the heart (1875), the spondylolisthetic pelvis (1839), acute yellow atrophy (which he named) (1843), perforating gastric ulcer, lardaceous disease, and so on. He was a master at the autopsy table and worked out a method of performing autopsies which still is used in slightly modified form. A profound observer and recognized authority, he was so great-minded that he willingly acknowledged the validity of the young Virchow's criticisms of his unfortunate theory of " krasis," which disease concept disappeared from the later editions of his manual (1855–61). Rokitansky must be credited with having permanently established the line of pathological thought begun by Benivieni, Bonetus, and Morgagni, so that diseases were thereafter considered not merely as groups of symptoms or other fancied

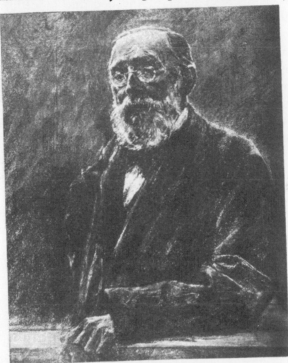

345. *Rudolf Virchow.*

changes, but from the solid point of view of the accurately observed and correlated structural changes found at autopsy. To him more than to anyone else is due the reputation of the new Viennese school, which drew pupils from all parts of Europe.

Rudolf Ludwig Karl VIRCHOW (1821–1902) is not only one of the most representative figures in the history of the medicine of the nineteenth century, but also one of the greatest pathologists of all time. Pupil of Johannes Müller, he taught pathology at Berlin until 1849, when, on account of his freedom in political utterances, he was forced to leave Berlin and accept a call to Würzburg as Professor of Pathology. There, during seven valuable years before his recall to Berlin, he laid the basis for his epoch-making book on cellular pathology. In 1856 he returned to Berlin as Director of the Pathological Institute of the Charité Hospital, where he accomplished and supervised an enormous amount of work in the performance of autopsies, in the collection of some twenty-three thousand specimens for the museum, and in the prosecution of pioneer investigations in microscopic pathology. He was the founder of the doctrine of cellular pathology, which not only removed the limitations imposed by the study of gross material only, but replaced the ancient structure of humoral pathology which had dominated medicine for more than twenty centuries and had found a belated champion in Rokitansky with his theory of krasis. According to Virchow's theory, which is based on his phrase: *Omnis cellula e cellula*, the seat of disease should always be sought in the cell, and the morphologic products and morbid phenomena of disease are nothing but the manifestation of the reaction of cells to the causes of disease. It is an essentially solidistic pathology. As explained by him (1895): " The essence of disease, according to my idea, is a modified part of the organism or rather a modified cell or aggregation of cells (whether of tissue or of organs). . . . Actually every diseased part of the body holds a parasitic relation to the rest of the healthy body to which it belongs, and it lives at the expense of the organism."

This concept has had to be considerably modified, as we shall see later, by more recent studies in experimental pathology, immunology, and endocrinology, which have brought back into the picture a modified humoral concept. It is no less true, however, that Virchow's revolutionary contributions should be regarded as among the most significant in the history of medicine. The pathologist-historian W. H. Welch believed that " the establishment by Virchow of the principles of cellular pathology marked the greatest advance which scientific medicine has made since its beginning." The career of Virchow, an ardent democrat and fiery adversary of Bismarck in the Reichstag and in the press, coincided with those of the radical reformers who brought about the fall of the reactionary governments in Germany, Italy, and France, just as Paracelsus' career coincided with that of the reformer Luther.

The doctrine of cellular pathology announced by Virchow in his epoch-making book, *Die Cellular-pathologie in ihrer Begründung auf physiologische und pathologische Gewebelehre* (1858), was based on the cellular theory of living structure and the observation that the microscopic appearance of living cells was profoundly changed in disease. If one admits that normal life comes from the normal functioning of the body cells, it is evident that changes in form and therefore in function should give rise to disease. Virchow maintained that pathology should abandon all hypotheses founded on metaphysical constructions, diatheses, and dyscrasias and should be based exclusively on the positive investigation of visible changes. " The cell doctrine," he wrote, " applied to all living structures, leads to a cellular physiology and a cellular pathology, which is always based on histology — that is, on the anatomic knowledge of the structural elements." Virchow's book outlined a new and important orientation for scientific medicine, although, of course, he was not able to solve all the problems of pathology or always to arrive at accurate generalizations. Virchow demonstrated that cells were reproduced by division of nucleus and cytoplasm rather than from Schleiden's unorganized cytoblast. This proliferation of cells by division, first observed by Mauro Rusconi in 1826, had been clearly understood by Goodsir, to whom Virchow gives proper credit, and by M. Barry, who as early as 1840 stated: " reproduction of cells by . . . division of the nucleus of the parent cell is universal " (*Philosophical Transactions*, 1841, p. 207). Virchow's doctrine of cellular pathology added to almost every field of pathology and especially to that of inflammation. Already in 1824 Dutrochet had clearly described the passage of the white corpuscles through the vessel wall, and in 1843 William Addison had advanced his theory of the identity of pus cells with the white corpuscles of the blood — observations which were not firmly established until Cohnheim's classic experiments on the frog's cornea and mesentery (1867–73). A long and acrid discussion between the adherents of the cellular and humoral theories of inflammation followed, the former aided by Metchnikoff's discovery of phagocytosis, and the latter by the recognition of the various antibodies active in the process of immunity. Eventually, however, the truth was reached in a compromise between the two theories, in which both are recognized as playing their important roles in this fundamental pathological process. Knowledge of the microscopic appearance of various malignant tumours, begun by Johannes Müller in the thirties, was of course greatly advanced by the application of the principles of cellular pathology. Virchow however, wrongly held that cancer cells developed in unorganized mucoid substance from a pluripotential connective-tissue corpuscle, an error that was later rectified by Remak and Waldeyer. Virchow undoubtedly went too far also in his tendency to ascribe all disease processes to cells. He never recognized life in intercellular substances. He stated that fibrin was not to be regarded as an excretion from the blood but as a local product resulting from local cell activity; yet he recognized that " amyloid " (his own term) was an infiltration of an organ from without. He brought to medicine many new pathological concepts that are still in use. At the same time as Hughes Bennett, he gave the first description of leukemia (*Weisses Blut*, 1845); he established the true nature of thrombosis and embolism; defined cloudy swelling, fatty degeneration, and amyloid change, agenesia, heterotopia, ochronosis, and many other pathological concepts. It is wrong to criticize him for not having recognized the importance of pathological physiology, as is shown by the title of the famous journal founded by him in 1847, *Archiv für pathologische Anatomie und Physiologie und für klinische Medizin*. Its first volume speaks of pathological physiology as the "very citadel of scientific medicine, of which pathological anatomy and the clinic are only outworks." In regard to his emphasis on the cell, no one today would regard the cell as the ultimate unit of vital activity, yet it still remains the all-important structure from which concepts and studies of normal and diseased form and function must proceed. This is not the place, however, to give further details of his essentially localistic doctrine, of the opposition that it encountered, of the modifications that this opposition required, and of the commanding position that it has now held for many decades.

5. Clinical Medicine

Pathology and clinical medicine, by separating themselves from metaphysical concepts and doctrinal systems, at this time entered a period of investigative progress that created a new world in symptomatology, diagnosis, and the understanding of the nature of disease. The great French and English schools maintained the Hippocratic trend in clinical medicine. The Germanic schools turned toward a more analytical method that led to a purely materialistic concept of vital phenomena, to scepticism in treatment, and to the construction of a new dogmatism. [It is but fair to add that therapeutic scepticism had its deserved place at a time when the true knowledge of the nature of disease was still in its childhood; and, as has subsequently been shown, drugs were usually given uselessly or even harmfully. It is pleasant to observe that with a better knowledge of the nature of the disease and of the action of drugs, clinical investigation is now turning more and more toward therapeutic problems. "Therapeutic nihilism," which should be considered more correctly as often an unwillingness to indulge in an unreasonable use of drugs, has now been replaced by a rational drug therapy. *Ed.*]

The history of clinical medicine in the early part of the nineteenth century centres in FRANCE, which under Napoleon had dominated almost all Europe politically, and, according to a general tendency that has already been noted, therefore progressed scientifically at the same time as its social and economic order prospered. One can hardly find a better example in history of the development in a single country of many great scientific figures at the same time as great men developed in politics, warfare, and other fields of human activity. It is in the France of this period especially that the change from the theoretic systems of the eighteenth century to modern clinical concepts can be observed.

An extraordinarily interesting figure, vigorous, authoritative, conservatively obstinate, and faithful to the ancient scholastic traditions, was that of F. J. V. BROUSSAIS (1772–1838), of Saint-Malo, pupil of Bichat, surgeon of the armies of France, physician-in-chief at Val-de-Grâce, and from 1831 Professor of General Pathology at Paris. According to Broussais, vital phenomena depended on external stimuli, especially heat, and produced chemical changes which in turn modified the normal functioning of the tissues. When these stimuli were moderate, the body remained healthy;

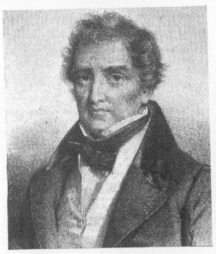 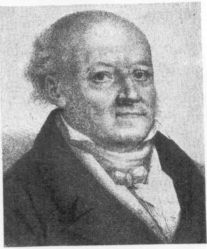

346. *François Joseph Victor Broussais.*

347. *Baron Corvisart, Napoleon's physician.*

when they were too weak or too strong, disease ensued. All diseases were local and were transmitted from one organ to another by sympathy or by means of the gastro-intestinal mucosa. All excessive stimuli produced hyperæmia and thus inflammation. The basis of all pathology was gastro-enteritis. Broussais called his doctrine "physiological medicine," in order to emphasize that disorders of function were more important than structural changes. His best-known works are *L'Histoire des phlegmasies ou inflammations chroniques* (1808) and *L'Examen des doctrines médicales* (1816).

In therapeutics Broussais believed that the physician should dominate nature and not merely try to assist it, as the Hippocratists maintained. He thought an antiphlogistic or debilitating treatment was necessary for almost all diseases. His favourite remedy was the application of leeches to the stomach or to the head with the aim of preventing or curing gastro-enteritis. An idea of the number of leeches used by Broussais, who was the most sanguinary physician in history, is afforded by his custom of ordering hundreds of leeches daily and by the enormous number of these animals that were imported into France in the early days of the century, when his system had its greatest vogue.

The last of the great blood-letters was J. B. BOUILLAUD (1796–1881), who called Broussais the "Messiah of medicine." However, he was an able and skilful physician who played an important part in establishing the connection between rheumatic fever and heart disease; he also recognized the value of digitalis às "the opium of the heart" (1835). He was the first to localize the speech centre in the middle of the left cerebral hemisphere (*Traité . . . de*

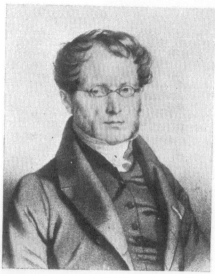

l'encéphalite, Paris, 1825). Like Broussais he was an enthusiastic phrenologist. The leader and first master of the brilliant school that brought medical primacy to France was J. N. CORVISART (1755–1821), among whose pupils were Bretonneau, Dupuytren, and Laënnec. He was Napoleon's chief physician and one of the most celebrated physicians of his time in all Europe. Acquainted with Auenbrugger's discovery of percussion as early as 1760, he resurrected this forgotten method and published it in a French translation, *Nouvelle Méthode pour reconnaître les maladies internales de la poitrine* (1808). His lectures, often improvised at the Collège de France or in the Anatomical Hall, were celebrated for their elegance of form and

348. *P. C. A. Louis.*

exactness of logical thought. He was chiefly concerned with diseases of the heart, and his book on the subject, *Essai sur les maladies et les lésions organiques du cœur et des gros vaisseaux* (Paris, 1806), is one of the classic texts of cardiac literature and the best on the subject since the time of Senac.

The intensive study of tuberculosis was initiated by the Provençal Gaspard Laurent BAYLE (1774–1816), whose *Recherches sur la phthisie pulmonaire* (1810) recognized six kinds of consumption, of which the commonest would be correctly designated as tuberculosis today. He successfully correlated tuberculosis of the lung with the same disease in other organs, and obviously recognized tuberculous meningitis (Obs. 8), a discovery often attributed to Papavoine (1830).

The greatest of the French clinicians of the period was René Théophile Hyacinthe LAËNNEC (1781–1826), of whom Thomas Addison said: "Laënnec contributed more toward the advancement of the medical art than any other single individual." His discovery of the stethoscope and its use in auscultation, together with Auenbrugger's rediscovered percussion, permitted the development of physical diagnosis far beyond anything previously attempted, an advance that was not greatly amplified until the days of the X-ray and the various instruments of diagnostic precision. The story of Laënnec's discovery of mediate auscultation, and his use first of cylinders of paper and later of hollow wooden tubes, copying the game

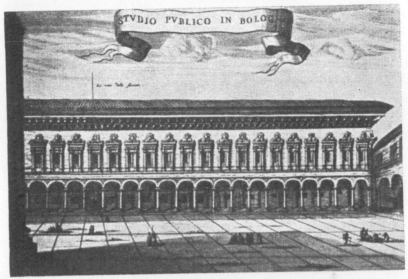

349. *The University of Bologna in the eighteenth century.*

played by urchins of listening to the sound of taps on hollow logs, should be read by all who are interested in the history of medicine. Thoroughly aware of the importance of pathologic anatomy for clinical medicine, as early as 1803 he began a course on the subject that aroused the fierce opposition of his friend and co-pupil Dupuytren. A keen observer and endowed with great intelligence and a remarkable critical spirit, this one man practically created the physical diagnosis of cardiac and pulmonary diseases, giving excellent descriptions of phthisis, bronchiectasis, pneumothorax, cancer of the lung, emphysema, and so on. His description of pneumonia was so excellent that Osler frequently recommended it to his students for study. By the irony of fate his name in medical terminology is attached, not to any of these great achievements, but to a short account in a description of chronic pleurisy (Observation XXXV, 1826 edition) of the hobnail liver, which had been recognized more or less clearly since the days of Hippocrates. On account of its yellowish colour, he proposed the name

" cirrhosis " (*kirrhos*, yellow). His immortal work *De l'auscultation mé-diate* . . . (Paris, 1819) was published only two years after his discovery of the stethoscope. The second enlarged edition (*Traité des maladies des poumons et du cœur*, 1826) gives the pathology, diagnosis, and treatment of each disease encountered, as well as the physical signs elicited, as in the first edition. We quote his classic description of the vesicular murmur and of crepitant rales: " Pulmonary respiration. On applying the cylinder . . . to the breast of a healthy person, we hear, during inspiration and expiration, a slight but distinct murmur, answering to the entrance of the air into, and its expulsion from, the air cells of the lungs. This murmur may be com-pared to that produced by a pair of bellows whose valve makes no noise, or, still better, to that emitted by a person in a deep and placid sleep, who makes now and then a profound inspiration. The moist crepitous rattle has evidently its site in the substance of the lungs. It resembles the sound produced by the crepitation of salts in a vessel exposed to a gentle heat, or that produced by blowing into a dried bladder, or it is still more like that emitted by the healthy lungs when distended by air and compressed in the hand — only stronger. Besides the sound of crepitation, a sensation of humidity in the part is clearly conveyed. . . . It is the pathognomonic sign of the first stage of peripneumony, disappearing on the supervention of hepatization and reappearing with the resolution of the inflammation " (Forbes's translation).

Henceforth bronchial breathing, vesicular respiration (Andral's term), cavernous respiration, pectoriloquy, egophony, crepitant, mucous, bubbling, and sonorous rales, metallic tinkle, became expressions that were as necessary a part of the physician's terminology as the subdivi-sions of the variations of the pulse had been earlier, and infinitely more useful.

One of France's greatest clinicians was P. C. A. LOUIS (1787–1872), who devoted many years to clinical study, especially of tuberculosis and typhoid fever. His introduction of the statistical method into clinical medi-cine, by which he was able *inter alia* to demolish Broussais's system, was of prime importance to the progress of medicine. A master of objective observation, he agreed with Broussais that " the truth is in the facts and not in my opinion that estimates them." In the wards and autopsy rooms of the three great Paris hospitals he made accurate observations on the nature of phthisis (1825), based on 358 autopsies and 1,960 clinical cases. A similar analysis of typhoid fever definitely established this disease entity, though it remained for his students to differentiate it from typhus. Among the other eminent French clinicians of the period were Baron Antoine

PORTAL (1742–1832), A. F. CHOMEL, and P. A. PIORRY (1794–1879), the inventor of the pleximeter and author of a very popular textbook.

Close at the heels of this eminent French school, and reflecting their influence, followed a group of noted ENGLISH clinicians, whose achievements were characteristic of the essentially clinical British school of thought. Again we note a connection with a flourishing period of English history,

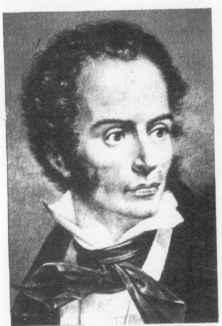

350. *René Théophile Hyacinthe Laënnec.*

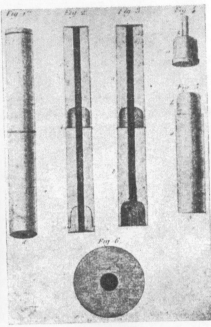

351. *Laënnec's stethoscope.*
(*From* De l'auscultation médiate,
Paris, 1819.)

the Victorian era, when a time of great economic and literary prosperity followed a victorious peace. First among these great English clinicians was Richard BRIGHT (1789–1858), one of the " Great Men of Guy's " for more than thirty years, and the describer of the chronic disorders of the kidney still known under the name of " Bright's disease." Under the modest title of *Reports of Medical Cases* (1827), Bright included his description of nephritis and the differentiation of renal from cardiac dropsy in a book that is one of the most important in the history of medicine.

As physician, teacher, and man, Bright can be regarded as the prototype of the great English physician of his time. Botanist, geologist, naturalist of the first order, lover of artistic engravings and himself no mean artist, a tireless traveller, always on the search for new sensations, a penetrating observer of the customs and monuments of the countries he visited, and a brilliant writer, Bright exhibited throughout his life an exemplary modesty and simplicity. His success as a clinician and medical investigator did nothing to spoil his tranquil, serene existence. In regard to his great discovery, albumin in the urine had already been observed by Dekkers, Cotugno, and others; hardened kidneys had been as-

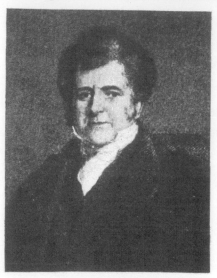

352. *Richard Bright.*

sociated with dropsy by Saliceto; Morgagni had described clinical and post-mortem findings in kidney disease. But it remained for Bright so to correlate his clinical observations in the wards set apart for the purpose, with the various changes found at autopsy, that " Bright's disease " permanently entered the category of diseased states. The subdivisions of the various forms of chronic, non-suppurative renal disease are still matters of debate, and of course much knowledge has been gained in the century that has passed about their various points of difference; the term " Bright's disease," however, still remains useful and necessary for the clinician today. Bright's reports also contain valuable observations on many clinical conditions, such as diabetes, acute yellow atrophy. Jacksonian epilepsy, status lymphaticus, laryngeal tuberculosis, and other original observations frequently credited to others.

A colleague of Bright's at Guy's Hospital was Thomas ADDISON (1793–1860), whose name is permanently connected with pernicious anæmia and chronic disease of the adrenal glands. In his introduction to *The Constitutional and Local Effects of Disease of the Suprarenal Capsules* (1849) he gives a brief description of a severe " idiopathic " form of anæmia, which under the name "pernicious anæmia" has long been recognized as the most important primary disease of the blood. It was often known as "Addisonian anæmia," a more correct term than "Biermer's," whose description was made twenty years later. The disease of the adrenal glands described in this monograph, and now known as "Addison's disease," is a clinical syndrome resulting from any one of several lesions of these bodies. By an accident not unique in the history of medicine, Addison was not widely acclaimed during his lifetime, and even among his admirers the importance of his two great discoveries remained unrecognized.

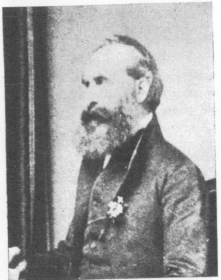

353. *Thomas Hodgkin.*

Thomas HODGKIN (1798–1866), pathologist to Guy's Hospital, in 1832 published his original description of the enlargement of the lymph nodes and other lymphatic tissues which was called "Hodgkin's disease" by Wilks in 1865. Though Hodgkin included instances in his series of reported cases that were of a different nature, the majority were truly examples of the disease that bears his name, as may be seen in the specimens still preserved in Guy's Hospital museum. Without the aid of the microscope some confusion of diagnosis was inevitable, but this does not detract from the clinico-pathological skill that made his discovery possible. Knowledge of "rheumatism" was promoted by John HAYGARTH's (1740–1827) clear description of the acute disease and the chronic forms indicated by nodosity of the joints, in the first part of his *Clinical History of Diseases* (1805). The recognition of the connection of acute rheumatism with one of the most important forms of heart disease is chiefly due to English acumen. The mere association of the two conditions, to be sure, had been observed by Morgagni, also by Ferriar of Manchester, but had been regarded as accidental. In 1789 Jenner reported to the "Fleece" or Gloucestershire Medical Society his clinico-pathological observations on a disease of the heart following acute rheumatism. Baillie in the second edition (1797) of his *Morbid Anatomy* (end of Ch. 2) connected rheumatism with "morbid growths" of the heart and noted that "Dr. Pitcairn has observed this in several cases," according to Wells, "about the year 1788." In 1810 William Charles WELLS (born in Charleston, South Carolina, 1757; died, London, 1817) gave a clear account, twenty-five years before Bouillaud, of cases of rheumatic fever that developed cardiac disease (palpitation and, at autopsy, cardiac hypertrophy). He also recognized rheumatic nodules on the tendons. In another field, James PARKINSON (1755–1824) rests securely in medical history for his *Essay on the Shaking Palsy* (1817), the classic description of paralysis agitans ("Parkinson's disease"). A reformer and political agitator, geologist and palæontologist, he also gave an important early account of appendicitis (1812). Thomas WATSON (1792–1882) was the leading clinician of his day and the author of one of the most widely read books in English on clinical medicine (1843). It was justly popular through the English-speaking world for more than three decades — a long life for a medical textbook — on account of its clarity of exposition and lucidity of style.

Important contributions made by English physicians to the study of tropical disease, especially in the service of the East India Company, should be noted here. Patrick RUSSELL (1727–1805) wrote a well-known book on the poison of snakes, especially of vipers; and Joseph FAYRER (1824–1907) was the author of other important works presenting his long and patient investigations on the poisonous animals of India. The studies of J. MACPHERSON on cholera, of E. HARE on dysentery, and of I. G. MALCOLMSON on beriberi are but a few of the valuable British contributions to knowledge of tropical medicine during this period.

With the gradual dimming of the brilliancy of the Edinburgh school of clinical medicine, there arose in IRELAND in the early part of the century a remarkable group of clinicians — Graves, Stokes, Cheyne, Corrigan, Adams, Colles (of "Colles's law" fame), Wallace — known as the Irish or Dublin school. Never before or since has this locality attained such medical eminence, drawing students from many parts of the world. Though preceded chronologically by Cheyne, the real leaders were Graves and Stokes.

Robert James GRAVES (1796–1853), after receiving his degree in 1818 and visiting various European centres, became physician to the Meath Hospital and a founder of the Park Street School of Medicine, where he introduced the best type of clinical teaching. Though not the first describer of the type of goitrous disease that bears his name, he was the first to give a full picture of it, recognizing the rapid heart, protruding eyes, and nervousness, as well as the enlarged thyroid. His other great achievement was a reversal of the universal custom of always starving fever patients. Stokes's biography of Graves tells of his request, while visiting a hospital convalescent ward, that his epitaph should be: "He fed fevers." His colleague at the Meath Hospital, William STOKES (1804–78), son of a Dublin Regius Professor of Medicine, was a pioneer in the new methods of clinical diagnosis. His warrants of immortality are his descriptions of the peculiar type of breathing known as Cheyne-Stokes respiration, and of the combination of slow pulse and cerebral attacks known as Adams-Stokes syndrome, both first described, less adequately to be sure, by the other member of the team. Though he had the antiquated attitude toward fever — that it was a disease *per se*, with accidental lesions in individual cases (1874) — he was a leader in the new study of cardiac and pulmonary diseases. His *Treatise on . . . Diseases of the Chest* (Dublin, 1837) and his *Diseases of the Heart and Aorta* (Dublin, 1854) are both works of great historical value. John CHEYNE (1777–1836), the oldest of the group, was a Scotsman who in 1811 joined the staff of the Meath Hospital, later to retire to England. His description of Cheyne-Stokes respiration occurs in the second volume of the Dublin Hospital *Reports* (1818). He is not to be confused with the earlier George CHEYNE (1671–1743), who wrote on the gout (1720), from which he himself suffered, and on the "English malady" (1733), later known as neurasthenia. Robert ADAMS (1791–1875), though famous for his original account of cerebral attacks with permanently slow pulse, now known to be due to heart block (Dublin Hospital *Reports*, 1827, IV, 396) and earlier recognized by Morgagni and others, was widely known as an able physician, who also wrote an excellent account of rheumatic gout (1857). Sir Dominic CORRIGAN (1802–80) is remembered today in connection with aortic regurgitation, though his masterly description (Edinburg M. & S. *Journal*, 1832) was preceded by those of Cowper, Vieussens, and Hodgson. "Corrigan's pulse" in this condition is well known to medical students.

AMERICAN medicine of the period had able physicians whose care of patients compared favourably with that found in the world's centres, though the habit of contributing to progress by research and the opportunity for doing so were not conspicuous. Exceptions to this generalization of course existed. In 1803 J. C. OTTO (1774–1844), of Philadelphia, definitely established the clinical entity hemophilia, though occasional references to "bleeders" can be found here and there for centuries earlier. Otto traced a family of "bleeders" through several generations and recognized "that males only are subject . . . and although the females are exempt, they are still capable of transmitting it to their male children." The name "hemophilia" was given by Schönlein (1828); discovery of the delayed blood-coagulation time in hemophilia is credited to J. H. WRIGHT

(1894). Prominent in the early half of the century was the Virginian, Philadelphian by adoption, John Kearsley MITCHELL (1798–1858), an excellent practitioner, teacher, and writer. His *Cryptogamous Origin of Malarious and Epidemic Fevers* (1849) was an important contribution to the parasitic concept of infectious diseases. In New England, Nathan SMITH (1762–1829), who had practised several years under the pioneer conditions of New Hampshire before taking his M.B. at Harvard as the sole member of the class of 1790, established a medical department at Dartmouth in 1798, himself teaching anatomy, surgery, chemistry, and medicine for several years. He was " concerned in bringing forward " three other schools, Yale, Bowdoin, and Vermont. From 1813 till his death he taught medicine, surgery, and obstetrics at Yale, as the most distinguished member of its first faculty; he lectured at the University of Vermont, where he helped establish the medical school in 1822; and taught medicine at Bowdoin (1821–6). In 1825 he helped McClellan start the Jefferson Medical College; but after moving to New Haven in 1813, his main activities were centred at Yale. He was one of the first ovariotomists (1821), made an important study of necrosis that is a classic for the surgeon (1827), and published a masterly essay on typhus fever (1824), of which Welch said: " Never before had the symptoms [of typhoid fever] been so clearly and accurately pictured." His decided stand for the specificity of the various infectious diseases had an important influence on the understanding of fevers at a critical time. Elisha NORTH (1771–1843), of Connecticut, was a strong American advocate of vaccination for smallpox (1800); he published the first book on epidemic meningitis (" spotted fever," 1811) and established the first American eye dispensary (1817). James JACKSON (1777–1868) was a co-founder, with J. C. Warren, of the Massachusetts General Hospital and its first physician. It was there that he introduced the first clinical teaching in Boston. His *Course of Lectures* (1827) is one of the earliest American texts on the subject. He is credited with being the first to describe alcoholic neuritis (" *arthrodynia a potu*," 1822) and was an important factor in establishing in this country understanding of the nature of typhoid fever (1838), and in reorganizing the Harvard Medical School and the Massachusetts Medical Society. His *Letters to a Young Physician* (1855) and his *Memoir of James Jackson, Jr.* (1835), are among the best of American essays in medical literature.

The Dublin school had a marked effect on American medicine; but even more important was that of Pierre C. A. Louis, whose American pupils assumed leading positions along the Atlantic seaboard. One of the most promising was the above mentioned James JACKSON, Jr. (1810–34), who even in his short career completed a valuable essay on cholera and recognized a prolonged expiratory sound as diagnostic of early phthisis.

Best known of Louis's American pupils was the Philadelphian W. W. GERHARD (1809–72), who is properly credited with the definite differentiation of typhus and typhoid fevers (*American Journal of the Medical Sciences*, 1836 and 1837). Of Gerhard's other writings the most important were his study of tuberculous meningitis in children (1833–4) — ac-

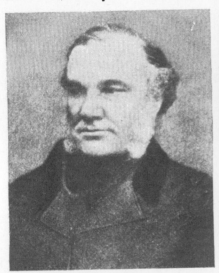

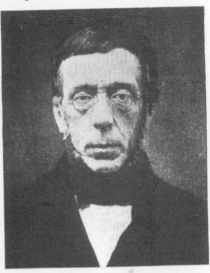

354. *Thomas Addison.* 355. *William Wood Gerhard.*

cording to Osler, its first accurate clinical study — and his book on *Diseases of the Chest* (1842). The intestinal lesions of typhoid had already been recognized (Huxham, Pringle, Bretonneau), and Louis had written an excellent description of the disease entity (1829), which apparently was commoner than typhus in France at the time. In Great Britain and America typhus was common (see Nathan Smith's excellent account of the Philadelphia epidemic of 1812–13); but the two diseases were generally regarded as one until Gerhard's study of the typhus epidemic of 1836. His clear differentiation of the two, on lines of the best clinico-pathological tradition, was the first breach in the wall of the mysterious continued fevers. Other pupils of Louis, George Cheyne SHATTUCK (1813–93), of Boston, and William POWER (1813–52), of Baltimore, like Laënnec an early victim of consumption, Caspar Wistar PENNOCK (1799–1867) and Alfred STILLÉ (1813–1900), of Philadelphia, contributed to this problem — one of the most important of its day. While Henry Ingersoll BOWDITCH (1808–92) followed his master in the study of pulmonary tuberculosis, he insisted on the importance of low, damp climates in its causation and was the first, before Dieulafoy, to tap pleural effusions with a pump (invented by Eyman) trocar, and cannula (*American Journal of the Medical Sciences*, 1852 and 1863). Jacob BIGELOW (1787–1879), of Watertown, Massachusetts, a great medical botanist, in 1835 wrote *An Essay on Self-limited Diseases*,

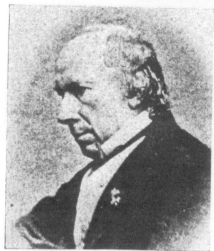

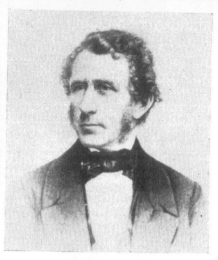

356. *William Stokes.*   357. *Daniel Drake.*

which, in O. W. Holmes's opinion, did more than any other publication in English to rescue medicine " from the slavery of the drugging system."

In the development of the medicine of the Middle West, the outstanding figure was that of Daniel DRAKE (1785–1852). Taken as a child from New Jersey to Kentucky, Drake was apprenticed to William Goforth, from whom he received the first diploma to be granted west of the Alleghenies. He was the peregrinating professor par excellence, serving at Transylvania, Cincinnati, back at Lexington, at Jefferson, back at Cincinnati again, Louisville, back again to Cincinnati, at Louisville, and finally at Cincinnati again, founding medical schools as he passed. His greatest achievement was his remarkable book on the *Diseases of the Interior Valley of North America* (2 vols., 1850–4), a veritable encyclopædia of the whole biology of the Mississippi Valley in its relation to the various diseases encountered there. His *Practical Essays on Medical Education and the Medical Profession in the United States* (1832), a *rarissima* of American medical literature, is a beautifully written presentation of medical ethics and duties, as well as a description of medical education and needed reforms.

Toward the middle of the century, after the glorious periods of the French and English schools, VIENNA became the centre of clinical medicine in Europe. Josef SKODA (1805–81), born at Pilsen, was the greatest clinician in the new Vienna school. He was the first to teach there in German (1847). His *Abhandlung über Perkussion und Auskultation* (Vienna, 1839) forms the scientific basis of modern physical diagnosis. A man of genius in the rapidity and acuity of his observations and in the rigour of his criticism, he was the first in the Germanic countries to apply Laënnec's discoveries, teaching that observable physical phenomena are of the greatest importance in the diagnosis of disease. Skoda's treatise is the first systematic attempt to be based on physical laws in distinguishing different categories by the sounds perceived in the examination of the thorax. His observations were brilliantly confirmed through the following century and still constitute an important part of the treasure of practical medicine.

Skoda's skill as a diagnostician made him one of the best-known physicians of his time. To be sure, his diagnostic skill sometimes led him to make too rapid or too detailed diagnoses which were not always confirmed by the subsequent course of the disease or by the autopsy. Skoda initiated the so-called " therapeutic nihilism " that was characteristic of the Viennese school. Once the diagnosis was established, he regarded his essential task as completed, and often did not concern himself further with the case. Another prominent member of the Vienna school was the Bohemian Johann von OPPOLZER (1808–71) who, after following Schönlein as head of the clinic at Leipzig (from 1850) for a short time, spent most of his career in Vienna. Oppolzer also was an able diagnostician, beloved by his pupils and his patients. He introduced into the Viennese school a middle road between the therapeutic nihilism of Skoda and the polypharmacy that was prevalent at the time, maintaining the necessity of basing treatment on chemico-physiological experience.

In GERMANY the leading figure in clinical medicine was Lucas SCHÖNLEIN (1793–1864), the founder of the so-called natural-history school, as opposed to the fanciful nature-philosophy school of the Bavarian Lorenz OKEN (1779–1851), who however is gratefully remembered as the editor of the journal *Isis* and originator of the German Congress of Nature Investigators and Physicians (1822). Schönlein is better known for his clinical teaching and his general influence on German medicine than for his individual contributions to medical progress. However, he was the first to describe peliosis rheumatica (1837), called " Schönlein's disease " in Germany; he discovered the micro-organismal cause of favus (*achorion Schönleinii*, 1839) and proposed the terms *typhus abdominalis* and *typhus ex-*

anthematicus, which are still used in Germany to differentiate typhoid from typhus fever. Another famous German clinician was Karl August WUNDERLICH (1815–77), Oppolzer's successor at Leipzig. This able student of physiological phenomena and intellectual philosopher not only wrote an excellent short history of medicine (1859), but also contributed an important study on body heat in disease (Leipzig, 1868). As Garrison observes, Wunderlich "found fever a disease and left it a symptom." Clinical thermometry, which had been attempted by Sanctorius in the early seventeenth century, was first established in medicine by Wunderlich, though the mercury thermometer had been invented by Fahrenheit a century earlier (1714). From Wunderlich's time it became a necessary part of the physician's armamentarium and was one of the first instruments of precision to aid medical practice.

Outstanding among the ITALIAN clinicians of the first half of the century was Maurizio BUFALINI (1787–1875), of Florence, one of the hardiest adversaries of the theories of Rasori. While still a student, Bufalini wrote an *Essay of the Doctrine of Life* (1813), in which he maintained that life was such a complex phenomenon that it could be interpreted only by the sum of as many of its manifestations as possible, and that the doctrine of simple dynamism was an absurdity. His *Fondamenti della patologia analitica* (1819) emphasized the importance of factual observations as the basis of medical science. Giovanni SEMMOLA (1793–1865), a pupil of Magendie and head of the Neapolitan school, made important clinical and experimental studies on the blood of cholera patients (Naples, 1837). His most important work was his *Trattato di farmacologia e terapia generale* (Naples, 1854). A leader of Italian clinical medicine was Salvatore TOMMASI (1813–88), of Naples, who was also an able opponent of the Rasori school. Tommasi maintained from the beginning of his teaching (1844) that Morgagni was the lighthouse of the clinic, and experimental pathology its compass. He was a capable and learned physiologist and was the founder of modern clinical medicine in Naples.

6. Surgery

The surgery of the first half of the nineteenth century is characterized by the increasing number of daring major operations, performed with an astonishing rapidity necessitated by lack of anesthetics. The evolution of surgery, as the result of scientific study of the subject, had at last raised it to an equality with the other branches of medicine. The surgeon was regarded as the equal of his medical colleagues by the public and the profession alike, and toward the end of the century acquired the confidence of the public even to a greater degree than that held by his medical colleagues. No longer was the art practised by empiricists and barbers, as in the eighteenth century, but by illustrious physicians who had carefully studied anatomy and pathology before taking up surgery. It no longer sufficed to be a skilful technician; an adequate scientific preparation was necessary. This change was reflected in the character of the teaching: special schools which gave diplomas without requiring preparation in other branches of study still existed in the middle of the century, but were rapidly disappearing, so that by the second half of the century throughout most of the world the right to practise surgery was given only after completion of an adequate course of study.

Two factors of the greatest importance which are discussed later in this section were the introduction of anesthesia by Morton and Long, and the discovery of antisepsis by Lister. As will be seen in the next chapter, these two fundamental aids brought to surgery a rapid and decisive development unequalled in the history of medicine. A further developmental factor was the progress in anatomy and pathology, which explains the supremacy of the French school in the first half of the century. Surgical specialties had not yet broken away from the main stem. Gynæcology, orthopedics, otology, and so on were still practised by the general surgeons.

In FRENCH surgery the most famous operator and ablest diagnostician of his time was the Baron Guillaume DUPUYTREN (1777–1835), who attracted to his clinic at the Hôtel-Dieu pupils from all countries of the world. An eloquent teacher and man of wide culture, he held a high position in the social life of his time. He was one of the stoutest upholders of the importance of pathologic anatomy as a basis for surgery, as is to be seen in his endowment of the Paris chair of pathological anatomy.

An ardent student of anatomy, Dupuytren became a prosector at the age of eighteen, in 1808 was appointed adjunct surgeon to the Hôtel-Dieu, and in 1812 Professor of Operative Surgery. He soon acquired an enormous fortune and was able to put a million francs at the disposition of the exiled Charles X. Among his numerous works, of which the most important was his volume of lectures on surgery (1839), should be mentioned his publications on the surgical treatment of aneurysms, on the ligation of the external iliac and the subclavian arteries. His descriptions of varicose aneurysms, of fracture of the lower end of the fibula (Dupuytren's fracture, 1819) and the characteristic flexion of one or more fingers due to contraction of the palmar fascia (Dupuytren's contraction, 1831, but described earlier by A. P. Cooper) are classic. In spite of his unbounded ambition and his rude treatment of his rivals, he was greatly admired by his colleagues and patients.

J. M. DELPECH (1777–1832), professor at Montpellier, is one of the first orthopedists worthy of the name. He created an orthopedic institute there out of his own resources, and was one of the first to realize the

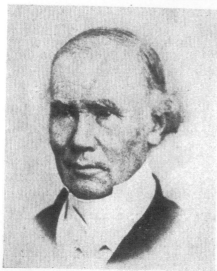

358. *A. A. L. M. Velpeau.*

importance of Pott's disease, recognizing its tuberculous nature. He was the first to practice subcutaneous section of the Achilles tendon. He was murdered by a patient upon whom he had operated for varicocele, who blamed his loss of a rich marriage on the indiscretion of the operator.

J. D. LARREY (1766–1844) was the surgeon-in-chief of Napoleon's Grand Army, adored by the soldiers and held in great esteem by the Emperor, who left him a legacy of a hundred thousand francs, saying that he was the most virtuous man that he had ever known. Larrey took part in all the campaigns of the Republic and the Empire, was wounded three times, and followed Napoleon to Waterloo. It is said that in one day after the battle of Borodino he performed more than two hundred amputations. His books were particularly concerned with military surgery. To him is due the creation of the Flying Ambulance, the precursor of the modern method of treating those wounded in battle.

Among other famous French surgeons was A. A. L. M. VELPEAU (1795–1867), who, though belonging to the old school of empirical surgeons, was an operator of the highest order. His three volumes on operative surgery (1832) were important contributions to this subject; Velpeau's arm bandage for fracture of the clavicle is still taught to medical students. J. F. MALGAIGNE (1806–65) was an expert operator whose manual of operative surgery (1834) went through a number of editions and translations. He was an excellent medical historian, whom many critics regard as the most profound French writer in this field. His edition of Paré's works (1840), containing an ample biography and historical introduction, is especially noteworthy. Auguste NÉLATON (1807–73), physician to Napoleon III, was a celebrated surgeon of the period, especially known for his skill in ovariotomy. He was the first to introduce the flexible rubber catheter that bears his name (1860) and is still the preferred instrument for permanent use. He also invented a porcelain-tipped probe for the lo-

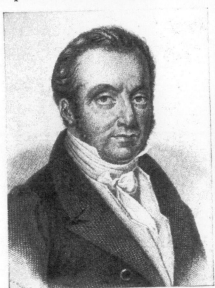

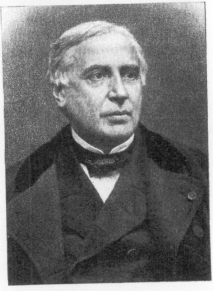

359. *Guillaume Dupuytren.*   360. *Auguste Nélaton.*

cation of lead bullets, which has additional interest as having been first used to sound Garibaldi's wound at Aspromonte.

P. J. ROUX (1780–1854), Dupuytren's successor at the Hôtel-Dieu, was a bold operator in the fields of amputation and staphylorrhaphy (repair of cleft palate) and other plastic operations. Jacques LISFRANC (1790–1847) was celebrated for his operations for amputation of the jaw and of the shoulder and foot at the tarso-metatarsal joint (Lisfranc's amputation). Paul BROCA (1824–80), surgeon at the Necker Hospital, is deservedly regarded as the founder of the modern surgery of the brain. An able anatomist, he was one of the first to attempt surgical intervention in the brain and to diagnose the site of cerebral tumours by the localization of the functional changes found. He established that the centre of articulate speech was in the third convolution of the left frontal lobe (Broca's area). He was one of the greatest French anthropologists, inventing instruments for the determination of the brain and skull ratios (craniometry), standardizing bone measurements, and classifying colours of the hair and skin.

We note also the work of J. Z. AMUSSAT (1796–1856) for his studies on urethral stricture and his attempts to reintroduce into surgery the torsion of arteries recommended many centuries earlier by Lanfranc; of A. J. de LAMBALLE (1799–1867), noted for his plastic operations and intestinal sutures; of J. R. GUÉRIN (1811–86), especially in orthopedic surgery; of L. A. MERCIER (1811–82), for his studies of the hypertrophied prostate.

Leading ITALIAN surgeons of the period were A. VACCÀ-BERLINGHIERI (1772–1826), founder of the Pisan school; T. VANZETTI (1809–88), who

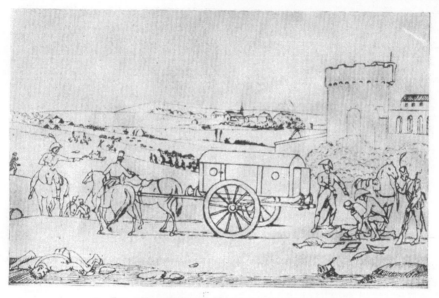

361. *Larrey's ambulance. Sketch by Duplessis-Bertaux.*
(VAL DE GRÂCE MUSEUM.)

performed the first Italian ovariotomy (1848); F. RIZZOLI (1809–80), father of Italian orthopedics; L. APPIA (1818–98), one of the founders of the International Red Cross; P. LANDI (1817–95), and F. PALASCIANO (1815–91), organizer of military surgery and the first to recommend the neutral treatment accorded the sanitary corps in warfare; B. LARGHI DA VERCELLI (1812–77), who made use of nitrate of silver in the treatment of wounds before the days of Lister; and G. SILVESTRI, who in 1862 was using the elastic bandage at Padua before the days of Esmarch. P. M. R. BARONI (1799–1854) was one of the first to practise lithotripsy; L. CINISELLI (1803–78) is credited with being the first to use electric acupuncture in the treatment of aneurysms; L. AMABILE (d. 1892) was one of the first to attempt skin grafts; and T. RIMA (1777–1843); as Giordano has shown, was the first to treat varicosities of the leg with ligation of the saphenous vein, an operation generally credited to Trendelenburg.

ENGLAND played an important role in the development of the surgery of the period under consideration. In the earlier part of the century its chief representative was John BELL (1763–1823), whose studies in surgical pathology had an important influence on the development of English surgery and especially of the surgery of the blood vessels. Bell and his brother, Charles, were excellent artists, making their own illustrations for his books on the *Anatomy of the Human Body*, *Engravings*, and *Principles of Surgery*. An enthusiastic admirer of Italy, where he died, he left a monument of his love for that country in a magnificent book entitled *Observations on Italy* (1825), which for its vivacity of style and extensive knowledge of Italian art thoroughly merits the praise given it by Garrison, who regarded it as one of the best books of travel ever written by a physician. Sir Astley Paston COOPER (1768–1848), pupil of John Hunter, was one of the most skilful and active operators of his time, enjoying an international reputation and being showered with honours by his profession and by his government. An industrious anatomist, operator, and practitioner, he rose at six in the morning, often received patients late into the night, and dictated his writings while making rounds in his carriage. He made a number of anatomical observations which are still remembered in " Cooper's fascia " of the spermatic cord, " Cooper's hernia " (femoral), " Cooper's ligaments " (of the breast, the abdomen, and the shoulder). He successfully ligated the common carotid and the external iliac arteries for aneurysm, and studied the effects of these procedures in experiments on dogs. He was one of the first to amputate at the hip joint (1824). Among Cooper's best-known followers were Benjamin TRAVERS (1783–1858), who wrote an excellent treatise on eye diseases (1820); Charles Aston KEY (1793–1849), who ligated the external iliac for femoral aneurysm (1822), and the subclavian for axillary aneurysm (1823); Sir William FERGUSSON (1808–77), a skilful and successful operator of lightning speed, who, however, emphasized the need for conservative surgery and planned all his operations carefully in advance. He is said to have operated for hare-lip more than four hundred times. Abraham COLLES (1773–1843), professor at Dublin for thirty-two years, is credited with the first ligature of the innominate artery and with several ligations of the subclavian. " Colles's fracture " of the radius was described by him in 1814, and " Colles's law " (that a mother may remain immune from syphilis while bearing a syphilitic child) appeared in his *Practical Observations on the Venereal Disease*

(1837).[1] Robert LISTON (1794–1847), a Scotsman who became Professor of Clinical Surgery at University College, London, was a skilful, rapid operator who suggested a number of new operative procedures and was the first in England to use the newly discovered anesthetic, ether. James SYME (1799–1870), of Edinburgh and London, was especially renowned for his amputations and joint excisions, showing that the latter method was to be preferred when feasible. Lister's father-in-law, he was one of the first to adopt antisepsis (1868) and also anesthesia (1847).

Approaching the inestimable gift of antisepsis to suffering humanity through the imperishable work of Lister, we must realize that though surgical infection had been fought against at various periods of medical history, it never was more rampant than in the early nineteenth century. Hippocrates and Celsus had recommended urine and vinegar for surgical wounds, and the Father of Medicine also recognized the value of cleanliness and of dry dressings. The great thirteenth-century surgeons had used wine to cleanse wounds and even fought the doctrine of laudable pus. In the seventeenth century M. Biondo and his followers, and in the early nineteenth Vanzetti, had practised a rational treatment of wounds and surgical incisions. Lawson Tait and John Ashhurst, post-Listerian " diehards," were to achieve excellent results without antiseptics by the use of simple cleanliness. However, none of the attempts mentioned had any permanent influence on surgical procedure. With the work of Lister, the situation was radically and permanently changed.

Joseph, Lord LISTER (1827–1912), born at Upton in the county of Essex, was one of the greatest figures in the history of surgery. He first applied himself to microscopic anatomy and physiology, studying such problems as the structure of the iris and its action in dilating the pupil, the pathogenesis of inflammation, and the mechanism of intravascular coagulation of the blood. A pupil of Syme, Lister in 1860 became Professor of Surgery at Glasgow. Profoundly impressed by the great mortality that he observed after amputations, often reaching forty-five per cent at that time, and by the prevalence of hospital gangrene, he demanded extreme cleanliness in his wards and made free use of Condey's fluid and other deodorants. He insisted that wounds need not secrete pus; nevertheless, infections and blood poisoning continued with but little change. Encouraged by Pasteur's discoveries, he began to study the possibility of sterilizing the operative field in order to prevent the development of patho-

---

[1] The converse, known as " Profeta's law," that a syphilitic mother may bear and nurse a normal child without giving it syphilis, was announced in 1865 by the Sicilian G. PROFETA (1840–1910).

genic bacteria. He correctly reasoned that by destroying the bacteria that caused suppuration one could obtain the healing of wounds by first intention. After trying various antiseptic solutions, he finally turned to the use of a carbolic-acid spray, in an attempt to sterilize both the operative field and the whole operating-room. This method was used for the first

time on August 12, 1865; his results were first published in the *Lancet* in 1867. They were so strikingly favourable that news of his discovery was rapidly spread throughout the world and his system widely adopted. It is said that it was Pasteur who first suggested the passage of the scalpel through a flame in order to sterilize it, thus beginning the era of *aseptic surgery* for " clean wounds," as opposed to Lister's antisepsis.

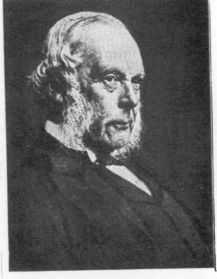

A man of great nobility of thought and character, a simple Quaker in his private life, Lister received the highest honours in England and on the Continent. He was the first physician to sit in

362. *Joseph Lister.*

the House of Lords, and on his death his remains were interred in Westminster Abbey. In 1869 Lister became Syme's successor at Edinburgh; and in 1877 Professor of Surgery at King's College, London. Part of the Glasgow ward in which he carried out his great work has been preserved in the Wellcome Historical Medical Museum in London. Among the publications celebrating his centenary, one of the most interesting is that of the Wellcome Museum (1927), which contains a catalogue of the exhibition organized for the occasion, a series of portraits of Lister and his collaborators, and the apparatus that they used.

It should be noted that Enrico BOTTINI (1835–1903), later professor at Pavia, in 1863 had begun experiments with carbolic acid at the Novara Hospital. His findings on its value as a disinfectant of the operative field were published the year before Lister's publication, in 1866 (*Dell'acido fenico nella chirurgia pratica* . . . in *Ann. Univ. di Med.*, 1866, CXCVIII, 385). Part of this has recently been reprinted by G. P. Arcieri of New York in the new medical history journal *Alcmeone*.

In the GERMAN-SPEAKING COUNTRIES also surgery attained notable successes. The Viennese school of Dummreicher and Schuh, and the Germans, von Gräfe, Dieffenbach, and Langenbeck, became the pioneers of modern surgery. Factors contributing to this development were the better organization of the German clinics and the superior discipline which emphasized recognition of the fundamental principles of modern surgery. In the Vienna school also, development of the various specialties, such as ophthalmology, otolaryngology, and dermatology, was fostered by Rokitansky's emphasis on pathology. Among the most famous German surgeons of the time was Conrad Martin LANGENBECK (1776–1851), Professor of Anatomy and Surgery at Göttingen, who, among other achievements, successfully performed the total extirpation of the uterus. To Karl Ferdinand VON GRÄFE (1787-1840), of Warsaw, and Professor of Surgery at Berlin, is due a number of surgical innovations such as improvements in the technique of blood transfusion, Cæsarean section, rhinoplasty, and repair of cleft palate. Johannes Friedrich DIEFFENBACH (1792–1847), von Gräfe's successor at Berlin, was another of the most important German surgeons of the period; first for his work in plastic surgery, and later in internal operations and orthopedics. M. J. CHELIUS (1794–1876), professor at Heidelberg and author of a well-known surgical textbook, and G. F. L. STROMEYER (1804–76), founder of modern military surgery in Germany and developer of subcutaneous tenotomy, were other well-known figures. Bernhard von LANGENBECK (1810—87), nephew of Conrad and successor of Dieffenbach, is remembered chiefly as the founder of the *Archiv für klinische Chirurgie* (" Langenbeck's *Archiv* ") and of the German Society of Surgery. The leading German surgeon and teacher of his day, he introduced various new operations, such as those for subperiosteal and subsynovial resection. Viktor von BRUNS (1812–83), professor at Tübingen, was another skilful operator and a pioneer in the surgery of the larynx. Gustav SIMON (1824–76) was a gifted practitioner of gynæcology, especially successful in the repair of vesico-vaginal fistula. He was the first to attempt total extirpation of the kidney (1869) and reintroduced the forgotten operation of splenectomy.

Among surgeons of other European countries should be mentioned the Swiss J. P. MAUNOIR (1768–1861), of Geneva, who made important contributions to the surgery of cystic tumours and to ophthalmology (construction of artificial pupil). The eminent Russian surgeon Nikolai PIROGOV (1810–81), was the greatest surgeon of his country, renowned for his knowledge and technical skill. He introduced the operation for the amputation of the foot that bears his name and was responsible for the induction of female nurses into the Russian armies of the Crimean War. The Swede Christian August EGGEBERG (1809–47), surgeon and gynæ-

cologist, the Finn Gustav Samuel CRUSEL (1810–58), a pioneer in the use
of galvano-cautery; the Belgian Antoine MATHIJSEN (1805–78), inventor
of the plaster bandage (1851), were all important figures in the surgery of
the day.

AMERICA produced a number of able surgeons during this period.
First among them was Philip Syng PHYSICK (1768–1805), often called
the Father of American Surgery, who in 1805 at the University of Pennsylvania became the occupant of the
first chair of surgery to be divorced
from the sister subject, anatomy.
Though averse to writing for the medical press, Physick was an able contributor to the advancement of his specialty: he is credited with being the
first to invent a tonsillotome; the first
after Monro *secundus* (1767) to use
the stomach pump; the first to give an
adequate description of rectal diver-
ticula; inventor of an operation for artificial anus; and a pioneer in the use of
absorbable ligatures. His most famous
operation was the successful removal
of several hundred stones from the
bladder of Chief Justice Marshall. In
Boston, John WARREN (1753–1815)
had a distinguished career during the
Revolution, and was for forty years

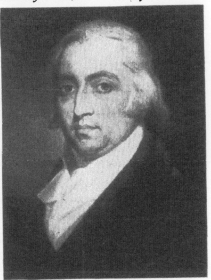

363. *Philip Syng Physick,*
"*the Father of American Surgery.*"
(*From the original portrait by Sully
at the* UNIVERSITY OF PENNSYLVANIA.)

the foremost surgeon in New England. He was a founder of the Harvard Medical School and its first Professor of Anatomy and Surgery. His
son, John Collins WARREN (1778–1856), was a founder of the Massachusetts General Hospital (1820) and its principal surgeon; he also helped
found the *New England Journal of Medicine and Surgery* (1811), the
oldest existing weekly medical journal in the world. He wrote effectively
on ether as an anesthetic and on various surgical topics (for example,
excision of the elbow joint, 1834), as well as on archæology. Valentine
MOTT (1785–1865) was a master of the surgery of the arteries, always
practising his technique on the cadaver before undertaking the operation
on the living. He was the first to ligate the innominate artery for aneurysm
(1818), though this was not successfully accomplished till 1864, by A. W.
Smyth. In 1821 he successfully ligated the common carotid; in 1827, the

common iliac for aneurysm; and in 1831, the external iliac for femoral aneurysm. His bone and joint surgery was renowned. Boldest of operators but extremely careful in his pre-operative and post-operative care, he performed "more of the great operations than any man living, or that ever did live," in the words of his teacher, Sir Astley Cooper. He was the chief founder of the New York University Medical School and Professor of Surgery there. Garrison (4th ed., pp. 502 and 503) gives a remarkable list of early American surgical achievements, especially in the fields of the ligation of arteries and of operations on bones and joints, most of the descriptions appearing in the *American Journal of the Medical Sciences* and the *New England Journal of Medicine and Surgery.* George Mc-CLELLAN (1796–1847), founder of the Jefferson Medical College (1825), where he served as Professor of Surgery, had one of the largest surgical practices in the country, and shared with J. C. Warren and Valentine Mott in establishing many new surgical procedures. The most successful surgeon west of the Alleghenies was the Virginian Benjamin Winslow DUD-LEY (1785–1870), who settled in Lexington, Kentucky. Especially skilled in the lateral operation for lithotomy, he lost only six patients in 225 operations, and was known even in England as " the lithotomist of the nineteenth century." He was a founder of the Transylvania Medical School (1817), where he was long Professor of Surgery.

When equipped to combat pain with anesthesia, and infection with antisepsis, in the middle of the century, surgery became well prepared for the phenomenal advances that are touched upon in the next chapter.

Anesthesia (a term suggested by O. W. Holmes) for surgical operations was America's greatest contribution to medicine. The story of its adoption is a good illustration of the view that the spirit of the times is an important factor in bringing about and recognizing scientific discoveries — a suitable ideology is required, in the jargon of today. As we have seen, soporifics of various kinds had been used sporadically from the earliest times: Homer's nepenthe, the hemp of the Chinese and Scythians, Dioscorides' potion, the soporific sponge of Salerno, the mandragora of the great thirteenth century surgeon Hugh of Lucca. None of these survived, however, and operations continued to be performed well into the nineteenth century without any attempt to relieve the agony of the patient other than perhaps with a stiff drink of whisky. Along with the increased knowledge of chemistry, acquired toward the end of the eighteenth century, the anesthetic properties of nitrous-oxide gas were discovered (1800) by Sir Humphry DAVY, who even suggested that " it may probably be used with advantage in surgical operations." Sulphuric ether, also, had been used in the treatment of pulmonary diseases, and was shown to have anesthetic properties by Faraday (1818), and the Americans Godman (1822), Jackson (1833), and Wood and Bache (1834). Mesmerism was being used to prevent pain with more or less success on both sides of the Atlantic, and Dupuytren is said to have purposely caused his patient to faint to avoid the pain of the knife-thrust. Ether was first used in surgical operations by Crawford W. LONG (1815–78), " discoverer of the use of sulphuric ether as an anesthetic in surgery on Mar. 30th, 1842 at Jefferson, Jackson County, Georgia," in the words of the inscription on Long's statue in the Statuary Hall in the national Capitol. A simple and modest country practitioner with but few surgical cases coming to him for treatment, Long did not publish his discovery to the medical world until 1849, though he continued its use in surgery and obstetrics throughout his life and had employed it successfully in eight operations before Morton's "Letheon" was published to the world in 1846. Long's discovery received but little recognition from the

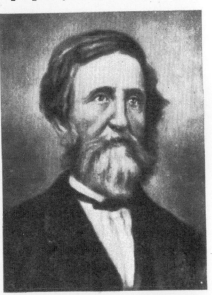

364. *Crawford W. Long.*
(From an oil painting by his daughter, now at the UNIVERSITY OF PENNSYLVANIA.)

medical world, however, until publicized by Marion Sims's article of 1877. In 1844 Horace Wells (1815–48), a Hartford dentist, had some of his own teeth painlessly extracted while under the influence of nitrous oxide (" laughing gas "); but having told his discovery to his temporary partner, W. T. G. MORTON (1819–68), he abandoned the practice after an untoward result. Ether had been suggested to Morton and supplied to him by the chemist C. T. JACKSON, who thus claimed his share in the great discovery. Morton had the good fortune to persuade John Collins Warren to be allowed to try it at the Massachusetts General Hospital, and he did so successfully on October 16, 1846. Within a month the success of ether anesthesia was published to the world by one of the witnesses of the operation, the eminent surgeon H. J. Bigelow; in another month it was being employed in London in dentistry by a Mr. Robinson, and in surgery by Robert Liston. Its use spread rapidly throughout Europe and within a year Sir James Simpson was using it in childbirth, though he shortly after switched to chloroform. Before the year was out, the Russian Pirogov had written a manual on the subject. During the unfortunate controversy which was carried on as to priority (in which Long refused to be entangled), O. W. Holmes, when asked to give his opinion, made the punning reply that the credit might well be given to "e(i)ther."

Within twenty years anesthesia was followed by Lister's equally important discovery of antisepsis, two of the greatest achievements in the whole history of surgery.

7. Obstetrics and Gynæcology

Obstetrics emerged from the sphere of general surgery early in the nineteenth century, successfully making for itself an independent position in university instruction. The rapid evolution of operative technique, the great improvement that followed the recognition of the contagiosity of puerperal fever, and the rapid development of histological and pathological studies were among the chief factors in determining the great progress of this branch of medicine. Gynæcology, also, began to emerge as a surgical specialty, though often united in the medical curriculum as in practice with obstetrics or general surgery, as in fact it still is in many places. It is difficult in a short general history of medicine even to summarize the development of these specialties about this time, a subject which has been ably treated and in considerable detail by medical historians. We shall limit ourselves therefore to noting only the most important names and events in gynæcology and obstetrics of the period.

Early in the century France held the primacy in this field. Among the successors of Baudelocque the most prominent was Antoine Dubois (1756–1837), an excellent clinician, who attended at the birth of Marie Louise, using version and the forceps to extract the posteriorly presenting head. The general surgeon A. A. Velpeau was the author of a treatise on the art of delivery (1835) which enjoyed a great reputation in its time. Mme Lachapelle (1769–1821), a renowned midwife and directress of the Paris Maternité from 1797 to 1821, held an honourable place among French obstetricians and wrote a highly valued book on the mechanism of childbirth. Among the German obstetricians the most celebrated were Adam Elias von Siebold (1775–1828), professor at Würzburg, and his son, Eduard (1801–61), an able practitioner and historian of his subject. His book (1845), later continued by Dohrn (1904), is one of the most complete texts that exist on the subject.

A great innovator in modern obstetrics and one of the greatest medical benefactors to humanity was Ignaz Philipp SEMMELWEIS (1818–65), of Budapest, whose work was the most potent-influence in overcoming the terrific mortality of puerperal fever that existed at that time. Semmelweis's views on the subject were so fiercely combated by many of the most illustrious obstetricians of his time that he was forced to resign from his position at the Vienna Krankenhaus. In 1845 he became Professor of Obstetrics at Budapest, where he published his great work, *Die Aetiologie, der Begriff und die Prophylaxis des Kindbettfiebers* (Budapest and Vienna, 1861). His courageous championship of asepsis in obstetrics, which ushered in a new era in the history of this discipline, did not prevent him, however, from becoming a victim of the persecutions of his enemies, a martyr to his discovery, dying in his prime in an insane asylum.

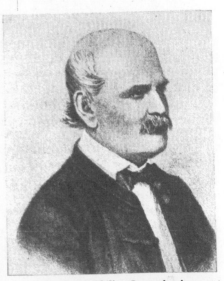

365. *Ignaz Philipp Semmelweis.*

The history of the contagiosity of puerperal fever is one of the most interesting in medicine. In no field of medicine were the disastrous effects of surgical infection more tragic than in obstetrics. Puerperal fever had rightly become the terror of women about to be delivered, particularly in hospital wards. The most extravagant theories had been proposed about its origin, even the suggestion that it was due to certain diets or the odour of certain flowers. Toward the end of the previous century, however, the infectious nature of puerperal fever was gradually becoming recognized, especially by the Britishers, Smellie, William Hunter, John Leake, Alexander Gordon (of Aberdeen), and Charles White (of Manchester). The last named, especially, recognized the need for cleanliness in all the surroundings of the delivery and for the segregation of febrile cases (*A Treatise on the Management of Pregnant and Lying In Women*, 1773). Still clearer were the exhortations of Oliver Wendell HOLMES (1809–94) in his article " On the Contagiousness of Puerperal Fever " (*New England Quarterly Journal of Medicine*, 1842–3, I, 503). Holmes's views also had met strong opposition: H. L. Hodge and C. D. Meigs, professors of obstetrics in the two

Philadelphia medical schools and leaders in their specialty, ridiculed the idea that the disease could be introduced by the hands of the attending physician or nurse. If the precautions recommended by Holmes and other Cassandras had been adopted, however, Semmelweis's great achievement would have been forestalled and thousands of lives saved. Semmelweis, being present at the autopsy of Kolletschka, Rokitansky's assistant, who had died of a dissection wound (1847), noticed that the lesions were similar to those found in women dying from puerperal fever. He also observed that puerperal death-rates were highest in those clinics where the students entered the obstetrical wards after coming from lectures on pathology and from the dissecting-room. He at once prescribed that all hands should be washed most carefully and that the room should be cleaned with calcium chloride. The mortality of his service diminished immediately and greatly, while it continued unchanged on all the other services. In spite of this evidence, and in spite of his affirmation that the cause of puerperal fever could be found in blood poisoning, a statement contained in his memorable communication to the Vienna Medical Society (1847), he was fought and persecuted by all the great obstetricians of Vienna. The publication of his book (1861) let loose a new campaign against him; even Virchow declared against him on purely theoretical grounds. There were only a few non-obstetrical physicians who supported his doctrines, such as Rokitansky, Skoda, and Hebra. It was not for twenty years that his doctrine was generally accepted; in 1894 a monument was erected to him at Budapest.

The discovery of the contagiosity and control of puerperal fever marks an advance of inestimable value from the point of view of social hygiene. To this discovery is chiefly due not only the rapid decrease in the mortality of childbirth but also the shift from midwives, who until then had mostly presided over childbirth, to well-trained surgeons and obstetricians.

Among the Italian obstetricians of the early part of the century should be noted F. ASDRUBALI (1786–1832), inventor of the embryotome (1812); P. BONGIOVANNI (1777–1827), of Pavia, and his successor T. LOVATI (1800–71); F. BILLI (1787–1866), of the Obstetrical School of St. Catherine at Milan; C. ESTERLE (1819–62), Director of the Schools of Trent and Novara; V. BALOCCHI (1818–82), of Florence; G. B. FABBRI (1806–75), of Bologna; and C. MINATO (1824–99), gynæcologist of Pisa.

The most notable figure among English obstetricians was Sir J. Y. SIMPSON (1811–70), who succeeded James Hamilton in the chair at Edinburgh when only twenty-nine years of age. He introduced the anesthetic use of chloroform (1847), which had been discovered by Liebig and Wöhler in 1837. Though an opponent of Lister, he advanced medicine in many ways (surgical instruments and diagnostic procedures, hospital improvements, medical history, etc.). A teacher revered by students, who came to his lectures from all parts of the world, he accumulated an enormous private practice. In 1869 he had received many testimonials of the high esteem in which he was held and was made an honorary citizen of Edinburgh. John BURNS (1775–1850) is recalled as the author of a popular textbook, *The Principles of Midwifery* (London, 1809), which went through fourteen editions and was translated into German and Dutch. A. G. BOZZI-GRANVILLE (1783–1871), an English physician of Italian origin, was celebrated for the high quality of his operative technique and

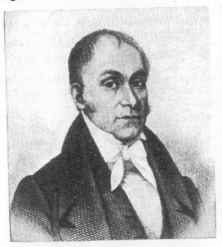

366. *Ephraim McDowell.*
(*From an original engraving at the*
COLLEGE OF PHYSICIANS OF PHILADEL-
PHIA.)

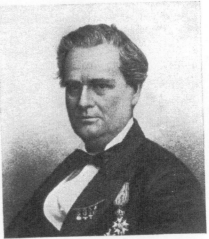

367. *J. Marion Sims.*
(*From an engraving by H. B. Hall,*
Jr.)

was one of the best-known gynæcologists of his time. Robert LEE (1793–1877) was the author of a number of investigations on the intestinal functions of the fetus and on version in cases of arm presentation. He was a prolific writer on various subjects, such as the pathology of the uterus and its adnexa.

AMERICAN gynæcology during this period made its first great contribution to medical progress with the introduction of ovariotomy for ovarian tumour, suggested by the Hunters and John Bell, but first performed by McDowell in 1809. Ephraim McDOWELL (1771–1830) was a Virginian who, after studying under John Bell, practised in Danville, Kentucky, then a village in the wilderness. He successfully removed an ovarian tumour under these primitive conditions without anesthesia or antisepsis, a crowd waiting outside anxiously for the result, and his patient, Mrs. Crawford, singing hymns while he worked. His publication of his first three cases, all successful, in 1816 (*Eclectic Repertory*) marks the beginning of modern abdominal surgery. In 1821 Nathan Smith independently performed an ovariotomy; but the operation was generally viewed with disfavour till the forties, when it was revived by the brothers J. L. (1799–1885) and W. L. ATLEE (1808–78), of Lancaster, Pennsylvania, who eventually performed some four hundred such operations with a relatively low mortality. Another great service to the suffering female was performed by the Carolinian J. MARION SIMS (1813–83) in the operative treatment of vesico-vaginal fistula. He discovered that a vaginal speculum — at first a bent spoon-handle — with the woman lying in a special position on her side (" Sims's position "), permitted' him to see " everything, as no man had ever seen before " (1845). Moving to New York, he demonstrated in the face of great local opposition that this common and practically incurable form of fistula was now amenable to surgical cure. His discovery, which he demonstrated abroad, was quickly taken up throughout Europe and brought him many honours. His assistant in New York, the Virginian T. A. EMMET (1828–1919), was another master of female pelvic surgery, whose operation for perineal repair is still familiar to medical students. Hugh Lenox HODGE (1796–1873), professor at the University of Pennsylvania, was the leading American obstetrician of his day and inventor of the first pessary of the type still in use. The first American textbook of obstetrics was published by Samuel BARD (1742–1821) in 1807.

Among the prominent FRENCH gynæcologists and obstetricians of the early nineteenth century should be mentioned J. C. A. RÉCAMIER (1774–1856), who in 1818 invented the vaginal speculum that bears his name; P. C. HUGUIER (1804–73), who especially studied hysterometry, ovarian cysts, and amputation of the cervix uteri; and J. H. DEPAUL (1811–83), author of an important treatise on clinical obstetrics.

In AUSTRIA, K. Braun FERNWALD (1822–91) held the greatest reputation in the Viennese clinic of the period. L. J. BOER (1751–1835) was a prominent teacher at the University of Vienna, where he was followed by J. SPAETH (1823–96). The most celebrated obstetrician in GERMANY was F. K. NAEGELE (1778–1851), called the Euclid of Obstetrics. He insisted that accurate knowledge of the mechanism of childbirth should form the basis of every obstetrical operation. He described the obliquely contracted pelvis that goes by his name (1839), and wrote a number of works, of which the most popular was his *Lehrbuch der Geburtshilfe für Hebammen* (1830). Karl SCHROEDER (1838–87) wrote an excellent and popular treatise on gynæcology that was much translated. F. A. M. F. von RITGEN (1787–1867) established the operation of symphysiotomy, which had been proposed by Assalini, condemned by Siebold and Killian, but supported by Galbiati (1832) and Morisani (1881).

During this period the principle of watchful waiting was accentuated in obstetrics, though the forgotten operation of Cæsarean section began to be revived. It is said to have been first performed in America by J. L. RICH-MOND of Newtown, Ohio (1827); and several repetitions on the same patient were reported in the pre-anesthetic period.

GYNÆCOLOGY, which, as we have seen, remained part of general surgery in the early part of the century, developed rapidly with the introduction of narcosis. New methods of gynæco-logical examination and treatment were developed by Sir James Young SIMPSON (1811–70). Thomas Spencer WELLS (1818–97), of St. Thomas's Hospital, London, and for a while Di-rector of the~Maritime Hospital at Malta, in 1856 introduced ovariotomy into the British Isles. He succeeded in reducing its mortality from almost 100 per cent to about 4 per cent. In the pre-Listerian era he was outstanding in his emphasis on the strictest cleanli-ness of instruments and hands.

About this time began the first studies of gonorrhœal affections of the female génitalia, and in fact all gynæ-cological study reflected the progress in pathologic and micro-organismal concepts. Gynæcology was becoming a surgical discipline in practice and teaching, and from the point of view of prophylaxis and social hygiene was assuming a notable importance.

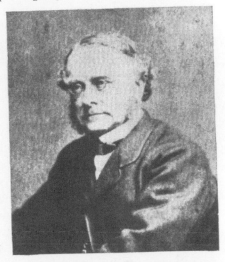

368. *Thomas Spencer Wells.*

8. Ophthalmology

The ophthalmology of the period registered notable advances based on the better knowledge of the anatomy and physiology of the organ of sight. A new era in the history of this discipline began with Helmholtz's inven-tion of the ophthalmoscope in 1850 (*Description of an Eye Mirror for the Examination of the Retina in the Living Eye*, 1851). His apparatus con-sisted of a triangular instrument with an acute angle at the top; two mirrors on the side of this triangle reflected the light into the eye of the patient at an angle of fifty degrees. This great invention made possible for the first time the examination of the retina during life, and opened up the whole physiology and pathology of the eye grounds. Helmholtz also was aware of the importance of his instrument in the diagnosis of refractive errors. An interesting precursor of the ophthalmoscope is the instrument of Charles BABBAGE (1792–1871), while Cumming at the London Hospital and Brücke of Vienna had caught glimpses of the human retina in the previous decade. Even before Helmholtz's discovery, however, ophthalmology had made its start as a surgical specialty in the first decades of the century.

The teaching of ophthalmology as a separate discipline in the university clinics was begun by Karl HIMLY (1772–1837) at Göttingen. Early in the century studies concentrated on the best method for removing cataract. At first attempts were made to crush the lens, as was recommended by W. H. J. BUCHHORN (d. 1814), after which the extraction of the lens through a large incision in the cornea was recommended by the English physician DE WENZEL (d. 1790), and successfully practised by F. JÄGER (1784–1871), one of the leaders of the Viennese school.

One of the greatest ophthalmologists of the century was Albrecht von GRAEFE (1828–70), son of the surgeon, Karl Ferdinand, and known as the master of ophthalmic surgery. Von Graefe, who received his degree in Berlin in 1847, founded in 1854, with Donders, the *Archiv für Ophthalmologie*, which contains most of his important publications. He became docent in 1852, professor in 1857. The most highly esteemed ophthalmologist of his period and founder of a great school, to which physicians flocked from all parts of the world, tireless in his activities and a man of high intelligence and profound culture, he died of tuberculosis at the age of forty-two, leaving a record permanently connected with the operation for cataract by linear extraction (1867–8). He is perhaps better recalled to medical students by the eye sign in exophthalmic goitre that bears his name (1864).

To von Graefe is owed a number of other important contributions, such as iridectomy for glaucoma (1857), recognition of papillary stasis as an important diagnostic sign in cerebral tumours, and of amblyopia. He thoroughly appreciated the importance of the ophthalmoscope, which he made the basis of many of his ophthalmic investigations. He firmly established sympathetic ophthalmia as a clinical entity (1866), a condition which had been known since classical times but was first adequately described by William McKENZIE (1791–1868) in 1830. Its exact nature, whether infectious, allergic, or of other obscure origin, is still an unsettled problem.

Another great figure, especially in the physiology and pathology of the eye, was F. C. DONDERS (1818–89), the greatest Dutch physician of the nineteenth century. First Professor of Anatomy, then of Physiology and Hygiene, he devoted himself to the eye at von Graefe's suggestion and founded an eye clinic at Utrecht. When named Professor of Physiology at Utrecht (1852), he confided the direction of the clinic to Hermann

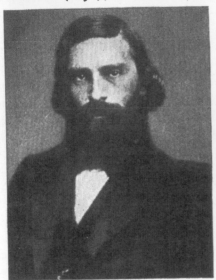

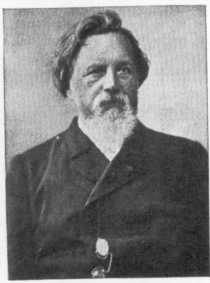

369. *Albrecht von Graefe.*   370. *Frans Cornelis Donders.*

SNELLEN (1834–1908), known to student and patient for his test types (1862). Donders's chief work was his treatise in English on *The Anomalies of Refraction and Accommodation* (London: Sydenham Society; 1864). No less important were his studies on the physiology of the eye (ocular movements, colour sense, and visual perception).

Donders was a co-founder with von Graefe of the *Archiv für Ophthalmologie*. It is to his initiative and tenacity that Holland owes the foundation of special eye hospitals and systematic instruction on the eye. He constructed a new form of ophthalmoscope with a mirror perforated in the centre, which is the model of the type still in use. The work of von Graefe and Donders had an enormous influence on the whole subject of ophthalmology, giving a sound basis for the many improvements that quickly followed in diagnosis, operative treatment, and the use of spectacles.

In GREAT BRITAIN, an eminent Scotsman who studied in London, James WARDROP (1782–1869), wrote his *Essays on the Morbid Anatomy of the*

Human Eye (1808), classifying inflammations according to the locality involved. His study of keratitis reflects the influence of Bichat. James WEAR (1756–1812) is credited with being the first to have described gonorrhœal ophthalmia (1795) and recognized its venereal origin. Benjamin TRAVERS (1783–1858) was a leading practitioner of the subject, especially known for his *Symposium of the Diseases of the Eye and Their Treatment* (1820), one of the earliest works in English to deal with the subject systematically. The first public hospital for the eye (Joseph Beer had a private hospital in his own house in 1786) was the Royal London Ophthalmic Hospital, founded under a different name in 1805. Popularly known as " Moorfields," it has long been the centre of influence for ophthalmology in English-speaking countries.

Ophthalmology in AMERICA was content to follow the lead of Europe during the first part of the century. George FRICK (1793–1870), of Baltimore, was one of the first specialists in the subject in the United States. He brought to this country the ideas and influence of Beer, under whom he studied, and wrote the first American book on the subject, *A Treatise on Diseases of the Eye* (1823). William GIBSON (1788–1868), a Philadelphia surgeon, was an early operator for strabismus (1818). This condition had been surgically treated by Eschenbach of Rostock in 1752, but it was not until Stromeyer cut the eye muscles of the cadaver in 1838 and Dieffenbach applied the operation to the living in 1839 that the operation was placed upon a firm foundation. Henry W. WILLIAMS (1821–95), a leader in early ophthalmology in America, gave a course of lectures devoted to the eye in 1850 and became professor of the subject at Harvard in 1871. His younger brother, Elkanah (1822–88), was one of the first to confine his professional work to the eye, ear, nose, and throat. He became Professor of Ophthalmology at Miami Medical College in 1860, and did much to spread knowledge of the ophthalmoscope in the United States. Cornelius Rea AGNEW (1830–88), after studying in Great Britain and France, specialized in ophthalmology, establishing an ophthalmic clinic at the New York College of Physicians and Surgeons in 1866, where he became Professor of Ophthalmology in 1869. He founded the Brooklyn Eye and Ear Hospital, and soon afterwards the Manhattan Eye and Ear Hospital. He was a prolific writer, an inventor of new instruments and of operative procedures, such as canthoplasty and the correction of external strabismus. The first eye infirmary in America was opened in New London in 1817 by Elisha North. The New York Eye and Ear Infirmary was founded in 1821; the Wills Eye Hospital of Philadelphia in 1833, following the demise of the earlier Pennsylvania Infirmary for Diseases of the Eye and Ear. The

Massachusetts Eye and Ear Infirmary was founded by E. Reynolds and J. Jefferies, Jr., in 1827; and the Baltimore Dispensary for the Cure of the Diseases of the Eye in 1823.

A precursor of the ITALIANS who dedicated themselves to this specialty was Antonio SCARPA, surgeon and anatomist (see pp. 601, 625), who made important discoveries concerning the anatomy of the eye and was an able, brilliant operator, gifted with great didactic powers. Other eminent Italians were F. FLARER (1791–1850), of Pavia; A. DE ROSA (1792–1855), of Padua, who succeeded G. J. Beer, the first occupant (1812) of the chair at Vienna; G. B. QUADRI (1780–1851), the first professor of the subject at Naples, whose *Lezioni* were published by his son, Alessandro. His *Annotazioni pratiche* (4 vols.) give the first clear description of excision of the iris in the construction of an artificial pupil.

F. C. BOLL (1849–79), of German origin, Professor of Physiology at Rome from 1873, in his memorable communication to the Accademia dei Lincei, *Sull'anatomia e fisiologia della retina* (1876), announced his discovery of the colouring matter in the rods of the retina, the visual purple (rhodopsin), which gradually fades in the presence of light.

The first professor of the subject at the University of Charkov was the Italian Vanzetti, who, after acquiring a great reputation in Russia, returned to Padua in 1855 to direct the surgical clinic.

FRENCH ophthalmology remained for a long time united to surgery, and the subject was practised and taught mostly by foreigners. Julius SICHEL (1802–68), of Frankfurt, founded the first private eye clinic in Paris. In 1838 he took as his assistant L. A. DESMARRES (1810–82), asking him to "help me in putting my German kitchen into French." Other French ophthalmologists were C. J. Carron DU VILLARDS (1800–60), who in 1835 founded the first eye dispensary in Paris; and A. Sarre D'UZÈS (1802–70), inventor of the opsiometer.

BELGIUM experienced a terrible epidemic of trachoma from 1825 to 1840, which appeared first in the army but spread rapidly through the civilian population after the Revolution of 1830. The study of trachoma and means of restricting its spread was energetically undertaken by L. S. FALLOT (1788–1872) and J. F. VLEMYNCKX (1800–76). Florent CUNIR (1812–53) was the founder of the first eye journal in French, the *Annales d'oculistique* (1838), which was edited by Belgian oculists up to the death of Evariste Warlomont.

Ascertaining the number of blind people in a country was first begun by the United States in 1830 and is now practised by most civilized countries. There is estimated to be about two and a half million blind people in the world, ranging from 476 per million in New Zealand to 13,251 per million in Egypt. Teaching the blind was first begun systematically by Valentin HAÜY (1745–1822), who founded at Paris the Institut National des Jeunes Aveugles (1784). He later embodied his principles in an essay on the education of the blind. Special printing for the blind, which had been known in crude forms since the sixteenth century, was not developed until Louis BRAILLE (1809–52) — himself blinded by an accident at the age of three — invented his compact alphabet of raised dots (1829). Today large libraries of books in many languages, composed on the Braille system, are available to the blind throughout the world. Institutions for the blind have existed since the time of St. Basil's at Cæsarea in the fourth century, and of the Hospice des Quatre-Vingts, which was founded by St. Louis in 1260 and still exists in Paris. However, it was not until 1791 that Liverpool founded England's first institute, with the Edinburgh asylum following two years later. Other cities followed rapidly: Vienna, 1804; Berlin, 1806; Prague, Amsterdam, Dresden, 1808; Copenhagen, 1811; the Perkins Institute of Boston, 1829; the New York Institute, 1831; the Pennsylvania Institute, 1833.

9. Otology and Laryngology

Otology can be said to have been initiated largely by the anatomical and pathological studies of Eustachius, Valsalva, Cotugno, and Scarpa. Among the great events that signalized the progress of otology was the catheterization of the Eustachian tube, first practised by E. G. Guyot, a postal official at Versailles (1724), and later improved by the English military surgeon Archibald Cleland. Among the other more important operations to be devised were: mastoidectomy, first practised by Petit in the eighteenth century, and the perforation of the ear-drum, first carried out by Cooper in 1800. The most important writers on the subject in the early nineteenth century were: J. M. G. ITARD (1775–1838), who in 1821 published the first scientific treatise on the diseases of the ear; W. KRAMER (1801–75), of Berlin, who devoted himself to the treatment of auditory disturbances, and F. von TROELTSCH (1829–90), whose treatise on otology was widely renowned, and passed through seven editions. It was published in English translation in 1874 by the Sydenham Society. Important otologists of the period were E. P. VOLTOLINI (1818–89), professor at Breslau and a founder of the *Monatschrift für Ohrenheilkunde;* Joseph TOYNBEE (1815–66), who published a descriptive catalogue of some two thousand specimens of the internal and middle ear prepared from the cadaver. Best known of the French otologists was P. MÉNIÈRE (1799–1862), who described the clinical syndrome that bears his name (1861).

Study of diseases of the larynx and the other respiratory passages was greatly stimulated by the invention of the laryngeal mirror (1855) by Manuel GARCIA (1805–1906), a gifted singing teacher who, wishing to observe the position of the vocal cords while singing, succeeded in examining his own larynx by the aid of two mirrors. Johann Nepomuk CZERMAK (1828–73) was conspicuous in developing these studies (1858). At the same time Ludwig TÜRCK (1810–68) published his discovery of the laryngoscope, having first examined the larynx with it in 1857. This gave rise to a violent polemic for priority between Türck and Czermak. Tracheotomy was first successfully performed for croup by Bretonneau at Tours in 1825. The first to do a tracheotomy in Paris (1831) was Armand Trousseau, who was especially concerned with tuberculosis of the larynx. Intubation of the larynx for croup was first carried out with a small thimble-like tube in the larynx (1856) by Eugène BOUCHUT (1818–91), but with such poor therapeutic results that it failed to replace tracheotomy. Intubation was first successfully practised by Joseph O'DWYER (1841–98), of New York, in 1884, after four years of experiments directed toward finding a satisfactory instrument. Within a decade the procedure was definitely established after less opposition than is usually aroused by radical innovations.

A snare type of tonsillotome had been invented by Physick in 1827. It was followed by procedures invented by a number of Americans in rapid succession, such as C. S. MATTHEWS (1828), and William B. FAHNESTOCK, who invented the guillotine form (1832). Voltolini was the first to use galvanocautery in laryngeal surgery (1867), and to operate on the larynx with the aid of external illumination.

10. Dermatology and Syphilology

The period under discussion is one of the greatest in this specialty, because it is the time when gonorrhœa, syphilis, and soft chancre were differentiated, and when the specific pathological and clinical pictures of these important diseases were first definitely fixed. Philip RICORD (1799–1889), born at Baltimore of French parents, is its most illustrious representative. He it was who definitely established the error of John Hunter's belief that gonorrhœa and syphilis were identical, a problem that had produced interminable discussions between the partisans of the unitary and dualist doctrines. Ricord showed by a series of experiments, involving 2,500 inoculations, that gonorrhœal pus could not cause syphilis. It was not until about this time that the term " syphilis " began to replace in general use other synonyms such as " lues venerea." Ricord was the first to establish the characteristic phenomena of the three stages of syphilis, giving masterly descriptions of the bone and muscle lesions. He was the author of a number of important monographs on venereal diseases. He

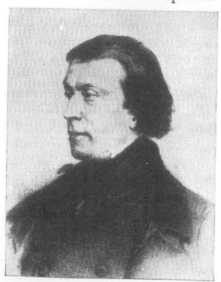

371. *Philip Ricord.*

had a reputation, not only as an eminent specialist to whom people came from all parts of the world, but also as a brilliant orator and caustic wit, epitomized by Holmes's description of him as the " Voltaire of pelvic literature . . . who would have . . . ordered a course of blue pills for the Vestal Virgins." He was the chief surgeon at the Hôpital du Midi, where students and physicians crowded to his lectures. His chief work was the *Traité pratique des maladies vénériennes* (Paris, 1838).

Prominent among ENGLISH syphilologists were Langston PARKER (1805–71), advocate of mercurial vapour baths, and Jonathan Hutchinson, whom we have already met. Among the ITALIAN venereologists were V. TANTURRI (1835–85), of the University of Naples; R. CAMPANA (1844–1919), professor at Genoa and Rome; P. PELLIZZARI (1823–92); C. SPERINI (1812–94), and T. DE AMICIS (1838–1924), of Naples, who made notable studies on mycosis fungoides, multiple idiopathic sarcoma, and hystricism (*ichthyosis hystrix*).

An important position in the dermatology of the period belongs to the English physician Robert WILLAN (1757–1812), the first to distinguish lupus from eczema. He introduced a rational nomenclature and made the best classification of skin diseases that had been proposed up to that time, dividing them according to their external appearance (papular, squamous, bullous, etc.). His *Description and Treatment of Cutaneous Diseases* (1798–1807) was completed by his pupil Thomas BATEMAN (1778–1821). For its beautiful illustrations and accurate descriptions, including many diseases that had been little known hitherto, it has long been regarded as a classic work of modern dermatology. One of the most interesting figures in the history of dermatology is the Baron Jean Louis ALIBERT (1768–1837), a classifier of skin diseases by the "natural method," whose clinic at the Hôpital St. Louis was for years the world's centre for this specialty. To him is owed the first description of "Aleppo button" (1829), of mycosis fungoides, and of keloids (1810). A keen observer, he taught his pupils the fundamental need for making the most careful examination of skin lesions. He was the author of a treatise on dermatology (1829) that, especially from the iconographic point of view, is a masterpiece. His pupil L. T. BIETT (1781–1840) abandoned Alibert's system for that of Willan, which was in turn supplanted by Hebra's pathological classification.

The Moravian, Ferdinand von HEBRA (1816–80), probably the greatest dermatologist of the century, was one of the best representatives of the Viennese school when it was at the height of its glory. Hebra was a careful and able pathologist, as well as a keen clinical observer, and was the first to establish the parasitic origin of many skin diseases. The nature of papular and marginate eczema, erythema multiforme, the lichens, impetigo herpetiformis (1872), rhinoscleroma, pitiriasis, and so on, was so well described by Hebra that he is properly to be regarded as the creator of a sound dermatology based on pathologic anatomy. His great atlas of cutaneous diseases (1856–76) is a monumental work of inestimable value.

Hebra was one of the most popular physicians in Vienna, noted for his often sarcastic witticisms, and for his finesse and goodwill. Founder of the great school of Viennese dermatology, he had as his pupil F. G. PICK (1834–1910), professor at Prague and Vienna, his son-in-law, Moritz KAPOSI (1837–1902), and Isidor NEUMANN (1832–1906), all of whom carried on the great reputation of his school.

In GERMANY F. W. F. von BAEHRENSPRUNG (1822–64), professor at Berlin, contributed to the knowledge of neurotrophic dermatoses. The NORWEGIAN school, especially, J. HJORD (1798–1873) and D. C. DANIELSSEN (1808–75), made important studies on the pathology of leprosy. The classic text on this subject, which was for the first time correctly described only in this period, was that of H. C. C. LELOIR (1855–96), *Traité pratique et théorique de la lèpre* (Paris, 1886).

11. Psychiatry and Neurology

The history of modern psychiatry can be traced, as we have already noted, to the work of such men as Valsalva, Pinel, and Chiarugi, who initiated the reform in the fundamental concept of psychopathology and in the more rational treatment of the insane. It is only in the nineteenth century, however, that the subject became founded on a solid basis of anatomical and physiological study. Neurology as a separate discipline came into being in this period, and solutions were found for several of the most important problems of the physiology of the nervous system. To this time belongs the splendid work of Charcot and his pupils and of the Italian precursors of Lombroso. It is in this historically important period that psychiatry took its place in university instruction and developed as an important factor in the field of hygiene and social medicine.

We have already mentioned the earliest efforts toward an essential change in the treatment of the insane at Milan, and those of Chiarugi at Florence, of Pinel in France, and of Howard and others in England. Italy was a leader in this field, together with Belgium, which surpassed all others in its famous village colony of Gheel. We mention especially the Asylum of Aversa, well described by Alexandre Dumas, Sr., who attended a festival of the insane there.

It is fitting to recall that the positive concept of insanity as an organic disease, as opposed to the more ancient psychologic and metaphysical concepts, was first announced by Morgagni in 1760. This fundamentally structural concept of mental change was developed by the almost forgotten Neapolitan SEMENTINI (1743–1814), and by Chiarugi, who defined madness as " a primary injury of the brain." The humane treatment of the insane was energetically supported by the Baron Pietro PISANI, Director of the Palermo Institute, in his *Istruzione per la novella Reale casa dei matti* (1827); also by Gaetano LA LOGGIA (1805–89), a Sicilian who was one of the most authoritative psychiatrists of the period. In the Italian school of anthropology Augusto TEBALDI (1833–95), of Padua, specialized in legal medicine; Antonio BERTI (1816–70) wrote a notable study on insanity and homicide (*Pazzia ed omicidio*, 1877); and F. R. BONUCCI (1826–66) courageously maintained the doctrine of the irresponsibility of maniacs, melancholics, and idiots in his book on legal medicine and in a volume entitled *Principi di antropologia e fisiologia morale dell'uomo* (1866). He was the first to maintain that in other mental conditions, such as hysteria, hypochondriasis, and epilepsy, the legal responsibility was greatly diminished.

Italy was the first country to make obligatory the public instruction of psychiatry (decree of Carlo Alberto of 1838, by which a chair of psychiatry was attached to the Insane Asylum of Turin). Teachers there were Bertolini, Bonacossa, Porporati, and E. Morselli, who was succeeded in 1890 by Lombroso. Italian psychiatry was worthily represented by the Milanese Cesare CASTIGLIONI (1808–73), one of the most energetic advocates of the modern treatment of the insane; by Serafino BIFFI (1822–90), of Pavia, a student of the anatomy and physiology of the brain and proponent of colonies for the insane; and C. F. BELLINGERI (1789–1848), of

Turin, founder of the theory of nervous antagonism. The name of A. VERGA (1811–95) is connected with the "ventricle of Verga" and the "ossicles of Verga." His "Psychiatric Appendix" (1852) to the *Gazzetta Medica,* which can be regarded as the first Italian periodical on this subject, energetically upheld the need for special psychiatric teaching. He also published an interesting study of the madness of Tasso (1845). Carlo LIVI (1823–77), who created a practical school of psychiatry at the Asylum of Reggio Emilia, was the author of an excellent book on the death sentence from the point of view of pathology and physiology.

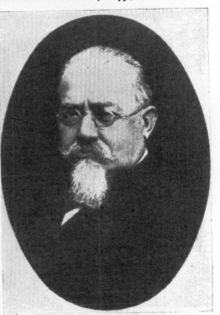

The greatest lustre was conferred on Italian psychiatry by the splendid work of Cesare LOMBROSO (1836–1909), of Verona, one of the greatest Italian investigators and teachers of the past century. A close student of the anatomy and physiology of the brain, he was the real initiator of the study of criminology. His books *Genio e follia* (1864) and *L'Uomo delinquente* (1876) were enormously successful, were translated into many languages, and quickly became the classic text for physicians and legisla-

372. *Cesare Lombroso.*

tors. His studies on cretinism and pellagra formed the basis for legislative measures against these diseases. His school at Turin was highly esteemed by physicians, who flocked to it from all countries. He is one of that small group that leaves an ineffaceable trace in medical history and opens new paths for scientific research.

In FRANCE, Jean Martin CHARCOT (1825–93) was one of the greatest neurologists of his time. It was perhaps his incomparable qualities as teacher, writer, and organizer that contributed most to the great reputation of this gifted clinician, whose profundity and clarity of observation joined with an admirable originality in pathological synthesis to visualize the broad aspects of clinical symptoms. He was the creator of the greatest modern neurological clinic, and a masterly describer of many disease pictures, such as hysteria, muscular atrophy, amyotrophic lateral sclerosis, multiple sclerosis, and paralysis agitans. He was a great clinician in the broadest sense of the word, careful of the patients committed to his care, wonderfully energetic and diagnostically acute, though in his examination of hysterical patients he is now thought to have sometimes produced symptoms by the suggestive nature of his questioning. Charcot brought to his clinic at the Salpêtrière a group of devoted pupils who were among the founders of modern neurology. In 1898 a monument was erected in front of this hospital in memory of one of the greatest figures in the history of French

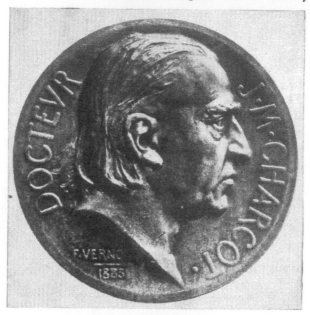

373. *Jean Martin Charcot.*

medicine. His masterly *Leçons sur les maladies du système nerveux* (Paris, 1872–83; published in translation by the Sydenham Society, 1881) and his magnificent *Iconographie de la Salpêtrière* (1876–80) are classics in the eloquence of their style, the value of their contents, and the clarity of their exposition.

Among the precursors of Charcot as pioneers in French psychiatry are to be mentioned Sylvestre BLANCHE (1795–1852) for his studies on hysteria, and his efforts toward the humane treatment of the insane; Alexandre BRIERRE DE BOISMOND (1797–1881) for his studies on suicidal mania; J. P. FALRET (1794–1870), director and clinical teacher at the Salpêtrière, for his original description of cyclical insanity; A. L. FOVILLE (1799–1878), author of a popular treatise on the nervous system; and J. J. MOREAU DE TOURS (1804–84), an energetic reformer of insane asylums. Most eminent for his studies on the pathology of the nervous system and one of the great pioneers in the budding specialty of neurology was Guillaume B. A. DUCHENNE (1806–75), the first describer of a whole series of hitherto unknown diseases of the nervous system, such as glosso-labio-laryngeal paralysis (later known as progressive bulbar paralysis), pseudo-hypertrophic muscular paralysis and the type of progressive muscular atrophy

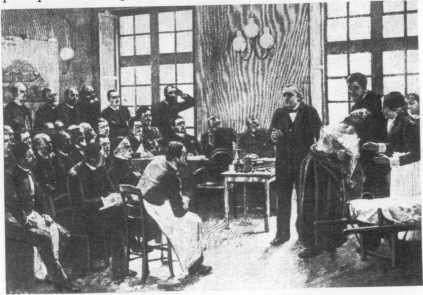

374. *Charcot's clinic at the Salpêtrière.*

that begins in the upper extremity (Duchenne-Aran's disease). He was among the first to make extensive use of electricity in the diagnosis and treatment of nervous diseases.

ENGLAND early recognized the need for new methods of treating the insane. Especial credit is due to John CONOLLY (1796–1866) for his courageous advocacy of the "no restraint" method of treatment (*The Treatment of the Insane without Mechanical Restraints*, 1856). After twenty years as director of the great asylum at Hanwell, which accommodated more than one thousand patients, he was able to announce that in twenty-four English asylums, harbouring more than ten thousand patients, all methods of mechanical restraint had been definitely abolished Samuel TUKE (1784–1857) was the grandson of Henry, the founder of the famous York Retreat, of which he wrote a description (1813). He was the author of a number of psychiatric works, and can be regarded as one of the founders of English psychiatry; his son, Daniel (1827–95), editor of the *Journal of Mental Science*, and co-author with J. C. Bucknill of the manual of psychological medicine (1885), was also eminent in English psychiatry. In 1885 he pointed out the tardy state of development of the American and Canadian asylums.

Among early AMERICAN neurologists and psychiatrists should be mentioned G. M. BEARD (1789–1883), a pioneer in electrotherapy, and W. A. HAMMOND (1828–1900), a Surgeon-General of the U. S. Army, the first to describe athetosis, and author of an able book on nervous diseases (1871). James Jackson's description of *arthrodynia a potu* (1822) is one of the best early accounts of alcoholic neuritis; and his colleague, John WARE (1795–1864), wrote a lengthy study of delirium tremens (1832) which is still a classic on this subject.

In GERMANY, the eminent clinician Wilhelm GRIESINGER (1817–68) was the apostle of the new psychiatric thought. His book on *The Pathology and Treatment of Psychic Diseases* (Stuttgart, 1845) offers accurate clinical syndromes based on pathological studies and objective psychological analyses. To the German school also belonged Theodor MEYNERT (1833–92), professor at Vienna and author of important studies on the anatomy and physiology of the brain; and Richard von KRAFFT-EBING (1840–1902), who was professor first at Strassburg, then at Graz and Vienna. He is especially noted for his book on *Psycopathia sexualis* (1876), a fundamental study in this line, which by 1924 had passed through eighteen editions.

German neurology also made important progress, though not as a specialty separate from general medicine. Especially noteworthy was Moritz ROMBERG (1795–1873), who was one of the first to collect in his book on nervous diseases (1840–6) extensive clinical studies on the physiology and pathology of nervous diseases. Among his original descriptions was that of so-called " ciliary neuralgia "; he is better known for the description of the ataxia that occurs in tabes when the eyes are closed (Romberg's sign). Robert REMAK (1815–65), an eminent histologist, brought also to the nervous system important microscopic studies, such as those on the pathology of tabes (1836–7), ascending neuritis (1861), Remak's ganglia of the heart, and so on. He was an important advocate of electrotherapy in nervous diseases (1858).

12. *Legal Medicine*

Legal medicine in the nineteenth century translated into practical progress the pioneer steps of the seventeenth century. This discipline developed illustrious representatives in ITALY, such as Francesco ROGNETTA (1800–57), who taught ophthalmology in Paris and wrote important articles in the French journals. He worked extensively in toxicology and especially on the medico-legal aspects of arsenic poisoning. The Florentine R. BELLINI (1817–78) wrote an excellent volume on *Lezioni sperimentali di tossicologia*. G. G. UTTINI (1741–1817) was the first Professor of Legal Medicine at Bologna, where he was followed by V. L. BRERA. Francesco RONCATI (1832–1906) was a well-known psychologist who also successfully pursued the study of legal medicine. An important contribution was made by Lombroso in his insistence on the use of the experimental method in legal medicine (1865). In his book *Medicina legale del cadavere* he published a number of interesting observations on the methods of identifying the cadaver. He deserves to be regarded as the initiator of the use of scientific methods by the police, a subject now well developed in all civilized countries. The studies of Lombroso and his school led to a new picture of crime and the criminal and exerted a notable influence on penal legislation. To them is owed in great measure the development of modern methods of crime-prevention.

Among the authorities on legal medicine at the beginning of the century in GERMANY, we note H. A. HENKE (1775–1843), the author of a highly valued textbook of legal medicine; Karl LIMAN (1818–91), whose handbook of legal medicine includes a number of important case studies; and J. G. MENDE (1779–1832), who especially studied the medico-legal aspects of pregnancy and childbirth. He wrote a treatise on legal medicine (5 vols., 1819–30), in which the historical side is amply developed. J. L. CASPER (1796–1864), of Berlin, was a leader in this field in Germany, insisting on a reform in legal medicine to keep it closely connected with scientific medicine in general. His books on medical statistics and state medicine (1825), on the probable duration of human life (1843), and on medico-legal autopsies (1850 and 1853) were deservedly popular, while his *Praktisches Handbuch der gerichtlichen Medicin* (2 vols., 1856) was long the classic authority on the subject. Among the FRENCH, A. A. TARDIEU (1818–79) was noted for the clarity of his writing and the logicality of his conclusions. The best-known ENGLISH authority on the subject was Sir Robert CHRISTISON (1797–1882), Professor of Materia Medica at Edinburgh. The AMERICAN T. G. WORMLEY (1816–94) is remembered for his excellent book on the microchemistry of poisons (1867). Early treatises on the subject in English were those of T. R. BECK (1823), Isaac RAY (1839), and W. A. GUY (1844).

13. Therapeutics

The therapeutics of the period reflect the stimulus received from physiological and chemical progress. While in some schools, like that of Vienna, therapeutics were put well in the background, there was elsewhere a genuine attempt to attain a rational therapy on the basis of clinical and physiological studies, and of pharmacological experiments on animals. Scientific study of the action of drugs constitutes the characteristic note of the time, when pharmacology passed largely from the hands of empiricists into those of the physicians and physiologists. As we have seen, it was in this period that the first attempts at immunization were successfully achieved in Jenner's vaccination, a concept that can be traced back to Robert Fludd's (1638) attempt to overcome tuberculosis with the sputum of cured consumptives. In this period, when experimental medicine was triumphantly asserting itself, but when ancient therapeutic ideas were still flourishing, we see the greatest contrasts in the history of therapy and pharmacology. On the one hand, the Viennese clinicians affirming that all treatment should be withheld in acute diseases; on the other, the disciples of Broussais, who continued to practise blood-letting on a vast scale. New therapeutic fantasies, such as magnetism and homeopathy, existed along with the return to ancient methods, such as hydrotherapy, dietetics, and other physiological methods. It was in the treatment of febrile diseases that the most violent contests ensued between those who favoured antipyretic remedies, the partisans of hydrotherapy, and those who tended toward therapeutic nihilism. Finally, it was in this period that the pharmaceutical industry began to develop, first in Germany and England and then in France and America. The introduction of a number of new drugs into the therapeutic armamentarium and the discovery of the active principles of many already in use were other factors in making this period important in the history of pharmacology. In 1806 Friedrich Sertürner (1784–1841) discovered morphine; in 1818 Pelletier and Caventou discovered strychnine, and in 1820 quinine, the active principle of cinchona bark; Geiger and Hesse isolated atropine from belladonna in 1833, and in 1859 Niemann first prepared cocaine. In 1853 C. G. Pravaz (1791–1853) published his description of the first hypodermic syringe, shortly to be improved by Alexander Wood (1853), thus opening up an entirely new field for the administration of drugs.

Therapeutic regimes and dietary cures now first began to be worked out on a scientific basis, as might be expected when one considers that the study of organic chemistry and metabolism began about this time. Hydrotherapy and the systematic medicinal baths at spas, chemical analysis of mineral waters and knowledge of their physiological effects, and the erection of scientific criteria for the proper control of such treatments, all had their true origin in the first half of the century.

Among the best-known ITALIAN pharmacologists were L. SCARENZIO (1797–1869), of Pavia, who instituted the first pharmacological laboratory; G. OROSI (1816–75), of Pisa, author of a *Farmacopea italiana* that was regarded as the best book on the subject up to the end of the nineteenth century; A. MOLINA (1830–1905), of Padua, author of a two-volume *Trattato di materia medica;* and F. COLETTI (1819–81), professor at Padua and founder of the pharmacological museum there, a prolific writer, especially on the effects of poisons.

Among FRENCH pharmacologists, especially worthy of mention is J. B. A. CHEVALIER (1793–1879) for his studies on the chemistry of food substances and their " falsification," and on the purity of drugs. The Minorcan, M. J. B. ORFILA (1787–1853), chemist and physiologist, indicated new paths in the study of the effects of poisons in his classic *Traité de toxicologie générale* (1813–15). E. F. A. VULPIAN (1826–81), a student of letters, then a technician in Flourens's laboratory, published the results of his vast experience in his *Leçons de physiologie générale* (1866), which contained important sections on toxicology and pharmacology. We note also E. SOUBEIRAN (1793–1858) for his studies on chloroform, and F. A. JAUMES (1804–68), author of a valuable treatise on pharmacology (1848).

Studies in the GERMAN-SPEAKING countries also advanced therapeutics and materia medica; W. BERNATZIK (1821–1902), professor at Vienna, especially promoted iodine therapy, and R. BUCHHEIM (1820–79) summarized in his textbook of pharmacology (1856) his own and his pupils' long experience at the Pharmacological Institute of Dorpat. K. G. MITSCHERLICH (1805–71) wrote a large textbook on the subject that went through a number of editions, which was based on his extensive personal investigations. D. von SCHROFF (1802–77) is especially remembered for his studies on belladonna and atropine.

Prominent among the ENGLISH pharmacologists of the first part of the past century were the celebrated Robert CHRISTISON (1797–1882), of Edinburgh, author of a well-known book on poisons; and Jonathan PEREIRA (1804–53), author of a celebrated book on materia medica. Among AMERICAN writers on materia medica was Joseph CARSON (1808–76), of Philadelphia, who also is locally remembered for his *History of the Medical Department of the University of Pennsylvania* (1869). Among the SWEDES we note F. FRISTEDT (1832–93), of Upsala, and P. F. WAHLBERG of Stockholm.

Among the best-known advocates of hydrotherapy was Vincenz PRIESSNITZ (1799–1851), a Silesian farmer, who was the apostle of treatment with cold compresses. Latin students of this subject were A. TARGIONI-TOZZETTI, G.

GARELLI, of Turin, L. TIMINELLI, of Bassano, and the Frenchman L. J. D. FLEURY (1814–72), author of a number of important monographs on hydrotherapy. In England, James Clark (1788–1870) popularized the bath treatment; J. M. GULLY (1808–81) wrote on and practised the water cure.. The old Roman town of Bath, in Somersetshire, had taken on such prosperity in the previous century in the bath treatment of gout and rheumatic disorders in the hands of William OLIVER (of Bath-Oliver biscuit fame) and others that in the early nineteenth century during the Regency it became one of the most popular resorts of England. The prevalence of gout among the English upper classes gave many physicians ample opportunity to study the therapeutic effects of various kinds of bathing. Of the Germans who especially advocated balneotherapy, the most prominent were A. VETTER (1799–1845) and H. BREHMERS (1826–89), the founder of the Goerbersdorf Sanitarium in Silesia, the model institute of Europe. Noteworthy was the book published by the Russian physician F. BEJAWSKI in 1834 which contained much information about artificial mineral waters.

14. Hygiene and Social Medicine

We have referred in the previous chapter to the first real attempts to protect the State against epidemics. Sanitary legislation against infectious diseases was to receive a new impulse from the terrible epidemic of cholera that spread throughout Europe in 1830. After the great plague epidemics in the fourteenth and fifteenth centuries, a marked progress in the study of hygiene had resulted, together with the appearance of sanitary legislation in the Italian cities that dominated commerce at that time. It is logical, then, that after the cholera epidemic of 1830 it should be England that made the greatest effort to combat diseases which endangered its maritime traffic and threatened one of the most vital of its economic resources. With the beginning of the Industrial Revolution at this time England also experienced a great movement of the population from the country into the cities. Those cities where commerce and industry were concentrated saw a rapid increase in their population, accompanied by all the phenomena that such movements imply. Just as the expansion of commerce and industry in the Italian cities of the Renaissance led to the foundation of hospitals and the creation of a system of sanitary legislation, so the same causes in England produced similar results in the first half of the past century. Important hygienic problems arose: the need for a sanitary defence of the great ports from the spread of diseases brought from overseas, the need for protecting cities from the dangers due to rapid overgrowth and increased industrialization.

In 1848 the British Parliament created a central office of Public Health, which at once began the study of methods to combat disease among factory workers. For the first time accurate statistics were collected to investigate the causes of mortality and to determine the differences between urban and rural disease and between the different trades and professions. The government took energetic steps to improve sewers, water supplies, and canals, to supervise markets and dwelling houses, all of which soon brought about noticeable improvements. One important factor to be appreciated by anyone studying the events that led to the improvement of hygiene at this time is the willingness to obey the law and the recognition of the importance of public health problems that is characteristic of the English. The English administrative structure contributed to these successes in creating a central office with provincial branches directly dependent upon it. Thus the public health administration which was organized in 1848 developed into the formation of a far-reaching Ministry of Public Health on July 1, 1919. The Acts of Parliament, registering the public opinion that preceded the various health acts, are important documents in the history of hygiene.

To name a few of the noteworthy English hygienists, we mention Neil ARNOTT (1788–1874), who was concerned especially with the heating and ventilation of houses and with prophylactic measures against typhoid; Alexander PARKES (1819–76), who was the first Professor of Hygiene at the Military School at Netley and author of a meritorious book on practical hygiene; Sir Humphry DAVY (1779–1829), who made a highly important early contribution to industrial hygiene, the invention of the coal-miner's safety lamp (1818); Charles HALL (1816–76), who studied especially the occupational diseases of steelworkers; Thomas Southwood SMITH (1788–1861), active in the struggle against epidemic diseases, inspector general of the alkali industries, and author of a series of valuable reports on the subject; Sir George BUCHANAN (1830–95), the illustrious president of the Public Health Office, who was one of the most valuable hygienists of the past century and accomplished important work in all fields of public hygiene. The lawyer Sir Edwin CHADWICK (1800–90) was perhaps the most important of all in initiating these developments in public hygiene, in demonstrating the value of the census and of bills of mortality in the control of public health, and for his valuable reports on the poor-laws (1834), the health of the labouring classes (1842), and on cemeteries (1843). It was his survey that stimulated a similar study in New York (1853) by J. H. GRISCOM (b. 1809), the first work of this kind to be undertaken in the United States.

Sidney, Lord HERBERT (1810–61), Secretary for War in the English Cabinet at the time of the Crimean War, was important to military hygiene, if only for the enthusiastic help that he gave to Florence NIGHTINGALE (1823–1910). The story of the brilliant achievements of the Lady of the Lamp (so called by the soldiers in memory of her nightly tramps through the military hospital) in creating a female nursing service in the military hospital at Scutari and then at Balaklava (Crimea) is well known by laymen and physicians alike. Her energy and her indomitable and disinterested spirit of sacrifice crowned her activities with such success that on her return to England the sum of fifty thousand pounds was collected to create a nursing school bearing her name at St. Thomas's Hospital (1860). This event is properly regarded as initiating a new era in the history of the care of the sick and wounded.

William BUDD's (1811–80) book on *Typhoid Fever, Its Nature, Mode of Spread and Prevention* (1873) was so important in promoting knowledge of that disease that it has recently been reprinted by the American Public Health Association (1931). In 1866 Budd assumed control of the campaign against a cholera epidemic, which he was successful in quickly stamping out. John SNOW (1813–58) was the first to demonstrate that cholera was transmitted by water, thus overcoming the London epidemic of 1854. He is said to have invented an early pulmotor for asphyxiated infants (1841). William FARR (1807–83) was one of the founders of the study of statistics of morbidity and mortality. His book on *Vital Statistics* (1885) presents the curve of incidence of a typical epidemic — early rapid ascent, slow rise to the peak, and an even more rapid fall (" Farr's law ").

T. R. MALTHUS (1766–1834), in his famous essay on *The Principles of Population* (1798), maintained on the basis of his statistical observations that poverty was in large measure due to increase in the population, and therefore proposed that there should be legislative provision for a proper proportion between the nutritional capacity of the State and the birth-rate. The term " Malthusianism " as applied to general methods for lowering the birth-rate was suggested by the philosopher Condorcet; as a matter of fact, this principle was condemned by Malthus.

In FRANCE, the modern organization of public health control began with the laws of 1789–91 and the foundation of the Council of Public Hygiene in 1802. The Superior Council of Health established in 1822 appears not to have been especially active; but the Revolution of 1848 produced a new and more efficient organization in the Consulting Committee on Public Hygiene, with a Council established in each department and arrondissement in 1889. Among those who concerned themselves with this subject at the beginning of the century was A. G. LABARRAQUE (1757–1850), known for his study of occupational diseases and for " Labarraque's solution," a disinfectant that is still in use. Numerous French treatises appeared on various aspects of public hygiene, especially during the forties. H. REVEILLÉ-PARISE (1782–1852) wrote an able treatise on the hygiene of old age (1843); Louis VILLERMÉ (1782–1863) was especially concerned with the hygiene of silk- and wool-workers, Tanquerel DES PLANCHES (1809–62) with lead workers, F. M. MÉLIER (1798–1866) with tobacco, DELPECH with the rubber industry; and finally, A. J. B. Parent DUCHATELET (1790–1836) devoted himself to the study of prostitution in Paris and initiated the governmental control of prostitutes.

Following the success of the British methods, GERMANY arranged an excellent governmental supervision in the field of public health. When the period of economic prosperity and industrial development began in Germany toward the middle of the century, university institutes developed rapidly, often under the protection of enlightened rulers, and the success of liberalism carried with it the breath of liberty through the activities of the great German universities. Among the most distinguished German hygienists was Max von PETTENKOFER (1818–1901), who early studied the chemical conditions of the atmosphere and its significance to proper ventilation and clothing, the relations between soil and drinking water, and later concentrated on metabolism. The Institute of Hygiene, founded at Munich in 1866, was the first great scientific institute where rigorously controlled experimental conditions permitted the fundamental investigation of hygienic problems. Pettenkofer's work on cholera and plague served as the basis of successful sanitary measures and soon other German cities created institutes based on Munich's model.

Pettenkofer was one of the most remarkable figures of his period. Convinced of the importance of chemistry in the development of hygiene, he was a tireless apostle of the study of the origin of infectious diseases and of the measures necessary to combat them. Sent by Germany to the International Sanitary Conference of 1874, he upheld the need for quarantine of travellers coming from the Orient, where plague and cholera were endemic. His interest in the problems of alimentation and metabolism has already been referred to in an earlier section. To his initiative is owed the publication of the *Archiv für Hygiene*, and of the *Zeitschrift für Biologie*, and the great *Handbuch der Hygiene* that he published with Ziemssen (1882). He can properly be regarded as one of the chief founders of modern hygiene whose work paved the way for the scientific hygienists of the latter part of the century. Among his precursors are to be noted Ignaz LORINSER (1796–1853), active in school hygiene; G. WARRENTRAPP (1809–86), who was concerned especially with the hygiene of prisons; K. M. FINKELBURG (1832–86), who was responsible for the German legislation supervising trade and the control of food substances, and finally J. UFFELMANN (1837–94), who was concerned especially with alimentation.

In the UNITED STATES sanitary legislation developed rapidly about this time. Already in 1836 child labour was forbidden in certain states of the Union and little by little admirable legislation was developed in this field. The report (1850) of the Massachusetts Sanitary Commission, under the leadership of Lemuel SHATTUCK (1793–1859), had an important influence in pointing out the unsanitary conditions of American cities, but it was not until 1869 that a permanent State Board of Health was established in Massachusetts. In 1855 a temporary State Board of Health had been created in Louisiana, and many other states followed during the seventies. In 1866 New York City established its Board of Health, which has been a leader in promoting public health measures and organization in American cities. In 1872 the great American Public Health Association was organized. The increasing prosperity of the country, combined with good methods of organization, has brought about the creation of many institutes for the investigation of problems of alimentation, child hygiene, and so on, which have greatly aided the work of the national, state and city public health departments.

Defence measures against infectious diseases were being promoted. Parkes, of London (1847), and Prunner, of Cairo (1851), for instance, proposed the improved sanitation of cities as the most efficacious measure against cholera. In 1851, a memorable date in the history of hygiene, all the countries of Europe convened at Paris in the First International Conference, to decide on common quarantine measures to take against the spread of plague, cholera, and yellow fever. Thus statesmen and the common people were acquiring the conviction that the successful struggle for public hygiene required an international solidarity, and the basis of modern sanitary legislation was laid.

15. History of Medicine

As a section on the history of medicine now appears in this volume separately for the first time, it is desirable to examine the development of this discipline from ancient times, recapitulating briefly the older periods to which we have made allusion. As already stated, Hippocrates should be regarded as the first medical historian because of the attempts that he made to interpret the work and concepts of the physicians of the schools of the preceding period, especially when one reflects on the difficulties made by the paucity of preserved data. His book on *Ancient Medicine* indicates the high regard in which he held the work of his predecessors.

This first attempt at medical history was followed by others which emphasized the biographies of famous physicians, "lives" or "eulogies," like those of the great soldiers and philosophers, from which we can sometimes obtain useful facts but rarely estimates that are worthy of consideration. To this category belong the biographies of Menon, disciple of Aristotle, and of Dionysius of Ephesus. Of the same sort was Hermippus' book (third century B.C.) on famous physicians. A. C. Celsus brought to the history of ancient medicine a very remarkable contribution. Soranus (second century of our era), author of a life of Hippocrates, also wrote ten books containing a series of biographies. In the chapter on Arabian medicine we mentioned Ibn Abi Usaibia and the accounts that he gave of the physicians of his period; his work is especially valuable for its bibliographical references. Guy de Chauliac in the fourteenth century had written penetratingly on the medical wisdom of the past.

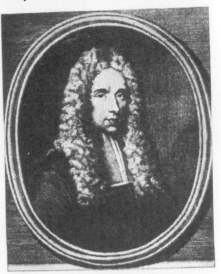

375. *Daniel Le Clerc.*

With full recognition of these early writers and of the valuable contribution of the Renaissance to the history of medicine, we must accept, however, that the writing of medical history really begins in the seventeenth century with the book of Daniel LE CLERC (1652–1728), of Geneva (*Histoire de la médecine*, 1696). This constitutes the first attempt at a synthetic survey of medical history from the most ancient times. From the point of view of modern historical criticism, to be sure, Le Clerc's work can be regarded only as a first and imperfect attempt, covering but little after the time of Galen and tending to include fantastic legends and all manner of subjective interpretations. Among the most noteworthy historical works of the eighteenth century are the bibliographies of the great Albrecht von Haller: the *Bibliotheca botanica, chirurgica, anatomica* (each 2 vols.) and *Bibliotheca medicinæ practicæ* (4 vols.). The care and industry exerted in their preparation make Haller an extremely valuable bibliographical source for those searching the medical records of the past.

During the first half of the eighteenth century an English historian, John FREIND (1675–1728), a man of affairs who was closely connected with the political activities of his time, wrote *The History of Physic from the Time of Galen to the Beginning of the Sixteenth Century* (London, 1725–6), which contains an interesting account of medicine, particularly of English medicine, during the Renaissance. But it was especially the Germans who became concerned with the history of medicine about this time, all the more because of the philosophic orientation of German science in the eighteenth century. Among these historical writers were K. W. Möhsen (1722–95) (medical numismatics); Gottfried Gruner (1744–1815) (a history of epidemiology); and E. G. Baldinger (1738–1804) (medical biographies). The best known of the French historical writers of the period was the surgeon Antoine Portal, who wrote a history of anatomy and surgery in seven volumes (Paris, 1770–3). After several less important efforts, such as the books of A. F. Hecker (1790) and Blach (with a French translation, 1797), there appeared a remarkable work by the German historian Kurt Sprengel (1766–1833), *Versuch einer pragmatischen Geschichte der Arzneikunde* (5 vols., 1792–9), which went through several editions and was translated into several languages. Sprengel's history still constitutes a valuable source for historians on account of the profound erudition of the author, who carefully examined original material that threw new light on various periods of the history of medicine. His work is based on a correlation of medicine and political events. It is divided into eight great periods; thus the period of the expedition of the Argonauts corresponds to the earliest periods of Greek medicine; the Peloponnesian War to Hippocratic medicine, and so on. This obviously artificial division necessarily handicaps the presentation. However, among the older works Sprengel's should be regarded as one of the very best, especially for the section on German medicine of the seventeenth and eighteenth centuries. Less important is the contribution of G. C. Ackermann (1792), whose study stops with Paracelsus, whom he was one of the first to regard as among the chief founders of modern medicine. An interesting but little known book, as Daremberg remarks, is Rosario Scuderi's *Introduzione alla storia della medicina antica e moderna* (Naples, 1794; French translation, Paris, 1810). Scuderi is perhaps the first writer to approach the history of medicine from the philosophical point of view. Especially valuable are his chapters on the development of chemical medicine, in which he denies to Paracelsus the important role attributed to him by the German school. Among the historians of the beginning of the century, were Cabanis, who published in 1804 a short study on *Les Révolutions et la réforme de la médecine;* Kieser, who divided medicine into Oriental and Occidental cycles; and J. F. K. Hecker, who wrote a valuable account of the devastating epidemics of the Middle Ages (English translation by the Sydenham Society, 1844). His *Geschichte der Heilkunde* from the third to the fourteenth century (2 vols., 1822) was followed by his *Geschichte der neueren Heilkunde* (1839), covering various aspects of eighteenth-century medicine. A little known work that contains a vast amount of historical information is Emil Isensee's *Geschichte der Medicin und ihrer Hilfswissenschaften* (6 books in 4 vols., Berlin, 1840–5). Ludwig Choulant (1791–1871) was an accurate student of medical history who composed valuable chronological tables and two carefully prepared bibliographies (1828–42). These works, which have been recently republished (New York, 1922; Munich,

1926), are indispensable aids to the student of medical history and especially on the phase of anatomical illustration. In 1825 appeared Leupold's history of medicine; in 1831 medico-historical essays by Schultz; and in 1838 those of Lessing, covering the period up to Harvey. The systematic history of Quitzmann (1843) considers the development of medicine like that of a plant from its seed to its ripe fruit; in 1838-9 Friedländer published a history, which however is somewhat obscure and confused. On a much higher level is the *Lehrbuch der Geschichte der Medicin und der epidemischen Krankheiten* (3 vols., Jena, 1845), by H. HAESER (1811–84), especially valuable for its account of epidemic diseases. This work in the richness of the material that it covers and the originality of the author's opinions is one of the most readable of medical histories and still may be studied with profit. Among the French writers of the period, RENOUARD published a history of medicine from the earliest times up to the nineteenth century (Paris, 1847); and A. C. SAUCEROTTE wrote on Bichat, on the historical relations of philosophy to medicine, and similar subjects. For the history of Renaissance medicine, the work of K. F. H. MARX (1796–1877), of Göttingen, is especially valuable. He was the first to show (1848) the importance of the anatomical studies of Leonardo da Vinci.

Toward the middle of the nineteenth century two Italians wrote memorable histories which still afford invaluable sources of material for the student. Salvatore DE RENZI (1800–72), of Paternopoli, in the province of Avellino, and professor at Naples, published a *Storia della medicina italiana* (5 vols., Naples, 1845–8), which is a model of accuracy and profundity of research, valuable for its clear description of historical epochs and for the copious notices of every phase of Italian medicine. De Renzi was the first to point out the grandeur of the ancient Italian schools, the importance of the school of Pythagoras, and the glorious role that the school of Salerno played in medical history. The documents gathered by De Renzi in his *Collectio Salernitana* (5 vols., Naples, 1852–9) represent one of the most complete studies in the whole field of medical history. This illustrious scholar deserves the place of honour among the Italian medical historians of all time. His books, which have now become rare, when studied with the respect that they deserve, will reveal an eloquent story of the best and most representative figures in Italian medicine, a story supported by the most careful documentation, without exaggeration and with a clear, calm objectivity. Francesco PUCCINOTTI (1794–1872), of Urbino, professor at Pisa and contemporary of De Renzi, published a *Storia della medicina* in two parts (4 vols., Livorno, 1850–66), which is one of the best Italian works on the subject. Puccinotti may perhaps be reproached for having let his judgment be influenced by the rigidity of his religious convictions;

but the admirable patience with which he discovered, copied, and published important ancient texts, thus opening up new horizons in a number of fields, gives to his book a lasting value.

Another notable Italian historian of medicine was the epidemiologist Alfonso CORRADI (1833–92), Professor of Pathology at Modena, then at Palermo, and Professor of Therapeutics and Pharmacology at Pavia, who wrote a monu-

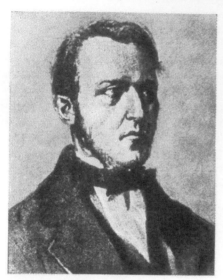

376. *Salvatore De Renzi.*

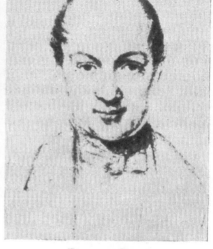

377. *Francesco Puccinotti.*

mental and minutely documented history of epidemics in Italy from the earliest times up to 1850 (7 vols., 1865–83). Among his other historical works the best known are his *Storia della chirurgia dagli ultimi anni del secolo scorso fino al presente* (1871), and his *Storia dell'ostetricia nei secoli XVIII e XIX* (1872). The teaching of medical history was begun in Italy in 1806 at Florence, the first chair being occupied by Giovanni BERTINI. At Naples the physiologist A. MIGLIETTA taught the subject from 1814 to 1821. After the Napoleonic period the Florence chair, transferred to Pisa, was held by C. PIGLI (1772–1845) until 1845, when it was occupied by Puccinotti, who had been Professor of Clinical Medicine. The chair at Naples was occupied in 1869 by De Renzi; that of Padua by G. MONTESANTO. Medical history was taught at Bologna by A. C. DE MEIS (1817–91), who followed G. CERVETTO. De Meis was forced by political trouble to flee from Naples, and through the influence of Claude Bernard and Trousseau obtained the chair of semeiology at Paris. Returning later to Italy, he accepted the chair at Bologna, where his historical studies were greatly influenced by Hegelian philosophy.

Two great French historians of medicine flourished in this period. The first of these was C. V. DAREMBERG (1817–72), whose profound knowledge of ancient texts produced excellent studies of Homeric, Hindu, and pre-Hippocratic medicine and translations and critical editions of *Oribasius*, the *Four Masters of Salerno*, the *Works of Hippocrates*, of *Galen* and *Celsus*. His *Histoire des sciences médicales* (2 vols., 1870) is one of the

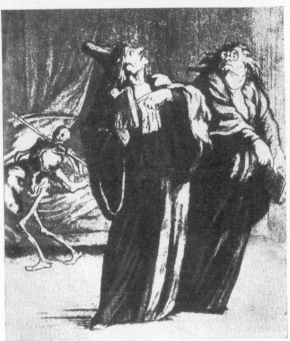

378. *The medical consultants. Caricature by H. Daumier.*
(COLLECTION PAQUEMENT.)

most interesting and well-written books that the literature of this discipline possesses. Daremberg's wide classical culture and clear vision of the historical evolution of medicine through the centuries brought together a series of admirable historical pictures, unbroken by an excess of bibliographical references and citations, in which the great figures of medicine, such as Paracelsus, Bichat, and Morgagni, are delineated in a masterly manner. In his criticism Daremberg is often severe, always strict, but never unjust; he loves the polemical style and brilliantly supports his point of view, which is always original, in a way that carries conviction through the authority of his erudition.

The second of the great French medical historians was the philologist Émile LITTRÉ (1801–81), a pioneer who brought new methods to the writing of medical history. His philological investigations, guided by his perfect knowledge of Greek and by his extensive culture and profound bibliographical studies, make this great French scholar one of the founders of modern historiography. Author of a well-known and popular dictionary, Littré also composed one of the finest and most complete editions of Hippocrates (10 vols., 1839–61). The Greek text, with the French translation opposite, constitutes the most important modern work in Hippocratic literature. He also published a valuable edition of Pliny (1848–50) and a number of biographical and bibliographical studies.

To this period, which was so rich in medical historiography, belong the works of CHINCHILLA (Valencia, 1841) and of MOREJON (Madrid, 1845) on Spanish medicine; that of BROECKX, on Belgian medicine (Ghent, 1847), and S. D. GROSS's *Lives of Eminent American Physicians and Surgeons of the 19th Century* (1861), *History of American Medical Literature from 1776 to the Present Time* (1876), and *A Century of American Surgery* (1876).

In this fertile period the study of the history of medicine definitely became part of the university curriculum. Soon, however, it entered a stagnant stage in most civilized countries during the period of materialism and of great microscopic and bacteriologic discoveries, when the attention of the medical world seemed to be concentrated solely on the present and on the new horizons of medical science.

16. The Teaching and Practice of Medicine

Summarizing the most important and characteristic facts of this period, we see that it exhibits the development of a positivist tendency, opposed to the often systematized idealism and romanticism of the eighteenth century. After having oscillated through centuries between religion and philosophy, alchemy and mysticism, dogmatism and rationalism, medical thought henceforth more and more relied on facts proved by experience; and only admitted the truths confirmed by objective scientific evidence. It is the laboratory that becomes the centre of medical activity rather than the clinic; it is in the laboratory that one solves or attempts to solve all the problems of disease and death. With the triumphs of cellular pathology and of bacteriology new horizons were opened and not only in the comprehension of the nature of disease. For the moment it was believed that even therapeutic problems could be solved with mathematical exactness. This is the essential note of the evolution of medical thought in this period — undoubtedly the most revolutionary and the most fertile in its fundamental concepts that the history of medicine records.

The consideration in the preceding pages of the development of medical sciences in this period clearly indicates the important changes that the nineteenth century brought to the evolution of the practice of medicine and to the social and intellectual position of the physician. In the eighteenth century the physician was still a characteristic figure, with a costume peculiar to his profession. He was often the victim of caricature in prose, verse, and illustration; the literature and engravings of former periods afford numerous samples of these caricatures. Toward the beginning of the century a notable change is apparent. With the orientation of medicine toward science, necessitating his careful study of the natural sciences, the physician loses this semi-miraculous, semi-charlatanesque character which he still held in the public eye at a time when the great clinicians were beginning to demonstrate the value of scientific experimentation, careful clinical observation, and a simple and rational therapy. In a predominantly positivist period charlatanism necessarily retreated, without of course

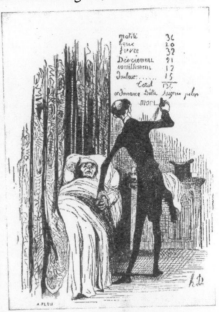

379. *Fate. Caricature by H. Daumier.*

entirely disappearing, as it is based on the ever present credulity of human nature. However, the ignorant and mountebanks were able to obtain public favour less easily; a stricter supervision was established, not only by the authorities but by public opinion, which, in spite of its many deviations, has generally recognized the merit of great physicians. Together with the robe and the wig, the ivory or gold-headed cane, and the three-cornered hat, the physician of the nineteenth century abandoned his Latin, with its redundant terms and sonorous metaphors, to return to the vernacular and the simpler habits of the bedside. Thus positivism of science found its immediate translation into practice, and the position of the physician was improved thereby. With the foundation of great hospitals, necessitating a greater number of physicians but reaching a far greater proportion of the population, with the great wars of the early part of the century, which required a large sanitary personnel, and finally with the epidemics, which constituted a grave menace to public health, there grew up a class of physicians richly endowed with a practical experience in medicine, surgery, and hygiene. Corporations and associations of physicians came into existence, which followed the ancient academies in their scientific tendencies, but were more mobile, more receptive to new ideas

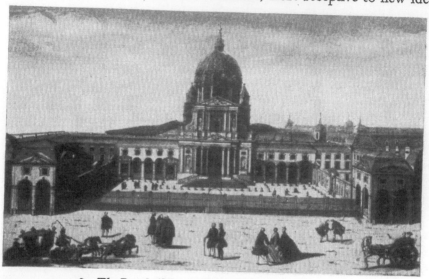

380. *The Royal Abbey of Val de Grâce, erected in 1665,*
now the school and museum of hygiene and military sanitation.

and discoveries, less bound to the essentially academic spirit that was characteristic of the earlier institutions of this sort. The same change was to be observed in medical journals, which quite suddenly took on an extraordinary development and became arenas in which not only the leading clinicians and teachers, but also the general practitioners came together for their scientific discussions. In this period dominated by the spirit of the French Revolution, the universities were representative of free research, places where men of the greatest intelligence formed radiating centres of scientific activity also in the field of medicine. No longer, as in the time of the Renaissance, was each university a closed school to which pupils came perhaps from distant parts, retaining no further connection with it, however, on their departure. The universities of the nineteenth century became highly integrated factories which, like the centres of the nervous system, rapidly reacted to receptive influences.

With the great diffusion of culture and of medical journals, with the increased facility of communication and with the political changes which brought people of different nations in frequent contact, medicine during this period lost much of its national character; though of course certain tendencies and intellectual orientations inherent in the mentality and living conditions of various peoples were retained and sometimes even accentuated.

Important scientific currents passed from Italy to the clinics of Vienna and vice versa. New ideas and technical improvements spread from France to Great Britain, Italy, and Germany, from Germany to Britain, and from Europe to America, bringing back from America in turn valuable contributions to medical thought and practice. The habit of young physicians of visiting foreign universities became more frequent; the world's medical literature became more easily available — indeed it grew to such proportions that critical reading of the important publications in many languages became more and more of an impossibility.

On the other hand, the political and social developments created new and important problems. The extension of commerce, the intensification of the relations of European countries with distant colonies, produced problems of naval hygiene and tropical disease. With the vast movements of troops, the great wars brought about unforeseen difficult problems of military hygiene. Finally, and this is undoubtedly the most important of these phenomena, the birth of new industries and the rapid growth of urban populations raised new problems of occupational disease and the need for legislation protecting the health of workers.

These events in turn forced new studies on the physician and increased to the same degree the importance of his position in society, necessitating his collaboration and advice in framing and carrying out public health legislation. The advent of political and social medicine became one of the most characteristic events in the history of medicine of the past century. The diffusion of culture by the introduction of obligatory elementary teaching spread knowledge of hygiene to ever increasing numbers of the people. The teacher, providing instruction for the most remote villages, opened the way for the physician and the hygienist. Popular superstitions, to be sure, were far from disappearing, but they played less of a role, especially in the great centres. The physician was called more frequently even in outlying districts. At the same time the rapidity and frequency of communication brought about by the railroads facilitated the transport of patients even from distant regions to the clinics and hospitals of the great cities, where this abundance of clinical material, reinforced by the resources of the laboratory, provided excellent opportunity for medical instruction and study.

Thus the physician occupied an important position in the social structure of the nineteenth century. He was honoured both by the government, which confided to him important functions, and by patients, who invoked his aid in increasing numbers. This had its important repercussion on the social and economic position of the physician, who in most countries occupied a leading position among the professions. Throughout the period considered in this chapter, physicians often played an important part in the cultural and political life of the country, so that we find them in the highest political offices and as leaders of great intellectual currents. Eco-

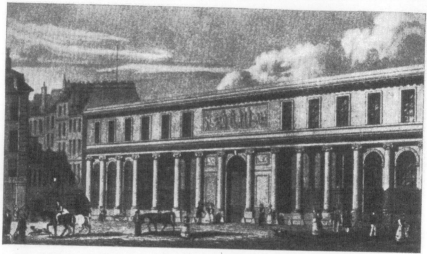

381. *L'École de Médecine of Paris at the beginning of the nineteenth century.*
(From a contemporary engraving in the BIBLIOTHÈQUE NATIONALE.)

nomically they achieved a high degree of prosperity. One can, to be sure, cite such and such a physician of a previous period who had made a great deal of money and reached important positions; as a whole, however, the medical profession was better appreciated in the nineteenth century than ever before, and a greater number of physicians attained to an adequate or even easy existence.

The period, then, that begins at the end of the eighteenth century with the revolutions of governments and individual consciences was dominated by an eminently positivist and incipient biological current which brought a new aspect to the career of the physician. He is no longer the sorcerer of remote ages, the priest of ancient times, the clerk of the Middle Ages, the astrologer or alchemist of the fifteenth century, the blood-letter of the seventeenth, or the philosophizing academician of the eighteenth. His costume is no longer that of white linen, or of red robe with silken bonnet.

His office is no longer in the temple, or in the pharmacist shop, or in the Academy. He no longer depends on the Church, or on the State, or on the conservative conventicles of bewigged academicians. The physician of the nineteenth century — typified by the great figures of Corvisart, Laënnec, Charcot, Rokitansky, Virchow, Bright, Lister, Lombroso, to name but a few — is simply the scientist, detached from the temple and the academy to take his proper place at the bedside of the patient. His costume is of the simplest, the street clothes of the ordinary civilian, the white gown in the laboratory and wards. He gives his service conscientiously and humbly but with the profound conviction of accomplishing his duty by following the way that nature has pointed out in the teaching of the biological sciences.

CHAPTER XX

THE SECOND HALF OF THE

NINETEENTH CENTURY

CLINICAL MEDICINE BASED ON THE FUNDA-MENTAL SCIENCES. GROWTH OF THE SPECIALTIES

1. Introduction

THE VARIOUS factors influencing the development of medicine that were considered in the previous chapter have continued to operate, many, in fact, at an accelerated tempo. As regards increased facilities of communication, the railroads and the telegraph, introduced in the first half of the century, began to affect social conditions to a considerable degree only in the latter half of the century. The telephone, invented in the seventies, became a potent factor in social existence only at the turn of the century, the automobile still later, while the airplane and radio were still in the early stages of their development. New medical discoveries and inventions were reported throughout the world within a few weeks of their first announcement. Patients were quickly and easily brought long distances to medical centres where they could profit by facilities unknown to previous generations. It is difficult to exaggerate the effect that such social changes have had on scientific progress, as well as on medical practice.

[762]

The political and social events of this period had a remarkable influence on the progress of medicine. During this epoch Germany was forging its way to leadership in European industry, commerce, and science. This was the heroic age of German medicine, and German medical schools were centres of medical learning. The teachings of Koch and Virchow and their schools had a prominent impact on the orientation of medicine at this time. Nevertheless, in other European countries, as in France, England, and Italy, medical science achieved remarkable conquests. It is during this period that the American medical schools began to establish their new programs of teaching and soon to assert an independent and fruitful activity, with the help of the great and generously endowed institutions that played an important role in the fostering of scientific research.

The limits of this historical period which extends from the beginning of biochemical and microbiological discoveries up to the end of the nineteenth century cannot be fixed with absolute exactness — a circumstance that of course applies to all historical periods and not only to the history of medicine. The beginning of the microbiological concept can be differently dated according to the values placed on the various discoveries that opened the paths. From the discovery of Bassi, which marked the beginning of bacteriology, to the contribution of Koch, which may be said to close the first stage of this discipline, three decades intervened. A new medical era started with the development of microbiology: the physician was forced to make an essential change in his method of thought and his concepts on disease, its causes and symptoms, and in his plan of treatment.

Another basic innovation upsetting long-established ideas was Virchow's doctrine of cellular pathology, which is sometimes regarded as initiating the modern period. Its fundamental influence on the concepts of etiology, nosology, and immunology brought immediate and remarkable application.

With the predominance of materialism we see spread through medicine the concept that it is in the realm of the infinitely small that the solution of the most important medical problems must be solved. The new discoveries in the field of cellular physiology and biology, as in physics and chemistry, accentuated more and more the tendency to place the centre of medical activity and research in the laboratory rather than in the clinic and to base medical progress on the results of these studies.

A mighty evolution in medical thought was initiated by the teachings of Claude Bernard. The principle that the results of physiological and biochemical experiment have to be applied to the explanations of the problems of life and death, of health and disease, had a tremendous influence on medical progress. It was a return to some of the concepts of Paracelsus and the chemoiatrists of the seventeenth century, but the definite change from metaphysical considerations to objective experiment enlightened and marked decisively a new trend of science.

The studies of the individual and his reaction to disease — his constitutional disposition — received much impetus from the evolution of microbiology; but at the same time they were closely connected with the traditional Hippocratic concepts of the constitution and its influence on the origin of disease. From the Hippocratic concept to the doctrine of the Italian schools, then to Kretschmer and the Americans, there is a dominant current of thought starting from this period which asserts that knowledge of the patient, his heredity and his environment, is fundamentally necessary for intelligent treatment. The concept of general pathology takes priority again over the local pathology advocated by Virchow. Studies on the vitamins, the endocrine organs, allergy, and metabolic disorders have opened new paths of medical thought, emphasizing the importance of the personality and the environment in the development of disease.

As a result of the new orientation and the rapid progress in medicine, we have seen an increasing tendency to specialization. The new task of the physician has obliged him to utilize long and complex laboratory studies, requiring special knowledge and special technical skill in one or another branch, and to achieve the difficult task of keeping up with the fruit of new scientific discoveries. It became necessary for more and more physicians to devote themselves exclusively to laboratory work; while, at the same time, the rapid progress in the specialties required intensive study and continued practice of those aiming at specialization.

These orientations, which brought remarkable success in all fields of medicine, had, however, neglected the social factors in the origin and course of disease. It was later during this period that the importance of social and economic conditions to public health were studied and appreciated, and that medicine began to assume its role as a social science.

The type of general practitioner who covered all branches of medicine became more rare. The family physician who in the past remained the friend and faithful counsellor of his patients, knowing their individualities as well as their history and their surroundings, has become, especially in the towns, less common and inevitably less able to accomplish such a vast task. The State, the community, the hospitals, the insurance companies, the schools, and the public itself asked for the aid of specialists. Even the small-town physician who still indulged in general practice was more and more frequently forced to summon the aid of a specialist colleague.

If such lines of thought may guide the consideration of this period of medical history, it has to be noted that an exact division between this and the following chapter cannot always be carried out. Many of the prominent scientists who exerted a great influence on the development of medical thought were active in both periods, and therefore the reader will often find in this chapter references to research that was completed later, and in the next chapter references to work that was begun at this time.

2. Biology

Biology — a term introduced almost simultaneously by Comte and Treviranus (1802) — is the study of living matter — of the different forms of organic life, of the laws that govern its existence, and of the conditions that influence its activity (Treviranus). From another point of view, it may be regarded as the sum of the forces that resist death; as J. Loeb has pointed out: " Death is not inherent in the individual cell, but is only the fate of more complicated organisms in which different types of cells or tissues are dependent upon each other " — a concept that has since been confirmed by the studies of tissue cultures *in vitro*. The fields of biology are numerous — its medical subdivisions include anatomy, physiology, biochemistry, pathology, bacteriology. General biology, the study of the progressive development of tissues and cells and the laws of their evolution, is as necessary a basis for the comprehension of medicine as are any of the applied specialties.

These studies received their greatest impetus in the second half of the nineteenth century, when the application of the cell doctrine, evolved by Schleiden and Schwann and brought to completion by Virchow, was made to newly developing fields. In the subject of heredity, both of the individual and of the species, which was brought into prominence by the work of Charles Darwin, new discoveries brought new points of view and led the way to many theoretical and practical advances. LINNAEUS' belief in the immutability of species was upheld by CUVIER, whose " catastrophe " theory proposed that existent species were eradicated with each geologic period; he did not discuss the creation of new species. The concept of evolution, which had begun to take definite form in the writings of Erasmus DARWIN, Lamarck (*Philosophie zoologique*, 1809), and Étienne Geoffroy SAINT-HILAIRE, found its definitive form in the theory of Charles Darwin. The variations in species depend, according to Darwin, on various naturally acting causes and especially on the struggle for existence and on its related

" natural selection." The consequences of this doctrine for the development of biology, and therefore for medical science, were of prime importance; because, obviously according to it, only the study of antecedent species, whether still or no longer in existence, could give an adequate explanation of the phenomena exhibited by living species. The fundamental " biogenetic " law, formulated in 1872 by Ernst HAECKEL, asserts that ontogeny — that is, the history of the formation of the individual — is but the repetition of phylogenetic history — the formation of the species to which the individual belongs.

This is not the place to trace the polemics produced by this doctrine; or the formation of two groups: (1) the *neo-Darwinists*, who maintained the inheritance of congenital characteristics and denied that of acquired characteristics, according to the continuity of the germ plasma theory of August WEISMANN (1834–1914), who combined it with " the omnipotence of natural selection "; and (2) the *neo-Lamarckists*, who maintained the inheritance of acquired characteristics — E. D. COPE (1840–97), Herbert SPENCER, and A. GIRARD (1846–1908). Nor will we speak of newer concepts in this field, such as the discontinuous variations or *mutations* of the Dutch botanist DE VRIES — spontaneous variations of specific hereditary characters that " breed true " (1886). It should be noted, however, that Darwin's theory of the origin of species has remained in spite of all attacks the fundamental basis of biological study.

Turning to CYTOLOGY (the study of cells), following the activity produced by the announcement of the cell theory, a second period of activity appeared in the seventies with the early researches on minute cell details, fertilization, and cell division; and again a third period, at the turn of the century, with the rediscovery of the Mendelian theory, the study of cytoplasm and of living cells, and the utilization of the experimental method in exploring cell function and somatic development. BRÜCKE's theory of the cell as an elementary organism has been modified by later studies. It remains, however, as the basic unit of life, because the supposed existence of cells without nuclei, able to survive and even to multiply indefinitely, was found to be wrong when a better microscopic technique revealed the presence of a nucleus, and when bacteria, at first thought to be without nuclei, were shown by nuclear stains to be practically all nuclei. Recent studies (1932–44) by Ethel B. HARVEY, to be sure, have shown that under appropriate conditions some cells, though deprived of their nuclei, but probably not of their centrospheres, may survive and even multiply to a limited extent, whether fertilized or not. To BIZZOZERO belongs the credit of being the first to show (1868) that even such nucleus-free cells as mammalian erythrocytes at one time had had nuclei and had lost them. Max SCHULTZE had already shown (1861) that a cell was not a hollow structure, but " a small mass of protoplasm endowed with the attributes of life." Thus the concept of the nucleus and protoplasm as essential to the cell remained unchallenged, and studies of the structure of the cell followed rapidly. The filamentous structure of animal protoplasm (Flemming, 1882), — thread-like masses (*mitoma*), with interfilamentous substance (*paramitoma*) — was suggested; then R. ALTMANN's granular structure, then BÜTSCHLI's alveolar or froth theory (1891). All these studies led to the fundamental concept that life is closely connected with the colloidal structure of protoplasm (see Graham's *Clinical and Physical Researches*, Edinburgh, (1876).

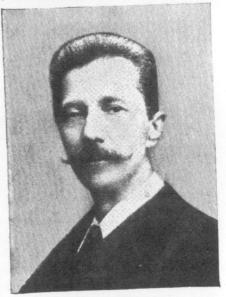

Studies of the structure of the cell nucleus, begun by Brown and Purkinje, led to the discovery of its granules and nuclear membrane, and to the distinction between *chromatin* (Flemming's term, 1879), the stainable material, and *achromatin*, the nuclear juice. Among other studies of prime

382. *Giulio Bizzozero.*

importance should be mentioned those of Weigert, Ehrlich, and others on the microchemistry (staining qualities) of the cell. To explain the multiplication of cells, Virchow in 1855 formulated the axiom: " *Omnis cellula e cellula*," [1] which was further refined by Flemming to " *Omnis nucleus e nucleo.*" Remak's (1858) studies on the division of cells, observations on the polarization of protoplasm, and on the indirect division of the nucleus, first observed by Schneider, further added to comprehension of the picture of cell division. The word " protoplasm " was first (1846) given by the botanist Hugo VON MOHL to the contents of the cell — " cell " being a term that in the etymological sense is correct for plant tissues only — though Purkinje had applied it to undifferentiated fetal tissue in 1839. Following the discovery of the centrosome by Flemming (1875) and, independently, by

[1] This well-known dictum, which Virchow put forth when he finally abandoned the theory of spontaneous generation of cells, has recently been ascribed to Leydig by C. Oberling (*Le problème du cancer*, 1942, p. 31). This, however, lacks supporting evidence and appears to have been due to a misinterpretation of a statement by Marc Klein in his *Histoire des origines de la théorie cellulaire* (1936).

E. VAN BENEDEN (1876), it was regarded by the latter and by Theodor Boveri (who named it) as an important and autonomous " dynamic centre " of the cell, which also divided with the division of the cell (1887–8). Eventually the four most important phases of indirect cell division (rearrangement of the chromosomes in prophase, metaphase, anaphase, and telophase) were observed; also the distinction between indirect division (*mitosis*, Flemming, 1882) and direct division of nucleus and cell (*amitosis*). The autonomy of the cell in the complete organism was established; it became regarded as an individuality with a life of its own, existing in a sort of social arrangement whereby all the cells were subdivided into regions and directed by a superior organization. But more recent studies have demonstrated that chemical, physical, and electrical phenomena of great biological importance are active outside the cell, thus demanding that the theory of the cell as the basis of vital activity be reinforced by a modern humoral doctrine.

Exploration of the structure and function of the cytoplasm — the nonnuclear portion of the cell — included the recognition of mitochondria by Altmann, between 1880 and 1890, and doubtless by earlier pioneers in cytology. Though the various forms and arrangements taken by these bodies in different species in health and disease have been satisfactorily determined and something learned of their chemical composition, it must be admitted that thus far their significance in the cell is still a matter of conjecture. The same may be said of the Golgi apparatus, first observed by the Italian neurologist in 1898, with the added disadvantage in this case that it cannot be studied in living cells as can mitochondria.

Studies on FERTILIZATION and HEREDITY logically followed the acquisition of knowledge of the finer details of cell form and nature. The origin and the constitution of the sperm cell and its motility were explored especially by SERTOLI and Merkel. The constitution of the ovum and its relation to fertilization were explored by Hertwig (1875), Merkel (1881), and Boveri. The ovum and spermatozoon, each known for many years, had been shown by M. BARRY (1843) to unite in the process of fertilization. The observations in 1875 of O. HERTWIG (1849–1922) on artificial fertilization of the ovum of the sea urchin showed that the head (nucleus) of the spermatozoon quickly penetrated into the protoplasm of the ovum and united with the female nucleus.

Parthenogenesis (the development of the female ovum into an organism without fertilization) is known to occur in some species. It was produced (1901) by J. LOEB (1859–1924) experimentally in sea urchins, normally incapable of developing without fertilization, by changing the constitution of the sea water in which the ova were immersed. Similar results have also been obtained by " needling " unfertilized ova. These studies, together with many others on the effects of various forms of physical energy on living matter, resulted in his theory of " tropisms " (1890), attributing all activity of lower forms of animal life to physical and chemical stimuli unaffected by volition. They culminated

in the exposition of a mechanistic theory of life in his book *The Organism as a Whole* (1916). In the fertilized ovum, the male and female nuclei come to lie side by side, to form the primary nucleus of the embryo, and the chromatin of each divides into a number of chromosomes (Waldeyer, 1888). This number differs in each species, being 48 in man, but is the same in each cell of a given animal and species. These chromosomes then, having arranged themselves in a spindle, split longitudinally (W. Flemming, 1879) and form separate asters, and thus the inheritance from each parent is maintained in the nuclei of the new-formed cells. In 1902 C. E. McClung (1870–1946) discovered the " x " or sex chromosome, which is combined with a " y " chromosome in the male, as compared to two " x " chromosomes in the female. Many lower animals are bi-

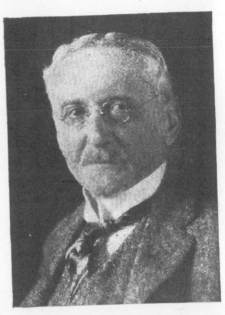

383. *Jacques Loeb.*

sexual, and even in man an occasional true hermaphrodite is found. In all mammals, however, certain anatomical and functional vestiges of bisexuality remain. The functional vestiges are manifested in the secondary sex characteristics, which by hormonal action can show such sex reversals as crowing hens, bearded ladies, and the like.

These and similar discoveries have given support to the mechanistic theory that life is merely a complicated physicochemical process as yet but partially understood. Though this has been a more productive hypothesis than the opposing " vitalism," the latter has not lacked adherents and has acquired new support in recent years. In H. Driesch's " dynamic vitalism," a theory of the autonomy of living processes, he raised four telling arguments against the mechanistic theory and proposed a quantitative modification of Aristotle's concept of entelechy, in an effort to give logical expression to biological realities. Details of the controversy, which is still unsettled, are far beyond the scope of this narrative.

SEGMENTATION OF THE OVUM had been observed and explained in 1826 by RUSCONI, who had correctly evaluated this process as the result of, and not the preparatory step toward, fertilization. These studies were furthered by the work of a number of scientists, such as that of NEWPORT (1853) on the ovum of the frog. A distinction was made between individual and hereditary elements, which led to the theory that the germ plasm was continuous from one generation to another. The botanist K. W. VON NÄGELI (1817–91) proposed the dis-

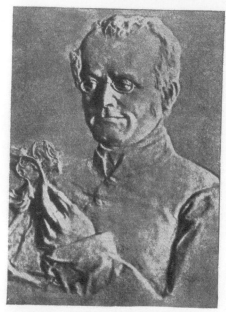

tinction between the vegetative *tropho-plasm* and the hereditary *ideoplasm*, in which was to be found every quality of the adult organism. A long discussion was opened on the hereditary nature of physical qualities and on the effect of various stimuli on hereditary tendencies. This led to new experimental investigations, especially on the *nature of hybrids*. According to the *Mendelian law*, the discovery of the Augustinian monk Gregor MENDEL (1822–84), when pure strains are cross-bred, the qualities inherited from the original parents occur in proportions subject to laws that can be stated with exactness. Though later discoveries have required a considerable amplification of Mendel's dominant-recessive ratio, the law remains one of the most important pillars of the genetic structure.

384. *Gregor Mendel.*
Bas-relief by T. Charlemont.

No less important were the results of these studies in explaining hitherto unknown phenomena of embryonal life, the formation of organs in the embryo and the development from embryonal cells. Ernst HAECKEL (1834–1919) evolved the theory of an original hypothetical structure called the *gastræa* as the ancestral form of all multicellular organisms (1884). Oscar HERTWIG (1849–1922) proposed the theory of the *cölom*, based on two mesodermic cavities that were found in higher animals during embryonal life, which grew between the two primary germinal layers, ectoderm and endoderm. Among the best-known of these students of embryonal life was Wilhelm HIS (1831–1904), who is often called the founder of modern embryology.

3. Anatomy

The anatomy of the later half of the nineteenth century, influenced by the work of the great microscopists of the earlier half, has been directed toward the microscopy of finer tissue details rather than to that general morphology which had constituted the most important part of anatomy up to this time. With the perfection of methods of study — the microtome, new staining methods, and improvements in the microscope — histologic and cytologic knowledge was greatly extended. The anatomists of this period were also great biologists — such as Max SCHULTZE (1825–74) and later W. FLEMMING (1843–95) — who successfully attacked many difficult problems of cell life.

Of basic importance was Schultze's concept of the cell — independently of Brücke — not as a membranous bag about a cavity, but as a jelly-like mass enclosing a nucleus. He also established the idea that protoplasm existed widespread through the animal and vegetable kingdoms. In addition to valuable contributions to zoology and embryology, he wrote important articles on the sense organs (ear, 1858; nose, 1863; retina, 1866), introduced new techniques, and founded the *Archiv für mikroskopische Anatomie* (1865). Flemming, whose work has already been noted in the section on Biology, further developed the knowledge of protoplasm and cell multiplication and of the structure of lymph nodes and other organs. Many anatomists were also embryologists, pupils of the great Johannes Müller and Kölliker, like W. HIS, Sr. (1831–1904) and Francis Maitland BALFOUR (1851–82), the author of a great *Treatise on Comparative Embryology* (1880–1), who did much of his work at the Zoological Laboratory at Naples. The tragic death of Balfour at the early age of thirty-one while Alpine mountain-climbing, was undoubtedly a major loss to British biology of the end of the nineteenth century.

Among the isolated discoveries of the period was that of the small parathyroid glands — by Ivar SANDSTROM (1852–89) in 1879 — the brief description by R. Owen in 1862 having apparently passed unnoticed. The cell groups scattered through the pancreas that are now known to manufacture insulin were first reported (1869) by Paul LANGERHANS (1847–88) in his inaugural dissertation.

The microscopic examination of tissues — virtually a new field initiated by the cell theory — was greatly aided by various technical devices, which have by no means become exhausted even now. It is difficult to realize that the all-important pioneer work of a century ago was accomplished largely on teased-out, unstained specimens, floated on to thick, uneven slides. In 1842 Schleiden, complaining of the lack of a book on histologic methods, suggested free-hand cutting of tissues with a razor. The sliding microtome, first used in the eighteenth century, made but little headway till aided by embedding material that permeated and held soft tissues firmly (such as soap, Flemming, 1873; turpentine-paraffin, 1876; celloidin, Duval, 1879; chloroform-paraffin, Klebs, 1881). Only with the last named did serial sections become possible. The rotary microtome was invented in 1885 by C. S. Minot of Harvard and Pfeifer of Johns Hopkins independently. To alcohol, oldest of the fixatives, A. HAN-

NOVER (1814–94) added chromic acid (1844); W. Flemming, chrom-osmic-acetic acid; K. Zenker, potassium bichromate and mercury bichloride. Osmic acid, as a fat-precipitant, was found especially valuable for the nervous system. When formalin was added to the list (F. and J. BLUM, 1893), various combinations, usually bearing the name of the combiner, were introduced, each with its special purposes and supporters. The cut sections were first stained with carmine, and it was with this that Virchow did most of his work. Though Corti had used it on the cochlea in 1851, its real introduction followed J. von GERLACH's (1820–96) fortunate oversight (1858) in exposing a hardened section of cerebellum to it overnight. Hematoxylin was introduced as a nuclear stain by F. BOEHMER in 1865; and when Fischer produced eosin as a counterstain in 1875, the groundwork for tissue-staining had been laid. Saffron is said to have been used by Vieussens and even by Leeuwenhoek in earlier centuries. New methods (such as von Recklinghausen's silver impregnation, about 1900), materials, and combinations have continued, and still continue, to be useful in differential staining of tissues and cell components, different modifications being required for the killed tissues and for the vital staining of still living cells.

Histologic details of the intricate nervous tissue invited many studies during this period, beginning with Virchow's description of the supporting tissue — neuroglia. Kühne investigated the end plates of the motor nerves (1862); Schultze, of the sensory nerves (1858–66); O. F. C. DEITERS (1834–63) demonstrated the connection of the nerve cell with the axis cylinder (1855); Wladimir BETZ (1834–94), the large "Betz cells" of the pyramidal area (1874); L. A. RANVIER, the structure of the nerve sheaths and the "nodes of Ranvier"; Franz NISSL (1860–1919), the characteristic granules of the ganglion cells (1894). Camillo GOLGI (1843–1926), of Cortona, a pupil of Bizzozero, began in 1870 his studies on the interstitial tissue of the nervous system, together with investigation of the grey matter of the cerebrum (1870) and the finer anatomy of the cerebellum (1874). He was the first to use the chrome-silver-nitrate staining method, which brought out new histologic details of the finer structure of the brain and spinal cord. In 1883 he demonstrated in the central nervous system multipolar cells with long and short axis cylinders and dendritic arborizations that are called "Golgi cells." Such studies, added to those of the earlier anatomists and the observations on the degeneration of the nerve fibre when severed from its nerve cell ("Wallerian degeneration") led to Waldeyer's important formulation of the neuron theory (1891). In this now universally accepted concept, which underlies all neurological study, the unit of the nervous system is the neuron, consisting of a cell with many branching processes, which are characteristically of two sorts: a single long discharging axone, or axis cylinder process, and a multiple network of short dendrites that establish connections with other nerve cells. Equally distinguished with Golgi was the Spaniard RAMÓN Y CAJAL (1852–1934), who worked in the same field with successful results.

Cajal's improvements on Golgi's staining method produced further cytological discoveries in various parts of the nervous system, collected in *The Degeneration and Regeneration of the Nervous System* (English translation, Oxford, 1928). The most celebrated of his pupils are Nicolás ACHUCARRO (1881–1918), Pio del Rio HORTEGA (d. 1945), who produced still further improvements in staining methods, which permitted the discovery of two new types of glia cells: mesodermal microglia and ectodermal oligodendroglia, and J. F. TELLO Y MUÑOZ (b. 1880), who studied the neurofibrillæ of lower vertebrates.

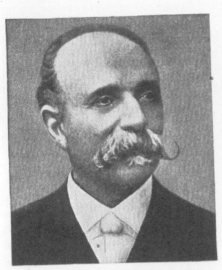

385. *Camillo Golgi, Nobel Laureate, 1906.*

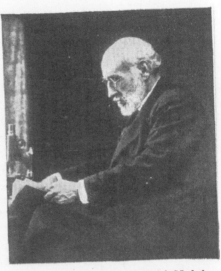

386. *Santiago Ramón y Cajal, Nobel Laureate, 1906.*

In hematology, new staining methods led to identification, chiefly by Ehrlich, of various types of leucocytes. "Plasma cell" was the name given by Waldeyer (1875) to a kind of connective-tissue cell. The cell known by that name today was first recognized by Cajal (1890), and named by Unna (1891). The "irritation form" of the lymphocyte was described in 1904 by W. TUERCK (1871–1916), and other forms by Naegeli. The basophilic mast cell goes back to von Recklinghausen. Recognition of the blood plates (thrombocytes), usually ascribed to Bizzozero, was probably achieved by the Frenchmen J. DONNE in 1842 and DENYS in 1887.

Thus anatomy, no longer a cold science limited to the observation of the dead body, had developed in close communion with biology and physiology into a consideration of the nature of all the elements that comprise the animal organism, in order to discover their origin and function.

Among the outstanding German anatomists of this period were F. G. MERKEL (1845–1919), noted for his studies of connective tissue; and Wilhelm HIS, SR.

(1831–1904), of Basel, who made contributions of the highest importance to knowledge of the origin of tissues and to anthropology. Details of his scientific work may be read in his *Lebenserinnerungen* (Leipzig, 1903). His *Die Häute und Höhlen des Körpers* (Basel, 1865) introduced a new classification of tissues for embryological study, while by the use of serial sections and three-dimensional models he made reproductions of microscopic anatomy of permanent value. His *Anatomie menschlicher Embryonen* (1880–5) presented the first study of the human embryo as a whole. In 1886 came his demonstration that the axis cylinder is a part of the nerve cell. He was one of the organizers of the Anatomische Gesellschaft; and founded the *Archiv für Anthropologie* and the *Zeitschrift für Anatomie und Entwicklungsgeschichte* (1876), which, as the *Anatomische Abteilung* of Du Bois-Reymond's *Archiv*, he edited from 1877 to 1903. His ability in this field is shown in the anecdote of his identification by comparative measurements of the remains of Sebastian Bach (1895). One of his pupils, F. P. MALL (1862–1917), greatly stimulated the scientific study of embryology and anatomy in America; pupils of Mall were R. G. Harrison, G. L. Streeter, W. Lewis; Streeter long directed the Carnegie Institute for Embryology at Baltimore, which was founded by Mall and has been an important centre of embryological research. Also to be noted are the names of Karl REICHERT (1811–83), for his studies on the acoustic macula and the germ layers, and on the development of amphibian crania; and T. Nathaniel LIEBERKÜHN (1711–56), who studied the eyes of vertebrates and discovered the intestinal glands that bear his name. Franz von LEYDIG (1821–1908) first described the interstitial cells of the testicle, which now are recognized as the source of a male hormone (ANCEL and BOUIN, 1923) and early (1856) recognized the nature of cell protoplasm. Wilhelm von WALDEYER (1836–1921), director of the Berlin Anatomical Institute, described the group of tonsillar tissue about the pharynx, known as "Waldeyer's ring." His discovery of the germinal epithelium and his already mentioned construction of the *neuron theory* were of prime importance. Emil ZUCKERKANDL (1849–1910), professor at the University of Vienna, was known for his studies of the anatomy of the nasal cavity and its accessory sinuses, and of the ear, and for the discovery of the small body still known as "Zuckerkandl's organ." The eminent pathologist Solomon STRICKER (1834–98) contributed useful studies on the anatomy of the tissues, the structure and proliferation of cells, and the anatomy of the cornea. Carl HEITZMAN (1836–96) is known for his *Anatomical Atlas*, which served for more than three decades in the teaching of anatomy in German universities; and Karl BARDELEBEN (1849–1918) for extensive investigations and anatomical works and especially for the monumental *Handbuch der Anatomie* (1896–1915), in many volumes, which he edited. Outstanding in comparative anatomy was Karl GEGENBAUR (1826–1903), who showed that the vertebrate ovum was a single cell, and that Goethe and Owen were wrong in regarding the skull as being a fusion of vertebræ. He wrote treatises on human and on comparative anatomy that went through many editions, and attracted many pupils (FÜRBRINGER, RUGE, MAURER, H. BRAUS, and a number of Americans).

French anatomists included M. F. C. SAPPEY (1810–96), A. A. VERNEUIL (1823–95), P. E. LAUNOIS (1856–1914), G. P. POIRIER (1853–1907), NICHOLAS, and G. E. LAGUESSE (1861–1927), founders of the Association of Anatomists. Among histologists, Louis RANVIER (1835–1922) studied the peripheral nerves ("nodes of Ranvier," 1878) and connective-tissue cells (clasmatocytes); and A. PRENANT (1861–1925) wrote a valu-able treatise on histology and an excel-lent book on embryology.

Among Americans, Charles S. MINOT (1852–1914), Professor of Embryology and Comparative Anatomy at Harvard, wrote various important books on em-bryology, which were translated into several languages. He invented im-proved forms of the sledge microtome, designed the rotary form that is in general use today, and made valuable anatomical studies, especially on the pla-centa (1891). His "law of cytomorpho-sis" (in *Age, Growth, and Death*, 1908) postulates that the ageing process is due to the constant change of protoplasm into less flexible form. G. H. PARKER's (b. 1864) *The Elementary Nervous System* (1919) presents the results of

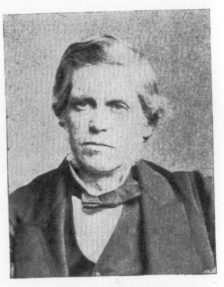

387. *Sir William Bowman.*

his studies on the persistence in higher vertebrates of primitive neuromuscular mechanisms, and his evidence that muscle differentiates in the embryo before the nervous system (cf. Galen's law that function determines structure). Mall and his pupils have already been mentioned.

In Belgium, P. J. VAN BENEDEN, Professor of Zoology at Liège and co-dis-coverer of the chromosomes, later (1883–7) showed that these bodies were de-rived equally from both parents, thus advancing knowledge both of cellular division and of the relation of the chromosomes to heredity. His pupil BRACHET, professor at Brussels, specialized in experimental embryology.

Among English anatomists of the period was William BOWMAN (1816–92), who discovered in the kidney the glomerular capsule that bears his name, and evolved a filtration theory of urine formation that is the most important element in the present concept of that process. Later in life he became an eminent oph-thalmologist.

Italian anatomy had as its chief representative in this period Eusebio OEHL (1827–1903), whose important treatise on the microscopic anatomy of the skin

(1857) was reproduced almost in its entirety in 1890 by UNNA of Hamburg. His histological and physiological studies have interesting relations with the later work of Pavlov. Among Oehl's pupils were E. Sertoli, remembered for his description of the " cells of Sertoli " in the testicle, and G. Bizzozero, undoubtedly the greatest Italian pathologist of the second half of the nineteenth century. At twenty-six Bizzozero was already Professor of General Pathology at Turin; in his laboratory there studied surgeons like BASSINI, clinicians like Forlanini and Bozzolo, pathologists like GRIFFINI and P. FOÀ, A. RUFFINI (1864–1929), author of important studies on gastrulation, and G. LEVI (b. 1872), distinguished for his investigations on the structure of growth. The foundation of the zoological laboratory at Naples by Anton DOHRN also had an important influence on biological studies in Italy.

The study of human PALÆOANATOMY and PALÆOPATHOLOGY began during this period, following the discovery of the Neanderthal man in 1856 and of the *Pithecanthropus erectus* by E. Dubois in the Trinil gravel beds of Java. The femur of the latter, now thought to be the oldest of human remains, is of " interest in that it is the site of a definite diseased outgrowth of bone." Prehistoric human bones have now been found in various parts of Europe, Africa, and Asia (Palestine, China) that have suggested many problems that are still under discussion (see Chapter xxi). The palæopathologic studies of M. A. RUFFER (1859–1917), Roy MOODIE (1880–1934), G. Elliot SMITH (1871–1937), and others on disease processes in Egyptian mummies reveal many bony diseases in man much as they exist today, while examples of repaired fractures, chronic arthritis, and other bony lesions have been found in animals as far back as the Permian Period.

ANTHROPOLOGY in this period was advanced by the studies of Broca, Virchow, Darwin, Huxley, Lyell, Spencer, and J. L. Q. DE BRÉAU (1810–92) on savage and fossil man. In 1886 Alphonse BERTILLON (1853–1914) established his method of identifying criminals by anthropometric measurements. In 1892 Francis GALTON demonstrated the identification value of fingerprints (dactyloscopy). In the many thousands of cases that have been examined, the prints of no two individuals have been found to be exactly alike. The method therefore has proved to be of great practical identification value in criminology and after mutilating accidents, and also in preventing confusion of the newborn in obstetrical hospitals. There is now an interesting movement under way in America to get all persons to have their fingerprints recorded. In Italy important studies of Italian crania were made by L. CALORI, founder of the National Museum of Anthropology (1869), and of the *Homo mediterraneus* by G. SERGI. LOMBROSO's contributions to the pathological and criminal side of the subject are world-famous (cf. *L'Uomo delinquente*, 1876).

4. Physiology

In the past century, physiology has undergone a development unsurpassed throughout its previous history. Research in this field is seldom conducted by single investigators, but by groups who have dedicated themselves to the solution of special problems. Every phase of physiology has flourished and new concepts and complex hypotheses have been proved by decisive results obtained from sound methods. The true foundations of gross and microscopic anatomy having been laid, science turned more intensively to the study of function. In all branches of physiology, with the aid of physics and chemistry, discovery followed discovery, new problems became manifest, and unsuspected interrelations between tissues and organs appeared, which gave rise to a new concept that we might call neo-humoralism. Let us summarize a few of the more typical and important results.

In the domain of the physiology of the BLOOD, the role of the leucocytes was established in inflammation, which together with cancer is the most important of pathologic phenomena. Though Thomas Addison had observed this (1843), and G. Zimmerman had recognized their importance in inflammation (1852), Virchow's *Cellular Pathologie* had denied that leucocytes were identical with pus cells. The experiments of Julius COHNHEIM (1839–84), however, established the correct view (1867) and, taken with Elie METCHNIKOFF's (1845–1916) discovery of phagocytosis (1892), overthrew Virchow's erroneous views on inflammation. The discovery of the blood platelets is ascribed to the gifted Bizzozero (1883). They appear to have been first described as a third blood particle by Alfred DONNÉ (1801–78) in 1842, and more fully by M. Schultze (1865) and Osler (1873). In 1878 they were shown by the founder of modern hematology, G. HAYEM (1841–1933), to be chiefly concerned with coagulation, and their origin from processes of the megakaryocyte in the bone marrow was described by J. H. WRIGHT (1869–1928). The general phenomena of coagulation were explored by Alexander SCHMIDT (1831–94), O. HAMMERSTEN (1841–1922), P. MANTEGAZZA (1831–1910), P. MORAWITZ (1879–1936), A. E. WRIGHT (1861–1947), W. H. HOWELL (1860–1945), and many others. Study of the resistance of the red blood cells to anisotonic fluids has been a fruitful method in both physiology and clinical medicine. Hypotonic salt solution was used for this purpose by Duncan in 1867, and again by L. C. A. MALASSEZ (1842–1909) in 1872, but this development received its chief impulse from the work (1903) of H. J. HAMBURGER (1859–1924).

The physiology of the CIRCULATION attained highly valuable discoveries with the aid of instruments of greater and greater precision. The studies of H. P. BOWDITCH (1840–1911), T. W. ENGELMANN (1843–1909), Gaskell, Luciani, and

G. FANO (1856–1930), Hugo KRONECKER (1839–1914), and Wilhelm HIS, Jr. (1863–1934), on the rhythmic activity of the heart, and the myogenic origin of the heart-beat; and the discovery by the brothers Ernst Heinrich (1795–1878) and Edward Friedrich WEBER (1806–71) of the inhibitory influence of the vagus on cardiac action gave a firm foundation for the later triumphs of cardiology. Albert von BEZOLD, who had discovered the accelerator nerves of the heart and their origin in the spinal cord (1863), showed that after they and the vagi had been cut, the heart still could be stimulated to contract by pressure.

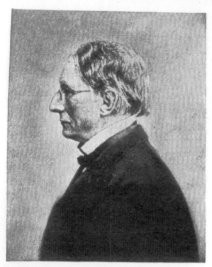

388. *Carl Friedrich Ludwig.*

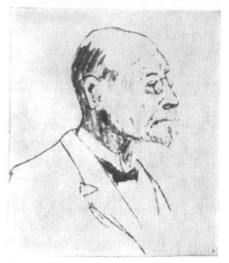

389. *W. Einthoven, Nobel Laureate, 1924.*
(Pencil sketch by K. J. Franklin, M.D.)

Moritz SCHIFF (1823–96), a pupil of Magendie, had already shown the presence of vasomotor fibres (vasoconstrictor) in the cervical sympathetic (1856). Quantitative estimation of the output of the heart was begun by A. FICK (1829–1901) on the principle of its estimation through the respiratory exchange (1870), and by N. ZINTZ (1847–1920) and O. HAGEMANN (1862–1926) in 1898.

Of the greatest importance in the physiology of the circulation and the basis of much future work were the studies of Carl LUDWIG (1816–95), one of the greatest masters of physiology of modern times. He was Professor of Anatomy at Marburg, then at Zurich and Vienna and for thirty years at Leipzig, where he founded a model physiological institute to which pupils came from all parts of the world. His major contribution, even above his own discoveries, is to be found in the education and stimulation that he gave his students. To him is owed the introduction of the graphic method of recording (especially of the kymograph [1847], the *Stromuhr*, the mercury manometer), the filtration theory of renal secretion, the discovery of the innervation of the submaxillary glands (1851), and the important observation that they could be made to secrete by stimulating the sympathetic system (1856). A vivid picture of Ludwig's personality and influence is to be found in the tributes of his pupils, von Kries, Kronecker, Burdon Sanderson and William Stirling. Aiming solely to advance science and to build capable investigators, yet furnishing them with problems, often even planning the details and carrying them out himself, he published much of his work under the name of or in collaboration with younger men. The list of these who reached eminence, too long to mention here, includes such names as Bowditch, Brunton, Cloetta, von Cyon, Dogiel, Lothar Meyer, Mosso, Schweigger-Seidel, Schmiedeberg. Many agree that he was " the greatest teacher of physiology who ever lived."

Fundamental for knowledge of the nature of the HEART-BEAT were the discovery (1893) of the auriculo-ventricular bundle by Wilhelm His, Jr. (1863–1934), the registration of the electrical impulses of the heart (1879) by J. Burdon Sanderson (1829–1905) and Page and (1888) by A. D. Waller (1856–1922) and G. Fano, which culminated in W. Einthoven's (1860–1927) electrocardiograph (a light and extremely delicate string galvanometer that reduced inertia and periodicity of the electrical deflections to a minimum). The sensitivity and precision of this instrument quickly produced a correct analysis of the various types of cardiac arrhythmias, especially in the hands of Sir Thomas Lewis (1881–1945), and has permitted progress in the study of the dynamics of cardiac action in health and disease that still continues undiminished.

The action of the isolated heart was illuminated by H. N. Martin's (1848–96) method of isolation (1880); by Kronecker's proof of the failure of the heart muscle to tetanize and its disorderly action when " Kronecker's point " is punctured; by Sydney Ringer's (1835–1910) combination of salts (" Ringer's solution ") that greatly prolonged the heart's survival time; by the " block " effects of the H. Stannius (1808–83) sinu-auricular clamp (1852) and the W. H. Gaskell (1847–1914) auriculoventricular clamp (1882).

The physiology of RESPIRATION. Knowledge of how the body used oxygen — most important of the materials that support life — was slow in accumulating. In the eighteenth century Lavoisier had recognized the analogy between respiration and combustion, but erroneously believed that the change took place in the lung; in the second half of the century J. H. Hassenfratz (1755–1827) had shown (1791) that the blood contains not only oxygen from the air, but carbon dioxide from the tissues. Gustav Magnus inferred from the relations of oxygen to CO_2 in the arteries and veins that respiration (i.e., exchange of O_2 and CO_2) occurred in the tissues (1837, 1845). This was confirmed by C. MATTEUCCI's (1811–68) discovery (1856) that isolated muscles respire (i.e., consume oxygen) and give off heat and Lothar MEYER's recognition (1857) that the oxygen was held by some kind of chemical union. This control was attributed by Hoppe-Seyler (1862) to hemoglobin, whose spectrum had been discovered by Ångström in 1855. The proof that the essential seat of respiration was in the tissues and not in the blood was furnished by the work of F. W. PFLÜGER (1829–1910) and his pupils on the gasometry of the blood (1866), on the mechanism of respiration (1868), and on O and CO_2 interchange in various experimental conditions (1875). The relation of atmospheric pressure to respiration was studied especially by Angelo Mosso (1846–1910), whose laboratory on Monte Rosa became an important centre for the study of the effects of high altitudes. His view, however, that the ensuing dyspnea was caused by acapnia (lack of CO_2) has been displaced by the demonstration by J. S. HALDANE (1860–1936), C. G. DOUGLAS, and Joseph BARCROFT (1872–1947) that it was due to the diminished oxygen pressure in the rarefied atmosphere. Mosso is also remembered for his concept of fatigue (1891), investigated with the ergograph, as due to an identifiable tonic substance produced by muscle activity; also for his demonstration of the reflex nature of deglutition. Luigi LUCIANI's (1842–1919) studies on intrathoracic and intra-abdominal pressure, and the researches of Schiff, Brachet, and especially Hering on the respiratory centre, were also important.

Study of the internal secretions (ENDOCRINOLOGY) has assumed the highest importance in recent times. The doctrine of internal secretion of certain ductless glands, first conceived by Claude Bernard, had been initiated by P. Mantegazza and supported by Brown-Séquard, who showed (1856) that removal of the adrenal glands caused death of the animal. Shortly before, Thomas Addison had brought these glands into relation with the fatal disease that bears his name (1849–55). Various disturbances had been observed by RESTELLI (1845) after extirpating the thymus, and deficiency phenomena found by the Swiss surgeon Kocher (1880) and the cousins Reverdin after extirpation of the thyroid gland. Among the contributions of the Italian school to this subject were Luciani's theory that the task of the thyroid was the disintoxication of the organism, and the work of Giulio VASSALE (1862–1912), a foreshadower of the discovery of insulin, on the fatal effects of removal of the pituitary and on the function of the parathyroid glands (use of parathyroid extract in tetany).

Diabetes·mellitus, known but not understood for centuries, was said (with but little justification, to be sure) to be connected with the pancreas as early as

1788 (Cawley, *London Medical Journal,* 1788, IX, 286). This connection was definitely recognized (1877) by Étienne LANCEREAUX (1829?–1910). The condition was produced experimentally by the clinicians VON MERING and MINKOWSKI by removing dogs' pancreas (1889); Minkowski having already studied the acidotic urine of diabetes (1884), and von Mering having produced glycosuria with phlorhizin (1886). The pathologic microscopic studies of OPIE (1901) connected the islands of the pancreas with human diabetes, and the na-

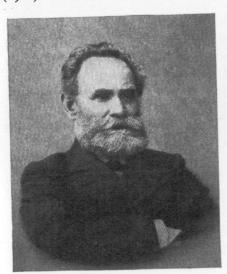 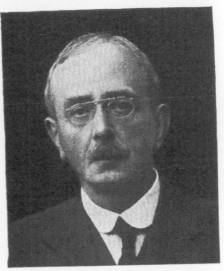

390. *Ivan Petrovich Pavlov,*   391. *C. S. Sherrington,*
Nobel Laureate, 1904.   *Nobel Laureate, 1932.*

ture of the disease was further elucidated by the chemical studies of NAUNYN. (who introduced the term " acidosis "), MAGNUS-LEVY, and others. The islands of Langerhans were first associated (1893) with an internal secretion by G. E. LAGUESSE (1861–1927). Exophthalmic goitre and myxœdema, which were known clinically since the first and third quarters of the nineteenth century, respectively, were connected with dysfunction of the thyroid gland (1859–84) by the dog experiments of Moritz SCHIFF (1823–96) (removal of the thyroid with subsequent thyroid grafts or administration of thyroid extract). Experimental surgery (Sir Victor HORSLEY) showed that post-thyroidectomy cachexia, myxœdema, and cretinism were all due to lack of thyroid secretion. The chemical nature of the active agent was established (1896) by E. BOWMANN's (1846–1896) discovery of iodothyrin and E. C. KENDALL's isolation (1914) of the actual crystalline substance, thyroxin.

In the physiology of DIGESTION, especially important was the work of Ivan Petrovich PAVLOV (1849–1936) on gastric and pancreatic secretion.

His technique of preparing lasting and freely accessible gastric pouches and pancreatic fistulæ, without injuring nerve or blood supply of the affected organs, thus produced uncontaminated gastric juice and afforded valuable new information about gastric and pancreatic digestion. Perhaps chief among these observations was the proof of the so-called psychic secretion — the production of gastric juice without the introduction of food into the stomach (1879). These experiments, followed on a vast scale with the aid of his pupils, especially CHISCHIN, demonstrated *inter alia* the innervation of the pancreas from the vagus and other important relations. From Pavlov's studies has come the highly important concept of the conditioned reflex: that from frequent repetition of definite stimuli, reflexes can regularly be obtained that have no direct connection with the given stimulus. Thus bell-ringing, after having been sufficiently associated with the exhibition of food to hungry dogs, can produce a flow of gastric juice even when no food is exhibited (see his *Work of the Digestive Glands*, 1897).

The study of the function of the liver and pancreas, begun by Claude Bernard, was further expanded by his pupils and successors. His pupil Willy KÜHNE (1837–1900), Professor of Physiology at Amsterdam and Heidelberg, who also conducted valuable investigations of the properties of muscle and of the peripheral terminations of the motor nerves (1862), was especially concerned with the intermediate products of gastric and intestinal digestion. He isolated trypsin (1874) and indole (1875) and practically founded the doctrine of enzymes (1878). Angelo Mosso demonstrated the essentially reflex character of the act of deglutition (1876) by showing that the peristaltic wave from the pharynx continues after section of the œsophagus, to be abolished, however, by section of the nerves. The independence of gastric motility from nerve stimulation was shown on the excised stomach by HOFMEISTER and SCHÜTZ, R. HEIDENHAIN, and W. B. Cannon, and in Carrel's ingenious extra-vital cultures of the excised stomach.

Knowledge of the physiology of the GALL BLADDER was advanced by the important studies of A. G. BARBERA (1867–1908). Gmelin's studies of the bile were continued by Berzelius's isolation of biliverdin (1840), HEINTZ's isolation of bilirubin (1851), A. STRECKER's (1822–71) identification of sodium glycocholate and taurocholate, and Max JAFFÉ's (1841–1911) discovery of urobilin in the urine (1868). It is only in recent times that the bile pigments have been conclusively shown to be formed from hemoglobin breakdown in the cells of the reticulo-endothelial system. Cholesterol, a prominent constituent of the bile and of gall-stones, is now known to be constantly present in the blood and of widespread though still obscurely understood importance in the body economy.

NEUROPHYSIOLOGY. In electrophysiology we note the studies of BIEDER-MANN (1895), HERING and WALLER, MATTEUCCI (1841) (secondary contraction), DU BOIS-REYMOND, BERNSTEIN, HERMANN. The studies of TÜRCK on the cutaneous distribution of the spinal nerves (1863) and of SETCHENOV on the central inhibition of spinal reflexes, with Cajal's correct inference that dendrites carried afferent impulses to the nerve cell, the axone carrying effector impulses from it, gave rise to the doctrine of synapses of the reflex arc, to which notable contributions were made by ERB, WESTPHAL, JENDRASSIK, and C. S. SHERRINGTON with his experimental studies (1895-8), leading to the concept of " reciprocal innervation " of muscle groups. By this is meant that when one set of muscles is stimulated (as in flexing the elbow), the opposing muscles are reflexly inhibited (i.e., the elbow's extensor muscles are relaxed).

Studies in *neurophysiology* led to investigation of the velocity of the nerve impulse (Helmholtz, 1850) and to a constantly increasing knowledge of the physiology of the spinal cord and its degenerative processes. The studies initiated by Charles Bell (1811) and F. Magendie were further developed in the doctrine of metameric division of sensory and motor roots, proved by Sherrington (1893) (see his *Integrative Action of the Nervous System*, 1906), and in the theory of reflexes, founded by Marshall HALL (1790-1857) and advanced by the work of Goltz, Schiff, and others.

Important progress was made in knowledge of the physiology of the BRAIN, beginning, as we have noted, with the early discoveries (1860) of Paul BROCA (1824-80). G. FRITSCH (1838-97) and E. HITZIG (1838-1907) were the first to show (1870) that excitation of single regions called motor areas, in the parietal lobe of the cortex, provoked localized movement of single groups of muscles. Luciani and Tamburini, together with Seppilli, further advanced knowledge of motor and sensory localization in the cerebral cortex. H. A. MUNK (1839-1912) asserted (1881) that there were also psychomotor and psychosensory centres; Bartolomeo PANIZZA (1785-1867) was the first to show the existence of a cortical visual zone. F. L. GOLTZ (1834-1902) also made important contributions to the problem of cortical physiology. Further impulse was given to these studies by the refinement in neurohistological technique of the Italian Camillo Golgi, and the Spaniard Ramón y Cajal. Cerebral localization was perfected by numerous other investigators, such as the Russian, Wladimir BECHTEREV (1857-1927) and especially P. E. FLECHSIG (1847-1929), who mapped out projection and association zones. It was this new knowledge that made possible the great development of cerebral surgery and also gave new impetus to the study of experimental psychology.

"English physiology," as Fulton puts it, "was Scottish born and London bred," and, it might be added, Dutch conceived, in view of Boerhaave's great influence. Andrew Sinclair, the first Edinburgh Professor of the Institutes of Medicine (so called because the course was based on Boerhaave's *Institutiones medicæ*), had such distinguished successors as Whytt, Cullen, and later (1848–74) J. Hughes BENNETT (1812–75), William RUTHERFORD (1839–99) from 1874 to 1899, and E. SHARPEY-SCHAFER (1850–1935) from 1899 to 1935. An Edinburgh graduate, William SHARPEY (1802–80), the first full-time English physiologist, and the first to hold the chair of physiology at University College, practically founded modern British physiology. Though his name today is perhaps better remembered for his anatomical studies — ear ossicles, the bone " fibres of Sharpey," and so on — his chief historical importance lies in the stimulation that he gave to the pursuit of the subject through his own activities and those of his pupils, Foster, Burdon Sanderson, and Sir Joseph Lister. Highly important contributions to the development of physiology were made by the English school at Cambridge, founded by Michael FOSTER (1836–1907), himself a zealous investigator of the heart (Cf. the inherent capacity of heart muscle to contract). He was author of an important textbook (which ran through seven editions and was translated into several languages) and also of a short but valuable history of physiology; was founder of the first Physiological Society (1876) and of the *Journal of Physiology* (1878) and instigated (1881) the formation of the first International Physiological Congress. He had many distinguished pupils: W. H. GASKELL (1847–1914) (physiology of the nervous system and the muscles and nerves of the heart); H. Newell MARTIN (1848–96), Professor of Biology at Johns Hopkins University, who studied the isolated heart and the effects of pressure and temperature changes on its rate; I. George ADAMI (1862–1926), the leading Canadian pathologist of his day, author of an important two-volume textbook on pathology, and student of heredity and of tumours; J. N. LANGLEY (1852–1925), Foster's successor as Professor of Physiology at Cambridge, noted for his work on the sympathetic nervous system. Among other eminent pupils of Foster were Sherrington, Sydney RINGER, Henry HEAD, and C. S. ROY (1854–97), in physiology; BALFOUR, in embryology; Milnes MARSHALL and SIDGWICK, in zoology; Francis DARWIN and VINES, in botany. Notable pupils of Gaskell and Langley, and thus continuers of the Cambridge school, were Gowland HOPKINS (1861–1947), Walter Morley FLETCHER (1873–1933), A. V. HILL (b. 1886), J. BARCROFT (1872–1947), G. R. MINES (d. 1914), Hugh ANDERSON (1865–1928), W. H. R. RIVERS (1864–1922), H. H. DALE (b. 1875), Keith LUCAS (1879–1916), E. D. ADRIAN (b.1889), G. Elliot SMITH (1871–1937). The Oxford school of physiology was founded (1878) by John Burdon SANDERSON

(1829–1905), a pupil of Sharpey's, who worked chiefly on the electric responses of irritable tissue with the use of the capillary electrometer. His successor, Francis GOTCH (1853–1913), was also an eminent electrophysiologist.

The physiology of the SENSE ORGANS was investigated by Lussana and by Luciani, while studies of the physiology of TASTE (begun by Malpighi's association of the tongue papillæ with taste), HEARING (see Helmholtz's monograph,

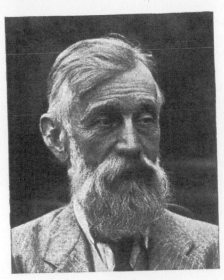

392. *Sir Michael Foster.*

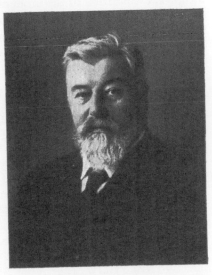

393. *W. H. Gaskell.*

1863), SPEECH (see Donder's monograph, 1870), and SMELL (Zwaardemaker) developed interesting and complex phenomena in the functioning of these organs. The physiology of VISION was so extensively pursued that we must content ourselves here with mentioning but a few items, such as Helmholtz's discovery of the ophthalmoscope, which was at the basis of much of the progress of modern ophthalmology. The theory of colour vision, earlier announced (1807) by Thomas Young with the assumption of three colour-sensitive elements in the retina, was amplified by the studies of J. DALTON (1766–1844) and A. F. HOLMGREN (1831–97) on colour blindness. New impulse was given by the theory of J. VON KRIES (1853–1928) of Frieburg that there were two active elements in the retina: the *rods*, which perceived light sensation, and the *cones*, which perceived sensations of colour. The physiology of ACCOMMODATION in man and animals was extensively studied by HELMHOLTZ (1854) and further amplified by BEER of Vienna (1899).

In this period also was begun a new discipline, EXPERIMENTAL PSYCHOLOGY (FECHNER, LOTZE, WUNDT, MACH, JAMES). At this time also were founded the psychological laboratories of the larger universities. Mosso's studies on fatigue and his work on fear (*La Paura*, 1884), together with investigations of normal and artificial sleep, and of the psychology of the sexual functions, initiated by Breuer and Freud, formed the basis for extensive studies, which have already opened new approaches to knowledge of disease and determination of normal physiological states. Such studies have given rise to principles of great social importance, such as the rational organization of labour on the basis of a psycho-technical examination of the productive powers of the labourer.

These physiological investigations also have stimulated investigation of the *psychology of children and adolescents*, of the attention, of fatigue of pupils and labourers, studies which form the basis of the most modern phases of public hygiene.

ITALIAN physiology of the period was well represented by the Turin school of Mosso and the school of Giulio FANO (1856–1930) and Filippo BOTTAZZI (1867–1941). Noteworthy studies were accomplished by G. CERADINI (1844–94) on the functions of the semilunar valves; by A. HERLITZKA (b. 1872) on the physiology of the aviator; and by C. FOÀ (b. 1880) on vasomotor innervation. Luigi Luciani (1842–1919) discovered in the isolated frog's heart the periodic movements that are known as " the Luciani phenomenon "; but his best-known work was on the *function of the cerebellum*. His textbook, in several volumes, which is especially valuable for its historical elements, attained wide renown and was translated into several foreign languages, including English (1911–17). In the field of the nervous system PAGANO studied the effect of injections of curare into the basal nuclei and discovered the important *carotid reflex*, later developed by Hering and others.

5. Biochemistry

The very brief account of the first one hundred years of modern biochemistry that space permits in this and the following chapter would fail in historical perspective if it did not stress the influences that directed the flow of events during the period.

Biochemistry at the beginning of the second half of the nineteenth century was dominated by three main influences: the stimulus of organic or " animal " chemistry afforded by the work of J. von LIEBIG (1803–73) and F. WÖHLER (1800–82), MAYER's Law of Conservation of Energy (1842), given universal application by H. L. F. von HELMHOLTZ in 1847, and the revolution of 1848 in Germany.

The possibilities of ORGANIC CHEMISTRY for the investigation of animal economy were quickly seized. Qualitative metabolic experimentation was inaugurated by the development of such tests as those of J. F. HELLER (1813–71) in 1844 and A. N. E. MILLON (1812–67) in 1849 for protein, M. von PETTENKOFER (1818–1901) for bile (1844), H. von FEHLING for sugar in urine (1848), and the method of Liebig for the estimation of urea (1853). It is not possible to overstress the importance of tests, methods, and techniques in the development of biochemistry. They are the tools of research and the arbiters of progress. Fehling's solution opened the way to a definitive chemical study of diabetes mellitus, a step that Graham LUSK (1866–1932) regarded as responsible for the study of intermediary metabolism and the development of the science of nutrition. The early test for sugar was as essential to the great accomplishment of Claude Bernard as its quantitative offspring, fashioned by the labor and thought of OTTO FOLIN (1867–1934) and Stanley R. BENEDICT (1884–1936), was to Banting's and Best's discovery of insulin.

It took nearly seventy-five years satisfactorily to adapt Fehling's basic principle, reduction of copper in an alkaline medium, to the quantitative analysis of sugar in small amounts of blood or other body fluids. Indeed, although bloodletting by venesection was an old practice, the hypodermic syringe was not introduced until 1845 by F. RYND; and well into the twentieth century it was usual to expose the vein before puncture. The study of cerebrospinal fluid in man had to await the introduction of lumbar puncture in 1895 by H. QUINCKE. The original publications upon blood sugar methods from Folin's and Benedict's laboratories, at Harvard and Cornell respectively, were made in 1913–15. Almost yearly improvements in the technique were reported in the following fifteen years by the friendly rivals.

The physiology of METABOLISM can be divided, according to von NOORDEN, into three phases: first, the *qualitative*, inaugurated by Liebig and Wöhler, in which were determined the products of animal metabolism and the conditions of their formation; second, the *quantitative*, based on the studies of VOIT and PETTENKOFER, in which were established nutritional equilibrium in terms of calories and the validity of the laws of the conservation of energy in living animals. This found particular development in the studies of RUBNER, GRAHAM LUSK, BENEDICT, and others. Third, the study of *intermediate products* of metabolism, in which were especially notable the researches of Friedrich MÜLLER (1893), Adolph MAGNUS-LEVY, MINKOWSKI (1884), G. EMBDEN (1874–1933), and W. FALTA (1913). In Italy good work on carbohydrate metabolism and on convulsogenic zones was done by Pietro ALBERTONI (1849–1933) and his pupils Ivo NOVI, SABBATANI, and PUGLIESE; and on the peptones by G. FANO (1856–1930).

Helmholtz's law of the conservation of energy, embodied in the first law of thermodynamics, had incalculable influence both in initiating a physicochemical approach to problems in physiology and in colouring viewpoints in all branches of thought. Thus, as early as 1849, in the work of H. V. REGNAULT (1810–78) and Reiset with their closed-circuit animal respiration apparatus, and with the great classic *Die Verdauungssäfte und der Stoffwechsel* (1852) by H. F. BIDDER (1810–94) and C. SCHMIDT (1822–94), there emerged the idea of the *balance sheet* in metabolism. This concept remained the philosophical basis for the interpretation of metabolic

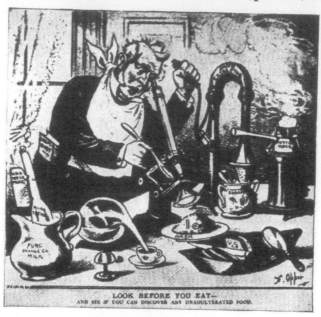

394. *"Look before you eat."*
(*Cartoon from* Punch, *1884.*)

phenomena for nearly one hundred years, until the recent revolution in thought resulting from the application of isotopes as tracer substances (see Chapter xxi).

The apparatus of Regnault and Reiset is the progenitor of modern closed-circuit equipment for the measurement of respiratory metabolism. The French investigators supplied preliminary information upon the relationship of dietary carbohydrate, fat, and protein to what A. F. W. PFLÜGER (1829–1910), pupil of Helmholtz, later called the "respiratory quotient" (R.Q.), and they foresaw the principle involved in the "law of surface area." This was more clearly envisioned by Bidder and Schmidt, who also established the idea of a constant pattern of metabolism: "This typical metabolism . . . is that of the fasting. It must be nearly the same in animals having the same body volume, surface, and temperature; the larger the body surface, the body volume and temperature remaining constant, or the higher the body temperature with surface and volume constant, the higher will be the metabolism as determined by the laws of static heat" (G. Lusk: *Nutrition,* Clio Medica). We see here an early, clear appre-

ciation of the application in the living organism of the science of thermodynamics. An earlier contribution, also of fundamental importance, was made by
Schmidt in 1850 in his study of epidemic cholera. Here a lucid description
(based on chemical studies) of the importance of the conservation by reabsorption of the salts and water of the intestinal secretions, and the relationship of loss
of water and salts to dehydration, laid the foundation for the modern understanding of *water balance*.

One physical technique leads to another. R. W. BUNSEN (1811–99), an outstanding inorganic chemist, who introduced spectrum analysis (1859) and the
use of the " extinction coefficient " (1857) in spectrophotometry, also perfected
GAS ANALYSIS. The quantitative measurement of respiratory gases led to the estimation of the gases of the blood, first made by Bunsen's pupil Carl Ludwig,
who devised a mercurial gas pump for this purpose. The original analyses of
the gases of the blood were published in 1859 by one of Ludwig's students, I. M.
SETSCHENOV. The spectra of oxyhemoglobin and methemoglobin were discovered (1862, 1864) by F. HOPPE-SEYLER (1825–95), who gave these pigments
their present names. The spectrum of reduced hemoglobin as well as of " reduced " hemochromogen, a pigment of much recent import, was first described
(1864) by the English physicist G. G. STOKES (1819–1903). " Blood crystals "
were mentioned by F. L. HUENEFELD (1799–1882) as early as 1841. Crystalline
hemoglobin was definitely reported by Otto FUNKE (1828–79) in 1851, and the
prosthetic group of the blood pigment was obtained as crystalline chlorohemin
by L. TEICHMANN (1823–95) in 1853. The name " Teichmann's crystals " has
persisted to this day. The original quantitative spectrophotometry upon hemoglobin derivatives was carried out by K. Vierordt, who published a pioneer
monograph upon this subject in 1876. Further early work in the spectrophotometry of hemoglobin was carried out by C. von NOORDEN in 1880, by
E. CHERBULIEZ in 1890, and particularly by G. von HUFNER (1840–1908) with
an improved spectrophotometer of his own design (1877–90). After the work
of Ludwig and Setschenov, further analytical studies on the gases of the blood
were carried out by Pflüger in 1864–6, by Paul BERT (1833–86) before 1878,
and by Leonard HILL in 1895. Both spectrophotometry and gas analysis did not
reach their full development, however, until the twentieth century. The latter
technique finds its full expression in the beautiful manometric procedures developed by D. D. VAN SLYKE (b. 1883) and his colleagues, a half-century after
Bert, for the accurate determination of the gases of the blood and many other
analytical reactions. Manometry as applied by J. Barcroft and O. WARBURG
(b. 1883) to the study *in vitro* of the metabolism of surviving tissue slices is another instance of these techniques, which have strongly influenced the development of present biochemical knowledge.

Carl von VOIT (1831–1908), Liebig's great pupil and founder of the
modern science of nutrition, was stimulated by, and still further developed,

the ideas of Bidder and Schmidt. In 1857 his first important publication demonstrated the phenomenon of "nitrogen equilibrium." With Petten-kofer, who constructed the best respiration apparatus of their day, he wrote classical papers, beginning in 1863, on the metabolism of animals and man, in the resting and the active state, in fasting, in diabetes, and in leukemia. Independently of Pflüger, who used a different experimental procedure (gasometry of the blood, 1866) they established the seat of metabolism in the cells and not the blood; oxygen requirement was the result, not the cause of metabolism, as Liebig had believed. This dictum of Voit's (1881) has a very modern ring: "The mass and capacity of the cells of the body determine the height of the total metabolism. . . . The requirement of protein is dependent on the organized mass of the tissues, that of fat and carbohydrate is dependent on the amount of mechanical work performed."

Graham Lusk epitomized the ideas of his teacher in a definition of metabolism as "all the chemical changes which substances undergo under the influence of living cells." Another pupil of Voit was the celebrated Max RUBNER (1854–1932), who originated the law of the proportionality of metabolism (measured as heat loss) to the surface area of the animal (fully expounded in his *Energiegesetze*, 1902), and evaluated the isodynamic values of carbohydrate, fat, and protein. Lusk idolized Rubner and rated him as Voit's greatest pupil; but Lusk himself was a greater investigator than Rubner. In 1890, in an important experiment upon himself in Voit's laboratory, Lusk established the protein-sparing effect of carbohydrate. This work not only served as the beginning of Lusk's many further experiments in metabolism, but to this day has great clinical value. It supplies the fundamental basis for "feeding, not starving a fever." As an example we have the high-calorie, high-protein diet (forced feeding) in typhoid fever (Warren Coleman and E. F. Du Bois, 1915). Also classical are the studies in Lusk's laboratory of phlorhizin glycosuria (beginning 1898). In Lusk's hands "phlorhizin diabetes" became a stimulating, valuable tool for the elucidation of INTERMEDIARY METABOLISM, fundamental to an understanding of the diabetic state.

A controversy that raged between the rivals Pflüger and Voit and was not settled during their lifetimes hinged on the concept that "organized" or tissue protein, in order to undergo metabolism, must first be converted into unorganized or so-called "circulating" protein. Though such a fundamental question is important, as the basis for lengthy controversy it illustrates the futility of argument when the facts at hand are insufficient. A solution of some of the difficulties in the understanding of protein metabolism is at length being approached through modern research methods which suggest that protein in the body is not static or stationary either in the circulating blood or in tissue cells, but is dynamic and constantly undergoing change (see Chapter xxi).

Lusk carried the tradition of Liebig and Voit to America, and, with such fellow workers as J. R. MURLIN, E. F. DU BOIS, R. J. ANDERSON, A. I. RINGER, H. V. ATKINSON, D. RAPPORT, H. J. DEUEL, and W. H. CHAMBERS, at Cornell and at the Russell Sage Institute of Pathology, he extended knowledge of metabolism by the most critically controlled experiments in animal calorimetry that have ever been carried out. His encyclopædic *The Elements of the Science of Nutrition* (4th ed., 1929) remains the fountainhead of information in the field of energy metabolism up to the date of its publication.

Two of Helmholtz's students require comment for their achievements and the influence that they exerted: Willy Kühne and Willard Gibbs — the latter, one of the truly great minds in science. Kühne, whose main fields were muscle and nerve physiology, worked on hemoglobin in 1865, and the digestion of proteins by pancreatic juice in 1867. In 1876 he discovered the proteolytic ferment, trypsin, and made early, fascinating experiments on " visual purple " (1877). With Claude Bernard he laid the foundation stones in the investigation of the digestive ferments, and was far ahead of his time in courageously and skilfully attacking such problems as those involved in the chemistry of vision. Kühne's greatest influence, however, was through his pupils, particularly Russell H. CHITTENDEN (1856–1943), the founder in 1874 of the first definite laboratory of physiological chemistry with a course of instruction in America, at the Sheffield School of Science of Yale University. Chittenden's early work (1883–8) on peptic digestion, with the isolation for the first time of various intermediates produced from substrates in the digestive process, such as peptones, bore Kühne's stamp. The Yale laboratory became the centre for the spread of physiological chemistry in the United States.

The history of this development has been written appropriately by Chittenden himself (*The Development of Physiological Chemistry in the United States*, 1930). His history of the American Society of Biological Chemists will be published posthumously. Chittenden survived most of his pupils, one of the greatest of whom, Lafayette B. MENDEL (1872–1935), surpassed his master and built up at the Sheffield School a veritable intellectual dynasty of biochemists (see Chapter xxi). Chittenden states that 540 papers were published by the laboratory's staff from 1880 to 1927, a remarkable productivity over a span of nearly half a century. The scope of individual pursuits in the laboratory was as varied as the later development of the individuals. Many of the younger men, however, originally worked with Chittenden on some phase of enzyme activity, thus becoming the intellectual descendants of Willy Kühne and Helmholtz. Mendel, later the prophet of the importance of " little things " in nutrition, reported *On the Proteolysis of Crystalline Globulin* (1894). A. N. Richards, later an important elucidator of the mechanism of kidney function, published with his master *Variations in the Amylolytic Power and Chemical Composition of Human Mixed Saliva* (1898).

Josiah Willard GIBBS (1839–1903) of New Haven, Professor of Mathematical Physics at Yale (from 1871), deduced by abstract reasoning from the laws of thermodynamics, of which science he was cofounder with his teacher Helmholtz, many of the fundamental principles of physical chemistry. His prophetic vision in this field is contained largely in a remarkable paper " On the Equilibrium of Heterogeneous Substances " (published in *Transactions of Connecticut Academy*, 1875–8), which opened the new subject of chemical energetics. Gibbs successfully applied to these new fields the second law of thermodynamics (that energy always flows or tends to flow from states of greater to lesser concentration), embodying the concept of THE POTENTIAL. The familiar Gibbs-Helmholtz equation, which states that the electromotive force (the useful work it can do) of a reversible voltaic cell is equal to its free energy per electrochemical equivalent of decomposition, contains " all that the laws of thermodynamics can teach concerning chemical processes " (Nernst). Reversible cells are the basis for the most accurate measurement of pH (acidity), of oxidation-reduction potential, and of free energy — all of great concern to the biochemist. These applications, involving the accurate measurement of electromotive force, have reached high development in the hands of W. Mansfield CLARK (b. 1884) and others, exerting a profound influence upon the physical trend of modern biochemistry (see Chapter xxi).

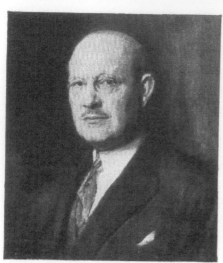

395. *Lafayette B. Mendel.*

F. G. DONNAN (b. 1870) in 1911, on the basis of thermodynamic reasoning, developed a theory of membrane equilibrium. A rediscovery of one of Gibbs's earlier predictions, it is now often called the " Gibbs-Donnan equilibrium." The theory was applied by Jacques LOEB (1859–1924) in his pioneer investigations of the colloidal behaviour of proteins, and since that time has had increasing physiological importance, particularly in elucidating diffusion phenomena across cellular membranes, " membrane potential," and the composition of " ultra-filtrates."

In the applications of physical chemistry to biology, osmotic pressure and " osmotic balance " occupy a position of prominence. Thomas GRAHAM (1805–

69) in 1854 defined osmosis as " the conversion of chemical affinity into mechanical power "; one may well start with Graham in formulating a better definition of the term " osmotic pressure " than that in common use at present. In 1861 Graham employed dialysis for separating " colloids " from " crystalloids." H. J. HAMBURGER (1859–1924), having in 1883 determined the range of fragility of erythrocytes in different concentrations of salt solution, concluded that hemolysis was usually a function of molar concentration. A similar method was applied (1887) by J. H. VAN'T HOFF (1852–1911) in his fundamental studies of osmotic pressure. S. J. Meltzer and W. H. Welch, on the other hand, had shown (1884) that erythrocytes could also be destroyed mechanically (in " a machine for shaking bottles " loaned by a manufacturer of mineral waters). BOTTAZZI's work on the osmotic pressure of animal fluids and on the colloidal state of living tissues (see also his hemocatatonistic concept of spleen function), GALEOTTI's on nucleo-proteins and R. HÖBER's on the physical chemistry of the cell (1902) are other examples of productive activity in this field. Modern elaborations in the same technique have served M. H. Jacobs over many years in his critical studies of the diffusion of various substances across the membrane of the red blood corpuscle. Finally, in 1895 E. H. Starling made his renowned contribution on the significance of the colloid osmotic pressure.

Chittenden mentions in his historical monograph that at the inception of their course in physiological chemistry at Yale the students used a text, *A Manual of Chemical Physiology, Including Its Points of Contact with Pathology* (1872), by J. L. W. Thudichum. This brings us to the influence of the German Revolution of 1848 in promoting the migration of men. It was in this way that Germany gave England her first biochemist, Johann Ludwig Wilhelm THUDICHUM (1829–1901), pupil of Liebig and Bunsen. A Hessian " nationalist," he did not adjust himself to Bismarckian unification. In 1853, taking with him a combustion furnace, a present from Liebig, he moved to London, to become a British citizen in due time. A man of boundless energy, Thudichum's interests were manifold. He wrote numerous erudite treatises on such varied subjects as the pathology of gall-stones and of the urine, chemical physiology and pathology, wines and viticulture, and cookery. Some histories of medicine credit him with being the first to use a two-stage operation for cholecystectomy, and with the invention of a nasal speculum that still bears his name; but they pass over his chemical accomplishments. His remarkable researches in this field stamp him as one of the most brilliant, courageous investigators in the history of physiological chemistry. Thudichum carried out pioneer investigations upon urochrome, the normal pigment of the urine (1864–93). He made early studies on the bile pigments (1862–76); but unfortunately he indulged in bitter polemic on this subject with Richard MALY (1839–94), the powerful editor of *Jahresberichte über die Fortschritte der Tierchemie*. Much of Thudichum's research was carried out in his capacity as chemist to the Medical Department of the Privy Council, which later evolved into the National Institute for Medical Research. Early in his career he became Professor of Pathological Chemistry at St. Thomas' Hospital — perhaps the first pathological chemist on record.

Under these auspices, in 1868–9, Thudichum published a classical paper on " luteins," yellow pigments found in corpus luteum (whence the name). This actually constituted the original discovery of the carotenoid type of pigments, and also established their widespread distribution both in animals and in plants. Thudichum's magnum opus as the " chemist of the brain," however, was too far ahead of his time for the biochemical fraternity to accept. His work, carried on in spite of such taunts from his detractors as that he " might as well give a chemical formula for bread and butter " or that he " obviously falsified," required the use of more than a thousand human and animal brains, and was possible only through a generous government subsidy. The starting-point of the work was the demonstration in 1874 that protagon, which Hoppe-Seyler's student O. LIEBREICH (1839–1908) had in 1865 discovered and claimed to be an entity, was actually a mixture of at least three groups of substances, lecithins, cephalins, and myelins. This kindled a controversy, which offended Hoppe-Seyler and continued into the twentieth century, but Thudichum was right. Lecithin and its structure had been discovered by C. Diakonow in 1867, but the cephalins and myelins were new substances, isolated and named by Thudichum. These he classified as phosphatides, which included nitrogenized constituents, such as sphingomyelin (isolated by him in 1878). In 1880–1 he discovered in the brain the " cerebrosides," which included the isolated phrenosin and kerasin, recognized by Thudichum to be galactosides. The mere naming and classification of these substances appear to be major achievements. Thudichum's researches on the brain were first published in the relatively inaccessible " Parliamentary Blue Books," then in accumulated form in English in 1884, and finally in the year of his death, 1901, in the belatedly acknowledged great classic *Die chemische Konstitution des Gehirns des Menschen und der Tiere*. Thudichum's contributions in this field have not been surpassed to this day, not even by the efforts along similar lines of that most skilful organic chemist, P. A. T. LEVENE (1869–1940). Otto ROSENHEIM, the distinguished lipoid chemist of the National Institute, London, having discovered samples of Thudichum's preparations, in a stable thirty years after his death, found them to be analytically reliable, many of the highest purity.

A century ago Claude Bernard had stressed that " the laws of science are the same in both physiology and pathology." His isolation of glycogen from the liver and recognition of the conversion of protein to carbohydrate furnished the proof that the animal body could build up from precursors — simple sugars and digested protein — such a complex substance as glycogen, and had a more profound effect upon metabolic thought than even Wöhler's isolation of urea. Paul Bert (1833–86), Bernard's favourite pupil, was an eminent student of atmospheric pressure who came to an untimely end because of his fierce, uncompromising anticlericalism. His interest was responsible for the fatal balloon ascension of Croce-Spinelli and Sivel. He left a monument to his memory in *La Pression barométrique* (1878), a book that has been republished in English during the Second World War as vitally important for aviation medicine. It contains Bert's pioneer investigations of blood gases, caisson disease, and the toxic effects of oxygen at high pressure.

By 1862 the exceedingly wide distribution of *cholesterol* in animal tissues and fluids as well as in plants had been recognized by F. W. BENEKE (1824–82). In 1861 Pasteur's studies of the butyric-acid fermentation of bacteria revealed anaerobic as distinguished from *aerobic metabolism*. The great man was wrong, however, in his insistence that living cells were necessary for fermentative activity. As early as 1858 the brilliant Moritz TRAUBE (1826–94) coined the word "enzyme" (ἐν ζύμη, leaven) for the hypothetical chemical substance that he regarded as responsible for fermentation in micro-organisms. Finally, in 1897, Eduard BUCHNER (1860–1917), Nobel laureate, who died of a wound suffered in the First World War, furnished ultimate scientific proof of the phenomenon of cell-free fermentation. The modern age of enzymes had begun.

In 1826, as part of the title of a small text, HÜNEFELD first used the term "*physiological chemistry*"; but it did not come into general use for another half-century. Liebig continued to speak of "animal chemistry" thirty years after the publication of his *Tierchemie* in 1842. The developments were such that it had become high time to recognize this applied branch of chemistry as a distinct discipline, a step accomplished by Hoppe-Seyler in founding in 1877 the journal which is still referred to as Hoppe-Seyler's *Zeitschrift für physiologische Chemie*. No other authoritative vehicle devoted primarily to biochemistry (in its physiological aspects) was established until 1906, although Thudichum made an abortive attempt (1879–81) to start one in English, the *Annals of Chemical Medicine*.

The early history of *acidosis* has interest. W. PETTERS found acetone in diabetic urine, and Kussmaul, of "fearful dyspnea" fame, demonstrated its presence in the blood. F. WALTERS in 1877, after feeding large amounts of hydrochloric acid to dogs, found changes in the blood, which he described as "acid intoxication." Ernst STADELMANN (1853–ret. 1921) in 1883, finding β-hydroxybutyric acid in diabetic coma, drew attention to its resemblance to Walters's "acid intoxication." The remarkable clinician, Oscar MINKOWSKI (1858–1931), whose work with von Mering on depancreatized animals is considered elsewhere, studied the acetone bodies in diabetic urine (1884), and also did pioneer work (1885) upon metabolism after excision of the liver.

Ehrlich's classical contribution on *The Needs of the Organism for Oxygen*

(1885) offered not only the first outlines of the " side-chain theory," but also a preview of the use of dyestuffs in the study of tissue respiration (oxidation-reduction processes in tissues).

Other important studies in this field were carried out by Mörner (cystin), Proust (leucin), Max Jaffé (urobilin), A. Ascoli (uracyl). Ascoli also wrote an important work on serology, which was translated into many languages.

Albrecht Kossel (1853–1927), Hoppe-Seyler's leading pupil and an eminent student of the chemistry of tissues, was the pioneer in the investigation of nucleic acids. It was he who originated the term " Bausteine " (building stones) for the amino acids, etc., in the metabolism of proteins. Kossel's work, emphasizing the need for a more exact understanding of the complex components of protoplasm, leads us to perhaps the greatest of organic chemists, Emil Fischer (1852–1919). In 1875 he discovered phenylhydrazine, the tool he used to advance the knowledge of sugars. Between 1883 and 1894 he had synthesized and supplied structural formulas for most of the common sugars and their isomers. In 1879–93 he synthesized numerous purines, including xanthine, and established the biochemical interrelationships of uric acid. In 1894 he supplied the " lock and key " concept for the specificity of enzyme activity. Having developed a hypersensitivity to phenylhydrazine, Fischer turned from sugar chemistry to the proteins. His work in this field established the structural nature of protein complexes, amino-acid units joined together by the " peptide bond." He proved his point by the creation of synthetic polypeptides. Fischer's accomplishments in this field, which have not been surpassed, were the harbinger of the great developments to come in the twentieth century.

In the past pages an attempt has been made to trace biochemical lineage. The direction of research in the twentieth century was established by the pathways opened up in the second half of the nineteenth. The pathways are different, though converging. Liebig is not the only progenitor; Bunsen and von Helmholtz also sowed their seeds, which bore lusty scientific progeny.

6. Pathology

The great development of pathologic anatomy in the second half of the nineteenth century was a natural consequence of the stimulus given it by the great masters of the first half of the century. The work of Rokitansky and Virchow pointed the way, which may be said to have been begun, as Virchow himself recognized, by Morgagni in the eighteenth century. The paths outlined by them gave pathology a constantly growing importance, and it became more and more recognized as a fundamental discipline of medicine. Leadership in the advancement in medicine, which about the middle of the century turned from France and Great Britain toward Germany in most of its branches, is nowhere better illustrated than in the field of pathology. As was only to be expected from the impetus supplied by the establishment of the cell theory by Schwann and Virchow, microscopic pathology cultivated an untilled field, with rich results. Whereas at the beginning of the century there were no chairs of pathologic anatomy in existence, in its second half we find many institutes and departments manned by physicians devoting themselves entirely to this subject. In university instruction pathologic anatomy played a part of great importance, and a steadily increasing knowledge of theoretical and practical aspects of the subject was demanded from students. Within this discipline we see developed special departments of study, leading to the construction of special institutes. Thus cancer, tuberculosis, tropical and other diseases have become the objects of specialized research in this way. Bacteriology (microbiology) has become an independent science and, as we shall see shortly, has assumed a highly important role in medicine.

CHAIRS OF PATHOLOGY were founded at Würzburg in 1849 and at Berlin in 1856, and in eighteen other well-known German medical schools in rapid succession. In Austria there soon were ten chairs, in Italy nineteen, pursuing the new pathology with an avidity that eclipsed the contributions to gross pathology of the older established chairs at Strasbourg (J. F. M. LOBSTEIN, 1777–1835) in 1819, and at Paris (J. CRUVEILHIER, 1791–1874) in 1836. The first pathological chair in England was established in 1827 at London University for J. F. Meckel, who did not serve, however; Carswell, appointed 1828, assumed his duties in 1831. Chairs in other countries followed later still, at the University of Pennsylvania, for instance, not until 1875 (James Tyson). The oldest society in this specialty is the New York Pathological Society, which celebrated the centennial of its foundation in 1844. The London Pathological Society was started in 1846 and the German Pathological Society, strangely, not until 1898.

Pathology has been well supplied with SPECIAL JOURNALS. The oldest pathological journal still in existence and the most celebrated is *Virchow's Archiv* (begun in 1847).

FUNCTIONAL PATHOLOGY. In addition to the natural emphasis on morbid anatomy, which persisted in many quarters well into the twentieth century, functional pathology and its handmaiden, experimental pathology, were developing their field, though necessarily overlapping the domain of physiology. The difference might be thought to be one of terminology, though one pathologist put it, " I'd naturally rather be a functional pathologist than a morbid physiologist! " However, the influence of the procedures at an investigator's disposal is always considerable in determining lines of work or classifying results.

Edwin KLEBS (1834–1913), though remembered more for his achievements in bacteriology, also made notable contributions to pathology, such as the experimental production of endocarditis (1876) and demonstration of its infectious nature (1878), the latter having been already adumbrated (1872) by H.

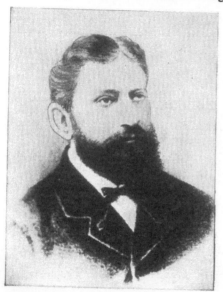

396. *Julius Cohnheim.*

HEIBERG (1837–97), of Christiania. Klebs noticed the large pituitary of giants before Marie, but failed to recognize the causal relationship. He observed (1870) hemorrhagic pancreatitis in sudden death before Fitz, and introduced (1869) the paraffin-embedding technique for microtomy that is still in use. F. D. von RECKLINGHAUSEN (1833–1910), though chiefly remembered today for his eponymic neurofibromatosis (1881), was one of the leading German pathologists and deserves the high appreciation that is given him in E. R. Long's *History of Pathology*.

Through Willy Kühne, Claude Bernard's influence was exerted on Julius COHNHEIM (1839–84), the pioneer and master experimental pathologist of the modern era. Virchow's most distinguished pupil, Cohnheim through his short active life illuminated the functional and experimental study of disease, both as assistant to Virchow at Berlin and as professor at Kiel (1868–72), Breslau (1872–8), and Leipzig 1878–84). His magnificent *Lectures on General Pathology* (1877) (available in English in the New Sydenham Society translation) remains a modern book, in a way that Virchow's *Cellular Pathology* and Rokitansky's *Handbuch* conspicuously do not. Cohnheim was " a bright and jovial student, full of drollery." His long hours with the microscope, under the guidance of Kölliker in normal and of Virchow in morbid histology, gave him the necessary structural foundation for his experimental work. In his study of the nature of inflammation he supported Virchow's tenet that the pus-corpuscle and the leucocyte could not be distinguished. With the ingenious use of dyes, however, he correctly derived the leucocyte from the blood, while Virchow believed that it might be a local tissue cell. According to Carswell, the formation of pus in the capillaries was first suggested by Dr. Simpson of St. Andrews in 1722. With his well-known frog mesentery experiment, Cohnheim actually saw the leucocyte escaping from the vessel wall, together with the widening of the lumen, slowing of the current, and diapedesis of erythrocytes — a forgotten observation of Addison (1849) and Waller. Cohnheim's view, contrary to Virchow's, that inflammation was impossible without blood vessels met a temporary obstacle in the changes found in avascular tissues such as the cornea. This, however, was overcome by Metchnikoff's discovery (1884) of the motile macrophage and microphage. Cohnheim also continued Virchow's studies on emboli and venous stasis and introduced valuable improvements in technique, such as frozen microscopic sections, staining muscle nerve endings with silver salts, and corneal nerve endings with gold. A congenital kidney tumour suggested to him the well-known theory that cancer might be due to misplaced embryonal rests. His successful inoculation of tuberculous material into the rabbit's eye was an early use of a method allowing continued observation of the development of a lesion. He produced good pupils — Lassar, Heidenhain, Litten, Ehrlich, Neisser, Weigert, and, of especial interest to Americans, William Welch, who while studying under Cohnheim at Breslau completed his study of acute œdema of the lungs, and W. T. Councilman. Other investigations by the clear-sighted Welch followed in this country (discovery of *B. aerogenes capsulatus* and exploration of its pathologic effects, further advances in the field of embolism and thrombosis, lesions of diphtheria toxin, and so on). More important to the progress of American medicine, however, was the dynamic concept of pathology that Welch brought to a profession overimpressed with the importance of pathologic anatomy, and his wise guidance not only of his department at Johns Hopkins but of the medical profession of the whole country throughout a long life, influential to the last.

Several important contributions to experimental pathology were made in Italy. PANIZZA's work on the optic nerve (1856) founded a doctrine of *descending degeneration*, later credited to Gudden, but correctly attributed by A. TAMBURINI (1878–1919) and L. CASTALDI (1890–1942). Panizza demonstrated a relation between the optic thalamus and sensation on the opposite side, discovered simultaneously by SWAN in the same year. The theory of nerve degeneration, however, owes most to the discovery by August WALLER (1816–70) that a cut nerve degenerates only in the part whose fibres are separated from their nerve cell — that is, distally in the case of motor nerves, centrally in the case of sensory nerves. L. PORTA's classical experiments on arteries (1848–59) demonstrated *collateral circulation* before Cohnheim. P. MANTEGAZZA's extensive and productive experiments on animal grafts (1862–6) opened the long road on which Carrel and others have since achieved so many triumphs. But also in the field of pathologic anatomy notable advances were made. Here, as in anatomy, microscopic research assumed the greatest importance. The study of various forms of anatomical anomalies, especially by Kölliker, Kundrat, Klebs, and KUSSMAUL, founded scientific teratology. In this field LOMBARDINI of Pisa was the first to perform decisive experiments on *teratogenesis* (1869), while DA-

RESTE's extensive researches entitle him to be regarded as one of the founders of *experimental teratology*, together with GIACOMINI, TARUFFI, and MARCHAND.

The DEGENERATIONS (a concept of Virchow's) were assuming something like their present arrangement in the framework of pathology owing to German work.

Von Recklinghausen described fatty and hyaline change; E. G. EICHWALD and H. J. Pfannenstiel, mucoid; Rey and Kaufman, calcification generally and the lesions in mercury poisoning; W. Ebstein, gouty urates; and F. A. Z. Zenker, waxy degeneration. Zenker is also said to have first described what is now called *Torula histolytica* meningitis. In the earlier study of the pigments and dusts, C. N. Nauwerck's name is associated with the bile pigments; those of E. Neumann and M. P. Perls with the blood; Armin Huber's with lipochrome; Zenker's with siderosis; R. Kobert's with argyria; J. A. Arnold's with dust. The nature of the necroses was explored by Carl WEIGERT (1845–1904) and Carl THIERSCH (phosphorus, 1867), and of infarcts by von Recklinghausen. Cysts, walled cavities of various kinds, with more or less fluid contents, have been known since antiquity and were classified in much the present style before the period covered in this chapter. Among brain cysts recognized later is porencephaly, a term proposed (1859) by R. HESCHL (1824–81). Virchow recognized (1867) its origin from softening of the brain tissue after thrombosis; and SEITZ showed (1897) that it might also be due to hemorrhage or infection. Mummification was distinguished from moist gangrene, which was properly ascribed to the action of putrefying bacteria. The first description of gas gangrene (1853) is usually attributed to J. G. MAISONNEUVE (1809–97), but this was preceded by more than two centuries by an account by Fabricius Hildanus in a letter (1607) to Horstius: the rapid spread following a wound of the leg, the stench, death in four days, and the sound " as if something hollow was underneath " leave little doubt that it was a true case of gas gangrene (Kellett). Pasteur was the first to identify one of the bacteria causing the condition — the gas-producing *Vibrion septique* (see section on Microbiology).

INFLAMMATION had its pathologic-anatomical basis rounded out in the work of Theodor LEBER (1840–1917) on the chemotaxis of leucocytes and dilatation of veins; in Boettcher's and Eberth's observations on giant cells; in E. Ziegler's exploration of the role of the tissue cells; and F. D. von Recklinghausen's synthesis of the various circulatory changes. We have already seen how recognition of the role of the blood vessels and phagocytes modified Virchow's purely cellular concept of inflammation, while Section 7 of this chapter, on Microbiology, touches on the part played by immunity. The long conflict between circulatory and cellular theories of inflammation was thus eventually settled by moulding the truths of each into a homogeneous whole.

Knowledge of the pathology of TUBERCULOSIS continued to advance in this period. Though Virchow taught that the nodular tubercle was an essential of tuberculosis and that phthisis and tuberculosis were different diseases, in the eighties it had become evident that the many and varied lesions of tuberculosis throughout the body were manifestations of the same disease. The erroneous concept that tuberculosis was always inherited *in utero*, held by Baumgarten among others, was successfully opposed by Georges Küss (1867–1936), of Paris, with the demonstration that " children of consumptives are not born tuberculous, but may become so." He was also the first, after Parrot (1876), to recognize (1898) the often silent lesion in the child's lung — the so-called primary complex, or Ghon tubercle (1912), named after the Austrian pathologist Anton GHON (1866–1936). Septicemic tuberculosis was first described by Yersin (1888). The almost constant presence of healed or active tuberculosis of the lungs in modern civilized communities was pointed out by O. Naegeli in 1900. Fortunately, the evidence of the tuberculin test shows that in some parts this is no longer the case, though the gains for mankind in this direction are not to be compared with the triumphs of veterinary medicine against bovine tuberculosis.

Silicosis became recognized as a special pulmonary occupational lesion (T. B. Peacock, and E. H. Greenhow, 1865); later asbestosis was also picked out as a harmful pneumokoniosis.

VISCERAL SYPHILIS had already been recognized for centuries (Massa, 1532; Morgagni, 1719; Lancisi, 1728); yet some varieties, such as syphilitic aortitis (F. H. Welch, 1876; P. Döhle, 1885) and aortic valvulitis (Herrick, Kiel dissertation, 1885), were not identified until much later (see Wilks, and also Lang's *Die Syphilis des Herzens*, 1889). Even up to the discovery of the *Treponema pallidum* by F. R. Schaudinn in 1905, statements as to the syphilitic nature of these conditions were guarded. Syphilis of the cerebral vessels was identified in 1874 by Otto HEUBNER (1843–1926). The relation of syphilitic aortitis to aneurysm was explained by Döhle in 1895. The syphilitic nature of paresis, progressive paralysis of the insane, first described by J. HASLAM (1798) and long regarded as a parasyphilitic disease, was established by NOGUCHI's demonstrations of the *Treponema* in the cerebral tissues. Locomotor ataxia, another " parasyphilitic disease," was renamed *tabes dorsalis*, on the basis of the wasting or degeneration found in the posterior columns of the cord (Remak, 1836–7). While its connection with syphilis is generally accepted on the basis of history, serological tests, and so on, its syphilitic pathogenesis remains obscure. The pathology of senile and presenile dementia was explored by Alois ALZHEIMER (1864–1915).

Diseases closely related to syphilis and mostly caused by Treponemata often indistinguishable from *T. pallidum* are found in various parts of the world under such names as yaws (framboesia), gangosa, goundou, bejel (Egypt), pinta (Latin America). The South American disease Oroya fever, first mentioned by Iago de Vasillo (1630), attracted but little attention until the epidemic of 1870 in the Oroya Valley. Its dermal manifestation, *verruga Peruana*, with a pre-Columbian history, was often represented on pottery. In his desire to add to the knowledge of this national disease, Daniel A. CARRION (1850–85), then a sixth-year medical student, had himself inoculated with verruga blood, and with his death proved the identity of the two diseases. Barton described (1905, 1909) the causative microbe, which in 1913 was named after him *Bartonella bacilliformis* by R. Strong *et al.* on the Harvard expedition to Peru, which expedition also fully outlined its pathological anatomy. It was first cultivated and Koch's postulates fulfilled by Noguchi and others in 1926. Elusive outbursts of the painful, but not serious epidemic pleurodynia (" Devil's grip," Bornholm disease) have been known in various parts of the world since it was first seen in Iceland by J. C. FINSEN in 1856 (pub. 1874). It was recognized in 1888 in America by W. C. Dabney, but its causative microbe still remains undiscovered.

PSITTACOSIS, a respiratory disease first recognized in the parrot family, was first detected (1879) by Ritter, a Swiss, in seven persons after contact with tropical birds. In 1892 two bird dealers, taking their stock from Buenos Aires to Paris, had 315 of 500 parrots die en route; both caught the disease themselves and spread it to others on arrival. Since then human cases have been recognized over much of the globe; in America, in the winter of 1929–30, 169 cases were found in fifteen states, with 33 deaths. Its virus cause (see Chapter xxi) and its occurrence in many bird species have been so well established that it is more properly called " ornithosis."

Throughout the world, study of MALIGNANT TUMOURS has been intensively prosecuted. The question whether the marked increase of cancer incidence is a true increase or an apparent one due to improved knowledge and diagnosis and to the greater longevity of civilized people in modern times has been illuminated by extensive statistical studies of an accuracy that has been greatly increased by improvements in pathological classification and diagnosis. The essential differences of epithelial and mesodermic tumours were established by R. REMAK (1815–65), who showed that skin cancer came from epithelium and not metaplastically from connective tissue, as Virchow had maintained. This was proved by the surgeon Thiersch's razor-cut serial sections, and extended to epithelial tumours of internal organs by Waldeyer. The nature of cancer metastasis, both by embolism in the lymph and blood channels and by direct extension, was solved by the great anatomist Waldeyer not long after.

Most of the tumours as we now know them had been identified histologically and named before the end of the century, not a few by Virchow; many had been known by their gross characteristics since the time of Morgagni and earlier.

Among *bony tumours*, the osteoclastoma or benign giant cell tumour had been first recognized (1850) by C. Robin (1821–85), better understood by Paget, by Nélaton (1863), and in America by Gross (1879), but not properly comprehended until the work of Bloodgood (1910). Multiple myeloma, called *mollities ossium* by McIntyre (1850), was recognized as a disease of the bone marrow by O. R. Rustizky (1873), who was the first to use the term "myeloma." Its association with a special proteose in the urine was established by Henry Bence Jones in 1848. The rather frequent tumour described (1922) by James Ewing as diffuse endothelioma, but now more generally known under the noncommittal name of "Ewing's tumour," was regarded as a variety of endothelioma. This group term was first proposed (1869) by Golgi for the tumour of the dura mater, now known as meningioma; and similar-appearing tumours had been called (1856) cylindromata by Billroth. Tumours of the synovial membrane (synovioma) were first described (1886) by Weir, and further studied by Adrian (1903) and Lejars (1910). The concept was widened (1927) to include tumours from related structures by L. W. Smith (b. 1895). Lymphosarcoma, the cancer due to the lymphocyte, was described by Hans Kundrat (1845–93), holder of the chair of pathological anatomy at the University of Vienna. He had followed Rokitansky's successor, R. Heschl (1824–81), and was succeeded by A. Weichselbaum (1845–1920), and then by A. Kolisko (1857–1918). Rokitansky's assistant, Hans Chiari (1851–1916), took the Prague chair, where the Czech and German universities managed to advance in spite of political complications. Carcinoma of the lung was found (1879) by F. H. Hürting and W. Hesse to be especially common in the Schneeberger mines — a new form of occupational disease; and this observation acquired further interest in the next century when it was found that the ore contained a high percentage of radium.

The complications of tumours — necrosis and ulceration, calcification, and so on — were being explored, again mostly by the German schools; and many different histological varieties were identified and named: fibroma, angioma, myeloma, lymphoma, myxoma, osteoma, chondroma, myoma, epithelioma, carcinoma, neuroblastoma, teratoma. It is fair to say that, although new varieties are still occasionally being described, the greater part of this phase of oncology had already been achieved by the end of the nineteenth century.

Knowledge of the causes of cancer and how it is produced made much less progress. The importance of Cohnheim's theory that it is due to the activation of dormant embryonic " rests " (1877) is still to be correctly evaluated; likewise. Hugo RIBBERT's (1855–1920) modification that adult cells might be similarly segregated by the irregular growth of adjacent tissue, later to develop as tumour cells. Virchow's emphasis on irritation as a cause is still upheld, but in a much more limited sense. External causes of cancer were demonstrated before the end of the nineteenth century, among others by Richard von VOLKMANN (tar and paraffin cancer, 1875); Hürting and Hesse (miner's cancer of the lung, 1879); R. H. Harrison (bilharzia cancer of the bladder, 1889); L. REHN (aniline cancer, 1895). Hosts of parasites (animal and vegetable) have been proposed as the cause of all cancer, which, however, have all been thoroughly discredited; but at least it can be said that the studies have been so actively pursued that constantly more facts are being brought to light which may aid in the solution of the problem.

Though much of the history of the special pathology of many parts of the body will be found later in this chapter in sections on the specialties, some phases are given here. Research on the histogenesis of the blood cells and the blood-forming function of the bone marrow by BIZZOZERO gave the necessary foundation for knowledge of the pathology of the hematopoietic organs and began a new era in the pathology of the blood. The hematopoietic role of the bone marrow was first described by E. NEUMANN in 1868, and the changes that take place in the bone marrow in pernicious anæmia were first observed by William Pepper in 1875. Disease due to a primary excess of red blood cells was established by Vaquez (1892) and also by Osler (1903); it is known eponymically today by their names, or as erythremia or polycythemia vera. Other bone-marrow diseases were coming to be recognized, such as osteosclerotic anæmia (marmorization of the long bones, first described by H. E. ALBERS-SCHÖNBERG (1865–1921), the X-ray martyr. The recognition of leukemia by Bennett and by Virchow has been described in the previous chapter; the changes it produces in the bone marrow were first detailed by Neumann in 1870.

The tremendous advance in microscopic technique in the past fifty years opened new fields in the special pathology of the blood, bones, and muscles, the circulatory organs, and the nervous system. We may note, in passing, Ehrlich's use of the aniline dyes, his division of polymorphonuclear leucocytes into three types according to the staining reactions of their granules, and his uses of intravital stains. Counting pipettes and slide-chambers also provided accurate determinations of hemoglobin, erythrocyte and leucocyte counts. The hematokrit (S. G. Hedin, 1891) determined the proportion of plasma and cell volume and thus gave indirect evidence of the volume of each cell. The plasma cell was established by Paul G. UNNA (1850–1929), and " stippling " of the erythrocytes by Grawitz (1899). New varieties of tumours were picked out by Waldeyer, von Recklinghausen, Grawitz, and others. Degenerations of the cells of the nervous system and their processes were made detectible by the methods of Weigert, Marchi, and Nissl.

Knowledge of the pathologic anatomy of the genital organs progressed, especially in regard to lesions of the testicles and ovaries. Myomata were recognized as benign tumours and accepted as a frequent source of uterine bleeding (von Recklinghausen, J. W. Williams, Pick). Like various lesions of the Fallopian tubes, they became more and more accessible to aseptic surgery. Early cancer of the uterus and cervical erosion were studied (1878) by J. VEIT (1852–1917); also extra-uterine pregnancy (1884). Cysts of the ovary (Waldeyer, Pfannenstiel), made familiar by the classic ovariotomies of McDowell and his successors, and ovarian tumours (Wilms), were subdivided into various types of different origin and significance. Appendicitis was divided into several varieties by Aschoff and others, and the various ways that it might be caused were elucidated.

In the pathology of the CARDIOVASCULAR system, as elsewhere, important progress was registered. In congenital heart disease, Henri ROGER (1809–91) described (1879) the patency of the interventricular septum, which is still known as " Roger's disease "; in 1888 E. L. A. FALLOT (1850–1911) demonstrated the frequently occurring group of lesions – pulmonary stenosis and the rest – that are known as the " tetralogy of Fallot." Peacock's great work on *Malformations of the Heart* appeared in 1858.

Though heart involvement in rheumatic fever had been recognized in the previous half-century, the characteristic subcutaneous nodules were not recognized until much later. Meynet is said to have made this observation on one case in 1875, and in 1881 Sir Thomas BARLOW (1845–1945) detected them in twenty-seven cases and reported their histologic appearance at the International Congress in 1881. Later (1893) he recognized their relation to the rheumatic valvular lesions. Barlow is more widely known as the original describer (1883) of the infantile (acute) form of scurvy, often known as Barlow's disease, which W. B. Cheadle had taken (1879) to be a combination of rickets and scurvy.

Myomalacia cordis was described (1881) by Ernst ZIEGLER (1849–1905), the author of one of the most successful works on pathology (in two volumes), and editor of the famous *Beiträge*. Myocardial infarction was recognized by Marie in 1896, the same year in which F. PICK (1867–1926) described the chronic pericarditis that goes by his name. This, however, had become well known in England, as P. D. White points out, following an original description by N. CHEVERS, of Guy's Hospital. The importance of fatty degeneration of the heart was first clearly recognized (1854) by William Stokes; of bacterial endocarditis by Sir Samuel WILKS (1824–1911); and its subacute form, with its tendency to give off emboli, by W. Senhouse KIRKE (1823–64) in 1852.

Arteriosclerosis as an independent condition chiefly responsible for incriminating the cardiovascular diseases as the group that today is the chief cause of death is a recent concept, due to Gull and Allbutt. Not only is it the direct cause of apoplexy, coronary heart disease, and nephrosclerosis, but it may add to the poor function of any viscus. Truly, as Osler said, " a man is as old as his arteries." The importance of Gull and Sutton's description (1871-2) of arteriocapillary fibrosis has only been appreciated in recent years as increasing emphasis is placed on the arteriolosclerotic form of Bright's disease.

The symmetrical blanching of gangrene of the extremities known as Raynaud's disease was described by M. RAYNAUD in 1862; periarteritis nodosa by Rokitansky in his *Diseases of the Arteries* in 1852, and again by Kussmaul in 1866. Its visceral involvement and unexpected frequency have only recently become established. Its allergic origin, originally suggested by G. B. GRUBER, has been ably explored (1942) experimentally and by clinico-pathologic correlation by Arnold R. RICH (b. 1893).

Comprehension of the pathology of the RESPIRATORY SYSTEM was furthered during this period by the observations on nasal lesions of E. ZUCKERKANDL (1849-1910), also the discoverer of Zuckerkandl's organ, and of Eppinger and others on emphysema and on pulmonary fibrosis, and by numerous other studies important more in the group than as individual contributions.

In the pathology of the DIGESTIVE TRACT we note R. H. Fitz's pioneer studies on appendicitis and on hemorrhagic pancreatitis with fat necrosis; also Zenker's on œsophageal ulceration and diverticulation; tuberculosis of the tonsils (Finger and others) and of the œsophagus (Birch-Hirschfeld); and on infected tonsils as spreaders of disease (Hodenpyl). Peptic ulcer, known since the time of Galen and Celsus, and more accurately outlined by Cruveilhier and by J. ABERCROMBIE (1832), without microscopic aid naturally was still frequently confused with cancer. L. Müller's monograph gives a good picture of the disease as it was understood in 1860; Virchow, Klebs, Boettcher, Rindfleisch, and most of the leaders of their day, all expressed their views, more or less supported by observation and experiment. Though the pathological histology and the possible outcome of the condition had become well understood by the end of this period, its nature still remained obscure, as in fact it still does.

The pathology of the ENDOCRINE SYSTEM progressed from Claude Bernard's prophetic studies and the earlier clinical descriptions of the more striking diseases to a scientific exploration of the tissue changes and in some cases of the mechanisms involved. It was not until the next century, however, that this important field really came into its own.

That loss of the *pituitary*, as chief regulator of the various glands of internal secretion, is often fatal has been known since Marinesco's experimental excisions (1892). When the eosinophil cells of the anterior (glandular) lobe are increased by hyperplasia or tumour (adenoma) in adults, the striking condition of acromegaly (P. Marie, 1895) results; giantism is produced if this happens while the

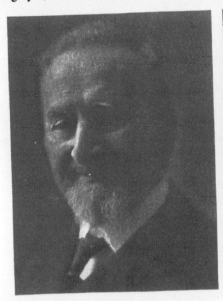
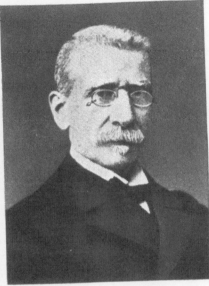

397. *Pio Foà.*   398. *Ettore Marchiafava.*

skeleton is still growing. This pituitary change can still be demonstrated in the pathologic museum, by the enlargement brought about in the *sella turcica*, the bony cup that surrounds the pituitary. Not long after Addison's description of the disease of the *adrenal* glands that bears his name, Brown-Séquard showed the fatal results of their removal in animals. Differentiation of cortical and medullary effects, however, and their various tumours and their results were mysteries that had to await exploration in the next century. *Thyroid* pathology was slower in correlating the histologic varieties of struma with the hyperthyroidism of the clinicians than in the correlation of diminished thyroid secretion (hypothyroidism) with cretinism and myxœdema. Here, too, excision was shown by the Swiss, M. SCHIFF (1856), to be fatal, and the role of the thyroid established by partial or complete thyroidectomy by the cousins, A. and J. L. REVERDIN (1882) and by Kocher's cachexia strumipriva. This had been found in human disease by T. B. CURLING in 1850, and in 1875 by Sir William W. GULL (1816–90). The importance of the recently discovered *parathyroid* glands became evident with E. GLEY'S discovery (1891), confirmed by G. VASSALE (1862–1912) and F. GENERALI (1896), of the fatal results of removing these small glands at the same time that the thyroid was excised. Their absence was found to cause tetany, the peculiar convulsive state associated with faulty calcium metabolism, which could be relieved by parathyroid transplants (von Eiselsberg, 1892).

The chief features of diabetes mellitus were produced experimentally (1889) by the excision of the *pancreas* by von Mering and Minkowski, the significant structure lost being shown (1901) by E. L. OPIE (b. 1873) and others to be the islands of Langerhans of this organ.

Among prominent ITALIAN pathologists was Pio FOÀ (1848–1923), professor at Modena and Turin, who accomplished notable work on the pneumococcus

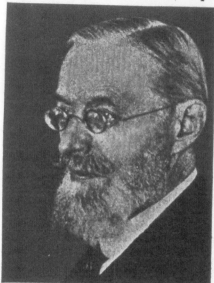

and on cytotoxic sera. He was a leader in the fight against tuberculosis and in sexual education. A. CARLE and G. RATTONE, pupils of Bizzozero, demonstrated (1882) the transmissibility of tetanus, while S. BELFANTI and T. CARBONE were pioneers in the study of hemolysis. B. MORPURGO studied osteomalacia and experimented with parabiosis. The *Diplococcus lanceolatus* (pneumococcus), whose discovery is usually ascribed to A. Fränkel (1884), was described in 1883 by G. SALVIOLI (1852–88) as found in the sputum, lung tissue, and pleural and pericardial exudates of persons dying of croupous pneumonia. Salvioli was also an early student of the phenomena of hemolysis and agglutination. A. CESARIS–DEMEL, a pupil of Foà, is known for his work on mammalian cardiac pathology and on the immature erythrocytes known as reticulocytes (*substantia granulosofilamentosa*).

399. *Guido Banti.*

In the pathologic anatomy of the nervous system, the name of Adelchi NEGRI (1876–1912) is celebrated for the discovery of those bodies in the brains of hydrophobic animals that characterize the disease rabies. Chief among modern Italian pathologists was Ettore MARCHIAFAVA (1847–1935), a highly esteemed teacher and investigator. A valuable contributor to many fields of pathologic anatomy, he is especially noted for his studies of the malarial parasite. In Grassi's opinion, Laveran, Marchiafava, and Celli cannot be separated in evaluating the steps in the discovery of the malarial plasmodia. Marchiafava's pupils BIGNAMI and Giuseppe BASTIANELLI continued this work, while GUARNIERI (1856–1918) described the peculiar corpuscles of smallpox and vaccinia that for a time were thought to be their causative agents. Guido BANTI (1852–1925) described the *splenic anæmia* (1882) that still bears his name, and was one of the early elucidators of typhoid septicemia, leukemia, and pneumococcic infection. A. LUSTIG

(1857–1937) is recognized as the founder of the modern Tuscan school of pathologic anatomy. The pathology of tuberculosis was constructively investigated by L. ARMANNI (1839–1903) and A. MAFFUCCI (1847–1903).

7. Microbiology[1]

Minute organisms only visible with the microscope had been observed by Leeuwenhoek (1675); their possible role in disease was visualized by Kircher, Spallanzani, and others. Marc Antony PLENCIZ (1705–86) in his *Opera medica physica* (1762) had maintained that contagion was due to a *seminale verminosum*, with a different kind of seed for each disease, a concept that was long denied by Klebs and others in the late nineteenth century; and Bassi had shown definitely that disease (of silkworms) could be caused by them (see Chapter xix). Henle's *Von den Miasmen und Kontagien* (1840) still further developed the concept that very small living structures were responsible for much human disease. It is in the period under review, however, that bacteriology acquired such an extraordinary development that it brought about a veritable revolution in the structure of medical thought. It caused an essential change not only in the concepts of disease and of contagion, but also in the whole method of medical thinking, to an extent that is difficult to appreciate for those who have grown up in the bacteriological era. With the work of Pasteur and Koch, the actual founders of the new science, there penetrated rapidly into all fields of medicine the idea that infinitely small beings, endowed with special pathogenic qualities, played a pre-eminent role in producing many diseases. The new concept made such a great impression that for a while it was believed that the cause of all diseases could be ascribed to microbes alone. The voice of pathology was muted; the clinic was subordinated to the reports of the laboratory and from it issued the standards for the legislator and the hygienist, for the obstetrician as for the dermatologist or pediatrician. Almost completely dominant, bacteriology at this period became the centre and goal of medical investigations; eventually, however, it became clear that it could not solve all problems of etiology and still less those of prognosis and treatment.

With the improved microscopes of the early nineteenth century and Amici's discovery of the oil-immersion lens, observations of micro-organisms were ac-

[1] The term "microbiology" is preferable to the more commonly used term "bacteriology," for the same reason as that given in the 1911 edition of the *Encyclopædia Britannica*: namely, that micro-organisms other than bacteria are included under this heading (protozoa and other animal forms, and the still unclassified filter-passing viruses). It seems hardly worth mentioning that only medical aspects are considered.

cumulating, all to be dumped by Linnæus into his botanical group "Chaos." However, Otto Frederik MÜLLER (1730–84), of Copenhagen, who coined the terms "bacillus" (little rod) and "spirillum," assembled micro-organisms into the group of Infusoria, with subdivisions of the low forms into *membranacea*, and *crassiuscula* (the lowest forms). This in turn led to C. G. EHRENBERG's (1795–1876) classification of *monadina, cryptomonadina, vibriona*, in his great folio *Die Infusionsthierchen* (1838) and to Dujardin's (1805–60) simpler division into *bacterium, vibrio, spirillum*. Shortly after began the pioneer work of Ferdinand COHN (1828–98), of Breslau, who was forced by the religious restrictions of his native city to go to the then more liberal University of Berlin. Here he had the good fortune to study under Johannes Müller and Ehrenberg. His *Untersuchungen über Bacterien* (1872), with its classified and accurate delineation and description of Micrococcus, Bacterium, Bacillus, Vibrio, Spirillum, Spirochæte, is rightly regarded by C. S. Dolley as ushering in modern bacteriology. Cohn also discovered the ability of bacteria to form spores and their multiplication by fission. Karl von Nägeli had previously grouped them, as they are today, as *Schizomycetes*. Stains (indigo, carmine) were first used in the study of bacteria by C. F. von GLEICHEN in 1778, and solid media (potato) (1863) by C. R. FRESENIUS.

The most representative and important figure in the whole field of bacteriology is without any doubt that of Louis PASTEUR (1822–95). The story of his life affords one of the most remarkable examples of successful achievement by a man whose genius was supported by an inflexible will and controlled by an enthusiastic, yet uncompromising critical sense. Pasteur, born at Dôle in the department of Jura, devoted himself early to chemistry, and was graduated from the École Normale of Paris in 1847. Professor first of physics, then of chemistry, at the Lycée of Dijon, then of chemistry (1852–54) at Strasbourg and later at Lille, he became in 1857 director of scientific studies at the École Normale of Paris. It is at this period that his important scientific work began. No other scientist has had to the same degree the pleasure of seeing the importance of his work so quickly and universally recognized and his ideas so enthusiastically accepted in their triumphal penetration, not only into the laboratory and the clinic, but also into the popular mind of the civilized world.

Though of less direct importance to medicine, his early chemical studies of the tartrates (DYSSYMMETRIC CRYSTALLINE FORMS with dependent differences of qualities) were of prime significance. They not only led to the development of the new specialty of stereochemistry (van't Hoff), but led Pasteur to his study of FERMENTATION, which in turn brought about his epoch-making studies of pathogenic bacteria and of successful ways of controlling their ravages. From his studies on the nature of the fermentation of beer and of lactic acid (1857) came the discovery of lactic-acid bacilli, and soon after of the bacteria causing butyric-acid fermentation. He showed that they could live without oxygen, in fact flourished in an atmosphere of carbon dioxide (thus introducing the concept of " anerobic " bacteria, as opposed to those requiring an atmosphere containing oxygen, " aerobic "). The perennial problem of SPONTANEOUS GENERA-

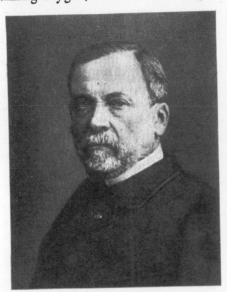

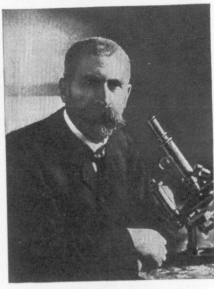

400. *Louis Pasteur.*   401. *Émile Roux.*

TION, which should have been decided by Spallanzani's successful refutation of Needham's contentions a century earlier, reappeared at this time, when Pouchet's infusion of hay bacteria survived the heat sterilization applied to it. However, in a number of reports to the French Academy of Science (1860–5) Pasteur produced convincing evidence that bacteria-free fluids remained permanently bacteria-free if properly protected. The final blow was given by John Tyndall's prolonged, and careful studies, which culminated in 1877 (in a letter to Huxley) with the demonstration of the superiority of discontinuous boiling to eliminate the resistant as well as the heat-sensitive germs. Thus for all time the delusion of spontaneous generation was disposed of. Discovering that the transformation of wine into vinegar was caused by the action of a microbe (*mycetum aceti*), Pasteur found that it could be killed by several applications of heat sufficiently low not to injure the quality of the wine (1863–5). This process, *pasteurization*, in wide use today in the preservation of perishable foodstuffs, has contributed immeasurably to the health and wealth of the civilized world. Later (1876) Pasteur applied the same methods to the protection of beer. In 1865, after the French silkworm industry had been seriously crippled by the disease *pébrine*, Pasteur was invited by the French government to study the situation Seeking for the cause, he found the offending germs not only in the silkworms but also in their moths and ova. He demonstrated a successful method of overcoming the plague by a systematic microscopic examination of ova with elimination of all those found to be diseased. Thus Pasteur confirmed Bassi's theory that fermentation is due to live organisms and consequently that decomposition and infectious diseases are due to germs that can be differentiated by their morphological and biological qualities. On these early basic discoveries by Pasteur followed his study of the causes of *anthrax* and of *chicken cholera*, in which field he was preceded by Casimir DAVAINE, who discovered the anthrax bacillus (1850–65), by Koch, who obtained it in pure culture (1867), and by Klebs, who showed that the disease agent was not filterable. Pasteur confirmed the anthrax bacillus as the sole cause of the disease (1880) and showed that a species (fowl) that is ordinarily not susceptible to anthrax could be made so by immersion in cold water, after which the disease progressed to a fatal termination. With Joubert he discovered the bacillus of malignant œdema ("*vibrion septique*"), the first anerobic organism found to be pathogenic, and though not especially concerned with the classification of bacteria, he was the first to describe staphylococci and streptococci (in puerperal septicemia) under the picturesque names of "*microbes en amas de grains*" and "*microbes en chapelet de grains*" (1879). His accidental observation of attenuation of virulent cultures of chicken cholera under unfavourable cultural conditions, together with passage through several generations of animals, led to his fundamental discovery of *preventive vaccination* against anthrax, which in spite of caustic opposition led to its successful application against the anthrax of sheep and cattle (1881). As Garrison emphasizes, "the principle that pathogenic properties of a virus can be attenuated or heightened by successive passages through the bodies of appropriate animals . . . led to one of the most luminous thoughts in the history of science — that the origin or extinction of infectious disease in the past may be simply due to the strengthening or weakening of its virus by external conditions, in some such way as the above." Finally Pasteur discovered the well-known treatment of rabies (hydrophobia) which bears his name. In July 1885 this was first successfully applied to a boy from Alsace, Joseph Meister, who had been bitten by a mad dog. The Pasteur Institute of Paris was founded and became the centre of a remarkable series of investigations to which the grand old man applied himself with tireless fortitude to the end of his days, gathering about him a school of illustrious pupils, among whom were Metchnikoff, Émile Roux, Yersin, and Calmette. Here under Pasteur's direction notable studies were conducted in all the varied fields of microbiology. Here, with poetic fitness, Joseph Meister for many years laboured in a humble capacity in the cause of the science that had saved his life. Before long, similar institutes were founded in various parts of France and her colonies, and centres for the distribution of the Pasteur anti-rabic treatment were established throughout the world. From all points of view, Pasteur will stand permanently as one of the highest examples of human virtue: his exceptional qualities as an investigator and leader, his intense and delicate goodwill toward all sufferers, his deep religious feeling, his pure and burning love of country, the nobility of his generous life, all centring in his scientific work, created about him an atmosphere of boundless affection and profound veneration. Even in his lifetime he became one of the great intellectual heroes of his time, who received from his own country and from the entire civilized world vivid proofs of gratitude. France bestowed on him, during life and after death, greater honours than have ever been given to a scientist before or since, recognizing the invaluable importance of his immortal work, not only in the field of hygiene and social medicine, but also in the economic benefits that it brought to the nation. It is said that in a widespread questionnaire undertaken some years ago by a Paris newspaper as to who was the greatest Frenchman, the votes for the humble chemist outnumbered those for Napoleon, Charlemagne, and all the rest. One can say without exaggeration that the civilized world correctly recognized in Pasteur one of the greatest and noblest pioneers of civilization.

Among the studies deriving from Pasteur's school are those of A. CALMETTE (1863–1933), who was director of the Pasteur Institute at Saigon, then at Lille. He introduced a protective serum against snake-bite, also the ophthalmic tuberculin reaction (1907), and invented the prophylactic antituberculous vaccination with attenuated live bacilli, known as B.C.G. (bacillus Calmette-Guérin) (1926). Émile ROUX (1853–1933), director of the Pasteur Institute of Paris, studied the experimental production of syphilis in monkeys and was one of the creators of modern antidiphtheritic serotherapy (1888). G. A. E. YERSIN (1863–1943) discovered the plague bacillus and prepared an anti-plague serum. To this school also belong L. MARTIN (studies on diphtheria and antidiphtheritic serum) and E. I. E. NOCARD, the veterinarian, who described (1888) bovine farcy, called after him nocardiasis (suppuration of the lymph nodes in cattle); in 1892 he discovered a bacillus associated with psittacosis. A genus of fungi was for some time known as Nocardia, but is now included with the Actinomyces.

The studies of Pasteur were followed by those of many other investigators, some of whom, like E. Klebs, the inventor of fractional cultures, and W. von WALDEYER, supported the truth of Pasteur's doctrines, while others, like the botanist E. HALLIER (1831–1904), cast doubt on his conclusions.

A great scientist who, with Pasteur, brought a very great contribution to the young science of microbiology and gave a new impetus to its advancement was Robert KOCH (1843–1910). Born at Klausthal (Hanover), Koch was graduated in medicine in 1866 at Göttingen, where he had Henle among his teachers. After serving through the Franco-Prussian War, he became district physician at Wollstein (1872), where in addition to his routine of country work he began his immortal bacteriological studies. Already in 1873 he had begun the study of the anthrax bacillus, having observed the frequent grave manifestations of that disease in his locality. He was able, for the first time in history, to work out the complete life cycle of the bacillus, transmitting it through many generations of mice and always producing the disease. He also was able to grow it on artificial media. His study of its spores threw new light on the question of how the infection occurred and how long it might last.

Koch's success in this work, confirmed by further experiments of Pasteur, though opposed by Paul Bert, led him in 1876 to seek an interview with Ferdinand Cohn, Professor of Botany at Breslau, to demonstrate his observations. Cohn and his colleagues and pupils, Auerbach, Weigert, Cohnheim, Welch, Traube, became at once delighted supporters of Koch's views. In 1878 followed Koch's studies on *Die Aetiologie der Wundinfektionskrankheiten*. Following the publication of this work, which was of fundamental importance in the problem of surgical infection, Koch was given an important post in the Imperial Health Department, with Löffler and Gaffky as his assistants. There he continued his studies that resulted in the constant improvement of technical methods — pure cultures, staining and microscopic examination of bacteria, and so on — work that he had first written about in 1877. With his technical innovations and photographic reproduction of bacterial preparations and unremitting search for further improvements, and with utilization of such advances in the microscope as the oil-immersion lens, he complemented the work of Pasteur in placing the new science on a firm basis. His ability as a patient and methodical investigator also found expression in his use of *transparent and solidifiable media*, such as gelatin and agar, which can be liquefied at temperatures sufficiently low not to harm the bacteria, yet solidify at room temperature. With suitable dilution single bacteria could thus be isolated and colonies grown in pure culture. By the use of this method most of the pathogenic bacteria were isolated and their properties gradually learned. In 1882, an outstanding date in the history of medicine, Koch presented to the Berlin Physiological Society his discovery of the tubercle bacillus, which was also cultivated by him. This discovery definitely established the infectiousness of tuberculosis, a concept that had been held by the physicians of the time of Hippocrates, reaffirmed by Fracastorius, and demonstrated (1868) by the experiments of the gifted J. A. VILLEMIN (1827–92), who transmitted the disease in animals by means of tuberculous material. The pathological picture of tuberculosis was now established in its broad lines. In this article also Koch first announced his famous Postulates — previously approached by Henle and Klebs — outlining the four steps necessary to prove that a given organism was the cause of a given disease. Though other criteria have since been found to be necessary in some cases and though certain organisms —

such as the *Treponema pallidum* and those of " virus " diseases — have been universally accepted as the causes of certain diseases without Koch's postulates having been fulfilled, nevertheless they remain today the foundation stone in the establishment of such a relationship. In 1883 Koch and his pupil Gaffky discovered the *Micrococcus tetragenus* and the *Vibrio choleræ* and demonstrated the transmission of the latter by food, but especially by drinking water. The previous year he had discovered the cause of infectious conjunctivitis (Egyptian

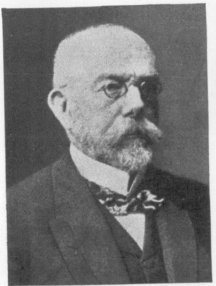

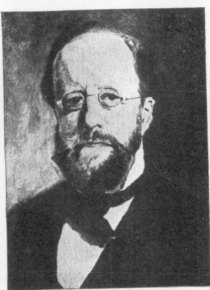

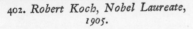

402. *Robert Koch, Nobel Laureate, 1905.*　　　　　　　403. *Edwin Klebs.*

ophthalmia, " pink-eye "), the Koch-Weeks bacillus — so called because of the 1886 contribution of the American ophthalmologist J. E. WEEKS. Koch's investigations covered most of the field of microbiology — malaria, recurrent fever, rinderpest, and so on. In 1890 he announced to the International Medical Congress at Berlin the discovery of tuberculin as a cure for tuberculosis. The success of this communication, coming from such a distinguished scientist, and one universally revered for his important investigations, was sensational, and great hopes for the conquest of the white plague were raised throughout the world. Clinical studies, however, soon showed that tuberculin was not to fulfil the great expectations for cure that had been raised. In its various forms and fractions, however, it has proved to be of diagnostic value, especially in the past decade. In 1891 Koch was made director of the newly established Institute for Infectious Diseases, where he worked out important methods of controlling water-borne infections by filtration. This had a striking effect in controlling the cholera epidemic in Hamburg (1892), during which his assistant, the American

W. P. DUNBAR, first recognized the existence of "carriers" of infectious diseases. At the 1900 Tuberculosis Congress in London and again at Washington in 1908 he maintained erroneously that the bovine type of tubercle bacillus — isolated by Theobald Smith in 1898 — was so different from the human variety that it was of little or no danger to man. This error, supported by Koch's authority (*summum jus, summa injuria*) retarded control of tuberculosis by a generation, until it was corrected by Theobald Smith. Koch headed investigating commissions to Rhodesia for the study of *Küstenfieber*; to German East Africa for the study of trypanosomiasis and other infectious diseases; and to Japan.

Robert Koch was one of the most famous men of his time and one of Germany's greatest scientists. By physicians, scientific institutes, and governments throughout the world he was given the highest honours and the most distinguished scientific awards. He gathered about him pupils who occupy illustrious positions in the history of bacteriology, among whom the best-known are Loeffler, Pfeiffer, Gaffky, Kitasato, Welch. Though possessed of the esteem and admiration of his colleagues, he did not acquire the popularity of Pasteur, partly because of his austere, distant manner, partly perhaps because of certain episodes in his private life that alienated the sympathy of many of his colleagues. Nevertheless, his great achievements in bacteriology and in hygiene, the vastness of his knowledge, and the importance of his investigations ensure for him permanently a leading role in the history of bacteriology.

This is not the place to enumerate all the discoveries in the field of bacteriology, a task that must be left to special histories of this discipline. As Koch said, "As soon as the right method was found, discoveries came as easily as ripe apples from the tree." We can only record the names and discoveries of some of the great pioneers. The accompanying table attempts to give in chronological order the names of some of the bacteria, the diseases they cause, and their discoverers. As many bacteria have been known by several names, in separate columns are listed the names recently given by Bergey's *Manual of Determinative Bacteriology*, that given by its first describer, and occasionally also another name that has had wide usage. Prominent among the early pioneers was one whose original studies in many fields pointed the way to much progress. Edwin KLEBS (1834–1913), who conducted important pathological studies at Bern, Würzburg, Prague, Zurich, Berlin, Lausanne, and Chicago, was led by his experiences in the Franco-Prussian War to undertake the study of the nature of traumatic infections. He was a precursor of Koch and Metchnikoff in the experimental transmission of syphilis to monkeys. He also made notable contributions to other fields of bacteriology, such as detection of the typhoid bacillus (1881), study of bacteria filtrates (1871), discovery of the diphtheria bacillus (1883), and so on. Another successful bacteriologist was Georg GAFFKY (1850–1918), who was Professor of Hygiene at Giessen and followed Koch as director of the Institute of Hygiene at Berlin. To him we owe important studies on rabbit

A CHRONOLOGICAL LIST OF DISCOVERIES OF SOME MICRO-ORGANISMS

Date	Present Name	Original or Common Name	Disease or Habitat	Discoverer
1849	Serratia marcescens	Monas prodigiosa	(a factor in certain miracles)	Ehrenberg
1850	B. anthracis	B. anthracis	anthrax	Rayer (Davaine, 1864)
1872	B. subtilis	B. subtilis	(soil organism)	Cohn
1873	Borrelia recurrentis	Spirochæta obermaieri	relapsing fever	Obermaier
1874	Micrococci	Micrococci	various infections	Billroth & predecessors; Koch (1878); A. Ogstor (1880)
1875	Mycobacterium lepræ	B. lepræ	leprosy	A. Hansen (b. 1841–d. 1912)
1875 (1879)	Clostridium chauvœi	B. Chauvœi	black leg (in cattle)	Bollinger (Arloing et al.)
1877	Clostridium œdematis maligni	Vibrion septique (B. œdematis maligni)	gas gangrene	Pasteur & Joubert (1879)
1877	Actinomyces bovis	Actinomyces bovis	actinomycosis	Bollinger
1878	Pasteurella aviseptica	B. choleræ gallinarum	fowl cholera	Perroncito, Pasteur (1880)
1879	Neisseria gonorrhoeæ	Gonócoccus	gonorrhœa	Neisser
1880	Eberthella typhi	B. typhosus	typhoid fever	Eberth (Gaffky, 1884)
1882	Klebsiella rhinoscleromatis	Rhinosclerombacillus	rhinoscleroma	von Fritsch
1882	Klebsiella pneumoniæ	Pneumoniecoccus	Friedländer's pneumonia	Friedländer
1882	Mycobacterium tuberculosis	B. tuberculosis	tuberculosis	Koch
1882	Staphylococcus pyogenes aureus	Staphylococcus aureus	pyogenic infection	A. Ogston, 1882
1883	Gaffkya tetragena	Micrococcus tetragenus	(inhabits respiratory tract)	Gaffky
1883	[Streptococcus pyogenes]	Erysipelkokken	erysipelas	F. Fehleisen
1883	Corynebacterium diphtheriæ	B. diphtheriæ	diphtheria	Klebs (Löffler, 1884)
1883	Vibrio comma	Kommabazillus (Vibrio choleræ)	Asiatic cholera	Koch
1884	Streptococcus pyogenes	Streptococcus puerperalis Streptococcus pyogenes	pyogenic infections	Rosenbach

The dates given are usually those of the publication of the discovery. See Bibliography, Chapter xx, VII, for references.

A CHRONOLOGICAL LIST OF DISCOVERIES OF SOME MICRO-ORGANISMS (continued)

Date	Present Name	Original or Common Name	Disease or Habitat	Discoverer
1884	Clostridium tetani	S. hemolyticus, Schottmüller (1903) B. tetani	tetanus	A. Nicolaier (J. Rosenbach, 1886)
1885	Proteus vulgaris	B. proteus vulgaris	rotting material, fæces, wounds	Hauser
1885	Aerobacter aerogenes	B. lactis aerogenes	(inhabits intestinal tract)	Escherich
1885	Pasteurella avicida	Micrococcus choleræ-gallinarum	fowl cholera	Zopf
1885	Salmonella suipestifer	B. suipestifer	hog cholera (secondary)	Salmon & Smith
1885	Pasteurella boviseptica	B. bipolare multocidum	hemorrhagic septicemia of cattle	Kitt
1886	Hemophilus conjunctivitidis	B. koch-weeks	epidemic conjunctivitis ("pink-eye")	Koch (J. E. Weeks, 1887) Salvioli
1886	Diplococcus pneumoniæ	Diplococcus pneumoniæ (Pneumococcus)	pneumonia	A. Fraenkel (b. 1848-d. 1916), Weichselbaum
1886	Erysipelothrix rhusiopathiæ	B. schweinerotlauf	swine erysipelas	Löffler
1886	Escherichia coli	B. coli commune	(inhabits intestinal tract)	Escherich (1885)
1886	Actinobacillus mallei	B. mallei	glanders	Löffler
1887	Neisseria intracellularis	Diplococcus intracellularis meningitidis (meningococcus)	cerebrospinal meningitis	Marchiafava & Celli (1884) Weichselbaum
1887	Brucella melitensis	Micrococcus melitensis	Malta (undulant) fever	Bruce
1887	[Streptococcus pyogenes]	Micrococcus scarlatinæ	scarlet fever	Klein (A. Dochez; G. F. and G. H. Dick, 1923)
1888	Salmonella enteritidis	B. enteritidis	food poisoning	Gaertner
1889	Hemophilus ducreyi	B. ducreyii	soft chancre	A. Ducrey
1892	Salmonella typhimurium	B. typhi murium	epidemic mouse typhus	Löffler
1892	Clostridium welchii	B. aerogenes capsulatus	gas gangrene	W. H. Welch & G. H. F. Nuttall
1892	Hemophilus influenzæ	B. influenzæ	secondary invader in influenza	R. Pfeiffer
1892	[Streptococcus pyogenes]	Strep. puerperalis (M. septicus puerperalis)	puerperal fever	Arloing (Chauveau, 1882)

Year				
1893	Salmonella psittacosis	B. psittacosis	(associated with parrot pneumonia)	Nocard
1894	Pasteurella pestis	B. pestis	bubonic plague	Kitasato, Yersin
1894	Clostridium novyi	B. novyi (œdematiens, Weinberg)	gas gangrene	Novy
1896	Neisseria catarrhalis	Micrococcus catarrhalis	inflammation of respiratory mucosa	Frosch & Kolle
1896	Hemophilus lacunatus	B. morax-axenfeld	diplo-bacillary conjunctivitis	Morax (Axenfeld, 1897)
1897	Brucella abortus	B. abortus	infectious abortion of cattle	B. L. F. Bang
1897 (1896)	Clostridium botulinum	B. botulinus	botulism	van Ermengem
1897	Salmonella icteroides	B. icteroides	(found in yellow-fever cadavers)	Sanarelli
1898	Shigella dysenteriæ	B. dysenteriæ	bacillary dysentery	Shiga & Kruse
1898	Salmonella aertrycke	B. aertrycke	food poisoning	de Nobele
1900	Salmonella schottmuelleri	B. paratyphi alcaligenes	paratyphoid fever (type B)	Schottmüller
1900	Shigella paradysenteriæ	B. dysenteriæ (Flexner)	dysentery, "summer diarrhœa"	R. Strong (Flexner)
1900	Escherichia communior	B. coli communior	(inhabits intestinal tract)	Durham
1902	Salmonella paratyphi	B. paratyphi A	paratyphoid fever (rare type)	Kayser
1903	Streptococcus viridans group (salivarius, etc.)	Streptococcus viridans (S. mitis)	subacute bacterial endocarditis, etc.	Schottmüller (Andrewes & Horder, 1906)
1905	Treponema pertenue	Treponema pertenue	yaws	Castellani
1905	Treponema pallidum	Spirochæte pallidum	syphilis	Schaudinn & Hoffmann
1906	Hemophilus pertussis	Microbe de coqueluche (B. pertussis)	whooping cough	Bordet & Gengou (Burger, 1883?)
1909	Bartonella bacilliformis	Bartonia bacilliformis (Strong, 1913)	Oroya fever (verruga peruana)	Barton (Noguchi, 1926)
1911	Pasteurella tularensis	B. tularense	tularemia	G. W. McCoy & C. V. Chapin
1915	Clostridium fallax	B. fallax	gas gangrene	Weinberg & Seguin
1915	Shigella paradysenteriæ (var. Sonnei)	B. dysenteriæ, group III	sporadic dysentery	Sonne
1916	Leptospira icterohemorrhagiæ	Spirochæte icterohemorrhagiæ	infectious jaundice	Inado & Ido

septicemia, cholera, and anthrax, and the first cultivation of the typhoid bacillus. In the new terminology, the genus Gaffkya was named after him for his discovery of the type species *M. tetragenus*. Friedrich LÖFFLER (1852–1915) was the co-discoverer with Klebs of *B. diphtheriæ* and differentiated it from pseudo-diphtheria organisms. He discovered several other bacterial causes of disease and demonstrated that foot-and-mouth disease was due to a filterable virus. As the table shows, the organisms that cause various diseases were being discovered with great rapidity. In 1879 A. NEISSER discovered the gonococcus. The meningococcus was demonstrated in the spinal fluid as the cause of epidemic cerebrospinal meningitis (1887) by Anton WEICHSELBAUM (1845–1920). It was first reported (1897) in the joints by R. FRANZ (b. 1881), and in the blood (1899) by Norman GWYN (b. 1875). The discovery of *B. pestis* as the bacterial cause of bubonic plague took place at Hong Kong in 1894, where the modern pandemic had been carried from its origin in Canton in the same year. S. KITASATO (1856–1931), coming from Japan, and G. A. E. YERSIN, from Indo-China, promptly isolated the same organism from human tissues. Spontaneous plague in rodents has been suspected off and on for centuries and demonstrated many times since the Canton epidemic. Its transmission through fleas was first suggested by M. OGATA (1897), the theory was developed by W. G. LISTON (1905), and the mechanism of transmission by A. W. BACOT (1914). Epidemic in rats as in man, plague is now taken to exist also endemically in reservoirs of rodents of the great continental plains.

Of *fungus diseases*, actinomycosis was first recognized by B. VON LANGENBECK (1845), and first effectively described by O. von BOLLINGER (1877), who recognized its fungus cause. Madura foot, recognized as due to a fungus (1860) by H. V. CARTER (1831–97) and named mycetoma, is now accepted as a form of actinomycosis. The names of C. O. HARZ (1877), A. PERRONCITO (1879), and S. RIVOLTA (1882) are also connected with this discovery. Blastomycosis was discovered by T. C. GILCHRIST (1896); sporotrichosis by B. R. SCHENCK (1898); leptothrix infections of the mouth by Brown KELLY (1896), of the eye by von Graefe (1855), and of the meninges by Ivy MACKENZIE (1931). The saccharomyces (cryptococcus, torula histolytica) infection, described by O. BUSSE and A. BUSCHKE in 1894, now known as torulosis or European blastomycosis, is a frequently fatal disease, especially in its cerebral form. Histoplasmosis, another fatal, though rare fungus disease, is caused by *Histoplasma capsulatum*, discovered (1906) and named by S. T. DARLING. It was later cultivated and recognized as a fungus by W. A. DE MONBREUN (1934). Its capability to produce calcified areas in the lungs in a considerable percentage of healed cases (C. E. PALMER, 1945) makes it a distinct source of error in the search for tuberculosis in military candidates. Infection by *Monilia albicans* (discovered in the disease of the mouth known as " thrush " by B. von Langenbeck, 1839) is a mild disease when on the skin, but more serious in pulmonary and other internal varieties.

IMMUNOLOGY is the study of the body's reaction to harmful agents. It had early been recognized that recovery from certain diseases conferred protection against later attacks. Thus, those pockmarked by smallpox were known to go unharmed through later epidemics; Pierre Chatard is said to have noted a similar immunity to yellow fever in the pioneers in the New World. Mithridates (132–62 B.C.) is said to have taken repeated small doses of poisons in order to build up resistance against possible attacks on his life

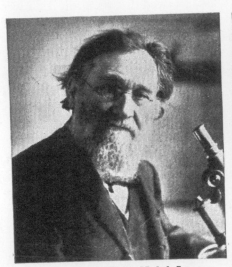

404. E. Metchnikoff, Nobel Laureate, 1908.

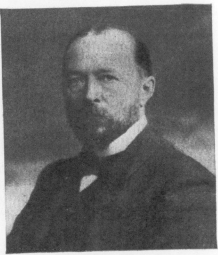

405. E. von Behring, Nobel Laureate, 1901.

by this means. However, the subject may be said to have had its effective start in such studies as those of Pasteur, Metchnikoff, É. Roux, and A. Yersin (1888), H. Buchner (1889), and von Behring and Kitasato (1890). As we have already noted, vaccination against smallpox seems to have been known by Orientals in very ancient times, and the importance to all mankind of Jenner's discovery of vaccination has already been emphasized. Metchnikoff's study of the origins of the blastodermic layers, and particularly of the mesoderm, revealed that the amœboid cells of this layer have the ability to ingest foreign material. Thus he arrived at the conclusion, first suggested by the work (1874) of P. L. PANUM (1820–85), and of K. ROSER (1856–1905) in 1881, that these cells play an important part in the process of inflammation. His study of infectious diseases from this point of view, the various steps being followed under the microscope, led to the establishment (1884) of the doctrine of PHAGOCYTOSIS (from the Greek, "to eat" and "cells"). The simplicity of this theory aroused a vast amount of discussion. For instance, E. Roux (1853–1933) and A. Yersin's demonstration of toxic substances in filtrates of broth cultures of diphtheria bacilli 1888), and Buchner's discovery of protective bactericidal substances in the blood (1886–90), albuminoids that he called *alexins*, produced a new and important rival to Metchnikoff's views in what was soon called the "humoral theory" of immunity. Bordet later (1898) showed that the protection was due to two substances, the thermolabile alexin, normally present, and a more stable substance produced by immunization, which he called *substance sensibilisatrice*. Toxins were first named and described in 1888 by L. Brieger (1849–1919) in the case of typhoid and tetanus. In 1895 R. F. J. Pfeiffer (b. 1858) discovered that the peritoneal fluids of immunized guinea pigs would dissolve cholera vibrios that had been introduced into the abdomen (bacteriolysins); in 1896 M. Gruber (1853–1927) and F. Widal (1862–1929) discovered bacterial agglutinins. In 1897 R. Kraus (1868–1932) discovered precipitins; in 1898 J. B. V. Bordet (b. 1870), perhaps the greatest of the later exponents of immunology, demonstrated bacterial cytolysis. This phenomenon had been earlier indicated by the work (1898) of S. Belfanti (1860–1939) and T. Carbone (1863–1904), and by L. Landois's (1837–1902) observation that animal serum would hemolyze human blood (1875).

The discovery by Emil von Behring (1854–1917) of the possibility of *passive immunization* of animals and man against tetanus and diphtheria, by the injection of serum from animals that had been actively immunized by repeated injection of tetanus or diphtheritic toxin (1890), led to the concept of antitoxins. The extracellular bacterial toxins, which were soon found to occur in only a few species, were called "exotoxins" as distinguished from the "endotoxins" that remain in association with the bacterial cell.

To these observations were added the brilliant discoveries of Paul Ehrlich (1854–1915), an outstanding scientist and genius of extraordinary activity, most accurate and profound in his researches, cautious and rigorous in his criticism. Experimenting with dye-stuffs and tissue-staining even as a student, to the detriment of his studies, he made many useful observations, such as the basophilic mast cell of the blood (1877), the diazo reaction in typhoid urines (1882), the fuchsin acid-fast stain of tubercle bacilli (1882), and intravital staining (1886). An attack of tuberculosis in 1887, following his experiments with this disease, required a long stay in Egypt. On his return, in 1890, he started a small laboratory, but the same year went to Koch's new Institute for Infectious Diseases, where he began his studies on immunity. In 1896 he founded the Institute for Serum Studies at Steglitz; and in 1899 he founded the Institute for Experimental Therapy at

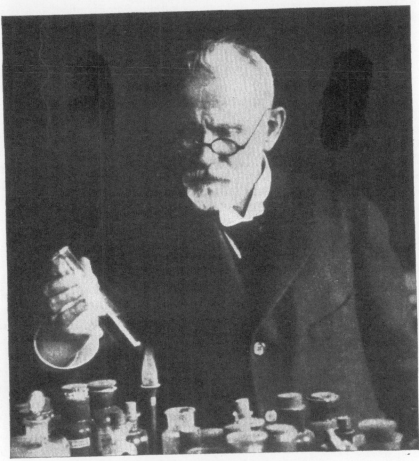

406. *Paul Ehrlich, Nobel Laureate, 1908.*

Frankfurt and in 1907 the Georg Speyer Haus for chemotherapy, both of which he directed.

Early in his immunological work he discovered that the specific antitoxic effect of immunizing serum could be demonstrated not only in experimental animals, but also *in vitro*. With J. MORGENROTH (1871–1924), he demonstrated (1899) many new facts about immune serum, largely based on the presence of a dissolving substance found in normal serum, which they called " complement," and a heat-resisting " immune body " produced by reaction to injected material. These corresponded to Bordet's " alexin " and " substance sensibilisatrice." Ehrlich also standardized experimental dosages with the concept of the Minimal Lethal Dose (the amount that would kill a 250-gram guinea-pig, characteristically in four days). There followed a series of studies that culminated in his SIDE-CHAIN THEORY, which conceived of the protein molecule as analogous to Kekulé's benzene ring with unstable side chains. These, acting as chemo-receptors, could combine with harmful materials to neutralize them; and, being manufactured under appropriate stimulus in excess (Weigert's law of overproduction), were cast off into the blood stream to protect the individual against similar harmful agents. Thus was explained the formation of antibodies under the stimulus of injected antigens. This so-called immunization can occur not only against harmful bacteria, but also against other substances, such as blood from other individuals of the same species. Ehrlich's concept of the mechanism of antibody-formation has been replaced by the concept that antibody globulins receive their specific combining affinities intracellularly under the impress of the specific configurations of the antigens. This "templating theory" was independently suggested by F. BREINL (b. 1888) and F. HAUROWITZ (b. 1896), by J. ALEXANDER (b. 1876), and by S. MUDD (b. 1893), and more recently has been advocated in slightly different terms by Linus C. PAULING (b. 1901). Ehrlich's concept of specific chemical combining sites on antigens and antibodies, sustaining to their counterparts a key-to-lock relationship based upon specific stereochemical configuration, has endured, however, and is the foundation of current immunochemistry. Specific configurational relationships, indeed, give promise of assuming similar basic importance in enzyme chemistry and in chemotherapy.

ACTIVE IMMUNIZATION with living pathogens was tried by Jaime FERRÁN Y CLUA (1849–1929) against cholera at Valencia (1881–5), and by W. HAFFKINE (1860–1930) against plague in 1895. Attenuated virus had of course been the underlying principle of Jenner's vaccination against smallpox in 1798 and of Pasteur's vacancies against rabies, anthrax, and swine erysipelas. Killed cultures were used against plague by A. LUSTIG (1857–1937), of Florence, and G. GALEOTTI (1867–1921), in 1897; against dysentery by K. SHIGA (b. 1870) and W. KRUSE (1864–1943), in 1901; against typhoid by Pfeiffer and W. KOLLE (1868–1935), in 1896; and finally bacterial extracts (tuberculin) by Koch against tuberculosis in 1891. The story of immunization against tuberculosis includes the work of A. MAFFUCCI (1847–1903), precursor of Calmette in the use of living organisms, and of E. Maragliano, who recommended the prophylactic treatment of tuberculosis by the injection of dead bacilli.

The most important steps in our knowledge of passive immunization were the treatment of diphtheria by antitoxin, begun by Behring in 1890 and amplified by Roux in 1894; the use of tetanus antitoxin by Behring (1892), and of anti-plague serum by Yersin and Calmette (1895). In 1913 Bela SCHICK (b. 1877) showed that those immune to diphtheria could be detected by their skin re-action to injections of diphtheria toxin. This has led to a number of similar valuable diagnostic tests. The combination of active and passive immunization was tried (1893) by G. LORENZ against swine erysipelas, and (1896) by A. SCLAVO against anthrax.

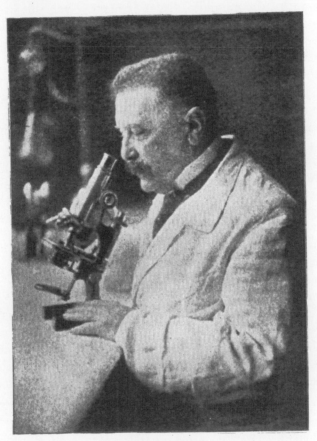

407. *Fernand Widal.*

Immunization against typhoid was attempted (1888) by F. WIDAL (1862–1929), working with A. CHANTEMESSE (1851–1919), but the former is much bet-ter known for his application of the agglutination test to the diagnosis of typhoid fever in the well-known "Widal test" (1896). This reaction had been discov-ered (1896) by the English bacteriologist H. E. DURHAM (1866–1945), working with his teacher, Max Gruber. Eye trouble, following expeditions to study tropical diseases, unfortunately removed Durham prematurely from the field.

Widal's name is also associated with the Hayem-Widal (acquired) type of hemolytic jaundice.

INSECT TRANSMITTERS (vectors) of micro-organisms that cause disease first came into prominence with Sir Patrick Manson's discovery (1877) that *Filaria sanguinis hominis* (*Wuchereria bancrofti*) was introduced into the human system by the mosquito, *Culex fatigans*. Even this had been preceded by Fedchenko's observation (1869) of the development of the guinea worm in *cyclops*. This principle shortly came into the greatest importance in establishing the cause and mode of transmission of malaria and yellow fever. Earlier, to be sure, a possible connection between mosquitoes and malaria had been adumbrated by the ancient Hindu, Susruta, just as Benjamin Rush at the end of the eighteenth century, J. C. NOTT (1848), and L. D. BEAUPERTHUY (1803–71) had casually linked yellow fever with the mosquito (1854). The possibility of such a connection was more definitely stated and some evidence was reported in 1882 in the case of yellow fever by Carlos Juan FINLAY (1833–1915), and in 1882 (pub. 1883) by A. F. A. KING in the case of malaria. Among other insect vectors, rat fleas as carriers of plague and typhus, and the louse as carrier of typhus, are referred to elsewhere; also the tsetse fly as carrier of African sleeping sickness. More recently the sand-fly (Phlebotomus) has been convicted as the carrier of Leishmaniases and of Oroya fever and pappataci fever, and various ticks and mites of rickettsial diseases.

PARASITIC DISEASES. The causative agent of malaria, a protozoal plasmodium, was first observed in living blood cells by Alphonse LAVERAN (1845–1922), a French Army surgeon working in Algiers, in 1880, and was more fully described, in the chief varieties as known today, by Marchiafava and Celli in 1885.[1] To Golgi belongs the credit of having traced the development of the parasites of tertian and quartan fever and the relation that exists between the developmental stage of the organism and the exacerbations of fever.

It was Golgi also who recognized the reason for the difference between the typical intermittent fever (tertian and quartan) and the grave pernicious type. In the former the parasites develop chiefly in the circulating blood; in the latter chiefly or almost exclusively in the internal organs (brain). Extending the search, Achille MONTI (Pavia) was one of the first to call attention (1894) to the localization in the viscera of the red blood cells infected with the parasites of estivo-autumnal fever. On the basis of this scientific progress, A. Celli inaugu-

---

[1] The statement that it had previously been seen in dried human blood by Joseph Jones in 1876 (pub. New Orleans M. and S. J., 1878) is not justified, as Jones obviously described merely the malarial pigment.

rated a systematic campaign against malaria, which achieved wonders in ridding Italy from this, one of its worst disease plagues.

Giovanni Battista GRASSI (1854–1925), of Rovellasca, near Como, Professor of Comparative Anatomy first at Catania, then at Rome, completed the picture of the life cycle of the plasmodium in birds and man. He had already done important work on the parasites of man and animals (cf. his studies on ankylostomiasis with the brothers Parona). In 1898 he demonstrated the special capacity of

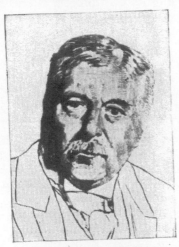

408. *Sir Patrick Manson.*

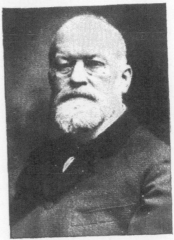

409. *C. H. L. Alphonse Laveran, Nobel Laureate.* 1907.

the genus Anopheles mosquito to transmit malaria from man to man by carrying the plasmodium in its digestive tract. The general problem was advanced in its various phases by pathologists, clinicians, and hygienists, such as P. MANSON (1842–1922), G. Bastianelli, A. BIGNAMI (1862–1929) (collaborator of Grassi), V. ASCOLI, W. S. THAYER, W. G. MACCALLUM, and others. It was Manson who proved experimentally the transmission of malaria to man by *Anopheles*, by exposing his son to the bite of an infected mosquito. W. G. MacCallum, as a student, first demonstrated (1897) the entrance of a flagellum into a " crescentsphere " (sexual conjugation of the malarial organism), provoking the outcry from Ross: " I have felt disgraced as a man of science ever since! "

Sir Ronald Ross (1857–1932), one of the most eminent and versatile of modern pathologists, who received the Nobel prize in 1902, demonstrated the life cycle of the parasite in the viscera of the infected *Anopheles* (1895–9). In 1898 he found also the sporozoites of the plasmodium in the salivary glands of *Anopheles*. After eighteen years in the Indian medical service, in 1899 he came to teach at the Liverpool School of Tropical Medicine; then, after devising and successfully applying methods of mosquito-extermination in West Africa, he became physician to King's Hospital (1912) and eventually (1926) director of the new institute that bears his name. A man of wide culture and untiring activity, he contributed to mathematics and wrote plays, poetry, and a notable autobiography. His verse beginning: " This day relenting God hath placed," commemorating his discovery of the malarial organism in the mosquito's stomach, is one of the noblest occasional poems written by a medical man. His principal work is entitled *Studies on Malaria* (1928).

Other important discoveries in the field of parasitology were those of the fluke, *Schistosoma hæmatobium* (Bilharzia), by Bilharz (1852); filaria found in elephantiasis by Manson (1877), and shown by him to be transmitted by mosquitoes (1878); transmission of yellow fever by *Stegomyia fasciata* (*Aëdes ægypti*), maintained by C. J. FINLAY (1881) and definitely proved by REED, CARROLL, LAZEAR, and AGRAMONTE (1900). Among intestinal parasites discovered in this period, Davaine first observed *Cercomonas intestinalis* (1857); P. H. MALMSTEM (1811–73), the *Balantidium coli* (1857); W. D. LAMBL (1824–95), the *Giardia intestinalis* (1859), later named after A. GIARD (1846–1908). Pathogenic *amœbæ* were seen by LOESCH (1875) and distinguished from the harmless forms; the several varieties and their role in producing amœbic dysentery were elucidated by a number of investigators: Koch, 1883; Kartulis, 1886; Osler, 1890; W. T. Councilman and H. A. LaFleur, 1891; Schaudinn, 1903; and others. Ankylostomiasis (hookworm disease) was shown by W. GRIESINGER (1866) to be due to the *Ankylostoma duodenale*, first found in the intestinal tract by A. DUBINI (1813–1902) in 1843. The devious route by which the parasite reaches the intestine after the larva has penetrated the skin — usually the sole of the foot — was shown by A. Looss (1898). The American variety, *Necator americanus*, discovered in Texas by Allen J. SMITH and later (1902) named by C. W. STILES, was found to be extremely common in the United States and in Puerto Rico (B. K. ASHFORD). The largely successful efforts of the International Health Board of the Rockefeller Foundation to eradicate this plague, and thus greatly to raise the level of existence among the lower classes of the Southern states, are one of the most brilliant examples of the contributions of richly endowed philanthropic foundations to the promotion of public health.

A number of trypanosomes have been found to be pathogenic. Though the earliest discovered (in the frog) and *T. lewisi* in the rat appear to be harmless, *T. evansi* (Griffith EVANS, 1880) was shown to be the cause of surra, a disease of ungulates. Sir David BRUCE (1855–1931) found that *T. brucei* (1894) caused the regularly fatal nagana, the animal disease transmitted by the tsetse fly (*Glossina morsitans*). In the equally fatal disease of man, *T. gambiense* (J. E. DUTTON, 1901) was found to be transmitted by another tsetse fly, *Glossina palpalis*. In addition to various other animal diseases, caused by *T. equiperdum*, *T. thei-*

leri, and *T. dimorphon*, we should record the South American disease named (1909) for Carlos CHAGAS (1879–1934), caused by *T. cruzi* and transmitted by biting insects of the family Reduviidas. Another group of parasitic diseases is represented by kala-azar, a tropical splenomegaly, caused by the flagellated body *Leishmania donovani* (1903). A cutaneous form — Aleppo or Delhi boil — is caused by *L. tropica* (J. H. WRIGHT, 1903). Still another group, *Babesia* (piroplasma), named after their Rumanian discoverer, V. BABES (1854–1926), has been found to cause a number of relatively unimportant diseases of man and animals. *Toxoplasma pyogenes* was reported by A. Castellani (1914) as the cause of a grave human disease — toxoplasmosis.

8. Internal Medicine

The student of the progress of clinical medicine in this period soon becomes aware of a special characteristic that underwent a marked development: namely, the improvement in the field of diagnosis, thanks to the steady improvement in research methods and accomplishments. This in turn brought about a closer connection between clinical medicine and pathology, which was largely responsible for these improvements. During this epoch, and especially in its earlier periods, which felt most profoundly the influence of the great revolutions in pathology and microbiology, the scientific clinician became essentially a pathologist. This tendency was especially marked in Germany, the most active centre of pathologic and microbiological investigations, where in a period of great economic prosperity there was an extraordinary development of well-equipped laboratories. Every hospital clinic had at its disposal the means and equipment necessary for the most delicate and complicated investigations. The great German clinicians of the period were, above all, excellent pathologists and often outstanding bacteriologists as well. Thus it came about that in the great German schools and clinics the highest importance was placed on laboratory studies, and less weight was given to bedside observations and especially to treatment. There were of course many exceptions, but there is no question that this trend dominated the German medicine of the second half of the century, as can well be seen in its scientific literature.

In Germany, in fact, the tendency reached such a point that laboratory research was in a fair way to overshadow clinical study in the productive activities of the clinic. The suggestion that acute rheumatic fever was due to allergy — the reaction of an individual sensitized to a foreign protein to intoxication by this protein — acquired many supporters in Germany and Russia, though the clinical picture of rheumatic fever obviously betrays its specifically infectious nature. Of course, in the sense, that the sensitizing antigens might be bacteria located at a distant site in the body, in which case the disease would still be classed as infectious, allergy may prove to be the factor that may produce the infectious process (Homer Swift).

In the advancement of knowledge of internal medicine in the second half of the century, when the laboratory specialties were making their most striking contributions, the GERMAN and AUSTRIAN universities took a very prominent part. Friedrich Theodor von FRERICHS (1819–85), successor of Schönlein at the Berlin clinic (1859), after occupying chairs at Göttingen, Kiel, and Breslau, was a leading exponent of the new learning. A pioneer in experimental pathology, he helped to explain the nature of acute yellow atrophy by his discovery of leucine and tyrosine in the urine of patients suffering from that disease. His clinico-pathologic studies of diseases of the liver (1858–68) and of Bright's disease (1851) and his monographs on digestion and on diabetes in Wagner's *Dictionary of Physiology* (1884) indicate the basis of his scientific fame. The clinical lectures of Frerichs were accepted as of classic perfection in the exact description of disease. His style of delivery, which was often dramatic, was imposing. His brilliant though opinionated diagnoses were usually intuitive, but always clear. Frerichs was revered by students and colleagues and he became one of the founders of the scientific teaching of clinical medicine, while his influence was prolonged through brilliant pupils such as Naunyn, von Leyden, Ehrlich, A. Fraenkel and von Mering.

Ludwig TRAUBE (1818–76), an outstanding student of morbid anatomy and physiology, a none too friendly colleague of Frerichs's at the Berlin clinic and like him a pioneer of experimental pathology, was concerned particularly with the pathology of fever and with the connections between diseases of the heart and kidney; he also worked on the functional effects of section of the vagus. He is recalled to students of physical diagnosis by " Traube's semilunar space."

Among other well-known German internists was the encyclopædist Hugo von ZIEMSSEN (1829–1902), whose greatest production was the seventeen-volume *Handbuch der speziellen Pathologie und Therapie* (English translation, 20 vols., 1874–81). Ernst VON LEYDEN (1832–1910), a pupil of Schönlein and Traube, followed the latter as head of the Berlin clinic in 1876. He founded with Frerichs the *Zeitschrift für klinische Medizin* (1879) and wrote numerous clinical studies (tabes dorsalis, poliomyelitis, etc.). Adolf KUSSMAUL (1822–1902), Professor of Medicine in various universities and finally at Strasbourg, first described periarteritis nodosa

(1866), progressive bulbar paralysis (1873), and diabetic coma with acetonuria, as well as various diagnostic and therapeutic procedures. He first observed the *pulsus paradoxus* and prescribed gastric lavage in dilatation of the stomach (1869).

Hermann SENATOR (1834–1911), head of the Berlin Polyclinic, was a celebrated clinician, noted especially for his studies on diseases of the kidney and diabetes, and for his introduction of the concept of autointoxication. Hermann NOTHNAGEL (1841–1905), a pupil of Traube, Virchow, and von Leyden, was Professor of Medicine at Hamburg, Jena, and after 1882 at Vienna. A man of brilliant culture, high ideals, and vast knowledge, he was the leading clinician of his time, venerated by his students and revered by his colleagues. He is best known as editor of the great *Handbuch der speziellen Pathologie und Therapie* in twenty-four volumes, which appeared between 1894 and 1905 and was shortly after translated into English (A. Stengel, editor). Numerous original observations in the domains of chronic diseases and gastro-intestinal and peritoneal affections are due to him.

Eminent among modern clinicians was Bernard NAUNYN (1839–1925), Professor of Medicine at Dorpat, Bern, Königsberg, and eventually Strasbourg. He will be remembered for his studies of gall-stones and diseases of the liver and pancreas. His book on diabetes still remains the most complete work on this subject, and also his general medical point of view was unsurpassed. In 1906 he coined the term " acidosis " for the condition underlying diabetic coma — a term that has since proved valuable in many other conditions. His *Erinnerungen, Gedanken und Meinungen* (1925), one of the best of many German works of this type and period, affords an interesting picture of the man and his time. Heinrich CURSCHMANN (1846–1910), a close student of bronchial asthma, is most remembered today for the " Curschmann spirals " found in that disease. Karl VON NOORDEN (b. 1858), professor at Frankfurt and later Nothnagel's successor at Vienna, is especially linked with the study of metabolic disorders. His influence has been continued by the widespread studies of his pupil Hans EPPINGER, JR. (b. 1879), professor at Freiburg and later at Vienna. Friedrich von MÜLLER (1858–1933), Professor of Medicine at Breslau, Marburg, Basel, and for many years at Munich, was one of the most eminent of modern German clinicians. Before World War I his highly organized and efficient clinic was the Mecca of students from many countries, affording opportunities to learn the best of the internal medicine of that day. Adolf STRÜMPELL (1853–1926) is best known today for his textbook of medicine, which went through many editions and was by far the most popular German text on the subject for many years. He was Professor of Medicine at several universities, finally at Leipzig; he described various new disease pictures, such as spondylitis deformans, acute hemorrhagic encephalitis, and the so-called Westphal-Strümpell disease. Friedrich KRAUS (1858–1936), of

Graz and Berlin, published important studies on diseases of metabolism and of the blood and lungs, and on the constitution in relation to fatigue and other factors. With Brugsch he edited a voluminous German *Handbuch der speziellen Pathologie und Therapie* (1919–25), in nineteen volumes. G. KLEMPERER (1865–1946), was a leader in the clinical medicine of Berlin; he published well-known textbooks on internal medicine and on diagnosis and therapy.

Among the clinicians of this time, which was called by A. MAGNUS-LEVY the "heroic age of German medicine," should be cited the names of O. MINKOWSKI; of Herman SAHLI, of Bern, well known for his books on percussion in children and on methods of clinical investigation, who first described acute rheumatism as an attenuated form of staphylococcic pyemia; and of C. A. EWALD (1845–1915) who was assistant of Frerichs and successor of Senator, to whom we owe a great work on disorders of digestion (1879–88). His pupil Ismar BOAS founded the first polyclinic for gastro-intestinal diseases in Germany (1886) and had a great fame as specialist in this branch.

ENGLISH clinical medicine flourished during the period under review as a worthy heritage from the masters of the first half of the century. The "Great Men of Guy's" were followed at that hospital by Gull, Wilks, Fagge, Pavy, and others. Sir William Withey GULL (1816–90) was a leader and one of the most gifted of the clinicians of his time, who fascinated his patients and pupils, though sometimes alienating colleagues by his imperious temper and sharp, even rude expressions. Some of his trenchant remarks have become traditional: "The road to a clinic goes through the pathologic museum and not through the shop of the apothecary"; "Savages explain, scientists investigate." He was eminently successful in practice, leaving an estate valued at £344,000, an unprecedented amount even in British medicine. Within a few years, however, this was surpassed by his rival, Sir William JENNER (1815–98), who was said to have left £375,000. Jenner was physician to Queen Victoria and taught at University College, London. He made an excellent clinico-pathological differentiation of typhus from typhoid fever (1850), ten years after Gerhard had published his study in the United States, which study, however, was not widely known in England. Gull was among the first to describe the lesions in the posterior portion of the spinal cord in locomotor ataxia and also the condition of thyroid deficiency known as myxœdema. Gull's and Sutton's concept of general arterio-capillary fibrosis (1871–2) was an important step toward better understanding of the so-called "degenerative" diseases that are becoming more and more important in modern life. In the kidney, as a noninflammatory form of Bright's disease, it is now known as nephrosclerosis.

Another prominent man of Guy's of the period was Sir Samuel WILKS (1824–1911), author of treatises on pathological anatomy and on the nervous system that enjoyed a great reputation; in fact, it was the influence of his writing that linked the names of Bright, Addison, and Hodgkin to the diseases that bear their names and went far to establish their nosological position. Sir Thomas Clifford ALLBUTT (1836–1925), an excellent clinician and student of disease, wrote ably on such subjects as the visceral neuroses and diseases of the heart, including angina pectoris, summarizing his knowledge of the circulatory system in a two-volume work on diseases of the arteries. He edited a voluminous *System of Medicine* that went through two editions. Allbutt was also, as we shall see, one of the most distinguished of English medical historians.

James MACKENZIE (1853–1925), of Edinburgh, brought an important new contribution to the knowledge of heart diseases, and devised the polygraph, an instrument that traced simultaneous records of the pulsations in the jugular vein, the apex beat, and the radial pulse. A comparison of the three tracings permitted an analysis of the different varieties of cardiac arrhythmias and their causes that established this important subject on a firm basis. In 1890 he discovered the cause of " dropped beat," the extra-systole; he recognized that the " perpetually irregular pulse " was due to lack of contraction of the auricle, which had gone into fibrillation. His followers, among whom Sir Thomas LEWIS (1881–1945) was the most eminent, brought a remarkable contribution to the knowledge of heart diseases, especially when the subject could be further explored by means of the electrocardiograph. Great as were Lewis's contributions to the knowledge of the arrhythmias and the nature of cardiac and muscle pain, however, he probably rendered even greater service in fighting the obsession that " useful discoveries are the prerogative of the laboratories " and in bringing the methods and standards of science to the patient's bedside.

No British clinician aroused the enthusiastic acclaim of colleagues and pupils more than Sir William OSLER (1849–1919), without doubt the finest and most representative figure of contemporary English medicine. Osler was a man of wide culture, a wise clinician, and a tireless student of medicine. Born at Bond Head, Ontario, Canada, he completed his medical studies at McGill University, where he later held the chair of clinical medicine. In 1885 he was called to a similar position at the University of Pennsylvania, where he actively pursued his clinical and clinicopathological studies. He afterwards referred to these few years, especially his experiences in the wards and deadhouse of "Blockley," as the most instructive of his career. In 1889 he became the first Professor of Medicine at the newly founded Johns Hopkins Medical School at Baltimore, one of the famous four with Welch, Kelly, and Halstead. There he was successful in reintroducing in

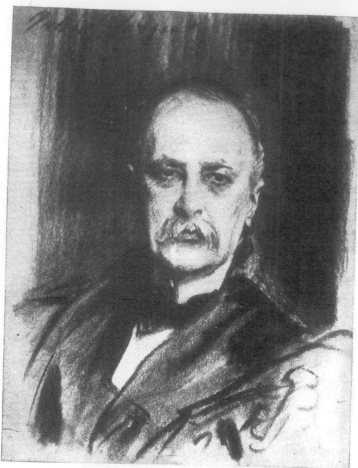

410. *William Osler. Charcoal sketch by Sargent.*
(COLLEGE OF PHYSICIANS OF PHILADELPHIA.)

this country a true bedside method of instruction, teaching in the wards where the students spent most of their time and acted as "clinical clerks." In 1904 he became Regius Professor at Oxford, and was the leading English clinician until his death, in 1919. Osler's *Principles and Practice of Medicine* (1892) struck a new note in medical texts, exposing at first hand a wide yet fresh store of information, so cunningly combined with pithy references to the recent studies of others and with intriguing literary allusions that it would seem impossible to have included the text in a single volume. Small wonder that it passed through nine editions in his lifetime, and still continues under the editorship first of Thomas McCrae and now of H. C. Christian. It is without question the leading one-volume textbook on the subject of our time, if not of any time, and has been translated into many languages. He also edited *Modern Medicine* (1910), a successful " system " that passed through three editions, and was the founder-editor of the *Quarterly Journal of Medicine* (1908).

Osler's contributions to medicine begin with his early studies on the blood platelets and include valuable monographs on *Cancer of the Stomach, Abdominal Tumours, Malignant Endocarditis* (Goulstonian Lectures), *the Cerebral Palsies of Children, Chorea and Choreiform Affections.* He described *Filaria osleri*, polycythemia with splenomegaly (sometimes known as Osler-Vaquez disease), hereditary telangiectasis with recurrent hemorrhage (also known as Osler's disease), and the Osler spots of malignant endocarditis. His numerous addresses and historical and biographical essays are preserved in *Æquanimitas, An Alabama Student*, and other works that are among the most attractive of their kind. He successfully taught the value of work for work's sake and the beauty of labour. His personality, like his writings, had an elusive charm that left an indelible impression on all who had the good fortune to know him. His cordiality and goodwill, his distinction of manner and profundity of historical and literary culture recall his own description of Boerhaave: " A warm-hearted, generous, sympathetic man, a great teacher, and indefatigable worker." His spirit of careful and accurate observation, his deep interest in everything beautiful and noble, and his passionate enthusiasm for his calling made him a most influential and beloved leader. Wherever Osler sojourned, renewed vitality of thought and productive work soon made itself manifest. The loss of his beloved only son, killed in Belgium in World War I, was a crushing blow from which he never recovered. He has been well treated by his biographers: his *Life*, by Harvey Cushing, is a great medical biography, and is well supplemented by Maude Abbott's *Appreciations and . . . Bibliography*. Osler's methods at Johns Hopkins have been worthily carried on by L. F. BARKER (1867–1943), a contributor to anatomy and neurology as well as to clinical medicine; W. S. THAYER (1864–1932), a leader in his specialty who contributed notably to the clinical study of malaria, typhoid, and acute endocarditis (especially the gonorrhœal form), and described the third sound of the heart; and W. T. LONGCOPE (b. 1877), the present incumbent of the chair, who has paid special attention to streptococcic infections and their relation to nephritis.

NORTH AMERICAN medicine in the latter half of the nineteenth century, with the steadily increasing population and wealth of the country, more than kept pace with its growing problems. Though pioneer conditions continued to exist until recently on the westward-moving frontier, physicians of experience and good training — often obtained in Europe — were numerous in the larger cities. In Philadelphia, a leading but no longer the accepted chief medical centre of the country, J. M. DA COSTA (1833–1900) was recognized as one of the most distinguished clinicians and diagnosticians of the country. The significance of his study of the "irritable heart" of Civil War soldiers was appreciated in World

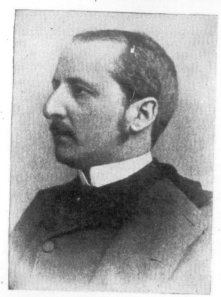

War I, when this condition under the names of "neurocirculatory asthenia" and "disorderly action of the heart" was found to be an important cause of disability. William PEPPER, Jr. (1843–98), son of the Professor of Medicine of the same name at the University of Pennsylvania, and himself Professor of Medicine and provost of that university, was a remarkable figure whose career testified to his preference for "the life of the salmon to that of the turtle." His vision, energy, and versatility accomplished important results in raising standards and improving methods of medical education, practically rebuilding his university as well as being responsible for such civic improvements as the city museum and free library. In his relatively short, crowded life he wrote many papers, including the first

411. *William Pepper.*

description of the hyperplastic bone marrow in pernicious anæmia, edited the first great American *System of Medicine* (5 vols., 1885–6), and conducted a large consulting practice. His school has been worthily carried on by a A. STENGEL (1868–1939), J. H. MUSSER (1856–1912), J. SAILER (1867–1928), D. RIESMAN (1867–1940), and others, whose achievements are too numerous to mention here.

Boston, like Philadelphia with its Norrises, Gerhards, Peppers, and Mussers, is noted for its medical families, such as the Warrens, Jacksons, Shattucks, Putnams — able physicians who have carried on the family tradition through generations. An outstanding achievement was the demonstration by R. H. FITZ (1843–1913) of the clinical importance of appendicitis (1886); he showed also that the old "inflammation of the bowel," or perityphlitis, was usually a peritonitis following appendicial rupture. His study of acute pancreatitis (suppurative, gangrenous, hemorrhagic, with fat necrosis) was also noteworthy.

A leader in the American medical profession for many years was Nathan Smith DAVIS (1817–1904), of New York. His experiences in his State Medical

Society led him in 1846 to call a convention to form the American Medical Association, which has now grown into the largest and most powerful medical organization that the world has yet seen. Called in 1849 to Chicago as Professor of Physiology and General Pathology, Davis later was a founder of the Chicago Medical College (now the Medical School of Northwestern University). A prodigious worker, he wrote extensively, edited several journals, and was a most stimulating teacher. Another leader of his profession in Chicago was Frank BILLINGS (1854–1932), the leading exponent of the still debated doctrine of "focal infection." The medical profession in New York was led for many years by Austin FLINT (1812–86), Francis Delafield, and E. G. Janeway. The first, born in Massachusetts of a long line of physicians, came to New York by way of Buffalo (where he was the founder of the Buffalo Medical College) and of the University of Louisville, where he was associated with S. D. Gross. He was a pioneer user of the binaural stethoscope, detecting the Austin Flint murmur in heart disease and introducing such terms as "cavernous" and "broncho-vesicular respiration." A unitarian, like Bayle, and Laën-

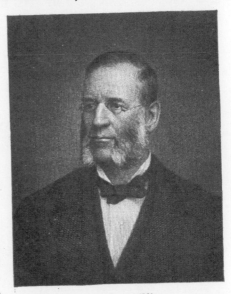

412. *Austin Flint.*

nec, he successfully combated the dual concept of pulmonary tuberculosis and such views as Niemeyer's that the worst thing that can happen to a consumptive is to become tuberculous. His *Principles and Practice of Medicine* (1866) was long a leading textbook on the subject. Francis DELAFIELD (1841–1915), trained in the newer pathology of Virchow, in 1872 wrote a *Handbook of Pathology*, which in expanded form in 1885 became the leading textbook on the subject in this country. Written in collaboration with T. M. PRUDDEN, it reached its 16th edition in 1936. As Professor of Medicine at the College of Physicians and Surgeons, he made important clinicopathological studies on the kidneys, the colon, and on the differentiation of lobar from bronchopneumonia. E. G. JANEWAY (1841–1911), Flint's successor at the Bellevue Hospital Medical School, stressed pathology as the proper basis for clinical diagnosis, and the necessity of becoming a specialist in internal medicine through a consulting rather than a family practice.

Among the eminent FRENCH physicians of the past ninety years, the Alsatian J. A. VILLEMIN (1827–92) holds a prominent position for his demonstration of the contagiosity of tuberculosis (1865–9). Professor in the Institute of Military Hygiene at Val-de-Grâce, he conclusively proved experimentally, before the bacteriological era, that tuberculosis could be transmitted by the injection of human tuberculous material into animals. One of the greatest masters of French clinical medicine was Armand TROUS-SEAU (1801–67), the first in Paris to practise tracheotomy, thoracentesis,

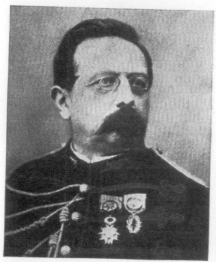
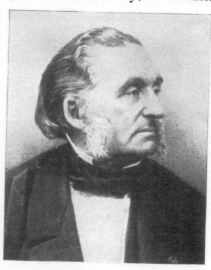

413. *Jean Antoine Villemin.*   414. *Armand Trousseau.*

and intubation. He gave the first adequate description of laryngeal tuberculosis (1837), and described the diagnostic sign in infantile tetany that bears his name — the artificial production of paroxysms by compression of the nerve trunks or vessels of the affected limb. His work *Clinique médicale de l'Hôtel-Dieu* (1861), from both the scientific and literary points of view, is one of the classical French texts of the period and long enjoyed a deserved popularity in many countries. The most illustrious of his pupils was Georges DIEULAFOY (1839–1911), who is remembered not only for his great treatise on *Pathologie interne* (1880–4), but also for his arresting personality at the bedside and as a teacher, and for various contributions to medical progress, such as his apparatus for the evacuation of pleural effusions. P. C. POTAIN (1825–1901) is an important figure in the domain of cardiovascular diseases, as the introducer of sphygmomanometry (quantitative estimation of the arterial blood pressure) being one of the first French clinicians to bring instruments of precision to the bedside. His contributions, which included the well-known apparatus for thoracentesis, were collected in *La Clinique médicale de la Charité* (1894); and were carried further by his collaborators HUCHARD, TEISSIER, VAQUEZ, and François-FRANCK. Georges HAYEM (1841–1933), Professor of Therapeutics and Clinical Medicine at Paris, was the most important French proponent of modern hematology. His books, *Du sang* (1889) and *Leçons cliniques sur les maladies du sang* (1900), are important landmarks, as is his description of chronic hemolytic jaundice (later known as the Hayem-Widal or acquired type). He was one of several independently to describe the blood platelets ("hematoblasts," 1877).

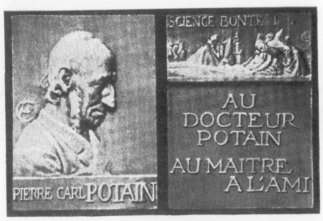

415. *Pierre Carl Potain.*

Among other French clinicians of note were C. G. BOUCHARD (1837–1915), whose text on general pathology was widely recognized, and J. J. GRANCHER (1843–1907), who upheld the unity of tuberculosis, described splenopneumonia and wrote on pediatric subjects and the pathologic and clinical effects of gastric ptosis. The name of F. GLÉNARD is even more closely connected with ptosis of the abdominal viscera. REQUIN and OLLIVIER studied hypertrophic cirrhosis, which was more fully described by V. C. HANOT (1844–96) in his well-known book (1876). It must be admitted, however, that though Hanot's cirrhosis still remains in medical terminology, its identity has never been definitely established. HUTINEL and SABOURIN advanced knowledge of fatty cirrhosis of the liver; and CHAUFFARD, the pigmented cirrhosis of bronzed diabetes. Chauffard's name is also linked with Minkowski's, as describers of the congenital form of chronic hemolytic jaundice. Syphilitic cirrhosis was elucidated by RICORD and LANCE-REAUX. Functional disturbances of the kidney were ably studied by ACHARD and WIDAL; AMBARD's coefficient (1910) has only in very recent years been replaced by more modern functional tests. Other French clinicians of note were: A. GRISOLLE (1811–69), whose book on *Pathologie interne* (1844) was especially strong in diagnostic measures; E. G. SÉE (1818–96), Trousseau's successor, who studied diseases of the heart and lungs; S. JACCOUD (1830–1913), especially known for his studies on albuminuria; H. HUCHARD (1844–1910), an eminent student of the cardiovascular system; L. BARD and A. PIC, investigators of primary cancer of the pancreas (1888); and H. VAQUEZ (b. 1860), a skilful clinician and investigator who first described erythremia (1882), which is also known as Osler-Vaquez disease. Among the best-known French textbooks are those by Brouardel, Gilbert and Thoinot, and by Charcot, Bouchard and Brissaud, and the *Nouveau traité de médecine* of Roger, Widal, Teissier, and Gouget.

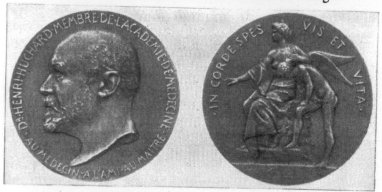

416. *Henri Huchard. Medal by Boucher.*

The leading figure of ITALIAN medicine of the period is without doubt Guido BACCELLI (1832–1916), whose versatility and energy recall the great Italians of the Renaissance. Pathologist, sociologist, poet, cardiologist, and malariologist, he was a good representative of the cultural and political as well as the medical life of his time. To him are owed the excavations in the Forum Romanum and the impulse to the sanitation of the Campagna and the Pontine Marshes. In semeiology he investigated the corpuscular nature of exudates, the laws governing the transmission of cardiac murmurs, and the type of pectoriloquy obtained in pleural effusion (Baccelli's sign). He promoted intravenous therapy, especially of quinine in malaria, of mercury in syphilis and echinococcus cyst, and of carbolic acid in tetanus (Baccelli's method). His most important publications are *La Patologia del cuore e dell' aorta* (4 vols., Rome, 1863–7); *Lezioni cliniche sulla malaria* (1869); *Di un nuovo metodo di cura per gli aneurismi aortici* (1856); *Sulla trasmissione dei suoni attraverso i liquidi endopleurici* (1877). Most of the important Italian clinicians of the end of the nineteenth century were his pupils. To A. CANTANI (1837–93), of Pavia and Naples, is due the first bacteriological laboratory attached to an Italian clinic, the first antirabic institute and laboratory of experimental pathology. He wrote an excellent treatise on nutritional disorders (1873, 1883), proposed a special diet for diabetics, and advocated enteroclysis in the treatment of endogenous intoxication, both of which procedures are known by his name. C. Bozzolo (1845–1920), of Turin, early described lethargic encephalitis (1895, 1900) under the term "*poliomyelitis superior acuta*"; with Perroncito and Pagliani he recognized *ankylostoma duodenale* as the cause of St. Gotthard anæmia (1879). Among his pupils in Turin were G. Mya, the founder of the Tuscan school of pediatrics, and F. Micheli, valued student of endocarditis and acute and chronic rheumatism. Mariano Semmola (1831–96),

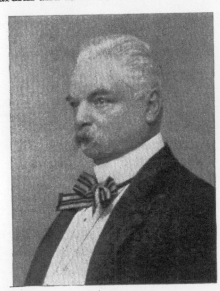

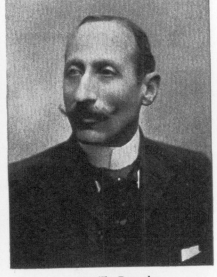

417. *Guido Baccelli.*   418. *Camillo Bozzolo.*

son of an eminent physician, was noted for his clinical and experimental study of Bright's disease (1850), and for his work in diabetes and in experimental pharmacology. Enrico de Renzi (1839–1921), of Genoa and Naples, to be distinguished from the historian Salvatore de Renzi, was concerned especially with diabetes, tuberculosis, and physical therapy; his successor at Naples, A. Cardarelli (1831–1926), and the latter's successor, P. Castellino (1864–1934), made important contributions to cardiology and early recommended the use of liver in the treatment of anæmia. At Padua an important anthropometric contribution was made by Achille de Giovanni (1837–1916), who distinguished three human types based on morphological criteria, which were later established by Ernst Kretschmer (b. 1888) as the leptosomic (asthenic), muscular, and pyknic. G. Viola (b. 1870), the Bolognese clinician, reduced these to two fundamental opposing types, the microsplanchnic and megalosplanchnic (corresponding to the broad and narrow thoracic types of the Berlin school, the lateral and longitudinal types of Stockard, the hyperontomorphs and hypo-onto-morphs of Beam). G. Rummo (1852–1917), student of circulatory dis-eases, and especially of cardioptosis, was the founder of *Riforma medica* (1885), a journal that has the unique distinction of having appeared daily for most of a decade. P. Grocco (1856–1916), professor at Perugia, then

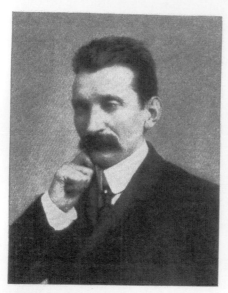
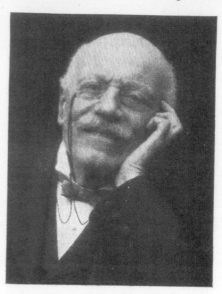

419. *Pietro Grocco*   420. *Augusto Murri.*

at Florence, where he organized a flourishing school, is remembered as the describer (1902) of the paravertebral area of dullness in pleural effusion (Grocco's triangle). A beloved Italian clinician was A. Murri (1841–1932), a pupil of Bouillaud, Traube, and Frerichs, assistant and the most illustrious successor of Baccelli. Murri brought Traube's functional patho-logical methods to Italian clinical medicine, was the first to recognize *hemo-globinuria a frigore*, and traced the mechanism of physico-pathological compensation in the heart (Murri's law). It was the experimental investi-gations (1882) of Carlo Forlanini (1847–1918) that led to the induction of artificial pneumothorax (1894) in the treatment of pulmonary tubercu-losis. His statement of the improvement that follows immobility of the lung in this disease was much opposed, but in recent years has thoroughly proved its worth.

His pupil S. Riva Rocci (1863–1936) was the inventor of the mercury sphyg-momanometer (1896), the model for the blood-pressure instruments in use throughout the world today. Other noted phthisiologists were A. MAFFUCCI (1847–1903) and E. MARAGLIANO (1849–1940), of Genoa, pioneers in the vaccine treatment of tuberculosis. Maragliano's studies on cardiac and renal affections and on malaria and tuberculosis were noteworthy, and his tenacious support, as a Senator of the Realm, of a broad sanitary program was of great practical value.

Though it is quite impossible to follow the rich and productive progress of medicine in the many countries in which it was profitably being studied during this period, some names must at least be mentioned. In Switzerland, G. M. D'ESPINES (1806–60), of Geneva, was particularly noted for his studies in epidemiology. The Belgian clinician B. van den CORPUT (1821–1908), professor at Brussels, was a distinguished pharmacologist and hygienist; the Dutchman VAN GEURS (1808–80), professor at the University of Amsterdam, was one of the greatest of Dutch clinicians, together with J. M. SCHRANT (1823–74) and G. B. SURINGAR (1802–74), Professor of Medicine at Leiden. Outstanding among Russian physicians were S. BOTKIN (1832–89), director of the Medical Clinic in St. Petersburg, and G. SACCHARIN (1829–97), of the University of Moscow. Among the Poles were J. DIETL (1804–78), a clinician whose name is still recalled in Dietl's crises of the kidney; T. CHALUBINSKI (1820–89), founder of the Medical School of Warsaw, an eminent clinician and hydrologist; and L. BIEGANSKI (1857–1917), author of numerous books on the history and philosophy of medicine, as well as on clinical subjects. Notable progress in scientific medicine has been made in Denmark, Switzerland, and Norway, especially during the present century, in fields that are too numerous and recent to be profitably retailed here. Among the early clinicians of note were the Dane W. RASMUSSEN (1833–77), who concerned himself especially with the respiratory tract; the Swedes Magnus HUSS (1807–90), best known for his studies on typhoid and on alcoholism; P. H. MALMSTEN (1811–83), one of the most celebrated of Swedish physicians, who discovered the parasites *Tricophyton tonsurans* and *Balantidium coli*; and J. A. WALDENTSTROEM (1839–79), professor at Uppsala, the first in Sweden to conduct clinical instruction in the dwellings of the poor.

9. Surgery

The study and practice of surgery was so expanded and advanced following the fundamental discoveries of anesthesia and asepsis that the time now under consideration unquestionably represents one of its most flourishing periods. With the need for great operative haste no longer existing, and with the knowledge that the most secret parts of the body can be explored without the introduction of infection, surgical technique has perfected difficult and complex operations undreamed of in earlier days. Surgical habit has changed also: " Observers no longer expect to be thrilled in the operating room," to use Cushing's phrase; today we find " the quiet, rather tedious procedures which few beyond the operator, his assistants and the timid by-stander can profitably see." With the advent of a proper pathological basis for the understanding of disease, the progressive surgeon, who hitherto had

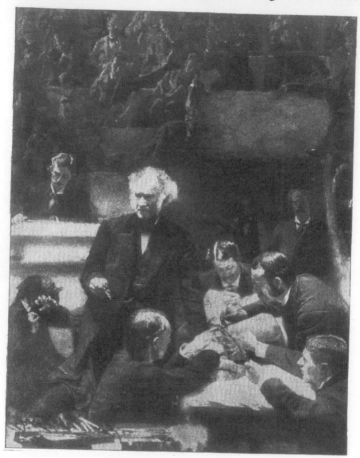

421. *The Progress of Operating-Room Technique. A. About 1870. S. D. Gross, who, like his assistants, is dressed in ordinary street-clothes. (Detail of Eakins's painting at the* JEFFERSON MEDICAL COLLEGE.)

relied chiefly on knowledge of anatomy as a basis for surgical efficiency, began to train himself in pathological anatomy as the foundation for his surgical career.

ANESTHESIA, since the discovery of the effects of ether by Long and Morton and of chloroform by Simpson, has been greatly developed, espe-cially in the twentieth century. Local anesthesia with cocaine, Schleich's infiltration anesthesia, Crile's block anesthesia (anoci-association), Bier's spinal anesthesia, and epidural, rectal, and intravenous variations have all contributed to lessen the discomforts and dangers of minor and major operations. Ether, which was long the preferred general anesthetic in America, and chloroform, preferred especially in England, are now given in less than half the major operations performed in progressive American hospitals.

Lister's antisepsis, with the damaging effects on the tissue of the chemicals used, has been universally replaced by ASEPSIS in all ordinary cases.

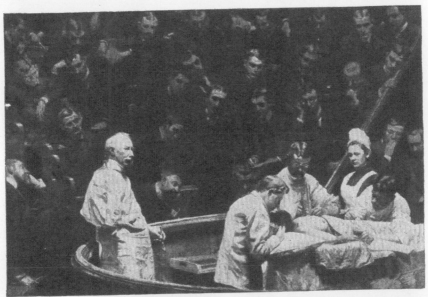

422. *The Progress of Operating-Room Technique. B. About 1890. D. Hayes Agnew, with assistants in gowns, but not gloves or masks.*
(*Detail of Eakins's painting at the* UNIVERSITY OF PENNSYLVANIA.)

Instruments, drugs, gowns, gloves, and so on are sterilized by dry heat or boiling, sterile masks are worn, observers are kept at a distance or behind glass screens, the air of the operating-room is perhaps sterilized by ultraviolet light, and the greatest care is taken in the avoidance of trauma, which lowers the resistance of the exposed tissues. Control of hemorrhage, both at the time of operation and after, is another item that has contributed to the successful performance of long and difficult operations.

CANCERS of various internal organs are often successfully attacked. Superficial tumours, to be sure, had long been legitimate objects of surgical attack. Furthermore, in 1833 J. LISFRANC (1790–1847) had resected nine rectal cancers by way of the perineum with but three operative deaths, and J. F. REYBARD (1790–1863) on May 2, 1833 had successfully extirpated a carcinoma of the sigmoid. It was not, however, until the seventies that, thanks chiefly to the gifted, thoughtful, and indefatigable work of Billroth, visceral cancer was systematically attacked by the surgeon. With increas-

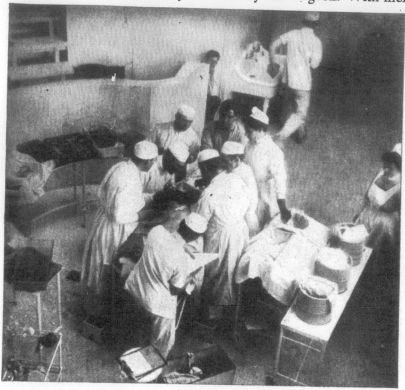

423. *The Progress of Operating-Room Technique. 1904. W. S. Halsted in the so-called " All-Star Operation." Assisted by his former assistants, Cushing, and Finney (opposite), Bloodgood (at his right), Young (at the instruments), Follis (leaving), Baetjer (seated), Miss Hampton (operating nurse). Note caps and rubber gloves, but no masks.*

ing ability to diagnose cancer in its early stages, and increasing recognition by doctor and patient of the necessity for its earliest possible extirpation, encouraging statistics are accumulating of apparently permanent cures of many types of cancer. In spite of the undoubted therapeutic value of X-ray and radium, surgery still remains the choice method of cancer treatment. Splenectomy, which began centuries earlier with Zaccarelli (1549), and Zambeccari (1680), was revived in the modern period by H. KÜCHLER (1828–73) in 1855 and Spencer Wells in 1866. It is now carried out with a low mortality not only in traumatic emergencies but more often in various chronic diseases of the hemolytopoietic system. Nephrectomy, performed by Gustav Simon in 1869, and resections of even large portions of the stomach and intestine have long been safe operative procedures.

PLASTIC SURGERY, dormant since the time of the Brancas and Tagliacozzi, was revived by J. L. REVERDIN in 1870, and again by L. X. E. L. OLLIER (1872), and Thiersch (1874), large raw surfaces being covered and mutilating scars avoided by skin grafts.

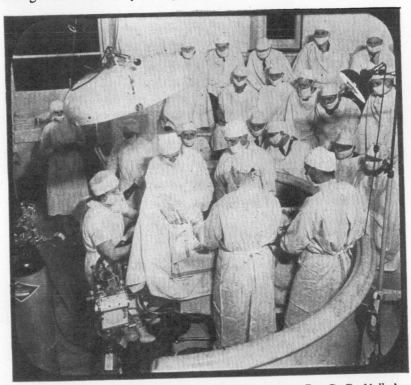

424. *The Progress of Operating-Room Technique. 1940. Dr. G. P. Muller's clinic (Lankenau Hospital, Philadelphia) showing modern technique. Note the caps and masks on both the surgical team and the spectators, the anesthesia apparatus, and the special lighting system.*

NEUROSURGERY began toward the end of the century with Bennett and GODLEE's operation on a brain tumour (November 25, 1884), and the similar operation by Francesco DURANTE in 1885. In 1873 Ernst VON BERGMANN (1836–1907) had described brain injuries (in the Pitha-Billroth *Handbuch der allgemeinen und speziellen Chirurgie*), and in 1888 he wrote a separate work on *Die chirurgische Behandlung bei Hirnkrankheiten*. In 1886 Sir Victor HORSLEY successfully removed some cerebral cortex in the relief of traumatic epilepsy and in 1888 extirpated a tumour of the spinal cord. In America W. W. KEEN (1837–1932), of Philadelphia, was a pioneer in this specialty: he successfully removed a meningioma (1888), tapped the ventricles (1889), and gradually acquired a wide experience in the extirpation of brain tumours. The subject has been further advanced, especially in the twentieth century, by Harvey CUSHING, of Baltimore, Boston, and New Haven; C. H. FRAZIER (1870–1936), of Philadelphia (trigeminal neuralgia, chordotomy for relief of pain); C. A. ELSBERG (b. 1871), of New York (surgery of the spinal cord); and W. E. DANDY (1886–1946), of Baltimore (ventriculography, hydrocephalus). In their hands the specialty has so developed as to require full-time attention.

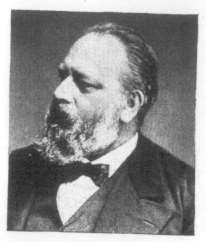

425. Theodor Billroth.

In the period under consideration the chief contribution to scientific surgery was made by the GERMAN-speaking countries. C. A. Theodor BILLROTH (1829–94), the founder of the Vienna School of Surgery, might also be called the founder of modern abdominal surgery. A graduate of Berlin and assistant at Langenbeck's clinic, later professor at Zurich and from 1867 at Vienna, Billroth was one of the first to introduce antisepsis into the Continental operating-room. His *Allgemeine chirurgische Pathologie und Therapie* (1863) was a classical surgical text, translated into ten languages. He was the first to resect the œsophagus (1872) and the pylorus for cancer (1881) and also the first to perform a total laryngectomy (1873). A man of high intelligence and ability, he was a friend of art and letters, an intimate of Brahms, and himself no mean musician. By his own work and through his many eminent pupils he was the most important single influence on the development of modern surgical knowledge. His pupil who made the most brilliant contributions to the surgery of cancer was Johann von MIKULICZ-RADECKI (1850–1905). Extirpation of cancer of the colon (1903), plastic reconstruction of the œsophagus (1886), and description of the symmetrical disease of the lachrymal and salivary glands known as Mikulicz's disease (1892) are his chief achievements. He advocated the use of cotton gloves in surgical operations, but these were soon replaced by Halsted's rubber gloves (1890). Another promoter of Listerism in Germany was Karl THIERSCH (1822–95), professor at Erlangen and

Leipzig, who advanced knowledge of carcinoma (*Der Epithelialkrebs,* Leipzig, 1865) and developed an excellent method of skin-grafting. Johann Nepomuk Ritter von NUSSBAUM (1829–90), professor at Munich, was one of the most skilful surgeons of his time, who contributed some eighty monographs on various aspects of his specialty. Richard von VOLKMANN (1830–89) described the contractures (1881) that bear his name and contributed notably to cancer study. He was the first to excise the rectum for cancer (1878) and among the first to publish follow-ups of the surgical treatment of cancer of the breast. Friedrich von ESMARCH (1823–1908), uncle by marriage of Kaiser Wilhelm II, was active chiefly as a military surgeon, introducing the first-aid package (1870) and the " Esmarch bandage " for controlling hemorrhage.

Among the leaders of the great Berlin and Vienna schools was Friedrich TRENDELENBURG (1844–1924), of Berlin, who proposed a sign, a symptom, a test, and an operation, all of which bear his name; he is best remembered for the " Trendelenburg position " (elevated legs and pelvis during and after pelvic operations). August BIER (b. 1861), von Bergmann's successor at Berlin, was a leader of German surgery, famous for the method known as " Bier's hyperemia." In recent years he has written chiefly on the philosophy of modern medicine, correlating it with Hippocratism and other medical doctrines of the past. Vincenz CZERNY (1842–1916), Billroth's assistant, and later professor at Heidelberg, where he founded the Institute for Experimental Cancer Research and the Samariterheim (1906), was an able contributor to both experimental and clinical surgery. Anton Freiherr VON EISELSBERG (1860–1939) was for many years Professor of Surgery at Vienna, where he was long recognized as the leader in neurosurgery in Austria and a bold and skilful operator.

AMERICAN SURGERY, which for many years following the establishment of anesthesia and asepsis was chiefly occupied in applying the new surgical knowledge that was being gained abroad, has so progressed, especially in the present century, that it now occupies a leading world position in surgical research and practice. The reasons for this cannot be stated in a few words, but among the contributing factors can be mentioned: the high and colourful position that surgery has attained in the United States, attracting many of the most active-minded to its pursuit, the prospects of high financial reward, the liberal provisions made by universities and private benefactors for the comprehensive study of the subject, both experimentally and clinically, and perhaps the practical American temperament, which likes to get early and decisive answers to its problems, individual and collective. Hospitals with good operating facilities are now within easy reach of ninety-five per cent of the people of this country. The surgical staffs of many, especially the larger hospitals, and of all the good medical schools, are actively pursuing surgical problems and collecting data, accurate for the most part, accounts of which appear monthly in the *Annals of Surgery*, the *American Journal of Surgery*, the *Archives of Surgery, Surgery*, and *Surgery, Gynecology and Obstetrics*. Surgical problems and individual operative failures are discussed at hospital, local, and national society meetings. These are but some of the ways in which better surgical knowledge and practice, often attained by the profession in innumerable imperceptible stages, have been steadily and notably advanced. Aided by the fellowships of the schools and philanthropic foundations, students come from many countries to profit by American surgical methods.

Most important of those who bridged over the anesthesia-antisepsis dividing line was Samuel David GROSS (1805–84), Professor of Surgery first at Louisville (1840), then at the Jefferson Medical College of Philadelphia (1856). In 1839 he published *The Elements of Pathological Anatomy*, the second treatise on the subject in the United States, which gave an especially good description of effusions, inflammatory and otherwise, and of the processes of granulation and healing. He was one of the first to open the abdomen for rupture of the bladder. His *Practical Treatise on Foreign Bodies in the Air-Passages* (1854), a pioneer synthesis of the knowledge of this subject, was accepted by Morell Mackenzie as " so complete that it is doubtful if it will ever be improved upon "! His *System of Surgery* (1859) was widely and deservedly popular; his skill as an operator was equalled by his ability as a teacher and writer. Historically valuable are his *Lives of Eminent American Physicians and Surgeons* (1851), *History of American Medical Literature* (1776–1876), and *A Century of American Surgery* (1876).

Henry Jacob BIGELOW (1818–90), of Boston, one of the greatest of New England surgeons, was concerned especially with the surgery of the genito-urinary tract. For bladder stone he advocated lithotrity (stone-crushing) with irrigation (1878) instead of the, more dangerous lithotomy; he was also the first in America to resect the head of the femur (1852). At the University of Pennsylvania, D. Hayes AGNEW (1818–92) and John ASHHURST (1839–1900) were interesting exemplifiers of the transition period: Ashhurst, who disdained the use of antiseptics, claimed operative results as regards infection as good as those of the more progressive Agnew and often got them unwittingly by maintaining great cleanliness. In Chicago, Nicholas SENN (1844–1908), a Swiss who came to this country in 1852, was an early exponent of scientific and experimental surgery; he was especially concerned with abdominal surgery (appendicitis, the pancreas, intestinal perforation). Christian FENGER (1840–1902) was another outstanding scientific surgeon of the Middle West, as well as being its first teacher of pathology.

ENGLISH surgeons were naturally among the first to profit by the increased opportunities offered by Lister's great discovery. They have always been noted for the sound anatomical foundation of their surgical skill, and have successfully correlated their specialty with pathology. Sir James PAGET (1814–99) was an able student of surgical pathology who wrote

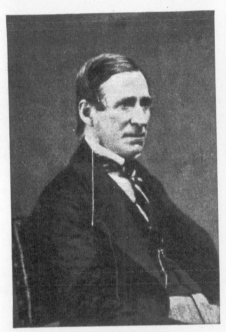 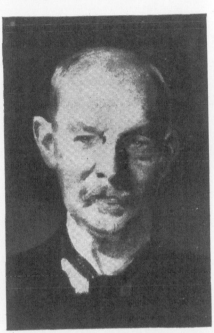

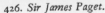
426. *Sir James Paget.*   427. *William S. Halsted.*

a valuable *Surgical Pathology* (1863) and *Lectures on Tumours* (1851). He was president of the Royal College of Surgeons, of whose museum he subsequently prepared a useful catalogue. Visitors there before its partial destruction in World War II could readily understand why the interesting exhibits and explanations were more utilized by British students than are the corresponding exhibits in other countries. Paget's name is associated with two eponymic diseases: *A Form of Chronic Inflammation of Bones* (*Osteitis Deformans*, 1877) and *On Diseases of the Mammary Areola Preceding Cancer of the Mammary Gland* (1874). Sir Jonathan HUTCHINSON (1828–1913) is especially known as a syphilographer on account of his description of the triad diagnostic of congenital syphilis — notched incisor teeth, interstitial keratitis, and sclerosis of the ear-drum. Surgeon to the London Hospital and professor at the Royal College of Surgeons, he also founded and edited the *Archives of Surgery*, the ten volumes of which were written largely by himself.

W. S. Halsted (1852–1922), first Professor of Surgery at Johns Hopkins, was a quiet but effective force in this country in transforming surgery from a series of dramatic incidents into a less conspicuous, painstaking, and scientific study of surgical types of disease. In addition to his introduction of sterile rubber gloves into the operating-room, his early use of silk ligatures and of infiltration anesthesia with cocaine, he devised numerous operative procedures and technical improvements, often based on previous experiments on animals.

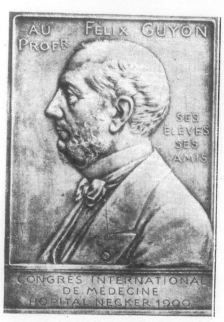

428. *J. C. F. Guyon.*

French surgeons of the period include many illustrious names, among whom only a few can be mentioned. J. C. F. Guyon (1831–1920) was a leader in the surgery of the urinary tract, who with his successor, Joaquin Albarran (1860–1912), made the clinic at the Necker Hospital a world centre for this specialty. Jules Péan (1830–98), a skilful ovariotomist and the first to extirpate fibroids *per vaginam*, was the inventor of the simple hemostat for the control of bleeding (1874) that plays such an important part today in operative surgery. C. E. Sédillot (1804–83) was the first to perform gastrostomy, though unsuccessful in both cases. Odilon Marc Lannelongue (1840–1911) was concerned especially with the pathology and surgery of bones, and was the first to transplant a (sheep's) thyroid for the cure of myxœdema (1890). Edmond Delorme (1847–1929), specially known for his work in lung and nerve surgery, was professor at Val-de-Grâce (1887) and wrote, *inter alia*, on the surgical lessons of First World War (1919). A. A. Verneuil (1823–95), a brilliant writer and founder of the *Revue de chirurgie* (1881), was one of the first to treat cold abscesses with iodoform injections. J. Lucas-Championnière (1843–1913), after studying with Lister at Glasgow, became the leading proponent of antisepsis and asepsis in France. As a pupil of Broca, he was interested in trephining and wrote an essay on *Les Origines de la trépanation* (1912) in prehistoric peoples.

Of the ITALIAN surgeons of the period, led by Enrico Bottini, Francesco DURANTE (1844–1934), the head of the Roman school, made important studies on the surgery of tumours and tuberculosis. He introduced the osteoplastic bone-flap in cranial surgery, a procedure later adapted by Bier for the amputated limb.

10. Obstetrics and Gynæcology

The OBSTETRICS of the period shared in the rapid advance of surgery, especially on account of the great reduction of puerperal morbidity and mortality and by the use of antisepsis and later of asepsis. Other factors in this development were the better organization of maternity institutes, and the use of anesthetics and the development of new surgical techniques.

Over a quarter of a century passed before the teachings of Holmes and Semmelweis were carried out, although as early as 1857 B. Fordyce BARKER (1819–91) in his *Remarks on Puerperal Fever* referred to the works of both. Gunning S. BEDFORD (1806–70) (*Principles and Practice of Obstetrics,* 1861) was one of the first American writers to accept their views on the contagiousness of puerperal sepsis.

Lister's work was slow in being applied to obstetrics. Henry J. GARRIGUES (1831–1913) is regarded by many as the father of antisepsis in midwifery because of his introduction of the use of bichloride of mercury into the New York Maternity Hospital. Garrigues's program of isolating sick patients, segregating the ante-partum from the post-partum and puerperal cases, ventilation of the wards, and the use of sterile caps, gowns, and bichloride of mercury solution in the delivery room, met with such success that it was promptly adopted by William LUSK (1838–96) at the Emergency Hospital connected with Bellevue and by W. L. RICHARDSON (1842–1932) at the Boston Lying-in Hospital. The use of chloroform as an anesthetic was begun in Great Britain, as we have seen, by James Young Simpson. It deserves to be remembered that he also contributed important papers on spurious pregnancy and the duration of human gestation. A leader in protesting against the unsanitary conditions that existed in the maternity wards of his day, he failed nevertheless to recognize the ætiology of puerperal fever.

Nathan KEEP (1800–75), of Boston, used ether for analgesia in labour for the first time in the United States on April 7, 1847, less than three months after Simpson had tried it on his first case. Keep was also a dentist, who was instrumental in founding the Harvard Dental School faculty (1868) and its first dean. The conviction of Harvard's Professor Webster of murder through Keep's identification of the charred remains of Professor Parkman by means of his dental work is one of the earliest of such cases on record.

It should be noted in passing that while Simpson employed ether and chloroform as an anesthetic, John SNOW (1813–58), who administered chloroform to Queen Victoria, and Keep advocated intermittent administration of the drugs, or what is now known as " obstetric analgesia." Snow was also the author of the first work on anesthesia: *Chloroform and Other Anæsthetics* (1858), and papers *On Asphyxia* and on the *Resuscitation of Newborn Children* (1841).

All the important problems of obstetrics have been notably advanced during this period. The indications for the proper use of obstetrical forceps were better worked out, while the axis-traction forceps (1877) of Stephen TARNIER (1828–97) considerably extended their field of usefulness. Cæsarean section was much more successfully and therefore more frequently used.

We have already seen how Cæsarean section was referred to in classical legends, and probably practised by the early Persians and Romans. (Some authorities think that the word " Cæsarean " was derived from a law of the Cæsars (*Lex Julia*) that every woman dying in advanced pregnancy should be operated on in order to extract the fetus. This procedure was revived during the Renaissance and was practised successfully on the living by Cristoforo MAINI (1540). A Swiss pig-gelder, Jacob Nufer, is said to have performed it on his own wife about 1500. In 1580 François Rousset was able to collect only fifteen successful cases. The first successful Cæsarean in America was done by Jesse BENNETT (1769–1842), of Virginia, in 1794 on his own wife. Other early Cæsarean sections in the United States were performed by Brodie, S. Herndon (1845), William G. Smith (1855), Charles Mills (1856 and again in 1857 on the same patient). During the first half of the nineteenth century Cæsarean section had produced a mortality of about seventy-five per cent, and the procedure was seriously threatened by the advocates of craniotomy, who favoured sacrificing the child rather than subjecting the mother to such a risk. As late as 1870 Virchow reported forty cases all fatal. In 1851 Reynale incised the cervix to facilitate the vaginal route. The prognosis became an excellent one for mother and child. The method was followed in 1854 by William A. PATTESON, an eminent practitioner in Virginia, who performed what he called " vaginal hysterotomy," using virtually Duehrssen's incision. Alfred DUEHRSSEN performed his first operation on November 10, 1887 (publ. 1895). A new era of Cæsarean section began with Edoardo PORRO's innovation of removing the uterus in infected cases (1876); the mortality was reduced from 66 per cent to about 25 per cent even including complicated cases. The results in clean cases were improved by the practice of closing the uterine incision with a suture that was introduced by Ferdinand KEHRER and Max SAENGER.

In the field of preventive medicine in obstetrics, the procedure of instilling a dilute solution of silver nitrate into the eyes of the newborn as prophylaxis for gonorrhœal ophthalmia, introducd by K. S. F. CREDÉ (1819–92) in 1884, was of the greatest importance, Credé will also be remembered for

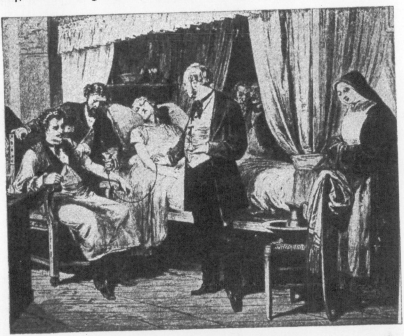

429. *Blood transfusion after childbirth.*
(Woodcut after Figuier, 1882.)

his popularization of the method of expressing the placenta (1861) that bears his name, although it had been recommended by John Harvie, in 1767, and others and is said to have been practised by the American Indians for generations.

Bedside instruction in obstetrics to supplement the didactic lectures given medical students in the United States was inaugurated against bitter opposition largely through the efforts of James Platt WHITE (1811–92), who held his first teaching clinic on obstetrics and gynæcology at the University of Buffalo in 1850, and Theophilus PARVIN (1829–99), of Philadelphia, in the last quarter of the century. As early as 1810 Thomas Chalkley JAMES began to conduct classes in midwifery in the Philadelphia General Hospital, and in 1822 a maternity hospital was established by the College of Physicians and Surgeons in Baltimore. B. C. Hirst stated that when he graduated in 1883 he had never seen a woman delivered and that in the early years of the twentieth century a committee had been organized in Philadelphia to set fire to the newly established University Maternity Hospital.

Among other notable advances in obstetrics was the podalic version by internal and external manipulation (1860, 1864), introduced by John BRAXTON HICKS (1823–97) of Guy's Hospital, whose name is also preserved in the sign of rhythmical uterine contractions. This manipulation, to be sure, had been preceded by the less well-known method of cephalic version advocated (1854) by Marmaduke Burr WRIGHT (1803–79), of Ohio. Hegar's sign of early pregnancy was reported in 1884 by C. Reinl, the first assistant of Alfred HEGAR (1830–1914), a German pioneer in gynæcological, especially abdominal, operations. Hugh Lenox Hodge and James Mathews DUNCAN (1826–90) added notably to progress on the mechanism of labour; and Simpson, Duncan, and Vinay on the toxemias of pregnancy. Carl Conrad Theodor LITZMANN (1815–90), who succeeded Gustav Adolf MICHAELIS (1798–1848) in the obstetric clinic at Kiel, carried on the studies of his predecessor on the bony pelvis and described his results in his *Die Formen des Beckens*, etc. (1861), which contains criteria for the modern conception of deformed pelvises. Induction of premature labour by mechanical dilation of the cervix (1892) is a valuable procedure introduced by Luigi M. BOSSI (1859–1919).

John C. W. LEVER (1811–58), of England, first noted the constant presence of albumen in the urine of patients with eclampsia or pre-eclamptic symptoms in 1843, and in 1859 Simpson wrote that "albuminuria, dropsy, and convulsions are successive effects of one common central cause — viz. a pathologic state of the blood, to the occurrence of which pregnancy in some way peculiarly predisposes." With the introduction of instruments for measuring blood pressure, Vinay in 1894 noted the regular occurrence of high systolic blood pressure in women with eclampsia. This observation was accepted very slowly, however, and as late as 1912 only Hirst and Polak in the United States stressed the point.

The importance of the contracted pelvis in practical obstetrics became better recognized, chiefly through the work of Gustav Adolf MICHAELIS (1798–1848), *Über das enge Becken* (1851). (The distorted pelvis of osteomalacia had been observed by William Hunter and the rachitic pelvis by Smellie; the obliquely contracted pelvis was described by F. K. Naegele in 1839; the *pelvis spinosa* by Kilian in 1854.)

Hodge's modification of Smellie's obstetrical forceps enjoyed widespread popularity in the United States in the nineteenth century, but was gradually supplanted by the long and short instruments designed by Simpson. In 1877 Étienne Stephane TARNIER (1828–97) introduced his curved axis-traction forceps, which were based upon the principle devised a century before by Van de Laar. They have survived with only minor changes to the present time. They were first used in the United States by Fordyce Barker in 1878.

By the middle of the nineteenth century GYNÆCOLOGY was beginning to emerge as a full-fledged special branch of surgery.

OVARIOTOMY. Thanks to the pioneer work of Ephraim McDowell, ovariotomy had been placed on a firm basis. McDowell's report of his case (he did thirteen additional cases with at least eight recoveries) sent to his old teacher, John Bell of Edinburgh, came to the hands of Bell's associate John LIZARS, who published the results of four of his own such cases (*Observations on Extraction of Diseased Ovaria*). As they were satisfactory in only one of the four, however, this report did little to win acceptance of the procedure in Great Britain. A successful operation in Great Britain was done in 1842 by Walne, Benjamin Phillips having had a fatal result two years before.

In England, ovariotomy was established through the work of Charles CLAY (1801–93) and Thomas Spencer WELLS (1818–97). Much of the latter's work is summarized in his *Diseases of the Ovaries* (1865–72). Wells operated on his first case in 1858 and became phenomenally successful in the surgery of the pelvic organs. His Scottish contemporary Robert Lawson TAIT (1845–99), in spite of a bitterly antagonistic manner, exerted great influence and was one of the most successful operators of his day. He boasted that he never used any antiseptic precautions such as Lister was introducing; through his emphasis on cleanliness, however, he was, as a matter of fact, a pioneer in aseptic surgery. He was the first to operate successfully (1883, pub. 1886) for ruptured tubal pregnancy (*Lectures on Ectopic Pregnancy*, 1888). Ovarian pregnancy was first observed (1897) by B. J. KOUWER (b. 1861).

In Germany, Chrysman performed an ovariotomy in 1819, and the operation was subsequently attempted by Dieffenbach, Heyfelder, F. A. Kiwisch von Rotterau, Nussbaum, Siebold, and Langenbeck, with poor results. About 1852 KIWISCH reported the results of fifty-four collected cases: fifty-one had ended fatally and he concluded that of all cases that had undergone operation at least half had died! Friedrich Wilhelm SCANZONI von Lichtenfels (1821–91) denounced the procedure in 1856 and advocated that it be abandoned, while as late as 1889 Skene regarded it as the most difficult operation in the whole field of surgery.

Ovariotomy was introduced into France by WOYERKOWSKI, August NÉLATON, and Eugene KOEBERLÉ (introducer of hemostatic forceps) in 1862, although it seems to have been attempted but seldom by other surgeons.

The classical American paper by Edward R. PEASLEE (1814–78), of New York, *On Ovariotomy* (presented 1864, pub. 1865) was influential in establishing various improvements and in evaluating the operation at that time.

UTERINE DISPLACEMENTS. Until 1864 when V. DENEFFE, a young Belgian just out of medical school, persuaded his chief, A. P. BURGGRAEVE (1806–1902), to permit him to try to shorten the round ligaments in the inguinal canals in a patient with a prolapsed uterus, operations to correct displacements of the uterus had not been attempted. Unfortunately at operation Deneffe was unable to identify the ligaments and Burggraeve was severely censured for permitting the experiment. Koeberlé, in 1869, stitched the ovarian pedicle in the lower angle of a laparotomy incision, and Lawson Tait performed a ventral suspension by including the fundus of the uterus in the sutures with which he closed the abdominal wall after he had done a bilateral salpingo-oophorectomy.

Chief reliance in correcting uterine displacements was placed upon the introduction of a pessary into the vagina, or, in desperate cases with complete prolapse, the passage was obliterated by elytrorrhaphy (*élytron*, uterus). One of the most popular of the innumerable pessaries then in use and the only one that has survived was that designed by H. L. Hodge, who, it is said, got his idea of the efficacy of the supporting curve from the design of the upright stand that held the shovel and tongs beside his fireplace.

Operations for the express purpose of correcting displacements of the uterus began with William ALEXANDER (1844–1919), of Liverpool, in 1881, although his report did not appear until 1883 after J. A. ADAMS (1857–1930), of Glasgow, had performed the same operation and published his results in 1882. A year later O. E. HERRICK (1849–1915) modified Amussat's technique, described in 1850, of cauterizing the posterior vaginal vault to produce adhesions that would hold the cervix back and tip the fundus forward by suturing the cervix to the posterior vaginal wall. Ventral fixation as an independent procedure was introduced by R. M. Olshausen (1835–1915) in Germany (1886) and Howard A. KELLY (1858–1943) in the United States (1885), and in 1886 W. C. WYLIE (1848–1923) reported his operation of intraperitoneal folding of the round ligaments, which was modified by Kelly, who carried out the same operation through the vagina (1888). D. T. GILLIAM (1844–1923) introduced (1900) the technique that bears his name, and in 1901 J. C. WEBSTER (b. 1863) introduced the operation now known as the Baldy-Webster suspension, although J. M. BALDY (1860–1934) did not do his work until 1902. The technique of suturing the broad ligaments in front of the uterus was introduced by Alexandroff in 1903.

We have seen in the previous chapter how the unhappy lot of the woman with a *vesico-vaginal fistula* was changed "almost with a magic wand" by Marion Sims, whose vaginal speculum (1845) led to the successful operation, using silver wire sutures.

To be sure, earlier operations had been attempted: Johannes Fatio had reported two successes in 1752 with the technique described by Hendrik van Roonhuyse (1672), and Jobert de Lamballe recommended an autoplastic procedure in 1845, which he performed on thirteen cases with but two deaths. De Lamballe's pupil Gustav Simon modified his preceptor's technique with success in thirty-five of forty cases. Also in the pre-Sims period (1840) John P. METTAUER (1785–1875) reported a successful case (1838), in which he used lead wire sutures, and in 1847 he described two additional successes. With the announcement of Sims's discovery (*American Journal of the Medical Sciences*, 1852), rapid progress followed. New and better needles, sutures, specula, and operating tubes were introduced (Bozeman, 1857), and improvements continued even up to the end of the century. By 1868 Emmet had operated on more than three hundred fistulas.

Other eminent gynæcologists of the Southern United States were J. C. NOTT (coccygodynia, mosquito theory of yellow fever), N. BOZEMAN, W. GIBSON, R. BATTEY, and T. GAILLARD THOMAS, whose *Practical Treatise on the Diseases of Women* (1868) held first rank for some years and was translated into five languages. It was at the first meeting of the American Gynecological Society (founded 1876) that the German-American Emil NOEGGERATH (1827–1925) read his famous paper on "Latent Gonorrhea," establishing it as an important cause of sterility in women. He was co-founder with Jacobi of the *American Journal of Obstetrics* (1868), which still flourishes with the addition of *Gynecology* to the title. Howard A. KELLY (1858–1943), Professor of Gynæcology first at the University of Pennsylvania and then at Johns Hopkins, was long a leader in the specialty in America. He was a pioneer in the treatment of uterine displacements, and in the establishment of cocaine as a local anesthetic and of X-ray and radium in gynæcology. He devised various operative and diagnostic measures, while his *Operative Gynecology* (1898) and *Medical Gynecology* (1908) are among the best books on the subject.

Outstanding among French gynæcologists and obstetricians were Jules PÉAN (1830–98), a skilful ovariotomist, S. L. POZZI (1846–1918), a pioneer in various gynæcological procedures, who was killed by an insane patient with a supposed grievance, L. DOYEN (1859–1916), E. K. KOEBERLÉ (1828–1915), an experienced ovariotomist, and G. SCHICKELÉ (1875–1927), an upholder of conservative forms of treatment. In Germany, Alfred HEGAR (1830–1914) is still recalled to us by "Hegar's sign"; H. FEHLING (1847–1926), inventor of the test for glycosuria, studied the functional pathology of the puerperium; E. BUMM (1858–1925), the first to cultivate the gonococcus, wrote a most successful *Grundriss zum Studium der Geburtshilfe* (15th ed., 1922); F. HITSCHMANN (1870–1927) demonstrated the normal cycle of histological changes in the uterine mucosa, thus dispelling the overemphasis on endometritis; F. von SCHENK (1849–1919) and E. WERTHEIM (1864–1920) devised successful radical operations for the extirpation of cancer of the female genitalia; A. DÖDERLEIN (b. 1860), author of a widely known treatise on obstetrics, described the acid-preferring vaginal bacillus that bears his name and was an early advocate of the radiation treatment of uterine cancer.

Among notable obstetricians and gynæcologists in South America were: from Brazil, Francisco de ANDRADE-PERTENCE (1823–86), "the best surgeon and obstetrician of his time" (Moll); the Cuban, ORTIZ-PEREZ, after whom a Cæsarean technique is named; the Argentinian, ZARATE, who also was the proponent of a well-known Cæsarean operation; in Mexico, J. M. RODRIGUEZ (1828–94), a pioneer in the diagnosis of pregnancy by combined palpation and auscultation.

11. Pediatrics

The diseases of children, as we have seen, had received special attention now and then since classical times, and in increasing measure since the Renaissance, and occasionally books had been written on the subject. But it was not until the nineteenth century that scientific observation of child life and increased knowledge of infantile nutrition and the causes of childhood diseases brought about a systematic study of this specialty, resulting in an enormous decrease in childhood morbidity and mortality. Soranus, for example, had written on the importance of proper diet and hygiene for the newborn; and from the fifteenth century on, we have noted books or chapters in larger works devoted to the subject. The eighteenth century was here also a period of preparation for the birth of a new specialty, which has proved to be one of the chief factors in the marked increase in recent years in the average duration of human life. Though for economic and other reasons families may now bring fewer children into the world, we have long since done away with the spectre of perhaps a quarter or even a half of the family failing to survive childhood. The progress of experimental medicine, the triumphs of bacteriology, the better preservation of foodstuffs, the development of the physiology of nutrition, the vitamins, the internal secretions — all have contributed to the scientific basis for the reduction of infantile morbidity and mortality. Slowly and tediously pediatrics acquired its position in university teaching; and, having become an important part of modern public health and social medicine, it has procured far-reaching legislation for the protection of infancy.

Among the most important of the sanitary regulations to safeguard the health of the young is K. S. F. CREDÉ's (1819–92) prophylactic treatment of *ophthalmia neonatorum* with silver nitrate. The application of asepsis to childbirth greatly diminished both maternal and infantile mortality; while the use of diphtheria antitoxin and the procedure of intubation (O'Dwyer, 1885) have saved thousands of victims of diphtheria (membranous croup).

INFANT FEEDING, a fundamental problem of pediatrics, was first put on a scientific basis during this period. P. BIEDERT (1847–1916) analysed the chemical composition of human milk as compared with that of other mammals and in 1880 gave a detailed classification of infantile diseases of the gastro-intestinal tract. The proper composition and quantity of food for the normal and athreptic infant were worked out by the physiological chemist Rubner. Otto HEUBNER (1843–1926), the best-known among German pediatricians, was the first to calculate infant diets on the basis of their caloric values. Other outstanding German contributions to the subject came from W. CAMERER (1894), Adalbert CZERNY, of exudative diathesis fame (1907), and Arthur KELLER (1906). While it has become increasingly clear that no infant food can equal mother's milk in ordinary cases, artificial foods, where maternal feeding is impossible or contra-indicated, have been so highly developed that the disadvantages of this form of nutrition can now in large measure be avoided.

Founders of the prolific GERMAN school of pediatrics were E. H. HENOCH (1820–1910), of Berlin, and Carl GERHARDT (1833–1902). Their lectures and treatises on the subject gave Germany a leading position in this field during the past century. Henoch's description of the purpura that bears his name appeared in the *Berliner klinische Wochenschrift* in 1874. In addition to those already mentioned, the disorders arising from nutritional errors have been explored by many investigators: M. VON PFAUNDLER (b. 1872), collaborator with Schlossmann in a huge *Handbook of Pediatrics* (1906; English translation, 1908), studied the motility of the stomach in nurslings; A. BAGINSKY (1843–1918), among many other investigations, explored the action of the glands of the gastric mucosa; T. ESCHERICH (1857–1911), the discoverer of *B. coli*, investigated the bacterial flora of the nursling and their modifications in disease (1886). The pathogenesis and treatment of these disorders was elucidated also by J. B. A. MARFAN (b. 1858), a leader of the French school.

Knowledge of the CONSTITUTIONAL DISEASES of childhood profited especially by the discovery of the widespread effects of vitamin deficiencies and endocrine imbalance. The treatment of rickets, studied by P. C. G. GUÉRIN (1839), A. Trousseau (1849), E. Beylard (1852), and others, was put on a firm basis by its experimental production in animals with deficient diets (Findlay, McCollum, and others); and by its successful treatment, experimentally and clinically, with cod-liver oil.

SEASIDE HOSPITALS have proved to be very helpful in the treatment of childhood diseases, and especially in the prophylaxis of tuberculosis. The first institute of this kind was founded at Margate in England in 1796, with sixteen beds. Recognition in Italy of the value of fresh sea air and sunlight in such hospitals is largely due to G. BARELLAI, who in 1862 founded the first hospital of this kind at Viareggio; Italy developed more than forty, with seven thousand beds, which compared favourably with the great English and French hospitals of the kind, such as Berck-sur-Mer. Hospitals devoted entirely to children have come a long way since George Armstrong's Dispensary of 1769; so that now they are accepted as necessary adjuncts to every first-class medical school or centre.

Credit for progress in pediatrics is largely due to two Frenchmen, A. C. E. BARTHEZ (1811–91) and F. RILLIET (1814–61), whose pioneer treatise on pediatric diseases (1843) is an important landmark. Among other French pediatricians of note are E. BOUCHUT (1818–91), author of a valuable book on child hygiene, and J. M. PARROT (1839–83), who wrote on athrepsia and on luetic pseudo-paralysis of the newborn. Cadet DE GOSSICOURT (1826–1900) collaborated with the best-known specialists of his country in a great *Traité clinique des maladies de l'enfance* (1897). Henri ROGER (1809–91) described the congenital heart syndrome known as Roger's disease and was the first to give systematic clinical instruction in pediatrics in France, though he was never advanced academically beyond the position of lecturer.

England was slower in developing pediatrics as a separate specialty. Its best-known representative was Charles WEST (1816–98), also a gynæcologist and obstetrician, whose *Lectures on Diseases of Children* (1847) is a classic, translated into German by Henoch, as well as into many other languages. He was active in the foundation (1852) of the Hospital for Sick Children in Great Ormond Street, London. Sir Thomas BARLOW (1845–1945) was the first to describe the infantile form of scurvy that bears his name (1882); and G. F. STILL (1868–1941) the form of chronic arthritis known as Still's disease. Another eponymic disease comes to us through W. J. LITTLE (1810–94), orthopedist and neurologist as well as pediatrician and a founder of the Royal Orthopedic Hospital. His *Influence of Abnormal Parturition Especially in Relation to Deformities* (1862) includes the description of the infantile spastic paralysis that goes by his name. S. J. Gee (1839–1911), of the Great Ormond Street Hospital and St. Bartholomew's, gave the original description of cœliac disease; and Clement Dukes (1845–1925) of the " fourth disease," a fourth acute exanthem to be differentiated from measles, German measles, and scarlatina. John Thomson (1856–1926) of Edinburgh attained international fame largely through his textbook, which, like its author, was popular and in wide demand.

The virtual founder of pediatrics in America was Abraham Jacobi (1830–1919), a German who came to New York after the Revolution of 1848. He began lectures on pediatrics at the College of Physicians and Surgeons in 1857, founded the first American pediatric clinic (1860), founded and edited the *American Journal of Obstetrics* (1868), wrote on numerous phases of his specialty (including a history of American pediatrics), and in general fostered its progress by constant precept and example. A contemporary, J. L. Smith (1827–97), of Stafford, New York, wrote a fine *Treatise on the Diseases of Infancy and Childhood* (1869), which passed through eight editions. Henry Koplik (1858–1927), of New York, de-

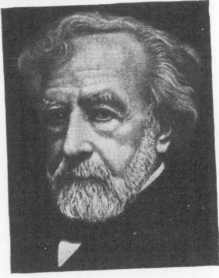

430. *Abraham Jacobi.*

scribed in 1898 the small spots in the mouth that are pathognomonic of measles.

12. Ophthalmology

The new paths in ophthalmology opened by the discoveries of Helmholtz, von Graefe and Donders were being explored by many followers throughout the world. Here, as in other fields, the progress in pathology and bacteriology brought powerful help, while anesthesia and asepsis permitted tremendous advances in operative procedures. Cataracts could be removed safely and surely; the fistula operations for glaucoma and cyclodialysis, introduced by Heine, afforded to the eye surgeon a choice of methods, while L. Laqueur's (1839–1909) use of physostigmin as a miotic has proved most helpful in treating this important disease. Plastic surgery has been successful in correcting traumatic and paralytic deformities of the palpebral fissure. The ability to correct errors of refraction and accommodation has steadily increased with the addition of new diagnostic methods of precision and skill in the manufacture of bifocal lenses and those of various combinations of curves.

Among the eminent GERMAN operators of the period was Alfred Karl VON GRAEFE (1839–99), nephew of the great Albrecht, who was noted as a skilful operator, and author of an important study on disorders of the movement of the eye. A. MOOREN (1828–99), director of the Düsseldorf Clinic, wrote on sympathetic disturbances of vision; R. FOERSTER (1825–1902), director of the Breslau Clinic, studied glaucoma and myopia and developed the perimeter for accurate outlining of the fields of vision; J. JACOBSON (1828–89), of Königsberg, the leading practitioner of eastern Europe, introduced numerous operative improvements for cataract and trachoma. Julius HIRSCHBERG (1843–1925), author of an authoritative and exhaustive *Geschichte der Augenheilkunde* (9 vols., 1899–1911) and editor of the *Centralblatt für praktische Augenheilkunde*, was the first to use the electro-magnet in the extraction of metallic foreign bodies from the eye. This technique has been improved by various investigators, especially William SWEET of Philadelphia. The brothers PAGENSTECHER (Alexander, 1828–79, and Hermann, 1844–1918), the last pupils of the school of von Graefe, enjoyed international fame at Wiesbaden. Best known of all this group was Ernst FUCHS (1851–1930), professor at Liége till 1885, then at Vienna. He was the author of several important monographs, and the famous *Treatise on Diseases of the Eye* (1889), whose many editions and translations helped to make Vienna the Mecca for students of the eye for many years.

The FRENCH school was led by the Greek Photinos PANAS (1832–1903), of Cephalonia. For many years professor at the Hôtel-Dieu, he was the author of a well-written textbook (1894) that contained excellent clinical descriptions. The Swiss E. LANDOLT (1846–1926) was one of the most active representatives of physiological optics, who wrote a meritorious treatise (1880). Other eminent French ophthalmologists were P. F. LAGRANGE (1857–1928), of Bordeaux, inventor of the fistulizing operation for glaucoma; F. de LAPERSONNE (b. 1853), Panas's successor; H. PARINAUD (1844–1905), describer of an infectious tuberculous conjunctivitis; and V. MORAX (1866–1935), who made important studies on trachoma and discovered (contemporaneously with Axenfeld) the diplobacillus of conjunctivitis that bears their name.

In SWITZERLAND, Jules GONIN (1870–1935) is important as the first to recognize the importance of lacerations in the production of detachment of the retina and to treat this condition with thermocautery. The importance of the retinal tear was known to Leber, who described and theorized at length about it. But it was Gonin's accomplishment to have revived Leber's theory and to have translated it into practice. How he started on his now world-famous operation is interesting. An old lady had a retinal detachment that had bothered her for many years, the movements of the detached retina, causing light-sensations, kept her in constant fear of losing the vision of her other eye. She wanted, therefore, to have the affected eye removed. Gonin thought that this was a good case where he could test his theory, since there was nothing to lose, and applied the thermo-cautery in the region of the retineal laceration with the intent of causing an ad-hesive scar where retina, choroidea, and sclera were matted together. The oper-ation had excellent results.

O. HAAB (1860–1931), of Zurich, is noted for his giant magnet for the ex-traction of foreign bodies (1892), and for his atlases of ophthalmoscopy and external diseases of the eye. The magnet is said to have been first used for ex-tracting fragments of iron by Fabricius Hildanus (1627). A. VOGT (b. 1879), professor at Zurich, has developed special methods of ophthalmoscopy and in-vestigations of cataracts in glass-workers.

Prominent among ITALIAN operators of the period were REYMOND of Turin, N. MANFREDI (structure of the retina, tuberculosis of the choroid), ALBERTOTTI, the Italian historian of the subject, GRADENIGO of Padua, A. ANGELUCCI of Na-ples, and G. CIRINCIONE and G. OVIO of Rome. L. BARDELLI of Florence was the leading Italian ophthalmologist of this time.

Among ENGLISH operators, William BOWMAN (1816–92) did the most toward the scientific advancement of the subject. Proceeding from his earlier histolog-ical studies, which included an investigation of the ciliary region (1847) and discovery of the basement membrane of the cornea, he devoted himself to the practice of ophthalmology, becoming the best operator on the eye in the United Kingdom and the first president of the Royal Ophthalmological Society. He advanced the treatment of lachrymal disorders, advocated iridectomy for glau-coma, and devised an artificial pupil when the pupillary space had been oc-cluded. His graduated digital tonometry in suspected glaucoma is still in use. His contemporary George CRITCHETT likewise improved the treatment of glau-coma and devised such a superior operation for the relief of strabismus (squint) by subconjunctival myotomy, that it remains practically unchanged today. Jonathan Hutchinson, the great syphilographer, recognized the syphilitic nature of interstitial keratitis, as opposed to von Graefe, who denied that syphilis could attack the cornea. Hutchinson established keratitis, the notched incisor teeth, and sclerosis of the ear-drum as the distinguishing external triad of congenital syphilis. Hutchinson was also one of the first to include tobacco among the causes of toxic amblyopia producing cerebral amaurosis (1865). Among other contributions, the internist Allbutt, prior to 1869, had observed that chronic lead poisoning could cause total blindness from atrophy of the optic nerve. R. H. ELLIOTT (b. 1864), first professor at the Medical College of Madras and since 1929 at the London School of Tropical Medicine, treated glaucoma by trephining the sclera and wrote a standard work on *Tropical Ophthalmology* (London, 1920).

In the UNITED STATES, ophthalmology has been vigorously and successfully pursued; errors of refraction were studied with especial vigour. Attempts to correct myopia and hypermetropia had been made since the earliest days of specialties, but it was not till the work of Donders in the nineteenth century that a scientific attack on the problem could be made. Prominent among his pupils were John GREEN of St. Louis, William THOMSON and William F. NORRIS of Philadelphia, who were pioneers in the United States in the systematic refraction of their patients' eyes.

Incidentally, the relief that refraction brought to "eye-strain" was found by S. Weir Mitchell to be an important aid in the treatment of headache and of functional nervous disorders (1874). This concept was further extended by G. M. GOULD (1847–1922) to include lowered resistance to disease and various psychoses. Astigmatism, which was first detected by Thomas Young in his own eye (1793), was first corrected, by cylindrical lenses, before 1854 by Isaac HAYS, for fifty-three years editor of the *American Journal of the Medical Sciences.* " Skiascopy " was established as a useful method in the estimation of refractive errors by E. JACKSON (1856–1942), of Philadelphia, who was long active in Denver, Colorado. Cases of toxic amblyopia had been recognized as the result of alcohol by Boerhaave, and of tobacco by Beer (1792). The subject was first thoroughly investigated, however, experimentally as well as clinically, by G. E. de SCHWEINITZ (1858–1938), long the acknowledged leader of the profession in this country. His textbook of ophthalmology was one of the most popular and widely known throughout the world of those written by an American medical author. The first case of wood-alcohol blindness to be observed in the United States was noted by RAY of Louisville (1896); with the bootleg liquor of the prohibition period this accident, which often resulted fatally, was not infrequent. " Heterophoria " (imbalance of the eye muscles) was so thoroughly analysed by G. T. STEVENS (1886) that he was able to detect weakness of any of the six pairs of eye muscles. American ophthalmology owes much to two German immigrants: H. J. KNAPP (1832–1911), a pupil of Helmholtz, became the leading ophthalmologist in New York, writing on numerous subjects such as corneal curvature and ocular neoplasm; he founded the *Archives of Ophthalmology and Otology* (1869). Karl KOLLER (b. 1857) in 1884 discovered the local anesthetic qualities of cocaine in the eye, the general principle of which had been observed by Anrep in 1876. Cocaine and its less dangerous successor novocaine have now for half a century greatly facilitated minor surgery throughout the body.

Ophthalmology in RUSSIA long remained under German influence, most of its leaders having been students in Germany, who copied German methods. Eminent in the specialty were MANDELSTAMM (Kiev), GOLOVIN, MAKLAKOV (Moscow), A. IVANOV, director of the Kiev Clinic, and E. ADAMUEK, director of the Kazan Clinic.

In SCANDINAVIA, ophthalmology was late in developing as a separate specialty, most of the university chairs being founded toward the end of the past century. Nevertheless, notable contributions to the subject have been made from Scandinavian countries. Johan WIDMARCK (1850–1909), of Stockholm, acquired international fame for his studies on the action of ultraviolet rays in the production of snow blindness, and on electric ophthalmia and solar erythema. Finsen's method of actinotherapy was based on Widmarck's studies. The Uppsala physiologist A. F. HOLMGREN (1831–97) was the first to recognize the importance of colour blindness as a source of accidents in railroading and in navigation. His test of carefully selected woollen skeins of different colours (1874) is still employed in detecting unsuitable applicants.

13. Otology, Laryngology, Rhinology

Though considerable knowledge of the anatomy of the EAR had been acquired already in the seventeenth century and Valsalva and Cotugno had early established an anatomical basis for some of its diseases, systematized knowledge of structure and function of the organ in health and disease was still scanty. The surgical treatment of otitis media and mastoiditis had been attempted in the eighteenth century, but was not well established till the middle of the nineteenth. Even perforation of the ear-drum, first practised by Astley Cooper (1801) for deafness following occlusion of the Eustachian tube, was not in general use.

The surgical approach to the treatment of diseases of the ear was renewed after the fundamental error was removed that arrest of the purulent process in the ear produced meningitis and brain abscess, so that continuation of the flow of pus from the ear had been regarded as desirable. Salomon Moos (1831–95) was an important figure in establishing the true relation of aural suppuration to cerebral lesions.

We have noted in the preceding chapter the importance of the work of the Provençal J. M. G. Itard in catheterizing the Eustachian tube and establishing criteria for puncture of the ear-drum; representatives of the school established by him were Amédée BONNET (1809–58) and P. MÉNIÈRE (1799–1862), the latter recalled by the eponymic Ménière's syndrome. The English school grew contemporaneously under the leadership of Joseph TOYNBEE (1815–66), writer of an early English treatise on the subject (1860), and the Irishman Sir William R. W. WILDE (1815–76), the father of Oscar Wilde. Sir William, after preparing at London, Vienna, and Berlin, studied especially the anatomy of the middle ear, which he recognized as the site of origin of most aural diseases. He also wrote on ophthalmology and was the founder of the *Dublin Quarterly Journal of Medical Science*. These men especially were responsible, according to Politzer, for stimulating the lagging German school into productive activity. Other English otologists were Adam WARDEN, inventor of an otoscope to illuminate the tympanum, and James YEARSLEY (1805–69), author of an important treatise on deafness, who was the first to establish that nose and throat disorders might cause deafness. He is said to have been the first English specialist in this field.

GERMAN otology in the latter half of the century contributed especially to the anatomy and physiology of the ear. Emil ZUCKERKANDL (1849–1910), the Viennese anatomist, and the otologists Joseph GRUBER (1827–1900) and G. RETZIUS (1842–1919), brought important contributions to the morphology of the muscles of the ear-drum, the Eustachian tube, and the ear ossicles. It was

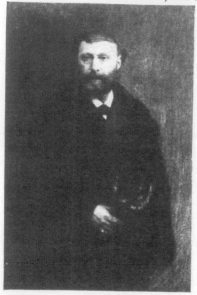

431. *Adam Politzer.*

Max Schultze who first described the nerve endings in the labyrinth (1858) and the connection of the nasal lymphatics with the meninges through the cribriform plate (1859) and in the Schneiderian membrane of the nose (1863). The functions of the ossicles and of the tympanum were investigated by Helmholtz, von HENSEN of Kiel, and Friedrich BEZOLD, of Rothenburg and Munich, who also gave an excellent early description of mastoiditis. The relation of the semicircular canals to body balance was explained by F. L. GOLTZ (1834–1902), a pupil of Helmholtz. Clinically, Adam POLITZER (1835–1920), professor at Vienna, was the accepted world's leader in his specialty. He was the author of a celebrated *Lehrbuch* (1878), and of a *Geschichte der Ohrenheilkunde* (2 vols., 1913) that is the best on this subject. Surgery of the ear was advanced by E. ZAUFAL (1833–1910), director of the Otological Clinic at Prague, who improved and popularized mastoidectomy and successfully ligated the internal jugular vein; M. F. TRAUTMANN (1832–1902), professor at Berlin; and L. STACKE (1859–1918), who first excised the ossicles of the middle ear.

The scientific study of DISORDERS OF THE LARYNX AND THE NOSE really begins in the second half of the nineteenth century. The University of Vienna was the centre for these studies, with such internationally famous men as Karl STOERCK (1832–99), author of a famous textbook of laryngology, L. von SCHROETTER (1837–1908), H. CHIARI (1851–1916), M. HAJEK (1861–1941), and Hans KOSCHIER (1868–1918).

Laryngology is usually combined with otology and rhinology as a clinical specialty, in university teaching, and in scientific publishing. These specialties made their most rapid growth — a truly remarkable one — in the two decades bordering on the turn of the century. Major contributory factors were the invention of the laryngoscope, the application of the discovery in 1884 of the local anesthetic effects of cocaine, and of X-rays in both diagnosis and treatment.

L. Türck (1801–68) and J. Czermak (1828–73), with his pupil Semeleder, advanced laryngoscopy, though they unfortunately became involved in long and jealous controversy. The eminent German Gustav Killian (1860–1921) was the first to view the bronchi through the natural passages (bronchoscopy) and devised numerous operations for diseases of the nose and throat passages. Viktor von Bruns (1812–83) initiated extirpation of laryngeal tumours through the mouth without external incision. In France, E. Isambert (1827–76) wrote ably on laryngeal tuberculosis, and Charles Fauvel (1830–95) was author of a useful book on diseases of the larynx. One of the most eminent throat specialists in the nineteenth century was Sir Morell Mackenzie (1837–92), who wrote and practised extensively on diseases of the larynx, including cancer, and was one of the earliest to use the laryngoscope routinely. His treatise (1880), together with those (1872) of J. Solis-Cohen (1837–1927) and (1881) F. H. Bosworth (1843–1925), placed the specialty on a firm literary basis (Delavan). The part that Mackenzie played in the fatal illness of the German Crown Prince Friedrich Wilhelm, later Emperor (1888) was bitterly criticized by German surgeons and was not without its political consequences. He was instrumental in founding the British Laryngological Society (1888). Of Americans, Joseph O'Dwyer's (1821–98) brilliant establishment of intubation in diphtheria (1885) has been referred to in the previous chapter. Laryngoscopy was devised by B. Babington in 1829 and independently in 1855 by Manuel Garcia, a teacher of singing in Paris. It was introduced to America (1858) by E. Krakowitzer (1821–75), a Viennese who had come to the United States after the political disturbances of 1848. Its steadily increasing use eventually brought a strong stimulus to the development of laryngology in the United States. The laryngoscope was popularized in this country by Horace Green (1802–66). He got an instrument from Krakowitzer and used it regularly, in spite of much opposition, to diagnose various lesions and to treat them with local applications. His *Treatise on Diseases of the Air Passages* first appeared in 1846. Packard credits him with being the pioneer laryngologist in the United States. The New York Laryngological Society, first of its kind, was founded in 1873, and the American Laryngological Society — the oldest national society — in 1879. The *Archives of Laryngology* was founded in 1880, by Elsberg, another pioneer in the use of the laryngoscope, Solis-Cohen, Knight, and Lafferts. The first special hospital was the Metropolitan Throat Hospital and Dispensary of New York, founded by Clinton Wagner (1837–1914) in 1873. Chairs for the specialty were established at Harvard and at the College of Physicians and Surgeons (New York) in 1875. The subject acquired a special section of the International Medical Congress of 1881.

The operation for the evacuation of pus from the MASTOID PROCESS had been auspiciously developed in the eighteenth century by J. L. PETIT (1774); also by the Germans J. L. JASSER (1782), J. G. H. FIELITZ (1785), A. F. LÖFFLER (1790), and in 1796 by the Dane A. KÖLPIN (1731–1801), only to be forgotten through half of the nineteenth century (Weber, 1825; Forget, 1860). A. F. von TRÖLTSCH (1829–90) – an important contributor to knowledge of the anatomy and pathology of the ear, introducer of the otoscopic mirror, and author of a good *Lehrbuch der Ohrenheilkunde* (1861) – successfully developed (1861) "artificial trephining" of the mastoid process. He was rapidly followed in 1862 by Lawrence TURNBULL (1821–1900), of Philadelphia; in 1863 by H. PAGENSTECHER and by H. SCHWARTZE (1837–1900); and in 1868 by James HINTON (1822–75), the first aural surgeon to Guy's Hospital. The radical operation is said by Sir Charles Ballance (*Surgery of the Temporal Bone*, 1919) to have been devised by E. ZAUFAL of Prague (1894) and STACKE of Erfurt (1897).

Removal of diseased TONSILS was slow in advancing on account of the fear – by no means unfounded – of severe hemorrhage. Improved methods and technique, however, supported by the views of F. H. Bosworth (1884) and others that all faucial tonsils were abnormal and should be removed, brought tonsillectomy into increasing favour, especially in America. By 1900, according to Wright, America " was producing nearly half of the laryngological literature of the world – much of it on tonsils and adenoids." The importance and frequency of ADENOIDS was established (1868) by Wilhelm MEYER (1824–96), the great Danish otologist, in his article *On Adenoid Vegetation in the Nasopharyngeal Cavity* (1870). Again to quote Wright: " It is difficult to find a report of a morbid process which so thoroughly in one essay exhausts the subject from almost every point of view." Whereas but few cases of adenoids had been previously reported, Meyer was able to detect 102 in eighteen months. Total excision of the larynx (suggested by A. M. KOEBERLÉ as early as 1856) was said by Foulis to have been carried out in 1866 for syphilis by Heron WATSON. It was performed successfully by Billroth in 1873 (reported 1874). By 1886 it had been performed and described many times.

In spite of the accessibility of the NOSE and the age-long recognition of such conditions as nasal syphilis and polyps, progress in this field lagged behind that of the throat. Not till the eighties were caustics and actual cautery revived with the help of cocaine and the snares of Fallopius and Hippocrates, improved by Jarvis (1880), and better instruments devised (for example, Bosworth's nasal saw, 1887). The nature of nasal polyps, known since Hippocrates, was better understood by Boerhaave and Morgagni than by Virchow, who started (1863) the stubborn error of calling them myxomas. This was first combated by C. M. HOPMANN (1844–1925) and by Chiari, who recognized (1887) the non-neoplastic nature of the changes in the mucosa.

The frequency of septal deviation was recognized as early as 1855 by Theile, though it was not until the 1880's that its etiology and varieties were much studied. In 1892 Potiquet, in accord with Morgagni's ideas on the subject, established the relation of the deformity, in non-traumatic cases, to the development of the facial bones in adolescence. Correction of the deformity was attempted by various surgeons throughout the century, to be replaced by the submucus operation, suggested by Burkhardt, and improved (1889) by R. KRIEG (1848-1933); in 1899 by Boenninghaus; in 1903 by O. T. Freer; and in 1904 by Gustav Killian.

Interest in disease of the accessory NASAL SINUSES was revived by the anatomical studies (1888-92) of E. ZUCKERKANDL (1849-1910), the great Viennese anatomist, and by F. E. R. VOLTOLINI's (1819-89) method (1887) of transillumination. Operations on the antrum had been done through the alveolar ridge, as the infection was thought to come from carious teeth, though Mikulicz had approached it from the nose (1877). Milestones along this road were: E. WOAKES (1837-1912) on the relation of ethmoiditis to nasal polyps (1887); F. H. BOSWORTH (1843-1925) on disease of the ethmoid cells (1891); Ludwig GRÜNEWALD (b. 1863) on frontal sinusitis (1892) and his *Die Lehre von den Naseneiterungen;* Max SCHAEFFER's (1846-1900) operation (1890) through the middle meatus; A. Q. SILCOCK (1855-1904) on trephining for frontal sinusitis and its relation to orbital disease (1892); R. SCHWENN (b. 1869) on malignant tumours of the accessory sinuses.

14. Urology

Up to the second half of the nineteenth century the surgery of the urinary organs had made but little progress. Surgical treatment of the kidneys and ureters was almost non-existent; the only operations performed, and these only sporadically, were incisions into perirenal abscesses or large pyonephroses that were capable of being diagnosed by external examination. Operations on the bladder were confined to lithotomy, lithotripsy, and the occasional removal of tumours, and these were usually mere attempts at palliation. Hypertrophy of the prostate was treated only by catheterization, and the only surgical intervention in this organ was the incision of abscesses.

During the second half of the nineteenth century much important progress was achieved. The surgery of the PROSTATE was greatly improved by the introduction of the perineal and the two-stage transvesical methods, and the demonstration by Albarran and Motz, and later by O. ZUCKERKANDL (1864-1921) and Tandler, that it was not a question of hypertrophy of the whole gland but of the lateral lobes or the periurethral portion. The more frequent radical operation that has naturally followed the lowering of mortality has saved countless elderly men from years of invalidism and the inconveniences and dangers of constant catheterization. Leopold DITTEL (1815–98), of the Vienna Clinic, in 1880 recommended the systematic excision of the median lobe. The perineal operation was proposed by Goodfellow (1891) and improved by Albarran, Proust and Gosset, Hugh Young and Wildbolz.

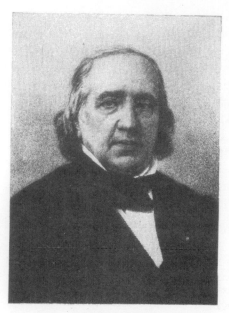

432. *Jean Civiale.*

Urological progress owes most to the French. In 1818 J. Z. AMUSSAT (1796–1856) began the first experiments on catheterization, with a technique that improved on the earlier work of Santarelli and Desault. Mercier's sound (1836) was a further improvement, as was Auguste NÉLATON's (1807–73) introduction of the rubber catheter.

Urethral stricture, treated with the cautery by Amussat, was investigated by I. G. MAISONNEUVE (1809–97) and his school; internal urethrotomy was practised by Maisonneuve and F. GUILLON (1793–1882). Lithotripsy, studied by FOURNIER (1783–1845) and Gruithuisen, was perfected by Jean CIVIALE (1792–1867) with the use of better instruments, which were still further improved upon by Mercier, Charrière, and Collin. Civiale, a master of his subject and a skilful technician, created the urological service at the Necker Hospital, where the school was founded from which emerged many of the world's greatest urologists, such as J. D. D'ÉTIOLLES (1798–1860) and C. L. HEURTELOUP (1793–1864). At the same time the English surgeon Sir Henry THOMPSON (1820–1904) and the American Henry J. BIGELOW were perfecting the technique of lithotripsy.

Endoscopy of the urinary tract began with the *Lichtleiter* (1807) of Philipp BOZZINI (1773–1809), of Mainz and Frankfurt, which, though rejected by the Viennese faculty as " a magic lantern in the human body," was revived in improved form (1826) by the Gascon P. S. SEGALAS (1792–1875). In 1885 Max NITZE (1848–1907) succeeded in constructing an electrically lighted cystoscope that proved highly useful in urological diagnosis. Felix GUYON, the greatest teacher of genito-urinary surgery of the century, and his pupil and successor, J. ALBARRAN, inventor of the cystoscope used for ureteral catheterization, were important in raising renal, vesical, and urethral surgery to a high scientific standard.

Among the successes of renal surgery of the period may be mentioned: nephrectomy, first practised by G. Simon, of Heidelberg, in 1869; nephropexy (E. Hahn, 1881); pyelolithotomy (Czerny, 1880); nephrolithotomy (Morris, 1880); renal decapsulation (R. Harrison, 1896; G. M. Edebohls, 1902).

15. Dermatology and Syphilology

DERMATOLOGY. Like most other medical disciplines, dermatology has made rapid progress in the period covered by this chapter. Its lesions being exposed to view, it has long possessed accurate and detailed descriptions of the great variety of clinical conditions encountered. With the advent of pathologic anatomy, also, it has examined these lesions microscopically — often, however, without finding characteristic changes that established the nosological status of the condition under examination. The terminology of clinical conditions, accurate for the period in which it was established, now is found to bring strange bedfellows under the same name and at times has been a hindrance to the proper evaluation of obscure conditions.

Following the great French school of the time of the Empire and the classical German and Austrian schools of Schönlein and Hebra, in Germany Koebner, Neisser, and Unna took the lead. Paul Gerson UNNA (1850–1929), of Hamburg, represents the highest development of the study of the microscopic pathology of the skin; his great *Histopathology of the Skin* (1894; translated into English, 1896), is still valuable for its detailed descriptions. In 1882 he founded the *Monatshefte für Dermatologie*. A leader in Norway was C. P. M. BOECK (1845–1917), whose description of *acne necrotica* (1889) and of a " benign skin sarcoid " (1899) brought him international reputation.

Among the numerous dermatological conditions described in this period were: acanthosis nigricans (Janovsky, 1890; Politzer, 1890); acrodermatitis perstans (Hallopeau, 1890); ainhum (J. F. da Silva Lima, 1852); alastrim (mild smallpox) (described by E. Jenner in 1798, earlier by Sydenham in 1771, and van Swieten, 1759, also by Izett Anderson, 1866); angioneurotic œdema (H. I. Quincke, 1882); blastomycosis (G. Busse, T. C. Gilchrist, 1894); dermatitis exfoliativa (E. Wilson, 1870); dermatitis herpetiformis (Duhring, 1884); erythema nodosum (E. Wilson, 1857); granuloma inguinale (D. Macleod, 1882); impetigo contagiosa (T. Fox, 1864); impetigo herpetiformis (Hebra, 1872); Kaposi's sarcoma (1872); lichen planus (E. Wilson, 1869); lichen ruber (Hebra, 1862); lupus erythematosus (P. L. A. Cazenave, 1851; also L. T. Biett, 1828); lupus erythematosus disseminatus (Kaposi, as erysipelas perstans faciei, 1872); morphea (Addison, 1869, and E. Wilson); ochronosis (Virchow, 1866); pityriasis rosea (C. M. Gibert, 1860); rhinoscleroma (Hebra and Kaposi, 1870); sarcoid (Boeck, 1899), J. F. Schamberg's progressive pigmentation (1901); sporotrichosis (B. R. Schenck, 1898); telangiectases, multiple hereditary (Rendu, 1896); urticaria pigmentosa (E. Nettleship, 1869); xanthoma (P. F. O. Rayer, 1836); W. F. Smith, 1869). The cause of many of these conditions still remains obscure.

Toward the end of the nineteenth century there flourished in FRANCE the school of E. VIDAL, E. BESNIER, H. HALLOPEAU (mycosis fungoides, erythroderma exfoliativa), L. A. BROCQ (parakeratosis psoriasiforme), F. J. DARIER (keratitis folliculare, 1889; White's disease, 1889), H. GOUGEROT (leprosy, the mycoses, Gougerot's tubercle), E. JEANSELME (leprosy, syphilis, medical history).

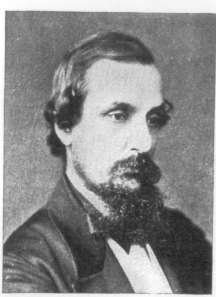

433. *Sir Jonathan Hutchinson.*

Among the most distinguished BRITISH dermatologists of the period were: Sir William F. Erasmus WILSON (1809–84), who left a superb collection of dermatological preparations to the Royal College of Surgeons, Jonathan HUTCHINSON, and the brothers Tilbury Fox (1836–79) and Theodore C. Fox (1849–1916). These are to be distinguished from Howard Fox (b. 1873), of New York, author of *Skin Diseases in Infancy and Childhood* (N. Y., 1928) and editor of the *Archives of Dermatology and Syphilology*, whose father, G. H. Fox (1846–1937), of New York, is particularly remembered for his *Photographic Illustrations of Skin Diseases* (1879–87, 1900–5). In the UNITED STATES, where dermatology had hitherto reflected European progress, figures of historical importance now began to appear. James C. WHITE (1833–1916), who first lectured on the skin at Harvard in 1858 and was professor there from 1871 to 1902, was especially important in building up his specialty and advancing dermatological education in this country. Louis DUHRING (1845–1913), the first Professor of Dermatology at the University of Pennsylvania (1875), a leader in his specialty, first described *dermatitis herpetiformis*, often known as Duhring's disease. Another prominent figure was J. A. FORDYCE (1858–1925), whose name is connected with a chronic disease of the mouth and lips (1896) and Fox-Fordyce's disease (1902), a neurodermatitis of the axilla.

VENEREOLOGY. Almost a century before the basic discoveries of Schaudinn and Hoffmann, of Ehrlich and Bordet and Wassermann, Ricord had

clarified the clinical picture of syphilis in masterly fashion and had put an
end to the confusion that had existed between syphilis and other venereal
diseases. The eminence of the French school was continued by his pupil
Jean Alfred FOURNIER (1832–1914), professor at Paris and director of the
internationally famous venereal clinic at the Hôpital St. Louis. Fournier
was the first to point out the relation of syphilis to the so-called parasyphilitic diseases (tabes dorsalis, paresis, 1876–94). He also emphasized
the importance of congenital syphilitic disease and wrote on its social aspects (*Syphilis et mariage*, 1890). Other important clinical students of
syphilis were Ernst FINGER (1856–1936), long the head of the second syphilis clinic of the Allgemeines Krankenhaus in Vienna; and the Moravians
Hermann VON ZEISSL (1817–84) and his son, Maximilian (1853–1925).

Venereology had already been advanced in the earliest bacteriological
periods with Neisser's discovery (1879) of the gonococcus as the cause of
gonococcic blenorrhagia (gonorrhœa). In 1889 Augusto DUCREY (b.
1860), Professor of Dermatology at Pisa and Rome, discovered in the pus
from a soft chancre the bacillus that bears his name. The etiology of the
venereal triad — syphilis, gonorrhœa, and soft chancre — was thus established.

16. Orthopedics

Although knowledge of orthopedic conditions and how to handle them
is already found in the *Corpus Hippocraticum*, this branch of surgery made
but little progress up to the eighteenth century. An exception was the construction of supportive and prosthetic apparatus, probably because of the
skill acquired by the makers of armour in earlier times. In the latter field
Fabricius of Aquapendente described various kinds of substitutions for paralysed or amputated members. Götz von Berlichingen, the famous German
soldier of fortune, is generally known as " Götz of the Iron Hand " because
of the apparatus he used to replace a hand lost in battle. Ambroise Paré described a mechanical hand made toward the middle of the sixteenth century
by a Parisian ironworker, and in his book on surgery he prescribed iron stays
for the treatment of scoliosis. These, however, were usually sporadic attempts of ingenious individuals, with probably a very limited practical
value.

The early source material of orthopedics is unusually rich, extending as
it does far into prehistoric times. Chronic arthritis has been observed in
reptiles of the Permian period; a bone tumour in *Pithecanthropus erectus* is
the earliest human lesion known; a healed fracture was found in the original

Neanderthal skeleton; osteomyelitis, tuberculosis, chronic arthritis, poliomyelitis, and various other lesions are present in the earliest Egyptian mummies.

The term "orthopedics" was first used by Nicolas ANDRY (1658–1742), in his book entitled *L'Orthopédie ou l'art de prévenir et de corriger dans les enfans les difformités du corps*, etc. (2 vols., Paris, 1741). The word is formed from the two Greek words *orthós* and *paideía*, meaning literally the straightening of children, though it has always been applied to deformities and other skeletal disorders of adults as well.

The specialty was chiefly restricted for some time to congenital defects of children such as lateral curvature of the spine, knock-knee, club-foot, the bony results of rickets, infantile paralysis, and ankylosed joints. It was gradually broadened, however, to include almost any lasting disorder of the skeletal system that had resulted in deformity.

Orthopedic surgery was late in becoming recognized as a separate discipline. It might be said to have started with the intervention of rigid bandages (at first glued together), as suggested by Tito Vanzetti (1809–88) in 1846, and perfected by A. M. MATHIJSEN (1805–78) in 1851 (plaster-of-Paris bandages). As in all other surgical disciplines the introduction of anesthesia and asepsis opened new horizons in this specialty also. At first orthopedics belonged to general surgery, and the operations were demolitionary rather than reconstructive.

The more conservative non-operative measures include a greater reliance on rest and reconstruction, on braces and physiotherapy (massage, gymnastics, hydrotherapy, heliotherapy). Braces, known since the time of the Egyptians and in frequent use by Glisson in the seventeenth century, were developed by J. G. HEINE (1770–1838), of Würzburg, the founder of German orthopedics, but brought to their highest development by H. O. Thomas, J. Hilton, and others, not only in supporting weak mechanisms but in promoting the healing of injured or diseased joints by prolonged rest. In the hands of W. SCHULTHESS (1855–1917), of Zurich, and of the Americans L. BAUER, L. A. SAYRE (1820–1900), E. H. BRADFORD (1848–1926) and R. W. LOVETT (1859–1924) of Boston, scoliosis has responded to various kinds of brace therapy. H. O. Thomas's static concept of foot deformities, being chiefly a problem of ligaments, to be combated by braces and supports, was opposed by Royal WHITMAN (1857–1946), who stressed the importance of muscle support and therefore of reconstructive exercises for the "weak" foot rather than the "flat" foot. The mechanics of this extremely common but complicated condition have been considerably elucidated in the past century by Arthur Keith, Joel Goldthwaite, Robert Jones, Royal Whitman, Robert Osgood, Steindler, and many of the most eminent men in this specialty. Mechanical and physical therapy has often been found preferable to operative measures, or useful where operations were not feasible. Sweden took the lead in the field of orthopedic gymnastics, in the work of Ling, who was the first to emphasize the great importance of physical exercise in orthopedic conditions. The great modern apostle of the Swedish school, J. G. ZANDER, was the inventor of a number of gymnastic apparatuses used in the cure of skeletal deformities. Jakob von HEINE (1800–79), of a family of eminent German orthopedists, was the founder of an orthopedic institute at Cannstatt which became one of the world's models of its kind through its director's wise use of the various forms of physiotherapy and surgical operations when necessary. Heine is most generally remembered as the first describer of " infantile spinal paralysis " (1840–60), more commonly known today as poliomyelitis. It is also known as Heine-Medin's disease, because of the Swede Oskar MEDIN (1847–1927), who established its epidemiology in 1887.

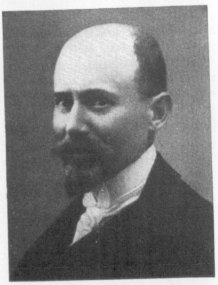

434. *Alessandro Codivilla.*

Among the most important advances in operative orthopedics, B. von LANGENBECK (1810–87) and F. KOENIG (1832–1910) popularized and improved the technique of osseous resection; K. NICOLADONI (1847–1902) was the first to undertake the transplantation of tendons (1880); Eduard ALBERT (1841–1909) invented the method of arthrodesis (surgical limitation of motion in a joint by fusion of bony surfaces) (1878); A. CODIVILLA introduced tenodesis (building of a joint by using tendon as a ligament); Payr and Putti introduced methods of arthroplasty.

ITALY has contributed illustrious figures to orthopedic surgery. F. RIZZOLI (1809–80), of Bologna, one of the first to recognize the need for the systematic study of diseases of the motor apparatus, founded the institute that now bears his name, from which have come many valuable studies. A. PACI (1845–1902), of Pisa, was the first to propose the " bloodless " (i.e., non-operative) reduction of congenital dislocation of the hip, later popularized by Lorenz, who realized the need for prolonged immobilization in the " frog position " if the dislocation was bilateral. Other notable figures were P. PANZERI, who recommended the forced straightening of knock-knee, and MARGARI and POGGI, pioneers in the operative treatment of congenital dislocation of the hip. The latter especially inaugurated the modern treatment of the condition by emphasizing the need for deepening the acetabulum, the socket that receives the head of the femur. An outstanding figure in modern orthopedics was Alessandro Codivilla (1861–1912), of Bologna, who made important contributions to many aspects of this discipline, establishing the prime importance of a good stump for prosthesis rather than the site of the amputation, the method of tendon transplantation including the tendon sheath in order to prevent adhesions, lengthening tendons to relieve contractures, operative treatment of infantile paralysis, operative treatment of congenital dislocation of the hip of long duration, traction on bones with the use of inserted nails to lengthen the shortening by disease, etc.

The idea of transplanting the tendon of a healthy muscle to substitute for the lost function of a paralysed muscle was first proposed in 1881 by Nicoladoni.

In GERMANY, the Hanoverian G. F. L. STROMEYER (1804–76), renowned for the successful subcutaneous section of the tendon of Achilles to correct club-foot, affords a good example of scientific internationalism. Influenced by Charles Bell and by the French surgeon Delpech, he set up his small hospital, whence his influence spread abroad. W. J. Little came from England to have his club-foot corrected and returned to become the pioneer of orthopedic surgery in England. Louis Bauer and William DITMOLD carried the new learning from Hanover to New York, where Lewis Sayre did much to establish the specialty in the United States. Sayre's vigorous Lectures on Orthopedic Surgery (1876) are still read. J. WOLFF (1836–1902) was a scientific student of the subject, also, who is chiefly remembered today for the so-called Wolff's law (1892), according to which every change in the use of a bone is followed by definite changes in its internal architecture and in its ability to stand new stresses. Albert HOFFA (1859–1907), like Wolff professor at Berlin, was a leader in orthopedics, known especially for his work on congenital dislocation of the hip, tendon transplantation, and the treatment of talipes valgus. C. BIESALSKI (1868–1930), of Berlin, devoted his chief attention to the reconstruction of the mutilated, bringing important improvements to the technique of prosthesis. F. LANGE (b. 1864), of Munich, has also contributed to the orthopedics of those wounded in war, and has written on the active and passive overcorrection of habitual scoliosis. A leader of the VIENNESE school of orthopedics was Adolf LORENZ (1854–1946), who is known for his studies on flat-foot, scoliosis, and spondylitis, and especially for his bloodless method of reducing dislocation of the hip. H. SPITZY (b. 1872), of Vienna, contributed to the orthopedic treatment of children and of the war-wounded and of the deformities of the vertebral column (1928). S. E. P. HUGLAND, of Stockholm, is known for his work on functional orthopedics and on deformities of the vertebral column. Jacques CALVÉ, of Berck, has been especially concerned with the study of paraplegias.

In FRANCE, A. BROCA. (1859–1924) was generally regarded as a founder of French orthopedic surgery and an eminent teacher. L. OMBRÉDANNE (b. 1871) Professor of Orthopedics at Paris, is known for his work in plastic surgery and on orthopedic surgery in infancy. E. KIRMISSON (1848–1927) is author of a meritorious work on diseases of the locomotor apparatus (1890); R. LERICHE specialized in the treatment of fractures; ROCHER, of Bordeaux, and MATHIEU, of Paris, are also prominent figures.

In ENGLAND, Hugh Owen THOMAS (1834–91), of Liverpool, is justly regarded as one of the founders of modern orthopedics. Coming from a family of bone-setters of good repute, he combined their special knowledge with the formal training of a surgeon. Long and careful study of the underlying principles of orthopedics and of bone surgery firmly convinced Thomas of the value of rest, " enforced, uninterrupted and prolonged," especially in the treatment, of fractures. He designed most of the fracture splints and braces now in use, the widely known " Thomas hip splint " having saved countless deformities and amputations after injury to the thigh. He is probably more responsible than anyone else for establishing the basic principles of modern orthopedic practice in many of its fields.

The interesting class of bone-setters — unqualified, unprofessional, yet legitimate manipulators of bones and joints (chiefly the knee and ankle) — has flourished in England for centuries: Sir Arthur Keith mentions a book, *The Compleat Bone Setter*, by a certain Friar Moulton, published in the middle of the seventeenth century. In fact, Keith states (*Menders of the Maimed*, 1919), that one of the chief reasons that Cheselden and the professional surgeons, who had been linked with the Barbers' Guild for centuries, wished to free themselves from this association was their desire to have done with " mystery." From the Guild of the Art of Surgeons thus founded in 1745, sprang the Royal College of Surgeons in the early nineteenth century. Nevertheless, bone-setters continued to flourish, presumably because the professionals had no greater success with the disorders being treated and but little more knowledge of them. The celebrated orthopedist W. J. LITTLE (1810–94) himself a sufferer from club-foot from infancy, failing to be helped by the bone-setters, was thus led to study medicine, had his club-foot rectified, learned from Louis Stromeyer to perform subcutaneous tenotomy, and thus became one of the chief pioneers of orthopedic surgery. Another of the strongholds of the bone-setters was the loose semilunar cartilage of the knee. " Internal derangement of the knee joint " had been skilfully manipulated (1782–1803) by William HEY and had been exposed and cured by ANNANDALE's operation (1883), which has long been a routine procedure. Yet H. A. BARKER, a celebrated bone-setter of the present time, wrote about and practised manipulations with sufficient success to have been knighted not so many years ago.

The development of special institutes for orthopedic cases has been an important factor in orthopedic progress. Though the Church had provided homes for the crippled for many centuries, the first hospital built specially to treat such cases was that of J. A. VENEL at Orbe, Switzerland, where he assembled accessories to treatment that would do credit to a modern hospital. Next in chronological order came Heine's institute at Würzburg (founded 1812), which has already been mentioned. This was followed in England by the Orthopedic Hospital of Birmingham (1817), and in France by those of Bar-le-Duc, Paris, and Montpellier between 1821 and 1828, and by Stromeyer's at Hanover in 1830. Holland's first institution came into existence when Heine moved to The Hague in 1833. Similar institutions were founded in Lübeck in 1818, in Copenhagen in 1834, in Florence in 1839, in Prague in 1845, in St. Petersburg in 1850, in New York in 1863 (Hospital for the Ruptured and Crippled), and in Philadelphia in 1867 (Philadelphia Orthopedic Hospital and Infirmary for Nervous Diseases), and the Rizzoli Institute in Bologna (1880).

17. Stomatology and Odontology (Dentistry)

Though the care of the teeth and the mouth as well as alleviation of their disorders is known to have existed since the most ancient times, the scientific development of the treatment of the teeth only began in the eighteenth century. We have seen that the Etruscans and later the Romans were skilled in the preparation of artificial teeth, in bridgework, and in making of partial dentures. Concern with various dental disorders and their alleviation is to be found in the works of Hippocrates (Epidemics), Galen, Oribasius, Celsus, Aurelianus, Paul of Ægina, and others of the classical period, as well as the Arabs, especially Avicenna, Abulqâsim and various Europeans. As might be expected, many causes were assigned empirically for caries, malocclusion, maleruption, and so forth. Until the beginning of the eighteenth century, however, the treatment of diseased teeth consisted mostly in extraction and was abandoned completely to barber-surgeons and surgeons, but also to empiricists and travelling mountebanks.

Renaissance and later medical writers often mentioned dental diseases. The first work devoted exclusively to the teeth was published anonymously in German in 1530, under the title *Artzney Buchlein wider allerlei Kranckeyten und Gebrechen der Zeen*, collecting in popular form the teaching of Galen, Mesue, and other ancient authors on teeth and their treatment. Johannes Arculanus (Ercolani), a Paduan surgeon, recommended for the first time in his *Practica* the filling of carious teeth with gold. In 1563 Bartolomeus Eustachius published his *Libellus de dentibus*, giving in thirty chapters the results of his anatomical studies. He was the first to assert that the second teeth have their own dental sac and do not originate, as Vesalius believed, from the roots of the milk teeth.

In 1557 a Spanish work on dentistry written by Francisco Martinez appeared in Valladolid, with a chapter devoted to dental prosthesis.

Ambroise Paré (1520–90) made an important contribution to oral surgery. He was the first to use obturators of gold or silver leaves to close defects of the palate. These obturators were held in position through a little sponge that was pushed into the nose through the defect. This same procedure was used later by Fabricius of Aquapendente (1537–1619), Fabricius Hildanus (1516–1634), and Matthæus Gottfried Purmann (1648–1711). These surgeons made an important contribution to the surgery of mouth and teeth, and remarkably improved the dental instruments. Purmann recommended the preparation of a model in wax before the execution of a prosthesis. The Englishman Nathaniel Highmore (1613–85) described the antrum or cavity that bears his name and was discovered by him upon the extraction of a tooth.

A very important treatise on the dental art, *Le Chirurgien Dentiste* (1728) was written by Pierre FAUCHARD, a Parisian dentist. This work, in two volumes, raising dentistry from a " handicraft of vagabonds " toward a learned profession, may be said to mark the beginning of modern dentistry. Fauchard made artificial dentures and gave a good description of an ingenious method of filling. Philipp PFAFF, dentist of King Frederick II of Prussia, published in 1756 a textbook that had a great influence on the practice of dentistry in Germany.

The first English book on dentistry was *The Operator for the Teeth* by Charles Allen (York, 1686). Thomas Berdmore is known to have prescribed trial filling with mastic before gold filling. John Hunter started the foundation of scientific dentistry with his work on *The Natural History of the Human Teeth* (1771). In his paper *A Practical Treatise on the Diseases of the Teeth* (1778) he asserted that a continuing pressure is able to change the position of a tooth.

At the end of the eighteenth century, the first mineral artificial teeth were perfected by DUCHATEAU and Dubois de CHEMANT. An Italian dentist, FONCI, improved them. His so-called " *dents ferro-métalliques* " were transparent and had clamps by which they could be attached to an artificial palate.

In England the art of dentistry was promoted by Sir John TOMES

(1815–95) with detailed microscopic studies of the normal and pathologic structure of the teeth. Great influence on the scientific development of the subject was exerted by Joseph Fox's *Natural History of the Human Teeth* (1803). In Germany a precursor of the scientific study of the subject was found in Moritz HEIDER (1816–66), who published, together with Karl WEDL, a popular atlas of the pathology of the teeth.

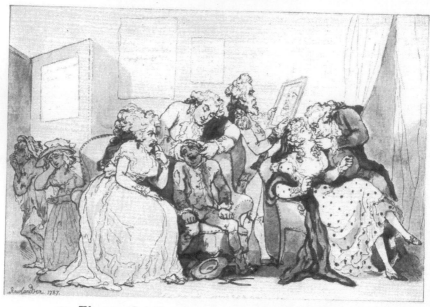

435. *The transplantation of teeth.* (*Caricature by Rowlandson.*)

Modern dentistry — that is, since the middle of the nineteenth century — has been largely developed in the United States. In Sigerist's phrase: " in one department of medicine America has led the way from the beginning." American dentists have been sought after abroad. Thomas W. EVANS (1823–97), founder of Pennsylvania's Evans Institute, was the dentist of Napoleon III and romantically brought about the escape of the Empress Eugénie from Paris at the time of the fall of the Third Empire. Among the artificial aids to the dentist, the outstanding landmarks were: the dental mirror (Bartolomeo RUSPINI, *c.* 1800); the rubber dam for keeping cavities dry (S. C. BARNUM, 1864); invention of better amalgam; the dental engine, at first foot-driven (MORRISON, 1870), then electrically, which is now used in most dental procedures; and porcelain and gold inlays (N. S. JENKINS). The work of Horace Wells and W. T. G. Morton, American dentists, in the 1840's, contributed in an important way to making the lay and medical public aware of the practicability of performing surgical operations under general anesthesia. Local anesthesia, infiltration and regional, by novocaine was accepted and developed far more eagerly in the United States by dentists than by physicians and surgeons.

The first constituted dental society in the world was the Society of Surgeon-Dentists of the City and State of New York (December 1834). The Pennsylvania Association of Dental Surgeons is the oldest dental society in continuous existence (since 1845). Dental journalism started in June 1839, with the appearance of the *American Journal of Dental Science*, which existed until 1860. *Dental Cosmos*, founded in 1859, continued as the leading journal in America until the 1930's, when it was taken over by the American Dental Association — founded in 1859 — under the title *The Journal of the American Dental Association* (being combined with the *Transactions of the American Dental Association*). The first International Dental Congress was held in Paris in 1889; the first session of the Fédération Dentaire Internationale (F.D.I.) took place in Paris in 1900.

The first American school — the first in the world — started in Baltimore as the Baltimore College of Dental Surgery in 1839, founded by Chapin A. HARRIS of Baltimore; in 1840 it gave the first degree of Doctor of Dental Surgery. In 1846 the Ohio College of Dental Surgery was established in Cincinnati. A number of excellent schools were established in America in the past century, which were especially praiseworthy for the capable practitioners that they produced. As a result, students have flocked to the American schools from all the countries of the world in considerable numbers for several decades.

18. Neurology and Psychiatry

Following the paths outlined by Duchenne, the forerunner of modern neurology, and by Charcot and his school, the specialty of neurology advanced rapidly in the latter part of the nineteenth century, establishing precisely the clinical and pathological pictures of many nervous diseases.

These advances were for some time accomplished chiefly by internists, and instruction in neurology was given in the department of internal medicine. In fact, in Europe today there are but few independent chairs of neurology. Chairs of psychiatry, on the other hand, were already in existence when these developments became manifest, with the curious result that in most European schools where neurology has any separate status at all, the existing title has been expanded to include neurology and psychiatry, even though the department may contribute but little to the younger specialty. In America, on the contrary, in very few medical schools are the two departments combined, and almost every school has had its separate department or chair of neurology for a generation or more. At Harvard, for instance, James J. PUTNAM was made Lecturer on Neurology in 1872, though the subject was not divorced from clinical medicine until 1895. At Pennsylvania, H. C. WOOD was appointed Professor of Diseases of the Nervous System in 1876, probably one of the earliest independent chairs to be established in this specialty. Whether the tendency toward greater specialization in this field is advantageous or not is a question that remains for the future to decide, as the small part of a big problem.

In the notable progress that has been made in the field of cerebral and spinal localization, establishing the sites in the nervous system where the manifestations of disease take their origin, a post of honour must be ascribed to the FRENCH school. Pierre MARIE (1853–1940), Charcot's greatest pupil, and professor at Paris from 1889, described many hitherto unknown forms of nervous diseases. Of these the best known are acromegaly (1886), the peroneal type of muscular atrophy, known as the Charcot-Marie-Tooth variety (1886), hypertrophic pulmonary arthropathy (1890), congenital cerebellar ataxia (1893), the so-called rhizomelic spondylosis (" Strümpell-Marie disease," 1898), psychasthenia (1903). His studies on aphasia, in which he found that Broca's area in the third frontal lobe apparently played no role in speech defects, have advanced the study of this important subject to a point where it is still awaiting final elucidation. H. OPPENHEIM (1858–1919), author of a number of important treatises on nervous diseases, was the first describer of amyotonia congenita (" Oppenheim's disease," 1900). His belief in the unfavourable prognosis of traumatic neurosis, the fallacy of which was shown during the First World War, prolonged over two decades unfortunate legislation that caused the payment of many unnecessary pensions to war invalids.

Wilhelm GRIESINGER (1817–68) was the most influential leader of German psychiatry in the struggle between the somatologists and the psychologists, in which the first won the battle. He wrote the first textbook on psychiatry (1845). Griesinger affirmed that all mental diseases were somatic diseases, specifically diseases of the brain, and he saw no difference between organic and functional disorders. For him each mental disease, whatever its apparent character might be, was only the manifestation of a brain disease. His influence guided German psychiatry definitely to anatomo-pathological conceptions. This viewpoint was the consequence of the splendid success of physiology and of Virchow's leadership in pathology.

In this period the number of classifications in psychiatry grew. Emil

KRAEPELIN (1856–1926), who in 1882 was assistant of Flechsig in his clinic at Leipzig and worked later with Erb and Wundt, in 1883 published the first edition of his well-known textbook of psychiatry. In 1896 he published his paper on the *Diagnosis of Dementia Præcox*.

The contribution of the French schools to the progress of psychiatry was outstanding. J. J. DÉJERINE (1849–1917), after heading the clinic at the Bicêtre, in 1901 became Professor of Clinical Medicine in the Paris faculty, and in 1911 director of the clinic at the Salpêtrière. In collaboration with his wife he published an important treatise on the *Anatomie des centres nerveux* (Paris, 1895–1901). His fame rests on his studies on tabes, muscular atrophy, interstitial neuritis, spinal radiculitis, the spinal arthropathies, the optic thalamus syndrome, and other eponymic syndromes due to lesions in the pons and medulla. Joseph BABINSKI (1857–1932), a Polish assistant of Charcot, is known for the great-toe reflex that bears his name (1896), and for his contributions to knowledge of cerebellar disorders (asynergia, 1899; adiadokokinesis, 1902) and his studies on hysteria. Georges GILLES DE LA TOURETTE (1857–1904) first described the jumping or saltatory spasm (impulsive tic, 1885). Maurice RAYNAUD (1834–81) first described the vasomotor asphyxia of the extremities (1862) that often leads to symmetrical gangrene. The study of myelitis was continued by Henry ROGER and other pupils of Marie's school. Other great French clinicians in this field were Charles FOIX (1882–1927), who studied the vascular topography of the brain; E. BRISSAUD (1852–1909), professor at Paris, collaborator with Charcot and Bouchard, and co-founder with Marie of the *Revue neurologique;* Fulgence RAYMOND (1844–1910), a veterinarian who later took his medical degree, became Charcot's successor at the Salpêtrière, and made worthy contributions to knowledge of the spinal scleroses, pseudo-tabes, the neuroses, psychasthenia, and progeria. Hypnotism as a form of mental treatment was practised especially by the Charcot school and at Nancy by A. A. LIÉBEAULT (1823–1904) and H. M. BERNHEIM (1840–1919). Now, however, it has been almost entirely replaced by various forms of psychotherapy. Paul Charles DUBOIS (1848–1918), of Bern, a pioneer psychotherapist, advocated the re-educational treatment of functional nervous disorders in his *Les Psychoneuroses et leur traitement moral* (1904), which today vies with psychoanalysis as the preferred form of treatment in these conditions.

In ITALY progress in psychiatry and anthropology was stimulated by the school of Lombroso. E. MORSELLI (1852–1929), of Genoa, was the founder of the *Rivista di psicologia scientifica*, and author of a manual of mental diseases (1885–94) and of an exhaustive treatise of general anthropology (1899). He founded the first laboratory of experimental psychology, where valuable studies were made on the clinical psychological nature of the individual and on the personalities of the insane. A. TAMBURINI (1848–1919) was responsible for important legislation on insane asylums and for many of the modern trends of Italian mental physiology and pathology. Among the outstanding Italian psychiatrists were A. TEBALDI (1833–95), of Padua (for his contributions to pellagra and legal medicine); A. VERGA (1811–95), founder of the *Archivio Italiano per le malattie nervose e mentali*, who advocated the improvement of insane asylums; and S. DE SANCTIS (infantile psychopathology). Giovanni MINGAZZINI (1859–1929), a leader of Italian neuropsychiatry, is chiefly known for his studies on the lenticular nucleus, recurrent paralysis of the oculo-motor nerve, encephalitis lethargica, and his published lectures on the pathology and clinic of nervous diseases.

Leonardo BIANCHI (1848–1927), one of the greatest masters of Italian neuropsychiatry, founded modern Italian psychiatric teaching at Naples (1890). He was the author of more than a hundred original memoirs and twelve scientific books on psychiatry, semeiology of the nervous system, hemiplegia, diseases of the brain, and cerebral localization. As Minister of Public Education he promoted the autonomy of the universities and brought about important modifications in the penal system.

Many of the neurological entities now recognized were established by GERMAN investigators in the earlier part of the period covered by this chapter. The most significant figure is that of the Bavarian W. H. ERB (1840–1921), who besides developing methods of electrodiagnosis and electrotherapy in Germany, established many valuable neurological concepts. More than anyone else he advanced the knowledge of the muscular dystrophies (classified by him in 1891); he was the introducer of the term " tendon reflex " for the so-called patellar reflex, first described by Westphal. He described myasthenia gravis (1878), and explored the relation of syphilis to myelitis, and the nature of tabes, brachial palsy, and spastic spinal paralysis. Erb's teacher at Heidelberg, N. FRIEDREICH (1825–82), is remembered in connection with the hereditary spinal ataxia that bears the name of Friedreich's ataxia; K. F. O. WESTPHAL (1833–90), Professor of Psychiatry at Berlin, in addition to describing the patellar reflex, developed the concept of agoraphobia, and advanced knowledge of the tract diseases of the spinal cord and of the affections of the nervous system in infectious diseases. H. I. QUINCKE (1842–1922) was the first to describe angioneurotic œdema (1882), and in 1895 introduced lumbar puncture into medical practice. P. J. MOEBIUS (1854–1907), of Leipzig, is remembered for his description of dysthyroidism (1886) and his monographs on the mental inferiority of women (1900) and the pathography of genius (1889–1900).

In the field of German psychiatry are to be noted such names as that of Karl WERNICKE (1848–1905), who composed two treatises on diseases of

the brain and insanity and also an excellent atlas of the brain. Emil KRAEPE-
LIN (1856–1926), Professor of Psychiatry in various German universities,
was one of the pioneers in experimental psychiatry; he introduced one of
the simplest classifications of psychopathologic disease, and established the
clinical pictures of dementia præcox and manic-depressive insanity. His
textbook was published in 1896. The Swiss P. E. BLEULER (1857–1939) also
brought an important contribution to the study of dementia præcox (schizophrenia) in the second volume of
Aschaffenburg's textbook, 1911. The
Dane A. J. T. THOMSEN (1815–1896),
of Schleswig, in 1876 described a new
form of disease, myotonia congenita
(" Thomsen's disease "), from which
he himself suffered.

The ENGLISH neurology of the
period owes its chief debt to the
Yorkshireman John Hughlings JACK-
SON (1835–1911), often known as the
father of English neurology, who was
induced to take up the subject by
Brown-Séquard shortly after the
foundation of the National Hospital
for the Paralysed and Epileptic
(1859). His concept of voluntary
movements being caused by nervous
impulses from the cerebral cortex was
one of prime importance; it was later

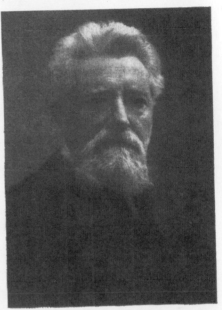

436. Leonardo Bianchi.

supported by the observations of James CRICHTON BROWNE (1842–1938)
and David FERRIER (1843–1928). Jackson's studies of aphasia and the unilateral convulsions that often follow brain injury or depressed fractures of
the skull established the syndrome universally known as Jacksonian epilepsy. Sir William Richard GOWERS (1845–1915) first described the superficial anterolateral funiculus in the spinal cord that is known as Gowers'
tract. He wrote an excellent treatise on ophthalmology (1896), illustrated
by his own hand, described ataxic paraplegia, and invented a hemoglobi-
nometer (1878) that is still in use. H. C. BASTIAN (1837-1915), an early
leader in English neurology, contributed valuable studies on diseases of the
brain, on the paralyses, on aphasia, word blindness, and word deafness.
Prominent among English psychiatrists were F. W. MOTT (1853–1926),

editor of the English *Archives of Neurology*, who studied the histological change in the brain in dementia præcox and its relation to the maldevelopment of the sexual organs (gonadal studies of psychoses), and author of a meritorious volume of clinical lectures on mental disease (1883). Hugh Crichton MILLER (b. 1877) has been one of the few scientific writers on hypnotism in recent years. W. J. LITTLE (1810–94) is remembered today

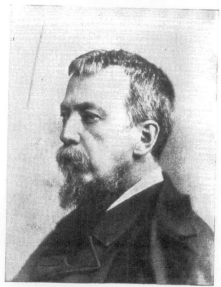

chiefly for his description of the cerebral spastic paraplegia due to birth injury (Little's disease, 1861). Leaders in English neurology were H. M. MAUDSLEY (1835–1918), the most influential psychiatrist and specialist in legal medicine, S. A. KINNIER WILSON (b. 1877), who described progressive lenticular degeneration, and Henry HEAD (1861–1940), who, among other things, ably analysed the varieties of aphasia.

A founder and spiritual leader of AMERICAN neurology was the Philadelphian Silas WEIR MITCHELL (1829–1914). During the Civil War, when he was given a special ward in the Military Hospital at Philadelphia, he made important studies of wounds

437. *S. Weir Mitchell.*
(*From a photograph by Gutekunst.*)

of peripheral nerves with Morehouse and Keen, which were later published in their book *Injuries of Nerves and Their Consequences* (1872). He was the first to describe causalgia (1864), postparalytic chorea (1874), and erythromelalgia 1878). With William Thomson he was the first to recognize the frequent causative relation of eye-strain to headache. He is best known medically, however, for his treatment of the functional neuroses by prolonged rest, known as the " rest cure " or " Weir Mitchell's treatment." The accounts of this appeared in his popular booklets *Fat and Blood* (1877), and *Wear and Tear* (1873).

In 1869 G. M. BEARD established the concept of neurasthenia, or nervous exhaustion, a functional condition that, under many names subsequently applied, has proved to be one of the commonest types of nervous disorder. The relief afforded by re-educational and other forms of psychotherapy is one of neurology's most important therapeutic contributions. This, in turn, has led to an increasing realization of the role of psychic factors in somatic illness, a point of view which many regard as a forward step of great importance in the practice of medicine today.

In 1872 George HUNTINGTON (1815–1916), a general practitioner in New York State, described the hereditary form of chorea, known to his medical father and grandfather, that is universally known as Huntington's chorea. American neurology has profited by its early segregation from internal medicine. At the University of Pennsylvania H. C. WOOD's chair passed in 1901 to Charles K. MILLS (1845–1931), who was one of the first in the United States to devote himself entirely to neurology. He created the great neurological service at the Philadelphia General Hospital (1877), where he discovered several hitherto unrecognized new conditions (unilateral ascending paralysis, 1900; unilateral descending paralysis, 1906; and macular hemianopsia, 1908). His successor, W. G. SPILLER (1863–1940), brought his intimate knowledge of neuropathology to bear in the identification of various neurological conditions. The operation that he devised with C. H. Frazier for the relief of intractable pain, spinal chordotomy (1899), has given relief to many hopeless sufferers. James Jackson PUTNAM (1846–1918), the first occupant of the chair of neurology at Harvard, wrote and taught ably on the pathologic anatomy and physiology of the nervous system, and on the differential diagnosis of its diseases, and was one of the first to describe the anatomical changes in poliomyelitis. Charles DANA (1852–1935), of New York City, also made notable contributions to neurology, as well as to public health and medical history (*Peaks of Medical History*, 1926), and, as a member of the Charaka Club, to the purely literary side of medicine (*Poetry and the Doctors*, 1916). F. X. DERCUM (1856–1931), professor at Jefferson, in 1882 described *adiposis dolorosa*, known as Dercum's disease. C. A. HERTER (1865–1910), the New York biochemist, was the author of a study of experimental myelitis (1889) and a textbook on the diagnosis of nervous diseases (1892). In 1888 he expanded the knowledge of Gee's cœliac disease, and in 1908 described the form of infantilism due to intestinal disease.

19. Legal Medicine

Legal medicine, or medical jurisprudence, is most commonly understood as that branch of medicine which deals with the " application of expert medical knowledge to the needs of law and justice," though the term is sometimes applied to the legal relations of the physician himself (Oertel). In the second half of the past century the field of legal medicine was considerably expanded, owing in great part to the marked progress in biology. Chemical recognition of poisons in the victim's body, the investigation of blood stains by microscopic and serologic tests, blood grouping in cases of suspected paternity, the microscopic identification of semen and other body fluids and of the incriminating bullet in gunshot wounds, are but a few of the special tests that have aided the medico-legal study of cases.

The teaching and pursuit of legal medicine has long had a greater development on the continent of Europe than in the English-speaking countries, where its pursuit is handicapped by lack of official contact of medical schools with legal authorities and by the neglect of the latter properly to utilize and evaluate the expert medical knowledge required in this field. In many European universities large independent institutes are devoted to this subject, equipped with special histological, bacteriological, chemical, hematological, and radiological laboratories, and engaged not only in teaching and investigation of the subject, but also in the performance of valuable official duties for the State. Among the English-speaking universities, only in Scotland is the subject taught in any detail, perhaps on account of the difference of the Scottish law from the English common law. Ever since legal medicine was first introduced at Edinburgh by Andrew Duncan (1791), the Scottish universities have had full-time professors of this subject and autonomous departments, sometimes housed with pathology in a separate building.

In Germany Fritz STRASSMANN (b. 1858), of Berlin, worthily continued the tradition of J. L. Casper and Karl Liman, writing numerous articles on legal medicine and its related subjects, especially legal psychiatry. He was the founder of the Berlin Society of Legal Medicine and a co-founder of the German Society of Legal Medicine (both in 1904). Most European universities have full-time chairs of the subject, occupied by specialists contributing to both the scientific and the practical development of the subject. In Austria, Eduard Ritter VON HOFMANN (1837–97) created the Vienna school, the greatest in the Germanic countries, even surpassing in fame the great school of Josef von MASCHKA (1820–99) at Prague. Von Hofmann was an able explorer of all phases of legal medicine; the vast material that was collected in his institute by him and his many pupils (Dittrich, Kratter, Haberda, M. Richter, and others) formed the basis of valuable contributions to the study of traumatic deaths, asphyxia, sudden death, and so on. His *Lehrbuch der gerichtlichen Medicin* (1878) is a classic and one of the best known on the subject; it was translated into many languages and shared popularity with that of Maschka on the same subject.

In France legal medicine was represented by a number of able specialists, outstanding among whom were Paul BROUARDEL (1837–1906) and A. LACASSAGNE (1843–1924), of Lyon. The close contact of French specialists in legal medicine with hygiene finds expression in the celebrated journal *Annales d'hygiène et de médecine légale*. The influence of Brouardel and Lacassagne is reflected in the prolific output of the Paris and Lyon schools, especially in the fields of general biology and immunology.

In Great Britain the impulse to the subject given in the early part of the nineteenth century by Robert CHRISTISON, one of the great medical jurists of his day, was continued by Francis OGSTON, and at Edinburgh by T. S. TRAILL, Sir Douglas MACLAGAN, and Sir Henry LITTLEJOHN. It was Christison and Newbigging who performed the autopsy on the victim of Burke and Hare in 1827 which brought about Burke's execution. Progressive legislation on mental disorders was promoted by C. A. MERCIER (1852–1919), who wrote a valuable textbook of insanity (1902). The best-known medico-legal expert in England today is Sir Bernard Henry SPILSBURY (b. 1879) lecturer in special pathology at St. Bartholomew's, and pathologist at Scotland Yard for the Home Office.

Legal medicine flourished in Italy, as would be expected from the country in which this discipline first arose, even though its supremacy was lost during the eighteenth century. Early in the nineteenth century Giacomo BARZELLOTTI (1768–1839), of Siena, founded the school from which came, even though indirectly, Giuseppe LAZZARETTI (1812–82) and Angiolo FILIPPI (1836–1905), of Florence. Both these men were especially successful in applying biological and clinical knowledge to medico-legal problems, the one through his precise knowledge of the legal aspects, the other through his mastery of pathologic anatomy and toxicology.

20. Pharmacology and Therapeutics (including Physiotherapy)

To those who have followed in the preceding chapters the evolution of medical science, it is obvious that therapeutics — the treatment of disease — is the oldest of its branches. It is only in the past century, however, that pharmacology, the study of the action of drugs, first became truly scientific, when with the aid of experimental investigations on animals, confirmed on man, it became able to recognize accurately the physiological and therapeutic effects of drugs. The study of medicines that had been in use through centuries proved the value of some and the uselessness of many more; while countless new drugs, mineral, vegetable, and biological, have more and more been submitted to scientific test before being admitted to the practising physician's armamentarium. As a result, "shotgun" prescriptions disappeared during the half-century covered by this chapter; but few drugs reached the standard required by the progressive physician, who got his results by more accurate diagnosis and the more efficient use of the few drugs that he could trust. The derogatory term: "age of therapeutic nihilism" was therefore unjustified. The trend is illustrated by H. HUCHARD's and N. FIESSINGER's La Thérapeutique en vingt médicaments (1910).

This scientific study of the action of drugs was foreshadowed by Magendie's study of arrow poisons (1809), which has been called the beginning

of experimental pharmacology, and by his introduction into medical practice, in his *Formulaire* (1821), of a number of potent scientifically studied
remedies. Another forerunner was his pupil Claude Bernard, in his experiments with curare (1850, 1856) and carbon-monoxide poisoning (1858).
The permanent, steady development, however, was largely initiated by the
Germanic countries. Rudolf BUCHHEIM (1820–79), professor at Dorpat
(Tartu) and Giessen, was one of the first to emancipate pharmacology
from traditional therapeutics and in the first exclusively pharmacological
laboratory to develop it on experimental lines as an independent part of
physiology. His studies of alkaloids, ergot, the solanaceæ, and the action of
various chemicals led to the production of his excellent *Lehrbuch der Arz-
neimittellehre*, which grouped drugs according to their chemical and
pharmacodynamic actions rather than according to their therapeutic effects.
His pupil Oswald SCHMIEDEBERG (1838–1921), of Kurland, professor for
two years at Dorpat and for many years at Strasbourg, was one of the greatest of modern pharmacologists. His experimental studies of digitalis, mus-
carin, and other drugs, and his early use of the frog's heart in the investigation of poisons, his physiological discovery of the formation of hippuric
acid in the kidneys, and his construction of the correct formulas of histamin
and nucleic acid, indicate the nature and versatility of his studies.

Schmiedeberg's path-breaking studies of the modes of detoxification and
excretion of drugs were further pursued by M. von NENCKI (1847–1901) and
have developed into an important branch of the subject. In 1873 Schmiedeberg
founded with Naunyn the *Archiv für experimentelle Pathologie und Pharmakologie*, long the most important pharmacological journal in the world. Carl
BINZ (1832–1913), a pupil of Virchow and Frerichs, was Professor of Pharmacology at Bonn, where he founded the Pharmacological Institute (1869). His
chief works were a textbook of materia medica (1866) and an interesting history
of anesthesia (1896).

The drug cocaine has an interesting history, of which a few high points
can be mentioned here. In 1858 A. NIEMANN isolated in Wöhler's laboratory the active principle of *Erythroxylon coca*, known since ancient times
by the South American natives as the " divine plant of the Incas." The alka-
loid was called by him cocaine. In 1884 Karl KOLLER (1857–1944) introduced cocaine as a local anesthetic; J. L. CORNING (1855–1923) of New
York, was the first to use it as a spinal anesthetic (1885), and August BIER
(b. 1861) in utilizing Quincke's lumbar puncture. C. L. SCHLEICH (1859–
1922) proposed its use in infiltration anesthesia in 1894; Halsted and Cushing in block anesthesia (1885–1902) (i.e., injection into a nerve trunk to
anesthetize its peripheral distribution).

Among the many new medicaments introduced into therapy during this period we note: carbolic acid as antiseptic (Lemaire, 1860), chloral (O. Liebreich, 1869), aspirin (1879), pilocarpine (Hardy, 1873), strophanthus (Frazer, 1885), salol (Nencki, 1886), ichthyol and resorcin (Unna, 1886), phenacetine (Kast and Hinsberg, 1887), sulphonal (Baumann, 1884; Kast, 1888), ethyl chloride (Redard, 1888), pyramidon (Filehne and Spiro, 1893), urotropin (Nicolaier, 1894), heroin (Dreser, 1898); and veronal and proponal (E. Fischer and J. von Mering, 1903–5), novocaine (Einhorn, 1904), pantopon (Sahli, 1909), shortly after. (A long list of drug discoveries arranged chronologically from ancient times can be found by those interested in D'Arcy Power's and C. J. S. Thomson's *Chronologia Medica*).

Among the FRENCH pharmacologists should be noted F. L. M. DORVAULT (1815–79), not to be confused with P. M. J. DORVEAUX (1851–1938), a student of the history of pharmacy. M. BERTHELOT (1827–1907) investigated the synthesis of organic compounds, especially animal fats, alcohol, hydrocyanic acid, and benzene. The work of Emil BOURQUELOT (1851–1921) on soluble ferments in fungi and the synthesis of glucosides was an outstanding contribution in these fields. G. DUJARDIN-BEAUMETZ (1833–95) wrote on the use of phosphorus and the experimental toxic effects of alcohol; his lectures on therapeutics at the St. Antoine Hospital at Paris were published in 1878–81. G. POUCHET (1851–1938) was a prominent French representative of the modern trend toward the scientific study of the action of drugs, together with the affiliation of therapeutics with pharmacology. The Dutchman Adolphe Pierre BURGGRAEVE (1806–1902) is remembered for his *Répertoire universel de médecine dosimétrique* (1876), in which he attempted to found the entire art of drug treatment on the use of alkaloids.

ITALIAN pharmacology was greatly helped by the foundation of the *Annali di chimica e farmacologia* by P. ALBERTONI (1849–1933) and I. GUARESCHI (1883); the *Archivio di farmacologia e terapeutica* (1893); *Archivio di farmacologia sperimentale e scienze affini* (1902). A prominent writer on Italian pharmacology was P. GIACOSA (1853–1928), of Turin, author of a *Trattato di materia medica*, who studied the oxidation of aromatic hydrocarbons and the transformation of the nitrates in the body, and was an outstanding historian. Passing in rapid review Italian contributions to clinical therapy, we recall Baccelli's introduction of intravenous therapy; Cantani's hypodermoclysis; Scarenzio's hypodermic injections of calomel for syphilis; P. Mantegazza's early attempts in opotherapy (injection of sperm) and his recognition that the sexual glands control secondary sex characteristics.

One of the most prominent among BRITISH pharmacologists was Sir Thomas Lauder BRUNTON (1844–1916), noted especially for his experiments on amyl nitrite and on digitalis and other cardiac stimulants, and for the application of the discoveries of the laboratory to his clinical practice. His best-known works are his textbook on pharmacology and therapeutics (1885), his lectures on the action of medicines (1897), and his monograph on the therapeutics of the circulation (1908). Sir Thomas Richard FRAZER (1841–1920), of Calcutta, Christison's successor at Edinburgh, was an early experimental student of the action of various drugs and alkaloids (physostigmine, strophanthus, arrow poisons, snake venoms) and one of the first to correlate chemical constitution with the physiological action of drugs (1867). The Scot A. R. CUSHNY (1866–1926), Professor

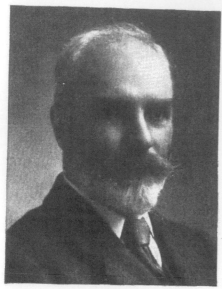

438. *A. R. Cushny.*

of Pharmacology successively at the universities of Michigan, London, and Edinburgh, was a leader in his field, especially noted for his studies on digitalis and on the antagonistic effects of optical isomers, and for his pathological studies on the heart and auricular fibrillation, and his development of Ludwig's filtration theory of urine-formation.

A pioneer in scientific pharmacology in the UNITED STATES was James BLAKE (1815–93), of California, who already in 1841 was investigating possible relationships between the chemical composition of inorganic salts and their biological action. The Philadelphian H. C. WOOD (1841–1920), whose textbook on *Therapeutics* (14 editions between 1874 and 1908) was long the standard work on the subject in English, was another path-breaker, who made free use of animal experimentation in his studies on the dynamics and toxicology of amyl nitrite, hyoscine, atropine, and many other drugs. His description of his own sensations following an overdose of hashish is particularly worth reading. Significant, too, was his influence on J. J. Abel, who was at one time his assistant and liked to acknowledge in public his debt to the older man.

TOXICOLOGY, the study of poisons, has contributed notably to the detection of crime and to protection against modern industrial hazards, as well as to the better knowledge of drug action. The medico-legal methods developed by men like A. A. TARDIEU (1867), G. DRAGENDORFF (1836–98), and R. A. WITTHAUS (1846–1915) have been considerably expanded by various microchemical and biological tests. The study of industrial poisons and hazards and their prevention has been led in recent times by Alice HAMILTON (b. 1869) and Cecil DRINKER (b. 1887) at the Harvard School of Public Health. Special laboratories for the study of industrial toxicology have been created by universities, governments, and enlightened industrial concerns, and already knowledge of how to control the hazards of many dangerous occupations is well developed.

PHARMACY, the art of manufacturing and dispensing medicinal drugs, has been greatly developed in the period covered by this chapter. The production of triturates and compressed tablets about the time that newly discovered active principles were replacing crude drugs, the many synthetic compounds — especially coal-tar products — that followed Perkin's discovery of the aniline dyes (1856), and the rapid development of organic chemistry, the so-called "biologicals" — vaccines, serums, animal tissues, and fluids having hormonal potency — all these have vastly changed and broadened the task of the pharmacist and the powerful pharmaceutical houses. Official pharmacopœias, beginning with the French Code of 1818 and the United States Pharmacopœia of 1820, and dispensatories, or commentaries on the official publications, have been published by most civilized countries, and frequent revisions have been issued. In the United States the National Formulary (1888) of unofficial substances has long enjoyed great authority. Pharmaceutical societies were founded in the past century in many countries (Great Britain, 1841; United States, 1851; etc.) to organize and control the members of the profession.

PHYSIOTHERAPY can be accepted as one of the first kinds of medical treatment to be established, presumably in prehistoric times. Hydrotherapy, special exercises, massage, sweat baths, have always held important places in the medical treatment of primitive peoples. The development of such methods also in the Hippocratic and Alexandrian periods, and especially in the Roman Empire, has been referred to very briefly. A few more notes on the earlier periods are added to lead up to the modern study of the subject.

Knowledge of the therapeutic virtues of water (HYDROTHERAPY), particularly of natural baths and mineral waters, is of ancient origin. We know that the temples of Æsculapius were built near healing springs, and that the Romans were well aware of the therapeutic qualities of the *aquæ Albulæ* of Tivoli, and those of Stabiae, Baiae, and Agnano, to name the most famous. In the Middle Ages the waters of Montecatini and Karlsbad were among the many that were in popular use. Of the Arabians, Rhazes and Avicenna attributed great value to balneotherapy. Ugolino of Montecatini wrote a treatise on mineral baths in the fifteenth century; eminent Italians, such as Pietro da Tossignano, Michele Savonarola, and Gentile da Foligno, have left valuable directions on hydrotherapy and the use of cold baths in fevers. *De thermis, lacubus, fontibus, fluminibus et balneis totius orbis* (1588), by Andrea Bacci, as its title indicates, gives exhaustive information about the baths known to antiquity and to his own times. Paracelsus' booklet on mineral baths and springs (published posthumously in 1576) highly praised many that he had visited in his own country, including the one now known as Baden-Baden. Lorenz Heister in Germany, and the Welshman

Charles Clermont and Robert Pierce in England, emphasized the therapeutic importance of baths in their writings and practice. Sir John Floyer, he who sent Samuel Johnson to be touched for the king's evil, advocated cold bathing in his *Enquiry into the Right Use of Baths* (1697), *The Ancient Psychrolusia Revived* (1702) and his *History of Hot and Cold Bathing* (1709). The ancient Roman city of Bath in the west of England regained its prosperity through the activities of such experts in the use of baths in gout as the two William Olivers (the elder born in 1659; the younger in 1695). In Germany the contributions of the Hahn family have already been referred to; also those of S. A. Tissot in Lausanne.

Toward the end of the eighteenth century William WRIGHT (1735–1819) revived the use of cold water in fever (1786), and James CURRIE (1756–1805) further developed this form of treatment, together with free draughts of cold water. Benjamin Rush applied cracked ice to the heads of fever patients and used cold water in the treatment of various diseases. In 1861 E. BRAND (1827–97), of Stettin, introduced the cold-bath treatment of typhoid fever, which was in vogue well into the twentieth century. L. J. D. FLEURY (1815–72) had already proposed the use of cold douches in intermittent fevers (1848). Great credit for the spread of hydrotherapy is due to William WINTERNITZ (1835–1917), who in 1892 opened at Kaltenleutgeben the first hydrotherapeutic clinic. It is said that in one of his experiments on the use of water, he applied to himself a " night pack " in an extremely cold basement. The water froze and he almost lost his life before he could be chopped out of the ice! He held the first chair of hydrotherapy at Vienna (1881), and wrote a treatise on the subject (1877–80) which was extremely popular. Winternitz's book was followed by a number of other texts in various languages.

Hydrotherapy, in the narrower modern sense — that is, the various applications of water with a therapeutic purpose — owed much, as we have seen in the preceding chapter, to the work of Vincenz Priessnitz. His establishment at Gräfenberg in Silesia enjoyed a great popularity, as did the establishment at Wörishofen of the priest Sebastian Kneipp. For some reason, however, the work of other deserving students of the subject, such as G. GIANNINI (1773–1818) in Italy, and J. C. A. RÉCAMIER (1774–1852) and LACORDIÈRE in France, failed to obtain the confidence of the profession and of the public.

Crenology (from κρήνη, a spring), the study of the use of mineral waters, was, as we have seen, especially advanced by Italian and English physicians. Friedrich Hoffmann was also an early and enthusiastic advocate of the use of mineral waters. The application of the new chemical knowledge and the analysis of these waters in the nineteenth century, and especially the discovery of the radioactive properties of a number of springs in the twentieth century, have given a marked impulse to the scientific study of this subject, which especially in Europe has become an important specialty.

We shall touch only briefly on thalassotherapy (sea therapy), the origin of which goes back to distant times. It was warmly advocated in the treatment of consumption by Roman physicians, who felt that it could bring about great improvement in this disease. In the present century, again, thalassotherapy, whether in the form of sea baths, sea voyages, or sojourns by the sea, has become popular and is given the credit for excellent therapeutic results. Thousands of bathers, many under medical supervision, annually throng the seaside resorts of the world.

MASSAGE as a means of medical treatment was used by the ancient Chinese and Egyptians, and we know that the Greeks and Romans attributed great importance to it. In the Renaissance, Paré prescribed massage especially in the treatment of fractures. In 1782 Tissot's book on medical gymnastics warmly recommended massage in various diseases and gave detailed indications for its use. Toward the middle of the past century some French physicians, especially Bonnet (1853), returned to the use of massage, but without having much influence on the profession at large. Massage and passive motion after injuries, especially fractures, were championed by Just LUCAS-CHAMPIONNIÈRE (1843–1913). His theories, at first neglected, received eventual recognition in the widespread use during the First World War of massage and early motion after fractures and gunshot wounds of the joints. The Dutch physician J. METZGER taught massage with considerable success at Amsterdam in the sixties. It was introduced into gynæcology by Thure BRANDT (1819–95), but in recent years its use in this field has much decreased. Neglected by the profession, partly on account of its very simplicity and its relatively high cost when carried out by specialists, this valuable form of treatment has only slowly made headway in becoming a therapeutic method in general use. Excellent modern expositions of the subject are to be found in Vinaj's book (2nd ed., Milan, 1903), and in *Massage, Its Principles and Practice* (1917), by the Britisher J. B. MENNELL.

GYMNASTIC EXERCISES have also been used in therapeutics since ancient times. The Italians of the Renaissance were well aware of its value and P. P. VERGERIO (1348–1419), of Capodistria, gives to physical culture an interesting chapter in his book on the education of the adolescent. Other Italian apostles of gymnastics were Vittorino da FELTRE (1378–1446), Francesco FILELFO (1398–1481), and Gerolamo MERCURIALE, whose *De arte gymnastica* (1569) is the first complete text on the subject and has served as a model for all subsequent works of its kind. We have seen that Sydenham was a strong advocate of horseback riding, influencing Francis Fuller (*Medica Gymnastica*, 1705) and Benjamin Rush, who, like the English Hippocrates, sent his patients on long horseback journeys to cure a variety of chronic ills. In the same vein is Theodor QUELLMALTZ's (1696–1758) rocking-horse, the progenitor of the electric horses of modern gymnasiums (*Novum Sanitatis præsidium*). S. A. Tissot and J. P. Frank were also enthusiastic advocates of gymnastic exercises for the young. The reviver of medical gymnastics was the Swede Per Hendrik LING (1776–1839), whose system used few mechanical aids and was based on the acquisition of increased mastery by the will over the movements of the body (see the section on Orthopedics). Though at first opposed by the medical profession, he eventually made the Stockholm Institute the centre of the theory and practice of medical gymnastics. To Ling's gymnastics without apparatus Zander added many mechanical devices (mechanotherapy) that seemed to him better calculated to develop special muscle systems (1865). German *Turnvereine*, important elements in Teutonic physical culture, arose from the *Turnhalle* gymnasium of F. L. JAHN (1778–1852), who devised exercises especially in order to fit German youth physically to rise above Napoleonic domination (1810).

ELECTROTHERAPY. Credit for the first use of electricity as a therapeutic agent (1744) is given by Duchenne, himself a pioneer in the field, to J. G. KRUEGER (1715–59), Professor of Medicine at Halle and later at Helmstadt; and by Priestley (*History of Electricity*, 1767) to C. G. KRATZENSTEIN (1723–95), who published a book on the subject in 1745. According to Vinaj, the first use of electricity in treatment was made in 1747 by the Paduan G. F. PIGATI, who attempted to introduce therapeutic substances into the systems of the gouty and the arthritic by means of the electric current.

HEAT as a form of medical treatment has been found useful since ancient times, not only by the use of blankets or sweat baths, but from " the lively vigorous warmth of young people." The virgin who lay in aged King David's bosom for this purpose had followers up to the seventeenth century, when Sydenham warmly recommended the practice. The modern rubber hot-water bottle had predecessors in the form of heated stones or jugs filled with hot water, which still are widely used. The most modern form of thermotherapy is the use of infrared rays or the electrical penetration of heat (diathermy), introduced (1898) by R. von ZEYNEK (b. 1869) and by C. F. NAGELSCHMIDT (b. 1875) in 1906.

These brief references may suffice to show the important position that physiotherapy has aspired to in recent times. Yet it lagged behind other forms of treatment in establishing and exploring the scientific bases for the methods used, with the result that it has fallen largely into the hands of cultists, such as osteopaths, chiropractors, naprapaths and the like. Fortunately, signs are accumulating that the tide is turning. In America the prominence given to new methods of treating poliomyelitis and B. Baruch's large gift for teaching and research in physical medicine offer legitimate hope for improvement in the near future. The ancient concept of the healing powers of nature has returned today in more ample and scientific form. The idea finds its application also in the wider diffusion of athletic sports, which are now followed with an enthusiasm that recalls the triumphs of ancient Greece, when the health of the individual and of the public, and the cult of beauty in harmony with physical and mental power, were regarded as the supreme goal.

21. Military Medicine

Wars have always been in past times breeders of pestilence as well as destroyers of the flower of a nation's youth. In the American Revolution dysentery and spotted fever, pneumonia, malaria, and other infectious diseases took a far higher toll in death and incapacitation than did the casualties of battle and the hardships of Valley Forge. In the eighteenth century the medicine of warfare gradually came under closer military control, with army hospitals and ambulance stations, schools, and even a special journal (1766). The Napoleonic Wars caused the loss of more than six million men to France and her allies in the first fifteen years of the century and are said to have dealt a blow to the physical standards of that country from which she never entirely recovered. The Crimean War demonstrated the need for placing military hygiene in a position independent of the bureaucratic control of the civil administration. The lack of an efficient nursing service in this war entailed such enormous losses to the allied armies, especially to the British, that it became the subject of a protracted investigation in the British Parliament. It was during this war, as we have seen in the previous chapter, that Florence Nightingale brought modern nursing into existence. In the American Civil War, anesthetics were used for the first time in warfare, but were not available in sufficient amounts. Sepsis still exacted its toll unopposed, with many fatal secondary hemorrhages from infection, and dysentery and the customary camp diseases were responsible for much death and disability. With an estimated 44,000 deaths in action and 32,000 from wounds, over 186,000 (61 per 1,000) died of disease. This medical story was published in great detail (six large volumes) in the official *Medical and Surgical History of the War of the Rebellion*, by J. J. WOODWARD *et al.* (1870–88), still valuable for its statistics, but, like most books of this kind, otherwise but little read. In the Spanish-American War also many more died from diseases, especially typhoid, than from battle casualties. An important development for all future wars was the foundation of the Red

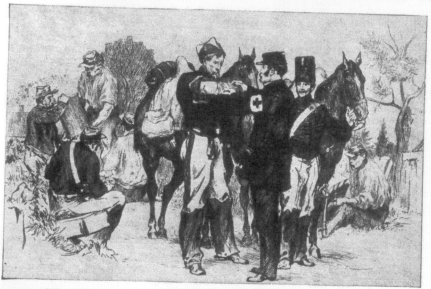

439. *A French aid station during the Franco-Prussian War of 1870, by A. Lançon.*

Cross. After the Italian Risorgimento in 1859, H. DUNANT (1828–1910), who was an eyewitness of the Battle of Solferino, wrote a widely popular and influential *Souvenir de Solferino*. This led to the International Conference at Geneva in 1863, and the Convention of 1864, by which fourteen powers solemnly promised to treat as neutrals the sick and wounded and the entire sanitary personnel when engaged in the exercise of their function. Red Cross societies now exist throughout the world, offering their invaluable services in times of earthquakes, flood, and famine as well as on the battlefield and to prisoners of war.

During the Franco-Prussian War the German sanitary organization functioned admirably. The Prussian army included almost four thousand physicians, as against the one thousand of the French. The wounded were properly and efficiently handled and infectious diseases were relatively few. An interesting fact brought out by Garrison in his *Notes on the History of Military Medicine* is that while the frequently vaccinated German troops had only 483 cases of smallpox, the French troops, of whom only a part had been vaccinated, had 4,178 cases, with almost 2,000 deaths.

The Sanitary Service of the Italian army can be traced to the institutions of ancient Piedmont. During the Regency of Maria Christina (1637–48) the rudiments of a sanitary service were begun; in 1701 the so-called *ospedali volanti* were created and a permanent military hospital was installed at the Villa Reale in Turin. The Sanitary Corps was again reorganized under Victor Emmanuel II by Alessandro RIBERI (1796–1861), the outstanding Italian surgeon of the period, who in 1851 founded the *Giornale di medicina militare*. With the establishment of the new Italian Kingdom, the *Comitato di sanità militare*, which had replaced the ancient *Consiglio*, was transferred to Rome in 1875, in turn to be replaced in 1920 by a *Direzione centrale di sanità militare*. In 1883 a *Scuola di applicazione di sanità militare* was opened at Florence.

In the period covered by this chapter military surgery was advanced by Esmarch and Billroth in the Franco-Prussian War, by Pirogov in the Russo-Turkish War, and by Appia and others in Italy in the Wars of Independence. Anesthesia and antisepsis especially have prevented untold suffering by the wounded soldier. Especially useful was the establishment (1910) by G. GROSSICH, of Fiume (1849–1926), of the routine treatment of war wounds with the tincture of iodine. Diagnostic roentgenology was applied to war conditions almost immediately after Röntgen's discovery: already, though crudely, by the British and Italians in 1896, to a greater extent in the Spanish-American War (1898), and still more in the Boer War (1899–1902). By the end of the century the medical corps had become an integral part of army and navy, its personnel governed by the same order of rank and regulations, and its prime duty to minimize the loss of efficiency from death and disease as well as to help the individual.

22. Public Health

The many advantages brought to humanity by the medical advances recorded in previous sections of this chapter at once suggest that public health and social medicine necessarily profited thereby. If the evolution of medical thought through the centuries permits us to recognize how the original concept of local disease has been developed slowly but surely toward the idea of general disease in the body, we may trace no less certainly the development of a community-health point of view along similar lines. From the concept of the sick individual as it first appeared in primitive civilization, " hygiene " came to include consideration of the welfare of the group, first of the family, then of the nation, and then of the world at large — a true social concept. Just as the physician acquired the conviction that disease was never limited to a single organ and that it concerned the entire individual in its origin, relationships, and results, so experience has taught us that every disease that strikes the individual has a direct effect on society as an organism. From this point of view the problems of " public health " have much in common with those of the health of the individual. When the discoveries of microbiology and immunology allowed the establishment of the laws of infectious diseases and evaluation of the various influences that determined and modified them, when the laws that governed heredity became known, when the effects of various toxic factors on man as an individual and as a group were revealed, then the necessity of considering the means of defence against disease as a social problem became more than ever obvious. At the same time the most modern investigations have demonstrated the truth of the ancient assertion that nature is the best of physicians. It is obvious, then, that it is with the increase of the individual's natural means of defence, and consequently in the improvement of the biological environment of the individual from the moment of his conception, that the supreme program of all public health should begin. The ancient Greeks understood this idea of physical betterment as part of an effort inspired by a constant striving toward beauty. The modern hygienists have returned to the essential lines of such a program, placing it on the sure basis of scientific research, and maintaining that beauty in the classical sense of the word represents perfect health, the eurhythmics of organic forces. But beyond and above the classical idea modern medicine has proposed and procured the safeguarding of the newborn and children still to be born; the protection of the weak and delicate, not in futile pity, but in an efficient attempt to reinvigorate them; and, finally, the temporary or permanent exclusion from social life of individuals stricken with diseases that are capable of constituting a danger to the health of the public. This evolution of the care of the individual into a national and social care, this legislative progress, which in the domain of health has ever more vast objectives, finally this essential transfer of medical activity from the field of the treatment of disease to that of prophylaxis, these are the characteristic and determining factors of the medicine of modern times, features that are especially well brought out in modern sanitary legislation and in the carrying out of public health assistance, prophylaxis, and hygiene.

At first in isolated attempts and then in a more thoroughly organized manner, legislation has brought the successes of bacteriology and of biological research into the practical domain of public health. Marked advances were achieved in the field of infantile diseases, as we have noted in a previous chapter. Improvement in the water supplies, the sewage system, the institution of medical control in schools, the provisions against

alcoholism, and the establishment of day nurseries (*crèches*) have combined with better knowledge of infantile diseases and special methods of
control greatly to lower infantile morbidity and mortality. Labouring conditions have been improved by legislation introducing shorter working
hours, the compulsory inspection of factories, the compulsory installation
of safety devices, the insurance of
workmen against industrial hazards
(started by Germany in 1884), unemployment compensation, and similar
measures designed to protect the labourer under conditions of modern
employment. In Britain a series of
Factory Acts have been passed from
1875 up to the present decade, raising
the age limits of child labour, protecting from industrial hazards, providing
first aid and standards of hygienic conditions. Especially in the control of
infantile diarrhœa and the four chief
diseases of childhood (measles, scarlet
fever, whooping cough, and diphtheria) has a favourable trend in infant mortality been evident, so that it
has been reduced more than fifty per
cent in many countries in the present
century and before the last war stood
at the lowest level known in history.

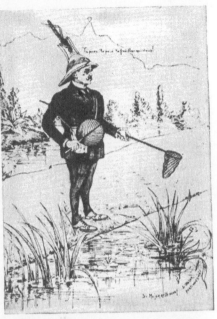

440. *French caricature of Ronald
Ross on his malaria survey in Mauritius.*

This improvement has been the chief cause of the lengthening of the average duration of human life from the fourth to the seventh decade in a few
generations.

Progress in the public control of infectious diseases, already contemplated in the earlier half of the century, is exemplified in the fight against
cholera, which began with the discovery of the cholera vibrio in 1884. At
the International Conference held in Venice in 1892, regulations were
adopted for an International Convention against cholera, standards that
were later augmented by the measures adopted against plague by the Paris
Conventions of 1903 and 1926. The campaign against endemic infectious
diseases has been so productive that the general mortality in Europe in the
two decades before World War I diminished almost one half. Epidemics
have occurred in less severe and less extended form and are usually recog-

nized in their early stages and restricted to their original foci. Influenza
and other epidemics brought about by the abnormal conditions of the First
World War are notable exceptions.

In Italy the struggle against MALARIA was highly successful. Following
shortly after the discoveries of the cause of malaria by Laveran, Ross, and
Grassi, the Italian campaign against malaria was begun chiefly through the

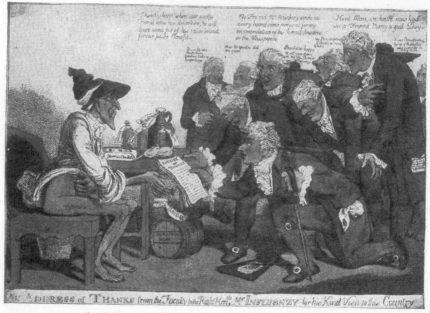

441. *An Address of Thanks from the Faculty to Mr. Influenzy.*
(*Cartoon by J. West.*)

efforts of Angelo Celli with the introduction of anti-malarial legislation and
State control of quinine (proposed by F. Garlanda in 1895), the free treatment of patients with quinine furnished by the communes, and the outlining
of malarial zones.

With the constitution of the Kingdom of Italy, the unification of the sanitary laws was undertaken and was brought about in 1888. The *Consiglio su-
periore di sanità* administered the public health of the country, with smaller
bodies acting for the provinces. The public health of the communes and of the
large cities was also better organized. Thus the modern sanitation of Naples,
which was begun in 1885 after the cholera epidemic, led to the rehabilitation of
the poorer quarters, improvements in the sewerage system and in the supply of
drinking water. Italian public health legislation has also included assistance to
the poor and hospital assistance in general. Such measures of course introduce

enormous difficulties in increasing the number of hospital cases and in balancing the budgets of these institutions. Rural and maritime hygiene have also been submitted to legislative control.

Campaigns against INFECTIOUS DISEASES that constitute a threat to public health, such as trachoma, leprosy, and hookworm disease, have been conducted on an extensive scale. Pellagra, which once had unfortunate notoriety as an Italian plague, especially in the rural districts of Venetia and

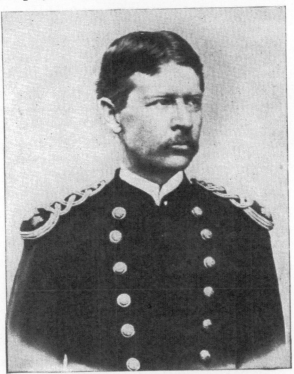

442. *Walter Reed.*

Lombardy, was reduced there to a few cases annually. The Italian mortality from pellagra decreased 98 per cent (from 115 per million inhabitants in 1887–9 to 2 per million in 1929–31). Similar success has been obtained in the United States, where the disease was found to be unexpectedly prevalent in the less prosperous districts. The recognition that it was chiefly due to lack of vitamins rather than to infection greatly contributed to the proper steps for its control. Ankylostomiasis (hookworm disease) has also succumbed to energetic control measures. The campaign in the southern United States conducted by the Rockefeller Foundation, both educationally and in the distribution of parasiticides, has greatly improved the hygienic status of this section. An interesting study in the epidemiology of measles was afforded toward the middle of the century by an outbreak in the Faroe Islands (1846), which had not been exposed to the disease for sixty-five years. An epidemic that attacked 6,000 of the 8,000 inhabitants was studied

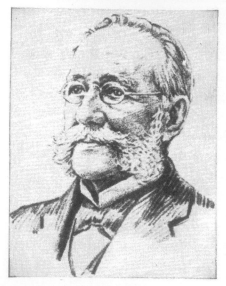

443. *Carlos Finlay.*

by P. L. PANUM (1820–85), when still an intern. With this splendid opportunity, form the epidemiological point of view, Panum was able to establish the period of contagiosity of the disease, the appearance of a rash on the thirteenth or fourteenth day after exposure, its independence of cowpox and smallpox, the immunity produced by a single attack, and similar valuable data. The study is famous in the history of epidemiology.

One of the greatest triumphs of modern hygiene has been the conquest of YELLOW FEVER by the United States Army Yellow Fever Board (1900), consisting of Walter Reed (1851–1902), James CARROLL (1854–1907), Jesse W. LAZEAR (1866–1900), and Aristide AGRAMONTE (1869–1931).

Following the suggestion (1881) of Carlos Juan FINLAY Y DE BARRES (1833–1915) that yellow fever was spread by a mosquito (*Stegomyia fasciata* or *Aëdes ægypti*), Reed and his board were sent to Cuba to investigate the problem. As no animals could be made to develop the disease, Carroll volunteered to be bitten by an infected mosquito, developed yellow fever, but fortunately recovered. Seven volunteers slept in the bedding of fever patients in mosquito-proof tents (fomites being then regarded as a probable mode of transmission) and failed to develop the disease, thus completing the proof that the disease was transmitted by the mosquito. Lazear, accidentally bitten by an infected stegomyia, died after a few days' illness. Having thus established that the stegomyia was the vector of yellow fever after it had bitten a patient in the first five days of his illness, and having determined the incubation period, the army under the able leadership of William C. GORGAS (1854–1920) succeeded, in a campaign of screening patients and destroying mosquitoes, in freeing Havana of yellow fever for the first time in a hundred and fifty years. The crowning achievement of the construction of the Panama Canal was made possible by the same methods. In fact, the Canal Zone, formerly almost uninhabitable by the white race, has become one of the most healthful areas in the world, malaria and various other infections having been almost eliminated.

Regulation of water supply to the large cities has become standardized either in the form of adequate filtration plants or, better still, by conducting pure water from distant regions many miles through aqueducts. Sand filtration was apparently first introduced in London in 1829, the London water supply still being mainly obtained from the Thames and Lea rivers. The bacteriological treatment of sewage was proposed by W. J. DIBDEN in 1896. New York City is supplied by aqueducts from the Catskill Mountains and the lakes north of the city, and also includes the use of several filtration plants. The importance of infected water in cholera and typhoid epidemics was well demonstrated in the Lowell and Lawrence epidemics of 1890 (W. T. SEDGWICK), and in the Hamburg cholera epidemic of 1892, when that city was supplied with unfiltered water, while its suburb, Altona, which was supplied with filtered water, had practically no cases of the disease. In Philadelphia and Washington the installation of modern filtration plants coincided with marked decline in the incidence of typhoid fever, which is now a comparative rarity in the United States, appearing usually in local country outbreaks or in individuals after the use of polluted milk, oysters, or water during summer travel.

The study of SCHOOL HYGIENE has produced a number of excellent regulations for the personal hygiene of schoolchildren and contributed notably to their collective health. Dental clinics detect and correct dental defects in early stages, deficient eyesight is promptly recognized and treated, good personal hygienic habits are established, and even special schools created for those handicapped by heart disease or retarded intelligence. The science of eugenics, though still in its early stages, can be regarded as contributing in broad lines to standards that should improve the physical and mental condition of the population.

An important impulse to all these hygienic activities and laws has come from the institutes of hygiene attached in some countries to the central sanitary administrations and to the universities, in which toward the end of the past century the teaching of hygiene was made obligatory. In the primary and secondary schools the practical teaching of hygiene has been established, an excellent stabilizing influence for the rising generation.

The greatest hygienic institute was that created by Koch in Berlin in 1885, and in the same year the first Italian institute of experimental hygiene was

founded by Crudeli in Rome. In Paris the Pasteur Institute was dedicated especially to bacteriological studies, which of course also have an important influence on practical hygiene. The Lister Institute was founded in 1891, the Liverpool and London Schools of Tropical Medicine in 1899.

The Scuola di Perfezionamento in Igiene, founded by Crispi in Rome, has
had outstanding teachers and scholars, and was praised by Koch as an example
of its kind. The various hygienic institutes of the universities have been centres
of the study of hygiene in Italy. At the University of Rome its director, G. Sana-
relli, conducted studies on yellow fever and enteric diseases, and his successor,
De Blasi, specialized in epidemiological studies of industrial and social hygiene.
The Turin Institute was founded by Pagliani; that of Padua by Serafini, and
was then under the directorship of Casagrandi. The model institute of Pisa was
directed by Di Vestea, who with A. Sclavo, director of the institute at Siena,
was an active propagandist for the hygiene of schools. An excellent *Trattato
d'igiene* (4 vols., Milan, 1933) is owed to D. Ottolenghi, of Naples.

One of the most remarkable features in connection with medical hygiene is its
great development in countries where organized instruction in modern medicine
has come into being only in the past century. Thus Japan has a number of scientific institutes and universities in which valuable investigations have been carried out. Among Japan's best-known physicians are Shibasaburo KITASATO
(1856–1931), founder of the Tokyo Institute for Infectious Diseases; Kiyoshi
SHIGA (b. 1870), discoverer of the dysentery bacillus that bears his name (1897);
Fujiro KATSURADA (b. 1868) and Akira FUJINAMI (b. 1871), discoverers of
Schistosoma japonicum; Ryukichi INADA (b. 1874) and Yutaka IDO (b. 1881),
discoverers of the *Leptospira ictero-hæmorrhagica*, the cause of Weil's disease
(1916); Kenzo FUTAKI (b. 1873) and Kikutaro ISHIKAWA (b. 1878), discoverers
of the *Spirochæta muris*, the cause of rat-bite fever, and a number of other
scientists, especially active in the field of parasitology.

Though MENTAL DISEASES have been more or less steadily increasing in
modern times, this was not appreciated as one of the most important of
public health problems until the beginning of the twentieth century. Mental hospitals, to be sure, had existed in the United States, for instance, mostly
as state institutions, since the Williamsburg, Virginia, Hospital was opened
in 1773. With the growth of the country, such hospitals naturally multiplied, though S. W. HAMILTON's list in *One Hundred Years of American
Psychiatry* shows that expansion was greatest in the seventies and eighties.
Psychopathic hospitals as such did not come into existence until the Boston
Psychopathic Hospital was opened in 1912. An out-patient mental clinic
was started at the Pennsylvania Hospital in 1885 and at the Massachusetts
State School in 1891; others followed slowly after the turn of the century.
Mental defectives were mixed with the mentally ill, as in fact they still are

to some extent. Special provision for their institutional care appears to have been started in France by Édouard SEGUIN (1812–80), who later came to this country, and was the first president of what is now called the American Association on Mental Deficiency (founded 1876). Special institutions for the care and education of the feeble-minded have increased but slowly. In many cases waiting lists are so long that parents may be advised to deposit their mental defectives in the public streets so that they have to be picked up by the police. Special institutions for epileptics are also an outgrowth of this period, the first in the U.S.A. having been established at Gallipolis, Ohio, in 1893.

23. The Study and Practice of Medicine

The characteristic figure of the American physician of the earlier part of this period is familiar to many older people even today. Among the well-to-do the urbane, rather majestic frock-coated figure, perhaps chop-whiskered, having left his top hat in the hall, brought with him to the sick patient a feeling of confidence and reliance that was worth many drugs. A faint whiff of iodoform and carbolic perhaps further conditioned the patient to profit by the important " bedside manner." An impressive " May I see your tongue? " followed by the pulse-taking ritual, and the newly intro-duced clinical thermometer were helpful preludes to a physical examina-tion well established by the earlier French school and only limited by Vic-torian reluctance to expose the female form. In many hospitals but few laboratory aids to diagnosis were in use — in fact, but few were available. In the early times in country districts conditions of practice were even cruder. Horse-and-buggy transportation over muddy roads limited the abilities of even the most persevering physician, so that many more than today, waiting in vain " until the doctor comes," died without medical aid or after it had arrived too late. Horseback was still often the best means of conveyance. Hospitals, primarily designed for the needy, had hardly begun to make suitable accommodations for private patients, and indeed good treatment was such a simple affair that the hospitals had little to offer be-yond the resources of the home.[1] Operations — more of an emergency or

[1] Some items illustrating the gradual development of the Pennsylvania Hospital may be detailed here as a sample of an American hospital's growth: Its contribution to early teach-ing of anatomy and obstetrics (Fothergill crayons and Shippen's lectures); its medical li-brary (for many years the best in the country), begun in 1762 with a gift from John Fother-gill; Benjamin Franklin's close association (*Some Account of the Pennsylvania Hospital*, 1754; president 1755; his inimitable inscription on the cornerstone); Thomas Bond's clinical lectures (begun 1766), " the beginning of systematic medical teaching on the continent "; gratis vaccination of the poor, 1809; Mental Department organized in West Philadelphia,

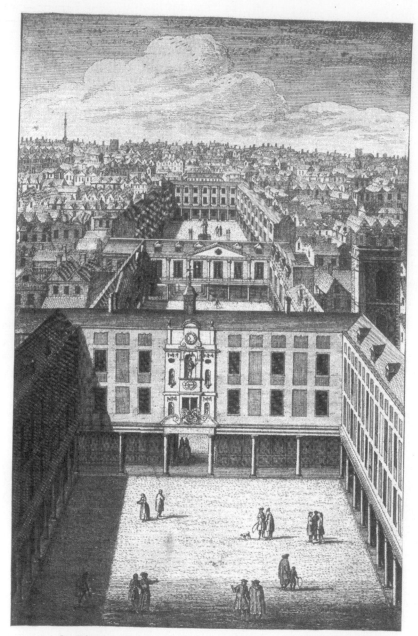

444. *St. Thomas Hospital, London.* (*Eighteenth-century engraving.*)

desperate nature than to improve the general health of the patient — were mostly done in the home, even if a room had to be changed into a temporary operating-room, with sheets covering the germ-infested draperies. Especially among the poorer classes, patients were taken to the hospital so often as a last resort that many refused to go at all, for fear of being carried out feet first in the "black box." Sufferers from mental disease, then fortu-

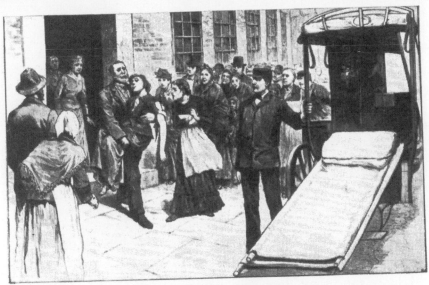

445. *Hospital ambulance, New York, 1882.*

nately much less prevalent than today, if requiring restraint were sent to insane asylums, with little hope for improving their condition or even attempts to do so. The patient perhaps succumbed to some disease then unknown, or to a disturbance of body functions then uncomprehended, but now well understood and often controllable. None was the wiser and all perforce resigned to the melancholy motto of " God's will be done! " Nevertheless, conscientious, intelligent men, possessing more of the available medical knowledge than is possible for the practitioner today, with highly developed powers of observation and imbued with a strong sense of their responsibilities, as a profession richly merited the well-known encomium given them by Robert Louis Stevenson.

1836; women nurses, 1848; Nurses Training School, 1878; X-ray service established, 1896; Social Service Department, 1910; affiliation with Philadelphia Dispensary (inst., 1786) and Philadelphia Lying-in Hospital (founded, 1828); University of Pennsylvania's Professor of Psychiatry becomes Medical Director of the Pennsylvania Institute, 1929. In the same year state aid was sought for the first time since 1796; and the keeping of weather records, started in 1766, was discontinued.

The COST OF MEDICAL CARE, which has always, like other commodities, tended to rise as the value of the currency unit depreciated through the centuries, had not begun to climb as disproportionately to the cost of living as it has in the twentieth century. A surgical example will illustrate: In America two generations ago, for a compound fracture of the femur, the general practitioner came to the house, gave the ether (or supervised its administration by one of the family), set the fracture and closed the wound with proper antisepsis and drainage, and paid several house visits to see that the family's care was satisfactory; total cost, twenty-five to fifty dollars. Today the patient is taken to a hospital, where the necessary charges for bed (or room), operating-room and anesthetist fees, X-rays before, during, and after operation, perhaps three private nurses, laboratory fees, and the surgeon's fee can easily mount to several hundred dollars, and even so, good hospitals are far from self-supporting. To be sure, the chances of survival, with a useful leg, are greatly increased; but who thinks of that? Ordinary visits, which about the year 1800 cost, say, one dollar, were still about the same around 1850; by the end of the century they had risen very little in the country, but were up to two or three dollars in the cities, and are now five dollars or more, with even higher increases for the specialists and consultants from the five and ten dollars then charged. Voluntary " honoraria," rather than payment for service rendered, were still maintained by some; one specialist, who lived till 1938, in his earlier career sent no bills; but each patient on leaving the waiting-room was expected to leave a five-dollar gold piece in the jar on the mantlepiece.

MEDICAL EDUCATION. In medical education the French and British emphasis on clinical instruction, with early admission to the wards, persisted, with corresponding lack of application of the growing contributions of research in ward and laboratory to the comprehension of disease processes. To be sure, great clinicians continued to observe acutely and to teach " sound " clinician medicine, though in France they were not to be compared with the earlier schools of Laënnec and Louis, or in Britain with Bright, Addison, Graves, Stokes, and others.

G. N. Stewart gives a picture of his medical education in the early eighties at the University of Edinburgh, then as usual one of the best undergraduate courses to be found anywhere. Gross anatomy, which with botany, zoology, and chemistry occupied the first year, was " well taught according to the old style," and a little of histology (with " a very fair laboratory course ") and physiology were also given. The latter consisted almost entirely of lectures to some four hundred men, with an occasional far-off demonstration of a frog reaction. The only laboratory work mentioned was one test of the urine for sugar, and a half-hour each with the laryngoscope and ophthalmoscope. Thus prepared, students started the second year with surgical lectures and ward dressings. Pathology, given in the third year, was acquired by watching autopsies and in "a fair course in pathological histology" — no bacteriology. Materia medica and pharmacology were covered by lectures only. The fourth year, except for a little instruction on skin diseases and more on legal medicine, was occupied by one hundred lectures on obstetrics (which included gynæcology). Of instruction in eye, ear, nose, and throat diseases there was none. Since that

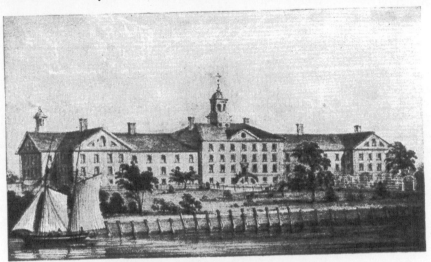

446. *Almshouse Hospital, Bellevue, New York, 1860.*

time, except for a fifth year added for sectional work in clinical subjects (including items like tuberculosis, children's and venereal diseases), the changes have been more in the way the subjects were taught than in the plan of the course.

On the other hand, in the Germanic countries medical progress was so rapid — part and parcel of the general burst of activity in Germany in the fifties and sixties — that it was not long before their research teaching led the world. Other causes for this renascence are not easily traced. Starting from the vague theoretical and metaphysical teaching of earlier years, such as *Naturphilosophie*, Germany and Austria entered this period far behind England and France. The professor continued his lectures "authoritatively expounding the traditional lore" (S. Flexner); yet before long, the whole type of instruction was transformed to the combination of lectures and practical work in wards and laboratory that still dominates medical teaching on both continents. This was due, according to Flexner's searching analysis, to the fact that the German professor was not merely a teacher of future practitioners but a lifelong scientific student of his subject, advancing through years of work in subordinate positions, and attaining eminence largely because of his success in investigation. This necessarily included close co-operation with and understanding of the laboratory as developed by men like Purkinje, Liebig, and Virchow, and naturally led to a type of clinical investigation more exacting in its methods than that based on simple clinical observation.

In the German Empire the chief professor of a department was chosen by the Minister of Education from names submitted separately by the faculty and the junior teachers. Other teachers, *Privatdozenten*, and assistants served long years, living on meagre pay or fees for voluntary courses, often with quite inadequate teaching and research facilities. A brief but vivid sketch of the Continental clinics in the earlier part of this period can be found in Garrison's *History* (4th edition, pp. 755 *et seq*.). The Germanic spirit of true investigative and teaching zeal is well seen in Billroth's *Über das Lehren und Lernen der medizinischen Wissenschaft* (1876).

In the United States formal medical education, which had started auspiciously on a university basis in the eighteenth century, had been overrun by the proprietary schools, starting with College of Medicine of Maryland in 1812. Most of these schools were combinations of " lecture, quiz, and cram," with short sessions and few expenses, self-appointed faculties, and no collegiate connections, degrees given *in absentia*, and even attendance not always being required. They were " diploma mills," which retarded medical education for most of a century. In the thirty years 1810–40, 26 schools had been founded; in the next 36 years (1840–76), 47 schools, and between 1873 and 1890 the incredible number of 114 more. The state of Missouri alone had 42 (Sigerist). Even the respectable schools had only two-year courses, obligatory for a few months per year, supplemented by voluntary courses or clinics with an associate faculty, or in privately conducted schools. Courses in dissections became required by the leading schools about the middle of the century. Organized bedside instruction — which had been begun by Thomas Bond at the Pennsylvania Hospital in the 1760's, but had fallen largely into disuse — was revived about the same time, starting with the Medical Department of St. Louis University, 1849. Clinical lectures and demonstrations had never been abandoned in hospitals, but must have been unsatisfactory indeed for classes that might number over four hundred. Bedside teaching did not become an important part of the course until the establishment of hospitals created for the benefit of medical schools, such as the hospitals of the University of Michigan (1869), owned and controlled by the state; of the University of Pennsylvania (1874); and of Johns

Hopkins (1889). Three-year courses were being established, though for some years a good part of the student's work might be as a " private pupil of a respectable practitioner "; and obligatory four-year courses were not established till the last decade of the century.

The curriculum was arranged much as described in G. N. Stewart's picture cited above. But American students, who had formerly gone to Edinburgh, then to Paris, now turned to Vienna and the German universities. The revelations of the new medicine — especially by the microscope and by new science of bacteriology — were combined with reforms from the top, such as those of President Eliot at Harvard (1871) and of Provost Pepper at Pennsylvania (1873–95), culminating with the foundation of the new medical school at Johns Hopkins in 1893. As O. W. Holmes quaintly expressed the situation at Harvard, " Our new President Eliot has turned the whole university over like a flapjack. There never was such a *bouleversement* in the Medical Faculty. The Corporation [of Harvard] has taken the whole management of it out of our hands. We are paid salaries, which I rather like. . . ." By 1892 Harvard had lengthened the course to four obligatory years. Students' fees had long been paid to the teachers of individual courses; tickets of admission, often on the backs of playing cards, are medical collectors' items. It was not until the seventies that teachers in American medical schools began to be paid salaries, and students' fees were established around $100 to $150 a year. These have risen, slowly at first, up to $400 to $600 a year in the best schools, though in state-supported schools fees are much less. Support by taxation, however, is not without its disadvantages, as when farmers of the agricultural state of Wisconsin protested to their legislators when university investigators found that margarine was just as nutritious as butter.

Better premedical training, a longer medical course, selection of the best possible faculty from other institutions at home and abroad, a good combination of the best of the foreign methods of instruction, and the generous support of the growing wealth of the country set the stage for the tremendous development, in North America even more than elsewhere, that took place in the next century. As Allbutt put it: " this new birth [of medicine] is nothing less than its enlargement from an art of observation and empiricism to an applied science founded upon research; from a craft of tradition and sagacity to an applied science of analysis and law, from a descriptive code of surface phenomena to the discovery of deeper affinities; from a set of rules and axioms of quality to measurements of quantity."

It may safely be said that while physicians in general have always earned a competence, very few have grown rich on their earnings in modern times any more than in previous centuries. Even for the few whose professional incomes are really large, the figures are less than some cited in earlier times; Richard Mead, for instance, charging a guinea for an office visit and two or more for outside, made £5,000 to £7,000 a year at a time when money had more than three times its present purchasing power. Physicians have made considerably less than men of equal ability, experience, and activity obtain in other professions or in industry.

PROFESSIONAL ORGANIZATION. Medicine is one of the most highly organized professions, not only in its literature, but also in the alignment of its members. The British Medical Association, founded in 1832, has held annual meetings since that date, and also had a publication, which since 1857 has been the weekly *British Medical Journal*. A truly national society, it has had branches and emulators in the various Dominions of the Empire. Together with the *Lancet* (a journal founded by Thomas Wakley in 1823), it has ably led medical progress, safeguarding the physician's proper interests and promoting medical reforms.

In the United States, medicine began to be " organized " in the county (New Haven, 1784) and state (New Jersey, 1766) societies. By 1800 there were seven state societies. The American Medical Association was not formed until 1846, and for a half-century was chiefly concerned with combating the evils resulting from the insufferable condition into which medical education had fallen. Reorganized in 1901 in its present form, based on the county and state societies, with state and federal houses of delegates, the association includes almost the entire medical profession of the country, each member getting the weekly *Journal*. The largest and most powerful of medical organizations, through its *Journal* and eight specialty journals, its various councils (on Medical Education, on Pharmacy and Chemistry, etc.), its medical *Directory* (U.S.A. and Canada), and numerous other activities, it takes an important position and exerts a tremendous influence on all aspects of medical life.

ETHICS. The highest attainable ethical standards have always been a necessity in a profession that has such intimate and confidential relations with others. As we have seen, beginning with the Code of Hammurabi, codes of ethics such as Thomas Percival's (1803) have been prepared since the earliest times. In 1847 the first official code was constructed by the American Medical Association for application to modern conditions; but the greatly changed conditions since that time, with practice becoming steadily more of a business, demanding closer connections with other applied sciences and businesses, this code has become more and more loosely interpreted. Personal advertising in the news columns of periodicals, treating patients and families in return for a company salary, group practice, fee-splitting, and abhorred evils of earlier days have, for better or worse, become more or less inevitable. Unfair practices, too, exist in the medical as in every other profession; yet the reputable physician continues in his dealings with colleagues and patients to abide by standards, often to his financial loss, which may be disapproved by and often incomprehensible to laymen. He continues to uphold the confidential nature of his knowledge about the patient, to refuse to take from another doctor a patient for whom he has been called in consultation, and to give of his best to rich and poor alike.

WOMEN PHYSICIANS have been with us since the time of Trotula, or since early Egyptian times, if we accept such evidence as the female figured in the famous stele of the boy with poliomyelitis. However, it required the protracted research shown in Dr. Hurd-Mead's *Women in Medicine* (1938) to demonstrate how continuous, if slender, has been the stream of trained women successfully practising medicine or even holding professional chairs through the centuries. Obstacles in the way of thorough medical education for women have been numerous in the past. When Elizabeth BLACKWELL (1821–1910) (not to be confused with Elizabeth Blackwell, 1712–70, who wrote *The Curious Herbal*), after having studied medicine privately in Nova Scotia, applied for admission to Philadelphia medical schools, she was refused by all four. Similar refusals were met elsewhere, until she was finally admitted to Geneva College, where she was graduated in 1849, the first woman to receive a medical degree in America. When her sister, Emily, was accepted at Rush Medical College, Chicago, the school was censured by the State Medical Society and a second term was refused her. Later the two sisters and Dr. Marie ZAKRZEWSKA (1829–1902), of Polish-gypsy ancestry, founded the New York Infirmary for Women and Children, the first hospital to be conducted wholly by women. Some excellent medical schools even today refuse, by decree or by custom, to accept women as medical students. More, however, admit at least a limited number and find these highly selected candidates industrious and competent. Harvard agreed to admit a few women of exceptional quality as late as 1944. In Britain most medical schools, except those of the London hospitals, are now open to women, as are most schools on the Continent, following Switzerland's lead (1876). Many hospitals accept women as interns; and, except for a considerable loss from marriage, they do well in regular practice, leaning especially toward pediatrics, gynæcology, and obstetrics and to the many positions now open in the social aspects of medicine.

The first medical school in the world solely for women was the Women's Medical College of Pennsylvania, incorporated in 1850 as the Female Medical College of Pennsylvania. This institution still flourishes in Philadelphia, its mixed faculty of men and women turning out annually classes of women educated in the best medical tradition. The London School of Medicine for Women was founded in 1874; the Women's Medical College of Baltimore in 1882. There are but few such schools in the world today, however, and with the more liberal admission policy of the regular schools, the need for many such special schools is small. As nurses and midwives women have played roles of waxing and waning importance in medicine from time immemorial. As trained nurses their great contribution to modern medical practice is acknowledged by all.

CHAPTER XXI

THE TWENTIETH CENTURY

1. Introduction

THE PERIOD covered in this chapter offers an extremely difficult problem to the historian, not only because it is so close to us, but also because progress has been so rapid and in some regards so revolutionary in all fields of medical science that it is almost impossible to form a synthetic judgment of all the factors that played an important part in the evolution of medicine. There have been in recent times several attempts, especially in the United States, to describe the medical historical events in the last fifty years, taking into consideration the influence that economic changes had on the development of medicine. Increasing understanding of the importance of medical history is proved by the fact that in almost all recent medical books devoted to different branches of medicine the introduction deals with a historical outlook. We think, however, that the evolution of contemporary medicine can be best understood in connection with the general history of medicine of the past. This may offer the opportunity to study not only the relation between events and the doctrines that have prevailed at different times, but also the gradual development of medical thought and of new concepts of the duties and rights of the physician and the part that he has to play.

The most important fact that influenced in a remarkable measure the development of medicine in recent decades was the political and social condition of Europe during this period. World War I, with its terrible destruction of human lives in Europe, and the economic and psychic depression that followed it everywhere, upset the collective mind of the civilized world. World War II brought about still more frightful conditions. We have witnessed the development of profound troubles, caused by the destruction of lives and of hopes, by the uprooting of moral principles that had been generally regarded as definitely accepted, and by the suppression of all freedom in the states that had been forced to accept the totalitarian regime. Many splendid treasures of culture were destroyed, scientists were killed or exiled, books were burned, and a number of universities had to suspend their activities. The care of the sick and help for the populations ravaged by famine and disease went back to the condition of ancient times. The harmful consequences of these catastrophes are still far from being realized, but will undoubtedly persist through generations.

At the same time, however, especially in the countries that were less directly affected by the immediate consequences of war and in which relatively normal conditions of life prevailed, exceptional advances in useful scientific discoveries were achieved. The necessities of war, the possibility given to a great number of physicians of studying many thousands of cases with the best methods and with almost unlimited support, the necessity and possibility of quick, intelligent co-operation by thousands of medical men following one accepted system — all these factors brought about a splendid development, especially in the field of surgery and of therapy. The mortality of the wounded was diminished in the Allied armies in an astonishing way; thousands of cases that only a few years ago would have been regarded as definitely lost were not only saved but brought to a quick recovery. The progress in medical organization, in transportation, in attendance on the wounded, has been of supreme importance in making this development possible.

During the last few years, at the same time as we were learning daily of a new terrible weapon or new systems to destroy humanity, we also learned daily of a new discovery, of new progress, of new research in the field of medicine to combat or compensate for this destruction.

The major development of the use of X-rays in medicine belongs to this period. It is true that chronologically Röntgen's discovery and its early applications were made in the last years of the nineteenth century, but the application of X-rays in medicine, in surgery, in all medical branches, as an invaluable help in diagnostics and in therapy, had its great development in the present century. Röntgen's discovery and its applications gave to the new developments of medicine a new direction on a solid foundation. It offered the possibility of making many diagnoses with an unprecedented sureness and it gave to the surgeon invaluable aid in penetrating the deepest recesses of the human body, guiding his hand with perfect reliability.

The progress of surgery as a science and an art was accentuated in this period through great achievements in all practical branches. The results of greatly improved technique in X-ray examination and treatment, the signal improvement in anesthesia and in blood transfusion and the powerful new drugs, gave the surgeon the ability to solve successfully many problems that up to our times appeared to be unsolvable. This progress was obtained through the combination of many factors: to those cited a few lines above must be added the improvement in microscopic and diagnostic chemical procedures, the better clinical diagnoses and methods of treatment that resulted from accumulated scientific experience and consultation with specialist colleagues.

The orientation of scientific studies toward biochemical research was evident in many signal discoveries, which have marked a new trend in research and in therapy. Biochemistry is, among all branches of medicine, the one in which the most significant progress has been achieved, and its revelations have had a direct influence on the conception and treatment of disease. This age has been called the age of proteins and enzymes, and it may be asserted that chemical studies and experiments have been predominant in the evolution of medical science and practice. Just as fifty years ago the physician was accustomed to start first from a microbiological concept and to consider microorganisms as the most important or maybe the only causative agents of a great number of diseases, now the trend is changed and we are convinced that a no less important and perhaps a more important role is played by conditions and occurrences that are to be regarded as chemical processes.

According to this concept and in consequence of it, the conviction had arisen that in the control of these facts and in the action exerted on them important and sometimes decisive help could be found in the fight against disease. From the theoretical concept and from experimental research on the chemistry of the cells, on secretions and excretions, and on the function of organs, modern medicine came to the conclusion that chemical agents could be greatly useful in this direction.

At the same time the enormous development of the chemical industry, the possibility of experimenting systematically with many new synthetic substances that were formerly unknown, and the great opportunities offered in clinics and scientific institutes set the stage for rapid and important developments in the field of therapy. From the first chemical studies of Pasteur and the first discoveries of Ehrlich to the most recent discoveries of the sulfa drugs and penicillin there is a long path of studies, trials, successes, and failures.

The evolution of pharmacology and therapy in the last period has been so unexpected and wonderful that to one reviewing the history of medicine throughout the past, the progress in this field in the last fifty years appears more significant and decisive than in all previous time. In fact, the whole concept of therapy, as has previously been said, has changed; not only has the number of remedies at the disposal of the physician grown beyond expectation, not only has their efficiency been proved by exact experiments, but our knowledge about the role of chemicals in the organism has revolutionized the orientation of modern therapy. The physician prescribes not merely to alleviate pain or other symptoms, but often with the assurance that he may be able to help directly and efficiently in attacking the cause of the disease. Experimental medicine has triumphantly entered the field of therapy, and for nearly every remedy we are able to determine with approximate exactness the reaction that it provokes. As a result, a great number of remedies have become no less popular than the universal remedies of olden times. Individual and collective suggestion also played a great part in this development. On the other hand, the tremendous amount and insistence of advertising often given to this or that pharmaceutical product or patent remedy, sometimes of little or no value, with exaggerated stories of wonderful cures, has often proved to be a distinct menace to the public health. Influencing a public opinion always dominated by suggestion, it recalls the power of astrology and magic in distant times. One may often listen to propaganda for this or that pharmaceutical product which seems to repeat the same words with which in ancient times the virtues of mandrake, of treacle or other miraculous medicines were extolled.

While the facts mentioned mark a new trend in the practice of medicine and of surgery, another revolutionary conquest of knowledge has taken place in the field of psychology and psychiatry. The doctrine of Freud has illuminated from a new angle the whole problem of the diseases of the psyche. It has offered a solution to some important problems, and changed the view of the physician and of the psychologist as to the causes of many psychoneurotic conditions. Many problems that seemed mysterious to doctors, priests, philosophers, and psychologists in olden times appear today in a new light. It is too early to appreciate the decisive importance of Freud's doctrine on modern medicine. The principle and findings of psychoanalysis met with universal contradiction in the beginning and still cause outbursts of indignation. Only in recent times has adequate recognition been accorded to the work of the great Viennese psychiatrist. His approach to the problems of the psyche stressed the important part that the subconscious plays in human minds. The cause of many psychoneuroses he traced to repression beneath the level of consciousness of previous experiences, often of a sexual nature. According to his method of prolonged exploration of details of the patient's past, these forgotten impressions were brought again to the field of consciousness, thereby, according to Freud, losing their capacity to prolong mental disturbances.

Finally, another extremely important factor that notably influenced the medicine of recent times was the evolution of modern industry and the strong organization of the working classes. Thanks to the recognition of the rights of the labouring classes and to their powerful organization, labour in many countries has obtained special laws ensuring prophylaxis of industrial hazards, defence against disease, insurance against physical misfortune, and protection from the handicaps of old age. Although these problems are being met differently in different countries and are still in the course of solution, there is no question of their great importance to the whole structure of modern medicine and to the place of the physician in the society of tomorrow.

The multiple bonds of medicine with other sciences, which have found practical expression in university teaching as well as in actual practice, constitute an important factor in the ever increasing penetration of medical knowledge among widespread classes of the population. Never before had medicine entered to an equal extent into the individual and social life of the time. From this period dates the supervision of the child, beginning with the day of his birth and continuing through his school life. His diet is controlled, his medical and mental hygiene cared for, and his mental aptitudes tested psychologically. The physician has entered the factories and controlled the installation of industrial safety devices and the prevention and treatment of industrial diseases. To this period belongs also the great development of public health statistics, which now constitute a specialty by themselves. In similar ways medical practice and supervision have entered the world of commerce with the creation of a real commercial hygiene; it influences maritime life in the promotion of naval hygiene and prophylaxis among the men. In the latest conquest of human intelligence and technical progress, in the air, medicine has had to map out proper regulations for the individual who is to operate at high altitudes; and a new branch of medicine, aviation medicine, has had a considerable development. Never before in history has medicine been so decisive in war, not only controlling the individual and collective hygiene of soldiers, but rapidly introducing for their benefit the latest discoveries and their most practical use. The increase in general culture and the enormous influence of the press and of the radio — another characteristic of this period — were further contributing factors. The efficiency with which the medical and lay press and the radio spread knowledge of medical discoveries and principles of hygiene has certainly been important in forming and increasing what may be called the hygienic consciousness of the people.

A remarkable fact in the evolution of the history of medical research in this period concerns the extension of medical studies in countries that in earlier times were unimportant in the progress of medicine. We have seen that during the Renaissance the impulse to the development of experimental medicine started from the Italian, and later from the French schools; that after the discovery of the New World and the development by the western European countries of traffic with America, the centre of medical studies was in Holland and England; that in the first half of the nineteenth century France was important in many fields of research, while later the German schools were the leaders in medical research. In the last fifty years the centre of medical research seems to have been transferred to the United States. The immense resources of North America, the great evolution of industry, the conception of a new trend in medical education, and the work of a great number of eminent scholars brought about the institution of medical schools that were equipped in the best way and opened their doors generously to the ideas, the teachers, and the pupils from other countries. With the help of richly endowed foundations and of splendid laboratories, the United States could not only equal, but not infrequently surpass the achievements of other countries.

An important contribution to the progress of medicine has been made in recent times by the Soviet Union, where a revolutionary change in the whole system of medical education and of public health has taken place, so that Russian medicine has attained a prominent place in the history of contemporary medical progress.

At the same time it should be stated that a considerable development of medical studies has taken place in Central and South America, where some great institutes were founded and important contributions were made, especially in the field of tropical medicine.

The attention of the reader is called to the fact that in this chapter the attempt is made to emphasize the outstanding features of the evolution of medical thought and the progress of medicine. It was obviously impossible to include many names of illustrious physicians and of important publications in a period when medical literature has reached enormous proportions. In a historical survey of modern medicine it is important for the reader who likes to have a comprehensive concept of the scientific currents and of the practical achievements of recent times to be acquainted with fundamental new concepts, with the interrelations between different branches of medicine, and with the facts that have been important in influencing the events.

While on the one hand it is necessary to divide the story into sections on the various disciplines, as otherwise it would be impossible to give any intelligent account of the situation, on the other hand it quickly becomes obvious that the story of each medical specialty frequently overlaps that of other branches. For this reason the reader will occasionally find the names of certain leaders repeated in the various sections of this chapter, as for instance when the clinician has made notable contributions to bacteriology, or the pathologist has advanced the progress of surgery.

In this chapter particular and detailed attention has been given to the sections on biology, physiology, biochemistry, and microbiology, the outstanding progress of which in the present century is less known in their historical development than are the advances in the practical disciplines. From the historian's point of view and for the full understanding of scientific progress in general, the steps in this rapid evolution deserve the close attention of students and practitioners, the more so as up to the present time such matters have not been presented in general medico-historical books. The reader who desires more details or more exhaustive bibliographical information must hunt them in the larger books devoted to the specialties. Here there is presented a summarized picture, within the limits above outlined, of the progress of the art and science of medicine in a period packed like no other before with discoveries and new concepts.

2. Biology

While the rapid development of the biological sciences was bringing new light to many obscure fields, physics and chemistry were also progressing in ways that had valuable results for medical thought and practice, as will be mentioned in many of the sections that follow. In this most important chapter of scientific history, indirectly connected with medicine, mention can only be made of some of the most striking discoveries which were noteworthy also for medical history. Such was Emil FISCHER's work on the *proteins*, and A. KOSSEL's and I. F. MIESCHER-RUESCH's on nucleins; also the studies of carbohydrates, which furthered knowledge of metabolism and of pathogenic bacterial action, and in the field of physics the discovery of *electrons* by Sir J. J. THOMSON (1897). From this grew the highly important study of radiant energy and *radioactive substances* (see Section 21). W. CROOKES had described the cathode rays and RÖNTGEN discovered (1895) the rays that bear his name, which have the power of passing through substances impermeable to light-rays. BECQUEREL's discovery in 1896 of the radioactivity of uranium led PIERRE (1859–1906) and MARIE CURIE (1867–1934) to the isolation from literally tons of pitchblende (1898) of minute quantities of a particularly strong radioactive substance. This Mme. Curie was able by the most painstaking study to identify as a new element, radium. After the tragic death of her husband she continued so to explore its characteristics and possibilities that not only were results of the greatest importance to medicine produced, but a new concept of the relations of energy to matter was demonstrated. A daughter, Mme. IRÈNE CURIE-JOLIOT, and her husband, Frédéric JOLIOT, have continued investigations in this field and in 1935 received the Nobel prize in chemistry for their work in transmitting radioactivity to materials that ordinarily do not possess this quality. The fascinating life of her mother, written by another daughter, Éve, who also made notable contributions by word and deed in the Second World War, illustrates in another field the superb intellectual endowment of this extraordinary family (see pp. 1073–4).

Various domains of physics have contributed importantly to progress in biology, as can be noted in many of the following sections. Relations between molecular size and structure and cell function are being profitably pursued; nuclear fission has begun to be constructively applied to physiological problems and to therapeutics. Technical advances have considerably improved the magnifying and resolving powers of the microscope, with the development of the dark-field microscope and ultraviolet-ray photography.

A new and as yet mostly unexplored field of knowledge of the form of the very small has been opened up by the development of the *electron microscope*, first by the mathematician and physicist H. BUSCH (*ca.* 1926) and his German compatriots, and later in practical electrostatic and magnetic types in this country. These powerful tools can produce useful electron micrographs at magnifications up to 40,000 to 60,000 diameters (enlargeable by photograph to more than 100,000), whereas photographs (with the light microscope), on account of the limitations of the wave length of light, stop at about 1,800 magnification (a photograph using ultraviolet rays reaches about twice this figure). The significant item, however, is not the magnification but the limit of resolution, as secondary magnification, though theoretically limitless, like the enlargement of a snapshot, provides no further detail. With the present electron microscopes, the limit of resolution is about 3 to 10 milli-micra (each a millionth of a millimetre), as compared to the .1 micron (a ten-thousandth of a millimetre) of the light microscope. In the biological field it has already become possible to electrongraph the hitherto invisible filter-passing viruses, whose size had previously only been calculated by indirect means. Formerly unseen details in bacteria, which up to now have been the smallest visible particles, have now been brought to light. Thus, our illustration shows the vaccinia bodies that protect against smallpox: a bacteriophage (the kind of virus that preys on bacteria); and antibody films, which are so important in protecting against harmful bacteria. Antibodies hitherto had been known only by their actions, and in a very crude way by their chemical composition. A few viruses had been detected, especially by PFEIFER (South Africa) using the dark field in strong direct sunlight, but no

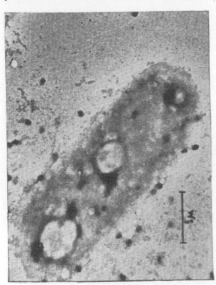 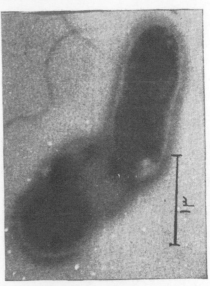

Electrongraphs of bacteria (reduced from original magnification of about 30,000). The scales indicate the length of one micron (one thousandth of a millimeter). Bacteriophage and antibody, though studied for years, had never been seen until the advent of the electron microscope.

447. *"Ghost" of a colon bacillus partially dissolved by bacteriophage — the small, round, dark particles in and on the edge of the bacillus.* (*S. E. Luria et al, Fig. 15, J. Bact., 46, 75, 1943.*)

448. *A typhoid bacillus with its margins and whiplike flagellae coated with antibody, i.e., protein from the specific antiserum.* (*S. Mudd and T. F. Anderson, Fig. 48, J. Am. Med. Ass'n., 126, 570, 1944.*)

details of form or structure could be observed. With sufficiently thin tissue sections, the instrument should also reveal unknown details of normal and pathologic histology. Already this need has stimulated invention of a new type of microtome capable of cutting sections down to .15 micra in thickness. On a different line of study, motion pictures have been used in the continuous observation and recording of physiological and pathological action and the fixation of characteristic moments, in both clinical and laboratory investigations. Pharmacology also has been greatly stimulated by chemical progress, which has led to the discovery of many useful drugs.

R. G. Harrison's demonstrations (1907), that bits of living animal tissue could grow under suitable conditions *in vitro* opened up a new field in the study of EXPERIMENTAL CYTOLOGY. This subject has been profitably developed by many investigators, so that now an excellent journal is devoted entirely to this specialty. Much valuable information has been obtained about the principles of cell growth, such as their nutritional requirements, potential immortality of successive generations, growth stimulants such as Carrel's trephones, the need of certain types for a framework to grow on, persisting differences of cancer strains from their normal prototypes (W. Lewis), origins and transformations of various types, the nature of included granules, and so on. By long series of successive microphotographs, with projection speeded up to simulate motion pictures, WARREN and MARGARET LEWIS have produced direct visual evidence of cell activities — such as the types of motion of different cells, and details of cell division and the cell in-gestion of solids (phagocytosis) and liquids (pinocytosis). This method has already been of value in the differential diagnosis of obscure tumours or as a dynamic aid to the traditional stained (dead') sections. Today it is pos-sible with a very precise micro-dissector (R. CHAMBERS, T. PETERFI) to produce minute non-fatal lesions in single cells growing in tissue culture and to study the structural results and the reactions of the damaged cell to various physical and chemical stimuli.

Another important chapter of cytology is the *genetic study of chromo-somes*. On such foundations as the individuality hypothesis (1888) of The-odor BOVERI (1862–1915), Professor of Zoology at Würzburg, extensive studies have been made by E. B. WILSON, H. S. JENNINGS, E. G. CONKLIN, and T. H. MORGAN in America, Richard GOLDSCHMIDT in Germany, Cesare ARTOM in Italy, and many others. The gene, or unit character, was recog-nized about 1902 as the element in the chromosome essential for heredity by the Dane W. L. JOHANNSEN (1857–1927); it has actually been photographed in recent years.

We now touch on a few high spots in EXPERIMENTAL EMBRYOLOGY, an important discipline that has developed for the most part during the present century. In the nineteenth century the opportunities in the field of descrip-tive embryology were so great that few investigators were led to approach the problems of development experimentally. The interest in Darwin's the-ory provided a powerful impetus to the study of comparative anatomy, and Haeckel's law of biogenesis (that ontogeny recapitulates phylogeny) in-duced many ardent supporters to search for evidence in the structural devel-opment of the embryo. Yet the mechanics of these changes in form remained unknown.

Wilhelm ROUX (1850–1924) was the first to recognize the importance of this field of investigation, to define its subject matter, and to outline methods of study. He began this work in 1880, aiming to explain phylogeny through study of ontogenic development, and trying by experimental interference to find how early organs and tissues become predestined to assume their prospective form and function. In 1895 he founded the well-known *Archiv für Entwicklungsmechanik der Organismen*. (In English, usage has made the term " experimental embryology " synonymous with developmental mechanics.) This experimental approach supplemented the work of the teratologist E. GEOFFROY SAINT-HILAIRE (1772–1844) and C. DARESTE's classic work on abnormal development in the chick (first published 1877).

Influenced by Weismann's theory of the continuity of the germ plasm, Roux believed that mitotic cell division provided the means for the distribution of the manifold potencies included in the fertilized ovum. He found support for this hypothesis in the production (1888) of a half embryo from one of the first two blastomeres (the earliest subdivisions of the fertilized ovum) of a frog's egg, the other having been killed by pricking with a hot needle. Roux's experiment, however, appeared to be contradicted when H. Driesch discovered (1891) that each of the first two or even four blastomeres of a sea-urchin egg, when separated by shaking, can develop into a whole embryo. Similar results were obtained by C. HERBST (1900) by immersing ova in calcium-free sea water and in other species by E. B. Wilson (1893), L. ZOJA (1896), T. H. MORGAN (1866–1945), and others. In O. SCHULTZE's experiment (1894), when the fertilized frog ovum was held firmly between two glass plates to prevent rolling, then inverted, a whole embryo developed from each of the two blastomeres. A. PENNERS, of Würzburg, found (1929) that twins could be obtained, even if the ovum were not inverted, until the four- or eight-cell stage had been reached, and concluded that many areas have the capacity to initiate gastrulation (the infolding of the vegetal pole of the spherical mass of cells known as the blastula). Despite these contradictory results, Roux's theory received experimental support in the field of the invertebrates; notably from the American investigators E. B. Wilson, T. H. Morgan, and E. G. Conklin. Most invertebrate eggs appear to have a mosaic pattern in which the destiny of the blastomeres and even regions of the unfertilized ovum can be predicted.

A modification of these experiments was reported by Hans SPEMANN (1869–1941) in 1901–3: by tying a hair loop about a newt's egg and producing varying degrees of constriction, he obtained a series of malformations ranging from anterior axial bifurcation to the production of autonomous twins. Thus Spemann and Falkenberg (1919) were able to explain the frequent occurrence of complete situs inversus (i.e., the occurrence on the left side of organs normally found on the right, and vice versa) in certain monsters and identical twins.

Gastrulation had long been recognized as a significant step in the sequence of events associated with organization of the embryo. It was known that a large portion of the ectoderm (the outermost of the three primitive layers) of the blastula swept downward to the blastopore (the mouth of the primitive gut, or archenteron), where it invaginated to produce the mesoderm and roof of the archenteron. Attempts at tracing the subsequent fate of different regions of this presumptive mesoderm were at first confined to the production of an injury in a single region, until W. Vogt mapped out the fate of the different surface areas of the amphibian gastrula (1929), by staining circumscribed regions with vital dyes and tracing their subsequent migrations.

The fate of exchange transplants between blastulæ or early gastrulæ of amphibians was extensively investigated by H. Spemann, beginning about 1918, along lines developed by Ross Harrison about the turn of the century. It soon became evident that before gastrulation had begun, the fate of the parts of the amphibian embryo had not been determined; thus if a piece of blastocele roof (presumptive skin) is excised and transplanted into the area of the presumptive neural plate of another blastula, it will form neural plate, not skin. Likewise presumptive neural plate will form skin if transferred to that region. Similar results are obtained even if the transplants are between regions that later belong to different germ layers (ectoderm, mesoderm, entoderm): thus, presumptive skin transplanted to the dorsal lip of the blastopore (presumptive mesoderm) is invaginated along with the surrounding tissue and forms mesodermal somites and notochord.

After completion of gastrulation the results of exchange transplantations are quite different. At these later stages the fate of various regions has been determined. Thus a presumptive eye region, if placed in the belly wall, becomes an eye, not skin or muscle. The fate of the presumptive mesoderm in the dorsal lip of the blastopore is determined first. Warren Lewis observed that if it is transplanted to a region of presumptive epidermis it does not form skin, but sinks beneath the surface, where it may produce somites or a notochord (1907). The experiment was repeated by Spemann and Mangold (1924) with one important difference: if early gastrulæ were used as hosts, instead of Lewis's older larvæ, the fate of the transplant was similar to that observed by Lewis, but the response of the host was very different. Now the overlying ectoderm produced a neural plate, and in some instances a secondary embryo.

When the presumptive mesoderm in the dorsal lip of the blastopore invaginates to form the roof of the archenteron and comes to lie immediately beneath the presumptive ectoderm, it " induces " the formation of a neural plate. It has therefore been called the " primary organizer " of the amphibian embryo. The nature of the substance that acts as the organizer was ardently studied during the decade preceding World War II. Crushing or boiling the cells had no deleterious effect upon their inducing activity. In fact, Spemann, Bautzmann, J. Holtfreter, Waddington, and Mangold observed that, after boiling, parts of the egg that formerly possessed no capacity for induction had now acquired it.

The absence of species specificity in the organizer (Geinitz, 1925) was confirmed by Holtfreter's discovery (1933) that adult tissues will induce the formation of secondary embryos if implanted into the amphibian blastocele. It is now thought that even some plant tissues have a similar effect. Neural inductions have been obtained by the injection of cell-free filtrates as well as by numerous synthetic organic compounds (Needham and Waddington). Needham has concluded that the natural evocator is a steroid (1942).

Several secondary and tertiary organizers have been identified, as, for instance, in the eye, where the effect of organizer activity has been most completely studied. The primary organizer induces the formation of a neural plate which has long been known to become the central nervous system; it is also known that the optic vesicles develop as lateral evaginations of the forebrain and subsequently invaginate and are known as the optic cups. In 1901 Spemann excised the presumptive eye-cup in a frog larva with the result that no lens was formed in the ectoderm; yet when Warren Lewis (1905) displaced the eye-cup so that it lay beneath a portion of the ectoderm that normally became skin, a lens was formed. Here, then, the optic cup was the secondary organizer of the lens. A tertiary organizer is found in the lens and is responsible for the induction of changes in the overlying ectoderm leading to the formation of the transplanted cornea. Needless to say, the field is still being cultivated.

From the above story it appears to be no exaggeration to say that never before have scientists of all countries and specialties combined in such a united, lasting, and well-organized effort as in this century to aid in the solution of biological problems.

3. Anatomy

Just as the major task of gross anatomical study had been largely completed early in the nineteenth century, so by the end of the century the major histological discoveries by routine methods had been achieved. As always, however, new methods led to further valuable discoveries. Especially by the use of new stains, the microscopic anatomy of the nervous system was further explored by Cajal and the Spanish school. More efficient microtomes permitted the preparation of thinner, more even sections, approaching a single cell's thickness, thus greatly clarifying the cytological picture. Very recently (1943), in response to the need for even thinner sections for electron microscopy, H. C. O'BRIEN and G. M. McKINLEY have developed a " cyclone knife " microtome, where a rapidly revolving knife cuts and flings off sections, as thin as 0.1 micron. Micro sections of whole organs, capable of being studied under the high powers of the microscope, revealed unsuspecting topographical details, both in normal and pathological structure. One has only to examine E. CHRISTELLER's (1889–1928) *Atlas der Histopographie* (1927) to appreciate the value of this advance.

After Sir Richard Owen (see p. 670) Sir Arthur KEITH (1866–1944) was the most popular representative of his specialty in Great Britain. In ad-

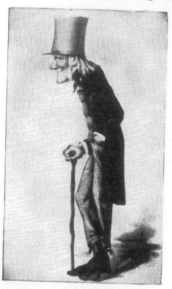

449. *Sir Richard Owen,*
a caricature.

dition to his discovery of the sino-auricular node, he illuminated the complicated mechanics of the developing mammalian heart, and various aspects of anthropology and comparative anatomy. A special muscle bundle connecting the right auricle with the ventricles of the heart, discovered in 1893 by W. His, Jr., was traced to its connection in each ventricle with the "fibres" described by Purkinje and erected (1906) by S. TAWARA (b. 1873) into a special conducting system for the cardiac impulse toward contraction. This system was completed by the discovery (1907) by Keith and Flack of a similar bundle of embryonal-like muscle lying between the superior vena cava and the right auricle, in which bundle the heart-beat normally arises.

Even in gross anatomy some progress, if less conspicuous than formerly, can be recorded. Maceration of heart muscle so unrolled the ventricular layer for J. B. MacCALLUM (1876–1906), that the dynamics of contraction could be better comprehended, and the way was opened toward the solution of such problems as the nature of the various cardiac arrhythmias and the form and distribution of myocardial infarcts. Further study of the anatomy of the living was made possible by motion pictures and the X-ray, and regional anatomy was better disclosed by accurate mechanical sectioning of frozen or formalin-fixed cadavers. The ancient method of arterial injection has been used to illuminate, by the use of different colours, the distribution of the coronary circulation in health and disease — a matter of considerable present clinical interest and importance.

An interesting generalization resulting from the combined use of the newer approaches of investigation is the theory of neurobiotaxis (1929) proposed by the distinguished Dutch investigator Ariens KAPPERS (b. 1877). According to this concept, the biological demands of the growing body may pull nerve cells or cell groups to a locality distant from their site of origin.

Special functions have been suggested by finer differences in structure, such as the alpha and beta cells of the islands of Langerhans in the pancreas, their individuality brought out by the use of special stains by R. R. BENSLEY (b. 1867). The carotid body (known since 1743) and aortic body are small structures lying in the bifurcation of the carotid arteries and touching the innominate artery and the arch of the aorta (A. BIEDL, 1902). Their function long remained unknown, but they have now been shown to be important sense organs regulating arterial blood supply through their sensitivity to chemical changes, producing the opposite effect of that of nerve endings in the vessel walls, which react to pressor stimuli (F. DE CASTRO, 1928; C. HEYMANS, 1930; and C. SCHMIDT and J. COMROE, 1939). Similarly in the kidneys the juxta-glomerular apparatus described by N. GOORMAGHTIGH in 1932 appears to control, in some species at least, the amount of blood flowing to the kidney glomerulus. Cells in the intestinal wall with chrome-salt affinities and in intimate connection with nerve fibrils were demonstrated (1897, 1906) by W. KULTCZYCKI and A. CIACCIO (1906). Such cells, by the use of silver impregnation studies, have been considerably explored by Masson. Further understanding of the finer anatomy of the brain followed the introduction of special stains — at first by Golgi, later by Ramón y Cajal (gold sublimate, 1913) and his pupil Pio DEL RIO HORTEGA (silver carbonate, 1919) — which disclose the intimate details of the apparently structureless mass of the interstitial tissue. Instead of a dual system of the large astrocytes and a separate syncytium of supporting interlacing fibres, these investigators showed that there were three types of cells, each with ramifying dendrites connected with the cell body: the astrocytes (macroglia, spider cell), the oligodendroglia, numerous but apparently unimportant smaller cells with, as the name implies, fewer shorter processes, and the microglia, which have, surprisingly, been shown by the Spaniards to be of mesodermal origin — angular cells with many short branches.

Circulation of blood in the SPLEEN — Galen's many-functioning organ of mystery — has had a tortuous history in modern times. The peculiar arteriolar sheaths were described (1861) by Franz SCHWEIGGER-SEIDEL (1834–71), but not recognized as sphincters till much later. The blood was thought by Billroth, Kölliker, and others to pass from artery to vein by a " closed " circulation (i.e., always inside of continuous lined channels); whereas W. MUELLER (1865) conceived of an " open " circulation whereby the arterial capillaries poured blood into the splenic pulp, which it returned to the venous sinuses, whose walls were permeable like those of barrels with some of the staves removed (MOLLIER). M. H. KNISELY (b. 1904), after studying living transilluminated mammalian spleens (1936), concluded that in normal spleens there was no interruption in the continuity of the blood channels, but that the vessels are so delicate that agonal changes could easily convert the picture into that called " open."

The PITUITARY GLAND, located in the centre, best-protected part of the brain, was well described by Vesalius, though it was long thought to secrete the mucus of respiratory catarrh until the idea was refuted by Schneider and Lower in the seventeenth century. It has been known for some time to be composed of separate parts that have different embryological origins. Microscopically, the anterior lobe cells have been known for some years to be of three types: the chief or chromophobe, the eosinophil, and the basophil. Their significance is considered in the sections on pathology and physiology. According to Rasmussen, the chromophobes constitute about 52 per cent of the population, the acidophils 37 per cent, the basophils 11 per cent.

The cartilaginous INTERVERTEBRAL DISKS have been intensively studied in the past two decades, starting with C. G. SCHMORL's (1861–1932) observations (1925) that they are frequently the site of lesions. These may be in either the central *nucleus pulposus* or the marginal cartilage, and they may herniate into the body of the vertebra or into the spinal canal, with hemorrhage. Thus they have been found to be a frequent cause of backache, fortunately of a kind that can usually be relieved by surgical means.

With the shift of investigative value in recent years away from normal gross and microscopic anatomy, much of the research interest of professional anatomists has turned to related biological fields such as experimental cytology and embryology, comparative anatomy and anthropology. Yet strong departments of anatomy are necessarily maintained in the good medical schools, and much of the student's time is required for the subject in his first year.

In the ANTHROPOLOGICAL field, in the same Trinil formations in Java in which Dubois found *Pithecanthropus* almost a century ago, R. von KOENIGSWALD has found two more skulls of the same type (1937, 1938) and in 1939 an upper jaw with human-like teeth and a brain case, both more massive than any known human remains. These, with a huge mandible found by him in 1941, led him to create the class *Meganthropus palæojavanicus*.

Extinct human giants in China also are suggested by the huge molars of *Gigantopithecus blacki* (now regarded as human by Weidenreich and renamed *Gigantanthropus*) as well as by the earlier discovered *Homo rhodesiensis* and the Heidelberg jaw. Is this, then, support for the conjecture that some of the myths of early times may be explained as the dim memories of vanished species, like the Komodo dragons; or, in the case of mythological monsters, as the analogies suggested by actual pathological specimens?

Durable special SOCIETIES appeared during the eighties (Anatomische Gesellschaft, 1886; Anatomical Society of Great Britain and Ireland, 1887; Society of American Anatomists, 1888; the French Société Anatomique de Paris, 1826, which lapsed in 1914 but was started again in 1924). Though combination journals, such as the *Journal of Anatomy and Physiology* (founded 1866), the *Journal de l'anatomie et de la physiologie*, etc. (1864), and *Archiv für Anatomie und Physiologie* (1877), were of earlier origin, strictly anatomical journals are, with some exceptions (*Anatomischer Anzeiger*, 1886) of twentieth-century origin: *American Journal of Anatomy*, 1901; *Anatomical Record*, 1906; *Archivio italiano di Anatomia*, 1902; *Zeitschrift für angewandte Konstitutionslehre*, 1913–21; *Russkyi Archiv Anatomii*, the 1920's; *Archive d'anatomie humaine et d'embryologie*, 1922; *Folia anatomica Japonica*, 1922.

4. Physiology

In none of the special fields included in this narrative has activity been greater in recent times than in physiology. The publication of literally thousands of articles annually has produced the inevitable breaking up of the subject into several subordinate fields, both for the individual investigator and for society meetings. Here especially have the review journals, such as *Physiological Reviews*, been of great help. With increased knowledge of the workings of the mammalian body has come the further development of the study of general physiological processes (that is, those common to living organisms in general), like Claude Bernard's *Physiologie générale*. This took form in the original outlook expressed by W. M. BAYLISS (1860–1924) in his *Principles of General Physiology;* in R. HÖBER's *Physical Chemistry of Cells and Tissues* (1945); and in the *Journal of General Physiology*. Surface action, the colloidal state, permeability, osmotic pressure, secretion, contraction, neural activities, electrical changes, together with many of the processes considered in the section on biochemistry, are the elements comprising this field. L. J. HENDERSON's (1878–1942) analysis of the physicochemical changes in the blood, J. Loeb's studies of electrolyte balance in

tissue fluids, R. Höber's (b. 1873) elucidation of the general principles of
cell permeability, M. H. Jacobs's (b. 1884) quantitative studies of this phenomenon, and the Swiss W. R. Hess's work on blood viscosity and its relation to circulatory changes come to mind in this connection.

The transplantation of blood vessels and whole organs with preservation of
function was vainly attempted from early times. Though the success achieved
by Alexis Carrel brought him the Nobel Prize in 1912, the method did not prove
of practical use except in the case of some endocrine glands after Halsted's
" physiological deficit " had been established. Very recently (1944) N. P. Sinit-
sin, of the Gorky Medical Institute, is said to have shown that the whole heart
can be transplanted in frogs with survival for as long as 130 days in normal
condition with normal electrocardiograms. V. A. Negovsky and other Russian
physiologists so constructively explored (1937–43) the act of dying that
wounded men and experimental animals have been brought back to life as much
as six to twenty minutes after clinical death has been officially recorded. With
the help of the Hooker-Drinker aerator (or the Gibbon apparatus devised in
1939), the introduction of blood saturated with oxygen has been an important
adjunct. The critical point apparently is reached when the tissues of one of the
vital organs have actually degenerated as the result of anoxia to such an extent
that their revival is no longer possible.

Of all the divisions of physiology none has been more steadily and consistently pursued than that of the organs of the CIRCULATION. The cause,
nature, and control of the heart-beat, the nature of heart muscle, the cardiac
output and its regulation, and the velocity and pressure of the blood flow in
arteries, capillaries, and veins have been explored by continually more accurate methods in such successful volume that the knowledge of even a generation ago has usually become obsolete, and even the important steps of
this progress are impossible to record adequately.

The " isolated heart " was elaborated into better and more durable material
for study in the heart-lung preparation of E. H. Starling and his associates,
which produced Starling's " Law of the Heart " (1918): a greater force of contraction follows greater filling, all nervous connections of course being severed;
with failure developing if the optimum filling is exceeded (see the 1918 Linacre
Lecture). Starling also developed useful theories of fluid balance in capillaries
dependent on colloid osmotic pressure and related this to tissue fluid and lymph-
formation. This work culminated in E. M. Landis's (b. 1901) quantitative studies on capillary exchange (1934) and those (1933) of C. K. Drinker (b. 1887)
and P. D. McMaster (b. 1891) on lymph. A. Krogh's (b. 1874) studies (1922
and earlier) of capillary capacity and intermittency of blood flow, and of the
control mechanism of the circulation, have been expanded by the work of J. T.

WEARN (b. 1893) and A. N. RICHARDS (b. 1876) on the kidney and also were the basis for the work of Landis. Krogh also elucidated the regulation of venous return and, with J. LINDHARD (b. 1870), developed (1912) the Fick principle for the measurement of cardiac output by respiratory exchange, using foreign gases such as N_2O. From this has arisen the modern development of methods for clinical estimation of blood flow. The experimental study of blood flow has been much advanced beyond Ludwig's historic *Stromuhr* by the development (1928) of the *Thermostromuhr* by H. REIN (b. 1898).

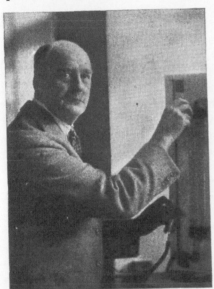 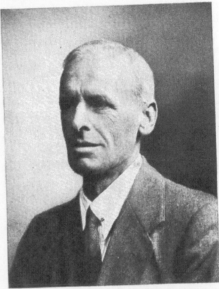

450. *Joseph Barcroft.*   451. *Ernest H. Starling.*

The nervous control of the circulation was clarified by the demonstration of its axone reflexes and of the importance of vasomotor functions of sensory nerves by A. Ninian BRUCE and William M. Bayliss. The use (1890) by L. FREDERICQ (1851–1935) of crossed-circulation experiments for demonstrating chemical effects was developed (1928) by C. HEYMANS (b. 1892) for the analysis of the circulation demonstrating the controls exerted by the carotid sinus (*Le Sinus carotidien*, 1933). This field has been further developed by D. W. BRONK (b. 1897) through the application of Adrian's methods of nerve-impulse registration.

The reservoir function of the spleen, whereby stores of red blood cells can be rapidly added to the circulation on demand, was definitely established (1923–5) by J. BARCROFT and his associates at Cambridge, England. The " circus movement " of the excitatory wave of muscle contraction was first observed (1906) by Mayer in the bell of the jellyfish. It was demonstrated in heart muscle in 1913, independently by G. R. MINES (*ca.* 1885–1914) and W. E. GARREY (b. 1873), and soon after was established as the basis of the clinical arrhythmias, auricular flutter, and auricular fibrillation, by Thomas Lewis and others.

Knowledge of the variations of blood pressure in both man and animals in health and disease has been promoted by numerous and various precision methods and instruments. S. RIVA ROCCI's indirect method (1896) (amount of external air pressure required to obstruct arterial flow) was quickly developed by von Recklinghausen, J. ERLANGER (b. 1874) D. HOOKER (b. 1876), and (oscillatory) M. V. PACHON (b. 1867), (auscultatory) KOROTKOW (b. 1874), and others, with return for investigative purposes to Stephen Hales's earliest of methods (1733) – direct communication of the manometer with the arterial blood flow. Puncture of the human artery for blood samples, a procedure now in common use, was introduced (1919) by W. C. STADIE (b. 1886) in a study of cyanosis developing in pneumonia, though puncture of the radial artery had already been shown (1912) by J. HURTER (b. 1878) to be a safe procedure. Venous pressure, measured indirectly by J. E. EYSTER (b. 1881), with the increased frequency of venepuncture, is now also measured in this direct manner. Capillary pressure has been likewise measured both indirectly (pressure required to blanch skin made semitransparent with an oil, as in the loops at the root of the nail) and directly by Landis (see *Physiological Reviews*, 1934) by insertion into a capillary of a fine-pointed pipette. One of the remote parts of the human body most recently to come into the field of direct quantitative observation is the right side of the heart. Analysis of the blood of the right auricle was first performed (1924) by W. FORSSMANN (b. 1904) on himself, by insertion of a long catheter into an elbow vein. It has recently (1941, 1944) been developed by A. COURNAND (b. 1895) to permit graphic registration of blood-pressure fluctuations as well as analysis of blood samples taken over considerable intervals under varying conditions. Thus he has found that auricular pressure ranges normally from o to 22 mm. of mercury and that in *cor pulmonale* it may rise as high as 80 mm.

Present concepts of the physiology of the ALIMENTARY TRACT were largely initiated by Pavlov's improvement on his master Heidenhain's pouch of the stomach. This produced a noteworthy planned experimental advance in gastric physiology similar to Beaumont's studies resulting from Alexis St. Martin's accident. W. B. CANNON's (1871–1945) early X-ray studies (1898) on the relation of gastric movements to hunger (1912), on the mechanical factors of digestion (1911), and on the relation of acidity of gastric contents to pyloric control (1907) illustrate the new progress; also those (1916) of A. J. CARLSON (b. 1875), such as the "Mr. V." studies, and of Boris BABKIN (b. 1877) on the origin of gastric secretion, digestion, and the movements of the alimentary tract. Hunger has been usefully analysed by such methods, Carlson showing (1917 and earlier) that the sensation was due to stomach contractions, which in protracted starvation so diminished as to account for the well-known disappearance of hunger in such a state. A. C. IVY (b. 1893) and his colleagues have added notably to this field by studies based on various modifications of gastro-intestinal pouches, also by their investigations of the hormones of the alimentary tract, and the function of the gall bladder, and by his application of the results to clinical problems. Bayliss's and Starling's " Law of the Intestine " (1899–1901) illustrated the useful ability of the gastro-intestinal tract, when stimulated by a bolus of food, to relax below the position of the bolus, while the part above contracts. Thus the vigorous contractions explain the colicky pains caused (1918, 1929) by W. C. ALVAREZ's (b. 1884) balloon when held fixed by a string in the lumen of the gut.

The long-standing conflict between Carl Ludwig's mechanical theory of KIDNEY FUNCTION and R. Heidenhain's secretory theory has been largely solved, and in the direction of Bowman's original combination concept based on anatomical differences of glomerulus and tubules. Progress toward the solution began with A. R. CUSHNY's (1866–1926) compromise hypothesis (1926) of filtration of a protein-free filtrate by the glomerulus with reabsorption of certain substances from the tubules.

Much direct evidence of the validity of this view has been furnished by the studies (1922–39) of A. N. RICHARDS (b. 1876) and his colleagues, especially with Wearn's method of procuring analysable urine by tapping a single glomerulus of the exposed amphibian kidney. By using urine collected from identified levels of the tubule and tubular perfusion fluid, it was found that reabsorption of glucose, for instance, occurred in the proximal tubule, and reabsorption of water in the proximal part of the distal tubule, and that increased concentration of phosphates in the urine was due, not to secretion, but to reabsorption of water. The possibility still remains, however, that some substances may be secreted by tubules in some species (E. K. MARSHALL [b. 1889] et al., 1924; H. L. SHEEHAN, 1936). Glomerular filtration rate in man was first measured (1926) by P. B. REHBERG. The limitations of this method have been controlled by the use of the plasma-clearance method, especially since inulin was shown by Richards and, independently, by Homer SMITH, using diodrast, to have the same clearance as the glomerular filtration rate. The " plasma clearance " concept (i.e., the amount of plasma cleared of a substance, such as urea, in a given period of time) was developed by Van Slyke in 1928, from the studies measuring renal function by comparison of the amount of urea in the plasma and the urine. First attempted by N. GRÉHANT (1838–1910) in 1904, this comparison developed into L. AMBARD's (b. 1876) well-known " coefficient " (1910) and F. C. McLEAN's (b. 1888) " index " (1916) and has since progressed to the exploration of the action of different parts of the nephron. It became possible to measure excretory power of the kidney as a whole when, in 1909, Abel and L. G. ROWNTREE (b. 1883) discovered that phenolsulphonephthalein was excreted almost entirely by the kidney (see Rowntree's and Geraghty's clinical test, 1912). The same principle was applied by Rowntree, Bloomfield, and Hurwitz to phenoltetrachlorphthalein (1913), which had been found to be excreted almost entirely by the liver. This, in the modification proposed (1925) by S. M. ROSEN-THAL (b. 1897) and Edwin C. WHITE (b. 1871), is still regarded as one of the best liver-function tests.

The history of ENDOCRINOLOGY is a matter of the past one hundred years and, with a few notable exceptions, of the present century. Its name is also young, coming from the Greek ἔνδον, within; κρίνειν, to separate. This branch of science deals with those glands that have no ducts, but pour their vitally important secretion directly into the blood stream. The principle that body functions can be regulated by chemical products of the body as well as by nervous control was proclaimed by Bayliss's and Starling's discovery (1902) that the flow of pancreatic juice was stimulated by a substance, which they named " secretin," that was manufactured by the intestinal mucosa and carried by the blood to the pancreas.

Secretin was eventually obtained in crystalline form in 1934 by G. AGREN. Though Starling's term " hormone " (ὁρμάνειν, to arouse, 1905) does not now apply strictly to all the endocrine products, it has outlived other suggested names, such as " chalone " and " autacoid," and seems destined to survive. The known organs that comprise this system are the pituitary, thyroid, parathyroid, adrenals, pancreatic islands, gonads, placenta and intestinal mucosa, and possibly also the pineal, thymus, spleen, and kidney. Comprehension of their proper function, which is in most cases necessary for health or even life itself, is complicated by their many interrelationships, especially with the pituitary, which acts as " the conductor of the endocrine orchestra," as Cushing aptly phrased it. It is still further complicated by the belief of Collip and others that, in addition, " anti-hormones " can be formed. The pituitary was thought by Paulesco (1906) and Cushing (1932) to be necessary for life; later investigators, however, have demonstrated that life can be maintained indefinitely, under proper precautions, in spite of the complex changes that follow its complete removal.

In the anterior lobe of the pituitary, the three cells normally found (chief or chromophobe, eosinophil, basophil) were first regarded (1908) as having different functions by A. GEMELLI (b. 1878), as in hibernation (Gemelli, 1906). As the chromophobe is a non-functioning, undifferentiated cell, the other two varieties, though capable of but few structural changes, are held responsible for many of its functions: regulation of growth, carbohydrate (fat) metabolism, and production of thyrotrophic, adrenotrophic, gonadotrophic, and lactogenic hormones. As to growth control, removal of the gland from animals was shown (1902) by G. VASSALE (1870–1924) and VECCHI (b. 1877) to produce a *cachexia hypophyseopriva*. The dwarfism produced by deficiency was named by Erdheim *nanosomia pituitaria*. Effects in man are considered elsewhere. The growth hormone, isolated by H. M. Evans and C. H. Li in 1944 in crystalline form, was shown by them to be potent even in doses of .01 mg. in producing rats of giant size. The thyrotrophic influence first appeared in N. ROGOWITSCH's observation (1889) of pituitary hyperplasia after thyroidectomy; and was demonstrated, the other way round, when P. E. SMITH (b. 1884) found (1922) thyroid atrophy and lowered oxygen-consumption after removal (hypophysectomy) and thyroid repair after administration of pituitary extract. A parathyrotrophic hormone has also been suggested by pathological and experimental physiological observations. Adrenotrophic influence appeared in the adrenal hyperplasia often found in acromegalics and in Cushing's basophilism (see Surgery). The rich story of the pituitary's gonadotrophic influence can be picked up with the enlargement found in pregnancy (L. Comte, 1898) and Erdheim's now neglected " pregnancy cells " in the anterior lobe (1909). In 1910 Crowe, Cushing, and Homans abolished sex function in dogs, with atrophy of the sex organs, by partial extirpation; and, in reverse, P. E. Smith and S. Aschheim and B. Zondek (in 1926) showed that anterior-lobe implants in immature rodents produced premature sexual development. This has been further broken down to a " follicle-stimulating " and a " luteinizing hormone." The lactogenic property of the anterior lobe was studied by I. OTT (1847–1916) and J. C. SCOTT (b. 1877) in 1911, and by Schafer and Mackenzie in the same year, and explored (1932) by O. RIDDLE (b. 1877) under the name " prolactin " (C. W. TURNER's [b. 1897] " galactin," 1932). It was connected (1933) with the stimulation of maternal instincts by B. P. WIESNER and N. M. SHEARD. The history of the intermediate and posterior lobes is more obscure, as the two are intimately connected topographically, and the latter is now known to be histologically and functionally connected with the hypothalamus. Posterior-lobe extracts were early shown to contain substances that raise blood pressure (Oliver and Schafer, 1894; Howell, 1898), and to contract the uterus (Dale, 1906) and other muscles. Zondek proposed that the *pars intermedia* secretes a true hormone — intermedin — which expands the melanophores (pigment areas in the skin of certain fish and amphibia). A transient diuretic effect of posterior extract was observed by R. Magnus and E. A. Schafer in 1901; however, it soon became recognized that the direct hormonal effect was antidiuretic. S. W. Ranson and others have shown (1935, 1936) that this in turn was in close functional relationship to the adjacent hypothalamus, the " pituicytes " (P. C. BUCY, 1930) that are present in both areas being thought to do the secreting.

THYROID physiological progress in the preceding half-century left less of significance to be gleaned in this period. E .C. KENDALL's (b. 1886) production in crystalline form (1915) of the active principle, which he named " thyroxine," was of prime importance for future study; also C. R. HARRINGTON's (b. 1856) construction (1926) of its structural formula, and its synthesis (1927) by Harrington and G. BARGER (b. 1878). J. F. GUDERNATSCH's (b. 1881) demonstration (1914) that thyroid substance hastens maturation and differentiation in tadpoles, at the expense of growth, has become a classic. PARATHYROID physiology was illuminated by Collip's isolation (1924) of the active principle, parathormone (see also Hanson and Berman). Its protein nature and approximate molecular weight have since been established, and its function in the mobilization of calcium and promotion of phosphorus excretion (F. ALBRIGHT) brought into line with the pathology and the clinical disorders of these minute glands. Prog-

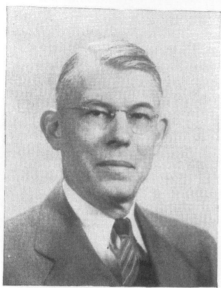

452. E. A. Doisy, Nobel Laureate, 1943.

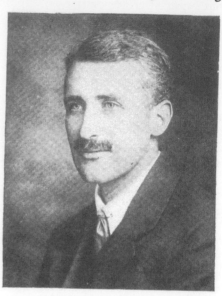

453. A. V. Hill, Nobel Laureate, 1922.

ress in knowledge of ADRENAL function, which had languished since Addison's and Brown-Séquard's classical discoveries, was resumed when J. J. ABEL (1857–1938) isolated (1898) its active principle, adrenalin (and TAKAMINE independently in 1901), and again when A. BIEDL established (1913) that it was the cortex (actually the interrenal body of the skate) that was necessary for life. By 1927 F. A. HARTMAN (b. 1883) and others had produced a cortical extract, "cortin," of some potency; and in 1930 W. W. SWINGLE (b. 1891) and J. J. PFIFFNER (b. 1903) produced an extract capable of maintaining life indefinitely after total adrenalectomy. The signal functional significance of this substance has been found, by observing the effects of, or relieving, a deficiency, to be manifold; but its normal function in the positive sense has not yet been satisfactorily explored and no one substance isolated that can be called the active principle of the cortex.

The GONADAL HORMONES have been an especially active field of exploration in recent years, much of which emphasizes that mammals, including the human, still retain some of the bisexual nature of lower organisms. The long-known female traits that develop after castration or persist in maldeveloped youths and such freaks as the bearded ladies of the side-shows began to receive their scientific explanations. Female hormones were shown to be obtainable from male sources and vice versa, and certain functioning tumours were found to produce pronounced secondary sex characteristics of the opposite sex. Ovarian endocrinology has profited by the already mentioned pituitary relationships; it also offered experimental proof of the role of the corpus-luteum secretion (progesterone) for the implantation of the ovum in the endometrium (L. FRAENKEL, 1901–10). Discovery (1923) by E. ALLEN (1892–1943) and E. A. DOISY (b. 1893) of estrogen in the follicular fluid was an event of major importance that has already had important results in medical treatment as well as in elucidating the physiology of sex life. The male hormone product of the cells of Leydig was foreshadowed by the testicular grafts in fowl of Brown-Séquard (1889), E. STEINACH (1861–1944) (1913), and A. LIPSCHÜTZ (1924). An active principle was first extracted (1927) by L. C. McGEE (b. 1904) and an active material isolated (1931) from men's urine in crystalline form by A. BUTENANDT (b. 1903), who gave it the name " androsterone." This was synthesized by L. RUŽIČKA (b. 1887) in 1934.

The physiology of the MUSCLES and muscular action has been a much discussed problem. The studies of Helmholtz, Matteucci, Du Bois-Reymond, and Marey threw light on the motor force of contraction, and on the electrical changes and the heat-production in the muscle fibre. Ludimar HERMANN (1838–1914) and Eduard PFLÜGER (1829–1910), studying muscle metabolism, confirmed Spallanzani's experiments on frog muscle, in which the muscle that no longer contained oxygen could still contract in an atmosphere of hydrogen and produce carbonic acid. To their observations were added those on heat-production (Fick), and on oxidation and reduction, which are at its basis; and W. M. Fletcher's and F. G. Hopkins's classical paper (1907) on lactic-acid formation. These investigations culminated in the quantitative studies (1919–35) of G. EMBDEN (1874–1933), A. V. HILL (b. 1886), and O. MEYERHOF (b. 1884), which established the origin of muscular force in carbohydrates, with the formation of lactic acid. This concept has been further modified by demonstration by C. LUNDSGAARD (1883–1930) of muscular contraction without the formation of lactic acid by splitting creatine-phosphoric acid, while R. MARGARIA maintains that lactic acid is formed only under conditions of anoxemic work. The Hill-Meyerhof concept is now thought to be concerned with the later phase of contraction, the early phase being due to alkalinization.

NEUROPHYSIOLOGY. In this important branch of physiology, early in this century, the British school of Cambridge became prominent with the clear-visioned and mechanically distinguished work of Keith LUCAS (1879–

1916), killed in his prime in the First World War. From this stimulus resulted the studies of E. D. ADRIAN (b. 1889) and G. R. Mines in England and of Erlanger and Gasser and others in the United States on various types of conduction in nerves and in the spinal cord.

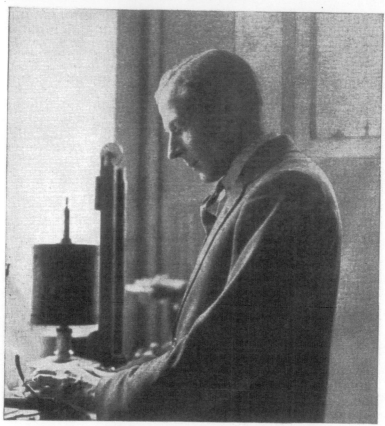

454. *E. D. Adrian, Nobel Laureate, 1932.*

Exploration of the conduction of the nerve impulse, Sherrington's " universal currency of the nervous system," was aided by Adrian's development of a method of nerve-impulse recording and the amplified cathode-ray oscillograph of J. Erlanger and H. S. GASSER (b. 1888) (see their *Electrical Signs of Nervous Activity*, 1937).

Various types of nerve fibres were analysed so constructively that these authors were able to predict by histological examination of a nerve the form of action potential that it would produce. The patterns of activity of single fibres were demonstrated by Adrian, B. H. C. MATTHEWS (b. 1906), D. W. BRONK and

K. HARTLINE (b. 1903), and others. M. L. LAPICQUE (b. 1866), and Mme. LA-
PICQUE developed (1909–25) the concept of chronaxy (the minimum time required to produce excitation of an irritable tissue) and considerably clarified the
nature of the excitatory process. The source of energy of the nerve impulse was
shown — by the work (1926) of H. DAVIS (b. 1896), A. FORBES (b. 1882), and
others on the recovery of size of the action current after passing from damaged
to normal nerve fibre — to lie in the nerve fibre itself.

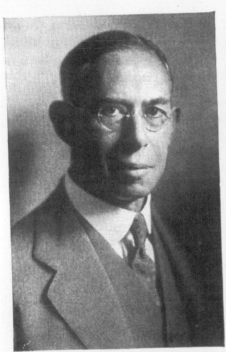

455. *Joseph Erlanger, Nobel Laureate, 1944.*

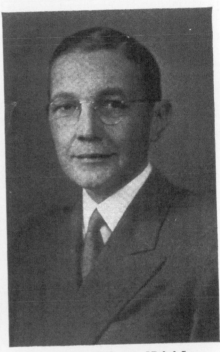

456. *Herbert S. Gasser, Nobel Laureate, 1944.* [PHOTO, BACHRACH]

Our knowledge of chemical factors in the transmission of the nerve impulse
began with the demonstration (1914) by T. R. ELLIOTT (b. 1877) of the identical effects of adrenalin and sympathin. In 1921 Otto LOEWI (b. 1873) established that when a frog's heart had been stopped by vagus stimulation, a " vagus
substance " was formed which induced similar effects in another heart. This was
shown by Sir H. H. DALE (b. 1875), with W. FELDBERG (b. 1900), to be acetyl-
cholin (see 1937 Harvey Lecture); he also showed (1936) that in a similar way
stimulation of cardio-accelerators produced adrenalin and suggested that " cho-
linergic " nerves were mostly parasympathetic, and "adrenergic " mostly sympathetic. The chemical concept has been further developed (1924–37) by W. B.
Cannon and A. S. ROSENBLUETH (b. 1900). Thus may be explained the phenom-

enon of the transmission of excitation from nerve to organ, and that of inhibition of activity by nerve stimulation.

Among the important advances in this field was the foundation of modern concepts of reflex action started by C. S. Sherrington and his school, notably J. C. ECCLES (1903) and D. E. DENNY-BROWN (b. 1901). Sherrington's analysis (1892 et seq.) of the rigidity of " decerebrate " animals and of the reciprocal in-nervation of antagonistic muscles (on excitation of one, the other is simultane-ously inhibited) culminated in his *Integrative Action of the Nervous System* (1906), setting forth the functioning of the nervous system as a unit. Postural reflexes have been elucidated by R. MAGNUS (1873–1927), in *Körperstellung* (1924), and by his pupil A. P. KLEIJN (b. 1883), J. G. DUSSER DE BARENNE (1885–1940) (1934), and G. G. RADEMAKER (b. 1871) in *Das Stehen* (1934).

The world-famous work of I. Pavlov on " conditioned reflexes " (i.e., reflexes brought into existence as a result of experience) and his experimental methods for their analysis are noted elsewhere in this work. It is perhaps less well known that such reflexes can inhibit as well as stimulate action — an important aspect for various functional diseases. His work on nervous irritability — experimen-tally producible in dogs when taxed with problems beyond their capacity — is also of practical significance, perhaps even in medical education!

The concept of " referred pain " (i.e., pain arising internally, but referred to some remote region on the surface) was established (1920 et seq.) in the studies of Henry HEAD (1861–1940) and his colleagues. This field has recently been further explored, and on a more fundamental basis, by Max FREY (1852–1932) of Würzburg.

Localization of sensory areas in the brain has undergone considerable re-vision during this period, due to the studies of Henry Head and Gordon M. HOLMES (b. 1876) on cortical lesions and on the thalamic syndrome, and to expansions and modifications (1916–31) by J. G. Dusser de Barenne and (1931–6) by Otfrid FOERSTER (1873–1941), P. BARD (b. 1898), W. H. MARSHALL (b. 1907), and C. N. WOOLSEY b. 1904). The mechanisms of the motor areas and their localization in the cerebral cortex and the interaction of various areas have been more fully explored by many investigators, including those just men-tioned and by N. A. BUBNOFF (1851–84) and R. P. H. HEIDENHAIN (1834–97), Sherrington and A. S. F. LEYTON (1869–1921), W. S. McCULLOCH (b. 1898), M. HINES (b. 1898), and S. S. TOWER (b. 1901).

What is commonly known as the sympathetic nervous system (i.e., the " ef-fector " neurons that connect the central nervous system with the viscera) was originally (1723, Winslow) so called because it was thought to deal with the " sympathies " of the body. It was named (1916), for obvious reasons, the involuntary nervous system by W. H. Gaskell and was shown by him to emerge from the spinal cord in three distinct groups: cranial, thoraco-lumbar, and sacral. J. N. LANGLEY (1852–1925), who added much to the knowledge of this system, renamed it the autonomic nervous system, placing, because of their functional relationships, the thoraco-lumbar group under the ancient name, sympathetic, and the cranial and sacral groups in a new category — parasympathetic. Although Langley was himself aware that " autonomic " carried an inaccurate implication of independence, it is of interest semantically that he thought it " more important that new words should be used for new ideas than that the words should be accurately descriptive." Conspicuous in the contributions to this important system is W. B. Cannon's demonstration of such activities as the emergency function of the adrenal in promoting bodily efficiency for meeting vital threats (1929) or maintaining " equilibria," Cannon's " homeostasis " (1932). Helpful knowledge has also emerged from the studies on central autonomic mechanisms by J. G. KARPLUS (1866–1933) and A. KREIDL (1864–1928) and by S. W. RANSOM (b. 1880) and others on the hypothalamus (1917–37), by C. M. BROOKS (b. 1905) on the brain stem (1931–3), and by J. F. FULTON (b. 1899) and his associates on cortical relationships.

A new field of electrophysiology — *electroencephalography* — has been opened up recently with the discovery by H. BERGER that characteristic action currents of brain activity càn be registered graphically (1929). Like electrocardiograms, these show constant significant differences for each individual — awake or asleep, calm or excited (H. Davis), and progress has already been made in linking various patterns with certain nervous diseases. In epileptic seizures, for instance, dramatic changes may occur in the alpha waves before clinical signs appear, and H. H. JASPER (b. 1906) has shown (1937) in some cases the location in the cortex where the attack originated.

With the turn of the century there began a new urge toward vitalism with Driesch's revivification of the Aristotelian *entelechies* and BERGSON's *élan vital*. In spite of the steadily increasing number of physicochemical explanations of vital phenomena, the discussions between materialists and vitalists became increasingly sharp before the First World War, while after that war the political and social upheavals and general intellectual confusion in many quarters very naturally promoted an urge toward philosophic speculation and the replacement of logical reasoning based on sound experiment by a metaphysical revival of earlier lines of thought. Fortunately, the majority of vitalists, however, like J. S. Haldane, have continued to seek all possible scientific explanations for vital phenomena, without expecting to solve the whole problem of life.

In FRANCE, C. RICHET (1850–1935) is best known for his introduction of " anaphylaxis " and his studies of the regulation of animal heat; M. and Mme. Lapicque for the doctrine of " chronaxy." Eugène GLEY (1857–1930) is known for his demonstration of the existence of iodine in the blood and thyroid gland

and for other contributions to the knowledge of internal secretions. In the field of biologic physics, J. A. D'ARSONVAL studied calorimetry and explored the effect of high-frequency currents.

Among AUSTRIAN physiologists may be mentioned A. KREIDL (1864–1928) (studies on the central nervous system), W. PAULI (b. 1869) (biologic physico-chemistry), E. STEINACH (1861–1943) (sexual rejuvenation), and A. BIEDL, professor at the German University in Prague (functions of the ductless glands).

In the NETHERLANDS, G. A. VAN RIJNBERK (b. 1875) studied cerebral locali-

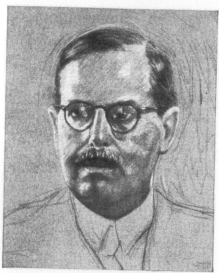

457. B. A. Houssay.

zation and the function of the cerebellum; BOCK (1866–1930) was a worthy embryologist, morphologist, and biologist; and DE BOER investigated the general physiology of muscles.

Among GERMAN physiologists, in addition to those already mentioned, important work was done by BIEDERMANN (Jena) in electrophysiology; by Embden (Frankfurt) on fat and carbohydrate metabolism, and the origin of lactic acid; by Otto Meyerhof of Berlin on muscle metabolism and lactic-acid preservation; by HÜRTHLE on the physiology of the circulation and muscle contraction.

American physiologists and biochemists have been constructively active. In addition to the studies on vitamins and endocrine and tissue cultures, already mentioned, we note the earlier work of H. P. BOWDITCH (1840–1911), the dean of American physiologists, who was a pupil of Ludwig's, under whom he described the " all or none " law of the heart muscle, and the staircase (*Treppe*) phenomenon. At Harvard he established the first teaching laboratory of physiology in America (1871). S. WEIR MITCHELL (1829–1914), though more widely known as a neurologist, poet, and novelist, also made important contributions to American physiology by stimulating activity in this field as well as through his own contributions. After studying with Claude Bernard, he investigated the action of various poisons with Hammond (1859), especially snake venoms (with E. T. Reichert), work which was later continued under his influence by Flexner and Noguchi (1909). W. H. HOWELL (1860–1945), of Baltimore, is known for his work on the effect of salts, venous pressure changes, etc., on cardiac action; his long-continued study of blood coagulation (antithrombin and thromboplastin); and his studies of various blood cells and fluids. A. J. Carlson's studies and W. B. Cannon's method of observing gastric and intestinal motility by Roentgen-ray photographs and his experiments on the effect of the emotions on animal behaviour, together with his concept of homeostasis, have already been mentioned.

In Belgium prominent physiologists were L. FREDERICQ of Liége (physiology of the circulation), J. DEMOOR (b. 1867), of Brussels (sialogogic effect of stimulating the *chorda tympani*), E. V. ZUNZ, of Brussels (physiology of the tissues), and C. HEYMANS (b. 1892) (physiology of the carotid sinus).

Swiss physiologists include L. ASHER (b. 1865), of Bern (glandular physiology), A. F. BATTELLI, of Geneva (tissue respiration), E. CRISTIANI, of Geneva (function of thyroid), and the previously mentioned W. R. Hess of Zurich.

Finally there should be mentioned the work of Sir Jagadis CHANDRA BOSE (1858–1937), of Calcutta, on the electrophysiology of plants; of B. A. HOUSSAY, of Buenos Aires (b. 1887), on hypophysial hormones; and of G. VIALE (1889–1934), of Rosario and Genoa, on the function of the adrenal glands.

5. Biochemistry

In this first half of the twentieth century biochemistry has come of age. As is natural in a developing science, there has been a tremendous increase in the number of active biochemists and the new information that they have elicited and published. With due regard for events so close at hand and for such important advances as those in the fields of the hormones and vitamins, the dominant trend of this period in biochemistry can properly be epitomized by the phrase " the Age of Proteins and Enzymes " — a direction foreshadowed by E. Fischer's work on peptides and E. Buchner's discovery of cell-free enzymes. There are numerous reasons for assigning such a prominent position to proteins: they are essential architectural components of protoplasm; their roles as enzymes (biocatalysts), hormones, immune bodies, and viruses; their activity in the transport of oxygen and carbon dioxide (the hemoglobins); and their participation in osmotic regulation and blood-clotting (the plasma proteins). Their very complexity of structure, their species specificity, and their relative instability have served as a challenge, which, in this mechanical age, was met by the invention of new physical devices for the separation of proteins and for the study of their large molecules and their behaviour in solution. To this interest, for instance, we owe the ultracentrifuge and apparatus to study electrophoresis. The intimate molecular structure of proteins has been brought to view by means of spectroscopic, magnetic susceptibility (LINUS PAULING and colleagues), and X-ray diffraction measurements. The application of stable and radioactive (" tagged " compounds) isotopes has disclosed hitherto unappreciated or unestablished details in intermediary metabolism and has revealed the fact that the *proteins in the body are not static but dynamic molecules, constantly undergoing change*. This remarkable discovery is one of the bases for the revolution in metabolic thought. The "balance-sheet" concept (that protein foods merely replace the rather small "wear and tear," the excess being eliminated largely as the end product, urea) had dominated the viewpoint for some eighty years. For example, in nitrogen equilibrium normally but little nitrogen was required for replacement of body protein, the nitrogen in the urine representing the nitrogen of the diet. The increase in nitrogen elimination following an increase in protein intake was the type of phenomenon that led to Otto Folin's concept (1905–6) of "exogenous metabolism" as opposed to "endogenous," the latter characterized by the constant excretion of creatinine. Useful and plausible in their day, these ideas were on the whole misconceptions, which have given way to the concept of *The Dynamic State of Body Constituents* (1942), an important monograph by Rudolf SCHOENHEIMER (1898–1941), one of the pioneers of the newer biochemistry. The modern viewpoint visualizes a kind of metabolic reservoir, the maintenance of its level being an expression, not of stagnation, but of "steady states" in numerous equilibria, most of which are under the control of biocatalysts, themselves specific proteins susceptible to change. Thus is explained the hitherto mysterious ready production of specialized proteins, structural as well as hormonal and enzymic; and, more significantly from the philosophic aspect, they appear to be the crystallization of a general principle, dynamic equilibria thus ensuring the "fixity" of Claude Bernard's "internal environment" in a way he could not have foreseen. Constant, controlled change, not fixity, is the body's secret of gaining the needed degree of freedom from its external environment. With expanding facts and broadening horizons there has also come a shift from the century-old insistence on the "need of oxygen for life" to the "need of energy." It has been made clear that in obedience to thermodynamic laws the needs of cell work are met by parcelling out from suitable stores free, useful energy, not heat. Useful work is obtained from many reversible steps (cf. the Gibbs-Helmholtz theorem) in which metabolites and biocatalysts participate, which are interposed in an essentially irreversible process, such as the breakdown of carbohydrates to carbon dioxide and water. Oxygen has more uses in the body than the direct oxidation of carbon. The unravelling of the mechanisms of protein and carbohydrate breakdown, and of reversible oxidation — reduction systems in this process of energy storage and utilization — form perhaps the most important chapter in this period of biochemistry.

The marring of this very fruitful period by two world wars has had at least one result: Germany has lost, perhaps permanently, her pre-eminence in biochemistry. This is due not alone to losses caused by the two wars, but also to the natural growth of the science in other countries, and to the forced emigration of hundreds of outstanding German investigators. Such biochemists as OTTO MEYERHOF, H. A. KREBS, Carl NEUBERG, Otto LOEWI, R. SCHOENHEIMER, and F. LIPMANN have found a haven in England or the United States. It is interesting that in the midst of the war J. K. PARNAS, of Poland, not only was given a laboratory by the Russians, but has been highly honoured by them. G. EMBDEN, on the other hand, died in Frankfurt under most unhappy circumstances; while the eminent Otto WARBURG was permitted to stay on at Berlin-Dahlem. In World War I, unfortunately, ample demonstrations in humans were available of the effect of food deficiencies — particularly the rarer and costlier animal fats and proteins — such as blindness due to xerophthalmia (vitamin A deficiency), and war œdema due to hypoproteinemia. In World War II provision against such deficits was widely made by the vitamin enrichment of flour for bread and by greater attention to proper protein diet.

If the literature of a subject reflects its growth, the modern development of biochemistry has been tremendous. Almost simultaneously three major periodicals came into being and have continued to flourish. The *Journal of Biological Chemistry* first appeared in 1905–6 under the editorship of J. J. Abel and C. A. Herter. The *Biochemical Journal* was created in Great Britain in 1906 (edited by B. MOORE and E. WHITLEY). The *Biochemische Zeitschrift* (1906) started with an imposing list of editors: C. Neuberg, E. Buchner, P. Ehrlich, C. von Noorden, E. Salkowski, and N. Zuntz. It has not maintained as high a standard of scientific presentations, however, as have the British and American journals.

Emil ABDERHALDEN (b. 1877), an inveterate editor with the characteristic German propensity for encyclopædic documentation, produced an important *Handbuch der biologischen Arbeitsmethoden* (1910) in twenty-four volumes, and a fourteen-volume *Biochemisches Handlexikon* (1911–32). In the same category is Carl Oppenheimer's *Handbuch der Biochemie* (1909). Increasing demands have brought forth new thriving journals — in America, the *Journal of Nutrition*, edited by J. R. MURLIN, now by G. R. COWGILL, and *Archives of Biochemistry* (1942), edited by F. F. NORD and C. H. WERKMAN; and in Russia, where such outstanding biochemists as W. L. ENGELHARDT and A. E. BRAUNSTEIN were making important contributions, *Biokhimiya* (1936). Journals like the valuable *Annual Review of Biochemistry* (1932, J. M. Luck editor) meet the essential need of digesting and correlating several thousand articles annually. The first volume of *Enzymologia* appeared in 1937. Nord and Werkman issue *Advances in Enzymology* (1941), which replaces the *Ergebnisse der Enzymforschung*. Two additional review publications are *Vitamins and Hormones* (1943) and *Advances in Protein Chemistry* (1943), edited by M. L. Anson and J. T. Edsall.

MANOMETRIC TECHNIQUES and apparatus have had a profound influence upon the direction of biochemical progress. The gastrometric, vacuum extraction procedures for blood, developed in D. D. VAN SLYKE's (b. 1883) laboratory (1913–24) have been important tools in the development of our ideas of electrolyte (acid-base) and gas equilibria in body fluids. In 1917, with G. E. CULLEN (1890–1940), Van Slyke introduced the concept of "alkali reserve," and with other colleagues, notably A. B. HASTINGS (b. 1895), F. C. McLEAN (b. 1888), and M. HEIDELBERGER (b. 1888), he gave substance to the interpretation of the blood as a physicochemical system, as originally formulated (1921–4) by Harvard's renowned L. J. HENDERSON (1878–1942). Henderson's name is permanently linked with that of K. A. Hasselbach in their "buffer equation" (1908–17). The acidification effect of oxygen upon blood was observed (1914) by C. CHRISTIANSEN, C. G. DOUGLAS, and J. S. HALDANE. Another important contribution by Henderson is an early (1911) appreciation of the role of the kidney in "base economy," further extended by J. L. GAMBLE, S. G. ROSS, and F. F. TISDALL in a classical paper on the *Metabolism of Fixed Base during Fasting* (1923).

The study of the respiratory (oxidative) metabolism of tissue slices surviving in media of known composition has materially extended the knowledge of intimate phases of metabolism and the activity of enzymes in numerous metabolic reactions. Joseph Barcroft's studies (1908) on the dissociation curve of hemoglobin (see his *Respiratory Function of the Blood,* 1914) and Otto Warburg's direct method illustrate the value of respirometry in permitting experiments when only small amounts of valuable material, such as enzymes or isotopically labelled organic compounds, are available. K. LINDERSTRØM-LANG's application of the Cartesian diver principle in an ultramicromanometer will doubtless foster further progress.

ISOTOPIC TRACER TECHNIQUES. A compound containing isotope, whether radioactive or not, retains its chemical and physiological properties, but it can at once be traced in mixtures or molecules in or out of the body. The enormous possibilities of this tool in research in intermediary metabolism were foreseen by Georg von HEVESY, before either stable or artificial radioactive isotopes were available, in a study of the course of radium D (the natural radioactive isotope of lead) through plant organisms (1923). Stable isotopes have become available largely through the work (1932–9) of H. C. UREY (b. 1893), their rapid introduction into biochemistry being due mainly to the clear planning of Schoenheimer. Unstable radioactive isotopes of many elements also have been employed in tracer studies, particularly of inorganic metabolism. For instance, Hevesy and E. Hofer (1934) demonstrated in man that half of ingested "heavy" (ergo, labelled) water is still within the body at the end of ten days, thus permitting estimation of the volume of total body water. By feeding (1935) labelled fatty acid to mice, Schoenheimer and Rittenberg show the fairly rapid turnover of "storage fat" (i.e., fat does not stay put). The Russians A. E. Braunstein's and M. G. Kritzman's concept (1937) of "transamination" was established by following labelled amino acids into body proteins, which, like the lipids, are in a condition of constant flux. Carbon dioxide, formerly regarded as an "end product," has been shown to participate in synthetic reactions in the animal organism — one of the most unexpected findings of the newer biochemistry (H. G. Wood and C. H. Werkman, 1942; E. A. Evans, Jr., and B. Vennesland and A. B. Hastings).

Oxidation-reduction systems and precise measurement of hydrogen-ion concentration have been the special province of William Mansfield CLARK (b. 1884). The fundamental contributions from Clark's laboratory since 1923, as well as the work of L. MICHAELIS (b. 1875) and J. B. CONANT (b. 1893), have emphasized the importance of reversible oxidation-reduction systems in the supply of free energy for cellular work. Measurements of potential upon various systems of biological interest have been contributed by E. S. G. BARRON and A. B. HASTINGS (1934), T. THUNBERG (1925), H. BORSOOK (1937), L. MICHAELIS and C. V. SMYTHE (1936), and E. G. BALL (1938).

The physical techniques of ultracentrifugation, developed by T. SVEDBERG and colleagues (1926–40) and J. W. BEAMS (1935–8), and of electrophoresis, contributed by A. TISELIUS (1930–40), H. THEORELL (1934–5), and L. G. LONGWORTH and D. A. MacINNES (1939–40) have notably advanced knowledge of proteins.

It is worthy of mention that W. B. HARDY (1864–1934) carried out pioneer investigations in this field as early as 1905, and recognized the influence of pH upon the speed of migration of proteins. X-ray diffraction studies (1933–40) upon crystalline and fibrous proteins, in the hands of W. T. ASTBURY, J. D. BERNAL, D. CROWFOOT, M. PERUTZ, I. FANKUCHEN, and R. B. COREY, have also disclosed important details in the structure of these complex molecules.

SPECIALIZED PROTEINS. The foundations for the physical chemistry of proteins were laid by labours of Sir William B. Hardy, Thomas B. Osborne (1859–1929), Jacques Loeb, and P. L. SØRENSEN (1868–1939). In the practical application of proteins to nutrition Osborne and L. B. Mendel began their joint researches on "synthetic diets," and in 1914 made the great discovery that lysine and tryptophane are indispensable for rats. This work has been carried virtually to completion by Mendel's pupil W. C. ROSE (b. 1887), in whose ample department of biochemistry all of the known amino acids have been evaluated. Rose and his associates have thus established (1931–44) that ten amino acids are "essential" for the rat, and only eight amino acids for adult man. The work (1940–3) of M. S. MADDEN, G. H. WHIPPLE, and their colleagues, using the technique of plasmapheresis combined with nitrogen-balance studies, has established the concept that the *plasma proteins are in equilibrium with tissue proteins* (i.e., further support for the " dynamic state ").

The site of urea-formation has been established (1924) in the liver by the hepatectomy experiments of J. BOLLMAN, F. C. MANN, and T. B. McGATH, that of urinary-ammonia production in the kidney by S. R. BENEDICT and T. P. NASH (1921), H. A. KREBS and K. HENSELEIT (1932). The separation (1941–5) of plasma proteins into five main fractions by E. J. Cohn and his colleagues has already proved to be of great practical and probable commercial importance in the treatment of shock and hypoproteinemia (albumin), in hemostasis (fibrinogen and thrombin), and in immunological prophylaxis (gamma globulins). Knowledge of the chemistry of the porphyrins and metalloporphyrins, which by Richard WILLSTÄTTER (1872–1942) and his successor, Hans FISCHER (1881– form the prosthetic groups of the respiratory proteins, has been furnished largely 1945). Willstätter's belief that enzymes are actually small molecules attached to a large inert carrier protein has now been disproved by J. H. NORTHROP's (b. 1891) crystallization of pepsin (1929) and, with M. KUNITZ, of trypsin and chymotrypsin (1931–3). Since the first crystallization of an enzyme — that of urease by J. B. SUMNER (1926), who also crystallized catalase (1936) — about twenty-five crystalline enzymes have now been obtained. They are all proteins. F. C. CORI's (b. 1896) crystallization (1942) of muscle phosphorylase led to a major achievement by Cori and his colleagues — namely, the synthesis *in vitro* of glycogen (1943). This is the first example, nearly one hundred years after Claude Bernard's isolation of glycogen, of a large molecule of this type being synthesized in the absence of living cells. The important coenzyme I (cozymase) was discovered in yeast (1904) by A. HARDEN (1865–1940) and W. J. YOUNG, pioneers in the critical study of fermentation. Their discovery (1911) that inorganic phosphate accelerates the fermentative process thus set the stage for the establishment of the relation of phosphate to carbohydrate metabolism. Otto Meyerhof's discovery of the same coenzyme in animal tissues such as muscle and brain was a demonstration of the essential identity of metabolic processes in all living matter, and introduced the picture of carbohydrate metabolism that Meyerhof was destined to develop.

HORMONES. Outstanding in the early chemistry of the hormones were the isolation and synthesis of adrenalin (J. J. ABEL; J. TAKAMINE; T. B. ALDRICH, 1899–1905), and of thyroxin (E. C. KENDALL, 1919–27; C. R. HARRINGTON, 1926–8; HARRINGTON and G. BARGER, 1927).

The chemistry of the hormones of the adrenal cortex has claimed a good deal of attention, and a number of active steroids have been isolated (O. WINTERSTEINER; T. REICHSTEIN; E. C. Kendall, 1935–6). No single compound effects complete replacement for the destruction of Addison's disease. Desoxycorticosterone is primarily concerned with the retention of sodium, whereas the hydroxycorticosterones appear to exert their influence mainly on carbohydrate metabolism. The female (estrogens) and male (androgens) sex hormones have been widely investigated and their structures established. They, too, are sterolic in nature. E. Allen and E. A. Doisy were the pioneers (1923) in this field. The investigations of Doisy and his colleagues (1923–33) have been concerned largely with estrone (theelin) and its derivatives. Important contributions on the chemistry of the sex hormones have also been made by A. BUTENANDT (1930–3), E. DINGEMANSE (1930), and G. F. MARRIAN (1929–33). An outstanding achievement in synthetic chemistry, which has contributed materially to our knowledge of these structures, was the conversion by L. Ružička and his colleagues (1934) of a derivative of cholesterol into androsterone, one of the male hormones. The work of J. W. COOK and E. C. DODDS (1934) upon synthetic compounds bearing some resemblance in structure to estrone has indicated that estrogenic activity is highly unspecific. This led to the synthesis of the very active artificial estrogen, stilbestrol (Dodds, 1939). The variety of functional uses to which the sterolic structure is put is indeed remarkable; the same skeleton is found also in the bile acids and in the antirachitic vitamin. The structural chemistry of the bile acids, explored for years by A. WINDAUS and H. WIELAND, remained unsolved until O. ROSENHEIM and H. KING, British investigators, supplied the key to the puzzle (1932).

Among the protein hormones, whose story is told in several other sections of this chapter, definitive chemical studies have been carried out mainly on insulin, which was crystallized by J. J. Abel and co-workers in 1926; on chorionic gonadotrophin, the hormone of pregnancy urine (S. GURIN, C. BACHMAN, and D. W. WILSON, 1940); and on the lactogenic hormone of the anterior pituitary (obtained in crystalline form by A. WHITE and C. N. H. LONG (1937–42)).

VITAMINS. Experiments in normal nutrition offered the first clear evidence of the existence in natural foodstuffs of essentials for normal nutrition other than the main nutrients: protein, carbohydrates, fats, water, and salts. To Sir F. Gowland Hopkins (1906–12) goes the honour for first demonstrating conclusively that young animals (rats) failed to grow on purified nutrients, but could be maintained if to these milk or alcoholic extracts of milk were added. Foreshadowings of the existence of what he called " accessory food substances " are found in earlier writings (N. LUNIN, 1881; C. A. PEKELHARING, 1905) as hypotheses, unsupported by experimental evidence. Independent investigations in the United States (E. V. McCollum and A. Davis, 1913; T. B. Osborne and L. B. Mendel, 1913) established the need for two such substances, a fat-soluble A and a water-soluble B, both needed for growth, one (A) antiophthalmia, the other (B) antiberiberi. A third, water-soluble C (antiscorbutic), was shortly added. The term " vitamine " (or correctly " vitamin," as they are not amines) was coined by C. FUNK in 1911; to the term " vitamin " the alphabetical letters

THE PRINCIPAL KNOWN VITAMINS, WITH THEIR DISCOVERERS

Name	Discoverer of Existence	Discoverer of Chemical Constitution	Synthesis
Vitamin A	McCollum, E. V., & Davis, M., 1913; Osborne, T. B., & Mendel, L. B., 1913	Karrer, P., et al., 1931	Fuson, R. C., & Christ, R. E., 1936; Kuhn, R., et al., 1937
Provitamin A (carotenes)	Moore, T., 1930	Karrer, P., et al., 1930	Milas, N. A., during the war; announced 1945
B vitamins			
B₁ (F, thiamine)	Eijkman, C., 1897; McCollum, E. V., & Davis, M., 1915	Funk, C., 1911; Jansen, B. C. P., & Donath, W. F., 1926 ("aneurin"); Williams, R. R., 1935 (thiamine)	Williams, R. R., & Cline, J. K., 1936
B₂ Complex			
B₂ (G, riboflavin)	Sherman, H. C., & Bourquin, A., 1931	Kuhn, R., et al., 1933	Kuhn, R., et al., 1933
Nicotinic acid (niacin, P-P or pellagra-preventive)	Smith, M. I., & Hendrick, E. G., 1926; Goldberger, J., et al., 1926	Huber, C., 1867; Funk, C., 1913	Harris, S. A., & Folkers, K., 1939
Pyridoxine, B₆ (filtrate factor I, H factor, "Y" factor)	György, P., 1934	independently by Lepkovsky, Szent-Györgyi, Emerson, Keresztesy, Kuhn, Ichiba, 1938; Williams, R. J., 1939	Williams, R. J., & Major, R. T., 1940
Pantothenic acid (pantothen)	Wildier, E., 1901	Kogl, F., & Tonnis, B., 1936 (Germany)	
Biotin (vitamin H, coenzyme R)	Boas, M. A., 1927; Parsons et al., 1931-40; György, 1931-40; MacLeod, J. J. R., & Best, C. H., et al., 1924-32;	von Babo & Hirschbrunn, 1852; Strecker, 1862	Szent-Györgyi, V., du Vigneaud, V., et al., 1940
Choline		King, C. C., & Waugh, 1932; Szent-Györgyi, A., & Svirbely, 1932 (hexuronic acid, 1928)	
Vitamin C (ascorbic acid, cevitamic acid)	Kramer, 1720; Lind, J., 1757		Haworth, W. N., Hirst, E. L., et al., 1933
Vitamin D	Mellanby, E., 1918-19; McCollum, E. V., et al., 1922	Hess, A. F.; Steenbock, H.; Windaus, A., et al., 1922-7; Rosenheim & Webster, 1927	
D₂ (activated calciferol)			
D₃ (activated dehydrocholesterol)			
Vitamin E (tocopherol)	Evans, H. M., & Bishop, K. S., 1922	Evans, et al., 1936; Fernholz, E., 1937, 1938	Karrer, P., et al., 1938
Vitamin K ("menadione," etc.)	Dam, H., 1929-35	Dam, H., & Karrer, W., et al., 1939; McKee, R. W.; Doisy, E. A., et al., 1939	K₁, synthesized in several laboratories

began to be added in 1920. The alphabetical nomenclature has been loosely retained, but both chemical and functional names for many of the vitamins have been added.

Subsequent work has been in the discovery of new vitamins by differentiation (e.g., the B vitamins), or in course of experiments in normal nutrition (e.g., vitamins E and K, pyrodoxin, biotin, etc.), in vitamin assay of foods, in isolation and identification of vitamins, and in their synthesis. Vitamin research has been enormously stimulated since 1933 by discovery of the relation of many vitamins of enzymes in animals, plants, and micro-organisms, with those working in the field of vitamins.

There are now more than thirty known vitamins. Fifteen have been isolated and identified, and a number synthesized. In the accompanying table is a list of the principal vitamins identified and isolated.

Vitamin A, a derivative of carotenoid pigments, is not a single substance. It is a constituent of the visual purple of the retina, functioning in light-perception. Epithelial structures appear to have an active vitamin-A metabolism.

The B vitamins are a large group of unrelated substances discovered in the course of differential purification of the original antiberiberi water-soluble vitamin B. At least three are related to respiratory enzyme systems (B_1, thiamine; B_2, riboflavin; and nicotinic acid). Others are B_6, pyridoxine, pantothenic acid, biotin, choline, folic acid). Thiamine (B_1) is related to co-carboxylase in carbohydrate metabolism. Its function in the prevention of beriberi has somewhat overshadowed its importance in the metabolism of tissues other than nerve and muscle. B_2, riboflavin, is the active group of Warburg's " yellow ferment." Nicotinic acid, the principal pellagra-preventive, is a constituent of co-zymase.

Vitamin C, ascorbic acid, was isolated in enzyme research (1928, A. SZENT-GYÖRGYI) as a hexuronic acid before its scurvy-preventive character was known. In 1932 the vitamin was isolated by W. A. WAUGH and C. G. KING and its identity with Szent-Györgyi's hexuronic acid was established. Its behaviour is that of a cell catalyst though its relation to known enzyme systems is not established. It is necessary for the maintenance of intercellular substances (bone matrix, collagen, etc.).

Vitamin D's antirachitic function is the attribute of a number of sterols, activated by ultraviolet light. Its mode of action is not understood, but it is concerned with the metabolism of calcium and phosphorus, and prevents rickets and osteomalacia.

Vitamin E, alpha-tocopherol, first discovered as an antisterility factor (differing in the two sexes), appears to have a much more general function than the prevention of sterility. It is an important antioxidant, and exerts a marked protective effect upon other vitamins.

Vitamin K (" menadione ") was discovered in 1935 by the Dane H. DAM, who assigned the letter K (for *Koagulation*) to it. Its activity is found in a number of naphthoquinones. The formation of prothrombin in the liver requires the presence of this vitamin, though it is not a component of prothrombin itself.

The number of biochemists to whom credit should go for their contributions toward the isolation, identification, and synthesis of the vitamins is too great to include in a volume of this character. Mention should be made, however, of some not otherwise included, such as Harriet Chick, L. J. Harris, S. S. Zilva, J. C. Drummond, R. McCarrison, and B. Sure.

THE NEWER ENERGY METABOLISM. A multiplicity of investigations, many already indicated, have converged to explain the role of oxidation-reduction processes, enzymes, and vitamins in changing food into useful energy.

Carbohydrates may be broken down for mammalian use in two ways — anaerobically to lactic acid in the steps of the Meyerhof cycle or aerobically to carbon dioxide and water in the steps of the tricarboxylic-acid cycle. The liberation of CO_2 (decarboxylation) in the aerobic as well as the anaerobic processes is enzymically controlled by carboxylases (E. AUHAGEN, 1932), the prosthetic group of which (co-carboxylase) has proved to be thiamin pyrophosphate, derived from vitamin B_1 (K. LOHMANN and P. SCHUSTER, 1937; S. OCHOA and R. A. PETERS, 1938). In polyneuritis due to thiamin deficiency, pyruvic acid is not decarboxylated and accumulates (R. A. Peters, 1937). Oxygen is transported by hemoglobin and myoglobin (H. THEORELL, 1932–4) to the tissues, where it meets a key substance, cytochrome oxidase (the " respiratory ferment " of Warburg, 1925–8). This has been shown to have the power to oxidize the catalyst below it in the scale of potential, cytochrome c (D. KEILIN and P. H.-S. HARTLEY, 1925, 1935–9; H. Theorell and Å. ÅKESSON, 1939–41), but also is unique in that it is oxidized by molecular oxygen. The oxygen ion finds its way to meet hydrogen and form water in an oxidation-reduction process that proceeds through cytochrome c to the flavoproteins — whose prosthetic group contains the essential structure of the vitamin riboflavin (Warburg and W. CHRISTIAN, 1932–3; H. Theorell, 1934; R. KUHN and T. WAGNER-JAUREGG, 1934; F. B. STRAUB, 1939; J. G. DEWAN and D. E. GREEN, 1937) — and to coenzyme I, which contains a close relative of the antipellagra vitamin (H. von EULER and K. MYRBACK, 1921–32). The studies by the Swiss V. HENRIQUES, the Britisher F. J. W. ROUGHTON, and the American W. C. STADIE on carbhemoglobin and carbonic anhydrase are important in elucidating the mechanism whereby CO_2 is eliminated from the body.

The storage of potential energy is one other factor to be mentioned in the " storage-battery concept " of the supply of energy. Since the time of Harden and Young (1904), phosphates have assumed a dominant importance in energy exchange. " Transphosphorylation " has been established

as an important mechanism, the main participators being phosphocreatine
(C. H. FISKE and Y. SUBAROFF, 1927; P. and G. P. EGGLETON, 1927) and
adenosine di- and tri-phosphate (K. Lohmann and O. Meyerhof, 1934) and
possibly an enzyme in the muscle protein, myosin (W. A. ENGLEHARDT,
1940–2). The concept of the storage of energy in the organism owes much
to the brilliant demonstration (1941) by Fritz LIPMANN of the role of the
high-energy phosphate bond in the above compounds and in acetyl phosphate and the pyruvic- and glyceric-acid phosphates.

Thus it may be said that at least a sound thermodynamic foothold has
been provided in the understanding of energy exchange and that biochemistry has here arrived at a significant meeting-place of oxidation-reduction
processes, enzymes and vitamins. The paths onward should be interesting.

6. Pathology

While pathologic anatomy in the present century has remained as important as ever in teaching the nature of disease and in the study of individual cases, in pathology's contributions to medical progress the emphasis has
shifted increasingly to the functional and experimental aspects. With the
interest now centred on mechanism rather than structure, British and American pathologists appear to have been able to adapt more successfully to this
new trend than those of continental Europe. This may be attributed, at
least in part, to the custom in Great Britain and America of concentrating chairs and departments under the general term Pathology, whereas on
the Continent, especially in Germanic countries, they have been divided
between Pathological Anatomy — the larger part — and *Allgemeine Pathologie*.

Though specialization in the practice of medicine increases in the science of medicine, the traditional boundary lines are tending to break down
with increasing overlap of different fields. This trend is reflected in the narrative of our two final chapters. Thus such pathological topics as acute
yellow atrophy and other liver lesions, and vascular lesions such as periarteritis nodosa and Buerger's disease, clinico-pathologic aspects of Bright's
disease, hemolytic jaundice, pernicious anæmia, and other hematologic conditions, and various endocrine, metabolic, and eponymic disorders illustrating both structural and functional pathology are considered in our clinical
sections, and some clinical aspects are to be found in this or in the microbiological or physiological sections.

In the field of pathologic anatomy new techniques, especially in neuropathology, have permitted further progress, and the old techniques have continued to detect some previously unrecognized diseases, or after recognition have placed them on a sound basis.

"Spreading factors," such as tissue extracts that enhance the action of infectious agents, were described (1928) by F. DURAN-REYNALS (b. 1899). It was not until 1939 that their mechanism was established, when it was found (1939, 1940) by E. B. CHAIN and E. S. DUTHIE that the intercellular cement substance, hyaluronic acid — a polysaccharide isolated (1934) by K. MEYER (b. 1884) and others — could be dissolved by an enzyme, hyaluronidase. Thus the bacteria that secrete hyaluronidase facilitate the spread of the infection they produce, and it has even been suggested that malignant tumours may in the same way facilitate their infiltration through adjacent tissues.

INFLAMMATION. Recent developments in this basically all-important phenomenon are the role of local and general allergy, that of the lymphatics and of mechanical fixation of an irritant in the tissues (Menkin), and the nature of the stimulant to the circulatory response (T. Lewis's "H substance").

While the etiology and pathologic anatomy of inflammation may be fairly well understood, there is still much to be learned about its pathogenesis and the far-reaching consequences of its functional effects on the organism. In inflammatory exudates Menkin has demonstrated substances of differing, though not exactly analysed, chemical nature, such as necrosin (1943) and pyrexin (1945), which he regards as responsible for the "basic pattern of injury" and the induced fever, respectively, and thus as important factors in the inflammatory process.

The number of morbid processes the nature of which is still unknown is much less than it was even a generation ago. Prominent in this category are Hodgkin's disease — still being discussed as to whether it is a granuloma or a neoplasm — and the leukemias, which the accumulating experimental evidence is gradually bringing into the group of neoplasms.

The concept of a *reticulo-endothelial system* (L. Aschoff, 1913), scattered through various organs but performing an important scavenger function, has led to practical results. Earlier studies by RANVIER, BIZZOZERO, METCHNIKOFF, MARCHAND, RIBBERT, KIYONO, GOLDMANN, and others had demonstrated special cells that had a marked avidity for engulfing foreign bodies. These have now been shown to be concerned in various other normal and pathological processes, to have their characteristic neoplasms, to develop a special type of leukemia (monocytic), and to be especially concerned in a group of diseases due to disorders of lipoid metabolism (Gaucher's, Niemann-Pick's, Hand-Schüller-Christian's disease, xanthoma, etc.).

Among what might be called "new" diseases, appearing since 1900, was lethargic encephalitis, described (1917) by C. von Economo (1876–1931). Appearing like a bolt from the blue toward the end of the First World War, as if connected with the influenza epidemic, it soon disappeared, leaving only its scars, with etiology and pathogenesis still obscure. No other disease has behaved in this way in modern times to remind us of some of the clearly described but now unrecognizable epidemics of the ancients. It was not until another score of years that it reappeared in less dramatic form and with a different stage setting, when it was recognized as due to any of two or more related viruses.

Granulomata, more or less resembling tubercle and gumma microscopically, have been identified from time to time, such as the condition known as sarcoidosis. This disease of unknown etiology was apparently first described by Hutchinson in 1869, designated by the name of his patient as "Mortimer's malady," and again by Besnier as *lupus pernio* (1889); it was called sarcoid by C. Boeck (1899) and as lymphogranulomatosis benigna, linked with the uveo-parotid syndrome, by J. Schaumann (1914). Another disease with a similar lesion is tularemia, identified (1919) by Edward Francis (b. 1872), who demonstrated its mode of transmission to man. According to Garrison, it was first observed (1925) in Japan by H. O'Hara, who experimentally inoculated his own wife. Brucellosis, shown (1918) by Evans to include both undulant or Malta fever and the contagious abortion of cattle, may give a baffling pathological picture. San Joaquin Valley fever (coccidioidomycosis) is another disease that has assumed importance in recent years, especially in the western United States. First observed (1892) by A. Posada in the Argentine, it was shortly after (1894) identified in its dermal form by E. Rixford. It was shown (1900) by W. Ophüls to be due to a pathogenic mould, *Coccidioides immitis,* and is now recognized as a self-limited, chiefly respiratory, infectious granuloma that sometimes may be fatal.

Tórulosis, though recognized in the central nervous system by Zenker as early as 1861 and classified as a fungus disease by Busse and Buschke (1894), has been explored chiefly in the present century by Stoddard and Cutler, who gave it the name *Torula histolytica* (1916) and others. A recently detected disease that is apparently of virus origin is lymphocyte choromeningitis, described (1925) by A. Wallgren as "acute aseptic meningitis." A disease of considerable variability in manifestations and seriousness and transmissible to many species, its pathologic changes are chiefly those indicated by its name (C. Armstrong, 1941).

The peculiar disorder of carbohydrate metabolism, wherein histologically demonstrable glycogen accumulates in the viscera, was described in 1929 by E. von GIERKE (b. 1877). Doubtless still more granulomata will be identified before many years.

In the field of *cancer*, D. HANSEMANN's (1872–1920) concept (1902) of " anaplasia " — that tumour cells may become more embryonic in appearance and grow more rapidly — was another important addition to the understanding of the nature of cancer. Many different varieties of tumours were described by investigators too numerous to mention here, all of which knowledge was assembled and evaluated in the masterly work of James EWING (1866–1943) on *Neoplastic Diseases*. The difficult borderline between anomalies and new growths was illuminated by E. ALBRECHT's concept of *hamartoma* and *choristoma*, structures having the microscopic appearance of tumours, yet differing from them in that they are congenital and of limited size rather than possessing powers of unlimited growth.

A number of new varieties of tumours have been established during this period. The " chocolate cyst " (1924) of J. A. SAMPSON (b. 1873), a tumour of misplaced endometrial cells, is found not infrequently in various parts of the abdominal cavity. Like the parent tissue, the tumour bleeds at the monthly periods, hence the chocolate-like appearance. Carcinoids (Argentaffine tumours), relatively benign abdominal tumours with the microscopic picture of malignancy, were apparently first recognized by Lubarsch (1888) and described (1913, 1924) by Pierre MASSON (b. 1880), whose new staining methods have been much employed. He demonstrated their connection with nerve cells (Kulchitzky) and a similar neural connection for nevi. He also established (1924) the peculiar glomus tumour, a neuro-myoarterial structure that appears to be concerned with temperature regulation of the extremities, the tumour often being found beneath the nails. The bone-marrow tumour that O. J. von RUSTIZKY in 1873 named " myeloma " had been earlier recognized by H. B. Jones (1848), Macintyre (1850), and Weber (1867); it was not until 1900, however, that J. Homer WRIGHT identified the plasma cell as the cell concerned in most cases of multiple myeloma. The very surprising increase in the number of primary cancers of the lung in recent years, like the problem of the increase of cancer in general, hangs on the dilemma of increased professional awareness (" *Was man weiss, man sieht* ") versus some changed environmental factors as yet unknown.

The differentiation of several types of glial cells (*q.v.* in the section on histology) gave P. BAILEY (b. 1892) and Harvey Cushing the opportunity to establish (1926) a dozen varieties of glial tumours, with their relative frequencies and survival periods. As their incidence and malignancy varied greatly in the different cells, and as glial tumours constitute almost half of all brain tumours, this was an advance of great importance for neurological prognosis and neurosurgery.

Attempts to advance with the cancer problem by experimental research are now being made throughout the world along many lines, but the new knowledge acquired has not as yet been synthesized to be of great practical value. The production of skin cancer with repeated applications of tar (1916) confirmed older clinical observations of the etiological relationship of certain chemicals to tumour incidence. The ingenious and patient work of J. FIBIGER in obtaining gastric carcinoma in rats by feeding spiroptera in infested cockroaches (1913) proved that "spontaneous" (that is, not transplanted) cancer could be produced at will in experimental animals under appropriate conditions, and opened an entirely new field for the experimental study of cancer.

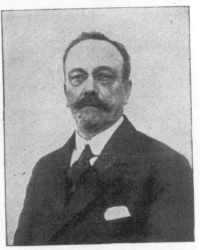

458. *Johannes Fibiger, Nobel Laureate, 1926.*

In the present century the outstanding contributions to cancer knowledge have been in the field of experimental cancer: the transmissible tumours of animals (A. HANAU [1858–1900], in 1889; H. MORAU [b. 1860], in 1894; Leo LOEB, 1901; C. O. JENSEN [1864–1934], in 1902); artificial production of cancer: nematode gastric cancer of rats (FIBIGER, 1913), tar cancer of the skin (K. YAMAGIWA [1863–1930] and K. ICHIKAWA [b. 1887]), in 1916, cysticercus sarcoma of the liver (F. D. BULLOCK [1878–1937] and M. R. CURTIS [b. 1880]), in 1915; the production of tumour by cell-free filtrates of viruses (in fowl, P. ROUS; rabbits, R. E. SHOPE; frogs, B. LUCKÉ); its production by chemicals of known composition (E. L. KENNAWAY, L. F. FIESER [b. 1899], and others), some of the substances being related to body products such as bile salts and estrogens; genetic studies by G. WOOLLEY (b. 1904), E. C. McDOWELL (b. 1887), M. SLYE, C. C. LITTLE, and many others; the effect of Roentgen rays and radium on various kinds of neoplastic tissue, exploration of manifestations of resistance and adaptation, and Warburg's demonstration of the peculiar fermentative type of metabolism of the cancer cell.

Among very recent finds are the observations, beginning (1933) with those of Murray and Little, that the incidence of mammary cancer in hybrid mice was determined by the degree of cancer susceptibility of the mother, suggesting that an extra-chromosomal factor was at work. J. J. BITTNER (b. 1904) found further (1936–44), highly susceptible from birth, mice nursed by a resistant foster-mother developed relatively few tumours. The nature of this milk factor, which has implications of great practical importance in human cancer of the breast, is still under investigation. A clue to the reason for the invasiveness of malignant tumours is offered in the quantitative determination (1944) by Dale COMAN (b. 1906) that cancer cells stick together much less tenaciously than do cells of benign tumours or normal tissue.

Thus, as in some other fields of medicine, the past hundred years, perhaps even the present century alone, have added more to our knowledge of cancer than have all the preceding centuries, and the accumulation of facts about cancer is progressing more rapidly today than in any previous generation. While the way that cancer is produced, in the sense of the precise mechanism that makes the normal cell become cancerous, still remains unknown, a number of causes (carcinogenic agents) of certain cancers — both clinical and experimental — are known, and each decade sees a noteworthy increase in the formidable array of evidence bearing on the nature of the condition. It is not presumptuous, then, to hope that adequate knowledge of its essential cause, and therefore probably of its control, will not be long in forthcoming. Thus it has become increasingly evident that genetic and hormonal influences, together with external factors — chemical, physical, and biotic (viruses) — all play important parts in cancer development.

In genetics, manipulation of closely inbred strains (i.e., strains essentially uniform genetically) has provided a tool adapted to many kinds of experimental procedures. In this way strains highly susceptible or highly resistant have been obtained (M. Slye). Genetic influences can be included or excluded in evaluating constitutional factors associated with tumours; and, using such " marker " gene characteristics as colour of coat or tail peculiarities — characters that have been located in sixteen of the twenty chromosomes of the mouse (C. C. Little) — genes influencing tumour-formation can be determined. Genetic influences have been demonstrated in mammary cancer (L. Loeb and others), leukemia (McDowell), lympho-, fibro-, and reticulum cell sarcoma (Little and Murray), and carcinoma of the lung (Lynch, Bittner).

The influence of hormones on cancer development was first shown in the case of estrogens and mammary cancer. E. LACASSAGNE was even able to produce (1932) carcinoma in the breasts of all of three male mice by injecting " folliculin," a cancer that does not occur spontaneously. Administration of ovarian hormones has also been shown capable of producing uterine cancer and fibroids, pituitary tumours, interstitial cell tumours of the testes (some metastasizing), leukemia, and invasive lymphoid tumours. Castration of mice at birth can produce tumours of the adrenal cortex, and an obvious relation of undescended testicle to testicular cancer has been established.

The carcinogenic effect of pure chemical compounds is a product of the past two decades, starting from the interesting but unsolved problems raised at the beginning of the century by the injection of scarlet red and similar dyes, and from the Japanese production of skin cancer with tar. After E. L. KENNAWAY had got a tarry extract from human skin that had tumour-producing qualities, W. V. MAYNEORD and I. HIEGER produced (1930) the first carcinogenic hydrocarbon, 1:2:5:6 dibenzanthracene. New compounds, which now number 169 (Hartwell), have been developed especially by J. W. COOK, HEWETT, and L. F. FIESER. Similar compounds having the opposite (inhibitory) effect on tissues have been developed (1935) by A. HADDOW.

In the pathology of the *endocrine system*, the added knowledge that was accumulated from the correlation of human pathological changes in form and function, augmented by the methods of experimental pathology, has placed the subject on a high if uncompleted level of accomplishment.

The story of PITUITARY pathology begins at least as far back as Bonetus's description (*Sepulchretum*, 1679) of a pituitary cyst, though the next landmark did not appear until 1840 — Mohr's description of obesity with pituitary tumour. Pituitary insufficiency, whether from destruction by tumour, cyst, or other cause, was found (1901) by A. FRÖHLICH (b. 1871) to produce the condition known as adipose-genital dystrophy, and this was shortly after reproduced experimentally by Harvey Cushing and others. The pituitary also was shown (1924-30) by B. HOUSSAY to be capable of promoting diabetes through its influence on carbohydrate metabolism. Important new understanding of the role of the pituitary and adrenal in the pathogenesis of diabetes has been furnished (1935-44) by C. N. H. LONG (b. 1901) and F. D. W. LUKENS (b. 1899). Premature senility (progeria) was linked with a pituitary lesion by HUTCHINSON and GILFORD (1904), and the condition established (1914) by the Dane Morris SIMMONDS (1855-1925). Through unbalance of its stimulatory effects on other hormones (thyrotropic, adrenotropic, gonadotropic), the pituitary has been shown by H. M. EVANS (b. 1882) and others to contribute to thyroid, adrenal, and gonadal disease. Pituitary basophilism (increase of the basophil cells of the anterior lobe) was shown (1935) by Cushing to be involved in the masculinization of women, as in the case of the bearded women of side-shows; a similar syndrome also being caused by a " functional " tumour of the adrenal cortex.

One of the functional tumours of the OVARY — the arrhenoblastoma (ἄρρηνος, male) was found by A. G. Pick (1905) also to produce a similar picture; whereas its opposite — the granulosa cell tumour of the ovarian follicle (first described by VON KAHLDEN, 1895, and named by VON WENDT, 1914) — produces premature sexual maturity in children or return of sexual activity in the aged. The follicular hormone has one effect on the uterus, lutein another, both being under the control of the pituitary, and still others have been identified in the placenta.

Recognition of the thyroid role of accelerating heat-production by its use of iodine in the synthesis of thyroxin has furthered the correlation of its morbid processes with the various disease pictures found. Simple goitre, known for centuries to occur in certain localities, is recognized as the glandular reaction to iodine deficiency. It can be produced experimentally, relieved or prevented by feeding iodine, and may occur in any except marine animals. The opposite extreme, thyrotoxicosis (exophthalmic goitre), results when excessive thyroxin is formed, either by a toxic adenoma or by diffuse hyperplasia. Conditions that do not fit into this simple classification are the various types of carcinoma, the maligneous thyroiditis of unknown origin (described by RIEDEL, 1896), and the struma lymphomatosa described by HASHIMOTO (1912).

PARATHYROID pathology, limited in the previous century to tetany following extirpation, has been explored in several ways. Tetany was shown by MacCallum and Voegtlin (1909) to be due to the fall of blood calcium below a critical level, thus revealing the role of calcium in lessening irritability at neuromuscular junctions. In the opposite direction, in 1904, Askanazy found in a case of osteitis fibrosa cystica (von Recklinghausen, 1891) a tumour of the parathyroid, and in 1925 (pub. 1926) Mandl of Vienna found and removed a similar tumour, with relief of the patient's condition. As the excessive excretion of calcium in the urine stopped at the same time, it was clear that the oversecretion of the parathyroid hormone (parathormone, Collip, 1924) had mobilized calcium from the bone with resorption of the skeleton and fibrous-tissue replacement; that is, it is no more an osteitis than is the " milk fever " of cattle (due to excessive loss of calcium in milk) a fever.

The ADRENAL cortex was shown experimentally (1924) by G. B. WISLOCKI (b. 1892) and S. J. CROWE (b. 1883) to be the part necessary for life. Later, histological studies demonstrated that it was the cortical damage that was responsible for Addison's disease. In fact, cortical extract, first prepared (1931) by W. W. Swingle (b. 1891) and J. J. Pfiffner (b. 1903), has been helpful in the treatment of this fatal disease. The tumours of the adrenal are of interest as well as importance. In addition to the cortical tumour producing precocious puberty or virilism and its histologically identical but functionally silent counterpart, the adrenal medulla may produce tumours of nerve-cell origin (neuroblastoma), with characteristic disease pictures (W. PEPPER, JR., 1901; R. HUTCHISON, 1907). It also produces chromaffin tumours, in common with other sites of the chromaffin system. These cells are thought to secrete adrenalin, and appropriately, therefore, many such tumours are accompanied by hypertension. The various lesions that cause Addison's disease had been known for many years, but only in recent times has the mechanism of the disorder been established as due to hypofunction of the cortex; as a result, sodium, chlorides, and CO_2 are decreased in the blood serum, potassium rises, and the urine output is decreased (R. F. LOEB, 1933–42). Clinical improvement has been obtained by administering sodium chloride and cortical extract. A dramatic lesion of the adrenal — massive bilateral hemorrhage with sudden death — was described in 1911 by A. WATERHOUSE (b. 1873) and again by C. FRIDERICHSEN in 1918, mostly following meningococcus infection.

In the PANCREAS, adenoma of the islands of Langerhans was first described (1902) by A. G. NICHOLLS (b. 1870), the first carcinoma by SAUERBECK (1904), though he took it to be a metastasis from the breast. Functioning tumours were described — first by R. WILDER (1927), and W. McCLENAHAN and G. W. NORRIS (1929) — which caused dangerously low blood-sugar levels through an over-secretion of insulin. Many have been removed, with relief of symptoms. The concept of hyperinsulinism was advanced (1924) by Seale HARRIS (b. 1870) on the basis of five cases observed. An important new tool for the experimental study of diabetes was brought to light (1937) by H. S. JACOBS in the ability of alloxan to produce hypoglycemia in rabbits. This was later (1943) found by DUNN and his colleagues to be associated with a necrosis of the islands, apparently due to a direct toxic action on the beta cells (C. C. and O. T. BAILEY, 1944) and not to their exhaustion by the hyperglycemic stimulus.

Various combinations of endocrine disturbance have been reported, but none more peculiar or provocative than F. ALBRIGHT'S (b. 1900) triad (1937) of osteitis fibrosa, skin pigmentation, and precocious puberty, and sometimes associated with diabetes mellitus and thyrotoxicosis. Gargoylism, Morquio's disease (familial osseous deformity and rarefaction, sometimes with added cerebral changes), and other eponymic diseases have also been ascribed to endocrine disorder.

The pineal gland, thymus, and spleen are other organs that, on the basis of experimental studies and occasional findings at autopsy, have been suspected of having endocrine activity, but adequate proof remains lacking.

GASTRO-INTESTINAL HORMONES continue to be added to Starling's original secretin (1902), such as gastrin (J. S. EDKINS, 1906), pancreozymin and A. C. Ivy's better-known cholecystokinin (1928); also possible hormones affecting the circulation, such as carotidin (C. D. CHRISTIE, 1933) and renin (R. Tigerstedt, 1898). The concept of antihormones was proposed (1934) by J. B. Collip, though their nature — antibody, neutralizing substance, or some other mechanism — is not yet understood.

FOOD-DEFICIENCY DISEASES (avitaminoses) have been known for some time, but without much knowledge of what substances were deficient. Hippocrates is said to have prescribed liver for the cure of night blindness. Scurvy had ravaged the sailors of Vasco da Gama and of Cartier, who in 1536 learned from the Indians how to cure his sailors with the juices of the almeda tree (Hakluyt). Fruit juice had been used to advantage since the sixteenth century (RONSSEUS, 1564); Kramer, an Austrian army physician, had used orange or lime juice (1720), and James LIND had established fruit juice in the British navy as a preventive of scurvy (1757), hence the nautical term " lime-juicers," or " limeys." CASAL, a Spanish physician, in describing pellagra in 1735, sensed the relationship between the disease and a maize diet. TAKAKI had greatly decreased the ravages of beriberi in the Japanese navy (1882–6) by adding variety to the almost pure diet of polished rice, which was later shown to be deficient in vitamin B_1. By 1889 it had become accepted that rickets was due to some qualitative deficiency in the diet. To EIJKMAN and GRIJNS is given the credit of first producing a deficiency disease experimentally (beriberi in fowl) and of discovering in the husks of the rice grain the important substance that was lost in the polishing process (1897–1900). Here we see introduced a new concept of disease as resulting from the absence of an essential nutrient, in contradistinction to the idea of disease as the exclusive result of agents acting positively to produce injury to body tissues. Other deficiencies were later produced experimentally. Theobald Smith's observation (1895) of a hemorrhagic disease in oat-fed guinea-pigs, was not properly evaluated until A. HOLST (1860–1931) and A. FRÖHLICH recognized (1907) scurvy in their guinea-pigs that were being fed on a deficient diet. Thanks to the studies of numerous scientists working in several specialties — biochemists, physiologists, pharmacologists, pathologists, and clinicians — a number of vitamins in pure form have been shown to cause disease experimentally when withheld from animals or to cure human disease arising from protracted deprivation of food sources of the vitamins or from failure to absorb or utilize those ingested. When there is not enough vitamin present for any of these reasons, diverse results may follow in independent systems of the body, yet they have usually been traced to one or two missing links in the biological chain.

Thus lack of vitamin A produces most of its effects by over-keratinization of epithelium. The B-vitamin group plays an important role as co-enzymes in intermediary carbohydrate metabolism. Lack of vitamin C was shown (1926) by S. B. WOLBACH and P. R. HOWE to inhibit the activity of certain formative cells and the production of intercellular substances, thus promoting the hemorrhage seen in scurvy. Vitamin D acts (as we have seen) by regulating phosphate and calcium metabolism; yet in excessive amounts it can produce harmful deprivations and metastatic calcification. When vitamin K, the coagulation vitamin, is deficient, the liver does not form sufficient prothrombin, and blood coagulability is thereby lessened. It should be noted that thus far the pathology of the vitamins has been mostly limited to specific diseases caused by gross lack; we may hope that, as knowledge accumulates, less severe deficiency (hypovitaminosis) may be shown to play a less obvious, but in the sum total perhaps a more important contributory role in a wide variety of disease conditions.

The great achievement in the field of *disorders of the blood* (hemolyto-poietic system), Minot's and Castle's discovery of the cure and nature of pernicious anæmia, is described in a later section. It had been preceded by increasingly diminishing returns from detailed studies of blood-cell morphology, and it was followed by a realignment of the concepts of the anæmias in general. In the first twenty years of the twentieth century it was customary to consider a few " primary " anæmias and group all the others in an omnium gatherum of " secondary " anæmias. These latter have now been arranged in logical classifications according to size, depth of colour, degree of immaturity, fragility of the erythrocytes, and response to different therapeutic agents that are nosologically useful to the pathologist and clinically valuable to the patient in determining the best form of treatment. No longer is the occasional severe anæmia of pregnancy called pernicious because it has many large cells like true pernicious anæmia, even though both may be helped by extracts of liver. No longer are all anæmias treated indiscriminately with iron; now it is known when to give it and why it helps. The mysterious " chlorosis " of previous generations has disappeared, not only because nutritional and hygienic conditions have improved, but also because when such conditions occur, the causative factors are recognized and efficiently dealt with. To be sure, as always, much still remains to be learned; but the progress in this field stands second to few and has raised knowledge and treatment of the anæmias to a high scientific level. Lack of space prevents even the briefest consideration of the many single varieties of anæmias due to congenital deficiencies, such as chronic hemolytic anæmia (spherocytosis), sickle cell, ovalocytic, and Cooley's anæmia, hemophilia, essential thrombopenia, or to nutritional lacks or to the numerous conditions causing increased blood loss or destruction.

The " target-cell " (as named by BARRETT, 1938) was first seen by R. L. HADEN and F. D. EVANS (1937), a red cell appearing as a bull's-eye of deeper width in the centre (i.e., in profile like a Mexican hat, instead of a dumbbell). As it has recently (1945) been produced experimentally by W. N. Valentine and J. V. Neel in hypertonic plasma, it is regarded as an erythrocyte whose envelope form is reversible and larger than its contents. Infectious mononucleosis, though described in the previous century by the Russian N.F. FILATOV, remained unnoticed for a few decades. Its peculiar blood picture was described (1920) by D. H. SPRUNT (b. 1900) and F. A. EVANS (b. 1889), who also named it. A peculiarity, the antibody response to foreign, or heterophil, antigens, was detected by J. R. PAUL (b. 1893) and W. W. BUNNELL (b. 1902) and has proved highly useful in diagnosis. An interesting sidelight is thrown on hematological progress by the steps of advancing knowledge of the frequently fatal disease of infants: *erythroblastosis fœtalis*. Long recognized only by its gross clinical signs, examples of the one disease were spread over three unrelated terms: icterus gravis, hydrops fœtalis, and hemorrhagic disease of the newborn. Then, blood-cell studies having shown that erythroblasts were greatly increased in all three of these conditions, they were grouped under the hemotologic name given above. Only recently has it become recognized that this also is secondary to destruction of fetal blood due to an incompatibility between the Rh factor of the fetal erythrocytes and the maternal blood plasma.

Classification of the neutrophil leucocytes according to their age by ARNETH (1904) and others, by the shape of the nuclei, and of old and young lymphocytes, has helped in evaluating their disease processes, especially when correlated with bone-marrow and lymph-node changes, and with classification into degenerated, hypoplastic, or cytolytic groups. Malignant neutropenia (agranulocytosis, P. K. BROWN, 1902; SCHULTZ, 1922) has declined in interest and importance since it has been shown (Kracke) to be mostly due to abuse of certain coal-tar drugs and thus has come under control.

The cumulative work of many investigators has identified the leukemias as malignant neoplasms of the blood cell involved, whether myeloid, lymphatic, monocytic, plasmocytic, or even eosinophilic or basophilic. It is also recognized as often masquerading with low leucocyte counts, the paradoxical " aleukemic leukemia." An apparently precancerous condition, "giant follicular hyperplasia " of spleen and lymph nodes, was described by N. E. BRILL, G. BAEHR, and N. ROSENTHAL in 1925. It has since been found frequently to terminate as leukemia or sarcoma of the lymphocyte or monocyte.

Knowledge of the *pathology of the heart*, as in other parts of the body, has more and more overlapped the progress in clinical medicine, in which section some of this progress will be referred to. Maude ABBOTT's (1869–1940) life-long cultivation of the field of congenital heart disease culminated in an *Atlas,* collecting and classifying over one thousand cases. Some of the twentieth-century landmarks in this field are the " EISENMENGER complex " (1897) (like Fallot's tetralogy except that the pulmonary artery is dilated); R. LUTEMBACHER's syndrome (interatrial defect associated with mitral stenosis (1916); A. SPITZER's (b. 1868) theory of incomplete torsion of the developing heart, giving a logical basis and new terminology (replacing Rokitansky's) for the various transpositions of the four heart valves.

The predominant role of coronary sclerosis in the production of angina pectoris was established by findings at autopsy and by animal experimentation. However, as C. S. KEEFER was among the first to emphasize (1928), angina is a functional state caused by myocardial anoxia, and thus may have various causes.

Though the cardiac arrhythmias are all examples of functional pathology, they are more suitably considered in the section on internal medicine; only the heart-blocks have shown demonstrable lesions — and then not always — such as fibrosis of His's bundle, gumma, thrombosis of the nutrient artery. In the WOLFF-PARKINSON-WHITE syndrome (1930) the opposite is found: namely, a shortening of the P-R interval with the ECG signs of bundle branch block. In some cases, as F. C. WOOD and others have shown, this may be due to an accessory bundle of conductive tissue bridging the auriculo-ventricular gap. The long known but little understood skin disease *lupus erythematosus* has in recent years become recognized in an important systemic or " disseminated " variety (W. H. GOECKERMAN, 1923). Its cardiac manifestations, not unlike those of rheumatic fever, were identified by Libman and Bernard Sachs in 1924.

Intracranial aneurysms have only been properly evaluated in recent years. H. M. TURNBULL (1918), C. P. SYMONDS (1924), and M. SCHMIDT (1931) have established their non-syphilitic origin, also their chief distribution in the mid-cerebral and basilar arteries, and their frequent production of intracranial hemorrhage in the young. The long history of aortic dissecting aneurysm (a long cylinder of blood in the middle coat of the aorta, which has been known to extend throughout the aorta's entire length) has had a new turn in the present century. This dramatic picture was first described in England by F. NICHOLLS in 1763 in the body of King George II, who died from a ruptured heart. Earlier (1728) experiments on aortas of cadavers led Nicholls to the erroneous conclusion that the condition was produced by a great increase of blood pressure tearing the intima, the blood being contained in the aortic wall by the tougher adventitia. Recognized by Morgagni (*De Sedibus*, 1761) and named by Laënnec, it was first diagnosed during life by W. P. Swain and P. M. Latham. Emphasis on the importance of the medial coat of the aorta, first raised by Henderson (1843), increased gradually following endorsement by Rokitansky and T. B. PEACOCK (1812–1882). C. W. Pennock's (1799–1867) experiments (1838), like Nicholls's, are examples of logical work retarding progress by reaching erroneous conclusions. The nature of the condition was explained (1910) by V. BABES and T. MIRONESCU on the basis of a preceding lesion in the media and established by J. ERDHEIM's (b. 1874) description (1930) of the cystic degeneration of media that is often found. Hemorrhage from the vasa vasorum has also been incriminated as a cause (M. D. TYSON, M. C. WINTERNITZ, 1937).

The pathology of the liver has been illuminated in recent years by increase in the knowledge of different types of sclerosis. To the hobnail liver described by Laënnec, the *hepar lobatum* of syphilis, and the sclerosis resulting from bile-duct obstruction or cardiac congestion, there have been added the various pigment and silicotic cirrhoses, the scarred livers of postnecrotic cirrhosis (B. MOORE, 1944), and the obscure, symptomless cirrhosis of Wilson's Disease. Much has been learned, too, but much remains to be learned, about the constellation of causes that produce them. V. C. Hanot's hypertrophic variety has been practically abandoned as an independent variety. The recrudescence on a large scale of epidemic hepatitis in World War II has explained most phases of this disease, and incidentally shown that the ordinary " acute catarrhal jaundice " is a sporadic variety of a condition whose epidemicity is peculiarly associated with wars. Instead of being due to a largely imaginary duodenal catarrh (Virchow, Frerichs) that temporarily obstructs the bile ducts — imaginary as cases did not come to autopsy — it has been shown (B. Lucké, 1944, and others) to be due to specific, seldom fatal infection that destroys the liver cells in large numbers. As W. G. MacCallum and G. H. Whipple demonstrated some years ago, liver and bile-duct cells have great powers of regeneration, and especially here, where the stroma is spared, so that their restitution is usually complete.

A better comprehension of *renal diseases*, the classification of which has proved troublesome since the time of Richard Bright, has followed the work of F. Volhard and T. Fahr (1914) on the nephroses and the nephroscleroses, and of M. Löhlein (1911) on non-suppurative embolic nephritis, such as follows subacute endocarditis; as a result, the simple grouping, of the previous generation, of large and small white and red kidneys into acute and chronic parenchymatous and interstitial nephritis has been replaced by a more accurate if more cumbersome classification. The term " Bright's disease," as H. A. Christian and others advocate, however, is wisely retained to indicate the heterogeneous group of chronic kidney disorders that tend to produce renal insufficiency and uremia. The true inflammatory glomerular nephritis has become accepted as relatively uncommon and usually recognized in the late fibrotic stage; but pyelonephritis, in its chronic form, has become an able substitute as a contributor to the Bright's-disease group (Soma Weiss, 1939). Another large group is that of the nephroses (a poor term that has served a useful purpose since introduced by F. Mueller, 1905). These degenerations of the tubules have been divided into several kinds — simple albuminous (T. Fahr, A. Epstein), lipoid (F. Munk, 1913), amyloid, cholemic — which give characteristic clinical pictures. The influence of Sir W. W. Gull's and H. G. Sutton's arteriocapillary fibrosis is especially seen in the development of knowledge of the other great contributor to Bright's disease — namely, arteriolar nephrosclerosis (Fahr). In this picture — whether slowly developing in the benign form or rapidly in the malignant — high blood pressure shares the field with the renal symptoms. It is in this group, too, that the experimental method has been especially helpful: H. Goldblatt (b. 1891) has produced in animals a similar picture by cutting down the blood supply to a kidney, thereby developing in the tissue an excess of pressor substances, which raise the blood pressure much as happens in man (I. H. Page, 1901). These substances were first detected by R. Tigerstedt in 1898. Intercapillary glomerulo-sclerosis, found so consistently associated with diabetes mellitus was described by P. Kimmelstiel (b. 1900) and C. Wilson in 1936. Recently a number of accidents (such as crushing injury, incompatible transfusions, snake venoms, sulfonamide poisoning, etc.) have been shown by various investigators to cause destructive lesions in limited areas of the kidney, which have been grouped under the appropriate term: "lower nephron syndrome" (hemoglobinuric nephrosis).

Among the twentieth-century pathologists who have attained recognition, one turns in the earlier part of the century to the eminent but waning influence of Germany and Austria for such names as: L. Aschoff (1866–1942), M. Borst (b. 1869), H. Chiari (1851–1916), A. Ghon (1866–1936), W. Hueck (b. 1882), W. Löhlein (b. 1882), O. Lubarsch (1860–1933),

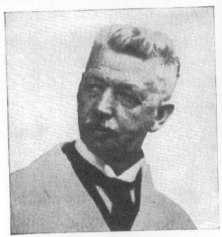

459. *Ludwig Aschoff.*
(Snapshot in autopsy room, Philadelphia General Hospital, 1926.)

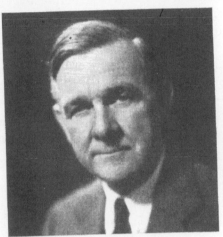

460. *George H. Whipple, Nobel Laureate, 1934.*

F. Marchand (1846–1928), J. Orth (1847–1923), G. Schmorl (1861–1932), O. Stoerk (1876–1926). Germanic pathology, like its other specialties, never recovered from World War I, and its recovery from the effect of World War II will be even more difficult. In Great Britain, where research resources have been more freely applied to other disciplines, in addition to those already mentioned, A. E. Boycott, E. H. Kettle (1882–1936), Sir Robert Muir (b. 1864), and M. J. Stewart (b. 1885) are representative of sound teachers and students of the subject. In France, C. Oberling (b. 1895), G. Roussy (b. 1874); in Switzerland, M. Askanazy (b. 1865), R. Rössle (b. 1876); among the Spaniards, G. Marañon (b. 1887); in Holland, H. T. Deelman (b. 1892), and N. P. Tendeloo (b. 1864) stand out. Several Italians have already been mentioned in the section on Anatomy. In America the older generation of pathologic anatomists, such as W. T. Councilman (1854–1933), James Ewing (1866–

1943), W. G. MacCallum (1874–1944), F. B. Mallory (1862–1941), W. Ophüls (1871–1933), T. M. Prudden (1849–1934), A. J. Smith (1863–1926), A. S. Warthin (1866–1931), and J. H. Wright (1869–1928) were succeeded by the more functionally and experimentally minded, such as Simon Flexner (1863–1946), L. Hektoen (b. 1863), O. Klotz (1878–1936), R. M. Pearce (1874–1930), H. G. Wells (1875–1943), F. C. Wood (b. 1869), G. H. Whipple (b. 1878), and others who founded the American Society of Experimental Pathology (1913). Worthy representatives of this trend today fill the chairs and senior positions of the leading medical schools of the country.

7. Microbiology

At the turn of the century, bacteriology was found to be progressing along the lines established by the pioneers of the previous quarter-century, but not at the same prodigious speed. Chief among discoveries of specific organisms causing disease was that of *Spirochæta pallida* (*Treponema pallidum*), which in 1905 was shown by Fritz Schaudinn (1871–1906) and Eric Hoffmann (b. 1868) to be the cause of syphilis. Hideyo Noguchi (1876–1928), a tremendously active investigator, demonstrated the relation of *T. pallidum* to neurosyphilis, explored the cutaneous reactions in syphilis, and developed special methods for the difficult cultivation of spirochetes. He cultivated *Bartonella* from Oroya fever and verruga peruana; but erroneously claimed to have discovered bacterial causes of trachoma, poliomyelitis, and rabies. Searching for the cause of yellow fever in Mexico, he unfortunately isolated the *Leptospira* of Weil's disease from cases harbouring both diseases. Having vaccinated himself against the supposed cause, which he had named *L. icteroides*, he proceeded to West Africa, without the protection that he expected, and succumbed to an attack of yellow fever.

The ripe apples of the previous period had mostly fallen, but some further specific organisms connected with specific diseases were isolated, such as T. Bordet's and Gengou's *B. pertussis* (whooping cough, 1906); Bruce's *B. melitensis* (Malta fever, 1907); B. L. F. Bang's (1848–1932) *B. abortus* (infectious abortion of cattle, 1897); G. W. McCoy's (b. 1876) and C. V. Chapin's (b. 1856) *B. tularense* (tularemia) (1911). Scarlet fever was definitely linked with streptococci in 1923 by the work of A. Dochez and (independently, 1923) of George (b. 1881) and Gladys H. Dick (b. 1881), though various strains of streptococci are capable of producing the disease and may under appropriate conditions produce various other lesions. However, a few obvious and important infections, even when the so-called virus diseases have been accounted for, still remain unexplained — rheumatic fever, for example.

IMMUNOLOGY. Investigation of the nature of the body's reaction to harmful invaders — already initiated by the work mentioned in the previous chapter — has grown to such degree that it almost constitutes a medical specialty of its own. In addition to natural and acquired resistance to diseases — immunity — it was found paradoxically by Portier and Richet that exposure to certain animal poisons produced increased sensitivity to infection (1902), a condition called anaphylaxis (ἀνά, here used as again; φυλάξις, protection), as distinguished from prophylaxis and immunity. Such sensitivity was soon found to occur in the case of many other proteins than those of bacteria — drug and food idiosyncrasies, sensitivity to pollen (rose cold and hay fever), to animal proteins such as horse dandruff, and in serum sickness (here a

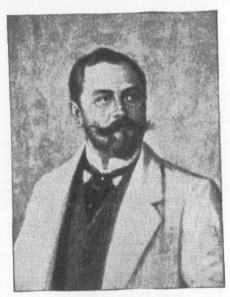

461. *Fritz Schaudinn.*

reaction occurs after administration of foreign serum such as diphtheria antitoxin). All of these have been grouped together (1907) by C. von PIRQUET (1874–1929) under the term " allergy " (ἄλλος, other, ἔργον, activity). The discovery was made (1903) by N. M. ARTHUS (b. 1862) that gangrene and ulceration are caused at the site of a second injection of horse serum. The " Arthus phenomenon " is now recognized as a form of allergy. Other important steps in the development of this field were the work of von Pirquet and Schick on serum sickness (1905), and that (1906) of M. J. ROSENAU (1869–1946) and J. F. ANDERSON (b. 1873). Skin reactions have afforded useful diagnostic tests such as the application of tuberculin by scarification (von Pirquet), by inunction (Moro), or subcutaneously (Mantoux). Another local skin reaction to bacterial filtrates was observed (1927) by G. SCHWARTZMAN (b. 1896), wherein injection of a filtrate from a bacterial culture into the skin of a rabbit, when followed in twenty-four hours by an intravenous injection, the skin showed severe hemorrhagic necrosis. The more general fact has been established by V. MENKIN (b. 1901) that substances circulating in the blood stream tend to effuse into sites of local inflammation, there to produce protective or harmful effects according to circumstances.

The intracellular "Donovan bodies" of the venereal disease *granuloma inguinale* were found (1905) by Major C. DONOVAN (b. 1863) packed in the cytoplasm of phagocytes. Though accepted as a true cause of the disease and apparently cultivated by some investigators, their true nature has not yet been determined.

Sir Almroth Edward WRIGHT (1861–1947), Professor of Pathology in the British Army Medical School at Netley, advanced the whole subject of vaccination by the use of autogenous vaccines (that is, vaccines prepared from the very bacteria that were being harboured by the patient) and by antityphoid immunization with cultures of typhoid bacilli killed by heat (1896–1909). When the exact minimum lethal temperature for the bacilli was established, this method proved very successful, so that when applied on a huge scale in the First World War, it practically eliminated military epidemics of typhoid and was a large factor in making this the first war in which fewer died from infectious diseases than from missiles. This was first successfully demonstrated on a large scale by Major F. F. RUSSELL (b. 1870) in 1912, during the mobilization of the U. S. Army on the Mexican border. Wright also discovered " opsonins " (1903), substances in the blood that " butter," or prepare, harmful substances for ingestion; he also introduced the " opsonic index " as a measure of the individual's resistance to pathogenic bacteria.

A milestone in serological diagnosis was the introduction of the Wassermann reaction, invented in 1906 as a complement-fixation test for the diagnosis of syphilis, by August von WASSERMANN (1866–1925), director of the Institute for Experimental Therapy at Berlin (in the suburb of Dahlem). True complement-fixation tests have been useful in various other diseases; and other simpler serum tests for syphilis have since been devised. The discovery (1902–43) by Karl LANDSTEINER (1868–1943) that normal human blood can be divided into four or more blood groups, some of which will hemolyze others, first permitted the extensive use of blood transfusion on a rational basis as a valuable, often life-saving form of therapy.

Recently (1940) Landsteiner and Wiener have demonstrated another factor, common in human blood (called the Rh factor because it is present in Rhesus monkey blood), which has iso-immunizing properties. This explains many of the transfusion accidents in supposedly " compatible " blood and also establishes the nature of the blood disease called *erythroblastosis foetalis*. In very recent times it has been found that blood can be kept outside the body for long periods, even many weeks, without deterioration, and the establishment of " blood banks " has further extended the usefulness of this method. Landsteiner, a member of the Rockefeller Institute of New York, also made important contributions on the virus of poliomyelitis, on the pathogenesis of paroxysmal hemoglobinuria, and on fundamental phenomena of antigens and of anaphylaxis.

The destruction of bacteria by an invisible but reproducible agent, bacteriophage, was discovered by F. W. TWORT in 1915, and again by F. D'HE-RELLE (b. 1873) in 1917. The several varieties of bacteriophage are now accepted as belonging to the rapidly growing class of filterable viruses and have actually been made visible by the electron micrograph as minute bodies adhering to the bacterial cell wall (see section on Biology).

An important bacterial phenomenon in human disease is the existence of " CARRIERS," apparently normal individuals who, however, liberate pathogenic organisms over indefinite periods and thus may be important factors in the dissemination of disease.

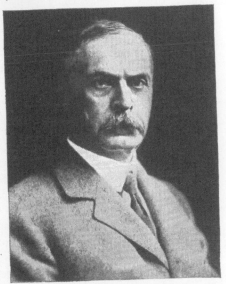

462. K. Landsteiner, Nobel Laureate, 1930.

Diphtheria carriers had been found in the nineties; and P. GUTTMANN showed (1892) that cholera vibrio persisted for a time after recovery from Asiatic cholera. After typhoid fever, especially, virulent organisms may continue to be excreted in the faeces (from foci in the gall bladder, or less often in the intestine) throughout life. The control of " Typhoid Mary," a cook whose trail was marked by numerous typhoid outbreaks (G. A. SOPER, 1908), presented interesting and difficult complications, as might easily be imagined. Among other diseases in which carriers play a role should be mentioned cerebrospinal meningitis (H. Albrecht and A. Ghon, 1901), and bacillary dysentery (H. Conradi, 1903; G. A. Charleton and L. Jehle, 1904.)

True-breeding VARIANTS (mutants?) of bacterial forms, though known for many years (Neisser, 1906; Massini, 1907, B. coli mutabile), have only recently been recognized as important, both theoretically and practically, in relation to virulence of infection (J. A. Arkwright, 1921; P. de Kruif, 1921). " Rough " and " smooth " colonies and other variant colony forms, with corresponding differences in cultural and immunological reactions, motility, and so on, are opening new vistas beyond the rigid bacteriology of earlier days and have already illuminated some of its unsolved problems.

Profitable knowledge of theoretical and practical value about the chemical composition of bacteria has been acquired in recent years. Starting with the discoveries by A. Dochez, O. T. Avery, and their colleagues (1913–17) of the antigenic relations that led to the many types that we now know, a stable " specific soluble substance " was isolated by them from the blood and urine and the culture fluids of rabbits and persons infected with the pneumococcus, and similar substances were found for other bacteria (H. Zinsser and J. T. Parker, 1923). Avery and various collaborators next found (1923–7) that they were polysaccharides, which in the case of pneumococci showed type specificity and that the capsule was largely carbohydrate. They have demonstrated (1944) that F. J. GRIFFITH's conversion (1928) of one biologically specific type of pneumococcus into another was due to the action of a " transforming principle," with nucleic acid as the fundamental unit, and that once the conversion was effected, the newly acquired character was transmitted without further addition of the transforming principle. It is unfortunate that consideration of a possible analogy with the origin of new species and the pathogenesis of cancer cells (A. HADDOW, 1944) is inappropriate in a historical study.

The role of lipoid and protein fractions of the tubercle bacillus had been considerably elucidated in recent years. For instance, Florence R. SABIN (b. 1871), working on the lipoid fractions characterized by J. F. ANDERSON (b. 1873), has identified the phthioic acid of the phosphatide fraction as the stimulant toward tubercle-formation. The protein fraction, studied especially by Florence SEIBERT (b. 1897) and E. R. LONG (b. 1890), contains two proteins with differing antigenic specificities which are thought to be responsible for the tuberculin reaction.

Further progress was made in establishing the role of *insect vectors* in transmitting disease; it has become known, for instance, that not infrequently more than one vector may be responsible for a given disease. The role of vectors has been especially prominent in the *Rickettsial diseases*.

Charles NICOLLE (1866–1936), director of the Pasteur Institute of Tunis, was a philosopher, a poet, and an outstanding scholar who accomplished important work in leishmaniasis, and was the first to show that the infecting agent of typhus fever was transmitted by the body louse (1909). Nicolle also claimed to have accomplished a successful immunization against trachoma and was one of the first to establish the prophylactic value of serum obtained from convalescents in typhoid and in measles. Louse transmission was demonstrated in 1910 for Mexican typhus (*tabardillo*) by H. T. RICK-

ETTS (1871–1910), who died of this disease in that year. Four years earlier this brilliant investigator, who was one of the many martyrs to the diseases that they were investigating, had shown that Rocky Mountain spotted fever (caused by *Dermacentroxenus rickettsi*) is transmitted by the wood-tick (*Dermacentor occidentalis*). The name *Rickettsia* has been appropriately given to this whole group of micro-organisms whose position in the scale seems to be between those of " viruses " and bacteria. It is now known that the rat flea can (as in the case of bubonic plague) transmit the New World or murine type of typhus and that rat lice and dog ticks (*D. variabilis*) are also incriminated. Murine typhus may exist endemically in mild form; and the epidemic (classical) variety, under the name of Brill's disease, has been seen in mild, sporadic form in Jews recently immigrating to America. The " trench fever " and " Wolhynian fever " of World War I and " Tsutsuga-mushi fever " and " scrub " or " mite typhus " of World War II are other varieties of this protean disease, which constitutes one of the most " griev-ous visitations of mankind, by war, famine and misery," as Hirsch puts it. " Q fever " (Q standing for Queensland) is the latest of the Rickettsial dis-eases to assume some world wide importance. First described in 1937 by E. H. DERRICK, it was shown in the same year by F. M. BURNET and M. FREEMAN to be caused by a *Rickettsia*, since known as *R. burneti*. It is another agent capable of frequently causing so-called " atypical pneu-monia."

FILTERABLE VIRUSES. A most actively progressing field at present is the study of the so-called viruses in relation to disease. The word " virus " for many centuries has signified the poison from a living being causing an in-fectious disease. It now is usually conferred specifically upon the group of very small, mostly filter-passing micro-organisms, at present known as " virus bodies." This is not a satisfactory term, either. Indeed, criteria (such as size, filtration, mode of transmission and cultivation, appearance) for es-tablishing the virus cause of a disease are still multiple and variable in dif-ferent instances (see table).

These minute bodies, so small that they pass through porcelain filters and are mostly invisible under the ordinary microscope, have now been convicted as the cause of literally hundreds of diseases of man (the exanthemata of child-hood, mumps, smallpox, rabies, poliomyelitis, influenza, several types of encepha-litis, yellow fever, and so on) and of lower animals and plants. In fact, the stream of new discoveries of virus causes of infectious diseases, of the structural and functional properties of the virus bodies and their methods of cultivation, has reproduced in this century an exciting and brilliant situation comparable to the state of bacteriology at the end of the previous century. Viruses were first

CHRONOLOGICAL LIST OF SOME "VIRUS" CAUSES OF DISEASE AND THEIR PIONEER INVESTIGATORS

Date	Name of Virus	Disease	Investigators
1892	V. of Molluscum contagiosum	Molluscum contagiosum	EB: McCallum (Lipschuetz, 1907). IB: Henderson, 1841 F: Juliusberg, 1905
1892	V. of mosaic disease	mosaic disease of tobacco	Ivanow, W. P. T.: A Mayer, 1886. S & crystals: Stanley, 1935. EM: Kausche & Ruska, 1939
1898	V. of foot & mouth disease	foot & month disease	Loeffler & Frosch. C: Hecke, 1933. EM: M. von Ardenne & G. Pyl, 1940
1905	V. of rabies	rabies	IB, F: A. Negri. C: Webster & Clow, 1936. S: Galloway & Elford, 1936. T: Pasteur, 1881
1907	V. of warts	infectious warts	F: Ciuffo. T: Jadassohn, 1896
1907	V. of vaccinia & variola	vaccinia & smallpox	EB: Paschen. C: Steinhardt, 1913. IB: Guarnieri, 1894 (1892).
1907	V. of trachoma	trachoma	EM: R. H. Green, T. F. Anderson, & J. E. Smadel, 1942 IB: L. Halberstaedter & S. von Prowazek. EB (T?): K. Lindner, 1910; D. Thygeson, 1935. T(?): Hess & Römer, 1906. F: Nicolle et al, 1912
1907	V. of dengue	dengue	F: Ashburn & Craig. T: Cleland, Bradley, McDonald, 1916; (?) Graham, 1903. C, IB?: Shortt, Rao & Swaninath
1909	V. of poliomyelitis	poliomyelitis	F: S. Flexner & P. A. Lewis
1911	V. of chickenpox	varicella (chickenpox)	IB: Aragao; Gins, 1918. T: Rivers, 1928
1911	V. of measles	measles	T, F: Anderson & Goldberger. EB: Coles, 1937
1911	V. of fowl sarcoma	fowl sarcoma	T, F: P. Rous. C: Rous and Murphy, 1912
1913	V. of sacbrood	sacbrood in honey bees	F: G. F. White
1915	Bacteriophage group	(virus destroyers of bacteria)	F: Twort; d'Herelle, 1917. M: Schlesinger, 1933. EM: S. E. Luria & T. F. Anderson, 1942
1920	V. of herpes	"fever blister"	T: Grueters; Lipschuetz, 1921. C: Parker & Nye, 1925
1923	Virus III	(found in rabbits)	T: Rivers & Tiller. S: Bechhold & Schlesinger, 1933. C: Ivanovics & Roscoe, 1936
1926	V. of dog distemper	dog distemper	F: G. W. Dunkin & P. P. Laidlaw. IB: Lentz, 1909; de Monbreun, 1937. T: Carre, 1905
1928	V. of yellow fever	yellow fever	Contagious: A. Laosson, 1882 T, F: Reed et al, 1901. T: A. Stokes et al, 1928. IB: Margarinos, 1928. S: Bauer & Thomas, 1932. C: Haagen & Theiler, 1932; Elmendorf & H. Smith (egg, 1937)
1929	V. of common cold	"cold"	T: Kruse, 1914. F, C: Dochez et al, 1931; Hyde & Chapman, 1937

Date	Virus	Disease	References
1930	V. of ectromelia	(a disease of mice)	Marchal; Ledingham, 1931. *EB*: Barnard & Elford. *C*: Paschen & Nauck, 1936
1930	V. of psittacosis	psittacosis (ornithosis)	*T, F*: Bedson, Western & Simpson. *EB*: Coles, Lewinthal, 1930. *S*: Lewinthal, 1935
1931	Virus of swine influenza *H. influenzae suis* (symbiosis)	swine influenza	*T, F*: R. E. Shope. *EM*: A. R. Taylor et al, 1944
1931	V. of equine encephalomyelitis	equine encephalomyelitis	K. F. Meyer; Haring & Howitt. *EM*: A. R. Taylor et al, 1942
1932	V. of *Lymphogranuloma venereum*	*Lymphogranuloma venereum*	*T, F*: S. Hellerstrom & E. Wassen (reported 1930). *C, EB*: Miyagawa et al, 1935
1932	V. of louping ill	louping ill of sheep	*T, F*: Greig. *S*: Elford & Galloway. *C*: Rivers & Fite, 1933
1933	V. of influenza	influenza	*T, F*: Smith, Andrewes & Laidlaw. *C*: Francis & Magill, 1934. *EM*: *A & B strains*: Francis, 1937. *S*: W. J. Elford et al., 1936. *EM*: L. A. Chambers et al., 1943; A. R. Taylor et al., 1943
1933	V. of rabbit papilloma	papilloma of rabbits	*T, F*: R. E. Shope. *EM*: D. G. Sharp et al.
1933	V. of St. Louis encephalitis	epidemic encephalitis (type A)	*T*: R. S. Muckenfuss et al. *S*: Bauer; Fite & Webster, 1934 (cp. v. Economo's lethargic encephalitis, 1917), and Japanese encephalitis (*T*: Kawamura, 1936)
1934	V. of choriomeningitis	choriomeningitis (?)	*T, F*: C. Armstrong & R. D. Lillie; Scott & Rivers, 1935
1934	V. of frog carcinoma	renal carcinoma in *Rana pipiens*	*T, IB*: B. Lucke. *F(?)*: Lucke, 1938
1934	V. of acute meningo-pneumonitis	(respiratory disease of man)	*T*: Francis & T. P. Magill
1936	V. of mammary cancer(?)	mammary cancer in mice	*T*: J. J. Bittner
1942	V. of epidemic hepatitis (?)	epidemic hepatitis	*T*: H. Voegt; G. M. Findlay & N. H. Martin; J. D. S. Cameron, 1943; F. O. MacCallum et al., J. R. Neefe et al., 1944. *F*: Brit. Off. of Health; W. P. Havens, 1944

The date is usually that of publication. An earlier date in parentheses is that of discovery or report.

? – Probably a "virus disease," but not yet adequately demonstrated.
C – Cultivated artificially.
EB – Elementary bodies described by.
F – Filterability established by.
IB – Inclusion bodies described by.
M – Morphology observed (usually by electron microscope).
EM – Electron micrograph (includes size).
S – Size (estimated or measured).
T – Transmitted by infective material.
See Bibliography Chapter xxi, VII, for references to the work cited in this table.

detected in animals by Loeffler and Paul Frosch (1860–1928) in foot-and-mouth disease (1898), and in plants by W. P. Ivanow in the mosaic disease of tobacco (1892). The virus of tobacco mosaic has been shown (1935) by W. M. Stanley (b. 1904) to be a rod-shaped nucleoprotein " macromolecule " that retains its pathogenicity and reproductive power even after repeated washing and crystallization. This extraordinary observation is so widely divergent from traditional views of the living nature of the causes of infectious diseases that it suggests interesting speculations as to the lowest forms of living matter, and even as to life itself.

The obstacle that viruses, unlike bacteria, demand living material in which to be propagated (i.e., were obligate intracellular parasites) was overcome when Ernest Goodpasture (b. 1886) found (1931) that this could be readily supplied in the form of fertile eggs, in which viruses grew luxuriantly after introduction through a window cut in the shell. This soon was found to be a good source of smallpox vaccine, to be followed shortly by F. M. Burnet's (b. 1889) growth, in Australia (1935), of different strains of influenza virus, thus permitting the preparation of influenza vaccines in large quantities. By the use of this method, instead of inoculation into mouse brains, the Rockefeller Foundation has accomplished large-scale production of yellow-fever vaccine. Another important step was made by Herald R. Cox (b. 1907), of the U. S. Public Health Service, in demonstrating (1938) that Rickettsia, the cause of the devastating typhus fever and the tick-borne Rocky Mountain spotted fever (described, 1903, by J. F. Anderson [b. 1873]), could also be grown by the egg method. Though drugs have thus far been impotent against virus diseases, potent sera appear to have been prepared against some of these diseases; fortunately there has not yet been good opportunity to try out their value. Though many virus diseases confer lasting immunity, it is widely believed that immunity persists only as long as living virus is present in body cells, and artificially produced immunity to them is still in the stage of history in the making. Viruses were until recently of interest in medicine as disease-producers so small that they were invisible with the light microscope and could pass through porcelain filters. They have already become an important group of pathogenic microbes which have several characteristic properties in common, some already showing detectible structural organization, and some tending, like bacteria, to form classifiable groups. Thus the group of psittacosis, trachoma, inclusion blennorrhea, and lymphopathia venerea have in common certain properties such as unusual staining reactions, antigenic relationships, and (except psittacosis) response to sulfonamides.

Size. The approximate size of the " elementary bodies " (the unit corresponding to a single bacterium) until recently had to be estimated from the size of the filter pores through which they could pass or from the velocity of sedimentation in an ultracentrifuge; now they can be directly observed and measured in the electron microscope. They vary in size from those just visible in the light microscope, such as that of Psittacosis (275 mμ), about one third the diameter of *B. prodigiosus*, down almost to those of macro-molecules. The smallest of these virus bodies have diameters (louping ill of sheep, 19 mμ; poliomyelitis, 12; foot and mouth disease, 10; S 13 and bacteriophage, 10) that approximate those of protein molecules such as serum globulin (65 mμ) and egg albumin (3.9 mμ). It is difficult to picture such a small body as being a living organism, especially as various viruses are known to have various chemical constituents; and it is quite premature as yet to assign them a position in the biological kingdoms. At present they stand between the molecules of the chemist and the organisms of the bacteriologist. With recognition of the great variation in size of these virus elementary bodies, the importance to function of structure rather than size is emphasized. Possible shifts in such fundamental concepts as the microbial and cell theories are suggested, a state of affairs that seems to be characteristic of present-day science in general.

The " cell inclusions," characteristic of many virus diseases, were first described (1844) in *molluscum contagiosum* by Henderson, and again in fowl pox by Rivolta (1865). They were seen by G. GUARNIERI in smallpox (1894) — called *cytoryctes variolæ* — and in brain cells in hydrophobia (1903) by A. NEGRI (1876–1912).

Yellow fever, which had been controlled through suppression of its mosquito vector in the Canal Zone, has had many organisms proposed as its cause — all eventually to be abandoned until its specific virus was demonstrated (pub. 1928) by Adrian STOKES (1887–1927), J. H. BAUER (b. 1890), and N. P. HUDSON (b. 1895). They not only succeeded in infecting monkeys with the disease, but showed that the infectious agent was a true virus readily passing through dense porcelain filters, thus confirming the earlier work of Reed and others. It was later shown to have a diameter of 22 mμ (i.e., extremely small even among the virus bodies).

Influenza had long been thought to be due to Pfeiffer's *Hemophilus influenzæ*, but this, like Olitsky's *Bacterium pneumosintes*, is now known to be merely a secondary invader. The virus nature of influenza was first suggested by Nicolle's successful experiments (1919) on monkeys and human volunteers; but the virus was not finally isolated until 1932 (date of publication) by W. SMITH (b. 1897), F. W. ANDREWES (1859–1932), and Sir Patrick LAIDLAW (1881–1940), who were fortunate in finding first the ferret and then mice to be suitable for virus transmission. The related swine influenza — first recognized clinically in 1918 — was shown (1931) by R. E. SHOPE (b. 1901) to require the combined attack of a virus, which alone was harmless, and a small bacillus (*H. influenzæ suis*), which produced the characteristic disease after the virus had prepared the way. Analogies with human influenza and the common cold are readily suggested. The *common cold*, the commonest of all respiratory infections and the greatest cause of absenteeism due to illness, has been widely accepted, since the work of A. Dochez and others (1929), as due to a virus that often paves the way for secondary invaders, not only of more severe upper respiratory infections but also of pneumonia, poliomyelitis, meningitis, and the like. Such considerations, however, are not yet suitable even for history in the making.

Virus diseases in birds have been shown to be of interest and importance (fowl plague, fowl pox, the Rous chicken sarcoma, psittacosis, etc.). The last named has in recent years acquired especial interest as being common in several species such as the pigeon and thus as the cause of many mild pneumonias in man, called " atypical " because of the difference in the disease picture from the traditional varieties and absence of the usual bacteria.

The part played by many foreign microbiologists has been indicated in the preceding pages. Some further notice follows of a few leading men in the United States and the British Empire, to which countries the role of leaders in this field seems now to have fallen.

First among British microbiologists should be mentioned Sir Patrick MANSON (1844–1922), whose work and influence, covering fifty years in two centuries, led to his designation as the " father of tropical medicine " (Professor Raphael Blanchard). His greatest discovery came while working as a young man in China (1879) — the mosquito transmission of filaria to man. This had been preceded by earlier confirmation (1877) of the presence of filaria in elephantiasis. His *Manual of Tropical Diseases*, which still continues through many editions, includes of course his own numerous original observations. He was said to be a man of great charm, interested in younger men and " helping lame dogs over stiles," yet insisting that most people had to learn to think and that the way to write well was to " know what you have to say and say it." His influence undoubtedly led to Ross's achievements in malaria, a disease that Manson is said to have produced in his son by mosquito-bite in order to convince sceptics. Returning to England in 1889, he taught tropical medicine at Livingstone College, Charing Cross and St. George's hospitals, and the Royal Free Hospital for Women, arousing the necessary interest for the foundation of the great London School of Tropical Medicine (1899). He retired in 1914, continuing to " warm both hands before the fire of life," together with fishing and " making things grow," yet maintaining to the end a constructive interest in tropical diseases. Sir Almroth Edward WRIGHT (1861–1932) also exerted great influence and was responsible for many, especially technical advances in this field. A versatile Irishman, he studied at Dublin, Leipzig, Strasbourg, and Marburg, taught at Cambridge and Sydney, was Professor of Pathology at the Army Medical School at

Netley (1892–1902), then became Professor of Experimental Pathology in the University of London. He is best known for his work on opsonins and the opsonic index (1903), the promotion of typhoid vaccination in the British army (1896–1904), and vaccinotherapy in general (1902–7). The name of Sir William Boog LEISHMAN (1865–1926), one of the many distinguished army medical officers, is perpetuated in the genus *Leishmania*, protozoa that he first saw in a case of Dumdum fever (Indian Kala azar). Major C. DONOVAN described the organism in the same year, 1903, and it was thus appropriately named *Leish-*

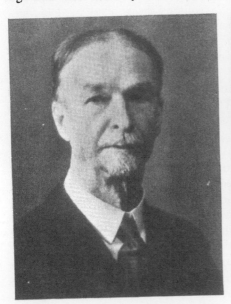

463. *Theobald Smith.*

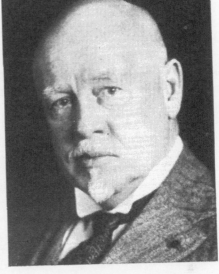

464. *William H. Welch.*

mania donovani by Laveran. Leishman finished his army career as a lieutenant-general, having succeeded Almroth Wright at Netley, was Chief Consultant and Director of Pathology in the Army Medical Department in World War I and Director General of Army Medical Services, where he was responsible for the widespread use of typhoid vaccine. Sir David BRUCE (1855–1931), another distinguished army surgeon, showed *B. melitensis* to be the cause of Malta fever (1886, pub. 1887), a problem to which he returned as head of the Malta Fever Commission, 1904–6. In 1894 he found that nagana, a fatal disease of horses and cattle, endozootic in Africa, was caused by a trypanosome, named after him *T. brucei*, which was transmitted from antelopes by the tsetse fly (*Glossina morsitans*). J. A. ARKWRIGHT (1864–1944), a martyr to the African form of relapsing fever caused by *T. duttoni*), M. H. GORDON, HORTON-SMITH, J. C. G. LEDINGHAM, F. S. LISTER (South Africa), W. J. TULLOCH, and F. W. TWORT are among other British scientists who brought lustre to this field.

Among the best-known American pathologists and bacteriologists is William Henry WELCH (1850–1934), first Professor of Pathology at Bellevue Hospital Medical College, New York, then one of the four founders of the celebrated Johns Hopkins Medical School and for many years Professor of Pathology there. He was the discoverer of *Staphylococcus epidermidis albus* and of *Bacillus aerogenes capsulatus* (which often bears his name), and he advanced our knowledge of embolism and thrombosis (1899). Still more important, however, was his influence in producing soundly trained pathologists and clinicians, who have occupied many important chairs throughout the country, and his wise guidance of the numerous institutions that sought his advice. In 1916 he became director of the newly created School of Hygiene and Public Health at Johns Hopkins, which position he relinquished after ten years to become Professor of Medical History in the same institution.

An even more eminent contributor to scientific bacteriology was Theobald SMITH (1859–1934), of Albany, New York. Before the publications of Roux and Behring, he showed that filtrates of the killed bacillus of hog cholera conferred immunity on injected animals (1886); while his demonstration (1893) of the transmission by the cattle tick of the cause of Texas cattle fever (*Pyrosoma bigeminum*, which he discovered in 1889) was an important early step in the recognition of insect vectors in disease. He discovered the highly important sensitization to specific proteins on reinoculation (1903), called " the Theobald Smith phenomenon " by Ehrlich, which was named and studied as " anaphylaxis " by Richet (1902). This has brought about the development of a separate condition: " allergy " (a term introduced by von Pirquet). Smith's differentiation of bovine from human tubercle bacilli is but one more of his many important contributions to his specialty. His modest attitude toward research in general, as well as toward his own contributions, revealed a true scientific philosopher. " Discovery," he once wrote, " should come as an adventure rather than as the result of a logical process of thought " (a variant of Pasteur's " Chance favours the prepared mind "). " A fact is worth more than theories in the long run: the theory stimulates but the fact builds."

Among other eminent American bacteriologists are V. C. VAUGHAN (1851–1929), a student of the poisons of bacteria and protein split products; Simon FLEXNER (1863–1946), first director of the Rockefeller Institute, eminent contributor to knowledge of venoms (1901), of epidemic meningitis (1909), of poliomyelitis (1910 ff.), and stimulator of productive research in many fields; Ludvig HEKTOEN (b. 1863), long Professor of Pathology at the University of Chicago, where he developed a number of eminent students of disease and himself contributed to numerous aspects of his field; William H. PARK (1863–1939), head of the New York City Health Laboratory, where he evolved the best methods of diphtheria prophylaxis; Hans ZINSSER (1878–1940), of New York and Harvard (Rickettsia), and others too numerous to mention.

We have witnessed a continuous and magnificent progression of enthusiastic and constructive investigations. Pupils and followers of Pasteur and Koch in many countries have explained many problems of the causation of infectious diseases, and have pointed the way to the successful defence against them by the organism — both individual and social. The return in very recent times to a basically clinical concept, according to which bacterial research is not sufficient to explain the disease picture always and entirely or to illuminate all disease problems, places the study of bacteriology and immunology in its proper position in the disease picture. The microbiologic concept can exert its greatest influence only if the importance of various other factors, such as the individual's constitution and environmental relationships, is given due weight. If these are recognized and investigated in their various connections, microbiology will appear in its true light as an increasingly valuable adjunct in the study of disease.

Thus in the twentieth century medical microbiology has been considerably extended in fields already outlined in the previous century. More disease-producing bacteria, and especially many filter-passing viruses, have been discovered. Progress continues to be aided by better instruments of precision, such as in very recent times the electron microscope, and by contributions from related sciences, such as the biochemical studies on the composition of the bacterial cell, and of the body fluids concerned in the resistance to infectious diseases. A considerable variability of "pure-line" strains of bacteria has been established, and in some cases correlated with changes in virulence of the organism, with obvious practical applications. Some evidence has been produced (F. Fuhrmann, 1906; R. R. Mellon, 1920; P. Hadley, 1927) that suggests even a life-cycle in these lowly forms of life. Ways of transmission of pathogenic organisms have been successfully explored, thus making possible the control of a disease by eliminating the insect carrier (vector) of the micro-organism. In the field of immunology much has been learned about the nature of both the host's protective cellular reactions to disease and all the humoral reactions to foreign protein that are grouped under the broad concept of allergy.

The pendulum has therefore swung from the optimistic expectation toward the end of the last century of a rapid conquest of all infectious diseases, to a later period of disappointment when progress was slow and the road to the elimination of many diseases remained uncharted and blocked, and now back to the present optimistic swing, less extreme than a few generations ago, but marked by much constructive activity in new lines of approach in this basic and important field of medical science.

8. Internal Medicine

The progress in the field of internal medicine during the period under consideration has been so manifold and so great that it is difficult to summarize even the most important facts. The connection of internal medicine with pathology, surgery, hygiene, and above all with physiology and microbiology has become so strong that a subdivision of the material into these

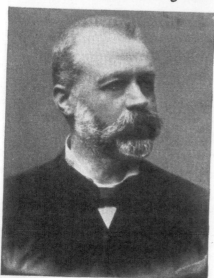

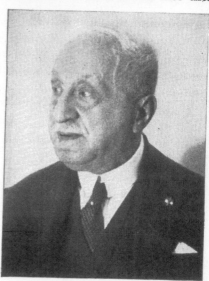

465. *Carlo Forlanini.*   466. *Edoardo Maragliano.*

sections is sometimes impossible. We cannot longer refer to internal diseases in the usual meaning of the term, because every case of so-called internal disease may call for the collaboration of the roentgenologist, the pathologist, the surgeon, or any other specialist, and its etiology, pathology, and prognosis be placed consequently in a very different light. We shall try to present in this section some of the most important progress in general medicine; to many diseases of which mention is made in this section the reader will find references in other sections.

A remarkable characteristic in general medicine during the last fifty years has been the shift in many etiological concepts of disease. Up to the end of the nineteenth century the germ was regarded as the foremost factor in the origin of disease, and this belief was the guide in clinic and therapy. With the greater knowledge of the chemical functions of the cell resulting from biochemical discoveries and general acceptance that " seed and soil " both were basic elements in normal and pathologic life, a new concept of constitutional pathology arose and a re-evaluation of the importance of chemical processes in the organism. Biochemical and pharmacological progress brought a real experimental knowledge of the reaction of organs to different chemical substances and a great number of scientifically evaluated new remedies, which effected both a revolution in therapeutics and a necessary revision of the accepted doctrines as to ways and means of healing.

The progress in diagnosis, due to the introduction of new and always better instruments of precision, illuminated the pathology of many diseases from a new point of view and opened the way to a deeper study of their origins and course. We shall try to give a summary picture of the outstanding progress in the most important groups of diseases, with occasional references to the prominent medical schools.

TUBERCULOSIS OF THE LUNGS. Artificial pneumothorax was advocated in 1882 by Carlo FORLANINI (1847–1918), of Pavia, a prominent scholar, who had devoted exhaustive studies to mechancial problems of disease. The first case was published by him in 1894, but only in later times was the value of this method recognized. In 1906 he published his results after twelve years of experience. This treatment is now universally accepted as the most efficient therapy of tuberculosis. The introduction of air into the pleural cavity for therapeutic purposes had been suggested as far back as 1822 by Carson of Liverpool. In the United States artificial pneumothorax, introduced by John B. Murphy of Chicago and his school, has become widely adopted. In 1910 Hans Christian JACOBÆUS (1879–1937), of Stockholm, worked out a method of crushing the adhesions of the chest wall. Many clinicians suggested different changes in the technique of the artificial pneumothorax, among them Maurizio ASCOLI, of Palermo, who performed bilateral pneumothorax. It appears from statistics published by Drolet that in recent years about fifty per cent of the patients in tuberculosis sanatoriums are treated by collapse therapy. If surgical methods are required, many doctors prefer lobectomy or pneumonectomy to thoracotomy. The most favourable indications are given by the cases of monolobar tuberculosis with infection of the bronchi in which an artificial pneumothorax will not be of much help.

In spite of the increased knowledge of the pathology and treatment of tuberculosis during the last fifty years, however, the decisive progress has been in public health measures, not in the field of medical therapy. The data on frequency and mortality of tuberculosis and the fight against them are to be found in the section on Public Health.

DISEASES OF THE HEART. As elsewhere, progress in the basic sciences and new methods of examination have greatly advanced our knowledge of heart disease and caused the establishment of a new specialty in the broad field of internal medicine.

Only in this century did sphygmomanometry become part of the routine physical examination; oscillometry (M. V. PACHON, b. 1867) and the measurement of venous pressure (F. MORITZ and H. von TABORA) were first introduced about 1909. After the first X-ray study of the heart (1896) by F. H. WILLIAMS (1852–1936), orthodiagraphy (outline of the heart shadow by parallel X-rays) was introduced by Moritz in 1902, and teleroentgenography by A. KÖHLER (b. 1874) in 1906. Graphic registration of the pulse was promoted when P. C. E. POTAIN investigated the venous pulse, and James Mackenzie combined the venous and arterial record in a polygram (1892), which was a fruitful analyser of the arrhythmias. The ballistocardiograph, introduced in 1937 by I. STARR (b. 1895), by recording graphically the impacts of the movement of the blood, permits calculation of the output and the work of the heart. The changes in the form of the record provide evidence of myocardial abnormalities not obtainable by any other method.

The electrocardiograph was constructed in 1903 by Willem EINTHOVEN (1860–1927) Professor of Physiology at Leiden. It consists of an extremely delicate silver-coated quartz fibre stretched between the poles of a powerful stationary electric magnet. Its very rapid response and lack of periodicity registered many previously undetected phases of the heart's action currents, with deflections that could be recorded graphically. In 1924 Einthoven was awarded the Nobel prize for this achievement. Although cardiac arrhythmias such as "intermittent pulse" had already been elucidated (1892) by Sir James MACKENZIE (1853–1925) and K. F. WENCKEBACH (1864–1940) (1903), we are indebted to electrocardiography and especially to the schools of Vienna (H. WINTERBERG and C. J. ROTHBERGER), London (Thomas Lewis), and Lyon (L. Gallavardin) for the rapid development of this field.

Electrocardiography not only detected additional kinds of arrhythmia, such as sino-auricular block and auricular flutter (W. T. RITCHIE, 1914), but also explained their nature and made possible their accurate clinical identification. It has also permitted detection of purely myocardial lesions, such as hypertrophy of one or more of the heart chambers, infraction, and trauma of the heart. Statistical analysis of electrocardiographic observations gave a sound basis to prognosis (F. A. WILLIUS). The routine use of chest leads (C. WOLFERTH and Francis WOOD, 1932; Frank WILSON, et al., 1926) further augmented our ability to diagnose and to locate myocardial lesions; the importance of electrocardiography in modern cardiology is well illustrated by the contribution of this method to the

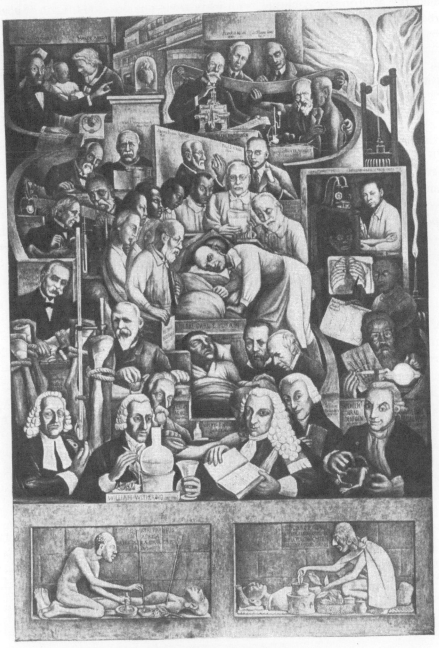

467. *History of Cardiology.*
(PANEL BY DIEGO RIVERA IN THE INSTITUTE OF CARDIOLOGY, MEXICO CITY.)

diagnosis of coronary occlusion with myocardial infarction (H. E. B. PARDEE, 1920), which was first proposed as a clinical entity by OBRASTZOV and STRASCHE-SKO (1910), and to its differentiation from angina pectoris being made possible during life by J. B. HERRICK (1912). Angina pectoris is now accepted as a functional state due to a temporarily insufficient nourishment of the heart muscle arising from coronary insufficiency analogous to the painful intermittent claudication in the leg (Thomas Lewis). Finally, the mechanisms of cardiac death have been investigated by the electrocardiographic method.

In the present century we have seen the decreasing importance of syphilis in the etiology of cardiac disease wherever modern procedures of prevention and treatment have been applied. On the other hand, the hypertensive and coronary cardiovascular diseases have increased in importance, being predominant as causes of cardiac morbidity and mortality in middle age. As for the common cause of heart disease in younger life, rheumatic fever, it is realized not only that the lesions may involve all the heart layers — endocardium, pericardium, and myocardium — but also that rheumatic carditis is the most serious disease of the adolescent.

RHEUMATIC HEART DISEASES. In 1904 Ludwig ASCHOFF (1866–1942), then pathologist at the University of Marburg, described a special kind of inflammatory nodule in the heart muscle, characteristic of the rheumatic process. A. F. COBURN (b. 1899), of New York, and others have shown (1932) that the Aschoff bodies are the late reaction following an initial hemorrhage and necrosis. The problem of the origin of rheumatic fever is not yet solved (Homer SWIFT), but it is admitted that a hemolytic streptococcus is probably the bacteriological agent concerned, though bacteria are not found in its lesions. The two most favoured interpretations of the disease, as a peculiar manifestation of streptococcic infection or as an allergic reaction, are not reciprocally exclusive, though the " constellation " of the causation of the disease still remains obscure.

The untiring work on *congenital cardiac defects* of Maude ABBOTT and others has recently produced a brilliant result in the successful ligature and section of the patent ductus arteriosus (R. E. GROSS, 1939). This treatment and pericardial resection (Beck, Schmieden, 1924) in chronic adhesive pericarditis — both good examples of the successful application to man of carefully planned animal experiments — are the best accomplishments of surgery in heart diseases. Sympathectomy (T. JONNESCO, 1910) and nerve injection (F. MANDL, 1925) and other arduous operations have been attempted, with less conspicuous success, for the relief of cardiac pain.

A warning against the tendency to subdivide internal medicine too much into independent specialized branches comes from the appreciation of significant cardiac involvement in such diseases as lupus erythematosus disseminatus, thyrotoxicosis, sarcoidosis, hemochromatosis, glycogenosis (E. von GIERKE's disease), and beriberi. In fact, even heart failure has been interpreted by some as essentially resulting from a metabolic disorder of the peripheral tissues (H. Eppinger, Jr., 1927) rather than the result of primary lesions within the heart itself. Although this extreme opinion has not been accepted as more than an occasional contributory factor, it is indicative of a sound tendency against artificial isolation of parts of the human body in the interpretation of diseases. Among those who contributed to the introduction into clinical medicine of modern ideas co-ordinating the metabolic requirements of the human body and the mechanical work of the heart, J. PLESCH and Jonathan MEAKINS may be mentioned. As noted earlier, Starling's " law of the heart " (1918) has considerably influenced concepts of cardiac function, modifying the ideas of the clinician as well as the physiologist. Already in the last century two different interpretations of the mechanism of heart failure were introduced: the " forward failure " theory (decreased cardiac output, with anoxia damaging to the heart muscle and rendering it unable to maintain the blood flow), emphasized in the present century by MacKenzie and many British clinicians; and the " back pressure " theory (obstruction to outflow increasing pressure in the venous system and heart chambers till the muscle becomes overtaxed), generally accepted in continental Europe. In 1913 H. VAQUEZ, co-ordinating opinions and observations of other pathologists and clinicians, established the doctrine of partial decompensation (i.e., of only one or two chambers) in contrast with the idea that the heart fails as a whole. While Lewis still maintained that digitalis essentially acts on atrioventricular conduction, the favourable influence of the drug on the failing heart muscle has been widely accepted. Although the mechanism of action of the glucosides is still a matter of discussion, the preparations, dosage, and methods of administration have been based on sound pharmacological investigation (S. FRAENKEL, Cary EGGLESTON). Other outstanding discoveries with regard to medical treatment are the antifibrillatory action of quinine and quinidine and the diuretic effect of organic mercurial compounds. Finally, the meritorious unremitting effort of the American school to standardize the methods of examination and the criteria of diagnosis and classification of heart diseases should be emphasized (Wyckoff, 1919; P. D. White, 1921; Committee of the American Heart Association).

DISEASES OF THE KIDNEY. Knowledge of chronic renal disease has been considerably advanced in the present century not only by recognition of the function of the different parts of the complex " nephron " (see Physiology); but also by a better classification of the clinical conditions, beginning with F. Volhard and T. Fahr, and by the elaboration of precise differential tests leading to better diagnosis and prognosis. Study of the functional state of the kidney, as indicated by such tests as its ability to excrete certain dyes (E. C. ACHARD, 1897; L. G. ROWNTREE and J. T. GERAGHTY, 1910), to preserve albumin in the body (detected by boiling urine or the Gmelin test) and to eliminate urea (D. K. MARSHALL, 1913; D. D. VAN SLYKE, 1914, 1928) have now been augmented by other tests that show the functional state of the various parts of the nephron during the developing stages of the disorder in question, when it is most susceptible to treatment. Thus the rate of glomerular filtration is measured by the clearance of inulin from blood; the effective blood flow by diodrast clearance; the excretory capacity of the tubules by the amount of diodrast excretion; the reabsorptive capacity of the tubules by glucose reabsorption, and by the concentrating power (maximum specific gravity) of the urine under controlled conditions in a given case (Volhard and Fahr). These procedures, to be sure, will be superseded in time and at present merely indicate the state of the pathologic functioning of the various parts; like the anatomical changes, they are but facets in the whole picture of Bright's disease. They do, however, permit better comprehension of the individual patient's condition, and therefore promote his well-being until further advances solve the whole problem. Hermann STRAUSS, of Berlin, emphasized the importance of the study of the blood chemistry as the most reliable index of renal function (1902). In 1912 Otto FOLIN, of Harvard, described a new colorimetric method for the determination of the nitrogenous constituents of the blood. From this and similar micro methods of determining minute quantities of blood and urinary constituents was derived important knowledge in the understanding of nephritis and its treatment. Another important step in the study of the diseases of the kidney was accomplished by Volhard's standard method (1918) for testing the specific-gravity concentration under controlled conditions.

GASTROENTEROLOGY. The twentieth century has seen the development of the scientific, biochemical, and radiographic basis for present-day gastroenterology. The contributions of such physiologists as W. B. CANNON (1896), H. B. WILLIAMS (1898), H. RIEDER (1904), and W. C. ALVAREZ (b. 1884), with his studies on the mechanics of the intestinal tracts (1922), are among the leading physiological additions to this field in the twentieth century.

Endoscopic methods have been popularized by Raoul BENSAUDE (1866–1938); by R. SCHINDLER, who developed the flexible gastroscope (1932) and popularized gastroscopy; by Herman STRAUSS (sigmoidoscopy, 1910), by E. B. BENEDICT, of Harvard, and others. The duodenal bucket was introduced by M. EINHORN (1908), facilitating studies on pancreatic secretion; B. B. Vincent LYON (1919) introduced the technique of biliary drainage; M. REHFUSS developed the technique of fractional estimation of the gastric contents (1914). In 1934 T. G. MILLER and W. O. ABBOTT, by means of their two-channel tube of small calibre, worked out a technique for the study of the secretory and motor functions of the small intestine in man. This procedure has been successfully applied to the diagnosis and treatment of a number of intestinal disorders, such as intestinal obstruction. These refinements have largely superseded the methods of gastric analysis used in the last century.

The concept of peptic ulcer has undergone considerable modification as to incidence, pathogenesis, and therapy. The present century is marked by the recognition of the greater frequency of duodenal ulcer, as popularized by the surgeon Berkeley, Lord MOYNIHAN (1910), far outranking gastric ulcer in numerical importance. The psychological concepts of Sir Arthur Frederick HURST (1879–1944) contributed much to the understanding of the course and nature of peptic ulcer. B. W. SIPPY's treatment of ulcer (1915) has become widely established; Einar MEULENGRACHT, of Copenhagen, introduced the clinical concept of liberal feeding of bleeding ulcers. The surgical treatment of peptic ulcer has also made noteworthy advances. Gastroenterostomy as a curative operation is discredited; subtotal gastrectomy, devised by H. von HABERER (b. 1875) and popularized by H. FINSTERER (b. 1877) and Jenö POLYA (b. 1876), and in America by A. A. BERG (b. 1872), marks a new era in the surgery of peptic ulcer. The relative merit of medical and surgical treatment is no longer a controversial subject, though many other aspects of the problem of peptic ulcer are still unsolved.

The visualization of the gall-bladder by means of dyes (tetraiodophenolphthalein) is due to the original idea of Evarts A. GRAHAM (b. 1883), of St. Louis, and its practical application (1924) by his associates, G. H. CO-PHER (b. 1893) and W. H. COLE (b. 1898). The incidence, diagnosis, and indications for surgical treatment of gall-bladder disease have been scientifically established, largely because of the simplicity and utility of the dye test. Liver functional tests, with various dyes, were introduced by J. J. Abel and L. G. Rowntree (phenoltetrachlorphthalein, 1910) and S. M. ROSENTHAL, of Montreal (bromsulfalein, 1925). In fact, the whole field of the complicated and numerous tests of the function of the liver has grown rapidly in the last few years. Regional ileitis was first noted (1932) by B. B. CROHN (b. 1884) and his associates as a clinical entity, a fact that has broadened the field of surgical usefulness in the abdomen by its approach to benign inflammatory diseases of the small intestine.

During recent years the concept of non-specific ulcerative colitis, its great frequency and its clinical importance, has been developed. Much of the clinical and pathological knowledge emanated from A. SCHMIDT (b.

1865) in Germany, and in the United States from J. A. BARGEN (b. 1894) and his medical and surgical associates in the renowned Mayo Clinic. W. C. ALVAREZ deserves special mention for his popularization of the nervous causes of many phases of indigestion and dyspepsia, for his simplified concept of the causation of such functional phenomena, and for his common-sense approach to this huge field of functional maladies. The period is also marked by the introduction of a new term: "psychosomatic" medicine, indicating organic visceral diseases resulting from chronic psychic trauma (Helen F. DUNBAR, 1934; Franz ALEXANDER; Eli MOSCHKOWITZ). Among the gastroenterological diseases that might be classified as psychosomatic in nature are included peptic ulcer, cardiospasm, and ulcerative colitis.

Functional tests of the liver, of the pancreas, and of the stomach have been markedly extended. The Miller-Abbott tube or balloon for overcoming intestinal obstruction is a typical example of the application of physiological principles to a mechanical device. Gastroenterology, which is half medical and half surgical, is marked in its progress by the very wide extension of the field of surgery. These advances include not only the now fully accepted subtotal gastrectomy for ulcer, but also total gastrectomy for new growths of the upper part of the stomach and of the lower œsophagus, and such massive procedures as removal of the head of the pancreas in one stage for carcinoma, and subtotal colectomies for colonic diseases.

DIABETES. In 1900 Eugene L. OPIE, then at Johns Hopkins, confirmed in man the earlier experiments on dogs (see Physiology) connecting the pancreas with diabetes mellitus. Studying histologically the pancreas of a child who had died of diabetes, he saw that the islands of Langerhans were so degenerated that they could hardly be identified. W. G. MacCallum later (1909) showed that ligation of the ducts destroyed all of the pancreas except the islands without causing diabetes; when the islands were also destroyed, diabetes promptly ensued. These observations led the British physiologist Sir Edward Schaefer (later Sharpey-Schafer) in 1916 to express the theory that the pancreatic island cells produce some form of internal secretion that controls the metabolism of sugar. In 1921 a young Canadian surgeon, Frederick Grant BANTING (1891–1941), prepared isletin, later called insulin, achieving one of the greatest discoveries in the field of modern medicine.

With the help of C. H. BEST he ligated the pancreatic ducts of his first dog on May 16, 1921, and soon obtained a dog with the acini that make the external secretion well atrophied, but with the islets well preserved. With the interfering acini thus disposed of, they then prepared a watery extract of the remainder, which they injected into the blood stream of a dog that was dying of diabetes, his blood loaded with sugar. Within two hours the sugar in the blood had fallen to one half — the extract of the islands of Langerhans had helped burn the sugar in the diabetic blood. Banting and Best continued in their experiments, with the help of J. B. COLLIP (b. 1892), perfecting the preparation of the extract. With their first human patient, Dr. Joe Gilchrist, a Toronto physician who had de-veloped a grave diabetes, they obtained a splendid result. The name " isletin," which Banting had first proposed, was changed to " insulin " at the suggestion of Professor MacLeod, in whose labo-ratory they worked. A clinic for dia-betics was soon instituted, and the good results were so decisive that insu-lin has been universally accepted and utilized in medical practice. A " sub-stitution therapy," it aids the patient in more ways than was orginally antici-pated, prolonging life and health, but not curing the disease. In 1923 the No-bel prize for medicine was awarded to McLeod and Banting, who shortly was appointed director of the Banting-Best Department of Medical Research at the University of Toronto. On February 21, 1941, while Banting was flying to England on a war mission for the Ca-nadian government, he was killed in a plane crash in Newfoundland.

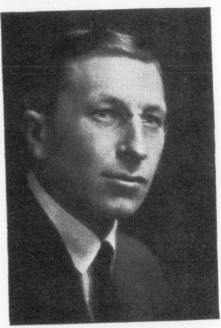

468. F. G. Banting, Nobel Laureate, 1923.

Less spectacular but very considerable progress has been made in com-prehension of the nature and control of Addison's disease of the adrenals. W. W. Swingle and J. J. Pfiffner's cortical extract, by restoring to mod-erate health animals whose adrenals had been removed, established the pri-mary site of the disease (1931). It was also discovered that there was an excessive loss of sodium chloride from the body and that excessive potassium had a detrimental effect. Control of these three factors has considerably improved the outlook for patients as far as the adrenal defects are con-cerned.

Other parts of the story of the endocrines will be found in the sections on Physiology and Pathology.

In the American schools, T. C. JANEWAY (1872–1917) represented the younger type of clinician who studied disease by physiological methods; he was selected as the first full-time Professor of Medicine at Johns Hopkins University when the chair was placed on this basis by a grant from the Rockefeller Foundation. These experiments in clinical pedagogy, though modified in various ways, cannot be said to have had more than a limited success. The notable contribution of E. LIBMAN (1872–1946), a clinician of international fame, to subacute bacterial endocarditis, Leo BUERGER's (b. 1879) description of thromboangiitis obliterans, A. S. EPSTEIN's (b. 1880)

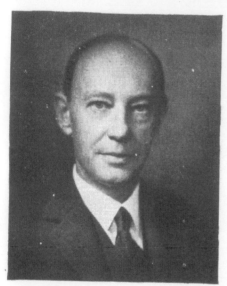

469. George R. Minot, Nobel Laureate, 1934.

of lipoid nephrosis, and Graham LUSK's (1866–1932) and E. F. DU BOIS's (b. 1882) studies on the metabolic disorders have contributed toward placing the United States in the forefront of medical progress. R. C. CABOT (1868–1939), a pious and unusually careful student of clinical medicine, especially emphasizing autopsy correlations, contributed to medical progress in his case-history method of teaching and still more by the inauguration of the " social service " system, which has greatly increased physicians' ability to care properly for the hospital and outpatient-department sick. G. R. MINOT (b. 1885) is the leading representative of today's Boston school of hematology, which has been one of the most successful in advancing this active field. His greatest achievement was his discovery with W. P. Murphy that pernicious anæmia, a hitherto uniformly fatal disease, could be consistently held in abeyance by feeding sufficient amounts of liver. The American school has been especially active in investigating this rapidly moving subject. In 1928 W. B. CASTLE extended Minot's studies on pernicious anæmia to explain the essential nature of the disease. He found that in pernicious-anæmia patients the gastric juice lacks the " intrinsic factor " that normally reacts with an " extrinsic factor " in the food to form an " anti-anæmic factor," which is normally stored in the liver. Thus, the life-preserving quality of Minot's liver-feeding is explained. Similar anæmia pictures, but secondary to other causes, have been produced in other conditions, where perhaps a faulty diet fails to supply enough of the " extrinsic factor," especially where pregnancy requires an extra supply; or, as in sprue, where the anti-anæmic factor is formed, but not absorbed through the gut. J. B. HERRICK (b. 1861) was the first to describe (1910) sickle-cell anæmia, a disease caused by a congenital anomaly of the erythrocyte, mostly in Negroes. Newly discovered anomalies of the red blood cell (other than the sphero-cyte of congenital hemolytic jaundice, and the sickle cell, which predispose to hemolytic anæmia, are the elliptical cell (M. DRESBACH, 1904) of the rare oval-cell anæmia, (H. VAN DEN BERGH, 1928), and the target cell (M. M. WINTROBE and W. DAMESHEK, 1940) as found in T. B. COOLEY's Mediterranean anæmia. The paroxysmal cold hemoglobinuria recognized in the previous century has been matched by a paroxysmal nocturnal hemo-globinuria (Marchiafava, 1911). Secondary anæmia, a diagnostic term for-merly used for all non-primary anæmias regardless of their nature, has now been replaced by descriptive classes such as " hemorrhagic," " hemolytic," " dyspoietic," etc., each with its recognizable characteristics. This in turn, together with grouping according to size and colour of the erythrocytes, has led to better comprehension and hence better ability to treat them. The ability of radioactive isotopes to " tag " erythrocytes has been utilized prof-itably to study their alterations from a new point of view, and they have also shown promise in the treatment of incurable conditions such as the leukemias.

Puncture of the bone marrow, where most of the blood cells are formed, was proposed by G. GHEDINI, of Genoa, in 1908. C. SAYFARTH suggested the sternum (1923) as preferable to the tibia; and with techniques based on M. I. ARINKIN's method (1929) much valuable information has been ob-tained as to the nature of various blood conditions (e.g., F. W. PEABODY's study of the bone marrow in pernicious anæmia, 1927) and in the diagnosis of obscure cases. Recently (1940) L. M. TOCANTINS has demonstrated that blood and various fluids can be introduced into the general circulation in large amounts by way of bone-marrow injection; and already this method has proved useful in various conditions.

In Italy, C. FRUGONI (b. 1881), a pupil of Grocco and a leading clini-cian in Rome, has devoted himself chiefly to the subjects of allergy, acute pulmonary œdema, and focal infections. He wrote an excellent book, Le-zioni di clinica (Rome, 1934). Luigi DEVOTO (1864–1936) is known as the founder of the first Italian industrial clinic (Milan, 1898); Devoto's pupil Maurizio ASCOLI (b. 1876), of Palermo, is associated with the " meiostag-min " surface-tension test of sera, and the use of adrenalin in the treatment of malaria. Aldo CASTELLANI (b. 1878), eminent specialist and writer on tropical diseases, while studying with Kruse discovered the so-called ab-sorption reaction (1902), used in the diagnosis of bacterial diseases. He is also famous for his isolation of new strains of fungi as causes of dermatoses, and his contributions to the etiology of African sleeping sickness. In 1901 J. E. DUTTON had found *Trypanosoma gambiense* in the blood of natives without connecting the parasite with the disease, and two years later Castellani independently found the same parasite in the blood and spinal fluid of patients suffering from sleeping sickness. Further links in the chain of evidence were supplied by Bruce and Nabarro in demonstrating that the tsetse fly was the vector (carrier) of the disease to man and that Gambia fever (Dutton and Todd, 1902), was a modified form of the same disease. At the Ceylon Medical School, Castellani discovered (1905) that *Spirocheta pertenue* was the cause of frambesia, a common disease on that island, and in 1906 isolated the cause of spirochetal hemorrhagic bronchitis (Castellani's disease). He has served as Professor of Tropical Medicine at the London School and at Tulane University and was the founder of the Tropical Institute at Rome.

Scientific medicine in LATIN AMERICA has been developed along the lines of biological studies, clinical observations, eradication of menacing diseases, and medical teaching. Many diseases were first identified in this period in various countries or brought under control, as, for instance, the elimination of yellow fever from São Paulo by RIBAS (1903), and from Rio by Oswaldo CRUZ (1909). The first Pan-American (fifth Latin-American) Scientific Congress at Santiago (1909) was a notable milestone in this progress. In the medical clinic at Buenos Aires, Mariano CASTEX (b. 1886) studied especially late hereditary syphilis, arterial hypertension, and the functional disturbances of the circulatory system. C. B. UDAONDO (b. 1885), Professor of Medical Semeiology and Clinical Propædeutics, is the author of an excellent *Treatise of Semeiology* (3rd ed., 1931); A. H. ROFFO (b. 1882) has conducted and supervised important clinical and experimental studies on malignant tumours in the Institute for the Study of Cancer. Internationally famous is B. A. HOUSSAY (b. 1887), until recently Professor of Physiology and director of the Physiological Institute of the Medical Faculty at Buenos Aires. His studies on the endocrine glands and particularly on the role of the hypophysis in diabetes mellitus and in relation to other endocrine organs, conducted by himself and his large corps of assistants, are among the most important additions to the knowledge of diabetes since the discovery of insulin. In Brazil, A. DE CASTRO (b. 1881), Professor of Medicine at his alma mater, the University of Rio de Janeiro, has contributed worthily to endocrinology and the study of nervous diseases. Brazil VITAL, having elaborated the principles of campaigns against snake-bite poisons, has placed Brazil in a leading position in this field. The name of Abel AYERZA (1861–1918) is well known for its connection with the disease of the *cardiacos negros*, due to sclerosis of the pulmonary artery (1901).

9. Surgery

The great achievements of modern surgery have been determined in increasing measure by the close unity of scientific work with the various medical disciplines. It is impossible today to conceive of a good surgeon who has not had adequate medical preparation — or a good physician, for that matter, who is not sufficiently acquainted with surgery to appreciate the need for surgical intervention as it arises. The clinician, surgeon, pathologist, radiologist, and the various specialists not only must collaborate on all obscure cases, but must know enough of the other fellow's job to make the collaboration intelligent and useful. Thus, while there is a marked tendency at present to an extreme degree of specialization and technical complexity in the various fields, there is at the same time an increased realization of the need for continuous and efficient collaboration. The narrow-mindedness apt to result from such extreme specialization certainly would endanger the further development of surgery along broad clinical lines. It is not merely by chance that even in the United States, where specialization has been highly developed, the academic leaders in surgery have remained general surgeons.

Modern surgery, passing beyond the repair of injuries and extirpation of diseased areas, frequently endeavours to restore one or another of the body's functional balances (Cannon's homeostasis) by surgical intervention, to promote normal function in surgical conditions with or without operative measures, and to utilize physiological methods in studying surgical problems; in other words, normal and pathological physiology has been added to the surgeon's stock in trade.

Among the factors that have contributed to surgical progress are the contributions of bacteriology and pathology toward more precise diagnosis and prognosis, and indications of the proper moment for surgical intervention and subsequent treatment. " Clinical pathology " has developed a separate specialty to furnish the clinician with information about biopsy material and the morphology, bacteriology, physics, and chemistry of the body fluids and excretions, important factors that often determine the management of a given case. The technique of X-ray examinations has been so developed that it is now diagnostically decisive in many surgical conditions. Biopsy, the removal and examination of tissues for diagnosis during life, has become a constant aid to the careful surgeon, especially when cancer is suspected.

Rapid frozen-section method for microscopical study was introduced by L. D. WILSON in 1905 and is today generally accepted. Endoscopy supplies accurate information about most of the hitherto inaccessible body cavities, and as a result of such developments surgery has recorded in the last decades so many notable triumphs that it becomes impossible even to allude to many of them in the following pages.

At the same time, progress in technique has been so remarkable that the surgeon of our times gives the picture of a wonderful combination of scientist and exquisite artist, who dares to face and is able to solve brilliantly the most difficult scientific and technical problems. In the hands of thoroughly trained men, the surgery of the brain, the lungs, the œsophagus, the heart, and all the abdominal organs, and plastic reconstructive surgery have made considerable progress. Operations such as those on kidneys, bile passages, stomach, and intestines, which a generation ago were regarded as dangerous, have become routine procedures for the skilled surgeon. Again, in other operations where the general condition of the patient is not affected by his ailment, as it is for instance in toxic goitre, intervention, as in joints and bones, is practically without mortality. Development of asepsis and chemotherapy assures the healing of incisions so perfectly that postoperative complications are mostly reduced to the "bad risks" and to postoperative pneumonia, phlebitis, and lung embolism.

With the recent developments of ANESTHESIOLOGY and with many physicians returned from military service experienced in a field that in leading medical countries had largely had its routine practice turned over to special trained nurses, progress was speeded considerably. Today many major operations are performed under spinal or local anesthesia, as well as general; and many different anesthetics are used, depending on the nature of the operation or the condition of the individual patient.

George CRILE (1864–1942), of Cleveland, is known for many ingenious contributions to surgery, especially his experimental and clinical investigations of surgical shock, and the reduction of operative shock by his procedure of "anoci-association," which, though not founded on an entirely sound physiological basis, has lessened mortality, especially in removal of thyrotoxic goitres. Crile also worked out an ingenious method of connecting the donor's artery with the vein of the recipient by means of a cannula, but it was far too difficult to be practical. In later years Crile turned to biologic-philosophic speculations, largely based on the work of specialized assistants.

Remarkable advances in surgery were brought about by the treatment of surgical shock by blood transfusion (treated also in the sections on Immunology and Therapeutics). The first method of overcoming clotting was devised (1913) by A. R. KIMPTON and J. H. BROWN, of Boston, conveying the blood directly into a large tube coated inside with paraffin and injecting it from the same tube into the patient's veins. By adding sodium citrate to the blood (R. LEWISOHN), the clotting of blood used in transfusion was eliminated. The method of transfusion was improved by E. LINDEMAN, of New York (1913).

After many attempts the latest development in the treatment of shock is the use of dried or lyophilized serum. Freezing serum or plasma with dry ice and proceeding to dehydration in a high vacuum (1909, by L. F. SHACKELL, of St. Louis [b. 1887]), has as the final result a yellowish powder which has only a fraction of the bulk of the original blood. It may be kept at atmospheric temperature indefinitely without degenerating and is quickly soluble in water. Our armed forces in World War II were supplied with large quantities of this dried plasma for immediate use at the very front in treating shock and hemorrhage. As a consequence of this progress modern surgery has greatly reduced the operative mortality of the most serious interventions. The treatment of infected wounds and open fractures, especially when there is much trauma to the tissues, was greatly improved during the First World War by the technique of *débridement* and Carrel's method of constant irrigation of the wounded part with a mild antiseptic. The treatment of the open wound with sulfa drugs and in most recent times with penicillin, by mouth and intravenously, has brought about a revolutionary change in surgical therapy and assured a favourable prognosis for a great number of cases that before would have been lost.

NEUROSURGERY has been one of the most remarkably successful fields in this period. Its astonishing progress in the United States is due chiefly to a small group led by Harvey CUSHING (1869–1939), of Johns Hopkins and Harvard. It was an outstanding example of the newer surgical trend to the combination of physiological, pathological, and clinical study of surgical diseases with a brilliant surgical technique.

At Johns Hopkins Hospital Cushing found that for the ten years before 1901 ante-mortem diagnosis of brain tumour had been made in only 32 cases of 36,000 admitted, and that only two of these had been operated on, both with fatal results. Cushing, who had become deeply interested in the experimental pathology of the nervous system, decided to devote himself to neurosurgery. He worked out a highly specialized technique for brain operations, based on the most painstaking care in the handling of tissues, an exact hemostasis, and the use of layers of interrupted sutures of fine silk in closing the wound. Using cotton pledgets for handling the tumours and minimizing bleeding, he obtained the greatest success. He took the greatest pains to avoid shock and introduced the practice of keeping a running record of the patient's blood pressure throughout the operation for the early detection of any alteration. In the following years Cushing perfected his method and did much to establish neurosurgery as a specialty in all the great clinics of the world. His operative mortality during the last years of his activity was only 8.7 per cent for a total of 635 operations, a success due chiefly to a brilliant, carefully executed surgical technique.

The world's leading neurological surgeon, Cushing wrote a series of brilliant monographs: *The Pituitary Body* (1912), *Tumors of the Nervus Acousticus* (1917), *A Classification of the Tumors of the Glioma Group*

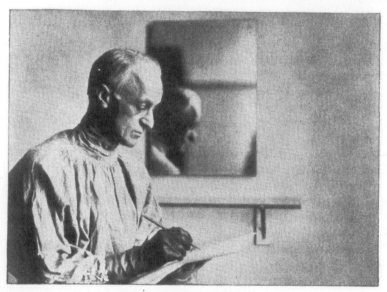

470. Harvey Cushing.

(1926, with Percival BAILEY), and so on, down to *Meningiomas* (1938). His *Life of Sir William Osler* (1925) obtained the Pulitzer prize; it is a classic in medical biography and a best seller. Even his *Reports* as surgeon to the Peter Bent Brigham Hospital in Boston are alive with pregnant reflections on medical problems. But beyond his special field of activities Cushing has set a splendid example to all physicians, and particularly surgeons, of how they should critically face their work. The account of his successes and failures was thorough and honest, and he was tireless in the observation of his cases for many years after operation.

SURGERY OF THE HEART. An Italian surgeon, Guido FARINA, was the first to suture a dagger wound of the heart (1896); the patient died, however, after a few days. In the same year Louis REHN, of Frankfurt (1840–1930), succeeded in suturing successfully a stab wound of the right ventricle.

About six hundred cases of successful operations have since been reported, with a mortality of thirty to forty per cent. Surgical treatment of heart-wounds actually is less sensational than lay reports would lead one to believe. Even the time factor often is not decisive. Rehn's patient came to the operating-table thirty-six hours after his heart was injured. In August 1938 Robert E. GROSS, of the Children's Hospital in Boston, operated upon and ligated an open ductus arteriosus in a child, aged seven and a half years. Since that first successful operation he has operated on fifty-six cases, with only two deaths. Others have confirmed these brilliant results. Improvement of the coronary circulation in patients with coronary insufficiency has been tried (1935) by grafting well-vascularized tissue (epiploon, muscle) to the epicardium (C. S. Beck, E. T. O'Shaughnessy). The results, though still under discussion, are promising. The left coronary artery was successfully sutured for the first time (1935) by C. S. Beck, who later tried with F. R. Mantz the effect of dusting powdered bone between the heart and the pericardium, in order to cause adhesions and lead blood vessels to the heart surface.

SURGERY OF THE BLOOD VESSELS has made great progress both experimentally and clinically. The Eck fistula has shunted portal blood experimentally around the liver to the vena cava since 1877; and Carrel in 1902 showed that arterial stumps could be successfully joined by end-to-end anastomosis, new functioning segments of arteries inserted, and even whole organs transplanted. The greatest difficulty in such procedures is the tendency for thrombosis to start at the damaged part of the vessel lining; but with the very recent introduction of continuous heparin administration to combat this tendency, it is possible that the near future will see Carrel's feats practically applied even to the transplantation of viscera in man. In 1902 Rudolph MATAS (b. 1860), of New Orleans, devised his operation of endo-aneurysmorrhaphy, for the radical cure of aneurysm by reconstructing the parent vessel by suturing its openings into the aneurysm.

Excision of the aorta for aneurysm has recently (1944) been successfully accomplished by J. ALEXANDER and F. X. BYRON. In a young man with but few symptoms, an aneurysm of the thoracic aorta three inches in diameter was removed without incident and without damage to his health, because of the richness of the existing collateral circulation. PAYR of Leipzig, HALSTED of Baltimore, and J. B. MURPHY of Chicago have been notable contributors to vascular surgery.

Sympathectomy has been used in essential hypertension, as first advised by F. KRAUS. Painstaking elaboration of the best method led to the combination of removal of the sympathetic chain and the splanchnic nerve in the lower thoracic and lumbar region. Though there is still no agreement as to the selection of cases and the standards of evaluation of results, it seems that the operation has a definite helpful result in some cases.

SURGERY OF THE CHEST. Ferdinand SAUERBRUCH (b. 1875), of Berlin, was among the first pioneers of thoracic surgery, which had lagged behind the surgery of other parts of the body. This lag was undoubtedly due to the difficulties produced by collapse of the lungs as soon as pressure was equalized by opening the thoracic cage, a condition only partly relieved by Sauerbruch's cumbersome cabinet. In 1909, however, S. J. MELTZER and J. AUER showed that respiration could be indefinitely maintained by air introduced intra-tracheally under positive pressure, a fact known to both Vesalius and Robert Hooke. With the use of these and other physiological methods in-trathoracic surgery could be practised as deliberately as surgery in other parts of the body without fear of pulmonary collapse or asphyxia. Sauer-bruch also had a large part in devising a new method of thoracoplasty, dividing the operation into stages and limiting the extent of the resection.

In recent times it has become possible to remove successfully whole lungs, or lobes, or even parts of lobes, for such conditions as abscess, bron-chiectasis, and early diagnosed lung cancers. Rudolph NISSEN (b. 1896), formerly of Berlin, now of New York, was the first to perform total pneu-monectomy successfully (1931). The patient was a twelve-year-old child with advanced bronchiectasis affecting the whole of one lung. The child developed normally, as is evident from a report eleven years later. Success-ful total pneumonectomy for cancer of the lung was performed by Evarts GRAHAM in 1933. The patient was a physician, who was still well ten years afterwards.

Other pioneers in thoracic surgery were, furthermore: T. Tuffier (1857–1929), E. L. Doyen (1859–1916), and E. Delorme (1847–1929) in France; J. E. H. Roberts and A. Tudor Edwards in England; P. Bull (b. 1869) and K. H. Giertz (b. 1876) in the Scandinavian countries; in Italy, Carlo For-lanini, of Pavia, who, though not a surgeon, laid (1884) the foundation of the surgical treatment of pulmonary tuberculosis with artificial pneumo-thorax; and in Canada, Douglas, E. W. Archibald, and N. S. Shenstone. Willy MEYER, the first American who was active in this field, has been followed by a large group of American surgeons devoted to thoracic sur-gery, such as A. Lilienthal, M. Thorek, L. Eloesser, J. Alexander, E. D. Churchill, and R. Overholt.

The ENDOCRINE GLANDS have furnished a fertile field for recent surgical prowess. Hyperthyroidism has been successfully treated by ligation of the thyroid artery or removal of parts of the thyroid gland. With proper precautions this operation can be repeated until a proper balance has been maintained; and if too much is removed, the patient can be indefinitely maintained on thyroid extract. Cushing's extirpations of pituitary tumours and his segregation of a new pituitary syndrome — basophilism — are among his most important contributions. Extirpation of parathyroid hyperplasias and neoplasms, begun by F. Mandl in 1925, has also explained the clinical entity *osteitis fibrosa* and shown how it may be cured. In cases of parathyroid deficiency, parathyroids have been transplanted. Various ovarian and adrenal tumours, betrayed by the secondary sex changes produced by the extra endocrine secretion, can often be removed in time to save the patient's life and bring him back to normal sexual existence.

Since the discovery of insulin occasional tumours of the islands of Langerhans have been found to cause severe hypoglycemia; these too have been successfully removed. A definite clinical syndrome has been laid to tumours of the chromaffin tissue of the adrenal glands (pheochromocytoma). Removal of the tumour completely cures this condition.

The founders of the world-famous Mayo Clinic, in Rochester, Minnesota, W. J. Mayo (1861–1939) and C. H. Mayo (1865–1939) not only themselves contributed notably to surgical progress in many fields, but established a private clinic for all branches of medicine (later the post-graduate school of the University of Minnesota), which in organization, scope, and performance is unexcelled anywhere in the world. The vast material at their disposal, excellently utilized, has formed the basis of an incredible amount of high-class work. Among their surgical assistants, E. S. Judd (1878–1935) promoted especially the surgery of the biliary and urinary tracts; and D. C. Balfour (b. 1882), the surgery of the thyroid, spleen, and abdomen.

Abdominal surgery had had a great revolution in the second half of the nineteenth century, thanks especially to the Viennese school. Theodor Billroth, as we have seen, was the founder of modern abdominal surgery, and the German school was important in its development. Improvement of details in the technical procedure of stomach, duodenal, and colon resections has succeeded in greatly lessening the danger of such interventions. Though technique in stomach resection still follows principles developed by Billroth, colon resection has been remarkably improved by the exteriorization method (Mikulicz). P. Kraske (1851–1930), with the resection of coccyx and sacral bones thus creating a good exposure of the rectum, brought about a decisive improvement in rectal resection. In 1907 William E. Miles (b. 1869), of London, introduced the abdomino-perineal method, which facilitates the radical resection of carcinomatous rectum by combining two approaches. This procedure has become the method of choice in the North American and British surgery.

These steady improvements in the results of intestinal resection have led to its application under certain conditions to benign ailments of the abdo-

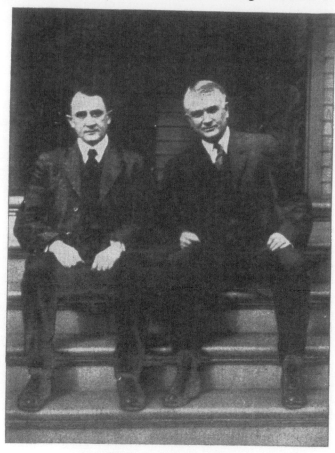

471. *Charles and William Mayo.*

men — above all, the resection of stomach and duodenum in peptic ulcers. In selected cases where surgical treatment is indicated, radical operation affords the greatest chance for complete cure.

PLASTIC SURGERY, dormant since the time of the Brancas and Tagliacozzi, was revived by Reverdin (1870), Ollier (1872), and Thiersch (1874), large raw surfaces being covered and mutilating scars avoided by skin grafts. The transplantation of tendons and muscles was later successfully carried out; and Vanghetti was even able to make use of the muscles in amputated limbs to increase the action of prosthetic apparatus (*cineprosthesis*). The First World War greatly advanced the use of implanted bones and transplanted skin muscles and areolar tissue in minimizing the functional and cosmetic effects of mutilating wounds (A. C. VALADIER, H. MORESTIN [1869–1924], H. D. GILLIES); while reconstruction of bones and joints (cranioplasty, rachisynthesis, nearthrosis) was furthered by TUFFIER, R. BASTIANELLI, E. LEXER (1867–1937), and other orthopedic surgeons. It was during the First World War that the large numbers of casualties focused attention upon the necessity of repairing these defects, with the result that governments organized groups to do this type of surgery, and many procedures were improved and others originated. In 1917 the tubed pedicle flap was devised by W. FILATOV (b. 1875), director of the Ukrainian Institute of Ophthalmology, and, independently, by Sir Harold GILLIES, of London. Its value lies in obtaining a better circulation in the skin and subcutaneous tissue and in allowing the flap to bridge over intervening skin so that the possibility of infection, seepage from the wound, and frequent dressings are obviated.

During the period between the First and Second World Wars plastic surgery came of age as an established specialty. When John Staige Davis of Baltimore, the first in this field, began his career as a plastic surgeon before World War I, no medical school, hospital, or clinic had a division or department of plastic surgery. Today there are many such, with scores of surgeons who devote all their time to this type of reconstructive work. In 1941 the American Board of Plastic Surgery was given the status of a major certifying board. The importance of the specialty is also indicated by the formation of the American Association of Plastic Surgery (1921) and the American Society of Plastic and Reconstructive Surgery (1931). The principles governing the shifting and rotation of tissue and the use of skin flaps still attached to the body for nourishment have been known and employed for centuries, and still form the basis of present-day plastic procedures, together with the discovery in the previous century that free grafts, especially of skin, could be made to live after complete severance from the body.

The dermatome, devised by E. C. PADGETT, of Kansas City (1939), has revolutionized the excision of sheets of free split-skin grafts, permitting the excision of skin grafts of uniform and predetermined thickness. It has greatly increased the number of available donor sites on the body by making possible the removal of split-thickness skin grafts from areas of the trunk and extremities that could not readily be utilized in the previous method of free-hand cutting of grafts.

Clinical and experimental evidence accumulated in recent years, chiefly by L. A. PEER of Newark and G. B. O'CONNOR and G. W. PIERCE of San Francisco, now provides information as to the fate of various types of cartilage grafts after transplantation in human tissues, allowing surgeons to make a judicious choice among autogenous, homogenous, and preserved-cadaver cartilage. Fresh autogenous-cartilage grafts have been found to survive successful transplantation as living tissue, whether transplanted with or without perichondrium, though they tend to become degenerated, with fibrous-tissue replacement. Of interest also is a new technique, devised by Peer, of grafting with diced cartilage for filling bony or cartilaginous defects. The experimental work (1941) of S. M. DUPERTUIS, of Pittsburgh, demonstrated the actual growth of young auricular and costal cartilage grafts in rabbits, suggesting the possibility that young human cartilage grafts might also continue to grow after transplantation and be useful in the surgical handling of saddle nose and other deformities in children.

In the application of plastic-surgery principles to ophthalmology, the work of J. M. WHEELER of New York was outstanding, and largely through the efforts of his pupil Ramon CASTROVIEJO of New York, and of A. ELSCHNIG (Vienna), W. FILATOV (Russia), J. W. T. THOMAS (England), and others, the use of corneal transplants has developed from a purely experimental into a practical procedure. Although entire transparent grafts have not been found to be more than temporarily successful, circumscribed or partial penetrating keratoplasty gives a reasonable expectation of permanently restoring sight in properly selected cases and with modern technique. Clinical use of refrigerated skin grafts was shown (1944) by J. P. Webster (b. 1888), of New York, to be successful if the recipient areas were suitable and if the grafts were autogenous and had not been refrigerated for more than three weeks. Recent years have seen a wider and earlier application of skin grafts to cover denuded areas in fresh burns, together with a much wider use of the split-skin graft rather than the small deep graft that was so frequently used.

The cineplastic operation, referred to in the previous chapter, had as its chief exponent during World War I Ferdinand Sauerbruch, and was perfected (1944) by Captain H. H. KESSLER, U.S.N.R., of Newark, New Jersey. The greatest advantage of this plastic operation is that it permits the application of a special type of mechanical arm or hand, manipulated by direct muscular control with the same muscles or groups of muscles that performed the action in the normal hand and with the retention of the same cortical psychomotor patterns.

Before World War I, fractures of the jaws had been treated by wiring the teeth by various methods; but refinements in technique have since been developed, notably by Robert IVY of Philadelphia (b. 1881) (twisted loop) and Fulton RISDON of Toronto (twisted wire, external arch wire, or a combination with an external labial arch wire to which the individual wires about the teeth are attached and the upper and lower wires connected by wires or elastics). The cast-metal splint about the teeth has been improved by the use of transparent acrylic (methyl-methacrylate) splints moulded to fit the teeth, Colonel Roy STOUT's open-bit splint being one of the most satisfactory.

Prosthetics as an aid to plastic surgery came into limited use after World War I, particularly in oral surgery, and has been utilized in the past twenty-five years in conditions that are inoperable or as an adjunct in intervals between operations as a functional or cosmetic aid. Gelatin compositions were used early, in many instances for replacement of a lost ear or nose; later, self-vulcanizing latex was substituted as providing a more durable material. Captain C. D. CLARKE, formerly of the Army Medical Museum, has done much valuable investigative work in this field. With the recent development of plastic and artificial rubber, the methyl-methacrylates and vinyl-resins have been found to be excellent materials for prosthesis, especially as they can be made pliable and offer a multitude of colours for the attainment of natural skin tints. Thus methyl-methacrylate head caps and vinyl-chloride " rubber " hands, fingers, ears, and noses have already been used on casualties in the Army Reconstruction Centers.

The Russians have been successful in a number of cases (1944) in reconstructing by the accepted methods the penis that has been shot away in battle. Not only can it be made so as to excrete urine satisfactorily, but also, by functional laws that have not yet been wholly explained, the new organ is said gradually to acquire the ability to become erect.

Among AMERICAN surgeons who decisively influenced clinical concepts and the technical procedures of surgery in this country W. S. HALSTED (see pp. 851–2) stands first. He was one of the big four who made Johns Hopkins Medical School world-famous. Halsted was quietly effective in this country in transforming surgery from a series of dramatic incidents into a less conspicuous, painstaking, and scientific study of surgical types of disease. In addition to his introduction of sterile rubber gloves into the operating-room and his early use of silk ligatures and of infiltration anesthesia with cocaine, he devised numerous operative procedures and technical improvements, often based on previous experiments on animals. By his meticulous technique, his strict asepsis, his clever clinical judgment, and his careful evaluation of surgical successes and failures, he became one of the greatest surgeons of this continent. The MAYO BROTHERS, who became world-famous, not only by their excellent achievements in surgery, but also by the systematic organization of a great medical centre, have already been mentioned. We have also to record the work of John B. MURPHY (1851–1916), who was not only an excellent surgeon but also an inspiring teacher, enlivening practically every field of surgery by new and successful methods. His international reputation was surpassed among American surgeons only by Cushing. Murphy was the first in America to induce artificial pneumothorax. The " Murphy button " used in the end-to-end anastomosis of the intestine was a familiar term a generation ago. The recent leader of Midwestern surgery was A. J. OCHSNER (1858–1925), whose popular writings and whose personal example were equally influential. In New York, Charles McBURNEY (1845–1913) acquired fame through his abdominal gridiron incision and the painful spot in the abdomen in appendicitis known as McBurney's point (1889); Robert ABBE (1851–1928) is remembered as an early user of catgut sutures and of radium in

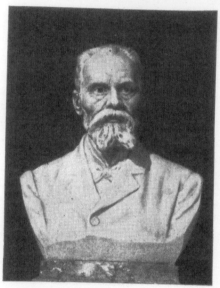
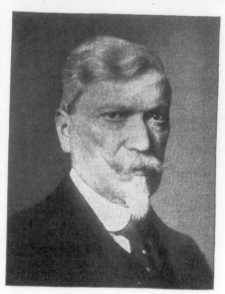

472. *Edoardo Bassini.*
(*Bust in the* PADUA CLINIC.)

473. *Antonio Carle.*

the treatment of malignant disease; G. M. EDEBOHLS (1853–1908) as the introducer of decapsulation of the kidney (1901) in various diseases of that organ; W. B. COLEY (1862–1936) for the use of erysipelas and prodigiosus toxins ("Coley's fluid") in the treatment of sarcoma (1891); and John B. DEAVER (1855–1931), one of the most skilful operators of his time, was a brilliant exponent of the "living pathology." He wrote on *Appendicitis* (1896), *Enlargement of the Prostate* (1905), *The Breast* (1917), and a *Surgical Anatomy* in three volumes (1901–3).

Among British surgeons Sir William MACEWEN (1848–1924), Regius Professor of Surgery at Glasgow, was one of the first to be active in the surgery of the brain (1893) and spinal cord and in orthopedics. Sir Victor HORSLEY (1857–1916), a British leader in the newer experimental and biological surgical trends, investigated especially the surgery of the nervous system and the endocrine glands. He improved the method of surgical approach to the brain and spinal cord and aided in the localization of function in the cerebral cortex. Sir Frederick TREVES (1853–1923) was a master of abdominal surgery. His *Elephant*

Man and Other Reminiscences (1923), together with entertaining accounts of world travel, are interesting medical borderline reading. Berkeley, Lord Moynihan (1865–1936), of Malta, and Professor of Surgery at Leeds, was one of the leading British surgeons of the present century and exponent of the " pathology of the living " (1910). He wrote prolifically, mostly on various phases of abdominal surgery. His clamp for intestinal resection is widely used.

Of recent French surgeons, Henri Hartmann (b. 1860) is the author of many surgical works, especially on abdominal, genito-urinary, gynæcological, and military surgery; his *Traité de chirurgie anatomo-clinique* (4 vols., 1903–13) is one of the most complete on the subject. F. Lejars (b. 1863), Professor of Clinical Surgery at the Hôpital St. Antoine, has written especially on military and emergency surgery; Paul Reclus (1847–1914) introduced the frequent use of local anesthesia into French surgery; M. T. Tuffier (1857–1929) acquired an international reputation for his pioneer work in experimental surgery, in the operative treatment of fractures, in renal surgery, and in the use of spinal anesthesia. Excellent texts on surgery have been published by Le Dentu and Pierre Delbet and by Duplay, Reclus, and A. Gosset.

In Italy Antonio Carle (1854–1927), a pupil of Billroth, did valuable work on the brain, the thyroid, and the gastro-intestinal and biliary tracts, but was still more important for the effect that his school at Turin had on the general progress of Italian surgery. Among Carle's distinguished pupils were R. Galeazzi, director of the Orthopedic Clinic in Milan, M. Donati (1879–1946) of Milan (surgery of parathyroids, abdomen, sympathetic nerves), O. Uffreduzzi of Turin (periarterial sympathectomy, hermaphroditism), and G. M. Fasiani of Milan (brain surgery). A. Ceci (1852–1920), a pupil of Durante and developer of scientific surgery at Pisa, was one of the first to practise splenectomy in Italy; he popularized the use of local anesthesia and was skilful in plastic surgery and in extirpating the larynx. G. F. Novaro (1843–1934), professor at Bologna and Genoa, made a remarkable contribution to laryngectomy and to intestinal surgery. Finally, Davide Giordano (b. 1864), a brilliant figure, emphasized the pathogenetic importance of the tetanus toxins, rather than of the bacteria themselves, made important contributions to the surgery of the abdomen, especially of the kidney and the liver, and has written scholarly essays on the history of medicine. From this school came R. Alessandri of Rome(surgery of the kidney and the biliary tracts), N. Leotta of Palermo (pulmonary surgery), and R. Bastianelli of Rome (abdominal surgery). E. Bassini (1847–1924), one of the masters of Italian surgery, is known especially for the operation on inguinal hernia that bears his name. He also devised useful operations for the extirpation of humero-scapular sarcoma, ileo-cæcal resection, and nephropexy.

Among the most illustrious names in modern Swiss surgery is that of Theodor Kocher (1841–1917), who was Professor of Surgery at Bern for almost a half-century. A leader in guiding the newer surgery into the experimental and physiological approach to surgical problems, Kocher attained such success in applying these methods to clinical surgery that through his pupils and by personal example he became one of the most important factors in establishing modern scientific surgery. His experimental studies, such as those on the coagulation of the blood and on the functions of the brain and cord, and his contributions to general surgery were overshadowed by his pioneer work on the thyroid

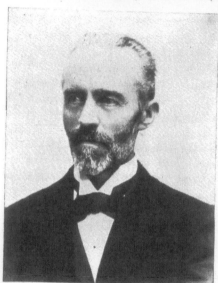

gland: the first to excise it for thyrotoxic goitre in man, he performed this operation in literally thousands of cases with an extremely low mortality, and this at a time when the operation, nowadays practically without danger, still belonged to the most difficult surgical interventions. Kocher's *Chirurgische Operationslehre* (4th ed., Jena, 1902; English trans., New York, 1894) enriched every branch of surgical art with painstakingly developed and self-practised methods. It may well be said that no surgeon of modern times had a more profound influence than Kocher. At a time when universality of surgery seems to be endangered by the growth of specialties, his powerful personality offers a brilliant example of a great modern surgeon.

474. *Theodor Kocher, Nobel Laureate, 1909.*

Surgery has reached a high level in various SOUTH AMERICAN countries, especially in the Argentine Republic, where J. ARCE (b. 1881) and P. CHUTRO (1880–1937) have attained international reputation.

10. Obstetrics and Gynæcology

The first four decades of the twentieth century have reaped the rewards of the teachings of Holmes, Semmelweis, Simpson, and their contemporaries in obstetrics and of McDowell, Sims, Lister, and their followers in gynæcology. The unhygienic conditions of the lying-in wards of the mid nineteenth century have become things of the past, and many of the technical procedures in gynæcology have become standardized as experience has accumulated. Physiologic concepts have replaced purely anatomic and mechanistic points of view and it is becoming increasingly evident that gynæcology is more than a surgical specialty as the trend deviates more and more away from operative procedures.

As in the field of general medicine, the armamentarium of the obstetrician and the gynæcologist has been greatly enriched by advances in other fields, such as Wassermann's test facilitating the diagnosis of syphilis; by blood transfusions, which have robbed tubal pregnancies and the hemorrhages of placenta prævia and the post-partum period of much of their dangers; Roentgen rays and radium for their value in diagnosis and in the treatment of such conditions as menorrhagia, uterine fibroids, and cervical carcinoma. New methods of physiotherapy have helped in the management of pelvic inflammatory diseases; and, finally, the advances that have been made in endocrinology have been of inestimable help.

CÆSAREAN SECTION., Prior to 1920 the Sänger or classical Cæsarean section was the method of choice, although Joseph B. DE LEE (1869–1942) and Alfred C. BECK (b. 1885) were becoming increasingly enthusiastic about low cervical section, originated by Frank of Cologne in 1907 and by Hugo Sellheim in 1908. In 1908 Veit and Fromme of Halle and Barton Cooke HIRST (1861–1935), of Philadelphia, independently and simultaneously described a transperitoneal cervical Cæsarean section with peritoneal exclusion, and in 1909 W. LATZKO (1861–1944) devised an extra-peritoneal approach, which has been improved by Edward G. WATERS (b: 1898), of Jersey City (1939).

ANESTHESIA. Anesthesia during labour has come into widespread use. Various methods are advocated, however, as will be seen in the section on Pharmacology and Therapeutics, but none have completely solved the problem.

PRENATAL CARE. As the importance of prenatal care in the prevention of the toxemias of pregnancy and the tragedies of delivery has become more and more widely appreciated, organized efforts have been made by the medical profession and governmental agencies to assure proper examinations and observation of parturient women in even the remotest communities.

Rösslin's sixteenth-century *Rosengarten* (translated in 1540 by Thomas Raynalde as *The Byrthe of Mankynde*) was the first book on obstetrics and maternal welfare written for the laity. In the early years of the nineteenth century William Buchan's *Advice to Mothers* (1803) enjoyed wide popularity.

The crowded condition of the Dublin Rotunda Hospital in the mid nineteenth century made it necessary for women to register and be examined some three months before the expected date of confinement. This led E. B. SINCLAIR (1824–82) and G. JOHNSTON (1814–89) to establish what was probably the first prenatal clinic in the world (1858). Their detection and treatment of patients with œdema, headache, vertigo, or albuminuria soon appreciably reduced the incidence of eclampsia in the hospital.

The first large-scale movement for prenatal care originated in Boston in 1912 when a public-spirited woman, a Mrs. Putnam, organized the Society for the Study and Prevention of Infant Mortality. Through the interest and efforts of Fred L. ADAIR (b. 1877), the work of the society was expanded about 1920 into the Joint Committee on Maternal Welfare, whose activities in turn were taken over by the American Committee on Maternal Welfare. From this committee has come the national, state, and local leadership in developing plans to conserve the health and lives of the mother, fetus, and newborn. One of the most picturesque and effective of these organizations is the Frontier Nursing Service that was established for the mountaineers of eastern Kentucky in 1925 by Mrs. Mary Breckenridge.

The age-long interest in MULTIPLE BIRTHS was stimulated by the well-authenticated birth in 1934 of the Dionne sisters. Probably identical quintuplets, all five survived in good health (A. R. DAFOE). Since then reports of quadruplets, and once of surviving quintuplets (Brazil), have multiplied. Chance suggests that females might be expected, if identical; for whereas there are but 96 females to 100 males in single births, in triplets the number rises to 101, in quadruplets to 156.

HOSPITALS devoted to the care of obstetrical and gynæcological patients have become increasingly numerous since the beginning of the twentieth century and have attained a high degree of perfection and luxury.

The first lying-in hospital in the United States was established in Philadelphia by William Shippen in 1765. Prior to 1799 New York City had no hospital for parturient women; but the yellow-fever epidemic of 1798 left so many pregnant widows without means of support that a lying-in ward was set apart in the Alms House in the following year. In 1801 this service was transferred to the New York Hospital. The New York State Hospital for Women (better known as the Women's Hospital) was established by Marion Sims in 1855 and soon became one of the gynæcological centres of the world. The Sloane Hospital for Women of New York City, erected in 1888 through the efforts of Edward Bradford CRAGIN (1859–1918), was one of the first specially constructed and adequately equipped maternity hospitals in the United States. At the University of Pennsylvania the first bedside teaching of obstetrics in the country was begun in 1889 by Barton Cooke Hirst; in 1897 an adequate maternity building was erected through his initiative.

The pathology and treatment of CANCER OF THE UTERUS have received considerable attention since the latter years of the nineteenth century, and T. S. CULLEN's (b. 1868) *Cancer of the Uterus* (1900) is worthy of inclusion in any list of the classics of gynæcology. While removal of the uterus for carcinoma of the corpus has long been accepted, radical hysterectomy for cancer of the cervix, introduced by Wertheim in 1900–1 and brought to its ultimate degree of technical perfection by Victor Bonney (b. 1872), has now been widely abandoned for local deep irradiation (H. A. Kelly, J. G. Clark, and others).

The introduction of UTERO-TUBAL INSUFFLATION as a non-surgical method of determining tubal patency by I. C. Rubin (b. 1883), of New York, in 1919, was an important contribution to the problem of sterility in the female. Rubin's work developed indirectly from previous unsatisfactory attempts to determine the patency of the Fallopian tubes by the injection of fluids that were opaque to X-rays. His method has received wide acceptance, although non-irritating radio-opaque substances are becoming increasingly popular.

FORCEPS. The twentieth century has thus far witnessed the introduction of three new designs in obstetrical forceps, of which two are of special value in the management of deep transverse arrests of the fetal head, while the third is used in the delivery of the aftercoming head in breech presentations.

The first of the forceps for rotating and delivering high transverse arrests were designed by Christian Kjelland (b. 1871) of Norway in 1915 and are almost identical in design with those described by Bethel in the nineteenth century. Lyman Barton, Sr. (b. 1866), of Plattsburg, New York, designed an even more radical modification (1924) of the conventional obstetrical forceps for the same purpose, which is considered by many to be more in accord with normal function in its action.

Forceps were applied to the aftercoming head by Smellie in 1755, and their routine use in such cases was advocated by Tarnier, Barnes, Meigs, and Busch. The instrument introduced by Edmund Piper (1881–1935), of Philadelphia, in the third decade of the twentieth century, was the first specially designed for the purpose.

Studies on pelvic architecture and mensuration were stimulated by the application of ROENTGENOLOGIC METHODS in the third decade of the century; important contributions have been made by Herbert Thoms (b. 1885) of New Haven, Connecticut, and E. W. Caldwell (1870–1918) and his associates, of New York. Their classification, by which pelves are divided into gynæcoid, android, anthropoid, platypelloid, and asymmetrical types, has done much to clarify the problem and the mechanism of labour.

Prior to the work of George W. Bartelmez (b. 1885), of Chicago, the sequence of events that took place in the uterine mucosa during the menstrual cycle were but poorly understood and the histological picture of tissue removed by curettage was frequently misinterpreted. *The Human Uterine Mucous Membrane during Menstruation* (1931) deserves a place of honour in gynæcological literature.

ERYTHROBLASTOSIS FŒTALIS (icterus of the newborn) has long been one of the most baffling problems in obstetrics, and efforts to treat the condition have been almost uniformly unsuccessful. In 1938 Ruth R. DARROW (b. 1895) suggested that it might be caused by sensitization of the mother to the fetal hemoglobin; but it remained for Philip LEVINE (b. 1900) and his associates, of Newark, New Jersey, to demonstrate in 1941 that both erythroblastosis and certain transfusion reactions were caused by the Rh factor (Landsteiner and Wiener).

OBSTETRICS has benefited by the many improvements in operative technique and more precise indications for their use. The great spread of the idea of prenatal and neonatal clinics has brought about a considerable decrease in maternal and infant mortality. Puerperal sepsis is under control, though the incidence is regrettably higher in the hospital than in the home, and there is still room for improvement. The tendency of some busy obstetricians, also, to see that the baby comes by the clock, an evil already noted by O. W. Holmes, is one requiring consideration. In those countries where many deliveries are still performed by midwives, standards for their selection and professional training have been much improved. Their close contact with all classes of society makes them valuable adjuncts to the physician, to whom they must turn for help in the various complications of pregnancy and childbirth.

11. Pediatrics

The splendid progress of pediatrics in the twentieth century may be said to be chiefly due to the basic aid received from preclinical sciences, especially biochemistry in the field of nutrition, to the improvement in diagnostic methods, and to the widespread and intelligent introduction of prophylactic measures. The more certain diagnosis of syphilis made possible by the Wassermann and other serological diagnoses, and the more potent remedies now available, such as Ehrlich's Salvarsan, have greatly reduced the ravages of congenital syphilis. Infantile tuberculosis has come under better control, owing to increased understanding of the disease processes (Albrecht, Ghon, Parrot, and Mantoux), which permits early diagnosis of infection in preclinical stages. The prevention of childhood tuberculosis, which is steadily receding as a main cause of disease and death in civilized countries, is being actively prosecuted by means of segregation of infected members of the family in the home, as well as of " open cases " in the population at large, by diminution of the spread of bovine forms in infected milk, and similar means.

PROPHYLAXIS OF THE INFECTIOUS DISEASES of infants is one of the brightest phases of recent pediatric progress. The long immunity produced by vaccination with cowpox has protected mankind from smallpox for over a century, and the shorter benefits resulting from tetanus antitoxin and typhoid vaccine have been known for more than a generation. More recent, however, is the discovery of the lasting immunity conferred by toxin-antitoxin mixtures and later by toxoids in diphtheria (Behring, G. Ramon, W. H. Park), those susceptible to attack being revealed by a positive cutaneous reaction (Bela SCHICK, 1913). Susceptibility to scarlet fever is revealed by the Dick test (1924), scarlet fever now being accepted as a streptococcic disease (A. DOCHEZ, George and Gladys DICK). The production, in the French army, of an active immunity to tetanus has had widespread application to pediatrics in the United States in the past few years. The discovery by Sauer that large doses of *H. pertussis* (phase I) vaccine would produce a high and fairly durable active immunity has greatly reduced the incidence and severity of whooping cough, the most fatal of the childhood contagious diseases, and has led to the development of hyper-immune human pertussis serum, an efficient passive immunizing agent.

The treatment of rickets with vitamin D (E. Mellanby, 1919), phosphates (H. C. Sherman and A. M. Pappenheimer, 1920), sunlight (Alfred Hess, 1921), or irradiated ergosterol (Hess, 1925; H. Steenbock, 1925), is now universally accepted and based on an established rationale.

The outstanding pediatric triumph in the endocrine field is the cure of cretinism, due to congenital thyroid insufficiency, by administration of thyroid extract. The relations of persisting infantilism to the pituitary and gonadal insufficiency, referred to elsewhere, still await complete explanation.

American pediatrics includes many well-known names, such as T. M. ROTCH (Philadelphia, 1814–1914), first Professor of Pediatrics at Harvard, who introduced the percentage modification of milk (protein, fats, and carbohydrates) for individual infant feeding. L. E. HOLT (1855–1924) and H. D. CHAPIN (1857–1942), both of New York and both authors of successful textbooks, were concerned with modified milk mixtures, pasteurization, and efforts to improve the purity of the milk supply in large centres (also H. L. Coit). Knowledge of infant metabolism in health and disease has been advanced by biochemical progress, especially in the studies of Fritz TALBOT (b. 1878), John Lovett MORSE (b. 1865), and others too numerous to mention. Among the younger generation, John HOWLAND (1873–1926) and his pupil W. McKim MARRIOTT (1885–1936) were particularly concerned with dehydration and acidosis, rickets and tetany. The latter's textbook, *Infant Nutrition*, is said to be the best presentation of modern infant feeding. The principles of the care of the premature infant have been well summarized by Julius HESS (b. 1876) and put into practice in his Premature Station in Chicago. E. A. PARK (b. 1877) not only has made important contributions to our knowledge of the functional pathology of rickets and scurvy, but has exerted a profound influence on the younger pediatricians in the United States. Disorders of the acid-base balance and water metabolism, postulated by L. J. Henderson and made applicable clinically by passing through the studies of D. D. Van Slyke, J. Peters, Glenn Cullen, and J. H. Austin, have been brought to pediatric therapeutics by J. Gamble, A. Shohl (b. 1889), W. McKim Marriott (and his student Hartmann), R. R. Darrow, and many others. The proper use of the principles laid down by these studies has saved innumerable infant lives. The White House Conference on Child Welfare called by President Hoover in the 1930's was an important milestone in summarizing existing knowledge and formulating programs for further investigation into the psychological, economic, and physical needs of children. The U. S. Federal Children's Bureau has also done a magnificent job.

J. M. KEATING'S (1852–93) *Cyclopedia* (1890), an important work in its day, is now of historical value only. Even the monumental *System of Pediatrics* (1922) of I. A. ABT (b. 1867) is already outmoded in many respects, so rapid have been the advances in this subject. A. V. MEIGS's (1850–1912) *Milk Analysis and Infant Feeding* was long regarded as a classic. Meigs, a shrewd thinker and able clinician, would never accept the germ theory of disease — a strange character! Joseph BRENNEMAN's *Loose Leaf Practice of Pediatrics* (Prior), in four volumes, is the outstanding reference work in this field. The upsurge of pediatrics in America is illustrated by such dates as the founding of the American Pediatric Society (1888); of the *American Journal of Diseases of Children* (1911); of the American Academy of Pediatrics and its organ, the *Journal of Pediatrics* (1932).

Twentieth-century British pediatrics has been fostered by such authorities as Sir Thomas BARLOW (1845–1945), a leader in all branches of pediatrics, Clement DUKES (1845–1925), John THOMSON (1856–1926), and J. W. BALLANTYNE (1861–1923) of Edinburgh, F. J. POYNTON (b. 1869), J. D. ROLLESTON (b. 1873), Harriet CHICK (b. 1875), Edward (b. 1884) and May MELLANBY, Noel PATON

(1859–1928), and Leonard FINDLAY (b. 1898) of Glasgow, and Leonard J. PARSONS of Birmingham. The *British Journal of Diseases of Children* was founded in 1904; the *Archives of Diseases of Childhood* in 1926 under the auspices of the British Medical Association. The British Pediatric Association first met in 1928, with G. F. Still as president.

J. J. GRANCHER, Armand de LILLE, ROUSSEL, J. COMBY, HUTINEL, and NOBÉCOURT are among modern French leaders in this specialty.

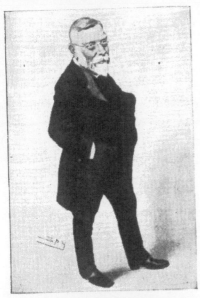

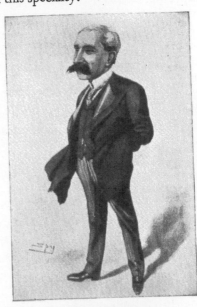

475. *Sir Thomas Barlow.*
(*Caricature by Spy in* Vanity Fair.)

476. *Sir Felix Semon.*
(*Caricature by Spy in* Vanity Fair.)

In GERMANY, H. FINKELSTEIN (1865–1939), Heubner's pupil and director of the Kinderasyl at Berlin, wrote an excellent and widely popular textbook. He introduced a new concept of alimentary disturbances and together with L. F. Meyer suggested the use of protein milk in the treatment of diarrhœa. A. SCHLOSSMANN (1867–1932), Pfaundler's collaborator and a famous teacher, studied the fasting metabolism of infants and recognized the great increase in metabolism following muscular action. A. CZERNY (1863–1941) wrote an outstanding work on nutritional disorders, and was responsible for the concept of the "exudative diathesis" (1907), which is still important in concepts of pathogenesis of children's diseases, although it is now usually classified among the allergies of childhood.

In HUNGARY, Johann von BÓKAY (1858–1937) is remembered as the founder of the Stephania Children's Hospital at Budapest. In Russia, C. RAUCHFUSS (1835–1915) founded a similar hospital at St. Petersburg; N. GUNDOBIN (1860–

1908) wrote a valuable textbook on the anatomy and physiology of childhood; and N. FILATOV (1847–1902), author of the famous book on children's diseases, did much to raise the scientific standard of pediatrics in that country.

The history of pediatrics in ITALY is short and recent. Though G. PALLONI was named Professor of Children's Diseases at Pisa in 1802, we must pass to the last two decades of the past century for the beginning of the real history of the subject. In 1882 D. CERVESATO (1851–1903) began teaching it at Padua, to be followed there by V. TEDESCHI (1852–1919). Teaching was begun by F. FEDE (1832–1913) at Naples in 1886; by G. MYA (1857–1911) at Florence in 1892; and by L. CONCETTI (1854–1920) at Rome in 1896. This triumvirate has produced numerous successful followers, especially Rocco JEMMA, Fede's successor, who made important studies on the leishmaniases. The Società Italiana di Pediatria was founded in 1894, and various pediatric journals have been published. Among the oldest and best known of these are *La Pediatria*, edited by Jemma, and the *Rivista di clinica pediatrica*, edited by C. Comba.

12. *Ophthalmology*

As in most specialties, remarkable progress has been achieved in the period under consideration by all branches of ophthalmology: the physiology of the eye, diagnostic technique, surgery, refraction, orthoptic training, prevention of blindness, and care of the blind.

The METABOLISM of the eye had been studied with all the available microchemical and microphysical methods, with the aim of throwing light upon the dependence of its metabolism on the circulation, and its importance for the maintenance of the intraocular pressure. The aqueous humour has been proved to be a secretion, and not a dialysate or a filtrate, by the studies of Jonas S. FRIEDENWALD, which are confirmed by D. C. COGAN, KINSEY and GRANT, and also by W. S. Duke ELDER and DAWSON. Its drainage plays the most important role in the normal function of the eye.

A better knowledge of the lens metabolism and its intricate oxidation-reduction process does not yet enable us to understand the intimate changes that take place in its substance, changes that, when deranged, lead to loss of transparency (cataract-formation). The scientists who deserve credit for these important studies are legion. Duke Elder has brought them well together in the effort to build a clear and logical picture of the complex phenomena of the physiology of the eye.

An outstanding development in ophthalmology was brought about by the application of new techniques in ILLUMINATION. One cannot overemphasize the importance of electric lighting and its progressive improvement for the increasing perfection of ophthalmologic diagnostic instruments, the self-illuminating devices representing the highest peak of achievement in this direction.

Among the new instruments the pride of place belongs to Gullstrand's "slit lamp." In 1911 Allvar GULLSTRAND (1862–1930), of Uppsala, whose work in dioptrics will be spoken of later, demonstrated a model of the slit lamp at a meeting in Heidelberg. The principle is not new; it is merely the principle of oblique focal illumination carried to its highest development. With this instrument such a wealth of detail of the eye tissues was disclosed in the clinical evaluation of eye diseases that a new branch of ophthalmology was created: BIOMICROSCOPY.

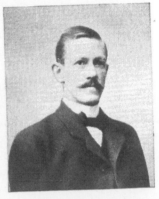

477. *Allvar Gullstrand, Nobel Laureate, 1911.*

Allvar Gullstrand made notable contributions to many problems of dioptrics. In 1911 he was awarded the Nobel prize for his mathematical physical studies of dioptrics in heterogeneous media (1891–1906). He also invented improved methods for estimating astigmatism and abnormal shapes of the cornea, for locating paralysed muscles, and for corrective glasses after removal of the cataractous lens. In 1889 he introduced a photographic method of locating the paralysed ocular muscle. In 1907 he stated that the yellow colour of the macula lutea is a cadaveric phenomenon, and in 1912 he devised the reflexless stationary ophthalmoscope.

Alfred VOGT of Zurich, L. KOEPPE, and F. E. KOBY, were among the first to publish notable works on this subject. Vogt's atlas summed up all the biomicroscopic knowledge of his period. The whole field has now been brought up to date and beautifully illustrated in M. L. BERLINER's book *Biomicroscopy* (1943).

Ophthalmoscopes have improved in optics and illumination, and many models were put on the market, some of the stationary type and many more hand models. Among the latter one must remember Jonas S. Friedenwald's opththalmoscope, which affords an unusually clear view of the fundus; it has a slit-like effect, three monochromatic light-filters, and increased magnification; it embodies the principles of slit-lamp microscopy to the fundus. Mention should be made of Nordenson's camera, with which beautiful pictures of the eye ground can be taken. More recently even coloured pictures have been taken. W. H. WILMER's (1863–1936) *Atlas Fundus Oculi* (1934), in which the illustrations are done in quadrichromy, gives the best representation of the eye ground in health and disease. Perimetry was refined especially by H. M. TRAQUAIR, who introduced the concept of isopters. Angioscotometry (mapping of visual defects from shadows of dilated vessels) was suggested and developed by J. N.

Evans, a Britisher now resident in Brooklyn, New York. A more detailed knowledge of the sclerochoroidal filtration angle has been made possible by gonioscopy. The outstanding work in this field is due to Uribe-Troncoso, a Mexican now working in New York, who used a focused beam of light and devised efficient contact glass. H. Schoetz (1850–1928), of Oslo, is internationally known for his ocular tonometer and a modification of Helmholtz's ophthalmometer.

The removal of cataract, the most frequent and important surgical operation on the eye, has been remarkably perfected. The difficulty of operating on a mobile field has been removed, thanks to better fixation, to Elschnig's forceps, and especially to suture of the superior rectus (*Zügelnaht*). The danger of sudden, spastic contraction of the orbicularis (frequent cause of loss of vitreous-end of the eye) is prevented through akinesia, a temporary paralysis of the muscle brought about by injection of novocaine in the muscle or the facial nerve. These improvements pave the way for the intracapsular extraction of the cataract. A. Knapp, A. Elschnig, H. M. Sinclair (a Scot working in England), and many others have proposed special types of forceps in order to grasp the lens without breaking the capsule. In this method the lens is seized by forceps, subluxated, tumbled, and delivered with the aid of pressure on the outside of the globe. The same result is obtained by other means: Ignacio Barraquer (Spain), for instance, has revived the use of a suction instrument (vibratory vacuum). Also the diathermic needle has been used for the removal of the lens *in toto* (Lopez Lacarrère, A. Jess).

An advance of great importance has been made in the operation for DETACHMENT OF THE RETINA by J. Gonin, a Swiss, which has been much improved by H. J. M. Wewe and W. Walter. This operation and its various improvements have rendered a hitherto almost hopeless condition amenable to successful restoration of vision in a large number of cases.

Corneal transplantation (keratoplasty) has been often attempted: first successfully practised by von Hippel in 1888 and by F. Salzer in 1900, then by S. Calderaro in 1908. A. H. Ebeling and Anne Carrel, operating on cats in 1921, obtained one clear graft; in 1922 J. W. Tudor Thomas, of Cardiff, succeeded in accomplishing attachment and healing in fifty transplants, employing grafts from animals of the same species. He has since obtained satisfactory results in human transplantation. Keratoplasty has now a definite place in eye surgery, thanks to the work of Ramon Castroviejo (New York) and V. P. Filatov (Odessa). The progress in this field has been so rapid and the results so outstanding that banks have been instituted for the utilization of the cornea of persons wishing to leave it to the bank after their death, or of those whose eye has been enucleated for a condition that left the cornea intact.

William MacKenzie had advised (1830) relieving increased tension of the eye by a paracentesis or sclerotomy. This had only a temporary effect. Definite results were obtained for the first time in history by Albrecht von Graefe's iridectomy. De Wecker had advocated the establishment of drainage through a filtering scar. Though he failed, his ideas bore fruit in the subsequent work of H. HERBERT at Bombay (1903, iris inclusion), and Sören HOLTH of Oslo (1863–1937) (1907, iridencleisis, locking iris in cornea), and culminated in the sclerectomy of P. F. LAGRANGE, of Bordeaux (1905), and the corneoscleral trephining of Colonel R. H. ELLIOT (1909).

The curiosity of a lawyer, Adelbert AMES, who asked himself if the two eyes see alike, led to the discovery of ANISEIKONIA, a condition in which the retinal image of one eye differs in size and shape from that of the other eye. The cerebral effort to fuse with two different images then causes headaches, nervousness, and even digestive disturbances. Aniseikonia cannot be considered a rare condition; more than two per cent of all patients with asthenopic symptoms are affected by it. A special instrument (the eikonometer) is used for its diagnosis, and special lenses to correct it, as evolved in the Dartmouth laboratories.

Skiascopy offers to the ophthalmologist the safest means of estimating refraction objectively. Edward JACKSON's (1856–1942) cross-cylinders represent the highest peak of subjective refraction and allow for the most careful evaluation of axis.

SPECTACLES, even at their best, represent only an approximate solution of the problem of correcting errors of refraction. The reason for this shortcoming has to be sought in the fact that it is an attempt to combine a stationary lens with the eye — an optical system that is in motion. The rational solution would be to put the correcting lens upon the eye adherent to it and following it in all its excursions. This idea has been realized with contact glasses, small shells of glass that are filled with saline and placed in close apposition to the eye. Since cornea, normal saline, and the contact glass have approximately the same index of refraction, the cornea loses its importance as a refracting surface and its role is taken over by the central part of the contact glass itself. Normal saline becomes thus a liquid lens whose shape and curvature are determined by the posterior surface of the contact glass. The principle has been known for a long time (Herschel, 1827), and many, but unsuccessful, attempts to make it practicable are on record. Only recently L. HEINE, of Kiel, in association with the Zeiss Optical Company, succeeded in putting on the market a rich series of ground contact glasses that afforded sufficient possibility of choice so as to fit most patients. The next step was to prepare moulds of the eyeball in order to obtain a better fit, and to make the contact glass, not of glass, but of plastic material in order to eliminate danger to the eye.

Study of toxic amblyopia was developed especially in the United States by Casey Wood and T. H. Buller (1904). Ethyl alcohol and tobacco amblyopia have been demonstrated to be due to vitamin B_1 deficiency and respond favourably to its supply.

Bernard Sachs (1858–1944), of New York, described prenatal degeneration of the macular region of the retina (1887) in amaurotic family idiocy, which had been observed in 1881 by Warren Tay (1843–1927), of London. This led to the discovery of other forms of abiotrophy of the retina, described especially by British ophthalmologists, of whom E. Nettleship and F. E. Batten were foremost. Familial retinoblastoma is another inherited disease of the eye — devastating in its consequences and one of the best examples of the occasional great importance of heredity in human cancer.

Notable progress here, as in other specialties, was connected with the growth of more intimate relations between ophthalmology and other branches of medicine. This has led to the application of advances in other fields, notably in pharmacology, to ophthalmology; and on the other hand ophthalmology has afforded constantly growing aid to general medicine and neurology. As such may be mentioned the studies on the retinal vascular changes associated with arteriosclerosis, by H. Friedenwald, J. S. Friedenwald, and Wagener.

In addition to the various British achievements considered above, we may note the work of R. W. Doyne (1857–1916), the founder of the Oxford Eye Hospital and the annual Ophthalmology Congress, whose name is associated with special forms of conjunctivitis, guttate iritis, family choroiditis, and discoid cataract. From Ida Mann, a surgeon at Moorfields, came two important works: *The Development of the Human Eye* (1928) and *Developmental Anomalies of the Human Eye* (1937). W. S. Duke Elder's *Textbook of Ophthalmology*, in several volumes (begun 1932), has been of great service, especially for its comprehensive bibliographies.

The greatest advances in ophthalmology in recent times have been in the direction of prevention. School inspection for infectious cases of conjunctivitis, adequate provision of spectacles for children with errors of vision, improved light-regulations in factories and schools, a rigid system of inspection of immigrants, all have brought important contributions to the prevention of eye diseases. It has been estimated that there are about 230,000 blind in the United States, and over 2,000,000 in the whole world at the present time, excluding those blinded in the World Wars. The ratio in census areas ranged from 478 blind per million persons in New Zealand to 1,325 in Egypt. Institutions for the blind have had an important development all over the world, but especially in the United States, where the education of these patients has made most remarkable progress.

13. Otology, Laryngology, Rhinology

In the present century oto-rhino-laryngology has grown so greatly that in the United States, for instance, the certifying board on this specialty has certified more men than has any other board, even including those on internal medicine and general surgery. This growth, however, consisted more in the application of the advances made in the previous century than in breaking historically important new ground. New and better techniques, to be sure, continue to replace earlier procedures, such as complete enucleation of the faucial tonsils, instead of incomplete amputation. Sinusitis, which in the eastern United States, at least, has almost replaced colds in the head in importance, is a problem still awaiting solution. Operation is approached more conservatively than a generation ago, and radiation has thus far offered little more than temporary relief.

In OTOLOGY more knowledge has been obtained of the functions of the oval window. Various " fenestration " operations for otosclerosis, based on the newer knowledge, have come into vogue, beginning with Maurice SOUR-DILLE's (b. 1885) three-stage operation opening a new window into a semi-circular canal. In 1938 J. LEMPERT (now of New York) elaborated a successful one-stage operation, which, in spite of its difficulties, has achieved some excellent results. Due to the brilliant work, chiefly by Americans, of such men as E. H. CAMPBELL, K. M. DAY, Walter HUGHSON (1891–1944), and J. R. PAGE, good results in suitable cases have been obtained in more than half the cases operated upon.

The method of audiometry, by which the individual's acuteness of hearing of sounds at various pitches is objectively tested and recorded, has contributed notably in localizing the site of the hearing difficulty and in recording the changes produced by treatment or by the progress of the disease. Pioneers in this field were the German A. HARTMANN, who devised an " acoumeter " in 1878, and the Englishman D. E. HUGHES, whose invention (1879), called an " audiometer " by Richardson, was said to be the first serviceable instrument. The method, however, was but little employed until the modern type of instrument was invented (1922) by the physicist C. C. BUNCH, of St. Louis, and by investigators in the Bell Telephone Company's laboratories. Devices to aid hearing have progressed far since the familiar ear-trumpet of earlier centuries. Bell's invention of the telephone (1876) was adapted before the end of the century to hearing aids of varying efficiency; it received considerable publicity through the use of the Alabaman Reese HUTCHINSON's " Acousticon " by Queen Victoria. Bone conduction, useful in certain kinds of deafness, started with R. S. RHODES's " audiphone " (1879), a fanlike device held between the teeth. Bone conductors of the electrically amplified telephone type were introduced in England (1920) by S. G. BROWN, and in America (1923) by H. GERNSBOCK (the " osophone "). With the development of vacuum-tube amplifying devices shortly after, hearing-aid instruments have become much more efficient, sightly, and easily portable.

Among the most illustrious of recent oto-rhino-laryngologists was H. NEUMANN (1873–1939), a skilful operator whose method for opening the labyrinth is the most in use today. The Rumanian T. GLUCK (b. 1853), professor at Berlin, has introduced various improvements in technique. Sir Felix SEMON (1849–1927) was the most famous English laryngologist (Semon's law).

RHINOLOGY made rapid progress early in the century with the introduction of the nasal speculum and head mirror to illuminate the entire nasal cavity; and again in the present century with improved X-ray technique, transillumination, and other procedures. Functionally the importance of the pharyngeal box and the accessory sinuses as resonating chambers was recognized, while inflammation of the latter structures, especially in superheated, arid American houses, is assuming formidable proportions.

Neoplasms of the nose, never common, had been reported in increasing numbers with the spreading study of pathologic histology. However, recognition of many varieties awaited the twentieth century: endothelioma, E. Althoff, 1907; chondroma, W. Uffenorde, 1908; lymphangioma, Hamm, 1903; glioma, J. P. Clark, 1905; rhabdomyoma, D. T. Vail, 1908; teratoma, L. A. Coffin, 1909.

Chronically enlarged and infected tonsils and adenoids (the pharyngeal tonsils) were found to be extremely common in most civilized countries. Their defensive role against bacterial infection has been weighed against their possible harm as sites of lowered resistance prone to repeated infections and as potential foci of infection causing trouble at distant sites in the body. In the case of adenoids, also, the bad effects of the resultant " mouth breathing " and of obstruction to the Eustachian tube have been taken into consideration. The problem is still under discussion. " Tonsils and adenoids " have been removed literally by the millions, especially in America, and though the vogue seems to have lessened, the operation still constitutes a mainstay of the specialist's budget. The tidal wave of literature on the subject began to recede as early as 1902; and though F. R. Packard pictured " the slaughter of the tonsils " as late as 1930, a better selection of cases is now the rule. Also, operations on the tonsils and for mastoiditis have been noticeably diminished already by the potent sulfonamides and penicillin.

PERORAL ENDOSCOPY. The methods of penetrating to various remote body cavities so well that lesions and foreign bodies can be not only seen but removed with appropriate instruments were brought to a high degree of efficiency, especially by Chevalier JACKSON (b. 1865), of Pittsburgh, in what may be called the new specialty of peroral endoscopy. We have seen how the larynx was laid bare by the laryngoscope, how early attempts were made by Adolph Kussmaul (1822–1902) in 1869 and by Sir Morell Mackenzie to inspect the œsophagus; and how Gustav Killian (1860–1921) had searched for foreign bodies in the bronchi through a rigid tube inserted through a tracheotomy wound (1898) and had removed an aspirated bone from the trachea by means of a modified œsophagoscope. From these crude beginnings a whole specialty has now developed.

A practical œsophagoscope was devised by Jackson with an accompanying source of light in 1902; and there slowly emerged an illuminated bronchoscope, introduced through the mouth, capable of exploring the whole bronchial tree, with its efficiency increased by accompanying scores of accessory instruments. Not only can the stomach now be thoroughly examined *per os*, but even photographs made of its mucosal lining. The far-reaching capabilities of peroral endoscopy in the diagnosis and treatment of respiratory and gastro-intestinal disease have been abundantly demonstrated, while Jackson's far-seeing policy of developing a maximum of skilled assistants has ensured the perpetuation of his methods. Successively filling six chairs in his specialty, most of them being created for him, he has been followed in each by a personally trained junior, with whom he has received and trained students from all parts of the world.

14. Urology

In the past fifty years genito-urinary surgery made rapid and outstanding progress, chiefly due to the discovery of the X-ray and to the improvements in anesthesia. New diagnostic methods were introduced which had a revolutionary effect in the development of the surgical intervention, not only permitting exact recognition of the nature and location of any lesion in any part of the urogenital tract, but also furnishing information of the functional ability of the organs. Thus the hematogenous origin of renal tuberculosis had been explored, and also the possibility of its treatment by removal of one kidney when the active process has been shown to be limited to one organ. The previous contention that renal tuberculosis was always caused by ascending infection from the bladder, suggesting that it was always bilateral and therefore not susceptible to surgical treatment, had been proved wrong.

The X-ray has permitted the precise and early diagnosis of reno-ureteral calculus with correspondingly better results in treatment. The first X-ray diagnosis of a renal calculus was made in 1897 by James ADAMS, a Glasgow surgeon, who operated on this case successfully. A pioneer in roentgenology of the urinary tract was James McINTYRE. Later the American Robert ABBE and the English FENWICK made further progress in the field of diagnosis. Charles J. LEONARD developed a technique by which he detected renal calculus in one hundred out of one hundred and thirty-six cases. In 1897 T. TUFFIER (1871–1929), of Paris, advocated radioscopy of the ureter after the passage of a middle catheter. F. VOELCKER and A. von LICHTENBERG recommended the injection of bismuth suspension, rendering kidney, pelvis, and ureter opaque to X-rays, suggesting this method for the diagnosis of hydronephrosis and of tumours of the kidney. In 1908 J. ALBARRAN published his experiences in this field, and later von Lichtenberg introduced the injection of collargol solution, thus successfully inaugurating ureteropyelography. There was a serious danger, however, which prevented a widespread use of the method: namely, that the substances to be injected were all toxic. In 1918 Donald F. CAMERON proposed the substitution of a twenty-five per cent solution of sodium or potassium iodide for the silver solutions, and later advised the use of a 13.5 per cent solution of sodium bromide, with excellent results.

In 1929 intravenous pyelography, advocated by ROSENSTEIN in 1924, was introduced with the practical method of Moses SWICK of New York. Various substances have been used, such as the selectan group, with a high iodine content and great solubility (uroselectan, iopax, skioden). Young and Waters have exhaustively treated the whole subject in their book on *Urological Roentgenology*.

A great success of modern urology was achieved in the treatment of enlargement of the PROSTATE GLAND by the two-stage method. Also Bottini's method of removing the obstruction to the urinary flow by thermogalvanic diaeresis of the prostate has lately been again taken up with improved modern instruments, especially in the hands of the Americans J. F. McCARTHY, Hugh YOUNG, T. CAULK of St. Louis, W. F. BRAASCH of Rochester, Minnesota, the German LICHTENBERG, and the French G. LUYS and M. HEITZ-BOYER. The differentiation of true neoplasma of the gland from the benign hypertrophies (apparently due to hormonal imbalance) has been actively and successfully investigated. In 1902 August SOCIN and Emil BURKHARDT reported about 109 operations with a mortality of thirty per cent. Extirpation of prostatic cancer was carried out with some success by Hugh Young and others, performing as radical a resection as possible. Also, modern studies on the control of the growth of the prostate by sex hormones have opened new horizons for the therapy of its tumours.

New methods of treating bladder tumour have been developed in recent times. In 1908 Edwin BEER, of New York, worked out a technique for burning the tumours with an electric sparking apparatus through the cystoscope (fulguration). Radium was also used for bladder tumours; diathermy has given satisfactory results, and ultraviolet light appears to be applicable in cases of urogenital tuberculosis. The surgery of renal tuberculosis is a twentieth-century development chiefly due to ISRAEL, ALBARRAN, and NICOLICH.

The first American urologists to achieve fame were Samuel D. Gross, author of a well-known textbook on genito-urinary diseases, and Henry J. Bigelow, who after studying in France became Professor of Surgery at Harvard and extended the influence of the French school in America. His *lithotrite*, an instrument for the removal of vesical calculus, is still in use, slightly modified.

Among the American contributions to the progress of urology we must refer to the modification of Nitze's cystoscope by Tilden BROWN, of New York. Very soon came the discoveries and modifications of Bransford LEWIS, L. BUERGER, McCARTHY, H. H. YOUNG, and Reinhold WAPPLER. Thomas J. KERWIN, of New York, a prominent American urologist who wrote the history of this specialty (New York, 1933) writes that Wappler showed an almost miraculous appreciation of the possibilities of instrumentation, putting into complete form the crude imaginings of impractical physicians or scientists.

L. G. ROWNTREE and J. T. GERAGHTY made an important contribution to urology with their dye test of renal function. In 1912 O. S. LOWSLEY published his research on the embryology of the prostate gland. A great number of clinicians and scientists working together in clinical laboratories have procured a continuous progress of urology in the advancement of scientific investigation and in the constant improvement of technique. The American schools have played a notable part in these advances. The American Urological Association was founded in New York in 1902, and the *Journal of Urology* (edited by H. H. Young) in 1907.

Among Italian urologists the best-known were G. NICOLICH, of Trieste (1852–1925), and G. LASIO, of Milan.

Urology is today a surgical specialty that is rapidly growing in importance. It is taught as such in most medical schools throughout the world and has its own special scientific societies and journals.

15. Dermatology and Syphilology

Dermatology in the twentieth century shows the increasing influence of the dynamic concept of cutaneous changes. Because of the rapid progress in medicine as a whole, there arose a feeling of dissatisfaction with the detailed, purely descriptive pathologic morphology of the nineteenth century. Recent developments attribute to the skin a much greater functional role than that allowed in classical times — merely of covering and mechanically defending the body. Above all, it is regarded as a large glandular structure, the intermediary between the external and the internal environment. It is also important in the regulation of body heat, in secretion, absorption of fats and various chemicals, sensation, and even respiration (this only to a small extent in man). The increasing awareness by other medical specialties of certain systemic dermatologic diseases, such as disseminated lupus erythematosus, sarcoidosis, and the lipoidoses, has stimulated the dermatologist to focus his attention again on systemic aspects of skin conditions. Thus there has arisen the tendency, especially in the American school, to designate dermatology as " cutaneous medicine." The enlargement of hospital centres for dermatology has made possible the complete study of the patient as contrasted with the superficial, almost casual study in the out-patient clinic. Stimulated by Josef JADASSOHN, the greatest clinician and teacher of the twentieth century, one of his pupils, Bruno BLOCH, of Zurich, may be said to have founded the school of dynamic dermatology through his researches, chiefly on cutaneous allergies and also on pigment-formation, endocrine dysfunctions, and carcinogenesis. The rise of this new functional phase of dermatology emphasized the need for physical changes in the dermatology departments of hospitals by the acquisition of their own laboratories of chemistry and pathology, and, through such influences as that of Raymond SABOURAUD, of their own laboratories of mycology and bacteriology. When this was not possible, the divisions of dermatology sought close collaboration with these other units of the hospital or medical-college group. Another practical result of the dynamic concept of dermatology has been the rise of industrial dermatology, supplying the increasing needs of industrial medicine.

Supplementing the descriptive and pathological aspects of dermatological progress, a physiological and experimental trend now seeks to explain the development and course of the disease in question. Micro-organismal causes of cutaneous diseases are being actively investigated, together with the reactions of the skin to a great variety of abnormal stimuli. Such studies as those of Finsen on reactions of light, of E. Hoffmann on œsophylaxis (protective influences from within), of B. Bloch on pigment-formation and cutaneous allergy, are gradually constructing a better knowledge of the functional pathology of the skin. On the basis of the physiological studies of A. Krogh, U. Ebbecke, E. Fischer, and many others, modern clinicians, such as W. H. Lewis and H. K. W. Schade, are elaborating new dermatological theories. Thus a real functional dermatology may be said to be coming into existence.

Many diseases of the skin, as for instance DARIER's (b. 1856) disease (1889), have been connected, according to recent studies, with the avitaminoses, on more or less valid grounds.

A new disease has been described recently by H. H. HAILEY, T. McCall ANDERSON, and others: namely, benign chronic pemphigus, which presents the same symptoms as malignant pemphigus, but is limited to the neck and the armpits and occurs in many members of the same family.

A great impulse to the study of *professional dermatoses* has been given by the two World Wars and the rapid development of war industry and new industrial procedures. Affections of the skin constitute today more than half of all professional diseases. Besides the dermatitis caused by irritation, new forms of allergic reaction, deriving from contact with different substances, have been described. A vast prophylaxis program is under way, including improvement of working conditions, protective apparel, inunctions with protecting substances that cover the exposed parts, substances resistant to the irritant agents.

In the field of dermatology as in all other fields of medicine, the sulfonamide drugs have assumed great importance. Local therapy of cutaneous infections has often given satisfactory results, and no less in seborrhœic dermatitis. The oral therapy is efficient in chronic ulceration of the legs, in erysipelas, and sometimes in pemphigus. As sensitization and also serious reactions may occur, however, dermatologists are convinced that caution is necessary in the use of these remedies.

A significant improvement in the diagnosis of skin diseases is given by the examination with Wood's lamp, which is especially important for the diagnosis of trichophytosis. In a recent epidemic in New York City the importance of this diagnostic method was amply illustrated.

A great number of new methods have been suggested for the cure of burns. The " sulfa " drugs in the form of emulsions, tannic acid, silver nitrate, and the so-called triple dye are some of the remedies that have been prescribed by different dermatologists.

A brilliant part of American dermatology is the work of Central and South

American physicians on those fascinating cutaneous diseases peculiar to the American tropics. These diseases include American onchocerciasis, American leishmaniasis, verruga peruana, and *el mal del pinto* and epidemic pemphigus. Many who have made significant contributions were not dermatologists. Professor Rodolfo ROBLES in Guatemala discovered (1915) the parasitic nature of American onchocerciasis. LINDENBERG, CARINI, PARANHOS, and RABELLO in 1909 described the organisms in American leishmaniasis and proved the identity of this lesion with Oriental sore. The young martyr to the disease he elucidated, Daniel A. Carrion, of Peru, in 1885 found the true relationship of Oroya fever and verruga peruana. Great contributions to another form of treponematosis of the New World, *el mal del pinto*, were made by S. GONZALEZ-HERREJON of Mexico and LEON Y BLANCO of Cuba. In Brazil, C. PAES-LEME and J. P. VIEIRA among others have done notable work on epidemic pemphigus. In addition the important and common fungous diseases of South America have been studied by PEDROSO, and O. da FONSECA, to mention only two of the outstanding contributors. Clinicians of the present time include such men as GONZALEZ-URENA and F. LATAPI in Mexico, Vincente PARDO-CASTELLO and Braulio SAENZ in Cuba, Julio OLIVARES in Costa Rica, and others. Central and South America, especially Peru, also have given to the field of medical history important collections of ceramics (*huacos*) with remarkable reproductions of pathological cases.

VENEREOLOGY. The efficacy of prophylactic measures in venereal disease was well demonstrated during the First World War, when the favouring circumstances of military discipline made it possible greatly to cut down the incidence of venereal disease among soldiers in camps and barracks. The campaign against venereal disease has been taking on increased force in recent years, especially in Scandinavia and America, countries that tend toward anti-venereal legislation such as compulsory examinations before marriage and childbirth. In other countries, such as England and Holland, apparently equally good results have been obtained by the less conspicuous methods of public education. Throughout the civilized world, however, the mystery attaching to the social diseases and the euphemisms employed in referring to them have been largely dispelled, so that the problem can be attacked without prudery, as can other important medical problems.

In the present century progress has been due especially to the achievements of the bacteriological, serological, and chemotherapeutic laboratories. The new trend began with the discovery of the *Spirochæta pallida* as the pathogenic cause of syphilis, jointly by the parasitologist F. Schaudinn (1871–1906), and the clinician Eric Hoffmann, in 1905. Serology, through the studies of Wassermann and of J. Bordet and O. Gengou, put the practising physician in possession of the important Wassermann test (1906, 1907), which, though not strictly a complement-fixation test as originally believed, has proved to be of the greatest value in the diagnosis of syphilis and in the estimation of the continued activity of the process. The third great step in this line of progress was the memorable discovery by Paul Ehrlich, with the collaboration of the Japanese Sacachiro Hata, of the therapeutic value of arsenobenzol (606, Salvarsan). Though this is not the *therapia magna sterilisans* hoped for by its inventor, it stands as the most valuable drug remedy for the disease, and if properly used, one capable of controlling its manifestations, perhaps even over long periods. Other valuable methods of syphilis therapy have been found in the heavy metal bismuth; and, especially for the parasyphilitic diseases, in the malariotherapy of Wagner von Jauregg. This and its modifications, hyperthermia produced in various other ways, have been especially valuable in the treatment of paresis, which had hitherto been accepted as an incurable disease. The serodiagnosis of syphilis has been enriched by a number of tests such as the sigma reaction of G. Dreyer, Noguchi's luetin test, R. L. Kahn's precipitin test, and those of R. H. Mueller, E. Meinicke, W. Hecht, and others.

In recent times a new treatment of syphilis with the so-called " massive dose " of neoarsphenamine (or, more safely, mapharsen) has been suggested by Drs. H. T. HYMAN, L. CHARGIN, and W. LEIFER, of New York. The intravenous treatment, kept up over a period of five days, has given very promising results. The studies of the efficacy of the much less toxic penicillin treatment of syphilis and of gonorrhœa are also very promising. Lymphogranuloma venereum (inguinale) was first fully described by Nicolas FAVRE and DURAND, in 1913, under the name " subacute inguinal lymphogranulomatosis," though it had long been known as climatic bubo and was first described some seventy-five years ago by Trousseau. It has become widely recognized since the specificity of W. Frei's diagnostic test (1925) became established. Various diagnostic tests, such as the serodiagnosis of gonorrhœa, and the use of various therapeutic measures, such as specific vaccines and sera, have contributed notably to the progress of venereology in the present century.

Syphilology has furnished practical evidence of the feasibility of the work of the international co-operative clinic, initiated by the League of Nations, for the critical evaluation of therapies and for the collection of other critically observed clinical data.

Signs of the separation of venereology from dermatology are becoming more evident. This appears to be due to the emphasis on the systemic aspects of syphilis, and perhaps the lessened intensity of its cutaneous reactions, the availability of the newer forms of therapy, and the need for greater public health measures.

16. Orthopedics

The specialty of orthopedic surgery, developing the principles laid down by the pioneers of the nineteenth century, may be said to have made more practical progress in this century than in any equivalent period. This can be attributed to such factors as the increased experience and confidence of its followers, their better knowledge of the basic principles of bone and joint structure and dynamics, and the time and ingenuity devoted to it by students of its problems. While it would be quite impossible, therefore, and also inappropriate, to attempt any thorough consideration of twentieth-century orthopedic progress, some illustrative aspects of the subject will be presented here in more detail than in previous chapters.

In no specialty has the stimulus of the two World Wars been more urgent than in orthopedics, with the need for prompt treatment of a great variety and profusion of wounds, in order to get the wounded back into service as rapidly as possible, to minimize the residual effects, and to rehabilitate the crippled. In the early years of the first war not only did the weaknesses of the handling of orthopedic cases become emphasized, but also the desirability of widening the scope of the specialty became manifest. Thus it was made to include the handling of fractures, injuries of nerves, brain, and spinal cord and resultant paralyses, deformities from scar contractions and muscle injuries, and functional disorders requiring re-education. The new and unexpected problems were met by the boldness of the operative surgeon or with complex mechanical devices or long-continued physio-therapeutic measures. Thus the figure of the modern orthopedist emerged, a bold and skilful surgeon, but also a patient and able observer and diligent re-educator, ready to correct the natural or acquired defects in the function of the organs of movement. It is only in this more recent period, when functional as well as anatomical repair was insisted upon, that orthopedics was forced into a rapid development. Furthermore, as many civilian orthopedic conditions are due wholly or in part to metabolic faults, the progressive orthopedist now must pay greater attention to the nature and causes of the disease in question and to non-surgical methods of prevention and treatment, either by himself or in close contact with an internist as partner. Thus divergent tendencies have been evident in the treatment of orthopedic conditions: one toward surgical intervention, the others toward non-operative forms of treatment and toward elimination of the causes. While every orthopedist must and does practise all these types of orthopedics, individuals and schools naturally tend toward one or the other. Considerable local differences in practice are often to be explained on this basis.

In the treatment of FRACTURES AND JOINT INJURIES, H. O. Thomas's splints (with and without traction) have proved very useful under both peace and war conditions; and his basic principles continue to influence orthopedic therapy, even though some details of his practice no longer find favour. For instance, his belief in rest " enforced, uninterrupted and prolonged " has been considerably modified, following the lead of Just LUCAS-CHAMPIONNIÈRE (1843–1913). The surprisingly early postoperative motion of joints (C. WILLEMS), active and passive, and early use of massage to prevent adhesions, muscle atrophy, and contractures, and even to produce quicker union through the irritation of the fragments, are now generally accepted principles. More accurate reduction of fractures and dislocations under anesthetic and fluoroscopic control lessens the frequency of malunion and the amount of deformity. The internal fixation of fractures, practically a twentieth-century development, was attempted with the use of wire by Lapoyède and Sicre (1775), by J. K. Rogers of New York (1827), by Malgaigne (1855), by E. S. Cooper of San Francisco (1861), by H. O. Thomas (silver wire, 1873), and by Lord Lister (1877). It first became of practical use, however, with the introduction of metal plates and bone screws (1905) by Sir William Arbuthnot LANE (1856–1943), who was regarded by many as the most skilful surgeon of his time, and Albin LAMBOTTE of Belgium. A bold form of external fixation of fractures was introduced after the First World War by H. W. ORR (b. 1877), the closed plaster-cast method, which even in cases of infected compound fractures found many adherents. Its value under military conditions was demonstrated by TRUETA in the Spanish Civil War. With the latest fixation appliance — the external metal splint rigidly holding the fractured fragments in place by pins driven through skin and bone (the Stader splint) — it is said that even broken femurs and tibias can be used in walking within forty-eight hours of the injury!

BONE GRAFTS, mentioned in Graeco-Roman times, were apparently first attempted by MacEwen; even autografts were used by Poncet in 1896; but they were first brought into practical use (1911) by F. H. ALBEE (1876–1945), of New York. Loosened cartilages in the knee joint were first recognized in 1879 by the Britisher Thomas ANNANDALE, Lister's successor at Edinburgh, and were removed by him in 1883. The treatment of this condition was brought into prominence in Germany by LAUENSTEIN (1890), in Italy by D. GIORDANO (1893), in France by BRAQUEHAVE (1896), and in America by Joel GOLDTHWAIT in the nineties. Loose particles in the joint ("joint mice") were known to Paré, and had been well described by A. Munro and John Hunter.

Operations for the support of the DISEASED OR FRACTURED SPINE are almost without exception a development of the twentieth century. In 1891 HADRA, of Galveston, Texas, had wired a fracture-dislocation of the cervical vertebræ, and he refers to an earlier case, of W. T. Wilkins, where silk ligatures were used. F. LANGE (b. 1864) of Munich also used both silk and silver wire and tried to immobilize spinal tuberculosis with celluloid plates. It was not until 1911, however, that an adequate support was forthcoming when R. A. HIBBS, of New York, removed the cartilage and periosteum of adjacent vertebral parts and thus procured bony fusion. The same year, ALBEE obtained similar results by fusing a section of a patient's tibia; since 1911 spinal-fusion operations have proved useful in a number of conditions.

Lateral curvature of the spine (SCOLIOSIS) has been studied since the time of Hippocrates, and various theories of its causation — such as congenital anomalies, poor posture or mechanical imbalance, occupation, rickets, or other diseases — have been proposed. Its treatment has been chiefly on the basis of immobility and relief from weight-bearing. " Almost every orthopedist of note has contributed something in the way of a bed, stretcher, or brace to the wide choice of appliances " (Bick). Sayre's plaster jacket (1877) was augmented by Bradford and Lovett, and by Codivilla's pupil R. Galeazzi, by combination with the frame treatment (1911). Mechanical correction has culminated in the " Risser " jacket (1931) — a hinged plaster jacket permitting gradual correction, with an opening for eventual spinal fusion. Postural exercises — as old as Galen — have been given a new direction by A. STEINDLER, toward developing compensatory curves to improve the body contour, rather than correcting the deformity of the spine. He believes that W. SCHULTESS, of Zurich (1855–1917), who studied intensively the pathology of scoliosis and precise methods of measuring and recording its deformity, was the " greatest clinical observer of scoliosis of all times."

The INTERVERTEBRAL DISK of the spinal column, with its central nucleus pulposus, important in the normal bending and twisting of the spine, has in recent years become recognized as a frequent cause of a severe form of backache and sciatica that is amenable to surgical operation. J. E. GOLD-THWAIT, G. S. MIDDLETON, and J. H. TEACHER in 1911 observed that the disk not infrequently ruptured into the spinal canal, thus exerting pressure on the spinal cord and nerve roots, and suggesting perhaps a tumour of the cord. Removal of the herniated disk or nucleus, or sometimes of an enlarged *ligamentum flavum*, usually brings dramatic relief. The pathology of the disk, which may also extrude into the bodies of the adjacent vertebræ and of the perhaps calcified nucleus, has been thoroughly studied by the Dresden pathologist C. G. SCHMORL (1861–1932).

LEGS OF UNEQUAL LENGTH were at first corrected by the surgically sound method of shortening the healthy leg (Rizzoli, 1847; J. A. Mayer, 1850; Codivilla, etc.); but for æsthetic reasons the operation found less favour than Codivilla's proposal (1905) that the short limb be lengthened (P. MAGNUSSON, 1908, 1913). In the hands of L. OMBRÉDANNE, V. PUTTI (1880–1940) (Codivilla's successor at the Rizzoli Institute, a brilliant surgeon and teacher of international fame) and L. C. ABBOTT, of St. Louis, a combination of osteotomy and prolonged skeletal traction has lengthened a long bone by as much as three or four inches with negligible displacement.

Reconstructive joint surgery (ARTHROPLASTY) has made considerable progress in the twentieth century, after a long period of marking time.

The operation to produce a new joint was started by John Rhea BARTON's (1794–1871) unintended production of a pseudoarthrosis of the hip (1826), following an osteotomy for the correction of an ankylosed (stiff) hip joint. The procedure was basically improved by OLLIER (1885), HELFERICH (1894), MIKULICZ (1895), and others by interposing various soft tissues or metals (V. KLUMSKY, 1900), but always under conditions that caused quick absorption of the interposed material. It was not until 1902 that the Chicago surgeon J. B. Murphy, and N. V. Quenu in France, produced satisfactory results with more durable tissues such as muscle and fascia. In the same year Robert Jones used gold foil for an ankylosed hip joint, which was found to have effective motion twenty-one years later. The authority of the German E. Lexer (1908) further established the fat-fascia procedure.

ARTHRODESIS, an operation to stiffen a joint whose movements have become uncontrolled, was introduced by E. Albert of Vienna in 1878. The operation was extended by Russell HIBBS (1911) to eliminate tuberculous joints, was applied to arthritis deformans by F. H. Albee in 1910, and to the neuroarthropathies, such as Charcot's joint, by D. CLEVELAND and E. N. SMITH (1921). Various improvements in the technique of the operation evolved from World War I, notably that of Putti (1922).

The ARTHROSCOPE, for the preoperative view of a diseased joint cavity, was first used by E. BIRCHER in 1922 and later by the American P. H. KREUSCHER (1925) and M. S. BURMAN and others (1931). In the nineties G. Vanghetti conceived the idea of " cinematic amputation " (the use of muscles in an amputated stump as motor units for artificial limbs). This was first performed in 1896 by his colleague A. CECI (1852–1920), and further pursued by R. GALEAZZI

(b. 1866), V. Putti, Sauerbruch, and G. Bosch Arana (1885–1939) (Argentine). In British and American hands the method did not produce as remarkable results with the casualties of World War I as it has in Italy, where it originated.

The problems of CONGENITAL AND OF RECURRENT DISLOCATIONS have required much attention through the centuries, and ingenious manipulations have been proposed. Open and closed methods of reducing dislocation of the hip both still have their advocates. Putti's triangular cushion and its substitutes, applied almost immediately after birth, have answers to the increasing difficulty of repair that attends a Fabian policy. Recurrent dislocation of the shoulder has been met by attempts (1902) to deepen the socket by O. Hildebrand (1858–1927), by wiring the head of the humerus to the acromion process (C. Beck, 1903), by strengthening ligaments J. P. Clairmont, 1917), and by E. Joseph's tenosuspension method (1917), later modified by Nicola (1929) and others. The knee-cap, whose dislocations also tend to recur, has been held in place by " reefing " the soft tissues, or by splitting its tendon and attaching one half so as to form a check ligament (Goldthwait, 1904), and malformations of the knee joint that predispose to the trouble have been corrected by bone insertions. It remains a problem.

While much of the non-operative treatment of orthopedic conditions falls under the head of physiotherapy (q.v.), C. L. Lowman's method (1927) of treating poliomyelitis is mentioned here. Lowman's underwater exercise of the weakened muscles is widely known in the United States through President Roosevelt's support of the Warm Springs Foundation. Lowman correctly worked out the principle that the higher specific gravity of water over air so supported the weakened limbs that they could function when less power was available, and so graded active exercise could be begun early. Sister Kenny's treatment of poliomyelitis is considered in the section on Neurology.

Tendon, fascia, and muscle surgery have been considerably developed in the present century, stimulated by war problems and the various poliomyelitis epidemics. Transplantation and lengthening of tendons, due to better attention to the functional problems involved and better technical attachment and sheath preservation, are now more uniformly successful; and for reasons not yet explained, it is found that the transplanted muscle may take on the action of the muscle it replaces, even though its original action was an opposing one. The value of fascial transplants was developed by Payr (1913), and by W. E. Gallie and A. B. Le Mesurier (1922), and tendons have been utilized as ligaments to strengthen joints (tenodesis). Nerve surgery is also in a new stage of progress. Nerve roots have been cut (ramisectomy) (O. Foerster, 1908), nerve ganglia and periarterial sympathetics removed, to eliminate pain and lessen spasm (R. Leriche, 1921), with results that are still *sub judice*. Severed nerves can be sutured

or transplanted with varying success, and undoubtedly the late war produced further advances in this, as in many other lines.

Diseases of cartilage and bone, grouped under the term OSTEOCHONDRITIS,
though of varying etiology, are mostly due to necrosis and fibrosis or seques-
tration. They have received various eponyms according to the part involved, such as A. Köhler's disease of the tarsus (1903), Osgood-Schlatter's
of the tibia (1903, 1908), Legg-Calvé-Perthes's of the hip (1909, 1910),
Kienböck's of the semilunar bone in the wrist (1910). The vexed subject
of chronic rheumatic arthritis, a term first used by R. ADAMS of Dublin
(1791–1875) in 1857, still awaits definite elucidation. A. E. Garrod's classification of chronic arthritis as two independent diseases, osteo-arthritis and
rheumatoid arthritis — the latter being of obscure infectious origin — is probably the favourite with most physicians. In America, Goldthwait's division
into hypertrophic and atrophic types (1904) and E. H. Nichols' and P. L.
Richardson's " degenerative " and " proliferative " types, with emphasis on
the soft-tissue changes, are still much in use.

In GREAT BRITAIN, H. O. Thomas's work was worthily carried on by
Sir Robert JONES (1858–1933), long the leader in this discipline in Great
Britain and head of the excellently organized British orthopedic services
during the First World War. N. Dunn, G. R. Girdlestone, E. W. Hey
GROVES, (1872–1944), A. H. Tubby, J. L. Hunter, and N. W. Royle in
Australia are among those who have also contributed. AMERICAN orthopedic surgery has been worthily represented by the Boston school of J. P.
Goldthwait, R. B. Osgood, and others; by the Philadelphians G. G. Davis
and De Forest Willard; by N. Allison of St. Louis, R. T. TAYLOR (1867–
1929), of Baltimore, and others too numerous to mention. In 1923 W. G.
STERN, of Cleveland, described the mysterious and fortunately rare condition arthrogryposis, in which the child is born with multiple fibrous ankyloses, often associated with other deformities in the joints.

In America, New York State in 1900 set the example for the care of
cripples in state hospitals, to be followed shortly by several other states.
World War casualties greatly increased the need: by 1929, the United
States had planned fifty-five special hospitals, mainly or entirely for orthopedic cases. Curative workshops were found not only to hasten recovery,
both physical and mental, but also to rehabilitate by teaching new trades,
and incidentally have produced many useful articles. In 1920 the Shriners
(a Masonic order) began a far-flung plan to erect hospitals for the care of
crippled children and to support study of their problems, which has penetrated throughout the United States and Canada. Associations for the aid
of crippled children, begun in New York City, are found in this and various

European countries and are active in their philanthropic aim of supplementing professional and hospital activities. In North America they are headed
by the International Society for Crippled Children (founded 1921). A census of crippled children was first accomplished by Massachusetts (1905) as
a basic step toward adequate public care, and similar censuses have been
made in Berlin, Birmingham (England), and elsewhere.

Eight special orthopedic journals, led by the *Archivio di ortopedia*
(founded 1884) had been established by the end of the nineteenth century.
They now number twenty-eight (see Bick's *Source Book of Orthopedics*,
Appendix A), all but three in America, England, France, Germany, and
Italy.

17. Stomatology and Odontology (Dentistry)

At the beginning of the twentieth century stomatology and odontology
were at an advanced stage of development, with many good schools in
Europe and the Americas teaching the various branches of these specialties.

In all the leading schools preclinical studies are pursued in co-operation
with the clinical. Anatomy, histology, physiology, physics, metallurgy,
and chemistry, bacteriology, and general pathology receive equal attention
with dental hygiene, oral diagnosis and medicine, operative and prosthetic
dentistry, orthodontia, maxillo-facial surgery, dental jurisprudence, and the
history of dentistry. The microbiological and biochemical studies of general medicine enter the dental field to explain the relations between local
and constitutional and systemic disease and lead toward treatment. The
bonds between dentistry and medicine are steadily becoming closer and
closer. In America and some European countries dentistry is still taught
separately from medicine, both because of the extensive special technical
and operative knowledge required, and because much of the medical curriculum today would be irrelevant. In Italy and several other countries the
degree in medicine and surgery is required. Even in those countries where
the subjects are taught separately and different degrees are given, however,
it is recognized that the specialty should be joined as closely as possible to
the other medico-surgical disciplines.

Recognizing the close connection of the dental apparatus with the rest
of the body, students of the normal and diseased structure and function of
the teeth have emphasized that they are not autonomous units, but depend
on the integrity of other systems, or vice versa, and exert an important influence upon them. Especial importance is attached today in dentistry to
the problem of oral sepsis and the relation between infections of the teeth

and tonsils and distant disorders of the body, whether produced by toxins, allergy, or the actual presence of bacteria. From this point of view has arisen, especially in America, the concept that periapical or periodontal infections, which can be diagnosed by clinical and radiological methods, may be a threat to the health of the entire organism and therefore should be removed. Though much exaggerated in some quarters, this trend can profitably be combined with more conservative methods, such as chemotherapeutic or surgical treatment of the necrotic dental pulp (e.g., apicoectomy, introduced by Carl Partsch).

The methods of ORAL AND MAXILLARY SURGERY, like most other specialties, have been greatly aided by the frequent use of the X-ray and of local and intra-oral anesthesia. Oral surgery has made great progress in the hands of such experts as the pioneer Americans Simon P. HULLIHEN (1810–57) and James Edmund GARRETSON (1828–95), " the father of oral surgery "; in the twentieth century as Leo Winter, Truman William Brophy, Vilray Papin Blair, Robert Henry Ivy, and Theodor Blum in America; Cavina and Sanvenero Rosselli in Italy; Alfred Armand Velpeau in France; Carl Partsch, Georg Axhausen, F. S. Esser, Christian Bruhn, F. Ernst, and Rosenthal in Germany; Hans Pichler in Austria; János Ertl in Hungary; Kostecka in Czechoslovakia. Pyorrhea alveolaris paradentosis is also known as Riggs disease after John M. RIGGS, who in 1876 first treated the symptoms by scraping. This, together with caries, represents the greatest affliction of the human mouth and has been extensively investigated from the point of view of etiology and pathogenesis as well as therapy. Here, also, advances can be recorded, though the problem is still far from solved.

Among the numerous modern students of dental histology we note Charles Francis Bödecker, Schour, Oskar Weski, Bernard Gottlieb, B. Orban, Hermann Euler, Wilhelm Meyer, Tohl Shimamine, Arturo Beretta, Fasoli, Silvio Palazzi, Oskar Römer, Guido Fischer, and Otto Walkhoff.

CARIOUS TEETH, still the greatest practical problem of dentistry, have been exhaustively studied by countless investigators, such as Willoughby Dayton Miller, G. V. Black, Joseph Arkövy, and Manicardi, without, however, actually settling the pathogenesis of the condition and the relative importance of such etiological factors as the diet, local care of the teeth, special infective organisms, constitutional diathesis, and so on. One of the most interesting of recent contributions to the problem of dental caries is the observation of an apparent protection by fluorides. F. S. McKAY, a dentist, noticed (about 1912) in certain districts in Colorado a condition of the teeth that he called " mottled enamel." He and G. V. BLACK established (1916) that this condition had a definite geographic distribution, determined by the water supply, and that the affected teeth were more resistant than normal teeth to dental caries, in spite of the enamel being obviously defective. It was later determined that such water supplies contain soluble fluorides in excess of one part per million, and that fluorides given to laboratory rodents produced enamel change, identifiable with the human lesions. The fluoride content of normal enamel was found to be less than that of mottled enamel and greater than that of carious teeth. Also experimental administration of fluorides decreased the incidence of "caries" in rats. Thus it appeared that dental caries might be controlled by adding soluble fluorides to water supplies, to foods or tooth pastes, or in other ways. Already topical application of fluoride solutions to freshly cleaned enamel surfaces is said to have reduced the number of new cavities in a given locality by something like forty per cent. The possibilities of such control for the future of dentistry are indeed far-reaching.

The materials and methods for FILLING CAVITIES have been improved. Various alloys and fused porcelain and gold may be used in the form of inlays, porcelain as jacket crowns and bridges for the restoration and preservation of the teeth.

Scientific DENTAL PROSTHESIS (artificial dentures) based on the mechanics of the articulation of the teeth may be said to have been founded by William Gibson BONWILL (1833–99), of Philadelphia, and chiefly developed by him and by the Swiss Alfred GYSI. Regarded a century ago as "the largest and most difficult part of dentistry" (C. A. Harris), it has receded as the progress in preventive dentistry has borne fruit, though it doubtless will continue as an important field for many years to come.

The development of ORTHODONTIA, the straightening of irregularities of the teeth, begun by Fauchard and John Hunter in the eighteenth century, has been largely an American contribution. Especially important in this respect was the work of E. H. ANGLE: A System of Appliances for Correcting Irregularities of the Teeth (2nd ed., Philadelphia, 1890), and Treatment of Malocclusion of the Teeth (7th ed., 1907) in establishing sound principles of dentistry, in inventing technical apparatus, such as the "ribbon arch," classification of the malocclusions of the teeth, the organization of the first postgraduate school of orthodontia (1900), the foundation of the American Society of Orthodontists (1901), and the establishment of the journal, the American Orthodontist (1907). Predecessors of E. H. Angle were E. C. Angell (1823–1903), who emphasized the importance of the first permanent molar; the "Father of Orthodontia," N. W. KINGSLEY (1829–1913), J. N. FARRAR (1839–1913), C. S. CASE (1847–1923), and S. H. GUILFORD. The subject has been developed in other countries by Oppenheim, Joseph Grünberg, H. Salamon, G. Korkhaus, L. Schwartz, d'Alise, Muzii, Arlotta, and Grandi.

DENTAL HYGIENE. One of the most brilliant phases of progress in dentistry has been social-hygienic prophylaxis, which is begun with schoolchildren and continued in industrial communities, armies, and hospitals. The apostle in this field, Ernst Jessen, began in 1902 the first dental clinic in schools, and his example was soon followed throughout the world. The experimental and survey work of the Philadelphia Mouth Hygiene Association, acting with the help of the Board of Education, is a good illustration of this type of co-operative, constructive endeavour. Today school clinics have greatly improved the treatment of diseased teeth in children; tomorrow will be the day of prevention.

THE X-RAY AND ITS APPLICATION IN DENTISTRY. The roentgenography of the teeth began with the work (published early in 1896) of W. KOENIG, in Germany, and W. J. MORTON's article, published in *Dental Cosmos*, June 1896. It was at first concerned only with impaction of teeth and their failure to erupt.

In recent years systematic examination of the teeth at regular intervals has made progress and much help has been provided to the busy dentist by the " dental hygienist," a woman trained in the care of the teeth, especially the removal of " tartar." This procedure was introduced in Connecticut by Dr. A. C. FONES, and about the same time in New York and New Orleans. His helper first went to the patient's house, but soon brought the patient to the dental chair, where better instruments were available and suspect caries could be shown to the dentist on the spot. As the procedure was called illegal in this form, systematic courses were started (Bridgeport, Connecticut, 1913) and in thirty-five states licensing examinations are now held.

The countries of the American continent have made especially good progress in this specialty. Thanks to their highly developed sense of physical hygiene, but still more to the gift of huge endowments, especially of the great benefactors, the Forsyth brothers, George Eastman, and the Guggenheims, research departments and magnificent dental clinics, such as Zoller's Institute at the University of Chicago, have been created in European as well as American schools, at the cost of many millions of dollars. London, Paris, Brussels, Stockholm, and Rome possess examples of such clinics. Even though every city has not had the fortune to receive these benefactions, still a great many have a regular dental service in schools, conducted at the expense of the cities and communities.

Thus it is clear that the practice of dentistry has reached a high degree of technical skill, aided by an ever broadening scientific basis. With increasing realization of the need for scientific investigation of its fundamental problems, in close co-operation with related sciences, the stage is being set for further advances, which may conceivably change the whole set-up of the practice of dentistry in the not too distant future.

18. Neurology and Psychiatry

Etiologic, pathogenetic, and clinical progress in NEUROLOGY in the present century has been aided by new methods of research. As will be seen presently, however, in this century it is psychiatry that has made the more important progress of the two.

The CEREBROSPINAL FLUID has been systematically and thoroughly studied from bacteriological, chemical, cytological, and serological points of view. The introduction of opaque material into the subarachnoid space for radiological examination, a discovery of the French neurologist SICARD, has permitted new lines of attack, such as encephalography, ventriculography, and rachiography; finally, cerebral arteriography (MONIZ) has assisted in the diagnosis of the various cerebral affections. These advances, as we have already seen, have contributed to the admirable progress of neurosurgery, which has become almost as important as the non-operative treatment of nervous conditions. Neurophysiology has contributed to practical neurology extensive researches on reflex activities and on the highly complex nervous autonomisms, already outlined by Hughlings Jackson. The subject has been further advanced by Magnus and his pupils, and by Sherrington's masterly studies, summarized in his *Integrative Action of the Nervous System* (1906). Pavlov's memorable researches on the function of the cerebral cortex and on conditioned reflexes have been of great importance in elucidating normal and pathological mental activities and their relations to the condition of the rest of the body.

The problem of POLIOMYELITIS is not definitely solved either for the source or for the mode of spread of the infection. The Kenny treatment, suggested by Sister Kenny, an Australian nurse, aims at combating spasms, inco-ordination, and pain as early as possible, with hot packs. Though this appeared revolutionary, it seems in the beginning that the results would be definitely encouraging. In certain cases, at least, when applied in the acute stages, it appears to be beneficial in lessening the amount of muscle paralysis.

The pathogenesis of MYASTHENIA GRAVIS has been the object of important research, especially by E. R. GONI and A. LANARI in Buenos Aires, stressing that the determining factor is lack of liberation of acetylcholine. Recent developments of knowledge about myasthenia gravis illustrate some of the ways in which medical science progresses. A physician, herself a sufferer from the disease, impressed by the similarity of the symptoms to those of curare poisoning, took physostigmine, a known antidote for curare poisoning, with dramatically successful symptomatic results. Further studies of the action of the drug and its relative, prostigmine, though they show that the action is definitely not the same as in curare poisoning, have thrown more light on the nature of the disease as well as providing the answer for its relief. Another nervous affliction, recurrent *familial paralysis* (Flatau), superficially a similar disease, has been shown to have a very different pathogenesis, connected with potassium lack. Bromides had been known to be sometimes effective in these cases and sometimes not, suggesting the obvious inference that success depended not on the sedative bromide but on the potassium when that was the base used.

A problem of great importance in our time is that of the SUTURE OF SEVERED NERVES with direct end-to-end suture by which nerve function can be restored. It is accepted that all nerves should be sutured at the earliest moment compatible with the patient's general condition and infection of the wound, to prevent formation of neuromas. In this connection the encouraging results of important experiments of nerve transplantation may be referred to.

These scientific developments, spreading beyond the limits of neurophysiology into psychology, have had important repercussions on the evolution of psychiatry. While psychiatry, like neurology, was for some time chiefly concerned with outlining various mental syndromes, it has been unable, with very few exceptions, to make the correlation with pathological anatomy that was so beautifully feasible in neurology. As a result, psychiatrists have become less interested in refinements of diagnosis and more concerned with psychologic states and practical responses to treatment. (See further details in the section on Public Health and Social Medicine.) Desire for more fundamental knowledge has not abated, however, and in a few instances improved investigative methods have already inaugurated new approaches to the understanding of the cause and nature of the psychic disturbances.

An important factor in the progress of PSYCHIATRY was given by the great development of the surgery of the brain. This subject has been dealt with in the section on Surgery, and here only the contribution that was made by Harvey Cushing and his school need be emphasized.

Of outstanding importance were the studies on the function of the *frontal lobes*. Egas MONIZ, of Lisbon, published in 1935 the results of his studies in this field, asserting that in the therapy of some psychoses it should be advisable to cut the communication between frontal lobes and thalamus. He invented an instrument (leucotome) that was introduced into the cavity of the skull through a hole in the prefrontal region. After the instrument had penetrated a certain depth and the sheath retracted, a series of cuts were made through the white matter. The results were very encouraging in many cases of troubles of the frontal lobes. Walter FREEMAN, of Washington, made a definite contribution in this field; he was the first to introduce postfrontal lobectomy in the United States. A large contribution to brain surgery was made by the Italians MARIOTTI, SCIUTI, SAI, RIZZATO, and BORGARELLO. The last two, operating on two hundred cases, obtained a recovery in fifteen per cent and marked improvement in thirty-one per cent of all cases.

One of the most signal successes of psychiatry in this period was the treatment of GENERAL PARALYSIS.

In 1910, when Salvarsan began to revolutionize antiluetic therapy, it was believed that a treatment of the disease was found. Shock therapy has been proved for a long time, artificial production of suppuration having been for a century believed to be beneficial in the treatment of mental diseases. Benjamin Rush had prescribed " a caustic applied to the back of the neck, or between the shoulders, and kept open for months or years, acting by the permanent discharge it induces from the neighborhood of the brain "; and we know that in ancient times it was believed that any serious illness might be influenced favourably by inducing another less dangerous. Hippocrates had observed that " persons attacked with convulsions recovered if a quartan fever supervenes."

In 1913 the actual etiology of general paralysis was demonstrated by Noguchi and Moore of the Rockefeller Foundation, who proved the presence of *Treponema pallidum* in the cerebral substance of the subjects.

Julius von WAGNER-JAUREGG's (1857–1940) fifty-year battle with general paralysis brought about one of the most stimulating discoveries in modern medicine. In 1890, following the discovery of tuberculin, he began to use it to produce fever in the insane with the hope that artificially induced fever might have the same effect as he had observed in a patient who had an attack of erysipelas. Later, by inducing malaria (1914), he found that among 86 paretics so treated, 21 were still alive and 7 were actually working after several years. After twenty years of effort he attained a degree of control over one of the worst afflictions of mankind. Recently more simple methods of producing artificial fever have been substituted for the malaria therapy.

The third method of shock therapy is the electric convulsive shock treatment, which surely has the advantage of being easy to apply. It was first used by CERLETTI and BINI, who published their result in 1938. Willis R. WHITNEY, of Schenectady, discovered that a powerful high-frequency electric oscillator would raise the temperature of those working near it, and other methods of raising the temperature by electrical devices have since been developed.

In 1937 Dr. Manfred SAKEL described for the first time a successful TREATMENT OF SCHIZOPHRENIA with hypoglycemic shock through insulin. This treatment had its origin in an attempt to alleviate withdrawal symptoms in morphine addicts, to whom were administered doses of insulin. This treatment was followed by the use of metrazol as a conversive agent, suggested by L. von MEDUNA (1938).

This treatment is now being used in many clinics and hospitals all over the world. It seems that today insulin shock therapy has been limited to certain types of schizophrenia, but it is generally accepted that the convulsive methods have to be considered useful in the agitated depressions and in states of manic or schizophrenic excitement. No adequate explanation has been found for the results of shock therapy. The astonishing results of this treatment, however, have served to encourage researchers, and it may be expected that they will make new and perhaps definite contributions to the solution of many important problems.

PSYCHOANALYSIS. An important part in the evolution of psychiatry in the twentieth century was played by the study of the field of consciousness and the subconscious. Art and literature in a time of predominant naturalism have stressed the importance of the fundamental instinctive drives. G. ZILBOORG in his *History of Medical Psychology* has called the new current in the evolution of psychiatry the Freudian psychiatric revolution. It was due to the achievements of the Viennese psychiatrist Sigmund FREUD (1856–1939). His first work was in neuroanatomy, and in his early writings he called himself a neuropathologist. He began as a research worker and became later a lecturer on nervous diseases at the University of Vienna. In 1885 he studied with Charcot in Paris; in 1886 he started private practice in Vienna. Deeply influenced by the school of Charcot and of Bernheim, he began a new approach to a rational treatment of the psychotic. The doctrine of psychoanalysis was founded by him in 1895 in collaboration with Josef BREUER (1842–1925). Their first book, on hysteria, appeared in 1895. This doctrine is based on the assumptions, first that the memory of previous events stored in the unconscious mind plays an important part in the mental life of the individual, and secondly that the mental conflicts often produced by such memories can be removed when they are brought to the surface and properly comprehended by a long process of search into the subconscious zone. Freud started on this line of interpretation with the thought that hysteria was due to psychic trauma of a sexual nature, and he was able to help many cases of nervous maladaptation, hysteria, and other functional disorders by the use of his analytical method. He placed the greatest importance on sexual stimuli and advanced the idea of the so-called Œdipus complex, which explains the situation of the individual who subconsciously attaches himself to the parent of the opposite sex. Freud rapidly became the head of a school, which has found adherents throughout the

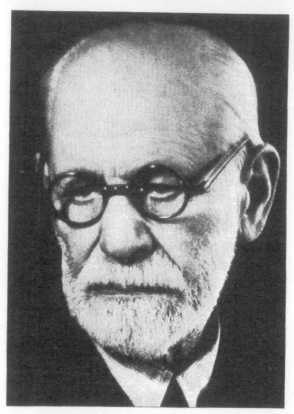

478. *Sigmund Freud.* (*Copyright, Marcel Sternberger.*)

world. His methods have been developed in modified form, with less emphasis on the sex factor, by his pupil C. G. JUNG (b. 1875), of Basel, and by Alfred ADLER (1870–1937), of Vienna and later of New York and Aberdeen.

The influence of Freud's work on medical psychology all over the world was immense. One of the most important contributions to this influence was the work of E. BLEULER on dementia præcox (1911). He introduced the term " schizophrenia " to denote a group of psychotic reactions, disproving the generally accepted idea of their incurability. His views of schizophrenia were accepted especially in America, and Freud's doctrine found large support in the United States, where A. A. BRILL was the most authoritative representative of psychoanalysis. He translated most of Freud's work and published a number of original contributions. In 1911 he founded the New York Psychoanalytical Society. The struggle for the recognition of psychoanalysis as the therapy of choice in psychoneuroses was very sharp, and it is still not ended. The value of psychoanalysis as a method of investigation and as an important part of general psychology, however, has already been proved.

The connection of psychiatry with other sciences for research purposes was the aim of the Institute of Human Relations of Yale University (1928). Many other centres of research have been recently instituted, among which may be mentioned the Psychological Clinic at Harvard University and the Institute for Juvenile Research in Chicago. Other groups of researchers are working at the University of Chicago, in Toronto, Cincinnati, St. Louis, and San Francisco.

The importance of psychiatry was well demonstrated in the past war when it became clear in the selection of men for the armed forces that latent or active neuropsychiatric disorders were among the most serious causes of military disabilities.

PSYCHOLOGY has had an enormous development in this period, which saw the first publications on the psychology of the newborn, the infant, and the adolescent. Eminent in this field is Pierre JANET (b. 1859), Professor of Psychiatry at the Collège de France, who developed the theory of psychological automatism (1889) and the concept of psychasthenia (1903). A. BINET (1857–1911) devised an intelligence test, widely known under the name of the "Binet-Simon test" (1914), which has introduced new trends into pedagogy and in the classification of soldiers and employees. Notable contributors to this field have been the Germans W. WUNDT, R. H. LOTZE, G. T. FECHNER, the French É. SEGUIN and J. A. É. CLAPARÈDE, the Americans G. Stanley HALL, William JAMES, and McKeen CATTELL, and the Italians S. DE SANCTIS, V. BENUSSI, and Maria MONTESSORI. Comparative psychology, by its study of lower organisms, has contributed to knowledge of human mental behaviour, especially in the work of the Americans H. S. JENNINGS, Jacques LOEB (theory of tropisms), and R. M. YERKES. In fact, in the hands of J. B. WATSON (b. 1878) it has led to the concept of Behaviourism (1914), a psychologic system that attempts to explain the activities of the human mind in the simple behaviouristic form of stimulus and response.

The INCREASE OF MENTAL DISEASES in this country has been proved by statistics. First admissions to all public and licensed hospitals for treatment of mental diseases in the state of New York show in the last twenty years an increase by 89.4 per cent. The state's general population increased only 29.6 in this period. The standardized male rate increased from 114.84 per hundred thousand general population in 1920 to 145.17 in 1940, whereas that of females decreased slightly between 1920 and 1930, but increased between 1930 and 1940. The most remarkable change in prevalence of mental diseases occurs in connection with psychoses with cerebral arteriosclerosis. General paralysis showed a downward trend, undoubtedly as a consequence of the decrease of syphilis. Alcoholic psychosis shows a steady increase, while the total cases of manic-depressive psychosis decreased despite a great increase in population (B. Malzberg).

The problem of this increase in mental diseases and of the hospitalization of the insane will surely be of major importance not only in this country, but much more so in Europe, where the terrible conditions of wars have created a depression of the individual and collective mind and have surely prepared a soil in which psychoneuroses are developing in a terrific number. The immense progress in the knowledge and treatment of mental diseases will undoubtedly have a decisive influence on this condition. However, what we have learned, especially in the last fifty years, about the origin of psychoses and the causes of their development, about the importance of collective psychosis, of their contagion, and of their consequences may have enlightened the men who will assume the task of preparing a lasting peace. Psychiatry and psychology will have to play a decisive part in the solution of this problem, which is a problem of the possibility of a social life. The historian of civilization will be able to prove how often the insufficient understanding of the psychology of different groups of people and of their leaders at different times may have contributed in creating a state of affairs of which actual war was the logical consequence.

19. Legal Medicine

The study and teaching of legal medicine has long had a greater development on the continent of Europe than in the English-speaking countries, where its pursuit is handicapped by lack of official contact by medical schools with legal authorities and by the neglect of the latter properly to utilize and evaluate the expert knowledge required in this field. In many European universities large independent institutes are devoted to this subject — equipped with special histological, bacteriological, chemical, hematological, and radiological laboratories — and engaged not only in the teaching and investigation of the subject, but also in the performance of valuable official duties for the State.

In the United States it is the coroner's office that mainly determines the standards of medico-legal jurisprudence. This was adopted from the English coroner system, which has been in practice since 1194 and has changed its functions but slightly during the centuries. The coroner continues to have juridical as well as medical responsibilities, being guided in the latter by " Coroner's physicians." In continental Europe no such office as that of coroner exists. In many European countries the theory and practice of the scientific detection of crime has been greatly advanced by the achievements of " institutes of legal medicine."

In Massachusetts the change was made in 1877; in New York City in 1918 (Dr. Charles Norris); and in Essex County, New Jersey, shortly after. In Maryland the medical-examiner system was established in 1940. Yet the above mostly changed before 1932. In 1932 the first chair of legal medicine in the United States was established at Harvard's medical school and Dr. G. B. Magrath was appointed to the professorship. After his death, in 1937, Dr. A. R. Moritz became his successor; he is also the chief medical examiner of the state.

In recent times the necessity for better organization in the scientific detection of crime in the United States has become increasingly evident. J. Edgar Hoover has stated that " each year sees 12,000 murders, 46,981 cases of felonious assault, 283,685 burglaries, and 779,956 larcenies." In addition to such crimes, the enormous loss of life due to accident must be added, and much of this loss is due to criminal carelessness. The importance of accurately establishing the cause of death in these cases, and the increased ability to do so when expert knowledge is available have led several states to change the coroner's office (which is an elective position, with frequently changing incumbents) for that of medical examiner (held permanently by an expert). In New York City there are about 80,000 deaths each year. Of these, about 15,000 must be investigated by the medical examiner's office to determine the cause of death; less than fifty per cent of the total number of the cases investigated are violent death. All deaths caused by occupational accidents and all deaths resulting from occupational diseases and industrial poisoning must also be reported to the medical examiner. A well-conducted medico-legal autopsy is the only reliable and accurate means of determining the exact cause of death, the time of its occurrence, and other often vitally important circumstances. Its proper performance requires not only a wide knowledge of general and special pathological anatomy, but also command of special technical procedures such as those of the toxicologist, histologist, serologist, and ballistician in detecting even the smallest quantities of various poisons. Dr. Alexander O. Gettler, the Chief Medical Examiner of the New York City office, has analysed since 1918 over 30,000 human bodies for poisoning. In all cases of fatal accident, the brain has to be analysed for alcohol to determine whether alcoholic intoxication was a contributory cause of the accident.

The Department of Forensic Medicine at New York University is led by Dr. H. S. Martland (1935). It is planned that an institute of forensic medicine as fine as any in the world for the scientific investigation of crime in one of the largest communities of the world should greatly stimulate the teaching and training in legal medicine.

One of the most interesting cases proving the part that an exact examination can play in the detection of causes of death was given by the radium poisoning cases of 1917–24. Some eight hundred girls were employed in a factory in New Jersey painting the dials of watches and clocks with luminous paint containing very small amounts of radium. Before the danger was recognized, for months they had " pointed " their brushes on their tongues and so swallowed infinitesimal amounts of radium, which lodged mostly in their bones. When several of these girls died, the true nature of these deaths was established by careful autopsy, and radium was demonstrated in their bones. The most heavily poisoned died of aplastic anæmia and necrosis of the jaw. The less heavily poisoned died later of osteosarcoma, the result of stimulation of the bone by the radium deposit.

The carcinogenic effect of radioactive substances on the body has recently assumed renewed importance both in the manufacture of the atomic bomb and in its mysterious effect after explosion.

In the development of forensic medicine in England, we may refer to the work accomplished by C. A. MERCIER (1852–1919), who wrote a valuable textbook on insanity (1902). The best-known medico-legal expert in England today is Sir Bernard Henry SPILSBURY (b. 1879), lecturer on forensic medicine at St. Bartholomew's Hospital and pathologist at Scotland Yard for the Home Office.

Legal medicine flourished in Italy, especially in the school of Filippi in Florence. Among the prominent scholars L. BORRI, and his pupil CEVIDALLI, who was in turn followed at Padua by his pupil PELLEGRINI, may be cited. Pupils of Filippi's Florentine school were DALLA VOLTA, professor at Catania; LEONCINI, Borri's successor at Florence; CAZZANIGA, professor at Milan; and BIONDI, professor at Siena. Lombroso's great school, emphasizing criminal anthropology, produced OTTOLENGHI, professor at Rome, and his pupil FALCO, professor at Messina, CARRARA and his pupils LATTES and ROMANESE. Other eminent students of the subject were DE CRECCHIO at Naples and ZIINO at Messina. G. PIERACCINI

(b. 1864), of Florence, is the author of a useful *Trattato di patologia del lavoro* (1905); he has also written an interesting and extensive medico-historical study on heredity in the Medici family.

Forensic medicine as a university subject is further advanced in Latin America than in the United States. The European system of establishing chairs is generally accepted at the universities and medico-legal institutes. Among the best-known teachers are N. ROJAS (Buenos Aires), J. BELBEY (La Plata), Dr. R. BOSCH (Rosario), R. DE CASTRO (Havana), A. FAVERO (São Paulo), and J. TORRES-TORIJA (Mexico City).

The increase of criminal delinquency during and after the war stresses the necessity of a scientifically organized fight against crime. It appears to be evident that in this fight research workers and pathologists, aided by the improved specialistic knowledge of all means of detection of crime, have an important part to play. In the attempt, also, to meet efficiently the enormous loss of life caused by accidents and criminal carelessness, the contribution that may be made by the Institute of Legal Medicine is certainly most important. It is therefore to be expected that in the program of social medicine of the future, forensic medicine will be conspicuous.

20. Pharmacology and Therapeutics

Modern pharmacological investigation has developed along two lines: one, the chemical, identification and synthesis of new preparations; and, two, the biological, study of the physiological effect of active substances. The latter has been so expanded as to include the action of a substance elaborated within a living body, whether exerted spontaneously within the same body or collected for use in others. This is illustrated in the definition given in Meyer and Gottlieb's well-known textbook: "Pharmacology deals with the reaction of living organisms to chemical agents," an interpretation that involves a wide overlap with physiology and other basic medical sciences. Pursuit of both these lines has greatly increased the number of valuable medicaments and comprehension of their pharmacological and therapeutic value, a development that without exaggeration can be regarded in sum total as one of the chief medical advances of the present century.

Estimation of the most important drugs has changed considerably in the course of this century. In the first decade a list of ten drugs thought to be most important consisted of: (1) ether and a few other anesthetics; (2) opium and its derivatives; (3) digitalis; (4) diphtheria antitoxin; (5) smallpox vaccine; (6) iron; (7) quinine; (8) iodine; (9) alcohol; (10) mercury. In 1945, when another such list was prepared, it began with: (1) penicillin, sulfanilamides, and other antibiotics; (2) blood plasma and its derivatives and substitutes; (3) quinine and its relatives; (4) ether and other anesthetics and opium derivatives; (5) digitalis; (6) the arsphenamines; (7) immunologic agents and specific antitoxins and vaccines; (8) liver extract; (9) hormones; and (10) vitamins — only four of which are represented in the earlier list. The implications of this trend away from many of the older drugs, especially those which could not be shown to have definite pharmacological action, are obvious.

Ehrlich's technique of CHEMOTHERAPY (the synthesis of many new drugs of slightly varying chemical formulas, each tested experimentally until one with a maximum therapeutic effect is obtained) has created a new and very important division of therapeutics. One of its earliest achievements was Ehrlich's introduction of Salvarsan in 1910, the six hundred and sixth arsenic compound to be prepared and evaluated by him in his search for a *therapia magna sterilisans* in the treatment of syphilis. This method of study has now been widely extended to many drugs, with results that are steadily increasing in value. In most recent times Gerhard DOMAGK's discovery (1932, 1935) of the therapeutic effects of sulphanilamide launched a new period in the drug treatment of infectious disease unsurpassed since the empirical discovery of cinchona bark.

The first of the group, sulfanilamide (prontosil, para-amino-benzene-sulfonamide) was synthesized by P. GELMO in 1908, but attracted so little attention that not much can be learned of the man today. Other related drugs (sulfapyridine, sulfathiazol, sulfadiazine, sulfamerazine, sulfamethyl guanidine) have been prepared, each with its special merits, and thousands of lives saved and illnesses shortened. Of pharmacologic importance, too, was the discovery of their mode of action, which consisted in halting growth and action of bacteria (bacteriostatic) rather than killing them (bactericidal). This in turn appeared to be connected with the fact that in bacteria susceptible to sulfonamides these drugs replace a certain chemical with a similar structural formula — para-amino-benzoic acid — which is essential to the multiplication of the bacteria in question, by what has been called " competitive inhibition of an enzyme reaction." Rare cases have been found where the infection proved resistant to a sulfonamide, or the individual sensitive, or the drug toxic; but for these the " antibiotics " have come to the rescue.

The concept of " ANTIBIOTICS " (meaning a chemical substance derived from living sources that is antagonistic to microbes) has been much expanded in recent years with the work of S. A. WAKSMAN (b. 1888) and his colleagues at Rutgers University, and of René DUBOS (b. 1901) at the Rockefeller Institute (gramicidin, 1939), and especially with the phenomenal success attendant on penicillin. However, the principle is found illustrated much earlier, as when Pasteur and Joubert showed (1877) that air-borne organisms inhibited anthrax; in Emmerich's and Loew's use (1889) of pyocyanase in the treatment of anthrax and diphtheria; and it is similar to W. B. COLEY's (1862–1936) combination in the nineties of the toxins of *Strep. erysipelatis* and *B. prodigiosus* to inhibit the growth of sarcoma.

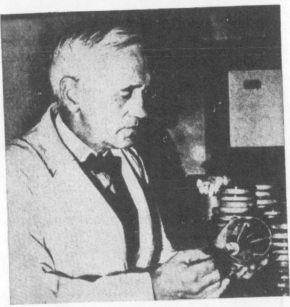

479. *Sir Alexander Fleming, discoverer of penicillin.*

Sir Alexander FLEMING (b. 1881), a pupil of Sir Almroth Wright, in 1922 discovered an antibacterial ferment in such substances as egg white, tears, and various microbes, which was capable of dissolving living bacteria, especially cocci. To this he gave the name " lysozyme." The most spectacular advance, however, was initiated by Fleming in his chance observation (1928, pub. 1929) that contamination of a plate culture of staphylococcus by *Penicillium notatum* caused colonies of cocci around the mould to become transparent, and even actually to dissolve.

Fleming was able to extract from this mould an active principle that he named " penicillin." Recognizing the antiseptic value of such a substance, he tried it successfully as a local application to infected surfaces with which he happened to be working, and found it superior to other potent chemicals, especially as it proved not to be toxic when injected into rabbits, and not to inhibit the action of leukocytes. Its apparent instability, however, and the unavoidable pressure of other work prevented Fleming from carrying his investigations further, and little more was done until the problem was further pursued (1938) by Sir Howard Walter FLOREY (b. 1898) and his group at Oxford, among whom E. B. Chain was notable. Conditions then were attained in which the substance was found to be more stable; its chemical and biological properties were explored, and sodium penicillin was crystallized. With Fleming's list of microbes, which he had divided into penicillin-sensitive and penicillin-insensitive, considerably expanded and explored by the Oxford group and others, it was shown that penicillin, like the sulfonamides, was chiefly a bacteriostatic (that is, it stopped the growth of organisms without killing them). In fact, with later products of greater purity, penicillin has become recognized as "the most potent weapon yet known to man in the war of science against disease" (A. N. Richards). The great difficulties of producing penicillin in adequate amounts proved insurmountable in an England engaged in the midst of a World War. This situation was met by the co-operation of British and American scientists with a number of pharmaceutical houses on this side of the Atlantic, under the guidance of the Committee of Medical Research of the U. S. National Research Council. With the elaboration of mass-production methods, in a few years it became possible to manufacture enough not only for the use of all the Allied armed forces, but also for civilians. G-Penicillin was synthesized by V. DU VEGREAUD et al. in 1946. Numerous antibiotics are now being actively studied, especially by the Rutgers group, and some (streptothricin, tyrothricin, streptomycin) give promise of being effective where sulfonamides and penicillin have failed.

Among the diseases not susceptible to treatment by the sulfonamides or penicillin or, in fact, any other known drug is the group of Rickettsial infections. Very recently Ludwig ANGSTEIN (b. 1891) and M. N. BADER at the University of Texas found that paraminobenzoic acid (PABA) was capable, when fed for several days, of preventing or aborting experimental typhus fever in guinea-pigs, with indications that the animals later were immune to reinoculation. PABA is the constituent of vitamin B that the sulphonamides block from entering bacteria, which thus lose the power of reproduction.

Thus the modern treatment of disease has received an important new orientation from the discoveries of modern biology. In addition to the "biologicals" already mentioned, we may recall the ever increasing importance of the prophylactic and active treatment of disease by SERUMS and VACCINES. These potent substances when best prepared and evaluated will also in all probability open up new wider horizons in the individual and social treatment of disease. Among the latest advances in this direction is the immunization against pertussis. After indifferent results with pertussis vaccine, I. Jundell (1867–1945) first used (1933) serum from persons inoculated with the vaccine as soon as possible after exposure. Pearl Kendrick (b. 1890) in 1936 used " reinforced or hyperimmune " serum prophylactically for exposed children. This was further developed (1937–44) by Joseph Stokes (b. 1896), S. Mudd (b. 1893), and their colleagues as a lyophiled hypcrimmune serum to the point of conferring significant passive protection and definitely lowering the mortality rate. For measles, one of the most fatal diseases for children under three, the gamma globulin fraction of blood from immune donors has been found not only to confer temporary protection if given within five days after exposure, but also to modify the attacks that it fails to prevent.

Among the NEW DRUGS that have probably been among the leading life-savers is carbon tetrachloride, formerly used only as a dry cleaner and fire-extinguisher. Maurice C. Hall (1881–1939), a veterinarian in the Bureau of Animal Industry in Washington, made the important discovery (1921) that this drug was the most efficient, practical eradicator of hookworm. This, together with its later modifications, according to S. M. Lambert (see *A Yankee Doctor in Paradise*) has put a spark into millions who would otherwise have been in their graves.

Cinchona bark and its products, which have played leading parts in the fight with malaria, acquired new significance when much of World War II spread to malarial-infested regions. The need thus made urgent, together with the early loss by the Allies of many of the sources of quinine, led to the development of atabrine (an alkyl-amino-acridine derivative), plasmochin (best against *Plasmodium falciparum* and for symptom-free carriers, and the latest addition, totaquine. And now, just as the need for quinine becomes less urgent, its long-sought synthesis has been achieved. When eighteen-year-old William Perkin discovered the first coal-tar dye almost a century ago, thus giving the start to the organic-chemistry industry, he was trying unsuccessfully to make quinine artificially. Since then many naturally occurring useful drugs have been synthesized; but quinine only succumbed in 1944, to the youthful American chemists Robert Woodward (b. 1917) and William Doering (b. 1918). After fourteen months' arduous work they succeeded in converting hydroxy-iso-quinoline, derived from either coal or petroleum, into quinotoxine, from which both quinine and the cardiac drug quinidine were readily produced. It is of course too early to tell what the therapeutic consequences of this discovery may be, but vistas of possibilities are unfolded. The anticoagulant heparin was isolated (1917) by Jay McLean (b. 1890) and named by Howell the next year. It has proved useful in threatened thrombosis (Best, 1929) and in various operations (Gordon Murray, 1940); and now has a synthetic — dicoumarin, isolated by Link and others (1941) — as a possible substitute.

TRANSFUSION of whole blood or plasma or blood substitutes (known since the seventeenth century) has been so greatly advanced in recent years that it constitutes one of the important therapeutic achievements of the twentieth century. The early attempts, in spite of frequent untoward results, had not been forgotten, though it was not until the nineteenth century that study of the subject was again resumed (Bichat, 1805; Blundell's indirect syringe method, 1824; Prevost's and Dumas's use of defibrinated

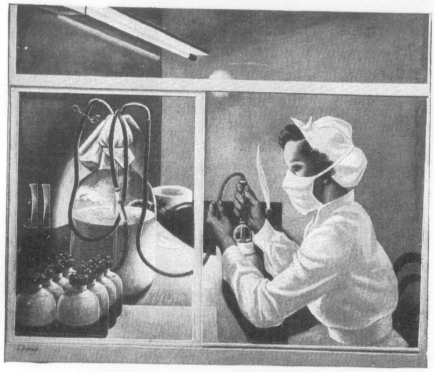

480. *Preparation of blood plasma in the laboratory. E. Fiene.*
(COURTESY OF THE ABBOTT COLLECTION, PAINTINGS OF ARMY MEDICINE.)

blood, 1821). Success with transfusions in animals kept alive human attempts until in the 1870's new enthusiasm developed. O. HASSE, regarding defibrinated blood as half dead, advocated whole lamb's blood (1874), and even whole milk had its supporters on both sides of the Atlantic. In the light of present knowledge one wonders how such fallacious and dangerous methods could even have found their way into the medical print of the period. Landsteiner's discovery (1900) of the four more or less incompatible groups of human blood explained previous disasters and first permitted a logical approach to the subject. Crile (1906) was one of the first to make practical use of this discovery with his direct method of suturing the donor's artery to the recipient's vein. However, when it was found by Albert Hustin (b. 1882), in 1914; Luis Agote, of Buenos Aires, in 1914; R. Lewisohn (b. 1875), in 1915, and others that blood coagulation could be harmlessly prevented by sodium citrate, the indirect method of drawing the blood into a receptacle and then injecting it into the vein soon came into general use. This in turn paved the way for storage of blood, first by Rous and Turner, (1916), later by D. N. Belanki (1928) of Moscow, and J. Tenconi and O. R. Palazzo (1934) of Buenos Aires. Conserved blood in human treatment was used by O. H. Robertson (1918), later by S. S. Yudin of Moscow (1930).

Following the lead of the Leningrad Institute of Blood Transfusion and, in America, of the Cook County Hospital in Chicago (1937), "blood banks" are now available in the United States and other countries in many hospitals where a refrigerated, glucose-citrated, "typed" blood mixture can be held for a number of days in readiness for emergencies. Sterile cadaveric blood and preserved erythrocytes have also been found useful under appropriate conditions. The needs of the two World Wars were urgent stimuli to a widespread development of the transfusion procedure that was made possible, in the case of whole blood, by Landsteiner's discovery of the human blood groups; and in the case of plasma, by different methods of vacuum desiccation and preservation in the frozen state (W. J. Elser [b. 1872] et al., 1935; S. Mudd and E. W. Flosdorf, 1935; M. Strumia, 1938). The use of plasma instead of whole blood was suggested by G. R. Ward and by F. W. Hartman in 1918. It was advocated again (1927) by M. Strumia (b. 1896) in order to avoid the dangerous antigenic properties of the erythrocytes, with the added advantage that the "leucocytic cream" and the erythrocytes could be used for other purposes. It was used by him, redissolved, in large quantities intravenously in 1938. The method of plasma desiccation permits indefinitely long storage, without deterioration, and convenient transportation of the dried powder. Readily redissolvable in sterile water, it can be given under field conditions, and already thousands of lives have been saved and convalescence shortened by "shots" of plasma given shortly after civilian injury or when the soldier was wounded and even still under fire. Not only is transfusion of value in other kinds of shock as well as after hemorrhage, but it has also been found extremely useful as an adjuvant in routine postoperative care, and in various infections, anæmias, and other non-surgical conditions. Fractionation of plasma, in the hands of E. J. Cohn (b. 1892), has produced a serum albumin component valuable in restoring blood volume as in shock; a serum globulin fraction that contains the well-known immunizing properties of serum; and a fibrin foam that has proved valuable as a physiological covering for raw surfaces and in staunching hemorrhage.

BLOOD SUBSTITUTES were also extensively studied and applied to needs of world warfare. Normal salt solution had been used in the nineteenth century, but was known to leave the circulation rapidly on account of its osmotic properties; the same held true to a lesser degree of " physiological " glucose and other substances. One of the first to appreciate the need for colloidal (large molecular) preparations, in order to be held in the circulatory system, was J. J. HOGAN (b. 1872), who proposed the use of 2.5 per cent gelatin (1915). This, however, had the disadvantage of accumulating toxic degeneration products and not being sterilizible. Following an extensive study by the British Medical Research Committee, Bayliss recommended a seven per cent gum arabic (acacia) in normal salt solution; but this later fell into disuse as dangerous unless very carefully prepared. In the Second World War there was a return to a better and safe variety of gelatin when whole blood or plasma was not available, as it was found to be neither contaminated nor toxic.

ANESTHESIA. With all the chemical and pharmacological developments that have occurred in the past half-century, it was to be expected that anesthesia would also become a complex field of scientific study and practical application. Instead of cocaine for local anesthesia and inhalation of ether or chloroform for general, there are now hundreds of chemical agents available, given in various ways depending on the individual circumstances. In many medical centres anesthesiology has taken its place as an autonomous specialty directed by a physician of sound physiological training who confines his activities to the one field.

Among the many important improvements in anesthesia that have taken place in recent years is the " closed " system of administration — nitrous oxide and cyclopropane or other combinations — conducted through a closed system of tubes through a mask fitting tightly over the face. The apparatus for the closed system was perfected in 1921 by Ralph WATERS of Wisconsin and has been shown to give excellent results.

Among the general anesthetics, ethylene, which has had a fluctuating history since first used as an anesthetic by T. NUNNELY (1809–70) in 1849, was established (1922, 1923) by A. B. LUCKHARDT (b. 1885) and his colleagues, and independently in 1923 by William E. BROWN (b. 1891). From this grew C. D. LEAKE's (b. 1896) production (1930) of the useful divinyl ether. Cyclopropane, an impurity of propylene, was found (1928) by G. H. W. LUCAS (b. 1894) and V. E. HENDERSON (1877–1945) to be a more potent anesthetic than propylene. Laughing gas (nitrous oxide) was mixed with oxygen for anesthesia in 1868 by E. W. ANDREWS. It was brought into the domain of practical anesthesia in the 1880's by Sir Frederic HEWITT, who was the first to construct a practical apparatus. With further improvements by the Cleveland dentist C. K. TETER and by E. I. McKESSON, J. GWATHMEY (1863–1944), J. S. LUNDY, and others, the method has obtained widespread favour.

INTRAVENOUS ANESTHESIA was practised by P. C. ORÉ as early as 1872, but only became popular with the introduction of the barbiturates by Fischer and von Mering in 1903, following Fischer's synthesis of veronal in 1902. It has attained a considerable vogue in the past decade, following its clinical exploration by J. S. Lundy (1934). Amytal (1929), nembutal (1930), evipal (1933) and pentothal are those receiving the widest support. Paraldehyde, intravenously, which was introduced in 1913 by H. NOEL and H. S. SOUTTAR, still finds users in restricted cases.

SPINAL ANESTHESIA. The development of regional anesthesia has in recent decades been especially great in its spinal applications. J. L. CORNING's early injection (1885) of cocaine into the lower dorsal spinal canal had produced anesthesia of the legs and urogenital organs. This was replaced by less toxic cocaine derivatives, such as stovaine in 1903 (so called after its introducer, E. FOURNEAU [French for stove] [b. 1872]) and procaine in 1904, and later butyn and tutocaine. An anesthetic in labour entirely without ill effects on mother and child is still being sought; none has thus far met the test of time and universal acceptance.

In 1899 Bernard KRÖNIG (1863–1918), of Freiburg, and Carl J. GAUSS (b. 1875) introduced "twilight sleep" (using morphine and scopolamine), but it soon became evident that it was not without danger from post-partum hemorrhage, and the baby was often asphyxiated. In recent years various barbiturates have gained widespread popularity, but like rectal anesthesia and J. B. DE LEE's (b. 1869) presacral novocaine, they have encountered serious objections. Scopolamine-morphine, used in Richard von Steinbüchel's twilight sleep (1903), was used intravenously (1916) by Elizabeth BREDENFELD of Switzerland.

Caudal anesthesia was advocated as early as 1901 by the Frenchman M. A. SICARD, and by M. F. CATHELIN (b. 1873) in 1905 in the second stage of labour. It was not for another generation, however, that a continuous procedure was developed (1940) by W. T. LEMMON and used for caudal analgesia in obstetrics (1942) by W. B. EDWARDS and R. A. HINGSON. It is now possible to paralyse the sensory tracts at such a high level that practically all abdominal and even some thoracic operations can be performed in this way. I. W. STOECKEL used this method in 1909, J. SCHLIMPERT in 1910 and 1911. Early proponents of the procedure in the United States were W. R. MEEKER (b. 1889) and M. L. BONAR (b. 1889) in 1927.

PARAVERTEBRAL ANESTHESIA was introduced by A. LAEWEN (b. 1880), of Leipzig, who blocked the nerves from the ninth thoracic to the third lumbar. In

1920 Gaston LABAT, of Paris, perfected the method of infiltration and nerve-blocking to induce insensitization to pain. Parasacral block, caudal block, trans-sacral anesthesia, and sacral block (that is, Labat's combination of caudal block with transsacral anesthesia) have proved to be useful methods.

RECTAL ANESTHESIA, described by Pirogoff in 1847, was unsuccessful until J. T. GWATHMEY (1863–1944) in 1913 used ether in a non-irritating mixture with carron oil. Avertin, rectally, which was proposed by F. Eichholtz in 1927, also has had its day of popularity.

ENDOTRACHEAL ANESTHESIA had been used on animals (1858) by John SNOW, of London, the first physician to devote himself entirely to anesthesia, and on man after tracheotomy (1869) by F. Trendelenburg. Its modern development began in 1907 with the introduction of insufflation anesthesia without tracheotomy by Barthélémy and Dufour, and two years later by S. J. MELTZER (1851–1920) and J. AUER (b. 1875) in the United States. Its application to clinical anesthesia is due to a number of investigators, such as F. J. COTTON and W. BOOTHBY (b. 1880) in 1911 and C. H. PECK in 1912.

REFRIGERATION is one of the oldest and newest of anesthetics: the effect of cold in dulling pain was known to primitives and was used by Marcus Aurelius Severinus (1646), and by Larrey in Napoleon's armies to aid in amputations; and now it returns in the hands of F. M. ALLEN (1941) and the H. E. MOCKS, Sr. and Jr. (b. 1880 and 1909), highly recommended for the same purpose.

The field of local anesthesia has broadened, especially in dentistry, and it has been extended to include laparotomies. In fact, more than once a reckless surgeon was said to have removed his own appendix in this way.

A leading pharmacologist in the earlier part of the century was Hans Horst MEYER (1853–1939), pupil and assistant of Schmiedeberg, who taught for twenty years at Marburg and twenty more at Vienna, retiring in 1924. Known in England and America by his numerous visits, Meyer was prominent in promoting scientific pharmacology by bringing it into a close relation with general biology, pathology, and clinical medicine. With his pupils he made numerous contributions on such subjects as the pharmacological effects of iron, bismuth, aluminum, and jaborandi, the nature of acute phosphorus poisoning, heat-regulation, diuretic and narcotic effects, and the influence of the sympathetic system normally and as affected by drugs. A good example of the tendency of pharmacologists to study physiological problems can be found in the important work of R. MAGNUS (1873–1927), Professor of Pharmacology at Utrecht, on postural reflexes (1924).

The leading pharmacologist in the United States in this period was J. J. ABEL (1857–1938), of Cleveland, who for almost forty years was professor at Johns Hopkins. His brilliant investigative work has been largely in the endocrine field: he was the first (1898) to isolate the active principle of the adrenal glands, which he named epinephrine. This was first obtained in crystalline form in 1901 by Takamine, who called it adrenaline. Abel and his co-workers also isolated bufagin and insulin in crystalline form. His investigations of histamin and similar substances and of the hormones of the pituitary were valuable in their fields; his ingenious method of vividiffusion (plasmapheresis), permitting him to isolate amino acids directly from the blood, has proved useful in various types of investigation. He was one of the first to use dye-stuffs as test materials of the functional efficiency of various organs. With Cushny he founded the *Journal of Pharmacology and Experimental Therapeutics*, of which he was editor from 1909 to 1932. His influence continues in the work of his many pupils, such as Reid Hunt, D. I. Macht, L. G. Rowntree, A. S. Loevenhart (1878–1929), and S. J. Crowe.

The Code of Ethics of the American Pharmaceutical Association (revised 1922) admirably sets forth the duties of the pharmacist to the public and to his colleagues. Such laws as the American Food and Drugs Act (1906) and the Harrison Anti-narcotic Act (1914) protect the health of the people from themselves and from unscrupulous purveyors. An International Pharmaceutical Federation was formed at The Hague in 1920; and several international conferences for the unification of formulas have been held since the opening Brussels Conference of 1902. The education of pharmacists has been given largely in special schools, in America a diploma, usually of Graduate in Pharmacy, being awarded after a two-year course. Now, however, four years of study are required for the baccalaureate degree, seven for the doctorate. Some universities (Michigan, 1868; Wisconsin, 1883; etc.) include pharmacy departments in their organization. Pharmaceutical journals have existed for more than a century, the oldest being the *Journal de pharmacie et de chimie* (founded in Paris, 1809, as the *Bulletin de pharmacie*) and the *American Journal of Pharmacy* (founded by the Philadelphia College of Pharmacy in 1825). Many pharmaceutical journals are now published throughout the world, some of high calibre, some frankly commercial. The *Archiv für experimentelle Physiologie und Pharmakologie* was founded in 1873; the *Archives internationales de pharmacodynamie* in 1895; the *Journal of Pharmacology and Experimental Therapeutics* in 1909.

21. Roentgenology, Radiology

The discovery of X-rays on November 8, 1895 by Wilhelm Conrad Röntgen (1845–1923) was first reported in his now classical *Preliminary Communication to the President of the Physical-Medical Society of Würzburg* on December 28, 1895. The sensational discovery was announced to the world on January 6, 1896 and greeted with universal enthusiasm as one of the most dramatic events in the history of science. These rays, called by their discoverer X-rays on account of their unknown nature, but now also known as Roentgen rays after their discoverer, are produced by the passage of an electric current through a special vacuum tube on the principle of the electrical phenomena described by Crookes and Hertz. They possess the property of penetrating dense bodies that are impenetrable to light-waves and giving an image on a fluorescent screen or photographic

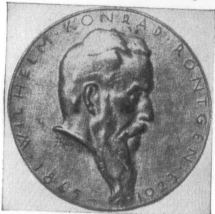

481. *Wilhelm Konrad Roentgen medallion.*

negative. They were soon found to be composed of three kinds of rays of different nature and powers of penetration. The alpha rays (identified as helium atoms by Rutherford, 1899) are stopped by a sheet of paper; beta rays (electrons, Giesel, 1899) penetrate about half an inch of animal tissue; whereas the hardest gamma rays (recognized as true waves by Villard, 1900) may pass through a foot of lead.

Immediately, the X-ray came into surgical use for the diagnosis of fractures and diseases of bone and for the recognition of foreign bodies. Roentgen-ray installations were shortly required in many hospitals. Soon the examination of internal organs was included when it was appreciated that rays are partly blocked by organs of lesser density or bone and that negatives with considerable differentiation of soft parts could be obtained. The examination of the lungs developed another large field for this activity. Foreign bodies in the bronchi and in the lung were exactly located. Chest X-rays as a routine part of a clinical examination have by now detected thousands of early symptomless cases of tuberculosis in schools and in the armed forces and are obligatory in most repeated health examinations. The radiology of the bones and joints has also been productive of a great amount of work: the diagnosis of vertebral variations under the influence of age and occupation, as well as the abnormalities of trauma and disease, was promoted by the work of A. W. GEORGE and R. D. LEONARD (1923), and a thorough exposition of the diseases of the vertebral body and the intervertebral disk was accomplished by W. A. EVANS (1932). Roentgenography of the teeth began with the work of W. Koenig in Germany (published early in 1896) and W. J. Morton's article in *Dental Cosmos* in June 1896. It was at first concerned only with impaction and failure to erupt. Renal and other calculi and pathological calcifications came into the diagnostic sphere of the rays in short order. They were used in obstetrical diagnosis as early as 1896 (Davis and Varmier). Cinematography, though partially achieved as early as 1897, by J. MacIntyre, has continued to progress in spite of the interruption of two world wars, though it still remains in the investigative state

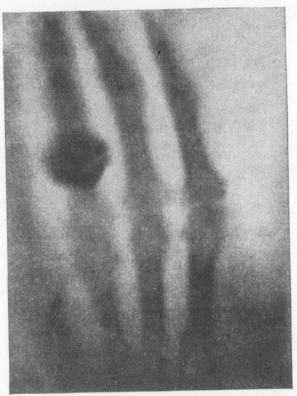

482. *The first Roentgen photograph. Mrs. Roentgen's hand with ring on ring finger.*

(R. Junker in Germany; R. Reynolds, of London; W. H. Stewart, of New York).

The applications of Röntgen's great discovery in the few remaining years of the nineteenth century were remarkable and to be expected. Though the developments in the twentieth century may have been less spectacular, in sum total they amount to greater advantage to the patient in diagnosis and treatment. Improved roentgenograms, and fluoroscopy, together with the increased experience of the operators, who already find it necessary to specialize in separate body fields, now detect much smaller or more obscure lesions than was previously possible. Aid from radio-opaque materials is obtained, not only in the digestive tract, but in almost all of the " external " cavities, in the urinary tract, and even in arteries and such remote vital regions as the brain and the spinal cord.

In 1897 W. B. CANNON (1871–1945), then a medical student and later Professor of Physiology at Harvard, introduced the use of bismuth, which is opaque to X-rays, in the roentgenological study of the gastro-intestinal tract of animals

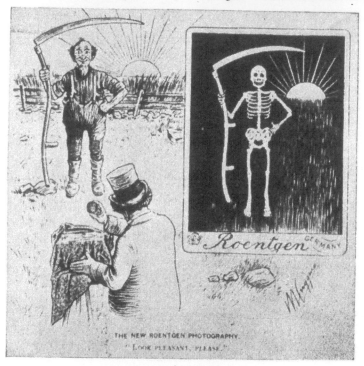

483. " Look pleasant, please."
(Cartoon from Life, 1896.)

(see American Journal of Physiology, 1898). In 1904 H. RIEDER (1858–1928), of Munich, and in 1906 C. BECK (1856–1911), of New York, applied the use of this material in the study of human disease; and later barium sulphate was substituted for bismuth. This method of investigating the gastro-intestinal tract proved to be enormously helpful in establishing the morphological and functional condition of the stomach and intestines and of diagnosing the presence of ulcers and tumours in early stages. It has now been extended to most systems of the body. In the respiratory tract, combined with the use of the bronchoscope, it has been of great value in the diagnosis of bronchiectasis and its extent, and in the early detection of pulmonary neoplasms. The roentgen diagnosis of gall-bladder disease was developed by L. G. COLE (1914) and others, and its "visualization" (rendering visible with X-ray by means of opaque material, 1924) by E. A. GRAHAM and W. H. COLE, of Washington University, with the use of tetraiodophenolphthalein, which is excreted through the biliary system and temporarily remains in the gall bladder, thus disclosing the outlines of the organ and the presence of gall-stones. The urinary tract was rendered visible by "retrograde pyelography" by W. F. BRAASCH (1910), Sir J. W. THOMPSON (1914), and others. "Excretory pyelography" began with the use of such opaque preparations as sodium iodide (Rowntree et al., 1923) and uroselectan, which shortly after intravenous injection is excreted by the urinary tract so that serial roentgenograms give accurate pictures of the condition of the kidney and its pelvis and of the ureters and the bladder. Lipiodol and other opaque materials are used for the outlining of enlarged bronchi in the lungs, or of the spinal canal, and also in the female genital tract for the diagnosis of tumours in the cavity of the uterus (C. Heuser, 1921) and to establish patency in the Fallopian tubes. Egas MONIZ, of Lisbon, was the first to introduce arteriography, injecting a solution of sodium iodide into the carotid artery. In 1929 he and his school reported successful localization on intracranial tumours. Finally we cite the progress in amniography through the injection of a solution of strontium iodide through the abdominal wall. By this method the fetal soft parts are visualized, the placenta is localized, and it is frequently possible to determine the sex of the fetus.

In 1913 E. WEBER injected air into the peritoneal cavity in order to outline more sharply the digestive organs by X-ray examination; and in 1918 W. DANDY introduced ventriculography (air in the cerebral ventricles) for the X-ray diagnosis of cerebral disease. Peritoneal insufflation was introduced to facilitate kidney and adrenal diagnosis in the same year, 1921, by H. H. CARELLI, an Argentinian publishing in France, and by P. ROSENSTEIN. Radiographic exploration of the brain and the spinal canal is performed by means of a contrast medium of low specific gravity, such as gas, air, nitrogen, or oxygen, introduced by lumbar puncture after the withdrawal of a certain amount of cerebrospinal fluid. Such methods have proved valuable in the localization of tumours and other lesions of the brain and spinal cord.

Advances have occurred, and are still occurring, in this field so rapidly that it has sometimes proved difficult to supply a sufficient number of well-trained personnel or to investigate the various suggested new procedures in a proper scientific manner. Today every reputable hospital of any size must have its X-ray department, equipped for both the diagnosis and the treatment of disease, just as surely as it must have a laboratory.

TECHNICAL IMPROVEMENTS by physicists and engineers have greatly contributed to the practical usefulness of X-rays. The fluoroscopic screen, which as a barium platinum cyanide coat on a bit of cardboard manifested the X-rays to

Röntgen on the memorable 8th of November 1895, has been frequently improved, beginning with Edison's substitution of calcium tungstate, and brought
to a high state of efficiency by C. V. S. PATTERSON, using cadmium tungstate
(1914). Other conspicuous improvements were: W. D. COOLIDGE's tube (1913);
Gustav BUCKY's diaphragm (1915); graded metallic filters, stereoscopic views
for the accurate location of lesions or foreign bodies (H. E. IVES, 1905), and the

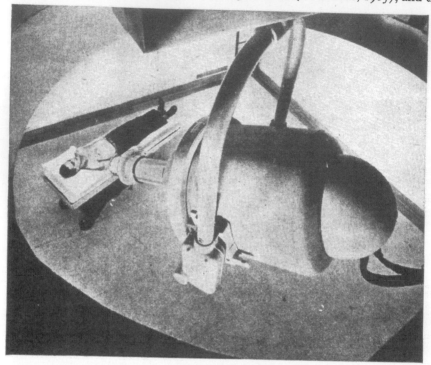

484. *The battle against cancer. A million-volt X-ray machine at the Walter Reed
Hospital, Chicago.*

development of more powerful therapeutic units. X-rays may now be used with
voltages in the millions, employing long-lived tubes that can stand the great
heat developed by means of " two-element vacuum tubes " immersed and cooled
in oil. Improved devices accurately control the voltage, current, and exposure
time, with accurate dosimeters that have made possible the internationally accepted unit, the " roentgen." Sure protection of patient and operator from dangerous currents and overexposure is provided, and numerous procedures and
instruments have been devised for more convenient and effective application
of the rays to diagnosis and treatment, in the most inaccessible parts of the body.
" Contact therapy " with low voltages is a recent development that has proved
to be most useful in various superficial lesions, of the kind treated, in a more
costly way, by radium. The method of " laminagraphy " (reproduction during

motion of a sharp edge of a thin layer of the object selected) was developed by several workers independently during the twenties for deep lesions such as lung cavities underlying much scar tissue.

The marked biologic effect of the Roentgen rays on body tissues was forcibly brought to the attention of the early investigators by the appearance on their hands and other exposed parts of chronic and painful skin ulcers, which were resistant to all forms of treatment and eventually turned into fatal cancer. Many of these early investigators, before this harmful effect was known, died from recurring cancers of the skin or from a fatal aplastic anæmia, as in the case of radium poisoning, before it was learned that harmful effects could be guarded against by the use of lead screens and glass that is rich in lead. Prominent among such martyrs to science were H. E. Albers-Schönberg (1865–1921), of Hamburg; Holzknecht, of Vienna; J. A. Bergonié (1857–1925), who was honoured on his death-bed by the President of the French Republic; the Britishers Spence, Blackall, and J. F. Hall-Edwards (1858–1926); the Americans F. H. Baetjer (1874–1933), of Johns Hopkins University, C. L. Leonard (1861–1913) and M. K. Kassabian (1870–1910), of Philadelphia, R. D. Carman (1875–1926), of the Mayo Clinic, and W. E. Caldwell (1870–1918), of New York.

Recognition of the effects of X-ray on the tissues led to its use in treatment, first of the dermatoses. John DANIEL (b. 1862), of Vanderbilt University, as early as April 1896 had produced skin reactions and loss of hair. L. FREUND (b. 1868), of Vienna, obtained a complete epilation in a case of a hairy nevus, and thus was led to the use of X-rays in the cure of sycosis. E. H. GRUBBE is said to have applied them to cancer of the breast and to lupus vulgaris in January 1896 and himself to have acquired an X-ray dermatitis; but he made no publication until 1933.

Roentgen therapy was given a quantitatively sound basis by the work of the physicist, B. KRÖNIG, and the gynæcologist W. FRIEDRICH, who found (1918) that the same doses to tadpoles of the same age regularly produced the same changes.

H. KÜMMELL first applied X-rays to the treatment of lupus vulgaris; others obtained good results in the treatment of skin cancer (T. A. U. SJOEGREN and J. T. STENBECK, 1899). The therapeutic effect of X-rays has been steadily extended to an increasing number of diseases. They were early used in the treatment of leukemias (W. A. PUSEY, 1902; Nicholas SENN, 1903; G. DOCK, 1904); they have also been found useful in retarding symptoms and prolonging life in Hodgkins disease, without, however, actually curing either of these conditions. The studies of J. A. Bergonié (1857–

1905), L. Tribondeau (b. 1872) (law of radio sensitivity), and Albers-Schönberg on the effects of the X-rays on the male sexual organs, and those of Halberstaedter (1905) on the ovaries, demonstrated their especially destructive effects on germinal and newly forming cells. This circumstance explains their usefulness in cancer, which is rich in young cells; another helpful feature being the general lowering of nutrition that the rays produce, especially through the destruction of capillaries and newly formed blood vessels. The effects of X-rays and radium on the cells of the blood, especially in diminishing the lymphocytes and granulocytes, have been brought out by Holzknecht and Bozzolo and many others. Deep radiation of tumours of the uterus (Albers-Schönberg, Dessauer, and others) dates from 1906–8 and signalizes the first steps in the use of the rays for the treatment of internal tumours.

Methods of dosage have now been perfected, and with the use of more penetrating rays even deep-seated lesions can be made the focus of large doses, which are divided into several portals of entry so that the intervening parts will not be damaged along any one avenue. In all the great surgical clinics and hospitals of the world, radiological departments and institutes are active in the routine lines of diagnosis and therapy and in exploring new fields of roentgenologic activity. In the treatment of malignant tumours X-ray and radium therapy constitute an invaluable method, especially in those cases where surgical intervention is no longer possible. We refer to the radiologic treatment of cancer of the skin by Tage SJÖGREN (b. 1859), a Swedish radiologist, of cancer of the stomach by I. Holzknecht, on permeation in mammary cancer by W. M. SAMPSON-HANDLEY (b. 1872). The monograph of Sir St. Clair Thomson (1859–1940) on cancer of the larynx (1930) is thought to be the best on this subject. Certain tumours are preferably treated by these means, while others can be delayed and the patient kept in comparative comfort by their use.

Among the many who have made valuable contributions to roentgenology we can name but a few. Guido HOLZKNECHT (1872–1931), professor at Vienna, was a leader in the scientific development of the subject, recognizing the early erythema effect, establishing the unit of X-ray intensity, inventing an instrument for measuring dosage, and developing methods of diagnosis and treatment in numerous departments of the subject. He was a prolific contributor to the literature of the subject from 1901 up to the time of his death. He was a typical martyr to the X-ray, dying after many operations for cancer, requiring repeated amputations of his right upper extremity. Among French radiologists we note A. BÉCLÈRE (1856–1939), who introduced the X-ray treatment of glandular tuberculosis; Foveau DE COURMELLES, BERGONIÉ, of Bordeaux; LEDUC, of Nantes;

and BORDIER. Prominent in Germany were H. HOLFELDER (b. 1891), of Frankfurt; R. GRASHEY (b. 1876), director of the Radiological Institute of Cologne and author of two radiological atlases; A. KÖHLER (b. 1874), first describer of Köhler's disease of the foot and author of a popular treatise, *Grenzen des Normalen*

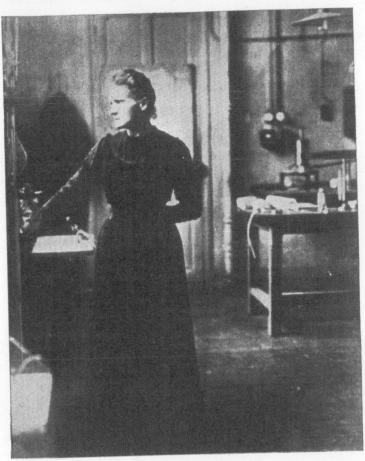

485. Mme. Curie in her laboratory.

und Anfänge des Pathologischen im Röntgenbilde (1910); Georg PERTHES (1869–1927), first to use deep X-ray therapy (1903) and to describe the disease of the hip that bears his name. In Italy, the first Italian institute was founded by M. GORTAN (1872–1937) in Trieste in 1904, to be quickly followed by others at Milan, Turin, and Rome. Among the outstanding Italian radiologists are F. GHILARDUCCI (1857–1924), A. BUSI, his successor at Rome, C. TANDOIA (1870–1934), M. BERTOLOTTI, of Turin, R. BALLI, of Pavia, and F. PERUSSIA (b. 1885), of Milan, author of a book on *Radiologia dell'apparato circolatorio* and of the first Italian treatise on radiotherapy. One of the first to develop the subject in America was Francis Henry WILLIAMS (1852–1936), of Boston, who in 1901 published a valuable book, *The Roentgen Rays in Medicine and Surgery*. To-day the subject is vigorously and profitably pursued throughout the country, attracting many of the best men in the profession.

RADIUM. The development of the biological uses of radium (discovered by the Curies in 1898) was similar to that of the X-ray. It was early shown to be more destructive of animal tissues than of bacteria lodged in them (H. Chambers, S. Russ, and others). Its first therapeutic use was for various skin diseases after Pierre Curie had purposely produced a burn on his arm, similar to Becquerel's accidental burn (1901). H. DANLOS (1844–1932) and R. G. BLOCK first used it in treating lupus in 1901; J. DANYSZ in the treatment of malignant disease in 1903. The general scientific exploration of its therapeutic value may be said to have been begun by L. F. WICKHAM and P. DEGRAIS (1906) and S. DOMINICI in the Biological Laboratory for Radium of Paris. Other pioneers in its therapeutic use were R. ABBE, M. BASHFORD, V. CZERNY, L. FREUND, H. A. KELLY, P. LAZARUS, and B. SZILARD. Like the X-ray, which has a similar effect on the tissues, its final place in the treatment of disease, and especially of cancer, remains to be evaluated. Suffice it to say that (in the form of " seeds," needles, bombs, and so on) either radium salts or their emanations (radon) continue to be used by many radiologists in the palliation of advanced cases of cancer, as a caustic, and in especially favourable localities, such as the interior of cavities.

The discovery in 1931 by Irène CURIE and her husband, F. JOLIOT, that radioactivity could be induced in a number of elements by isotope-formation has already proved highly useful in biological research and in the treatment of malignant disease. Such " tagged " elements can be traced in metabolic activities in the body — as, for instance, the role of " tagged " iron in anæmia and blood-formation. They have also shown promise, as in the case of " tagged " phosphorus in the treatment of leukemia (1939) and polycythemia (1944) by J. H. LAWRENCE and his associates.

The potentialities of the neutrons emitted by the hundred million volts of E. O. LAWRENCE's cyclotron in the treatment of malignant disease are still to be evaluated; still more in the mists of the future lie the biologic effects of cosmic rays and of the energy released by the recently achieved fission of the atom, i.e., nucleus.

22. Military Medicine

Shortly before World War I the introduction of various hygienic measures, and especially efficient vaccination against typhoid and tetanus, the

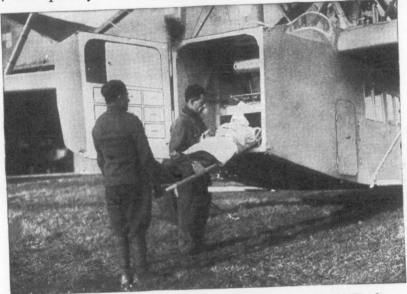

486. *Loading the wounded in an Italian Caproni airplane, World War I.*

conquest of insect vectors of disease, and the improved service of supplies
and provision of pure drinking water, were all advances that had results
of the greatest importance to the war. For the first time in history civilian
physicians of all the specialties gave their services by the thousands to the
armies in the fields and to the base hospitals. From the laboratory investigators of synthetic foods to those chemists who devised defences against
poison gases, from the physiologists who studied new functional problems
involved in aviation to the bacteriologists in the rear and near the front
line; from the investigators of new disease pictures and the problems involved in their treatment to the specialists in otolaryngology, ophthalmology, and psychiatry, who were given new war neuroses to study as well as
the shattering organic effects of war injuries — all contributed cheerfully
and to the best of their ability to the efficient handling of the vast and complex problems involved. Thus medicine in all its branches was mobilized
with all its resources to meet the problems of a type of warfare that was
hitherto unthought of in its destructiveness and horror. Abdominal, neu-

rological, and especially reconstructive surgery were eminently successful, in the hands of men like Harvey Cushing, G. W. Crile, Alexis Carrel, Arbuthnot Lane, C. Willems, H. Morestin, M. T. Tuffier, P. Chutro, R. Bastianelli, Robert Jones, J. P. Goldthwait, R. B. Osgood, N. Allison, H. D. Gillies, A. C. Valadier, to name but a few among many, for whose work in other fields of surgery we refer to the surgical sections. The assistance

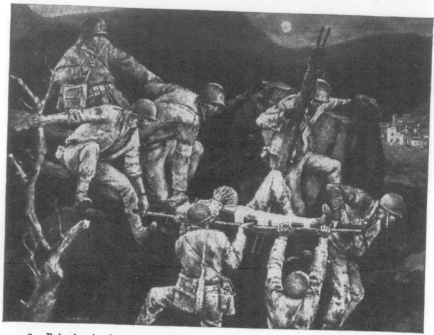

487. *Bringing in the wounded by moonlight in Italy, World War II. I. Hirsch.*
(COURTESY OF THE ABBOTT COLLECTION, PAINTINGS OF ARMY MEDICINE.)

given by the Red Cross reached a high degree of efficiency. Infectious diseases were controlled much better than had been expected, and for the first time in history the loss of life was less from disease than from combat wounds. Especially typhoid and tetanus were robbed of their wartime ravages by the prophylactic use of vaccines at stated intervals for typhoid, and immediately after being wounded in the case of tetanus. Thousands of lives were lost, to be sure, from epidemics of meningitis, measles, influenza, and other diseases that were promoted by the movements of such large numbers of the population, bringing many recruits into new surroundings from localities where they had had little or no previous exposure. The great pandemic of influenza of 1918–19 caused a great mortality among civilians and soldiers alike, in some parts of the warring countries greater than that produced by actual combat. The First World War amply demonstrated the need of an efficient hygienic organization in military medicine and of intensive training of all the sanitary forces. It demonstrated that an efficient hospitalization service can be established close to the front lines, and that if quick and proper assistance is given to the sick and wounded, a tremendous diminution in the morbidity and mortality figures can be obtained. The proper

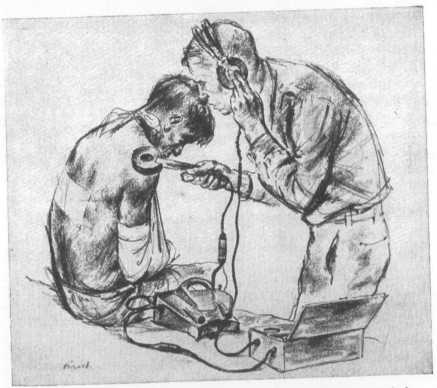

488. *A foreign-body locator, according to the principle of a mine detector, finds shell fragments in the flesh. I. Hirsch.*
(COURTESY OF THE ABBOTT COLLECTION, PAINTINGS OF ARMY MEDICINE.)

use of first-aid packages by the soldier himself, the rapid transfer to regimental aid stations, mobile hospitals, and base hospitals, with the use of ambulance trains, hospital ships, airplane transports — all these contribute notably to the reduction of the human ravages of war.

We want to refer here more fully to American military medicine during World War I, being more cognizant of the achievements in the American than in other services. Of the 4,000,000 soldiers mobilized in the American army, about 58,000 died from disease and 50,000 from battle casualties. Of the disease deaths, over 24,000 were due to influenza (J. S. Simmonds), which took a world toll of many millions. Medical officers, whether career men or recruited from civil life, were unselfish and often heroic in the performance of their duties, and sustained one of the highest mortality rates of any branch of the service. Their orders, in some cases appropriately placed above the orders of the combat officer, were often successful in preventing considerable loss of life and days of military service by the adoption of measures that avoided disease and epidemics.

The advance of general and medical science in the twenty-year interval between the two World Wars would have naturally been expected to produce much change for the better in the field of military medicine. Nevertheless, the results obtained in World War II compel one's highest admiration. In spite of the displacement of many more millions of the world's civilian and military population than in the First World War — a recognized fertile preparation for epidemics — and in spite of the many campaigns in heavily infested regions of the world, serious epidemics were conspicuously absent, much of which can properly be attributed to the precautions taken.

The following examples are taken from the American army as the only ones now available to us from official sources at the time of writing, but similar figures may be expected from the British and Russians. Every soldier was inoculated on induction against smallpox, tetanus, typhoid, and the paratyphoid fevers A and B. Those sent to areas where cholera, plague, typhus, or yellow fever existed were also immunized against them. Also, influenza vaccines were accumulated against a possible emergency. According to a War Department statement, in the first three years of World War II, the U. S. Army had "less than one death from disease per 1,000 men per year." In World War I the figure was about 19 per 1,000 (14.1 per thousand, according to another authority). In the Spanish-American War it was 26 per 1,000, and in the American Civil War 65 per 1,000. Of individual diseases, malaria, which early in the Pacific war claimed its hundreds per thousand men per year, was reduced to less than fifty chiefly by atabrine and DDT; the meningitis death-rate was 4 per cent (vs. 38 per cent in World War I) and the pneumonia death-rate 0.7 per cent (vs. 24 per cent in World War I). Avoidance of polluted water and cleanliness of latrines was never more successfully maintained. In this connection we wonder if it was a humorist who named the latrine fly *Fannia scalaris*. Disability from the exanthemata was negligible in World War II, and diphtheria, said to have been the most important infectious disease in the German army, caused practically no deaths. Venereal disease, the camp follower of war, remained a serious problem, in spite of the rapid cures procured with the new drugs; and emotional disturbances — the former "shell shock," now termed "battle fatigue" — reached an

" all high " in spite of better care based on better comprehension. The results with battle casualties were equally favourable to the medical situation. Of every 100 men wounded in battle, 97 survived and 70 returned to duty. This record result was due chiefly to the earliest possible treatment by skilled surgical specialists utilizing the most modern aids (plasma and blood transfusions, the pressure dressing of burns, free excision of necrotic tissue, sulfa drugs, penicillin,

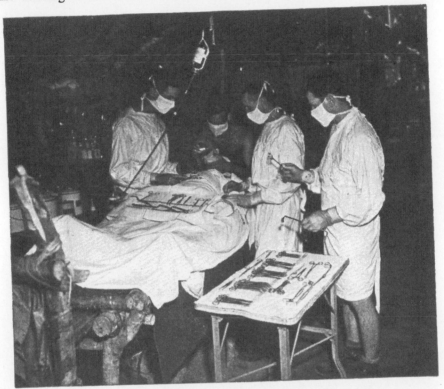

489. *Operation in a portable hospital, somewhere in New Guinea.*
(U. S. SIGNAL CORPS THROUGH SCIENCE SERVICE.)

X-ray and operating-room facilities), often in the very front line, and due also to the speed of the evacuation services, often by airplane. Perhaps the most important lesson learned was that military surgery cannot be carried out with the same care as civilian surgery. The lives of three quarters of those wounded in the abdomen were saved (as compared with much less than half in World War I); head and chest wounds also showed great if not quite so marked a reduction (15 to 50 per cent, according to Kirk). Severed nerves healed promptly after suturing, with recovery of function in the great majority of cases. Genital injuries from booby traps were a new development. Burns and blast injuries from aerial bombs caused important casualties. Rehabilitation received closer and prompt attention. Physiotherapy, perhaps even with extemporized home-made apparatus from salvage material, was begun at the earliest moment possible. Orthopedic specialists accompanied mobile troops as well as working at the bases at home and overseas. By early recognition and prompt, intelligent handling, a maximum number of the " battle-fatigued " were preserved for active service before the abnormal reactions had become firmly established. The pernicious connotations of World War I's term " shell shock " were avoided; and

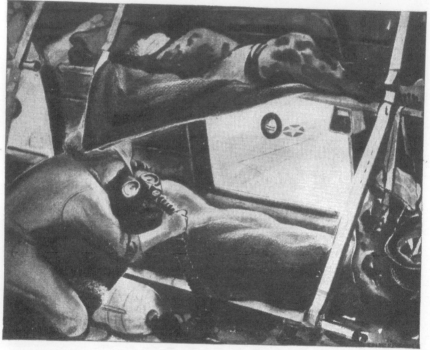

490. *A flight nurse administering oxygen to a wounded soldier in a plane bound for Australia. F. Boggs.*
(COURTESY OF THE ABBOTT COLLECTION, PAINTINGS OF ARMY MEDICINE.)

with the help of suggestion given in the semi-narcotized suggestible state, many serious cases were returned quickly to active service.

It is to such measures, pursued to a greater or less degree by all the warring countries, that death or disability in the military forces from disease or as the result of combat wounds was kept at a minimum. To accomplish these results, the American army alone utilized some 50,000 physicians, 90,000 nurses, and enlisted men who raised the total personnel to more than half a million. The individual soldier was given a better chance to help himself in his foxhole: his emergency food packet contained a more life-sustaining and better-balanced ration, the individual sulfa powder lessened the danger of infection, and the ingenious "syrette" enable him to give himself a pre-sterilized hypodermic injection of morphine. To a greater extent even than in World War I, army and navy medicine took advantage of civilian scientific resources. Through the three committees of the Office of Scientific Research and Development (those on General Science, Medical Reseach, and Aviation Medicine), contracts amounting to hundreds of millions of dollars were made with institutions of higher learning throughout the country, whereby its leading scientists were enrolled directly in the successful prosecution of a war that depended on science to an extent never before imagined.

AVIATION MEDICINE. According to Brigadier General E. G. Remartz, who has devoted an interesting study to the evolution of aviation medicine, it appears that the first book containing scientific data on aeronautics was written by an American, Dr. John Jeffries, in 1786, and was presented to the Royal Society in 1785. A Frenchman, Paul Bert (1833–86), published in 1878 an important contribution to aviation medicine. His book, *Barometric Pressure*, was ignored, however, and appeared in an excellent English translation by Mary Alice and Fred A. Hitchcock (1943), fifty-nine years after the death of the author. Bert was the first to make fundamental research in experimental physiology under the influence of barometric pressure and various phases of anoxemia.

Very remarkable are the British statistics after the First World War, showing that after the institution of a service known as care of the flier, the losses due to physical defects were reduced from 60 to 12 per cent.

The first school of flight surgeons was instituted at Hazelhurst Field, Long Island, in 1919.

The American Army Air Forces School of Aviation Medicine has accomplished a signal work. Experimental research and teaching of flight surgeons are its most important activity. Here medical officers are devoting their studies to all matters that concern the health and efficiency of the pilot and to the condition of his environment, and are able to make a decisive contribution to the progress of aviation medicine.

23. Nursing

The development of nursing in recent times has been so remarkable and nursing has taken such an important part in modern medicine that it becomes necessary to devote a special section to this subject, first summarizing some notices that may be found in previous chapters. The nurse has become a first-class co-operator with the physician in the hospital, in private practice, in the schools, in the factories, and in the laboratories; she plays an important role as social worker, and her position has greatly changed from olden times, when her work was regarded only as a work of charity.

The art of nursing obviously is of great antiquity — coeval, in fact, with the treatment of the sick and wounded. Even systematized nursing care, in some form, must have existed in the earliest hospitals. The Indian Emperor Asoka (*ca.* 250 B.C.) is said to have employed male attendants for nursing in his public hospitals, and the duties outlined for them suggest that they received some kind of training. The early Christian hospitals had women attendants called deaconesses, and the names of two, Macrina at the Basileion at Cæsarea (founded 370) and Olympia at Chrysostome's hospitals in Constantinople, have come down to us.

An important chapter in nursing history is found in the story of three great military and nursing orders that arose during the age of chivalry, one of which still continues in modified form. Each provided for a corresponding order of women. They were, in order of increasing importance: The Knights of St. Lazarus, the Hospitallers of the Teutonic Order, and the Knights Hospitallers of St. John of Jerusalem. The Order of St. Lazarus, founded about the middle of the twelfth century, was especially concerned with the care of lepers, so that it naturally dwindled and disappeared after the remarkable dying-out of leprosy in Europe in the sixteenth century. The Knights of St. John, expelled from Palestine by the Moslems in the thirteenth century, and again in the sixteenth century from Rhodes, were given the island of Malta, whence their power and possessions spread throughout Europe, with a considerable influence on hospital and nursing care. Long before the virtual destruction of the order in 1798, however, the nursing element had dwindled to insignificance. Its help in founding the International Red Cross Society and its resurgence as the St. John's Ambulance Association, which has rendered excellent wartime service, are not to be forgotten.

The Deaconess order took care of the sick in their homes — early visiting nurses. The numerous sisterhoods, such as the Ursulines (founded 1535), who figured prominently in the early trials of the Quebec colony, cared for the sick, the leprous, and the insane as a prominent part of their work during the Middle Ages and the Renaissance. In the latter part of the seventeenth century, however, a period of deterioration began that lasted for some two hundred years. The hospital nurses were generally of the charwoman type, unreliable and incompetent, slovenly, quarrelsome, and often hard drinkers. Dickens's portrait of Sairy Gamp in *Martin Chuzzlewit* is a vivid description of a nurse of his time.

The hospitals were terribly overcrowded. A leading Parisian surgeon complained in 1786 that the Hôtel-Dieu was to be rebuilt because " one could no longer see six unhappy patients heaped in a bed, annoying and frightening one another, infecting one another, and one throwing himself about and shrieking

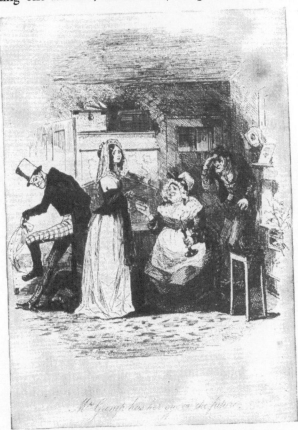

491. *Sairy Gamp, the disreputable nurse in* Martin Chuzzlewit *by Charles Dickens (London, Chapman and Hall, 1844).*

when the others had need of repose." Those dying at night might be left in bed with the living or on the floor near by till the day's routine began.

England was the first to recognize the need for a better class of nurses, as may be seen in Dr. Robert Gooch's recommendations (about 1825). In fact, it was on a visit to that country in 1822 that Theodore FLIEDNER, the pastor of Kaiserswerth, got the inspiration that in 1836 resulted in the foundation by him and his wife, Frederika, of the Diakonissen Anstalt, which may be said to have inaugurated the modern period of the nursing art. Before Fliedner died, thirty-two such deaconess houses had been founded, one at the German Hospital in

London (1846) and one at Pittsburgh (1850). Dock and Nutting say that modern training schools owe to the Kaiserswerth regime such practices as the probationary system, graded ranks from probationer to superintendent, class work and principles of discipline, etiquette and ethics, and absolute observance of the doctor's orders.

Florence NIGHTINGALE (1823–1910), born in Florence, a child of a well-to-do, cultured English family, was permitted to work at Kaiserswerth in 1850 and 1851 — a valuable prelude to her taking charge, in 1853, of an " Establishment for Gentlewomen during Illness." Before she could go further, however, the call came to her to organize a group of nurses to go to Scutari (1854) to take care of the neglected British sick and wounded of the Crimean War. The reforms instituted after a courageous propaganda by the Lady of the Lamp transformed the hospital and are said to have reduced the death-rate from 42 to 2 per cent. The Nightingale School, founded in 1860 at St. Thomas's Hospital, had from its start a great influence in the evolution of nursing, so that many training schools were started throughout Great Britain and Ireland in the next two decades. Public-health nursing in Britain may be said to have begun with the work begun by William Rathbone at the Royal Infirmary of Liverpool (about 1858). The British Nurses' Association (1887), the International Council of Nurses (1899), and the British Journal of Nursing (1893) were all founded by Mrs. BEDFORD-FENWICK, who has for nearly fifty years been the outstanding figure in British nursing.

In the United States, Bellevue Hospital of New York, which through the West India Company's hospital claims a foundation date of 1658 (or as an almshouse, 1735), and " Blockley " in Philadelphia (1731) were the first poorhouses that included care for the sick. The Charity Hospital of New Orleans (founded as a hospital and almshouse), the Pennsylvania Hospital of Philadelphia (the first to be founded solely as a hospital, 1751), and the New York Hospital of New York (chartered, 1771) were the first to be organized as hospitals. For some time the nursing conditions in all hospitals were very bad and only low-grade servants waited on the patients; the only good hospital nursing was done by the religious orders. The first systematic teaching of nurses began with Dr. Valentine SEAMAN, of New York, in 1798. The New England Hospital for Women in Boston was teaching nurses through the influence of Dr. Marie ZAKRZEWSKA about 1859 and was apparently the first to be granted a charter to teach nurses, but certificated graduates did not appear there for some years. The first school of nursing in the United States is generally said to be that founded by the Women's Hospital of Philadelphia in 1861 (fully organized in 1872). In 1873 important schools were started at Bellevue, the Connecticut Training

School at the New Haven Hospital, and the Boston Training School at the Massachusetts General. In the following years many great American hospitals founded nursing schools, more than a dozen in the seventies, about fifty more in the eighties. The first nurses' training school in a mental hospital was at McLean Hospital, Waverly, Massachusetts (1882). Nurses began to be trained as anesthetists in the first decade of this century — already in the First World War they were useful members of many American base-hospital staffs.

A great part in the development of nursing was played by the Red Cross (q.v.). In 1882 the United States became a member of the International Society and very soon instituted the Red Cross Nursing Service, which is the reserve of the army and the navy nurse corps. Early in the Civil War, Miss Dorothea Dix, who for twenty years had been doing a very important work to improve prisons, poorhouses, and mental hospitals, was appointed Super-intendent of Female Nurses for the army. At that time ward masters and orderlies helped with the nursing in hospitals, while the women nurses dressed wounds, gave medicine, and attended to diets. The value of trained nurses was proved by the Spanish-American War (1898–9), when about 1,500 trained nurses were active and gave valuable help. In the First World War the Army Nurse Corps numbered about 22,000 nurses. Army and Red Cross nurses together amounted to over 23,000, of whom 10,000 served overseas, many in base hospitals in the war zone or even nearer the front. Trained men and women served in these hospitals as also in the auxiliary hospitals, where splendid work was done. Hundreds of nurses from different countries died in the war, a number of them drowned in hospital ships that were torpedoed; nearly three hundred American nurses were among the dead.

In the Second World War the need of nurses everywhere in the world became of foremost importance. We cite the experiences of the army nurses who served in the siege of Bataan in the Philippines. There were 63 nurses for 3,000 patients, with medicines and supplies gradually giving out and constant attacks by the enemy. Some were made prisoners, some were wounded, and many killed. The nurses were unbelievably brave, and their heroism wrote an uncancellable page in the history of the war.

No less important is the part that nurses have begun to take in civil life, their social nursing activity has been an outstanding contribution to social work everywhere. In America public-health nursing was begun in 1877 by the Women's Branch of the New York City Mission, and about the same time in Philadelphia and Boston, extending in the nineties out into the Middle West and West, and before long to the whole nation. In 1942 there were 24,000 public-health nurses enrolled, and this number is continually growing.

An important branch of public-health nursing is the nurses' settlements, which originated in England toward the end of the nineteenth century. The first Nurses' Settlement in America was established in Henry Street, New York, in 1893 by Lillian WALD, a graduate of the New York Hospital, who went with a classmate, Mary BREWSTER, to live and work in the worst tenement districts of the metropolis. Their remarkable work was so efficient that it was generally acknowledged as one of the best in the world.

The public-health program requires that the public-health nurse make all the personal contacts necessary to educate the public in the prevention of disease, in infant welfare, in maternity care, and especially in the fight against tuberculosis, with a continuous supervision of active cases. School nursing has become effective through the co-operation of the nurses to whom the control is confided. In the field of industrial diseases nursing gives opportunity for much teaching in the prevention of accidents and disease. The university schools of nursing are largely an American development. With the opening of the Johns Hopkins Hospital (1884) and its School of Nursing (1889), the educational side of nurses' training was stressed. Beginning with the University of Minnesota in 1909, nursing training was raised to an academic level in a number of Midwestern universities. In 1924 Yale University established a school of nursing which set higher standards than the majority had ever had, with the express aim of preparing teachers and executives, and the school was later accepted as a permanent part of the university. In 1941 and 1942 the U. S. Congress appropriated $5,000,000 for the training of nurses, and the National Nursing Council for War Service was established.

The growth of the nursing profession in the United States during the last fifty years has been extraordinary; and during the war the number of nurses increased even beyond expectation. In 1883 there were in the United States 22 schools of nursing, which graduated a total of 600 nurses; in 1940, 1,300 schools had an enrollment of 80,000 student nurses. More than 400,000 nurses have been graduated in America since nursing training was instituted.

The development of nursing on the continent of Europe has remained more in the hands of the religious orders, the Deaconesses, and the Red Cross societies. Necessarily differing because of the different social customs pertaining to the status of women, and the general attitude toward education of women, it has lagged behind the advances in the Anglo-Saxon countries, though, until World War II started, it was making good progress.

In the south of Europe, which is largely Catholic, the religious sisterhoods were prominent in the development of nursing up to the end of the nineteenth century, while in the northern countries modern nursing was developed according to the English influence. In Italy lay nursing made great progress in the last thirty years. Many schools were organized under the patronage of the Red Cross, and the co-operation of nurses and doctors became close and constant.

Nursing in Soviet Russia had a splendid development after the Revolution. Before that event the lay nurse did not exist; there were only Sisters of Mercy, who were members of religious orders but had no scientific training. Now regular schools of nursing connected with hospitals have been established and two types of nurses are trained in two-year courses: medical nurses and nursery nurses. The nursery was outstanding in the sanitary system of Russia. For this institution's stupendous development, by 1937 there were more than ten million places for children in nurseries. The Soviet nursery has the aim of freeing the time and energy of the working woman, caring for the child, and educating the child as well as the mother. The director of the nursery is generally a woman physician, and the staff consists of doctors, psychologists, and nurses. In their daily contact close co-operation develops between the nursery workers and the mothers. A unique Soviet institution, as described by Sigerist, is the Rooms for Mother and Child in the railroad stations, staffed by a physician, graduate nurses, and technical personnel. Two nurses are stationed outside the Rooms for Mothers. The rooms care for hundreds of children every day; they are looked over by the doctor and washed, and their clothing is disinfected. They get meals, rest, and two rooms in which to play, with many toys and games. The whole service is free of charge. In all factories in the Soviet Union nurses supervise the health conditions of the workers and give them all possible information. Surely the picture of nursing in Russia deserves to be considered as an outstanding example of what nursing may do in modern sanitary welfare.

All over the world more and more are trained nurses required generally, not only to take care of the sick in their homes and in hospitals, but also to be responsible for teaching and administrative duties and for the routine procedures of the laboratory and X-ray departments. The need for less expensive nursing care, and more of it, has at times become so acute in the United States that a new class of less highly trained practical nurses has been developed. During the war, also, thousands of volunteer nurses' aides were of inestimable help in the care of the hospitalized sick.

From the first religious nurses of ancient Christian times up to the modern American or Russian nurse of today a splendid development has taken place. Contemporarily with the rise of women to a high place in the society of today, the work of nurses has covered a broader field, although the fundamental principles that have inspired and stimulated nurses of all times have remained the same. Through a well-organized educational system the nurse has become an indispensable collaborator of the physician, and in peace and war she is indispensable in the progress of practical and of social medicine.

24. Public Health and Social Medicine

Through all time the progress of medicine has been more or less closely linked, as we have tried to show, with cultural and economic conditions. The great change that occurred in this field in the last fifty years — the spreading of culture among large masses of people, the diffusion of knowledge of sanitary problems, and, on the other hand, the urge toward improvement of the conditions of life among the workers and the poorer classes brought about a new current toward social medicine. Medicine appeared no longer as a work of charity, but as a social duty. The problems of the conquest of diseases are facing today not only the scientist and the physician but also the statesman and the economist. The fight against disease today requires the co-operation of all citizens who are interested in the welfare of people, who know that the progressive improvement of public health is not only from a humanitarian, but also from the economic and social point of view a matter of national and international importance.

The history of INTERNATIONAL SANITARY LEGISLATION began with the first sanitary conference, which took place in Paris in 1851, but had very unsatisfactory results because of the endless discussions among the technical delegates. A second conference was called in Paris in 1859, a third in Constantinople in 1866. The Vienna conference of 1874 was of special interest because the German delegates were Pettenkofer and Hirsch, the two greatest epidemiologists of that time. This conference recommended new systems for the control of the spread of epidemics. At the fifth international conference, in Washington in 1881, the United States took part for the first time. This was chiefly a yellow-fever conference. One of the most important scientific discoveries was first made public at this conference by Dr. Carlos Finlay, the delegate of Cuba, who presented his views on the origin and mode of transmission of yellow fever. In the conference of Rome in 1885, Germany was represented by Robert Koch, and the most important problem was the spread of cholera. In 1903 a permanent international committee was appointed, which met for the first time in Paris in 1908, and began to function in 1909.

Two private institutions have been of the greatest importance in the field of international public health: the League of the Red Cross Societies and the Rockefeller Foundation. The League of the Red Cross Societies was constituted with the aim of encouraging and facilitating throughout all time Red Cross action for the relief of suffering humanity. The Rockefeller Foundation, endowed by John D. Rockefeller with one hundred million dollars, has been instrumental in dealing with some of the worst scourges of mankind.

A great part was played by the League of Nations in the modern international control of diseases. Article 23 of the Covenant of the League provided that all states, members of the League, " will endeavor to take steps in matters of international concern for the prevention and control of disease." An international health conference was held at Warsaw in March 1922 under the auspices of the League of Nations, and a provisional health committee was established at Geneva. The health organization of the League began its function in 1923, organizing the Epidemiological Intelligence Service, which has been the basis for every other important international sanitary activity. It became possible to obtain and make available exact information about the state of world health, building up local health services and facilitating the spread of information.

The last international sanitary conference before the war took place in Paris in 1938, in order to make some changes in the convention, which had been generally accepted by more than sixty governments. The utility of an international sanitary organization has been proved so decisively that it is to be expected that the United Nations will fully explore the possibilities of this service.

Compulsory HEALTH INSURANCE for workers has been provided in many countries, and a bewildering number of acts passed to promote mother and child welfare, compulsory notification of venereal and other communicable diseases, and so on. In America public-health expenditures have risen out of all proportion to the increase in the population. The United States government recently allotted ten million dollars for the study and eradication of cancer and large sums for the study of poliomyelitis, and at present it is engaged in a widespread campaign to reduce the ravages of venereal disease. Clinical examinations and laboratory tests for syphilis in those about to be married and in pregnant women are already compulsory in a number of states. The increase in government participation in health matters has been so rapid and so efficient that the question arises whether the basic relationship between the practitioner and the patient, already encroached upon by the factors stated above, will be lost in the transformation. About this special problem we shall take the opportunity of speaking in the section on the Study and Practice of Medicine.

In Great Britain *public health* emphasis shifted from the reforms of the previous century, directed chiefly at the control of infectious diseases, to the general prevention of disease in the individual and the community by the improvement of environmental hygiene and making the people " public-health conscious." Housing and town-planning acts and better laws governing industry were passed with the objectives of eliminating slums and overcrowding, improving ventilation, and reducing the risks in mines and factories. In the schools, the Ministry of Health started medical inspection in 1907; hygiene was taught, and milk and meals provided. The counties and boroughs were responsible for such individual services as maternal and child welfare, and aid to the poor for tuberculosis, cancer, venereal, orthopedic, and mental disorders. The cost is met by the State and the local rates, the Ministry planning, approving, and inspecting. The obligatory National Health Insurance Medical Service (1911) provides medical care by " panel " physicians, who in peacetime amounted to about 17,000, and also makes liberal financial allowance for associated research work. There is considerable diversity of opinion, here as elsewhere, as to the value of such systems. However, a White Paper was issued by the Minister of Health in 1944, based on Assumption B of the Beveridge Report, which promises a still more comprehensive medical service. The recent establishment of chairs of social medicine at the universities of Oxford and Birmingham is a good indication of the thorough way in which this important trend is being met in England. The health of the public has greatly improved: the death-rate in England and Wales, according to A. S. MacNalty, which was about 18 per thousand in 1900, had dropped to 12 per thousand by 1918, and stayed there up to the last war. The chief gain, as elsewhere, has been in tuberculosis (a decline of 49 to 69 per cent in various forms) and in infant mortality (down about 67 per cent).

At the beginning of the nineteenth century about one quarter of all children died before they reached two years of age, and more than one half before the age of ten. In London during the period from 1790 to 1809, 41.3 per cent of all children died before reaching the age of five years. The records of the foundlings' hospitals at that time were terrible. Of 10,272 infants admitted to the Dublin Foundling Hospital during the period 1775–96, only 45 survived, the mortality being 99.6 per cent.

In the United States the public-health program got well under way in the second decade of this century. Its progress has been due essentially, as L. I. Dublin puts it, to the realization of the need for " the remodelling of national life in the light of modern understanding of sanitary science." By means of such factors as increasing scientific knowledge of the subject, propaganda leading to an informed public opinion, and wise sanitary legislation, the advances in the United States have been, as elsewhere, most striking in the control of infectious diseases by extensive pasteurization of milk, elimination of bovine tuberculosis, widespread distribution of smallpox vaccine and diphtheria antitoxin, and similar measures. The steady rise of the standard of living up to the onset of the last war (shorter working hours, better use of leisure time, more nourishing and better-balanced diet, etc.) gave wage-earners, in Dublin's opinion, a living-level in 1935 equal to that of the wealthy in 1911. Industrial hygiene has greatly reduced occupational diseases and accidents, though automobile accidents still remain one of the major causes of death in this country. In the United States violence causes eight to ten per cent of all deaths.

Surgical progress (better diagnosis, earlier surgical intervention, better anesthesia and postoperative care) has been no small factor in the program of public health. Even in the case of cancer, which has increased relatively to other diseases, the known number of "five-year cures" is steadily increasing, and the true incidence of some varieties has actually fallen. Only in the diseases of later life has there been no improvement. The cardio-vasculo-renal diseases (coronary and chronic valvular disease, Bright's disease, hypertension, arteriosclerosis, apoplexy) now account for most deaths of those over forty-five years of age. Diabetes mellitus has also shown a true increase, insulin's help being limited to a longer and better life for the individual. Deaths from typhoid have been reduced to one tenth, from cirrhosis to less than half. Chronic syphilis, with about seven million diagnosed cases, accounts for about the same number of deaths as appendicitis, though both are susceptible to considerable reduction. The sharp reduction in INFANT MORTALITY in the United States began with this century. In New York City the infant death-rate, which was still 383.3 per thousand in 1870, fell to 213.6 in 1900, to 98.8 in 1915, and to 35.0 in 1940, a figure of which the most optimistic pediatrician of twenty years ago would never have dreamed. The great saving of lives of children had more than doubled the average duration of life. The most ancient statistics in the United States were drawn up 1789 by the Reverend Edward Wigglesworth for Massachusetts and New Hampshire. His table gave the expectation of life at birth as 28.15 years, a figure quite equal to that derived from European statistics. In 1855 a Massachusetts life table gave the expectation of life as 39.8 years. By 1901, according to the official life tables of the United States, the expectation of life at birth had risen to 49 years. Today it is over 60 years. It is necessary, however, to stress the fact that the increase in the average duration of life that has been achieved in recent times depends chiefly on the improvement of the mortality statistics for the younger age groups.

The net result of all these influences has been that in the twenty-five-year period 1911–35 in the U.S.A., the average duration of life, according to Dublin's study, has been extended from forty-six to sixty years. In spite of this progress, however, the need for better medical care necessitated by scientific progress and higher costs has led to various adjustments, especially in the past two decades. As long as " good medicine " reduces the cost of illness to society, " an impossible outlay by the individual may become a realizable economy to the nation " (A. M. Butler). Insurance for hospital care (the Blue Cross and similar activities), group practice (which obviates high individual specialist fees) with or without prepayment for service, the various schemes proposed for tax-supported medicine following the National Health Conference, all were significant indications of the trend being taken by American medicine.

In the sanitary legislation of modern times the problem of obligatory *sterilization* of the individual unfit to produce healthy children has attained increasing importance. The problem was emphasized in Germany by the concept of the hygienic defence of the so-called Aryan race contained in the program of the totalitarian regime. Granting the desirability of preventing as far as possible the birth of morons, epileptics, and future criminals, most hygienists recognize that with our present incomplete knowledge of the hereditary transmission of mental qualities and of the inherited combinations that go to make up the criminal, it is impossible to construct legislation to bring about such results without profoundly damaging the rights of the individual and the laws of nature. There are too many cases where individuals of the highest moral and mental capacity have arisen from the most unlikely origin and vice versa. Up to the present time the example of Germany in this field has not been followed by any other European state. The compulsory sterilization of habitual criminals, drunkards, and the insane is now foreseen, however, in some parts of the United States.

We have shown in the preceding chapter that already in the nineteenth century England and France were leading the way toward modern public-health legislation, and first in the protection of mother and child. In recent decades the United States has led in this kind of legislation. The results are shown in the most evident way by the statistics on the morbidity and mortality of infants.

The importance of SCHOOL MEDICAL SERVICE was generally accepted at the beginning of the twentieth century. In England a Royal Commission was appointed in 1902 to consider the importance of physical training of schoolboys. A definite system of inspection was introduced in Great Britain and a great benefit was observed as a result of this system in preventing epidemics and attaining a greater cleanliness, producing a better morale toward school. Defects of hearing and eyesight and also carious teeth were easily discovered. The question of feeding of schoolchildren was attentively examined, and the medical treatment of schoolchildren was legally provided for. Open-air and nursery schools had a great development in England and America, and in the following years a whole system of school hygiene was introduced in America and in many European countries, attaining in this way a definite improvement in the condition of health of the youth.

A consequence of these public-health trends is that the average age of the population in the countries in which the birth-rate is declining is increasing. From the tables of the Department of Health of the City of New York, it appears that the proportion of people over sixty-five years of age has almost doubled since 1900. The aging of the population has a great influence on the frequency of different diseases. Fifty years ago the diseases of youth — pneumonia, tuberculosis, and infantile diarrhœa and enteritis — were the chief causes of death. Today heart diseases and cancer, mainly diseases of old age, head the list. It is clear, however, that we cannot infer from the statistics that heart diseases and cancer are more frequent, in view of the fact that the number of living old people is greater.

The consequences of these factors, from the economic and social point of view, are remarkable. At the beginning of the nineteenth century the great problem of the hygienist was the conquest of the diseases of youth. This problem has been successfully solved, but the new problem is that the number of chronic diseases of old age has increased. There are many of them that do not kill, but disable. For instance, rheumatism, which is by far the most common of all chronic diseases. The number of invalids is increasing continuously and the progress in the therapy of these diseases has been very small. From the economic point of view, society has to face a very difficult problem.

Legislation against TUBERCULOSIS and the campaign to combat the spread of the disease have been widely developed, especially in America, thanks to private beneficence and to the efficient guidance of the state, national, and local anti-tuberculosis associations, aided as in the United States by Christmas seals and by private donations. Much has been done to make the public aware of the curability of this disease, no longer the Great White Plague, and of the importance of early diagnosis and treatment. A better public understanding of the rational treatment of the disease has resulted and efficient institutions for its control have been developed, in the form of research institutes, prophylactic dispensaries and hospitals, and sanitaria for treatment of the established disease. The poor economic and generally disturbed conditions during the World Wars, to be sure, led to a temporary rise in tuberculosis in Europe, but after the first war this was followed by a distinct drop that was only partly to be explained by the preceding elimination of susceptibles and chronic sufferers from the disease. This favourable trend has continued, so that in the United States tuberculosis has fallen from first to seventh in the list of the causes of death (from 224 per hundred thousand to 67 in the past twenty years, according to the figures of the Metropolitan Life Insurance Company).

The mortality-rate for tuberculosis in England in 1780 was 1,120 per 100,000 population; in 1930 the total mortality for all disease was only 1,140 per 100,000. In the United States in 1900 the mortality for all forms of tuberculosis was 201.9 per 100,000, and the proportion of tuberculosis deaths to the total mortality was 12 to 20.8. In 1937 the mortality from all forms of tuberculosis in the United States was only 53.6 per 100,000. In none of the more highly civilized countries, in normal times at least, does tuberculosis rank any longer among the first causes of death. Its eradication in man, as has already been accomplished for cattle in the U.S.A., is largely a matter of the efficient application of known procedures. The improvement of the hygienic conditions of the population, the early detection of cases by school physicians and application of hygienic measures, and the treatment of the sick in sanitaria have brought about general improvement of the condition all over the world, while the application of an intelligent and courageous treatment has saved many thousands of lives. What may happen in the postwar world is one of the great sanitary problems to be faced.

In 1928 there were in the United States 1,060 permanent and 2,555 temporary tuberculosis dispensaries. In 1940 there were over 600 sanitaria, with a total of about 100,000 beds. In a consideration of the frequency of tuberculosis, it is important to note that its apparent frequency was affected by the war. All drafted men were examined by fluoroscopy of the thorax. In this way many millions of men, and a great number of women who most likely would never have been submitted to a thorough examination of the lungs, have been observed and many early symptomless cases detected. The percentage of active tuberculous processes of the lungs was given by Shapiro as 0.87 per cent, by Ehrlich and Edwards as 0.38 per cent on many hundred thousands of cases examined. The mortality-rate of tuberculosis before the war was much lower in the United States than in many European countries (0.44 per cent in 1941). Italy now contains some 400 dispensaries, and the number of hospital beds for the tuberculous rose from about 14,000 in 1925 to 35,000 in 1932. Especially noteworthy is the new Instituto Clinico Carlo Forlanini, of Rome, named after the distinguished advocate of artificial pneumothorax, with 1,300 beds and large budgets for research and' for postgraduate instruction of physicians. The campaign against tuberculosis in nurslings and schoolchildren has resulted in open-air schools and summer colonies in the open air, which have now been adopted by all civilized countries.

The postwar economic distress and paucity of physicians and hospital facilities have already (autumn of 1946) overcome much of this gain in

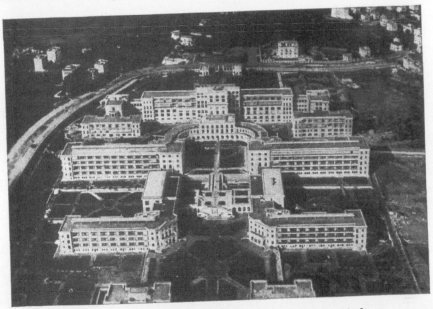

492. The Carlo Forlanini Institute of Rome seen from an airplane.

Europe. In Poland, for instance, the death rate from tuberculosis is said to be at least four times the prewar figures. In a certain medical school, seventeen per cent were suffering from active tuberculosis.

The problem of MALARIA is one of the most important. In the United States it is likely that there are annually 5,000 deaths from it. A new epidemiologic factor of the greatest importance was the problem of malarious troops transferred from tropical areas to the home country. Malarial survey was therefore a most important problem; this coupled with efficient use of the newly discovered anti-malarial drugs appeared to have eliminated this danger.

In Italy the incidence of the disease was reduced from 250,911 in 1924 to 208,557 in 1931; the mortality from 4,036 to 2,781. In the effort toward a better general hygiene, water supplies were improved. Angelo CELLI was the great leader in the fight against malaria. Large areas so unhealthy as to have been uninhabitable have been opened to colonization, and in them malaria has been greatly diminished. It is to be expected, however, that during World War II, and with the large migration of population, conditions have become worse, and it appears from the statistics at our disposal that the inci-

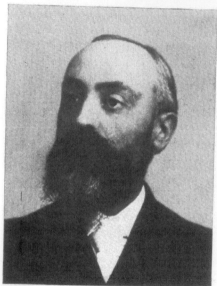

dence of malaria is again much higher. In Russia malaria is the greatest epidemiological problem, with three great centres and millions of cases every year. A systematic campaign was organized to fight the disease, and a Central Institute for Tropical Diseases was created in Moscow in 1920. Malaria stations were built everywhere. A large campaign was organized in 1936, the cases of malaria were reduced by 30 per cent, and deaths by 40 per cent.

Illustrative of postwar sanitary conditions in war-ravaged countries, the following statistical data from Italy, though far from complete, give a clear and desolate picture of the consequences for public health of the great economic destruction and suffering. During the war the general death-rate in Italy in-

493. *Angelo Celli.*

creased from 13.3 per cent in 1939 to 17.8 per cent in 1944; the mortality of infants (that is, of children in the first year of life) from 97 per thousand births in 1937, to 330 in 1945. Malaria, which was reduced to 55,000 cases in 1937, reached 363,547 cases in 1944, and 340,000 in the first six months of 1945. Such an increase can be easily explained by the fact that the system of irrigation was destroyed and the reclaimed Pontine Marshes were again submerged. Typhus fever, which had not appeared in Italy in epidemic form for fifty years, produced a sudden epidemic in Naples, with 5,200 cases and a high mortality-rate. It was probably imported by Italian soldiers returning to the country from Africa. An epidemic of smallpox occurred suddenly in southern Italy and was successfully conquered before grave damage resulted. The most serious problem was presented by the widespread increase in tuberculosis, especially among the people in the concentration camps and the returning soldiers. The average rate for the mortality from tuberculosis was 96 per 100,000 in 1932 and from the latest (1945) reports 320. All such sanitary problems are, of course, closely connected with the deficient food supply, inadequate housing conditions, and lack of medicines. In the typhus epidemic in Naples and in the malaria epidemic in Sardinia the use of DDT had a splendid success and has led the way to further experiments in this field.

Drainage of marshy lands appeared to be the obvious method of control, and in the United States this procedure was highly successful. L. W. Hackett, of the Rockefeller Foundation, in 1931 solved the problem of " anophelism without malaria," showing that in some regions the mosquitoes were concentrated in stables and not in houses and had the habit of biting cattle and not men.

The diffusion of malaria in other countries of the world was combated under the direction of the Ross Institute of Tropical Hygiene in London and the Rockefeller Foundation in New York, with the help of a series of legislative measures. Following the discoveries of Ronald Ross and of Patrick Manson, a combination of research and practical work was accomplished in Malaya, where the control of malaria was carried out by the government; in Singapore, where malaria has been stamped out; in Sumatra, Java, and the Philippine Islands, and later in India, Africa, and China. The knowledge of the modes of infection and the strong application of preventive measures brought about such a great success that it is reasonable to accept that this work has been of great benefit to the world and that it will be possible after the peace to achieve a systematic world-wide control of malaria and prevention of the disease.

The problem of YELLOW FEVER has entered a new phase. Hideyo No-GUCHI (1876–1928), who died of yellow fever while investigating it on the west coast of Africa, because of wrongly diagnosed cases given him for study, had for a time maintained that it was caused by a spirochete. Now, however, it is generally accepted as being due to a filterable virus. Paul A. LEWIS (1879–1929) and Adrian STOKES (1887–1927), a descendant of Sir William, were other martyrs to their investigation of yellow fever, the latter after having found that certain monkeys could be inoculated with the disease as experimental animals. The campaign undertaken by the Rockefeller Foundation attained the eradication of the disease in many countries of Central America; but in 1929 epidemics in the jungles of Colombia and Venezuela at points unrelated to any known centres of the disease proved that the conquest of yellow fever was still far from being achieved.

It has to be admitted that yellow-fever infection extends over vast regions of Africa and that monkeys or other wild animals are carriers of the disease. Only a permanent defence of the great centres of population can bring about a victorious progress in this fight. It is now recognized that several species of mosquito can transmit the disease and that they may be carried long distances by airplane. In this way a West African mosquito became established in Brazil, and a sizable epidemic resulted. It was only after strenuous and costly effort that the disease and the mosquito were eradicated; but the demonstration that eradication was possible more than repaid the effort.

BUBONIC PLAGUE assumed serious epidemic proportions in Hong Kong in 1894, and more than six million people perished from it in India in the next ten years. The problem was analysed by a plague commission appointed by the government of India, and the part that the infection of wild rodents played in the diffusion of the plague became evident. In the United States plague was introduced in San Francisco in 1900, and by 1940 rodent epidemics were occurring in California and in other states. The disease is still spreading among ground squirrels, in which it is now endemic and apparently not possible to be eliminated. Modern sanitary control has prevented it, however, from reaching epidemic proportions in man, though occasional cases are still found, as in San Francisco in 1907 and in New Orleans and Beaumont, Texas, in 1920. Rat surveys can efficiently establish the amount of plague in the rat population, which can be reduced by various measures and habitations protected by rat-proof devices.

The importance that rats or other rodents have as animal reservoirs of infectious diseases has been proved by the diffusion of RICKETTSIA and allied forms of this disease. It appears from recent studies that the Rickettsia group of organisms are widespread parasites of many insects. Zinsser proposed the hypothesis of the flea-rat cycle of infection. The fight against these diseases will be necessarily a fight against mosquitoes, rats, and lice, and only through a very strong control and a large measure of defence will it be possible to eliminate the dangers of this widespread infection. Modern sanitary control has prevented the diseases, however, from reaching epidemic proportions.

INFLUENZA has continued its periodic visitations in epidemic form through the period covered in this chapter, reaching pandemic proportions at the close of the First World War. It is estimated that in the United States alone it caused more than 500,000 deaths. It has also been noted that with each increase in speed of transportation, which now includes air travel, rapidity of the spread of an epidemic has correspondingly increased. The huge movement of the world population in the last few decades has also contributed to serious outbreaks of the disease in different parts of Europe. The ability to identify the causative virus, and some progress toward producing a potent vaccine for at least one of the known strains, lends ground for hope of better control of future epidemics. No serious outbreaks occurred in the last war.

In the fight against DIPHTHERIA the statistics of New York, where immunization with toxoid is compulsory before the admission of children to schools, are very important. In the decade 1910–19 there were 14,282 cases of diphtheria, with 1,290 deaths, as an annual average. In 1942 there were 413 cases, with seven deaths, in a population of seven and a half million.

The EPIDEMICS of infectious diseases have been of less importance in modern than in ancient times. *Smallpox*, for which vaccination has been known to be an efficient preventive for more than a century, continues to claim its victims among the ignorant and opinionated. In 1920 there were 4,486 cases reported in California, of which 92 per cent had never been vaccinated. *Typhus fever* has largely disappeared with the improved sanitation of the latter part of the nineteenth century. During World War I, with the prevalence of " cooties " imposed by the conditions of trench life, it made its reappearance under various names, such as " Volhynian fever " (H. WERNER, 1916) to recede again after the establishment of normal peace conditions. After World War II, due to better sanitary conditions and effective use of DDT, it became " virtually unknown " (E. L. Stebbins). The lessened severity of *scarlet fever* in recent times — a phenomenon that surely would have interested Sydenham — is something to be thankful for, though not explained.

Prophylaxis during pregnancy has reached in recent times a high degree, especially for the diet concerning the alimentation. Success has been achieved with the use of vitamin K during the last weeks of pregnancy through its action on the formation of prothrombin. Also very important was the discovery of the Rh factors (identified first by Landsteiner and Wiener) which are found in 86 per cent of the population of the United States. This Mendelian factor is transmitted to the fetus and is capable of determining an immune reaction so that with a positive Rh factor in the fetus and a negative mother the possibility of fetal erythroblastosis is established.

The campaign against MALIGNANT TUMOURS is in active progress in all the leading countries of the world. The increasing frequency of cancer has naturally led to an intensification, in both private and governmental hands, of investigative and clinical activities leading toward the conquest of this evil. In spite of considerable study of the point, it is by no means clear how much of the increase is merely apparent, due to the increased awareness of the profession and better means of diagnosis, and how much is an actual increase due to changed environmental factors. The remarkable rise in the recognized cases of primary cancer of the lung is one of the most striking features of modern cancer study, yet this also is thought by some to be due to the fact that " what one knows, one sees," but by others in chief measure to changes in the living-conditions of modern civilization. Special institutes and hospitals for the study of cancer have been founded in various countries, and are steadily contributing to diagnostic and therapeutic efficiency as well as producing valuable studies of the cause and pathogenesis of cancer in its various forms. Such are the Institute for Cancer Research at Dahlem, Germany, the Radium Institute of Paris, the Imperial Cancer Research Fund, the Radium Institute, and the London Free Cancer Hospital in London, the Crocker Institute and the Memorial Hospital in New York City, and the New York State Institute for Malignant Diseases at Buffalo. In addition, many well-equipped special departments of schools and hospitals devote themselves to cancer research, such as the Cancer Research Laboratories of the Middlesex Hospital, London, and the Yale Laboratories for the Study of Abnormal Growth. In Italy, the best-known are the institutes at Rome and Milan and the hospital centre in Turin.

Education of the laity for better control of cancer is an activity of the present century, apparently having been started early in the century by Georg WINTER, a gynæcologist of Königsberg. In the United States, the need having been realized by gynæcologists about 1905, the American Society for the Control of Cancer was founded (1913) on the recommendation of Dr. F. L. Hoffman, with the education of the public as one of its ten avowed aims. By such means cancer has been robbed of much of its mysterious terror, so that not only have earlier consultation, diagnosis, and treatment steadily increased the number of surgical cures, but also greater financial support and special institutes and journals for cancer research have been forthcoming. The great Cancer Institute of the U. S. Public Health Service, with its huge staff of physicians, chemists, and other Ph.D.'s, is a good example.

Though an adequate solution of the cancer problem must necessarily await more complete knowledge of its causes and how they act on the body cell, already good progress has been made in educating the profession and the public, with a gratifying, if not satisfying, increase in the number of surgically eradicated cases. There is little excuse today for the fatal outcome of " surface " cancers.

With changed dietetic habits and better recognition of the potential harm of alcoholic beverages, the mortality from chronic ALCOHOLISM has diminished in most civilized countries. The campaign against alcoholism has led to prohibition in some countries and to a none too fortunate temporary experiment in America. In European countries the mortality from alcoholism has declined considerably since World War I, and more sharply than has the general mortality-rate. In the United States, though the death-rate from alcohol is lower than in 1920, when national prohibition was started, the fall has been less marked than in European countries: in the

United States it has declined from about 6 per hundred thousand in 1900 to about 4 in 1930; in England from 11 to 0.2, and below 1 per hundred thousand since 1917. Norway has never exceeded 0.7 deaths per hundred thousand from this cause in this century (Dublin). The adverse social effects of alcoholism are of even greater importance than its effect on morbidity and mortality. Sir Arthur Newsholme states (1929) that " something like one fifth of the entire earnings of the wage-earners in Britain is still spent in alcoholic drinks," with a consequent deprivation of proper food and the necessities of life in many thousands of families and addition to the population of prisons. According to the Home Secretary (1925), " one fifth of the men who went to prison and one half of the women went for drunkenness." The magnitude of the problem of acute alcoholism is indicated by the fact that, according to the U. S. Bureau of the Census, in 1940 there were 11,987 first admissions to hospitals for mental disease of persons suffering from alcoholic psychosis or from alcoholism.

It has been stated that highly concentrated alcoholic drinks, providing a quick and cheap means of escaping distressing realities constitute the greatest danger. Reformed alcoholics appear to be best capable of helping sufferers from this disease, as may be seen in the success of such organizations as Alcoholics Anonymous, Inc.

The part that lack of education and poor living-conditions play as causes of drinking habits is evident from the example of Russia. In 1913 the consumption of vodka amounted to 8.1 litres (i.e., about two gallons) per person a year, and the average worker spent over a quarter of his wages on liquor. After the Revolution the consumption of alcoholic drinks dropped steadily. It was 4.5 litres in 1931, and 3.7 in 1935. These observations and a great number of studies in this field proved that the fight against inebriety has to be fought chiefly with the improvement of education. State action in regard to inebriety has been strengthened in a series of laws in all countries of the world. The attempt was made in 1920 to control the manufacture and sale of intoxicating liquors for beverage purposes in the United States under the Eighteenth Amendment to the Constitution, but the majority of the people being against such drastic control, after flagrant and increasing evasion the amendment was repealed in 1933.

The sale of habit-forming drugs and especially of morphine, heroin, cocaine, and marihuana has been controlled by national and international legislation. The illegal traffic in such drugs was important among the causes of the First World War in the Far East.

With the greater complexities of modern life and the increased tension of living-conditions, especially in cities, it is not surprising that there should be a considerable increase in MENTAL DISEASES, a topic already considered in the section on Neurology and Psychiatry. In the United States, for instance, where this increase has attracted the most attention, the number of mental cases in public and private hospitals is said to have risen from 83 per hundred thousand of the population in 1904, to 245 in 1923; in New York State, in institutions surveyed between 1909 and 1935, from 65 to 86 per hundred thousand. When such modifying factors as the better and earlier recognition of mental disease and more adequate institutional facilities are discounted, however, such figures need not be taken as indicating an alarming increase. The great majority of cases are due to six conditions: dementia præcox, manic-depressive insanity, alcoholism, paresis, arteriosclerotic psychosis, and senile dementia. Fortunately, the first four of these are already showing promising responses to recently introduced forms of treatment.

Rapid progress in mental hygiene in the United States was stimulated by a truly remarkable book by a business man, Clifford BEERS, of New Haven, Connecticut: *A Mind That Found Itself*. Beers had suffered a mental breakdown in 1900 and spent three years in three different mental hospitals subjected to callous treatment and countless needless humiliations. Having conceived a plan to form a world-wide movement for the reform of asylums for the insane, toward the end of his stay as a patient in a mental hospital he told his story and set down his observations in a book, which met profound approval by psychiatrists and in the press. Dr. Adolph MEYER, then director of the New York State Psychiatric Institute, the leading psychiatrist of America, suggested using the term, Mental Hygiene, which had first appeared as the title of a book (1843) by Dr. William SWEETSER (1797–1875). A nation-wide movement was launched: the Connecticut Society for Mental Hygiene was founded in May 1908, to be followed in 1909 by the National Committee for Mental Hygiene, and in 1917 by the journal *Mental Hygiene*. In 1930 the first International Congress was held in Washington, D.C. — at which time an International Committee was organized — and a second congress was held in Paris in 1937. In 1915 Dr. Thomas W. SALMON was made medical director of the National Committee, which gave a great impulse to the mental-hygiene movement and brought about a close collaboration between psychiatry and social work. Mental-hygiene clinics were established in connection with children's courts and institutions for juvenile delinquents. Mental hygiene as a morale factor in civilian and military life is receiving increasing public recognition.

The child-guidance movement received its early impetus from the psychologic clinic opened by Lightner WITMER at the University of Pennsylvania (1897) to treat retarded children. The first child-guidance clinic organized to meet the problem of juvenile delinquency was Dr. William HEALY's Chicago Juvenile Psychopathic Institute, which collaborated closely with the Juvenile

Court. Similar clinics soon appeared in various cities, with various emphases. The first to be specifically designated Child Guidance Clinic was established (1922) by the Mental Hygiene, with the aid of the Commonwealth Fund, which shortly after (1927) founded the *Institute for Child Guidance* in New York.

The campaign against VENEREAL DISEASE has been active in many countries. The rapid spread of venereal diseases in Russia after the First World War shows with what rapidity it can assume alarming proportions when released from the restraining influence of public opinion and morality, and from adequate economic and sanitary controls.

The problem was attacked by the Soviet Union in a rational way with a strong fight against prostitution and with the creation (1925) of a new type of institution, the prophylactorium which admits women suffering from venereal diseases. The results have been good so far and the control of the infected appears to be firmly established. In Italy, the prophylaxis of venereal disease, begun by Cavour in 1860, but subsequently amplified by various laws, especially the new regulations of 1923, has been successful in controlling gonorrhœa, syphilis, and other diseases of venereal origin. Dispensaries for the prophylaxis and free treatment of venereal disease have been established and visiting physicians and provincial inspectors employed by the State. As a result, the number of venereal patients has decreased rapidly: the incidence of soft chancre has declined from 90 to 95 per cent, and recent syphilis in various areas has diminished as much as 70 per cent. In the United States the syphilis mortality has shown a steady reduction, from 14.1 per hundred thousand in 1919 to 10.1 in 1935 (Dublin). The campaign initiated by Surgeon General Thomas PARRAN, of the United States Public Health Service, both in the education of the public and in the better diagnosis and treatment of existing cases, bids fair to reduce these figures considerably further.

The progress in sanitary legislation had been successful in improving the conditions of normal life before World War II. The hygiene of FOOD SUPPLIES, begun by such students as Pettenkofer, Voit, Rubner, and Lusk, has led to numerous laws controlling the production and transportation of food, especially milk, to veterinary legislation, involving the slaughter of infected cows, and to governmental inspection of the meat supply. In the United States the governmental use of tuberculin tests, requiring the slaughter of positively reacting animals, has reduced the percentage of infected cattle to insignificant proportions throughout the country. As a result, the bovine form of tuberculosis in man has practically disappeared.

Great research centres like the Pasteur and Lister institutes are the Rockefeller Institute (founded in 1901), the Brussels School of Tropical Medicine

(1906), and one of the latest, the Lester Institute at Shanghai. The Rockefeller Foundation, munificently established (1913) to promote the welfare of mankind, has expended hundreds of millions of dollars throughout the world to discover and eradicate preventable disease and to promote medical and public-health education.

Of similar importance was the development of medical studies in South America. We cannot enumerate all the names of these eminent Latin contributors to modern medicine; we note only the progress that has been made in the fields of hygiene, of university instruction, and of scientific research in recent decades. Outstanding were the two great Brazilian scientists Oswaldo CRUZ (1872–1917), Director of Public Health at Rio de Janeiro and reformer of the Brazilian sanitary service, and Carlos CHAGAS, the discoverer of the *Trypanosoma Cruzi*. From the Cruz Institute, founded in 1908, have issued numerous studies that throw new light on many problems of public health. The Butantan Institute at São Paulo (founded 1899), has been an important centre for the study of snake venoms and the production of anti-venom sera. In Buenos Aires leading hygienists were Carlos MALBRAN, first Professor of Bacteriology there, and his successor, José PENNA, founder of a chair of epidemiology and head of the bacteriological institute, and, in physiology, B. A. HOUSSAY, till recently director of the Physiological Institute. Other South American capitals have seen the development of good scientific medicine and sanitation in recent years.

Finally, we want to refer to an important problem connected with public health: that is, the increasing mortality produced by ACCIDENTS. Safety Council reports emphasize that a continuous campaign must be waged to bring down the figure of 94,000 persons killed, 9,750,000 injured, and a monetary loss through accidents of about $5,000,000 in a single year in this country. The motor-vehicle death toll of 23,800 in 1944, almost identical with that of the year before, represented a decline of about 40 per cent from the high figure of 1941, when nearly 40,000 persons were killed in traffic accidents. It must be noted, however, that during the latter part of the war period driving had been reduced at least 50 per cent.

It is not without interest to consider in this brief résumé of the progress of hygiene and social medicine how their essential lines are indicated in the pages of the Greek and Roman classics. The State is the supreme defender of the public and individual health; it, then, is responsible for the initiative through the agency of its medical functionaries: in the schools, the centres of physical education, considered as an essential factor in the well-being of the individual and of the nation; in public works, such as the water supplies, sewerage systems, supervision of food supplies, and so on. The hygiene of today has developed greatly within these basic lines because it is founded on the sanitary consciousness of the population, with its thorough belief in the efficiency of modern public-health methods. This faith in the validity of scientific systems and in the utility of hygienic measures, this sense of security in the work of the physician, which continues to penetrate further into localities distant from cultural centres, and which is creating a new individual and social life in our time, is the factor to which in the last analysis must be attributed the practical successes that have been obtained. Today an even greater diffusion of this sense of public health is the goal of the hygienist and legislatures engaged in the campaigns against infectious diseases, tuberculosis, and venereal disease, alcoholism, crime, cancer, and the so-called degenerative diseases of older life, such as chronic heart and kidney disease, all regarded as preventable social plagues.

25. *History of Medicine*

During the period of scientific reaction against mysticism and romanticism in the early nineteenth century, when materialism and positivism were dominant, the pursuit of the history of medicine was largely forgotten; the universities neglected the subject and only a few devotees continued its study. One might have thought that the new revolutionary medicine had nothing to learn from the past. But toward the close of the past century and at the beginning of the twentieth, when the need was felt for searching in the past for the story of medical thought through the centuries, medical men again returned to the study of the history of medicine.

It was a period when the European governments were adjusting themselves after exhausting wars and when the growing spirit of nationalism felt the need for establishing the historical importance of each country. At the same time the general diffusion of culture, the rapid increase in the number of medical publications, the enthusiasm for the subject of history, and the discovery of much invaluable material illuminating distant civilizations, all contributed to instil in medical scholars and students a renewed zeal for medico-historical studies. It is about this time that medical history societies were formed, the first medical history journals began to appear with regularity, imposing historical monographs were written, and the history of medicine resumed an honourable position in the universities. Medico-historical investigations multiplied; they extended to all historical periods and all branches of medicine. The great figures of the medicine of the past were redrawn in the light of modern historical criticism, which often disclosed the origins of apparently new original ideas in the works of forgotten scholars. At the same time the enthusiasm for collections of works of art expanded, recalling the time of the Renaissance, and the relations between art and medicine were again explored. This graphic documentation, this resurrection of ancient manuscripts and forgotten incunabula, formed the basis and the material for new, productive investigations. The iconography of the sick and injured and of epidemics, which begins with the earliest sculptures, drawings, and paintings and continues up to the more complete representation of modern moving pictures, has thrown new light on the history of disease. Finally, the exploration of new regions reveal in primitive medicine of isolated groups interesting analogies with the medicine of our ancestors. All these factors have contributed to a rapid growth in the study of the history of medicine, which has thus been removed from the isolation in which it existed a few generations ago as a study reserved to a small number of specialists or philologists. It is important to note the great contribution that physicians engaged in the active practice of their art have brought to modern studies. Some of the best-known historians of medicine are equally well known for their research or professional work in this or that specialty; a confirmation of the truth of the observation that to have an adequate grasp of medical history, which is both a science and an art, it is desirable to join a practical knowledge of medicine to historical studies.

In the following pages we shall attempt to cite some of the best-known students, writers, and teachers of the history of medicine and their more important achievements.

Throughout the past century and well into the first decades of the present the subject has been assiduously pursued in the GERMAN-SPEAKING COUNTRIES. Among the best-known German works on the subject in this period was that of J. H. BAAS (1838–1909) entitled *Grundriss der Geschichte der Medizin und des heilenden Standes* (Stuttgart, 1876; translated by H. E. Handerson, New York, 1889), which was followed by his *History of the Development of the Medical Profession and of the Medical Sciences* (1896). Theodor PUSCHMANN (1844–99), Professor of the History of Medicine at Vienna, planned the edition of a detailed three-volume *Handbuch der Geschichte der Medizin* (Jena, 1902), completed by Neuburger and Pagel, a work that still remains one of the fundamental authorities in this field. Puschmann also wrote a valuable *Geschichte des medizinischen Unterrichts* (Leipzig, 1889), which, however, necessarily does not include the important developments of recent times. His successor in the Vienna chair, Max NEUBURGER (b. 1868), has been a prolific writer on a wide range of historical subjects; his excellent *Geschichte der Medizin* (Stuttgart, 1906–11), carries the subject from the earliest times through the Middle Ages. It has been translated by Ernest Playfair (London, 1910–25). Undoubtedly one of the most interesting and thoughtful of modern textbooks of medical history, written with clear vision and an extensive knowledge of source material, Neuburger's work emphasizes especially the philosophic aspects of medical thought. Neuburger, formerly Professor Ordinarius at Vienna and now working at the Wellcome Museum in London, was the founder of the Vienna Institute of Medical History, which included an exemplary museum. A readable but none too accurate *Einführung in die Geschichte der Medizin* was published by J. L. PAGEL (1851–1912) in 1898; it was revised and improved by Sudhoff in 1915 and again in 1922. Karl SUDHOFF (1853–1938) was one of the greatest of modern

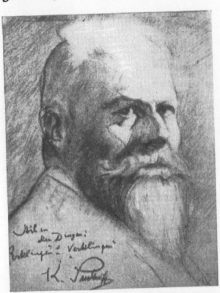 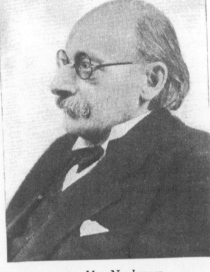

494. *Karl Sudhoff.*   495. *Max Neuburger.*

medical historians, who, after a long career as a general practitioner, devoted himself to the full-time study of medical history as the first director (1905) of the institute founded with a legacy by Puschmann at the University of Leipzig. Sudhoff was the founder (1908) of the *Archiv für die Geschichte der Medizin*, often known as Sudhoff's *Archiv*, and of the *Mitteilungen zur Geschichte der Medizin*, and was the editor of the *Arbeiten* of the institute and of *Klassiker der Medizin*. His individual contributions consisted of more than 500 monographs and articles and some 2,000 separate reviews and notes on medico-historical topics. His studies on Paracelsus extended over many years, eventually resulting in a magnificent edition of his medical works (1933). He contributed many new facts to the study of the origin of syphilis, strongly opposing the American origin of the sixteenth-century epidemic in Europe. His studies on the early literature of plague, the school of Salerno, and mediæval medicine are important contributions to these subjects. His institute was later under the directorship of W. von BRUNN, earlier professor at Rostock and author of a number of historical studies, notably a *Geschichte der Chirurgie* (Berlin, 1928). Among German histories of medicine should be noted the attractive lectures (3rd ed., 1930) of Ernst SCHWALBE, pathologist at Rostock; also the magnificent and exhaustive history of surgery from the earliest times up to the end of the Renaissance (3 vols., 1898) by E. J. GURLT (1825–99). Among the most recent German histories of medicine should be mentioned the useful five small volumes of the Göschen Collection by Paul DIEPGEN (b. 1878), Professor of the History of Medicine and director of the Institute at Berlin. G. HONIGMANN (1863–1930) was the author of a philosophical history of the evolution of medicine (1925); Richard KOCH (b. 1882), of Frankfurt, has also contributed a number of essays on the philosophic aspects of medical history. Among the histories of special subjects, J. HIRSCHBERG has contributed an exhaustive *Geschichte der Augenheilkunde* (9 vols., Leipzig, 1899–1918), and Max MEYERHOF (1874–1945), the most authoritative scholar on the subject, many excellent studies on Arabian medicine. Similar valuable histories by German writers on most of the specialties can be found listed in Section C of the general bibliography at the end of this volume.

Among biographical works, special mention should be given to E. GURLT's excellent *Biographisches Lexikon* (6 vols., Leipzig, 1884–8) in collaboration with A. HIRSCH. A completely revised second edition was accurately prepared (1929–34) by W. HABERLING. A continuation of this work with the biographies of prominent physicians up to recent times was published (2 vols., 1933) by I. FISCHER (1869–1943) of Vienna, who devoted a great deal of valuable work to the history of medicine and especially to obstetrics and gynæcology.

In ITALY toward the end of the last century the almost forgotten study of medical history returned to a place of honour. D. BARDUZZI (1847–1929), Professor of Dermatology at Siena, was one of the founders of the Società Italiana di Storia della Medicina and director of the *Rivista Italiana* on this subject. V. PENSUTI (1859–1925) taught the subject at Rome; C. FEDELI (1851–1927) concentrated on the history of surgical teaching; A. FAVARO (1847–1922) wrote many remarkable studies on Galileo and edited his complete works. D. GIORDANO, sometime president of the Italian Society and of the International Association, an excellent surgeon, has contributed notable brilliant studies on a variety of subjects, chiefly on the history of Italian surgery, collected in his *Scritti e discorsi*. Andrea CORSINI, a prominent hygienist, founded the historical museum of science in Florence, has contributed to a number of subjects, especially to the study of Tuscan Renaissance medicine, and has been for many years the editor of the *Rivista*. To Aldo MIELI, editor of *Archeion, Archivio di storia della scienza*, professor at Rome and later at the University of Santa Fé, Argentina, is owed a valuable bibliographical work on the history of science, a series of studies entitled *Scienziati Italiani*, and on history of chemistry (1923). He has more recently collaborated with Brunet on a *Histoire des sciences* (Vol. I, Paris, 1935) and is the permanent secretary of the International Academy of the

History of Science. To G. BILANCIONI (1881–1935) is owed a number of carefully documented monographs, especially on the history of otolaryngology. G. CARBONELLI (1859–1933) was the founder of a historical medical museum located in the ancient Hospital of Santo Spirito in Rome and has published some important mediæval texts. P. CAPPARONI was Professor of the History of Medicine at Bologna and wrote, *inter alia*, a valuable study on *Magistri Salernitani nondum cogniti* (London, 1925), and has edited the *Atti e memorie della Accademia di storia della medicina* (Rome). A. FERRANNINI and L. CASTALDI are other recent writers who have shed much light on early Italian contributions to medicine. Knowledge of the special disciplines has been advanced by such writers as G. Favaro, A. Monti, A. Valenti (anatomy); G. Martinotti (pathology); S.Baglioni, V.Ducceschi, G.B.Grassi (physiology); and V.Guerini (dentistry). F. La Torre has contributed a well-documented volume on *L'Utero attraverso i secoli* (Città di Castello, 1917); A. Pazzini has written on Italian folklore and the healing saints (Rome, 1939). Among clinicians who have contributed to medical history are G. Baccelli and A. Celli (malaria); L. Devoto and A. Maggiora (Ramazzini); V. Putti (history of prosthesis, ancient Italian surgery, and an excellent biography of Berengario). Other valuable contributors are: R. Ciasca (the guild of physicians and pharmacists, Florence, 1927); R. Messedaglia (Morgagni, Cotugno); A. L. Gualino (medicine at the court of the popes); F. Pellegrini (military medicine); M. Vallauri (Indian medicine); E. Morpurgo (epidemics, treatment of the insane); M. Cardini (Greek and Roman medicine, Malpighi); Viviani (Cesalpino); R. Simonini (pediatrics); Vedrani (psychiatry); G. Tanfani (the Paduan medical school); B. Pincherle (pediatrics, biography of Corti); and A. GAROSI (history of hygiene). Many of these special studies have been cited in the bibliographies of this history.

In FRANCE the history of medicine has had enthusiastic followers who have contributed to the subject in various important ways. Even such an outstanding clinician as M. Charcot found time to write on the *Iconographie de la Salpêtrière* (1876–80). L. MEUNIER's compact *Histoire de la médecine* (Paris, 1911) offers entertaining and valuable information, especially on the French clinics. E. JEANSELME (1858–1935), the eminent dermatologist, and P. E. MENÉTRIER (1859–1935), Professor of Pathology at Paris, were two leading writers on such subjects as Byzantine and Greco-Roman medicine, leprosy, syphilis, and mediæval epidemics. Among the modern French contributors we note CORLIEU's and LEGRAND's studies on the Paris Faculty (1896–1911); C. A. E. WICKERSHEIMER's *History of French Medicine in the Renaissance* (Paris, 1906) and his *Biographical Dictionary of French Mediæval Physicians* (2 vols., Paris, 1936); P. DELAUNAY's *Physicians and Medicines of the Eighteenth Century*, and a series of publications on mediæval French medicine; J. LÉVY-VALENSI's work on French medicine in the seventeenth century; and the numerous contributions of LAIGNEL-LAVASTINE, professor at Paris and one of the mainstays of the International Association of the History of Medicine, and editor of a voluminous and magnificently illustrated *Histoire de la médecine*, of which the first two volumes have been published. We note also such names as A. CABANÈS (1862–1928), who wrote a score of entertaining volumes on various curiosities of medicine; J. VIN-CHON, writer on pathology in history and art, a subject also studied by BORD, editor of *Æsculape;* BRUNON, the creator of the medical-history museum at Rouen; M. GENTY, librarian of the Académie de Médecine, editor of a series of *Biographies médicales* (Lyon, 1934–8), and author of important articles. An excellent *Histoire de la chirurgie française, 1790–1920* has been written by de FOURMESTRAUX. P. GUIART, Professor of the History of Medicine at Lyon, formerly taught the subject at Cluj in Rumania (1921–30), where he founded a medical-history museum. He has especially concerned himself with the medicine of ancient Egypt. The Société Française d'Histoire de la Médecine publishes an excellent bulletin, which provides an outlet for the activities of French medical historians.

The history of medicine is being actively cultivated in ENGLAND, many of the shorter articles appearing in the *Proceedings of the Section of Medical History* of the Royal Society of Medicine. Among modern writers on the subject, J. F. PAYNE (1840–1910) contributed an interesting study of Anglo-Saxon medicine. Sir Norman MOORE (1847–1922), a leader among British students of the history of medicine, wrote *The History of the Study of Medicine in the British Isles* (Oxford, 1908), a *Short History of St. Bartholomew's Hospital* (London, 1923), and a number of shorter articles. Sir William Osler, whose interest in medical history was manifested even in his ward teaching, was the author of a number of brilliant biographical and topical essays and addresses collected in his *Æquanimitas* (1905, 1910), *An Alabama Student* (1909), and many smaller articles. Sir D'Arcy POWER (1855–1941) wrote a number of interesting articles, a longer *History of Surgery, Chronologia Medica* (1923), and *The Foundations of Medical History* (Baltimore, 1931). To T. Clifford Allbutt (1836–1925), an eminent cardiologist, is due an excellent study on *Greek Medicine in Rome*. A leader in studies on the history of medicine and science in England is Charles SINGER (b. 1876), formerly Professor of the History of Medicine at Oxford, who also taught the history of the biological sciences at University College, London. In addition to numerous scholarly shorter articles, he has written a *Short History of Medicine* (1925), and *The Story of Living Things* (1931). He is the author of various studies, such as *Early English Magic and Medicine* (1920), *Greek Biology and Greek Medicine* (1922), *The Discovery of the Circulation of the Blood* (1922), and *Evolution of Anatomy* (1925), to some of which Mrs. Dorothy Singer, also an excellent medical historian, has collaborated. His two volumes of essays, *Studies in the History and Method of Science* (1921), have become rarities for bibliophiles. Among other contributors to the subject are E. T. WITHINGTON (*Medical History from the Earliest Times*), Sir St. Clair THOMSON, H. R. SPENCER, Sir Humphry ROLLESTON and his brother, J. D. ROLLESTON, Clifford DOBELL (*Leeuwenhoek and his " Little Animals "*); J. B. HURRY

(*Imhotep*); G. Elliot SMITH and W. R. DAWSON (*Egyptian Mummies; Egyptian and Assyrian Medicine*); and J. D. COMRIE (1875–1939), of Edinburgh (*The History of Scottish Medicine*, 2 vols., 1932). Douglas Guthrie, of Edinburgh, has recently written an attractive short *History of Medicine* (London, 1945).

The history of SPANISH medicine was fully covered by A. H. MOREJON (1773–1836) in his *Historia bibliografica de la medicina española* (7 vols., 1842–52). An excellent book on the same subject has been written by Eduardo GARCIA DEL REAL (1921), also author of a *Historia de la medicina contemporanea* (1935). To the school of Garcia del Real, professor at the University of Madrid, we owe a series of volumes containing essays and studies by his pupils. Among other Spanish historians should be mentioned Comenge, Oldmedella, and Cepero.

PORTUGUESE medicine has been recorded by M. LEMOS (the medical faculty of Oporto); MONTEIRO, Leite DE VASCONCELLOS (Portuguese medicine, 1925), R. JORGE (mediæval epidemics), L. DE PINA (Portuguese medicine), and A. da Silva CARVALHO, president of the Lisbon Society of the History of Medicine and author of a history of the Lisbon school of surgery and of a volume on Garcia d'Orta.

DUTCH medicine can boast of a number of students of medical history. Following such early writers as Jelle Banga (1786–1877), we note the names of H. F. A. PEYPERS (1855–1904), founder of the rejuvenated *Janus*, and of NIEUWENHUIS of Leiden, its present director. Other eminent students of the discipline are E. C. van LEERSUM (on Yperman); E. W. G. PERGENS (1862–1917) (ophthalmology); J. G. DE LINT (1867–1936) (*Rembrandt; Atlas of the History of Anatomy*, New York, 1926); M. A. VAN ANDEL; F. C. UNGER; B. W. T. NUYENS; J. B. F. VAN GILS.

In HUNGARY the most active historiographers were T. VON GYÖRY (1869–1937) (Morbus Hungaricus; Semmelweis) and I. von BOKAI (1858–1937) (pediatrics). The RUMANIAN Society of Medical History has been active under the directorship of V. GOMOIU, last president of the International Association. Medical history in POLAND has been concentrated in a medical history society presided over by W. SZUMOWSKI, professor at Cracow and publisher of a medico-historical journal. Active contributors to the subject were A. WRZOSEK (Poznán), and L. ZEMBRUSKI (Warsaw). Prominent in historical studies in YUGOSLAVIA has been Professor L. THALLER of Zagreb, president of the 11th Congress of the International Association. A leader in BELGIUM is J. TRICOT-ROYER, of Antwerp, the founder and honorary president of the International Association. His historical studies cover a wide range, but have been especially concentrated on leprosy. Other Belgian writers are VAN SCHEVENSTEEN, DENEFFE, and DE METS. Among the DANES outstanding are J. J. PETERSEN, J. W. S. JOHNSSON (1869–1929), and MAAR, who has contributed a number of important studies on Danish medicine. NORWAY has contributed a monumental production of the anatomical illustrations of Leonardo da Vinci by FONAHN, VANGEN-

STEN, and HOPSTOCK. The history of GREEK medicine has been especially studied by Adamanios KORES (*Corpus Hippocraticum*), KOUSIS, and KABBADIAS. In TURKEY a school of medical history has been founded and directed by A. SÜHEYL, who has published valuable studies on Turkish medicine and is teaching history of medicine at the University of Istanbul.

Interest in medical history in the UNITED STATES has been steadily rising in the past generation, after having passed through a lull similar to that experienced in other countries. A great impetus to the subject was given by the *Introduction to the History of Medicine* (1914) by Fielding H. GARRISON (1870–1935). This

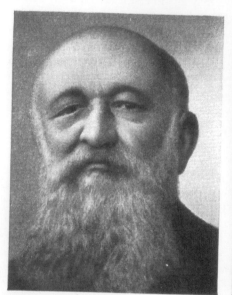

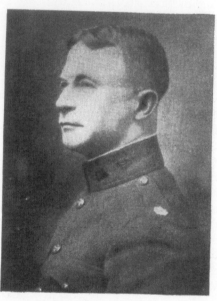

496. *Davide Giordano.*　　　　　497. *Fielding H. Garrison.*

excellent volume, which reached its fourth edition in 1929, presents a discriminating survey of the whole history of medicine, which is especially useful for its full treatment of the modern period and of Anglo-American medicine. It is written with an impartiality and a richness of detail that reveal extensive knowledge of the subject, and a freshness of style that is none too common in medico-historical writings. Paragraphs filled in every sentence with informative details of "who, what, and when," alternate with freer treatment of the more important topics, written with a characteristic lively touch that greatly adds to the readability of the book. A sensitive, versatile, and widely read scholar, Garrison was the author of a number of valuable medical studies, among them an important monograph on the history of military medicine, and was an incomparable "catalyzer" of historical studies among friends and scholars. In modern American medical history a place of honour belongs to the Johns Hopkins pathologist W. H. WELCH (1850–1933), a prominent scientist, who gave a splendid impulse to scientific research and was the founder of the Institute of the History of Medicine at Baltimore and of the medical library at that institution. Among other American medical historians may be mentioned F. R. PACKARD, editor of the now defunct *Annals of Medical History* and author of a valuable *History of Medicine in the United States* (2nd ed., 2 vols., 1931), and of a number of valuable monographs and books, such as those on Paré and on Macmichael's *Gold-headed Cane.* J. G. MUMFORD (1863–1914) was the author of a *Narrative of Medicine in America* (Philadelphia, 1903), and Howard KELLY (1858–1943) of a highly useful *American Medical Biography* (1920; 2nd ed., 1928). Earlier short histories by American authors were Robley DUNGLISON's (1798–1869) *History of Medicine from the Early Ages to the Commencement of the Nineteenth Century* (1872), Roswell PARK's (1852–1914) *An Epitome of the History of Medicine* (2nd ed., 1901), and M. G. SEELIG's (b. 1874) *Medicine, an Historical Outline* (1925). R. H. SHRYOCK's thoughtful and attractive *Development of Modern Medicine* (1936) exemplifies an interesting tendency — the entrance of the professional historian into medical historiography. Arnold C. KLEBS (1870–1943), an American of German origin, who lived at Nyon, Switzerland, the leading authority on medical incunabula, wrote on a variety of subjects, such as *The History of Vaccination* (1915), paleopathology, and Leonardo, and a valuable *Geschichtliche und bibliographische Untersuchungen* (1926). J. J. WALSH (1865–1942), of New York, was the author of a number of entertaining studies, such as the *History of Medicine in New York* (5 vols., 1919), *What Civilization Owes to Italy* (1923), *The Thirteenth, Greatest of Centuries; Medieval Medicine* (1920), *Makers of Modern Medicine* (New York, 1907), and so on. His brother Joseph has confined his historical studies especially to Galen. Among other American historiographers is C. N. B. CAMAC (1868–1940), of New York, who wrote an interesting historical work entitled *From Imhotep to Harvey;* his *Epoch-making Contributions to Medicine, Surgery and the Allied Sciences* (1909) was one of the earliest collections of annotated reprints of classical articles, a procedure that has since had a considerable vogue in the United States. Special mention is due to an outstanding scientist and book collector, J. F. FULTON (b. 1899), Professor of Physiology at Yale, to whom the foundation and the rapid development of the Historical Library at Yale is owed, and who has contributed a short *History of Physiology* (Clio Medica), *Selected Readings in the History of Physiology* (1930), and also accurate and well-documented bibliographies of Fracastoro's poem on *Syphilis* (with L. Baumgartner), the *Works of Robert Boyle* (1932), and of Lower and Mayow (1935). E. R. LONG (b. 1890) has written a capital *History of Pathology* (1928), and also has collected a useful *Selected Readings in Pathology* (1929). The latest series of reprints of landmarks in the history of medicine is the *Medical Classics* (beginning 1936) compiled by E. C. KELLY of Albany. These reprinted many classical essays, each accompanied by bibliographical and biographical notes about the author. Among American clinicians who have contributed to the history of medicine is Harvey Cushing, a brilliant writer with deep understanding, whose splendid collection of rare books forms the nucleus of the Yale Historical Library and who wrote numerous articles on Vesalius, W. Osler, and other subjects of historical and bibliographical interest. He belongs to the leaders of the medico-historical development in America. David RIESMAN (1867–1940) wrote *The Story of Medicine in the Middle Ages* (1935) and *Medicine in Modern Society* (1939). One of the few full-time American medical historians is Henry E. SIGERIST, professor at Johns Hopkins and director of the Institute of the History of Medicine there. Previously director of the Medical History Institute at Leipzig, he has followed in W. H. Welch's footsteps in making his institute a centre for the scholarly study of the subject in the United States. From his own pen have come a number of vigorous historical publications, such as his *Heliodorus* (1921), *Studies and Texts of Early Medieval Prescriptions* (1923), *The History of Medicine in Switzerland* (1921–3), *Einführung in die Medizin* (Leipzig, 1931, with English and French translations), a biographical volume of *Grosse Ärzte* (Munich; English edition, 1934), an excellent volume on Russian medicine (1937), and some volumes on social medicine, together with numerous smaller monographs and articles. At Sigerist's school are working L. EDELSTEIN, who has devoted accurate studies to the history of Greek medicine, O. TEMKIN, a diligent researcher in various historical fields, and Genevieve MILLER, who has published for many years a valuable bibliography of medical history in America. Among others who have been active in cultivating the history of medicine in the United States we like to refer to G. W. CORNER (*History of Anatomy*), E. E. HUME (many interesting volumes on the history of American military medicine), S. V. LARKEY, C. D. LEAKE, W. B. McDANIEL, 2nd; R. H. MAJOR (*Classic Description of Diseases*), Archibald MALLOCH, W. H. MILLER (1858–1939), E. H. ACKERKNECHT, V. ROBINSON (1886–1947), professor at Temple University in Philadelphia (*The Story of Medicine*), and G. ROSEN, author of a valuable book on *History of Miners' Diseases* (1943). Among the recent historical books we refer to the excellent *Progress in Medicine* and *Behind the Sulfadrugs* by Iago GALDSTON, and *Pioneers in Pediatrics*, by A. LEVINSON, which contains much important information. Harry FRIEDENWALD, a prominent ophthalmologist and a collector of rare books on the history of Jewish medicine, is the author of many important historical works (e.g., *The Jews and Medicine*, 2 vols., 1944), Logan Clendening (1884–1945), clinician at the University of Kansas, and a brilliant writer on various topics, published some interesting historical books, among which *Behind the Doctor* (1933) and *Sources in Medical History* (1944) deserve to be cited. To B. SPECTOR, professor at Tufts College, is due an excellent story of the Tufts Medical School. R. A. WINSLOW, Professor of Public Health at Yale, published a remarkable book on *Conquest of Epidemic Diseases*, and V. RICCI a valuable *Genealogy of Gynecology* (1943). We want to refer also to remarkable studies on history of PHARMACY by KREMERS and

George URDANG, founder and director of the Museum for the History of Pharmacy at the University of Madison, Wisconsin. A. A. MOLL's *Aesculapius in Latin America* is a valuable source for information about physicians, medical schools, and scientific developments in the Latin-American countries.

The study of medical history is centred in the American Association of the History of Medicine (founded 1925), which now has as its official organ the *Bulletin of the History of Medicine*, edited by Sigerist. This not only publishes the annual transactions and original essays but also correlates news from the various medical-history groups throughout the country. The stately *Annals of Medical History* (New York: Hoeber) appeared in quarterly or bimonthly issues from 1917 to 1943. Unfortunately, Victor Robinson's *Medical Life* has also suspended publication. Hoeber's series of *Clio Medica* (now 22 vols.) appears in duodecimo volumes devoted to the history of the various specialties or to medicine in single countries. The Chicago Society of the History of Medicine issues occasional volumes. The ten volumes of the *Transactions of the Charaka Club* (New York), some quite rare, constitute a charming and valuable collection of medical essays. The *Bulletin of the Medical Library Association*, edited by Thomas E. KEYS and Max H. FISCH, is one of the most lively and interesting medico-historical journals. A new quarterly review is the *Journal of History of Medicine and Allied Sciences* (edited by G. Rosen, a brilliant historian of deep culture), which began publication in 1946.

Medical history in CANADA has been described by W. B. Howell (Clio Medica, 1933), by J. J. Heagerty (*Four Centuries of Medical History in Canada*, Toronto, 1925), and by Maude Abbott (*History of Medicine in the Province of Quebec*, 1931). Elsewhere on the American continent, medico-historical studies have marked a great development in recent years. ARGENTINE medicine has been studied by E. Cantón, G. Maceda, and others, but the greatest impulse to these studies was given by Juan Ramón BELTRAN, who instituted the regular teaching of medical history at the University of Buenos Aires and was the founder of the Ateneo de Historia de la Medicina, a medico-historical society that became a centre of studies in South America. The school of Professor Beltran is publishing every year a volume of papers on historical subjects written by his assistants and pupils, and at the same time the *Revista Argentina de Historia de la Medicina*, edited by Beltran, presents papers of his collaborators which enlighten different chapters of medical history, especially in Argentina. PERUVIAN medicine has been studied by Hermilio VALDIZAN, and by C. E. PAZ SOLDAN, to whom we owe some important contributions to the history of Peruvian folklore. He is the founder of the Peruvian medico-historical society and the editor of its journal. Under his guidance historical studies are very popular in Lima. Dr. LASTRES has made an important contribution to them; his biography of Lope de Aguirre is one of the best books on the subject. In São Paulo the Sociedad Paulista de Historia da Medicina has given a great impetus to these studies. In GUATEMALA, Carlo Martínez DURÁN is the author of an accurate historical study on the development of medicine in that country; in VENEZUELA, a medico-historical society was founded in 1944 and has begun the publication of a journal. Joaquin Diaz GONZALES has published a valuable history of medicine in antiquity and many other papers on medical history. To the work of the society that is presided over by S. Dominici, professor at the National University, Diego CARBONELL (1884–1945) an eminent physician, historian, and writer who took an active part in the politics of his country, made a remarkable contribution. The history of MEXICAN medicine was written by F. A. FLORES (3 vols., 1886–8). Among the scholars devoted to historical studies we cite the names of J. J. IZQUIERDO (Mexico City) who wrote a good biography of Claude Bernard and many other papers on history of physiology. The history of medicine in HAITI was written by R. P. Parsons; of ABORIGINAL AMERICAN medicine by R. Pardal (Buenos Aires, 1938). R. Caballero (Rosario), Afranio Amaral (Brazil), E. Aldunate Bascuñan (Chile), F. Cannino (Peru), V. Delfino (Buenos Aires), and J. Tanca Marengo (Ecuador), are other Latin-American contributors to the history of medicine.

In most of the countries of Europe there have come into existence during the last fifty years societies devoted especially to the history of medicine. The International Society of the History of Medicine, with its permanent office in Paris, has tried to co-ordinate the work accomplished in different countries, and has already held eleven international congresses (Antwerp, Paris, London, Brussels, Geneva, Leiden-Amsterdam, Oslo, Rome, Bucharest, Madrid, and Yugoslavia). The war stopped its activity and it is difficult to foresee whether and when it can be resumed. National societies were flourishing in many countries and a number of them published their own bulletins. Besides those which we have quoted, special mention has to be given to *Janus*, the oldest of the medico-historical journals; *Isis*, the quarterly organ of the History of Science Society (founded and edited by George Sarton); the *Annals of Science* (published by Taylor & Francis of London); *Æsculape*, the official organ of the International Association, which suspended publication for each World War; and *Lychnos*, a valuable publication of the Swedish Medical Association, with a historical section. The *Mitteilungen zur Geschichte der Medizin und der Naturwissenschaften* (Leipzig), edited by Haberling, is the official organ of the German Society. The French Society also publishes an informative bulletin. In Holland the *Bijdragen tot de Geschiedenis der Geneeskunde* (in Dutch) and the *Opuscula Selecta Neerlandicorum de Arte Medica* are the chief medico-historical publications. The latter, which in 1939 had reached its fifteenth volume, reproduced bilingually the great classics of Dutch medicine. The *Arquivos de historia da medicina portugueza*, edited by M.

Lemos and Joao de Meira (Portugal) offered many valuable contributions. The Polish *Archives of the History and Philosophy of Medicine* was an excellent periodical, edited up to 1924 by A. Wrzosek.

Museums of medical history exist in many of the chief cities of Europe. Especially noteworthy is the private institute founded by Henry S. Wellcome, which in its new home near London University contains an astonishing number of valuable exhibits from all parts of the world: manuscripts, rare books, costumes, reproductions of works of art, ancient instruments, and even whole rooms lifted bodily from their original sites to represent various interesting phases of medical history. The museums of Rome, Paris, Vienna, and Leipzig are also noteworthy for their valuable exhibits.

Medical history is now taught in almost all the countries of the world. A model was set by Poland, where all five of its universities at least until recently possessed professors of the subject, with their institutes and their seminars; attendance at courses was obligatory, and examinations were held. In France there are chairs of the subject at Paris and Lyon. Germany had three professors *ordinarii*, seven *extraordinarii*, and four other lecturers; there are (or were) institutes of the history of medicine at Leipzig, Berlin, Jena, and Würzburg. In America organized teaching in the form of lectures or seminars or both is given in many of the best schools; medical history is also informally taught as part of the general preclinical and clinical instruction; this has been accomplished with especial success by men like Jacobi, Osler, Thayer, and Riesman. In many universities of Latin America, as in Mexico, Guatemala, Venezuela, Brazil, Argentina, and Peru, chairs of History of Medicine have been recently instituted. In Italy medical history is taught at present at Bologna, Siena, Padua, and Rome.

Any study of medical history necessitates the examination of contemporary documents and books. The large libraries of Europe have long possessed medical classics on their shelves, as well as a wealth of manuscript material. In America a number of medical libraries are adding constantly to their holdings, often benefiting by donations of fine private libraries, patiently compiled over the years by medical men engrossed in the history of their subjects. The Army Medical Library's great collection has proved an impetus to the study of medical history as to that of modern medical literature. The Boston Medical Library can boast an excellent collection of incunabula, as also can the College of Physicians of Philadelphia. The Institute of the History of Medicine, at Johns Hopkins University, is devoted primarily to works of reference valuable in historical research. The New York Academy of Medicine combines the older literature with historical reference tools. Sir William Osler's remarkable library is now at McGill University, and Harvey Cushing's fine collection has been incorporated in the new Medical Historical Library at Yale University, New Haven, with the precious collections of A. Klebs and of J. F. Fulton. No discussion of medical libraries would be complete without a word in behalf of the librarians whose efforts in organization and cataloguing have resulted in reference service indispensable to the historian. The librarians who devote their work to the great medical libraries have remarkably aided the progress of medico-historical studies — and deserve the gratefulness of all students interested in this subject.

Thus throughout the civilized world medical history has returned to a place of honour in our time; the work of professional medico-historians is amplified by a greater number of physicians who study and write on the subject *con amore*. The study of the past shows that the concept of the historical unity of medical thought is becoming more widely accepted; also the necessity of reviewing the road that has been traversed if one wishes to understand present facts and to evaluate present concepts. In a period when, as we have seen, study is being concentrated on biology — that is, on the investigation of the origin and nature of the species and of the individual — it is logical and necessary that the attention of physicians should turn zealously toward the origins of their art. It is only in this way that knowledge can throw light on many difficult and complex problems.

26. The Study and Practice of Medicine

The great progress of medicine in modern times has determined an essential change in the orientation of medical investigation and in preparation for its scientific study. With the profound modifications in the essential concepts of disease, and the extension of the physician's activities in biology, public health, and legislation, there has been also a necessary change in the individual and social conditions of his economic and intellectual existence. Let us attempt to note the most salient features of this evolution, which has been influenced not only by the great events in medical science but also very markedly by the political and social changes in the living-conditions in civilized countries, which in turn have provoked, directly or indirectly, new and different orientations in all branches of intellectual activities.

At the beginning of the twentieth century we find a more or less similar type of MEDICAL INSTRUCTION in all of the great countries of the world. For university studies a period of five or six years is required, or even longer if, as in the United States, two or three premedical years are required in addition to the four years in the medical school proper, with possibly one or two years in hospital internship. The method of examinations is much the same in the different European countries. Attendance is required at lectures on various topics and in the laboratories and clinics, to be followed by public examinations, which are conducted by the governments throughout continental Europe. Special topics can be pursued at the will of the student, all more or less covered by the general examinations. Britain is the only European country where medical teaching has a special character. In London various medical colleges, though nominally part of London University, are attached to the great hospitals which are especially concerned with clinical instruction. Oxford and Cambridge, on the other hand, deal chiefly with the preclinical subjects, though clinical instruction is given to a small number of students in the local hospitals and by the Regius professor and others. In England, the licence to practise is given after a special examination by various corporations, such as the Royal College of Physicians and the Society of Apothecaries, which acquired these privileges several centuries ago. For some time the College of Physicians and the College of Surgeons have had their examinations conducted by a Conjoint Board. The academic degree is that of M.B. (Bachelor of Medicine), the doctorate seldom being taken by surgeons; for this reason it is customary to address physicians as " Dr." and surgeons as " Mr." In America, the bachelor's degree was formerly followed by the doctorate after a certain lapse of time, accompanied by submission of an essay and a small fee. It has long since been abandoned, however, the doctor's degree being given on satisfactory completion of the medical course. This carries with it no licence to practise, which is acquired by passing another examination given by a State Board of Medical Licensure (with considerable reciprocity with other states) or by the excellent self-constituted National Board of Medical Examiners in recent years.

Various tendencies have manifested themselves in modern medical instruction. In some countries (Italy, Poland, Hungary, and Germany) a scholastic type of teaching may be said to predominate, relying in large part on formal lectures correlated with practical demonstrations. In French and English universities the greatest importance has long been given to practical instruction, so that the student begins early in his medical course to attend clinics and " walk " the wards of the hospitals.

In the great North American universities, as we have seen, theoretical instruction began to be reduced toward the end of the last century, a trend that made great progress in the first quarter of the twentieth. This was made possible by a considerable reduction in the number of students, which is limited to from fifty to one hundred and twenty-five per class in the best schools.

In clinical work the students are subdivided into several groups, which alternate in their courses under the direction of the professors and their assistants. This method of instruction, according to which almost all of the preclinical faculty and in some schools even the clinical professors devote their entire time to teaching and hospital demands (full-time professors), has brought a close

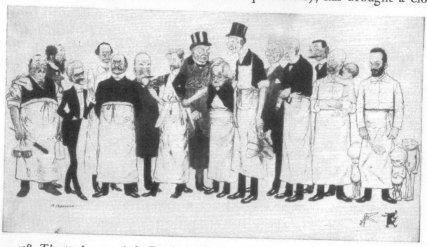

498. *The professors of the Faculty of Paris (1912). From left to right: Chantemesse; Pouchet; Poirier; Dieulafoy; Debove; Brouardel; Pozzi; Tillaux; Hayem; Cornil; Berger; Guyon; Launois; Pinard; Eudin.*
(Caricature by A. Barrère, Maloine, Paris.)

contact between the teacher and the student and combines the work of both in the laboratories and the wards. This North American method has been generally adopted by the better schools, most of which are attached to universities, and in many cases have at their disposition large staffs and considerable funds, whether from private sources or state appropriations. Undoubtedly medicine, especially in the United States, has experienced a period of rapid and extraordinary progress in the present century, radically changing a situation that as late as the beginning of the century left much to be desired in the way of medical instruction and opportunities for research. Since that time, owing largely to the efforts of educational reformers and of the American Medical Association, the number of medical schools in the United States has been notably reduced. In 1905 there were 160 medical schools, attended by 26,147 " students of medicine," from which 5,606 students were graduated. Now there are only 77 schools of medicine on the approved list for full four-year courses in medical science. Immediately preceding World War II, about 25,600 students attended these 77 schools, and about 5,700 of them were awarded medical degrees each year. The changes begun in the previous period have been greatly amplified by introducing educational methods and standards on a university level, and, in place of didactic clinical teaching, by giving students facilities for self-instruction in laboratories and as "clerks" in the hospital wards. Such methods are of course costly, so that, in spite of the great increase in students' fees, they meet a

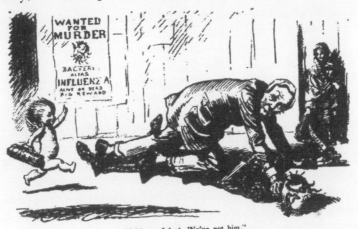

"Hold on, John! We've got him."

499. *The fight against influenza.*
(*Cartoon in* Life *by C. D. Gibson.*)

relatively small part of the cost of his education. The difference has been met by private gifts and endowments in private schools and by taxation in those state-supported, augmented in no small way by the aid of the great philanthropic foundations, such as the General Education Board of the Rockefeller Foundation. Key schools in relatively weak areas have been built up, weak departments in otherwise good schools have been strengthened; schools have even been founded or strengthened in foreign countries, and promising graduates brought from overseas on fellowships if they desire to become familiar with American methods.

Similar developments have taken place in Great Britain, under the wise leadership of the National Research Council, and aided by great private gifts, such as those of Lord Nuffield, of Morris-Oxford fame. In the Scandinavian countries, Switzerland, and Holland, similar trends were manifest, though in a smaller way. The growth of Soviet medical education between wars, as of all aspects of medicine, was prodigious. This can be expected to continue, even before war wounds are healed, in a state where the desires and pocketbooks of the public have as yet had but little weight. For the rest of Europe the ravages of war can hardly fail to retard for many years a form of education that depends so intimately on a prospering economy.

Though of course much will always remain to be accomplished, students in these countries no longer get their medical knowledge only from lectures and demonstrations, but now mainly from first-hand observation of laboratory material, experiments, and clinical cases.

A unique incident in the annals of medical education was the successful establishment during World War II of a displaced medical school in an Allied country. When Poland was overrun, its medical students and faculty were given classrooms, laboratories, and clinics by the University of Edinburgh. Classes taught by their own teachers in their own tongue proceeded to graduation, and true contributions to medical research were made.

Graduate schools and courses of medicine, too often in the past limited to " refresher " courses that refurbished forgotten undergraduate teaching, have been slower in improving their type of education. It was not until well into the present century that they began to develop an adequate university type of instruction capable of equipping the physician with the further special knowledge required in the specialties, and even today there are only two or three complete schools in the United States and Great Britain. In America there have been created fifteen Certifying Boards (starting with Ophthalmology in 1917), formed under the auspices of the American Medical Association and the appropriate national society of each specialty. These offer, after examination of the candidate's credentials and ability, to certify that he is properly equipped to carry on the specialty in which he is engaged, and thus far have certified some 25,000 specialists. The weaknesses of the self-styled specialists and the " 20-Gulden Spezialisten " of Vienna's prewar period are thus coming under control, until such time as they, like the general practitioner, have to obtain governmental licence. The present activity in medical science is indicated by the fact that there are in the United States 162 national and interstate medical societies, which support 80 journals for the publication of medical literature.

Medical education in Latin America continues to progress, the method of combining ward and laboratory work, as described above, having been introduced in some schools. Panama and Costa Rica are the only countries that lack medical schools today, though of the fifty-four schools in existence, only three have been founded in the twentieth century.

More than 3,000 students, who pay but small fees to the mostly government-supported schools, graduate annually; the numbers enrolled are surprisingly large, as a student may continue over many years, and many never graduate. Faculty salaries are low, but most are for part time only. Modern dentistry, introduced by the French, has been considerably promoted by American dental societies. There are now over fifty dental schools, with a course lasting from three to five years, and more than 2,000 dental degrees are granted annually. The special training of nurses has in recent years begun in sixteen countries; and public-health work has been especially fostered. In the past few years over fifty million dollars additional have been assigned to such work (more than half supplied by the U.S.A.), with some eighty laboratories for research. Chairs of Legal Medicine, often joined with Neuropsychiatry, have flourished, in several cases for over a century. The Pan American Sanitary Bureau, formed by international treaty in 1902, promotes in eighteen republics through its *Servicio Sanitario Cooperativo Intramericano de Salud Publica* all the various divisions of public-health improvement.

The profound changes in the development of medicine in the Soviet Union since the Revolution of 1917 are dependent on the basic concept that the goal of medical care and preservation of health of all citizens has to be controlled by the State.

The new system is based on the outgrowth of the ancient Zemstvo Medicine into a public service instituted in the rural districts of Russia in 1864. According to the Soviet system, all health services are free and available to everyone. All health activities are directed by central agencies that train the personnel they need and provide for its technical equipment. All physicians are in the service of the State and attached to some medical institution. Medical service is free and the prevention of disease is in the foreground of all health activities. The logical consequence of this principle, that the people's health is essential for the welfare of the nation, is that all phases of medicine become a public function of the State. The Public Health Commissariat of the Soviet Government — no such co-ordinating agency existed under the czars — thus assumed great importance in the life of the people, and within the first decade after the Revolution had made great progress. The Commissariat of Health was divided into eight departments: (1) sanitary-epidemic, with sections on tuberculosis, syphilis, malaria, etc.; (2) therapeutics; (3) sanatoria; (4) war sanitation; (5) railroads and steamships; (6) maternal and child welfare; (7) care of youth, sports, and physical culture; (8) scientific research (W. H. Gantt). Prostitution was prohibited and greatly diminished; employment was provided for all arrested prostitutes. Contagious diseases, especially malaria, were controlled by such measures as obligatory registration, opening of special stations for diagnosis and treatment, with free distribution of medicine. Instruction on personal hygiene and disease was spread through the medium of schools and factories, newspapers, radio, and movies. In 1913 there were 19,785 physicians in Russia; in 1941 the number was 130,348. In 1913 there were 13 medical schools with 8,600 students; in 1941, 106,000 students were being trained in 51 medical schools. Despite severe losses, medical education continued without interruption during World War II, and during its first two years 32,000 graduates took their places in the ranks of military and civilian medicine of the Soviet Union. The Committee on Higher Education of the Comissariat extended the medical course in 1935 to five years; lectures and recitations were increased, Latin was resumed for medical terms, and individual examinations and final board examinations were introduced. The medical course was gradually strengthened by increased time devoted to basic and clinical subjects and then to the medical specialties. Three faculties were established: general medicine and prophylaxis, hygiene and sanitation, and pediatrics, including maternity and child protection. Sigerist's book on *Socialized Medicine in the Soviet Union* exhaustively describes the part that the health centres have in the organization of medical services, and the way in which the system is functioning. In an analysis by the American Chemical Society of scientific articles on chemistry, in 1913 Russia was found to have contributed 2.5 per cent of the total in 1913, 0.7 per cent in 1918, 3.4 per cent in 1929; by 1940 the figure had risen to 14.1 per cent. This compared to a contribution by Germany of 34.9 per cent in 1913 (the highest of the lot), 26.9 per cent in 1929, 18.7 per cent in 1939, and 13.4 per cent in 1940 (the U.S.A. percentage at this time was over 33 per cent).

Medical research was for some time concentrated in the All Union Institute of Experimental Medicine (VIEM), which is said to include the largest collection of research laboratories in the world, with divisions in most of the capitals of the Soviet Republics. It is said to have been recently decentralized as the branches became better able to lead an independent existence.

SCIENTIFIC CONGRESSES, which are held at regular intervals throughout the world in many different fields, have contributed greatly to the diffusion of medical knowledge, which has now become international in the full sense of the word. National congresses on all the specialties have been held as a rule annually in all leading countries; international congresses usually meet every two, three, or four years. The first international medical congress was held at Paris in 1867, and since then similar congresses have met in the capitals of most of the countries of Europe and at Washington, D.C. (1887). The prewar congress at London in 1913 was followed by an intermission of several years, but they were then being held again regularly. Congresses on statistics, veterinary medicine, anthropology, and pharmacy, as well as on practically all of the medical specialties, have been held more or less frequently, even when the political horizons were overclouded, though of course they were suspended again by World War II.

In spite of the increased knowledge of disease and its treatment, and the greater interest of the public in health matters, irregular and irrational medical CULTS have sprung up in astonishing numbers, especially in the United States —

the most congenial of homes for fads in general. Homeopathy, to be sure, has gradually come more and more into line with orthodox medicine and appears to be on the way out. Not so Christian Science. A religion founded by the neurotic, Mary Baker G. EDDY (1821–1910) on the tenet that sickness and sin are human errors avoidable by proper thinking, it early developed a strong therapeutic element. Through the power of suggestion its healers have helped many thousands to better mental and physical states, though in the early days especially they undoubtedly were responsible for many avoidable deaths. Osteopathy, another cult founded in America in 1874 by A. T. Still, though based on a totally false principle, made such headway that in the United States it has several schools, with a four-year curriculum, and some 10,000 practitioners, who are required to take licensing examinations in some states. In England, however, a bill to legalize osteopathy (1937) was rejected by the House of Lords. A skilful use of manipulations and suggestion and an avoidance of conditions beyond their sphere has occasionally produced some benefits for their patients. An offshoot, chiropractic, based on much the same theory as osteopathy, is equally successful. Founded in 1894 by a groceryman, D. D. Palmer, of Davenport, Iowa, about the time of World War I, it had 79 schools in the United States alone. As in the case of homeopathy, Christian Science and these manipulative cults have had the useful effect of emphasizing the importance of psychotherapy and physical medicine. When this lesson is sufficiently assimilated, doubtless these cults also will dwindle. In the meantime, smaller profit-seeking cults and quacks come and go with a speed that would be bewildering if one had to consider them. In 1927 M. Fishbein's *New Medical Follies* described fifty-five cults based on variations of the themes described. On the other hand, popular superstitions, many passed down through the centuries from mouth to mouth, are definitely dwindling. Yet in the most highly civilized countries one still finds firm believers in the amulets and charms of primitive tribes, or in procedures based on mystic numbers, on the importance of colours or of the unusual or horrible, on "transference," the "doctrine of signatures," and so on. It is perhaps too much to expect that the child that is in man will ever wholly rise above the desire for cure by any means, whether reasonable or not.

An international award of the highest importance is the Swedish NOBEL PRIZE, given in several intellectual fields. The awards for the prize for physiology and medicine have been made as follows: In 1901, to Emil von BEHRING, of Marburg, for his work on serotherapy and especially in its use against diphtheria; in 1902, to Sir Ronald Ross, of University College, Liverpool, for his disclosure of the way that malarial organisms produce that disease; in 1903, to Niels R. FINSEN, director of the Royal Copenhagen Institute, for his treatment of lupus by concentrated light-rays; in 1904, to Ivan Petrovich PAVLOV, of the Military Academy of St. Petersburg, in recognition of his studies on the physiology of digestion; in 1905, to Robert KOCH, director of the Berlin Institute for

Infectious Diseases, for his work on tuberculosis; in 1906, jointly to Camillo GOLGI, of Pavia, and Santiago RAMON Y CAJAL, of Madrid, for their work on the anatomy of the nervous system; in 1907, to Charles Louis Alphonse LAVERAN, of the Pasteur Institute, for his recognition of the part played by protozoa in the causation of disease; in 1908, jointly to Paul EHRLICH, director of the Institute of Experimental Therapeutics of Frankfurt, and to Elie METCHNIKOFF, of the Pasteur Institute of Paris, for their studies on immunity; in 1909, to Theodor KOCHER, of Bern, for his work on the physiology, pathology, and surgery of the thyroid gland; in 1910, to Albrecht KOSSEL, of Heidelberg, for his studies on proteins and nuclear substances in the density of the cell; in 1911, to Allvar GULLSTRAND, of Uppsala, for his work on the dioptrics of the eye; in 1912, to Alexis CARREL, of the Rockefeller Institute, for his achievements in suturing blood vessels and transplanting blood vessels and organs; in 1913, to Charles RICHET, of the University of Paris, for his work on anaphylaxis; in 1914, to Robert BARANY, of Stockholm, for his studies on the physiology and pathology of the vestibular apparatus. From 1915 to 1918 the prize was not awarded. In 1919, it was given to Jules BORDET, of Brussels, for his discoveries in the field of immunity; in 1920, to August KROGH, of Copenhagen, for his discovery of the regulatory mechanism governing capillaries. In 1921 it was not awarded. In 1922, it was divided between Archibald Vivian HILL, of University College, London, for his elucidation of the thermodynamics of muscular contraction, and Otto MEYERHOF, of Kiel, for establishing the relation that exists between consumption of oxygen and the metabolism and lactic acid in muscles; in 1923, to Frederick G. BANTING and J. J. R. MACLEOD, of Toronto, for the discovery of insulin; in 1924, to Willem EINTHOVEN, of Leiden, for his investigations of the electric currents of the heart by means of the string galvanometer that he invented. In 1925 it was not awarded. In 1926, it was given to Johannes FIBIGER, of Copenhagen, for his discovery of spiroptera carcinoma; in 1927, to Julius WAGNER-JAUREGG, of Vienna, for his discovery of the therapeutic value of malaria inoculations in the treatment of paresis; in 1928, to Charles NICOLLE, of the Pasteur Institute of Tunis, for his investigations of exanthematic typhus; in 1929, to Christian EIJKMAN, of Utrecht, for his discovery of the antineuritic vitamin, and to F. Gowland HOPKINS, of Cambridge, for his "discovery of the growth-promoting vitamins"; in 1930, to Karl LANDSTEINER, of the Rockefeller Institute, for his discovery of the human blood groups; in 1931, to Otto WARBURG, of Berlin, for his discovery of the respiratory ferment; in 1932, to Charles SHERRINGTON, of Oxford, and Edgar Douglas ADRIAN, of Cambridge, for their discoveries regarding the function of the neurone; in 1933, to Thomas Hunt MORGAN, of Pasadena, for his studies of the chromosomes that transmit hereditary qualities; in 1934, to George H. WHIPPLE, of Rochester, New York, and George R. MINOT and William P. MURPHY, of Harvard, for their discoveries of the value of liver treatment in the anæmias; in 1935, to Hans SPEMANN, of Freiburg, for his discovery of the organizer effect in embryonal development; in 1936, to Henry Hallett

DALE, of London, and Otto LOEWI, of Graz, for their discoveries relating to the chemical transmission of nerve impulses; in 1937, to the Hungarian Albert DE SZENT-GYÖRGYI, for his chemical identification of vitamin C (ascorbic acid); in 1938; to C. HEYMANS, of Ghent, for his work on the carotid sinus; in 1939, to G. DOMAGK of the I. G. Farbenindustrie for his demonstration of the value of the sulfonamides in bacterial infections. This, however, had to be declined to conform with the 1935 regulations of the German government. No Nobel prizes have been awarded for the years 1940–2, but in 1945 they were given for 1943 to Henrik DAM, of Copenhagen, for his discovery of vitamin K and its role in blood coagulation, and to Edward A. DOISY, of St. Louis, for his investigation of its sources and methods of purification, its structure and synthesis; and for 1944 to Joseph ERLANGER, of St. Louis, and H. S. GASSER, now director of the Rockefeller Institute, for their development of a method to detect small changes in electrical potential of even single nerve fibres; in 1945, to Sir Alexander FLEMING, Sir Howard FLOREY, and E. B. CHAIN, for the discovery and development of penicillin; in 1946 to H. J. MULLER for his study of the influence of X-rays on genes and chromosomes. In the related field of chemistry, the prize was given for 1938 to R. KUHN, of Berlin, for his study of vitamin A, and in 1939 to A. BUTENANDT, of Berlin, and L. RUŽIČKA, of Zurich, but only the last named could accept the award.

The role played by WOMEN IN MEDICINE has been steadily increasing and became firmly established by the work that they accomplished during the two wars, when many men of the profession were in military service. They have not only carried on private practices in nearly every field, but many have proved to be good teachers, administrators, and investigators. In research, one has only to mention such names in North America as Dorothy Reed (Hodgkin's disease), Margaret Lewis (cytology), Maude Slye (experimental cancer), Alice Evans (undulant fever), Maude Abbott (congenital heart disease), Ruth Tunnicliff (streptococci, anerobes), Sara Brenham (meningococcus), Rebecca Lancefield (classification of streptococci), Georgia Cooper (types of pneumococci), Anna Williams (diphtheria), Josephine Neal (meningitis), Florence Seibert (chemistry of tubercle bacillus), Gladys Dick (scarlet fever), Florence Sabin (hematology), Catherine Macfarlane (uterine cancer), and Louise Pearce (experimental medicine).

Some idea of the development of MEDICAL LITERATURE in modern times may be obtained from the following figures. C. P. Fisher calculated that at the end of 1913 the world's medical periodicals amounted to 1,654 in number, of which there were 630 in America, 461 in Germany and Austria, 268 in France, 152 in England, 75 in Italy, and 20 in Spain (*Bulletin of the Medical Library*

Association). Since that time, although not a few journals stopped publication during or shortly after World War I, many more, usually of a specialized nature, took their place, especially in the Latin countries, so that the number doubtless was more than equalled before World War II. However, the appalling economic losses of this war will doubtless cause an even greater decrease in the number of medical periodicals. Damage to libraries has also been appalling.

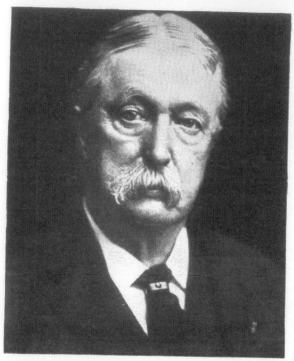

500. *J. S. Billings.*

E. R. Cunningham states that 50,000,000 volumes have been lost in Russia alone. On the other hand, medical publishing and library development is said to be progressing more rapidly than ever before in Latin America, with promising beginnings in Russia and the Orient.

In the ARMY MEDICAL LIBRARY (formerly the Surgeon General's Library) at Washington, which is the richest in the world in its collection of periodicals, in 1916 there were 1,895 being received annually; in 1921 this had been reduced to 1,240, but in 1925 had risen to 1,927 periodicals. In the Index Catalogue of the Surgeon General's Library, now midway in its fourth series, 4,020 different periodicals are listed for the period from 1880 to 1895; in 1916 the number had risen to 8,289, including a large number of defunct journals. In 1937, a list of 3,223 serials was published, to which 2,208 have subsequently been added. This greatest of published medical catalogues began to appear in 1880, and by 1945 there had been issued 57 large volumes, including 485,970 author titles and 2,796,-535 subject titles. It is a bibliographical tool that is valued in medical libraries throughout the world. Due mainly to the vision, energy, and general ability of John Shaw BILLINGS (1838–1913), this publication and the *Quarterly Cumulative Index Medicus* (a successor of the *Index Medicus* founded in 1879 by Billings and Fletcher) were cited by W. H. Welch as one of America's greatest contributions to medicine.

A characteristic of this period arising from the development of the specialties, which are still continuing to subdivide, is the appearance of RE-SEARCH INSTITUTES devoted to special lines of investigation. The various institutes of hygiene, tropical medicine, bacteriology, serology, radiology, experimental therapeutics, and so on, have taken an important place in the study of medicine.

A typically modern scientific institute is the Rockefeller Institute for Medical Research, of New York, founded in 1901 by John D. Rockefeller with an endowment of some seven hundred and fifty million dollars. It is not to be confused with the Rockefeller Foundation, which was created in 1913 "to promote the well-being of mankind throughout the world." This large organization has been far-sighted and liberal in its policy of promoting medical education in many countries of the world, especially China, by the creation of new schools, departments, and buildings, and in the support of traveling fellows, selected as promising standard-bearers of medical progress. Its International Health Board has promoted the campaign against hookworm throughout the world, and has supported exemplary rural health services in many American states and other countries. It has inspired research on the spread of yellow fever and malaria, and financed extensive preventive measures, sending important yellow-fever commissions to the west coast of Africa and to South America. It has fostered the development of public health officers and promoted nursing education and service in various countries. V. HEISER's *An American Doctor's Odyssey* gives an entertaining view of the far-reaching work of the Rockefeller Foundation in distant countries. The Rockefeller Institute is devoted more strictly to medical research along biological, pathological, epidemiological, and chemical lines, operating in conjunction with a hospital where are received a small number of patients suffering from the diseases under investigation at the moment. The valuable contributions of the Institute cannot be detailed here; suffice it to cite such items as the work of Noguchi on syphilis, of Simon Flexner on meningitis, poliomyelitis, and encephalitis lethargica; and of P. A. Levene on the chemistry of proteins, of D. D. Van Slyke on protein metabolism, blood gases and electrolytes, and renal tests; of Alexis Carrel, of Jacques Loeb, of Karl Landsteiner; and of Peyton Rous on filterable sarcoma and other cancer problems. The scientific work of the Institute has been recorded in a series of important monographs as well as in the *Journal of Experimental Medicine*, which it publishes. Scientific institutes, even if on a more modest scale, have arisen in all civilized countries, dedicated to scientific investigation and admirably complementing the work of the universities.

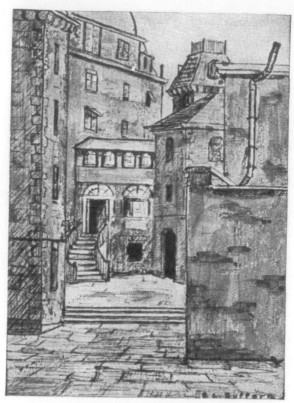

501. *A corner of old Bellevue Hospital, New York.*
(Sketch by G. L. Suffern.)

Modern HOSPITALS, which require a complicated administrative and professional service, often weigh heavily on the budgets of states, municipalities, or private charity and are presenting an increasingly grave and difficult economic problem.

Several trends combine to increase the importance of the hospital in the modern medical picture. First, the complex and expensive methods necessary for adequate study and treatment have more and more required the facilities of a well-equipped hospital; the various procedures can be accomplished with less delay, cost, and exhaustion under one roof than if multiple visits have to be made to or from the patient's or the nursing home; the attending physician knows that it is at the hospital that his patient will get the best and often the most satisfying care, and this knowledge has been more and more assimilated by the medically conscious public; the teaching hospital needs the very best in equipment and staff, men who are leaders in their profession, requiring special clinical

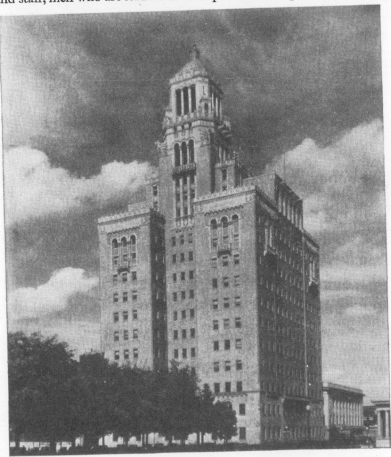

502. *The Mayo Clinic, Rochester, Minnesota.*

material, whether drawn from private or ward patients, both of whom, therefore, in increasing proportions must come to the hospital to profit by this situation. Much of this treatment has been free in the past, practically forcing staff members to seek their livelihood outside the hospital in a hurried part of their day's work. This, however, like so many aspects of medical practice, is also changing. Doctors are being more and more encouraged to have their offices in the hospital; free hospital treatment is being abolished and the attending doctors are being paid for their work out of fees collected from the patient or from his insurance or government subsidy. In 1934, Sigerist estimated that in the United States about 8,000,000 people applied for hospital treatment each year and that about 700,000 babies were born in hospitals. This requires the attention of an increasing number of the 150,000 physicians and almost half a million women engaged in nursing and social-service work. Yet even in normal times scarcity of physicians, nurses, and hospital beds may occur.

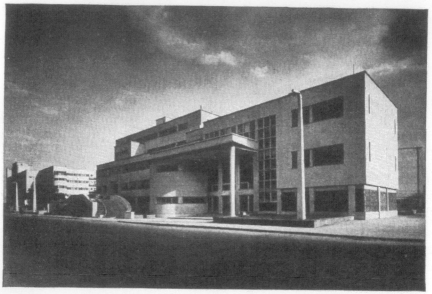

503. *The Institute for Cardiopathology, Mexico City.*

The organization of hospitals naturally varies in the different countries, as do their administrative system and architecture. The pavilion type of hospital has grown in favour in the present generation, where space is available, as in the Eppendorf (Hamburg) and Peter Bent Brigham (Boston) hospitals. Yet today hospitals in large cities tend more to be constructed in large units, as in the colossal structures of the two medical centres of New York and of the Mayo Clinic of Rochester. The increasing tendency to the skyscraper type is due not only to the limited space available in the central parts of big cities and its high cost, but also to the increased efficiency of elevator transportation and of the air- and light-giving qualities of the tall buildings, with the added advantage of being farther from the noisy streets. These huge structures, which accommodate many hundreds of patients in wards and private rooms and also permit the close concentration of wards, lecture rooms, and laboratories, symbolize in their way the idea of the concentration of all the medical disciplines. The prewar Italian hospitals compared favourably with those of the more powerful and wealthy nations in the efficiency of their plants and the nobility of their architectural lines. Such are the Hospital of the Policlinico in Rome, the Ospedale

Maggiore of Milan, the Hospital of San Martino of Genoa, the Policlinico San Matteo of Pavia, the Istituto Carlo Forlanini and the Eastman Institute of Rome. In Latin America, hospital construction in the twentieth century has proceeded apace with economic developments, the number now approaching 4,000. The great and affluent industries, social insurance, foreign populations desiring and supporting their own hospitals (there are seventeen in Argentina alone), and the increasing per capita wealth in the leading countries have all contributed to produce many hospitals, which make up in efficient appearance for their lack of the architectural charm of the ancient Spanish institutions. According to Moll, the proportions of those receiving hospital care has risen greatly — 40 per thousand in Argentina (as compared to 17 per thousand in 1900), and 60.8 per thousand in Chile. In addition to general hospitals, there are many for tuberculosis; also leprosaria and a considerable number of mental hospitals.

Another highly characteristic tendency of this important period in the evolution of medicine is, on the one hand, the close ORGANIZATION OF THE MEDICAL PROFESSION in scientific societies and professional corporations, which are constantly growing in strength; and, on the other hand, the division into as many groups as there are specialties. Thus we see the hygienist, the anatomist, the bacteriologist, the medical statistician, and the public-health official, who practically never come in direct contact with patients throughout their careers, all with their special societies and journals. Along with this tendency, however, we see clinicians turning directly to the aid of the chemist and the pathologist when the case requires special investigation, or to other specialists when their intervention seems desirable. The ensemble of medical knowledge has become so vast, the techniques of the specialties so complex, and laboratory tests so difficult, the preparation of sera and vaccines so delicate and weighted with responsibility, the scope of certain specialties like radiology so vast, that the approach to medical practice is subdivided into a hundred different paths, many of which, although having numerous possibilities for communication, touch but rarely.

Suggestive of the gatherings of the intelligentsia in the eighteenth century, the general public today is becoming increasingly curious about the " wonders of science " and particularly of scientific medicine, and becoming increasingly aware of the changed character of medical practice. No longer is the suave " bedside manner " able to cover ignorance of the patient's condition, as it was formerly forced to attempt to do when the means for reaching accurate evaluations were limited to history-taking and unaided physical diagnosis. Today the public wants to know and is being told the facts, the risk of a little knowledge as a dangerous thing being wisely accepted. The taboo on mention of tuberculosis has practically disappeared and cancer and syphilis are going the same way. Other evidences of lay interest in medicine are that novels about doctors and medical biographies have increased in popularity, moving pictures of medical "high spots" (Pasteur, Ehrlich, Harvey, the conquest of yellow fever) are deservedly successful, medical heroes' portraits have appeared on the postage stamps of more than one country, and medical congresses commemorated by special stamp issues. The example set by the hygienic exhibits at Düsseldorf and Dresden (1926) has been followed in the public museums and exhibitions of other countries. At the New York World's Fair (1939–40) the Hall of Man contained a number of accurate and entertaining biological and medical exhibits that were extremely popular. Not only does medicine continue to furnish subjects for great artists, as it has since the days of Rembrandt and the Dutch *genre* painters, of Velasquez and Goya, but also medical men turn frequently to art, as to literature, as an outlet for artistic self-expression. Physicians' art associations and exhibits are not uncommon. Conan Doyle, Somerset Maugham, Cronin, Bridges, Clemenceau, Sherrington, John McCrae, and C. L. Dana are but a few of the physicians who carry on the literary tradition of Keats, Holmes, and Weir Mitchell. Biographies and autobiographies of physicians have strongly attracted the attention of the reading public; among these books are some of the best sellers of the last years.

We may cite the biography of Osler, written by Harvey Cushing, a classic work which had immense popularity and won the Pulitzer prize, *The Odyssey of an American Doctor*, by Dr. Heiser, which emphasizes the splendid work of the Rockefeller Foundation, the autobiography *As I Remember Him*, of Hans Zinsser (1878–1940), the eminent pathologist and bacteriologist of Harvard, in which he gave a brilliant history of his life and his work and described with fascinating lucidity the phases of the leukemia that brought about his death. These and many other books, among which are some describing the life of American doctors in pioneer times, arouse extraordinarily the interest of the public in the life and work of doctors and in the progress of medicine. They helped in popularizing the physician and his work and in spreading the knowledge of the part that the doctor is playing in protecting the health of the individual and the welfare of society.

Medical ILLUSTRATION has progressed with the graphic arts. The semi-diagrammatic drawings of the previous century have been replaced by more accurate, artistic, and pleasing drawings, or by clear gross or microscopic photographs, moving-picture strips, and electrongraphs. A leader in artistic illustration was Max Brödel (1870–1941), who came to the United States from the Leipzig Art Academy and Carl Ludwig's laboratory. At Johns Hopkins, first as instructor (1907), eventually as director of the Institute of Art as applied to medicine, he taught the best of forms of medical illustration to medical students and would-be professional illustrators.

In modern medical research many problems appear to require attack along several different lines, best accomplished by a team of men with different training, and therefore presumably requiring a captain. This, together with greater appreciation of the responsibility of science to society to make known its discoveries to the public and to apply them to public welfare, has led to a growing movement to submit scientific research to central planning and control. This took form in the British Association for the Advancement of Science in Sir Josiah Stamp's presidential address in 1936, and in 1938 in its formation of a Division for the Social and International Relations of Science. Voices such as those of J. D. Bernal in England, and some Soviet views such as those of Academician Lysenko, deride freedom of inquiry in their advocacy of the totalization of science. They found unexpected support in the excellent results obtained by the centrally supported and controlled studies carried out in the recent war, culminating in the dramatic military result of harnessing the release of atomic energy. Other scientists, however, believing in the greater importance of an unrestricted search for truth, have combined to combat excessive regimentation, as in the British Society for Freedom of Speech, and point to the frequency with which the basic discoveries are made by individuals, though the useful applications may be worked out by groups.

It is certain that through all these paths, important though less frequented than formerly, passes the great highway of the general practitioner. Seeing patients in his office and in their homes, he must combine as best he can all the knowledge possessed by modern medicine; and if the responsibility for the public health of a community has been confided to him, this duty also must be discharged. Even for these men, however, the responsibility is lessened by the fact that they can always have recourse to the aid and advice of the institutes, state authorities, and their specialist colleagues. It is for such reasons that we must accept that the specialization of medicine constitutes one of the most important trends in the progress of medicine in our period.

From this situation comes the tendency, which is being constantly more accentuated in all civilized countries, to circumscribe this or that specialty with increasing precautions, demanding special examinations of those who assume the title of specialist. One unfortunate result of the growth of specialties is that the general practitioner sees his prestige gradually diminishing, though he is still recognized by the more far-sighted as the backbone of the profession.

Many factors have contributed to the increasing SOCIALIZATION OF MEDICINE in modern times. The old days when the simple relation of the individual doctor to his patient filled all requirements are gone beyond recall, whether for good or for bad. The increasing medical knowledge that brought specialization to clinical practice and to the laboratory demands many more doctors and the performance of many laboratory tests in many illnesses. The problem has been met in various ways with varying success. Group practice — each member of a group covering a different field of medicine, usually with pooled earnings — has found its greatest expression in the Mayo Clinic, the Cleveland Clinic, and the Ross-Loos Clinic of Los Angeles, but may consist of but a few specialists in private offices.

INDUSTRIAL MEDICINE. A procedure that organizes medical care has been set up successfully in many large industries. It provides easy access, much more economically, to expert consultations and laboratory studies; yet it has met opposition from " organized " medicine as impersonal and unnecessarily using expensive methods in a firm run for profit, and so on, and from an older generation that guards the individual patient-physician relationship at all costs. Prepayment medical groups have been formed here and there, but without gaining much headway; voluntary insurance against hospital and physicians' charges prospers, as one might expect, in insurance-conscious countries.

As the fields of industry have widened and machines became more complex, the increasing prevalence of occupational diseases and better means for detecting and treating them have led to a considerable development of industrial medicine.

Extensive studies have been made of the health of the coal miners and the conditions to which they are exposed (G. Rosen). In France a study was carried out among workers in brass and allied metals. Even earlier an interesting collection of pamphlets covering the period 1814–33 discussed the prevention of accidents in coal mines and various modes employed in the ventilation of collieries, the construction and application of safety lamps. As early as 1850, inspectors of mines had been appointed in Great Britain for the saving of life as well as for the better security of the mineral wealth of the nation.

By 1920, medical problems of industry had become so great and so extensive that many physicians began to specialize in this type of medicine. Industrial accident prevention received more and more attention. The United States Public Health Service began to play an important part in the study of industrial hazards and in stimulating the corrections of these hazards. Significant studies appeared dealing with pneumoconiosis, and the study of lead poisoning and its control was undertaken because of the widespread incidence of this disease. In 1927, scientific studies were being completed of gases and the principles of respiration governing their action. In 1928 Fritz Bauer contributed a study on *Aviation Medicine*. In 1929 Alice Hamilton described in detail the modern knowledge of industrial poisoning in the United States.

Many countries have developed official bodies to carry out inspections of the working-conditions, and laws were rapidly developed to protect the welfare of the workers. Larger industries and companies employ full-time physicians to improve the health and safety conditions of the employees, and the smaller industries call upon part-time physicians or occupational-disease clinics to help them with their medical problems. With the advent of World War II, laboratories had been developed to study the complex problems that developed in an expanding industry, in which many new compounds were being brought into use in production. The specially trained medical workers that were available were rapidly increased in number by special courses of training. Thus, with the end of the war, in many countries of the world, especially those containing the larger manufacturing companies, we find a specially trained group of men who have set up standards of protection for the worker. The development of social consciousness in the working classes has resulted in legislation that protects to a great degree the worker in both the large and small industrial plants as well as in the office and mercantile establishment. By the end of World War II, in 1945, a high degree of efficiency had been developed in the protection of the worker, and facilities made available for these measures to keep pace with the increasingly complicated development in manufacturing processes. The organization of international labour conferences for the discussion of the problems of labour, in most of the larger countries of the world, has permitted an exchange of experiences and methods that promises to be of increased value as a wider audience is gained for the transactions of this organization.

Protection of the public health has brought manifold government agencies into play — administrators, investigators, field men carrying out, with more or less efficiency as the case may be, work that would be impossible for the private practitioner to accomplish. The higher costs of medical service, to the individual as well as to the community, together with an increased realization of what the public owes to the poorer classes in health matters, have contributed to bring local and national governments more and more extensively into the public health field. The budgets and spheres of activity of public health services have been greatly increased in the present century: in addition to public health surveys and investigations, health centres and free dispensaries have been established in many cities, diagnostic tests are made, and sera and vaccines distributed gratis, salaried district surgeons visit patients in their homes without charge, and hospitals are reimbursed for their free care of the indigent (see the section on Public Health and Social Medicine). In America, notwithstanding the financial depression of the early thirties, public health expenditures have risen out of all proportion to the increase in the population. The United States Public Health Service has included in its scope a large division for the study and eradication of cancer, and engages actively in efforts to reduce venereal disease. The pros and cons of the problem of government participation in matters of health, one of the most important that faces the medical profession today, cannot be discussed here, nor can the various steps taken in the various countries toward meeting it even be outlined. This part of the general story is still very much in the future; perhaps before many years a more definite account can be given or definite trends at least recognized.

Hospitals on the European continent have long been supported by the government — in France and in most of Germany since the Napoleonic era, in Scandinavia similarly, and of course in Russia absolutely since 1917. Even in Britain and North America special hospitals for mental disease and for tuberculosis, and now for veterans, are mostly State-supported and undoubtedly will become more so. Compulsory sickness insurance was first started in Germany in 1883, and apparently benefited the insured, though at great cost of administration and producing inferior work by the underpaid, overworked physicians. In Scandinavia, sickness insurance became compulsory in Norway for low-salary groups in 1911 and in Denmark in 1933; in Sweden it is still voluntary, though with a fifty per cent subsidy by the State.

In England workmen's compensation acts had been passed in 1897 and 1906. In 1911 Lloyd George's National Health Insurance Act instituted an employer-employee-state partnership in compulsory sickness insurance for about a third of the population, with a large sum set aside annually for medical research under the supervision of the National Research Council. This " panel " system has continued in spite of considerable dissatisfaction, and has recently produced the " Beveridge plan " as an even wider extension of government health benefits. In Italy the Clinica del Lavoro, founded in 1898 by L. DEVOTO, has been an important centre for the experimental and clinical study of occupational diseases and for the promotion of legislation in this field. In the United States, governmental health insurance continues to meet obstacles. Workmen's compensation laws — beginning in New York and Wisconsin in 1911 — gradually were introduced in most states, but agitation for compulsory health insurance at that time died with the First World War. Voluntary hospital insurance — the Blue Cross and similar plans — has made considerable headway in recent years, with a tendency to include medical fees in the insurance as well. Now a National Health program has been the subject of proposed legislation for several years. The original Wagner-Murray-Dingell bill provided for " womb to tomb " security by a universal pay-roll deduction of six per cent on wages up to $3,000, with an equal amount put up by employers. With powerful public support, but emphatic disapproval of most of the medical profession, the bill has already been modified and improved, but the result is still in doubt. Arguments that many of the " underprivileged " do not get medical care under the present system are met by reference to the growth of the voluntary systems of relief (a better though slower change by evolution), and to the advantages of avoiding the evils of an abrupt, revolu-tionary method (bureaucratic waste, autocratic control, hampering the choice of one's physician, lowering the level of professional care, and so on). We may hope that the Anglo-Saxon genius for perseverance and compromise will yet find the proper key.

It is not the task of the historian to pronounce a judgment, or to fore-see the solution of a problem that is still being actively debated. But when we think that in the world of tomorrow the common man will certainly play a more important part than ever before in history and that the trend toward a new order is more directly based on the principle of equal rights for all, we may easily infer that the current that tends toward a socializa-tion of medicine will grow steadily stronger. We believe that it is of para-mount importance that physicians and their societies should be given an im-portant part in the preparation of the laws that must establish the sanitary service of the future; and that if legislative action is confided only or chiefly to politicians, economists, lawyers, or sociologists, it may easily be forgot-ten that medicine is not only a science, but also an art. No medical problem, whether it concerns the individual or the community, can be definitely solved according to a formula or a pattern. There are too many constitu-tional differences among individuals and groups to let us believe that it may be possible to establish a system that can solve these problems in a satisfac-tory way.

These problems raise the question of how much the physician should be made a functionary of the State. This development, which appeared earliest in the states with socialistic tendencies, though temporarily set back by the effects of the two World Wars and still far from solution, is in line with governmental steps to improve the condition of the labouring classes, the rise of infant hygiene, the tendency of medicine to turn toward prob-lems of public health, and the orientation toward industrialization. How far these steps can be applied without losing the essential personal relation of the physician to his patient may prove to be the crux of the problem.

While the new scientific discoveries and the consequent changed exigencies of practice have determined an increase in specialization, a unifying biologic concept has demonstrated the absolute need for the organic unity of scientific medicine. The concept of a purely local pathology can no longer be maintained; and every external stimulus is accepted as having an effect on the whole organism. This in turn suggests the need for a unitarian type of medical thought in the study of the prime causes of disease and of

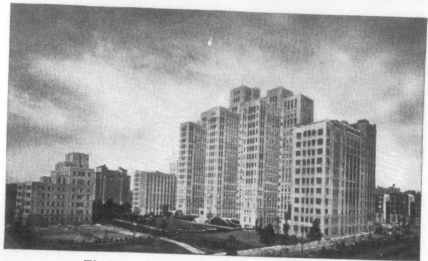

504. *The first medical centre, Columbia University, New York.*

the body's protective mechanisms. Ways must be sought to strengthen the whole organism because it is recognized that every affection, no matter how localized in appearance, constitutes a threat against the organism as a whole.

Trends that on the one hand have greatly increased the importance of the medical man to society in our time, have on the other hand reacted unfavourably on the economic condition of many physicians. This in turn suggested the idea, already proposed in some European countries, of establishing a *numerus clausus* for students in medical schools. Such a procedure, however, would seriously and probably harmfully limit the freedom of medical study and practice and seems less acceptable than the method of raising the standards of medical study and making examinations more strict, the method achieved in the great universities of North America. Racial laws, which existed in some European countries, limiting or suppressing the activity of Jews as students, teachers, research workers, and practitioners, and forbidding the issue of articles and books by them, created an important problem affecting the existence of many hundreds of physicians, but were necessarily suppressed by postwar conditions. Many excellent medical teachers and investigators, including several Nobel prize winners, were compelled to endure privation or seek a new livelihood in foreign countries, which will long continue to profit by their activities, just as France's neighbours, many years ago, profited lastingly by the expulsion of the Huguenots.

From such considerations it is obvious that the medical profession today is passing through a difficult period in which various opposing tendencies contend for supremacy, a period of transition, analogous to many others in the history of medicine, which directly reflects the political, social, and economic phenomena that dominate the time.

27. Conclusion

From the study of the history of medicine — that is, of the changes in the concept of disease, in the relation between doctors and patients, and in the position that doctors have assumed in society and toward the State — we may draw some conclusions. The history of medicine has to be considered as a chapter in the history of civilization, and is therefore closely interdependent with all the events in that history.

Historical thinking is today a fundamental requisite for the physician, and for the research worker no less than for the practitioner. It it obvious that just as the practitioner must unravel the medical history of each of his patients, so the good physician has to search for the origins of modern medical doctrines and pathological concepts if he wants to understand them clearly. Just as we can often disclose a hidden factor that explains the cause of a disease, so historical research may reveal in concepts and doctrines, in successes and mistakes that are regarded as quite modern, thoughts and hypotheses that had already been expressed by physicians or scholars of the past, but had remained forgotten, misunderstood, or sterile. Inquiry into the reasons for those mistakes and successes and for the bitter opposition that the great scientists often met forms one of the most fascinating chapters of medico-historical study.

Medicine, and this is one of the most valuable among the teachings of history, cannot remain equal to its great task without preserving for the physician his double character of scientist and *demiurgos*, worker for the people, according to the classic principle. If in the exercise of the art, he is guided by his knowledge of the laws of nature, then his technical knowledge, his calm judgment, his objective reasoning, and his personal intuition — which certainly plays a remarkable part in the make-up of the great physician — will suggest to him the rules that have to determine his activity. It is only thus that the clinician can be clinical in the true sense of the word — a matter far different from the mere calculation of figures or the counting of cells — in giving equal consideration, according to his experience, to all the endogenous and exogenous factors that can contribute to modify or to re-establish the normal state of health of the individual and the community. From the study of medical history we learn that the best physician is the one who constantly keeps in mind the welfare of his patient, looking not only at the manifest elements of his bodily illness, but also at his state of mind, which is a factor of utmost importance in the success of the treatment. He must be able to devote to his patient and his patient's condition all his attention, and he will be inspired by a strong confidence in his art and by the desire to help him. One would be blind not to recognize the historical fact that before and even after the advent of modern scientific medicine there were great and able healers who were not men of science, but who had the ability and the suggestive power to reassure the patient, to encourage him, to inspire faith in his recovery, and thus favourably to influence the course of the illness. It is no less obvious that there have been outstanding scientists who were very mediocre practitioners.

History teaches us that any division of the science from the art of medicine is necessarily harmful to practice. With an extreme swing of the pendulum, too much faith has sometimes been placed on the pronouncement of the laboratory when, forgetting the importance of the clinical picture, physicians have based their activities too exclusively on the laboratory report. For some time after the laboratory began to influence bedside practices physicians tended, through ignorance of the limitations and the possibilities of the new methods of research, either to place too much reliance on what came out of the four walls of the laboratory or not to take sufficient advantage of the information that it could properly give. They tended to pay more attention to the evidence of the microscope and of chemical reagents than to the information obtained by their own personal examination of the patient. Today, with a better knowledge of these possibilities and limitations, the expert physician tends to scrutinize sagaciously and objectively the information received from both sources. Clinical instruction in the Hippocratic sense fortunately never was completely neglected and voices continued to maintain the necessity of returning to the classical paths. All the marvellous discoveries of recent times cannot remove the physician from his post of honour in detecting morbid phenomena following the mysterious rhythm of life and death — a post, that is, at the bedside of the patient, watching no less carefully the individual than his surroundings.

Such principles indicate the orientation of modern medicine toward a Neohippocratism,[1] a return to some of the classical principles of medical thought. Modern medicine today turns to a dynamic, synthetic, unitarian direction after a period in which a morphologic analytical, localistic tendency dominated. It is a return to the classical concept of the ancient sage of Cos focused on the well-being of the individual and the improvement of the race, seeking for the cause of the disease, its prevention and cure, both in the individual and in his environment. The study of the nature and the cause of disease is progressing more and more along the lines of an " integrated pathology " — that is, using morphological, functional, physical, chemical, bacteriological, experimental, and, above all, clinical methods, in which the study of economic and social conditions also are important. It is significant that the best type of clinician is learning and teaching how best to utilize all the weapons at hand, in the laboratory as well as at the bedside, to focus more efficiently on the one vital item, the study and treatment of the patient.

Medical thought has returned to these principles, as we have seen in all periods of decisive progress, as a reaction against scholastic dogmatism and rigidified systems. In Alexandria it determined the peak of original research in anatomy and physiology; in the Renaissance the return to Hippocrates was accompanied by the renewed study of nature and of the classical traditions of learning; it stimulated the rebirth of clinical medicine with Baglivi in Italy, Sydenham in England, and Boerhaave in Holland. Clinical medicine, after the philosophical speculations of the eighteenth century, returned again to the fundamental Hippocratic concepts in the great French and English schools of the early nineteenth century. In our own time this current of thought begins to assert itself as a reaction against the overdogmatic trends of the laboratory. The careful physician is convinced that no test, however important and decisive it may be, can take the place of a synthetic clinical opinion and the personal judgment of an intelligent and experienced clinician as to the condition of the patient and of the community.

All these facts show clearly the new and important position occupied by the physician in society and in the State. In the ideal Republic of Plato the function of the physician was essentially political; today as ever the physician has the task of guarding the greatest of national assets. It is obvious that the improvement in the economic state of a country carries with

---

[1] The definition of Neohippocratism was first proposed by the author of this book in his work *Il volto di Ippocrate* (Milan, 1925) and has been accepted by many Italian, English, and French authors. The problem of Neohippocratism is treated in a number of modern works and essays (see Bibliography).

it a decrease in incidence of disease, a decrease in mortality, and a better physical condition of its citizens. With the principle once established that disease should be regarded as a disturbance in the harmony of organic functions and that every effort of modern medicine must converge on maintaining this harmony or re-establishing it when it is disturbed, it is evident that public health and governmental participation must play an important role. This transformation in the task of the physician, or rather the more extensive social application of the results of medical progress, should be recognized as being essentially based on principles similar to those of classical medicine.

Nobody can imagine that the medicine of our times has arrived at the climax of its development; on the contrary, the remarkable progress in the discovery of new and unknown factors, whose part in the origin of diseases and in their healing was hitherto unsuspected, merely opens new and, we may say, infinite horizons to research. The pessimism of those who speak of an increasing charlatanism and failing of public confidence in the regular profession is certainly not justified. As a matter of fact, history teaches us that a return to primitive mystic or superstitious medicine is a characteristic phenomenon of all historical periods when grave political upheavals or social changes have shaken humanity and led to great loss of human life and change of the economic structure. After all such experiences humanity finds itself in a state of economic and moral depression, in the need of an escape and in the expectancy of miracles. These are the sequelæ of severe illness and the symptoms of the loss of equilibrium of the collective mind, just as a return to primitive superstitions and the accessibility to all kinds of suggestion is characteristic of the individual who has suffered from a grave disease. But these are transitory events which disappear when the individual and the social organism are able to resume their normal function. Medicine, the art of preventing illness, of lessening pain, of averting death, and of returning the individual and the group as quickly as possible to good health, has obviously achieved scientific and practical triumphs that were not even hoped for in earlier times. We may expect that the role which social medicine will play in the world of tomorrow, after recovery from a terrible war, will be a decisive one. The disease of the collective mind will be a subject of study for the psychologist and psychiatrist no less than for the statesman and the sociologist.

It is yet too early to state objectively the consequences of World War II and the terrific destruction of human lives, of scientific treasures, and of moral values on the public health conditions in Europe and Asia. The terrific rise of mortality especially of children in many countries, the enormous increase in the frequence of tuberculosis and other diseases, the destruction of medical schools, hospitals, and welfare institutions, and, first of all, the lack of food and of fuel have contributed to create a situation that could not find an adequate remedy in the generous help that was offered by some countries and especially by the United States. It may be a long time before it is possible to assert whether, and to what extent, a recovery of public health conditions in Europe and Asia may be possible.

The evolution of medicine to a social science brought the splendid development that has taken place in the national and international organization of public health. Because of the importance of the problem of public health, the differences between classes and the frontiers between nations were subordinated, and sanitary measures tended to be generally accepted. The statistical data that have been collected, more exact than ever before, are good indications of the success in the fight against disease and constitute a new basis for the system of public health. The fact that the average duration of life has been extended recently from forty-eight to over sixty years in itself constitutes an important factor in the development of modern social medicine.

We have witnessed in recent times astonishing progress on one hand in knowledge of the biology of the individual and of his prenatal existence — the factors that determine and influence his life and his biological evolution — and on the other hand knowledge of the biological evolution of nationally and economically distinct groups. This research may still appear indefinite in its results; in fact, however, it is pointing the way to the medicine of the future. Progress in the knowledge of the individual and of his biological evolution has enlightened the understanding of the concept of disease at different times and under various conditions. Knowledge of the factors that influence social and interhuman relations and have a decisive impact on the well-being of humanity has emphasized the fact that the problems of individual and public health are intimately connected. The physician in the world of tomorrow will pursue the same fundamental aims that the classic writers of antiquity had designed and that history has formed. The physician will always be for his patients the magician from whom a wonder is expected, a priest to whom the sufferer confesses all secrets of his life and of his sins. He will always be the friend and the counsellor of the sick and of the healthy, of the individual, of the family, and of the community; and, above all, the expert judge and helper, guided by his knowledge and by his will to help and by his faith in his art.

When we consider the laborious path followed by medical science and medical art through the centuries, we may learn how this evolution has been brought about by a long series of events that have influenced medical progress and have been influenced by it. In a book on medical history the figures of the great scientists whose work exerted a predominant impact on the progress of science obviously take a prominent place. It should be recalled and stressed, however, that the architects of the extant structure of medicine were for the most part the millions of practitioners who lived their humble and modest lives giving their whole care and devoting their intelligence and their love to their profession. Their names are not remembered in history and live but a short time in the affectionate recollection of their patients and families, in the place of their activity. Nevertheless, the gratitude of all those who appreciate the wonderful progress of medicine is due to these unknown soldiers who fought courageously and sometimes heroically to protect the life and health of people entrusted to their care.

From the history of medicine we can elicit, therefore, not only useful information, but also valuable help and precious advice: like the traveller who, resting on his journey, can in the respite that is granted him take comfort in the lessons learned along the road. From them he can not only deduce the explanation and the comprehension of the phenomena that he has observed, but also predict some of the turns of the road that still remains before him; while others who follow him, strengthened by his experiences and his teaching, may confidently travel on in the assurance of fulfilling their high task.

BIBLIOGRAPHY

ABBREVIATIONS

Ac. – Accademia, Académie, Academy.

Aesculape – *Aesculape, Organ officiel de la société internationale d'histoire de la médecine*, Paris.

A.H.M. – *Annals of the History of Medicine*, New York.

Ann. – Annals, Annales, Annali.

A.G.M. – *Archiv für die Geschichte der Medizin*, Leipzig.

A.S.S. – *Archeion, Archivio di Storia della Scienza*, 1920–38, Roma; 1940–4, Santa Fé, Argentina.

B.H.M. – *Bulletin of the Institute of the History of Medicine*, Baltimore.

B.I.S.I. – *Bollettino dell'Istituto Storico dell'arte sanitaria (Atti dell'Accademia di Storia dell'arte sanitaria)*, Roma.

B.M.J. – *British Medical Journal*, London.

B.S.F. – *Bulletin de la société française d'histoire de la médecine*, Paris.

BULL. – Bulletin.

Isis – *Isis, International Review devoted to the History of Science*, Bruxelles; since 1941, Cambridge, Mass.

J. – Journal.

J.A.M.A. – *Journal of the American Medical Association*, Chicago.

Janus – *Janus, Archives internationaux pour l'histoire de la médecine et de la géographie médicale*, Leiden.

Med. Life – *Medical Life*, New York.

N.Y.A.M. – New York Academy of Medicine.

R.I.S. – *Rivista italiana di storia delle scienze mediche e naturali*, Siena.

Univ. – University.

Woch. – *Wochenschrift*.

Zeits. – *Zeitschrift*.

In this bibliography only historical writings have been cited. The first editions of original medical works by ancient authors have been cited in the text and are included in this bibliography only when the addition has special historical importance for its comments, annotations, etc.

For further bibliographical information about single subjects consult the excellent *Medical Bibliography* by FIELDING H. GARRISON, revised with important additions by LESLIE T. MORTON (London, Grafton and Coe, 1943). The bibliography of modern medical works will be found in the *Index Medicus* (1874–99 and 1903–27), continued now in the *Quarterly Cumulative Index*, and in the *Index Catalogue of the Library of the Surgeon General's Office*, U.S. Army, Ser. I–IV. These are the most complete world bibliographies of medical literature.

Added to the bibliography of some chapters are notes that may help to illustrate or to complete the text.

Excellent selections from the works of the CLASSIC MEDICAL WRITERS are to be found in the *Medical Classics* (5 vols., Baltimore, Williams & Wilkins Co., 1936–41); J. F.

FULTON: *Selected Readings in the History of Physiology* (Springfield, Thomas, 1930); R. H. MAJOR: *Classic Descriptions of Disease* (3rd ed., Springfield, Thomas, 1945); E. R. LONG: *Selected Readings in Pathology* (Springfield, Thomas, 1929); F. A. WILLIUS and T. E. KEYS: *Cardiac Classics* (St. Louis, Mosby, 1940); and L. CLENDENING: *Sources of Medical History* (New York, Hoeber, 1942).

The current literature on medical history is published regularly in *Isis, International Review devoted to the History of Science,* Cambridge, Mass. The bibliography on American current medical-historical literature, accurately edited by GENEVIEVE MILLER, appears regularly in the *Bulletin of the History of Medicine,* Johns Hopkins Press, Baltimore.

The names and dates of the origin of many periodicals can generally be found in *The Surgeon General's Index Catalogue of the Library,* supplementary volume to the first series (if before 1895); and in the second series under the heading: *Periodicals.*

CHAPTER I

The orientation of medical history in recent times and from different points of view has been discussed by many authors. Among them I should like to refer to H. E. SIGERIST, *B.H.M.,* 15:1, 1944. See also G. SARTON: The Problem of History of Medicine versus History of Art, *B.H.M.,* 10, 1941; G. ROSEN: Disease and Social Criticism, *B.H.M.,* 10, 1941; and B. ASCHNER: The Utilaristic Approach to the History of Medicine, *B.H.M.,* 13:3, 1943. See also this Bibliography, Ch. XXI, Sect. XXIV.

CHAPTER II

The literature on PRIMITIVE MEDICINE is very extensive, and in recent times many contributions have been made to it by leading anthropologists and psychoanalysts, among whom are S. FREUD, P. FEDERN, and E. ROHEIM. Exhaustive studies about primitive medicine have been published by E. H. ACKERKNECHT: Primitive Medicine and Culture Pattern, *B.H.M.,* 11 and 12, 1942; also: Psychopathology, Primitive Medicine and Primitive Culture in *B.H.M.,* 14, 1943. Important notices on the evolution of MAGIC MEDICINE are to be found in the excellent work of Sir J. G. FRAZER: *The Golden Bough* (3rd ed., London, Macmillan, 1910–15). The most important source for the history of magic and its relation to science is the works of LYNN THORNDIKE, especially his extensive study: *A History of Magic and Experimental Science* (New York, Macmillan, 1929–41); the richness of its original contributions and of the bibliography makes this book an indispensable reference work. A readable, interesting book is H. W. HAGGARD: *Mystery, Magic and Medicine* (New York, Doubleday, Doran, 1933). See also: A. PAZZINI: La medicina primitiva in *Trattato Enciclopedico di Storia della Medicina* (Milano-Roma, Arte e Storia, 1941).

For the relationship between individual and collective suggestion and magic medicine see A. CASTIGLIONI: *Incantesimo e magia* (Milano, Mondadori, 1934), and *Adventures of the Mind* (New York, Knopf, 1946). For the fight against epidemics, see G. STICKER: Vorgeschichtliche Versuche der Seuchenabwehr und Seuchenausrottung (in C. J. SINGER and H. E. SIGERIST: *Essays on the History of Medicine,* Zurich, Seldwyla, 1924).

An important discussion of the psychology of primitive people is in W. M. WUNDT: *Völkerpsychologie* (Leipzig, Engelmann, 1905–12), and Sir J. LUBBOCK: *The Origin of Civilization and the Primitive Condition of Man* (London, Longmans, 1911). An excellent introduction to ANTHROPOLOGY is found in M. F. ASHLEY-MONTAGU: *Introduction to Physical Anthropology* (Springfield, Thomas, 1945).

Remarkable contributions to the history of paleopathology have been made by A. C. KLEBS: Paleopathology, in *Bull. Johns Hopkins Hospital,* 28, 1917, and by R. L. MOODIE: *Studies in Paleopathology* (Univ. of Illinois Press, 1923).

PRIMITIVE SURGERY AND TREPANATION have been dealt with by K. JAEGER: *Beiträge zur frühzeitlichen Chirurgie* (München, Kastner, 1907); T. W. PARRY: The Prehistoric Trephined Skulls of Great Britain, *Proc. Roy. Soc. Med.* (Hist. Sect.), Vol. XIV, Suppl. (London, 1921), pp. 27–42; M. BRAUNE: *Geschichte der Trepanation* (Berlin, 1875); J. LUCAS-CHAMPIONNIÈRE: *Les Origines de la trépanation décompressive* (Paris, Steinheil,

1912); L. Manouvrier: Le T sincipital; curieuse mutilation néolithique, *Bull. soc. d'anthrop. de Paris*, 4 sér., 6–257, 1895; and *Rev. mens. de l'école d'anthrop. de Paris*, 13–431, 1903. See also: M. F. Ashley-Montagu: The Origin of Subincision in Australia, in *Oceania*, Vol. VIII, (1937); J. Busacchi: La trapanazione del cranio nei popoli preistorici (neolitici e precolumbiani) e nei primitivi moderni, *B.I.S.I.*, 2 ser., 1–65, 1935.

For the conception of BIRTH among the primitives see M. F. Ashley-Montagu: *Coming into Being among the Australian Aborigines* (New York, 1938), pp. 299 et seq., and Physiology and the Origins of the Menstrual Prohibitions, *Quart. Rev. Biol.*, 15, 1940.

A remarkable contribution on PRIMITIVE MEDICINE has been made by a series of essays by J. Wright: The Medicine of Primitive Man, *Medical Life*, 31:483, 1924; 32:137, 181, 237, and 316, 1925; see also: W. R. Dawson: *Magician and Leech, a Study of the Beginnings of Medicine* (London, 1929); and D. Mackenzie: *The Infancy of Medicine* (London, 1927).

The medicine of the AMERICAN INDIANS has been studied by J. L. Maddox: *The Medicine Man, a Sociological Study on the Character and Evolution of Shamanism* (New York, 1923); and N. E. Stone: *Medicine among the American Indians* (Clio Medica) (New York, Hoeber, 1932).

For PERUVIAN MEDICINE there is an attractive survey in J. F. Lastres: Medicina Aborigen Peruana, *B.H.M.*, Suppl. 3, 1944.

For primitive medicine in other areas see D. M. Spencer: *Disease, Religion and Society in the Fiji Islands* (New York, 1943), and G. W. Harley: *Native African Medicine* (Harvard University Press, 1941).

CHAPTER III

The most exhaustive study of ASSYRO-BABYLONIAN MEDICINE is B. Meissner: *Assyrien und Babylonien* (2 vols., Heidelberg, 1920–5); for the Code of HAMMURABI see: *The Oldest Code of Laws*, trans. by C. H. W. Jones (Edinburgh, Clark, 1926), and R. F. Harper: *The Code of Hammurabi, King of Babylon* (2nd ed., Chicago, 1904). The studies of von Oefele: Babylonian Titles of Medical Textbooks, *J. Am. Oriental Soc.* 37:250, 1917, Keilschriftmedizin, Abhandl. z. Gesch. d. Med., Heft 3 (Breslau, Korn, 1902); Materialien zur Bearbeitung der babylonischen Medizin (ibid., 1902), are important. The books of R. C. Thompson: *Devils and the Evil Spirits of Babylonia* (London, Luzac, 1903), *Assyrian Herbals* (London, Luzac, 1924), and *Chemistry of the Ancient Assyrians* (London, Luzac, 1925); and of L. W. King: *Babylonian Magic and Sorcery* (London, 1896), give much original information about magic and empiric medicine. See also an excellent survey by O. Temkin: Egyptian and Babylonian Medicine, *B.H.M.*, 4: 1936. For readers interested in a further knowledge of this period, the following books may be referred to: A. Boissier: *Choix de textes relatif à la divination assyrobabylonienne* (Genève, Kundig, 1905), and *Mantique babylonienne et mantique hittite* (Paris, 1935); G. Contenau: *La Médecine en Assyrie et en Babylonie*, pp. 227 ff. (Paris, Maloine, 1938); C. Fossey: *La Magie assyrienne* (Paris, Leroux, 1902); G. Furlani: *L'epatoscopia babilonese, Studi e materiali delle religioni* (Roma, Bardi, 1929); M. Jastrow, Jr.: The Signs and Names for the Liver in Babylonia, *Zeits. für Assyriol.*, 20:105, 1906; F. C. H. Küchler: *Beiträge zur Kenntnis der assyrisch-babylonischen Medizin* (Leipzig, Hinrich, 1904); H. F. Lutz: A Contribution to the Knowledge of Assyro-Babylonian Medicine, *Am. J. of Semitic Lang.*, 36:67, 1919; A. T. Olmstead: *The History of Assyria*, pp. 412 ff. (New York, Scribner, 1923); K. Sudhoff: *Die Krankheiten bennu und sibtu der babyloniseh-assyrischen Rechtsurkunde*, *A.G.M.*, 4:353, 1910; L. Waterman: Assyrian Medicine in the Seventh Century B.C., *Papers of the Michigan Acad. of Science, Arts and Letters, 1924*, 4:465, 1925.

CHAPTER IV

For the history of EGYPTIAN MEDICINE an extensive bibliography has been collected by M. Goldstein: *Internationale Bibliographie der altägyptischen Medizin, 1850–1930* (Berlin-Charlottenburg, Goldstein, 1933). An important contribution to this history was written by Sir W. M. F. PETRIE: *A History of Ancient Egypt* (London, Methuen, 1924). The best book on Imhotep is J. B. HURRY: *Imhotep, the Vizier and Physician of King Zoser* (2nd rev. ed., London, Oxford Univ. Press, 1938).

For the mention of medicine in the ancient P A P Y R I, the editions of *Papyrus Brugsch Major* (Leipzig, 1873), trans. by W. WRESZINSKI (1909); of *Papyrus Ebers*, ed. by G. M. EBERS (2 vols., Leipzig, Engelmann, 1875), trans. by H. JOACHIM (Berlin, 1880); and of *Papyrus Hearst*, ed. by G. A. REISNER (Leipzig, Hinrichs, 1903; Univ. of Cal. Publ. Egypt. Archeol., Vol. I), are indispensable as source material. Especially important is the work of J. H. BREASTED: *The Edwin Smith Surgical Papyrus*, with a scholarly introduction and an excellent facsimile reproduction of the original (2 vols., Chicago Univ. Press, 1930). For hieratic and demotic papyri, see F. L. GRIFFITH: *The Petrie Papyri, Hieratic Papyri from Kahun and Gurob* (2 vols., London, Quaritch, 1898), and F. L. GRIFFITH and H. THOMPSON: *The Demotic Magic Papyrus of London and Leiden* (3 vols., London, Grevel, 1904–9); also B. PEYRON: *Papiri greci del Museo Britannico di Londra e della Biblioteca Vaticana, Atti d. R. Acc. delle Scienze di Torino*, Ser. 2, 3:1, 1841. PROSPERUS ALPINUS: *De Medicina Aegyptorum* (Venetiis, F. de Franciscis, 1591), contains some remarkable observations by a great pharmacologist of the Renaissance who sojourned for a long time in Egypt.

Other aspects of Egyptian medicine have been discussed in the following works: E. VON BLOCH: *Die medizinischen Gottheiten der Aegypter, A.G.M.*, 4:315; W. R. DAWSON: *The Beginnings — Egypt and Assyria* (Clio Medica) (New York, Hoeber, 1930). See also: E. M. GUEST: *Ancient Egyptian Physicians, B.M.J.*, 1:706, 1926; E. HAGEMANN: *Zur Hygiene der alten Aegypter, Janus*, 9:214, 1904; J. G. DE LINT: *Beitrag zur Kenntnis der anatomischen Namen im alten Aegypten, A.G.M.*, 25:382, 1932; Sir M. A. RUFFER: *Studies in the Paleopathology of Egypt, J. Path. and Bact.*, 18:149, 1913–14; G. E. SMITH: *The Most Ancient Splints, B.M.J.*, 1:732, 1908; G. E. SMITH and W. R. DAWSON: *Egyptian Mummies* (New York, Dial Press, 1924).

On H E A L I N G G O D S, see W. A. JAYNE: *The Healing Gods of Ancient Civilizations* (New Haven, Yale Univ. Press, 1925).

CHAPTER V

The most exhaustive treatise on the history of J E W I S H M E D I C I N E is J. PREUSS: *Biblisch-Talmudische Medizin* (3rd ed., Berlin, Karger, 1923), which is today the most authoritative work on this subject. The history of Jewish hygiene has been dealt with accurately by M. GRUEN, ed.: *Hygiene der Juden (mit Bibliographie)* (Dresden, 1911). For Talmudic medicine see J. KATZENELSON: *Talmud und Medizin* (Berlin, 1928). Mystic medicine of the Cabalists has been studied by K. PREIS: *Die Medizin in der Kabbala* (Frankfurt, Kauffman, 1928).

An important contribution to the history of J E W I S H P H Y S I C I A N S has been made by H. FRIEDENWALD: *The Jews and Medicine* (2 vols., Baltimore, Johns Hopkins Press, 1944), in which the author examines the work and the lives of great scholars, translators, and research workers. See also H. ROSIN: *Die Juden in der Medizin* (Berlin, 1926), and I. MÜNZ: *Die Jüdischen Aerzte im Mittelalter* (Frankfurt, 1922). The development of ancient Jewish medicine is summarized in M. D. GORDON: *Medicine among the Ancient Hebrews*, in *Isis*, 33:4, 1941.

For the history of C I R C U M C I S I O N see J. ALMKVIST: *Zur Geschichte der Circumcision, Janus*, 30:86, 152, 1926, and D. SHAPIRO: *La Péritomie, étude générale et particulière, Janus*, 27:161, 241, 259, 1923; 28:120, 193, 1924. On the conception of P A T H O L O G Y see A. LODS: *Les Idées israélites sur la maladie, ses causes et ses remèdes* (Marte-Festschrift), Giessen, 1925. The prevention of contagious diseases has been studied by E. W. G. MASTERMAN: *Hygiene and Diseases in Palestine in Modern and Biblical Times, Quarterly Statement of Palestine Exploration Foundation* (London, 1918–19). Among the older historians whose works deserve to be consulted are T. BARTHOLINUS: *De morbis biblicis miscellanea medica* (Francofurti, Paulus, 1672), and R. MEAD: *Medica sacra* (London, Brindley, 1749). Other subjects in Jewish medicine have been treated by L. W. KOTELMANN, JR.: *Die Ophthalmologie bei den alten Hebräern* (Hamburg u. Leipzig, Voss, 1910); M. NEUBURGER: *Die Medizin in Flavius Josephus* (Reichenhall, "Buchkunst," 1919); L.. VENEZIANER: *Asaf Judæus* (2 vols., Strassburg, Trübner, 1916–17). On plague see O. NEUSTAETTER: Where did the Identification of the Philistine Plague as Bubonic Plague Originate? *B.H.M.*, 11:36, 1942.

The history of RITUAL FOOD regulations among the Hebrews has been studied by S. I. LEVIN and E. A. BOYDEN: *The Kosher Code of the Orthodox Jews* (Minneapolis Press, 1914).

CHAPTER VI

PERSIAN MEDICINE has been diligently studied by F. H. GARRISON: Persian Medicine and Medicine in Persia, *B.H.M.*, 1:4, 1933, and A. FONAHN: *Zur Quellenkunde der persischen Medizin* (Leipzig, Barth, 1910). Many passages dealing with medicine may be found in the work of the poet FIRDAUSI (Abu al Kasim ibn Sharaf Shah): *Shah Nameh*, trans. by A. G. WARNER and E. WARNER (9 vols., London, 1905–25, Trübner's Oriental Series).

The history of INDIAN MEDICINE has been treated by a number of Hindu authors, among whom are: Sir BHAGAVAT SINH JEE: *A Short History of Aryan Medical Science* (London, Macmillan, 1896); MUKHOPADHYANA (BHIZAGACARYA) GIRINDRANATH: *History of Indian Medicine* (3 vols., Univ. of Calcutta, 1923–9); and D. C. MUTHU: *The Antiquity of Hindu Medicine and Civilization* (3rd ed., New York, Hoeber, 1931). A remarkable contribution is that of J. JOLLY: *Medizin*, in *Grundriss der Indo-Arischen Philol. und Altertumskunde*, 3:10 (Strassburg, Trübner, 1901), and S. N. DASGUPTA: Die Medizin der alten Hindus, trans. by I. FISHER, *A.G.M.*, 20:80, 1928; also I. BLACK in PUSCHMANN's *Handbuch*, Vol. I, pp. 119–52 (Jena, 1901).

For MAGIC MEDICINE of the Hindus see W. A. JAYNE: *The Medical Gods of Ancient India* (Oxford, Clarendon Press, 1907). For the influence of the ancient traditions and laws on the development of Indian medicine an important source is *Institutes of Vishnu*, trans. by J. JOLLY (*Sacred Books of the East*, Vol. VII, Oxford, Clarendon Press, 1880), and the *Laws of Vishnu*, trans. and edited with comm. by I. G. BUEHLER (Oxford, Clarendon Press, 1886).

The fundamental sources of INDIAN MEDICINE are the *Atharva-Veda Samhita*, 2 vols. trans. with comm. by W. D. WHITNEY, ed. by C. R. LANMAN (Harvard Oriental Studies, v. 7–80, Cambridge, Mass., 1905), and *The Bower Manuscript*, ed. by A. F. R. HOERNLE (Calcutta, Government Press, 1893–1912).

For the original TEXTS consult *Charaka-Samhita* (collected works), English trans. by ABINASH CHANDRA KAVIRANTA (Calcutta, Dass, 1890); *Susruta-Samhita*, Latin trans. by HAESLER (1844); English trans. by A. F. R. HOERNLE (Calcutta, 1897); and by B. M. KUNJA-LAL (Calcutta, 1907–16); and *Vagbhata*, ed. by KUNTZ (Bombay, 1880).

The history and chronology of Indian medicine are presented by L. HELGENBERG and W. KERFEL: *Vagbhata's Astangah Raayasamhita* (German trans., Leiden, 1941), and NATH RAY DHIRENDRA: *The Principle of Tridosa in Ayurveda* (Sanskrit and English, Calcutta, 1937). For medical relief in southern India and the contribution of King Asoka see the paper of D. P. V. DEDDY, *B.H.M.*, 11, 1941. Much important information about ancient Indian medicine is to be found in A. F. R. HOERNLE: *Studies in the Medicine of Ancient India* (Oxford, Clarendon Press, 1907).

For single branches of Hindu medicine see U. C. DUTT: *Materia Medica of the Hindus* (Calcutta, Thacker, Spink & Co., 1877); A. ESSER: Beiträge zur Geschichte der altindischen Augenheilkunde, *Klin. Monatsbl. für Augenhlk.*, 80:254, 1928; R. H. ELLIOTT: The Indian Operation of Couching for Cataract, *B.M.J.*, 1:334, 1917 (also in *Lancet*, 1:361, 1917); and B. M. KUNJA-LAL: *The Surgical Instruments of the Hindus* (Calcutta, 1913).

CHAPTER VII

The most complete history of CHINESE MEDICINE is CHI-MIN WANG and LIEN-TÊ WU: *History of Chinese Medicine* (2nd ed., Shanghai, National Quarantine Service, 1936). The authors deal with Chinese medical history from the earliest times, beginning with magic medicine, plantlore, and folk medicine, and continuing up to the present day, taking into consideration the influence of Western medicine in China. A brief history, with a clear outline of the most important facts, is W. R. MORSE: *Chinese Medicine* (Clio Medica) (New York, Hoeber, 1934). See also C. GRUENHAGEN: Die Grundlagen der chinesischen Medizin, *Janus*, 13:1, 121, 191, 268, 328, 1908; C. GUETZLAFF: Medical Art among the Chinese, *J. Royal Asiatic Society*, 4:154, 1837, and A. BORDIER: La Médecine chez les Chinois, *Gaz. hébd. de méd.*, 2 sér., 9:833, 839, 1872; 10:1, 71, 678, 1873. On Chinese anatomy: *Anatomie mandchoue*, facsimile, ed. by V. MADSEN, trans. by V. THOMSEN (Copenhagen, 1928); W. COHN: Anatomie in China, *Deut. med. Woch.*, 25:496, 1899; and E. V. COWDRY: Taoist Ideas of Human Anatomy, *A.H.M.*, 3:301, 1926. A Chinese text on obstetrics, *Shou-Shi-Pen*, has been translated into German and published (Vienna, 1933) by F. HUEBOTTER, who also wrote a *Guide through Chinese Medical Writings* (Kumamoto, 1924).

The history of JAPANESE MEDICINE has been dealt with by Y. FUJIKAWA: *Medical Science in Japan* (Tokyo, 1912), and *Japanese Medicine*, English trans. by J. RUHRÄH (Clio Medica) (New York, Hoeber, 1934). These books show the influence of Chinese and later of Portuguese and Dutch medicine. On the same subject see L. ARDOUIN: *Aperçu sur l'histoire de la médecine en Japon* (Paris, 1884), and MONTEIRO: *De l'influence portugaise au Japon* (Lisbon, 1934). The history of Japanese ophthalmology has been treated by K. OGAWA: *History of Japanese Ophthalmology* (Tokyo, 1904).

CHAPTER VIII

The history of PRE-HIPPOCRATIC MEDICINE has been dealt with by C. V. DAREMBERG: *État de la médecine entre Homère et Hippocrate* (Paris, Didier, 1869), and *La Médecine dans Homère* (Paris, Didier, 1865); also Q. CELLI: *La medicina greca nelle tradizioni mitologiche e omeriche* (Roma, Casa ed. L. da Vinci, 1923). On Homeric medicine see H. FROELICH: *Die Militärmedizin Homers* (Stuttgart, Enke, 1879); O. KOERNER: *Die ärztlichen Kenntnisse in Ilias und Odyssee* (München, Bergmann, 1929), and *Wesen und Wert der Homerischen Heilkunde* (Wiesbaden, Bergmann, 1904).

On the cult and temples of ASCLEPIOS, see T. WEIGAND: *Bericht über die Ausgrabungen in Pergamon, 1927* (Berlin, 1928; repr. *Abhandl. der preuss. Akad. d. Wissensch.*, 1928, Phil.-hist. Klasse, nr. 3); *Zweiter Bericht, 1928–1932: Das Asklepieion* (Berlin, 1932; repr. *Abhandl. der preuss. Akad. d. Wissensch.*, 1932, Phil.-hist. Klasse, nr. 5). The best documented works on the subject are L. EDELSTEIN: Greek Medicine in Its Relation to Religion and Magic, *B.H.M.*, 5, 1937, and R. HERZOG: *Die Wunderheilungen von Epidauros* (Leipzig, Dieterich, 1931). E. J. EDELSTEIN and L. EDELSTEIN have collected in their excellent work: *Asclepius, a Collection and Interpretation of the Testimonies* (2 v., Baltimore, Johns Hopkins Press, 1946) all the documents concerning the myth of Asclepius, with a careful study of all the references.

On MAGIC MEDICINE: W. PATER: Dionysius Unveiled and Hippolytus Unveiled in *Greek Studies* (London, Macmillan, 1895).

For EARLY TEXTS see EMPEDOCLES: The Fragments, trans. by W. W. LEONARD, in the *Monist*, Chicago, 1907–17; H. DIELS: *Die Fragmente der Vorsokratiker* (3 vols., Berlin, Weidmann, 1922); and *Die Handschriften der antiken Aerzte* (in Auftrage der akad. Kommission, 2 vols., Berlin, 1905–6).

On the GRECO-ITALIC SCHOOL: A. MIELI: *Le scuole Ionica, Pitagorica ed Eleatica* (I prearistotelici) (Firenze, Libr. d. Voce, 1916); E. BODRERO: *Il principio fondamentale del sistema di Empedocle* (Roma, 1905); and *Eraclito, testimonianze e frammenti* (Torino, 1910).

CHAPTER IX

The history of GREEK MEDICINE has been dealt with in many historical books on the evolution of thought and science in Hellas. For a short history of the medical evolution see C. SINGER: *Greek Biology and Greek Medicine* (Oxford, Clarendon Press, 1922); R. FUCHS: Geschichte der Heilkunde bei den Griechen, in Puschmann's (Neuburger-Pagel)

Handbuch der Gesch. d. Med. (Jena, 1902). The schools of COS and CNIDUS have been the subject of many important studies, such as K. SUDHOFF: *Kos and Knidos* (München, Münchner Drucke, 1927). Some discoveries in Rhodes and Kos have been illustrated by G. JACOPI and L. LAURENTI: Monumenti di scultura del museo archeologico di Rodi e dell'Antiquarium di Cos, *Clara Rhodos*, Vol. V (1932).

HIPPOCRATES. Among a great number of BIOGRAPHIES of Hippocrates a good recent one is: H. R. MUCH: *Hippokrates der Grosse* (Stuttgart u. Berlin, Hippokrates Verlag, 1926). A pleasant book by a young Parisian physician, G. BAISSETTE: *Hippocrate* (Paris, Graisset, 1931), in a rather novelistic form, had great popularity.

The best English translation of the TEXTS is by W. H. S. JONES and E. T. WITHINGTON: *Hippocrates* (4 vols., London, Heinmann, 1923–31); the French ed. by M. P. E. LITTRÉ: *Œuvres complètes d'Hippocrate* (10 vols., Paris, Ballière, 1839–61), is a classic fundamental reference book with a scholarly introduction and an exemplary index. There is a German translation by R. KAPFERER: *Die Werke des Hippokrates* (15 vols., Stuttgart, Hippokrates Verlag, 1934).

For the chronology and the history of the HIPPOCRATIC BOOKS see LANDSBERG: Chronology of the Hippocratic Books, *Janus*, 2:107, 1853; J. J. A. LABOULBÈNE: Histoire des livres hippocratiques, *Gaz. d. hôp. de Paris*, 54:1033, 1051, 1059, 1067, 1075, 1881, and the excellent work of C. V. DAREMBERG: *Œuvres choisies d'Hippocrate* (Paris, Labe, 1855). An interesting modern appreciation of ancient scientific achievement is to be found in the book by W. F. PETERSEN: *Hippocratic Wisdom* (Springfield, Thomas, 1946).

On ANATOMY: A. HIRSCH: *Commentatio historico-medica de collectionis Hippocraticæ anatomia* (Berlin, Hirschwald, 1864), and R. KAPFERER: Der Blutkreislauf in den hippokratischen Schriften, *Münch. med. Woch.*, 86:295, 1939.

On OPHTHALMOLOGY: see J. HIRSCHBERG: *Geschichte der Augenheilkunde* (Leipzig, Engelmann, 1898–1918); H. F. MAGNUS: Die Kenntnis der Sehstörungen bei den Griechen und Römern, *Graefe's Arch. für Ophthal.*, 23:25, 1877; M. MEYERHOF: Die Operation des Stars in der griechischen Medizin, *Die Antike*, 1932.

On Hippocratic SURGERY: J. P. E. PÉTREQUIN: *Chirurgie d'Hippocrate* (2 vols., Paris, Baillière, 1878), and T. MEYER-STEINEG: *Chirurgische Instrumente des Altertums* (Jena, 1912). On obstetrics: H. FASBENDER: *Entwicklungslehre, Geburtshilfe und Gynäkologie in den hippokratischen Schriften* (Stuttgart, Enke, 1897).

On EPILEPSY: M. WELLMANN: Die Schrift *Perì hierès nósou* des Corups Hippocraticum, *A.G.M.*, 22:290, 1929; O. TEMKIN: The Doctrine of Epilepsy in the Hippocratic Writings, *B.H.M.*, 1:277, 1933; and *The Falling Sickness* (Baltimore, Johns Hopkins Press, 1945).

Other studies that may be consulted with profit are K. G. A. BIER: *Hippokratische Studien* in Quellen und Studien zur Geschichte der Naturwissenschaften und Medizin, Bd. 3, Heft 2, pp. 1–28 (Berlin, Springer, 1932); W. H. ROSCHER: *Die Hippokratische Schrift von Siebenzaftl* (Paderborn, 1913); the brilliant paper by W. OSLER: Physic and Physicians as Depicted in Plato, in *Æquanimitas* (Philadelphia, Blakiston, 1905), pp. 45–76; and an interesting essay by H. E. SIGERIST: Notes and Comments on Hippocrates, *B.H.M.*, 2:190, 1934. A recent contribution to the subject was made by W. A. HEIDEL: *Hippocratic Medicine, Its Spirit and Method* (New York, 1941). See also A. CASTIGLIONI: The Neo-Hippocratic Tendency of Contemporary Medical Thought, *Med. Life*, March 1934.

Hippocratic thought has been cleverly analysed by J. HIRSCHBERG: *Vorlesungen über hippocratische Heilkunde* (Leipzig, Thieme, 1922), and in J. WRIGHT: *The Legacy of Greece to Galen* (New York, 1927).

For the HIPPOCRATIC OATH, see the exhaustive study of L. EDELSTEIN: *The Hippocratic Oath*, text, translation, and illustration, suppl., *B.H.M.*, 1, 1943.

The so-called bench or SCAMNUM HIPPOCRATIS, used in the treatment of fractures, has been discussed and illustrated by many authors. On this subject see H. SCHRICKER: *Die Hippokratischen Geräte zur Einrichtung von Frakturen und Luxationen* (Jena, Kämpfe, 1911).

On MEDICAL STUDIES in classic antiquity, see J. E. DRABKIN: Medical Education in Greece and Rome, *B.H.M.*, 15:341, 1944.

CHAPTER X

Post-Hippocratic medicine. On Diocles of Carystos, see W. Jaeger: *Diokles von Karystos; die griechische Medizin und die Schule des Aristotles* (Berlin, de Gruyter, 1938). On Aristotle and his contribution to medicine, see G. Peirani: *La biologia nell'opera aristotelica* (Parma, 1866); A. Platt: Aristotle on the Heart, *Studies in History and Method of Science*, ed. C. Singer, 2:521, 1921; J. Geoffroy: *L'Anatomie et la physiologie d'Aristote* (Thèse de Paris, Chapelle, 1878); and D'Arcy Thompson: *On Aristotle as a Biologist* (Oxford Univ. Press, 1913). An important contribution to the conception of public health and its development according to Aristotle is P. Kalthoff: *Das Gesundheitswesen bei Aristoteles* (Berlin u. Bonn, Dümmler, 1934).

For the Alexandrian school, important sources are C. J. Singer: *Greek Biology and Greek Medicine* (Oxford, Clarendon Press, 1922), and *The Evolution of Anatomy* (New York, Knopf, 1925); C. J. Singer, ed.: *Studies in the History and Method of Science* (2 vols., Oxford, Clarendon Press, 1917, 1921).

On Herophilus see K. F. H. Marx: *Herophilus* (Carlsruhe u. Baden, Marx, 1838). On Erasistratus see R. Fuchs: *Erasistratea, quæ in librorum memoria latent, congesta enarrantur* (Inaug. Diss. Berlin, Leipzig, Fock, 1892), and J. F. H. Hieronymus: *Diss. exhibens Erasistrati Erasistrateorumque historiam* (Jenae, Maukianis, 1790).

Concerning the accusation that Erasistratus and Herophilus performed human vivisection, see Th. Meyer-Steineg: *Die Vivisektion in der antiken Medizin*, *Intern. Monatsschrift*, 1912. For an excellent review on the work of the Alexandrian school, see G. Sarton: *Introduction to the History of Science* (Washington, 1927), Vol. III, pp. 149–60.

CHAPTER XI

On ancient Roman medicine see the chapter in C. V. Daremberg: *Histoire des sciences médicales* (Paris, Baillière, 1870), and in P. Ducati: *Etruria antica* (2 vols., Torino, Paravia, 1925). For the history of malaria a scholarly work is A. Celli: *Storia della malaria nell'Agro Romano* (Città di Castello, Soc. Leonardo da Vinci, 1925), also in *Mem. R. Accad. naz. dei Lincei.*, Cl.,d. sc. fis., mat. e nat., 6 ser., 1, 1925 (English trans. London, 1933). On malaria see also E. Marchiafava and A. Bignami: *On Summer-Autumnal Malarial Fevers*, trans. by J. H. Thompson (London, New Sydenham Soc. Pub., 1894).

For the practice of medicine in ancient Rome interesting information may be found in G. von Rittershain: *Die Heilkünstler des alten Roms und ihre bürgerliche Stellung* (Berlin, Lüderitz, 1875); on Roman military medicine, W. Haberling: *Die altrömischen Militärärzte*, *Veröffentl. a. d. Geb. d. Militär-Sanit.*, no. 42 (Berlin, Hirschwald, 1910). On the Roman physician see also H. Gossen: The Physician in Ancient Rome, *Ciba Symp.*, Vol. I, 2, 1939. Medical references in the Latin poets are to be found in E. Dupouy: *Médecine et mœurs d l'ancienne Rome d'après les poètes Latins* (Paris, Baillière, 1891; English trans. by T. C. Minor in *Lancet*, January–May 1931). The development of public health has been discussed by R. M. Briau: *L'Archiatrie romaine, ou la médecine officielle dans l'empire romain* (Paris, Masson, 1877), and M. Cardini: *L'igiene publica di Roma antica all'età imperiale* (Prato, Giachetti, 1909).

The influence of Greek medicine in Rome has been dealt with by M. Albert: *Les Médecins Grecs à Rome* (Paris, Hachette, 1894); in the brilliant book by T. C. Allbutt: *Greek Medicine in Rome* (London, Macmillan, 1921), and in an attractive way by C. J. Singer: Science under the Roman Empire in *From Magic to Science* (London, 1928).

On Asclepiades see G. F. Bianchini: *La medicina d'Asclepiade per ben curare le malattie acute* (Venezia, Pasquale, 1769); L. Choulant: Der Rath des Asklepiades, *Allg. med. Ann.*, 1824, p. 577, and A. G. M. Reynaud: *De Asclepiade Bithyno medico ac philosopho* (Paris, 1862).

On Celsus one of the classic sources is G. I. Bianconi: *Lettere sopra A. Cornelio Celso al celebre abate Girolamo Tiraboschi* (Roma, Zempel, 1779). Very exhaustive is J. Ilberg: *A. Cornelius Celsus und die Medizin in Rom* (Leipzig, Teubner, 1907). The excellent edition with German translation by E. R. KOBERT: *Aulus Cornelius Celsus über die Arznei-wissenschaft*, contains an accurate historical introduction and good commentaries. The Eng-lish translation by W. G. SPENCER: *Celsus, De Medicina* (3 vols., Loeb Classical Lib., Cambridge, Mass., Harvard Univ. Press, 1935–8), is very reliable. The sources of Celsus have been studied by M. WELLMANN: *A. Cornelius Celsus, eine Quellenuntersuchung* (Berlin, Weidmann, 1913). Further observations on Celsus' works are in D. BARDUZZI: Curiosità celsiane, *R.I.S.*, 9:454, 1918.

The OPHTHALMOLOGY of Celsus was dealt with by J. HIRSCHBERG in *Die Augen-heilkunde des Celsus, Geschichte der Augenheilkunde im Alterthum* (Leipzig, Engelmann, 1899). For Celsus as a medical historian, see A. CASTIGLIONI: Aulus Cornelius Celsus as a Historian of Medicine, *B.H.M.*, 8, 1940.

The literature on GALEN is so abundant that only the most important recent works on this subject can be cited here. The most reliable edition of the Greek and Latin texts of Galen's works is by C. G. KÜHN, forming the first 20 vols. of *Medicorum Græcorum Opera quæ extant* (Leipzig, 1821–33). For the history of Galen's life see T. MEYER-STEINEG: *Ein Tag im Leben des Galen* (Jena, Diderichs, 1913); and J. ILBERG: *Aus Galen's Praxis* (Leipzig, Teubner, 1905). For commentaries on Galen's work see L. ENGLERT: *Untersuchun-gen zu Galens Schrift Thrasybulos* (Leipzig, Barth, 1929); J. WALSH: Galen's Clashes with the Medical Sects at Rome, *Med. Life*, 35:445, 1928; T. MEYER-STEINEG: Studien zur Physi-ologie des Galenos, *A.G.M.*, 6:417, 1912–13; E. WENKEBACH: *Beiträge zur Textgeschichte der Epidemiekommentare Galens* (Teil 1, Berlin, 1928; repr. from *Abhandl. d. preuss. Akad. d. Wissensch. Phil.-Hist. Klasse*, no. 4, 1927). An important contribution to the knowledge of Galen's work has been made by the recent publication of some books preserved only in the Arabic translation, the most important among them being R. WALVER: *Galen on Medical Experience*, Arabic version with English translation and notes (London and New York, Oxford Univ. Press, 1944). This text has a considerable importance for knowledge of the empirical medical school. See also M. MEYERHOF: Autobiographische Bruchstücke Galens aus arabischen Quellen, *A.G.M.*, 22:72, 1929, and *Über echte und unechte Schriften Galens nach arabischen Quellen* (Berlin, De Gruyter, 1928; repr. *Sitz.-Ber. d. preuss. Akad. d. Wissensch. Phil.-Hist. Klasse*, no. 28). These two papers by the most learned student of Arabic medicine illuminate the biography and bibliography of Galen with important original information. On Galen in English poetry see H. S. ROBINSON: Galen in Chaucer, Shakespeare and Jonson, *Med. Life*, 25:445, 1928.

On ARETÆUS THE CAPPADOCIAN see: *The Extant Works of Aretæus*, trans. by F. ADAMS (London, Sydenham Soc., 1860); E. J. LEOPOLD: Aretæus the Cappadocian and his contribution to Diabetes Mellitus, *A.H.M.*, 2:424, 1930.

For LUCRETIUS, the edition of W. E. LEONARD and S. B. SMITH: *T. Lucretii Cari "De rerum natura*," with introduction and commentary, is very valuable. On VITRUVIUS see C. D. LEAKE: Roman Architectural Hygiene, *A.H.M.*, 2:135, 1930.

CHAPTER XII

The history of BYZANTINE MEDICINE is dealt with in C. KRUMBACHER: *Ge-schichte der byzantinischen Literatur* (München, 1895); M. WELLMANN: *Die pneumatische Schule bis auf Archigenes in ihrer Entwickelung*, Philolog. Untersuch., Heft 14 (Berlin, Weidmann, 1895); and by Sir Clifford ALLBUTT in the *Glasgow Med. J.*, 70:321, 1913. An excellent survey of this period is R. BRUNET: *Médecine et thérapeutique Byzantines, Œuvres médicales d'Alexandre de Tralles* (2 vols., Paris, Geuthner, 1933–6); and see A. CORLIEU: *Les Médecins grecs depuis la mort de Galien jusqu'à la chute de l'empire d'Orient* (Paris, Baillière, 1885). On dietetics see E. JEANSELME: *Les Calendriers de régime à l'usage des Byzantins* (Paris, 1924), and Comment on traitait les obèses à Byzance, *B.S.F.*, 20:388, 1926. For the work of the great medical writers of this period, see the excellent English translation by F. ADAMS of *The Seven Books of Paulus Ægineta* (3 vols., London, Sydenham Soc., 1844–7).

CHRISTIAN DOGMATIC MEDICINE has been studied by S. D'IRSAY: Patristic Medicine, *A.H.M.*, 9:364, 1927.

CHAPTER XIII

The history of ARABIAN MEDICINE has been dealt with exhaustively by F. F. ARBUTHNOT: *Arabic Authors* (London, Heinemann, 1890); E. G. BROWNE: *Arabian Medicine* (Cambridge Univ. Press, 1921); G. SARTON: *Introduction to the History of Science* (Baltimore, Williams & Wilkins, 1927); in a brilliant chapter by M. MEYERHOF: Science and Medicine, *The Legacy of Islam* (Oxford, Clarendon Press, 1931), pp. 311–55. Dr. Meyerhof has made a great number of important contributions to the history of Arabic medicine. Noteworthy information on the subject may be found in C. BROCKELMANN: *Geschichte der arabischen Literatur* (2 vols., Weimar, Felber, 1898–1902), and in an excellent work by D. CAMPBELL: *Arabian Medicine and Its Influence on the Middle Ages* (2 vols., London, Kegan Paul, Trench, Trubner & Co., 1926). See also A. MIELI: *La Science arabe et son rôle dans l'évolution scientifique* (Leiden, Brill, 1939).

On AVERROES and his medical and philosophical work, a reliable source is E. RENAN: *Averroès et l'Averroisme* (Paris, Lévy, 1866). On AVICENNA: O. C. GRUNER: *A Treatise on the Canon of Medicine of Avicenna, incorporating a translation of the first book* (London, Luzac, 1930). On MAIMONIDES there is an abundant medical historical literature; see I. M. RABBINOWICZ: trans. of *Maimonides, Traité des poisons* (2nd ed., Paris, Lipschuetz, 1935), and M. MEYERHOF: *Un Glossaire de matière médicale de Maimonide* (Cairo, 1940). On ISAAC JUDÆUS (880?–932?), see S. JARCHO: Guide for Physicians (*Musar harofim*) by Isaac Judæus, trans. from Hebrew with introduction, B.H.M., 15:180, 1944. For the story of JÁBIR and his problematic personality, see J. RUSKA and P. KRAUS: *Der Zusammenbruch der Dschābir Legende* (Berlin, 1930), and P. KRAUS: *Jābir ibn Hanyan, contribution à l'histoire des idées scientifiques dans l'Islam* (2 vols., Cairo, 1942–3). This is a scholarly work with thousands of notes and an excellent bibliography, a veritable mine of information.

For Arabic OPHTHALMOLOGY a valuable source is J. HIRSCHBERG: *Die Arabischen Lehrbücher der Augenheilkunde* (repr. *Abhandl. d. kgl. preuss. Akad. d. Wissensch.*, Berlin, 1905), and Casey A. WOOD: *Memorandum Book of a Tenth-Century Oculist*, a translation of the *Tadhkirat* of ALI IBN ISA (Chicago, Northwestern Univ. Press, 1936).

For the discovery of the CIRCULATION by IBN AL-NAFÎS, a very interesting chapter in Arabic medical history, see the first publication by M. MEYERHOF: Ibn al-Nafîs (XII Cent.) and His Theory of the Lesser Circulation, *Isis*, 23:100, 1935, and *Ibn al-Nafîs und seine Theorie des Lungenkreislaufs* (Studien zur Geschichte der Naturwissenschaften und der Medizin, Vol. IV, Berlin, 1935).

An important contribution to the history of Arabic HOSPITALS was made by AHMED ISSA BEY: *Histoire des Bimaristans (hôpitaux) à l'époque islamique* (repr.: Congr. internat. d'hyg. méd. et trop., Cairo, 2:81). On Arabic medical schools see F. WUESTENFELD: *Die Academien der Araber und ihre Lehrer (Auszüge aus Ibn Schohba's Klassen)* (Göttingen, Vandenhoeck u. Ruprecht, 1837).

The great work of the TRANSLATORS who made Greek medicine familiar to the Arab world has been studied by many authors, among whom are H. FRIEDENWALD: *The Jews and Medicine* (Baltimore, Johns Hopkins Press, 1944), which contains a scholarly chapter on Moses Maimonides and exhaustive information on Jewish physicians and translators of Greek and Arabic authors. See also G. BERGSTRAESSER: *Hunain ibn Ishak und seine Schule* (Leiden, Brill, 1913). The whole subject has been studied in a masterly way by M. STEINSCHNEIDER: Die griechischen Ärzte in arabischen Übersetzungen, *Arch. f. path. Anat.*, 124:115, 1891, and in his book: *Die hebräischen Übersetzungen des Mittelalters* (Berlin, Kommissionsverl. des Bibl. Bur., 1893).

TURKISH MEDICINE was probably inherited from the Seljuk Turks, who preceded the modern Turks in Anatolia and carried on a remarkable development of medicine in the fourteenth and fifteenth centuries. In the hospital at Fatih, " there were innumerable doctors, surgeons, and oculists, up to two hundred men and women domestics." Silver probes were used by Altunizade; among the books written was a work on surgery by SERAFADDIN, and one by CELEBE on his operation for removing stones from the bladder. In 1555 a great hospital and medical school were founded at Istanbul, with special emphasis on anatomy. From the seventeenth century, Turkish medicine followed Western leads with dubious efficiency, until the overthrow of the Sultan, since which time progress has been rapid in this field. See the exhaustive studies of A. SUEHEYL: Zur Geschichte der Medizin und der Hygiene in der Türkei (in *Ciba Zeits.*, 1934), and many other valuable essays, published in the *Medico-Historical Archives of the University of Istanbul* (Turkish).

CHAPTER XIV

The history of the SCHOOL OF SALERNO has been studied first and in the most authoritative way by S. DE RENZI in his classic book: *Collectio Salernitana* (5 vols., Napoli, 1852–9). This work is still today a precious source of information and documentation. Among other works on this subject are P. GIACOSA: *Magistri Salernitani nondum editi* (Torino, Bocca, 1901), which is a signal contribution to the history of this school; P. CAPPARONI: *Magistri Salernitani nondum cogniti* (Terni, Stab. poligr. Altarocca, 1924; English, Wellcome Hist. Med. Mus., London, 1923); H. E. HANDERSON: *The School of Salerno* (New York, 1883); F. R. PACKARD: *The School of Salernum, Regimen Sanitatis Salernitanum*, English Version by Sir John Harington (New York, 1920); G. W. CORNER: The Rise of Medicine at Salerno in the Twelfth Century, *A.H.M.*, 3, 1931; and C. and D. SINGER: The Origin of the Medical School of Salerno in *Essays on the History of Medicine* (Zurich, Seldwyla, 1924). A recent exhaustive essay on Salerno, P. O. KRISTELLER: The School of Salerno, Its Development and Its Contribution to the History of Learning in *B.H.M.*, 17:2, 1945, contains an accurate original study of the documents and an important critical survey of the historical sources; the bibliography is excellent.

On SALERNITAN AUTHORS see H. E. SIGERIST: *Studien und Texte zur frühmittelalterlichen Rezeptliteratur*, Stud. z. Gesch. d. Med., Heft 13 (Leipzig, Barth, 1923); and G. CARBONELLI: *La Chirurgia di Rolando Capelluti Parmensis*, Riprod. Cod. lat., no. 1382 d. R. Bibl. Casanatense in Roma (Roma, Ist. naz. med. farmacol., 1927), a splendid facsimile reproduction of the text with Italian translation. See also H. E. SIGERIST: A Salernitan Student's Surgical Notebook, *B.H.M.*, 14:4, 1943.

Valuable contributions to the subject are D'IRSAY: The Life and Works of Gilles de Corbeil, *A.H.M.*, 7:362, 1935, and G. W. CORNER: *Anatomical Texts of the Earlier Middle Ages* (Washington, Carnegie Inst., 1927). On Benvenutus Grassus and Salernitan OPHTHALMOLOGY see N. SCALINCI: Benvenuto Grasso (o Grafeo) e l'oftalmiatria della scuola Salernitana, *R.I.S.*, 22:339, 1931, and C. A. WOOD: *Benvenutus Grassus' de Oculis* (San Francisco, Stanford Univ. Press, 1929). Karl SUDHOFF has contributed many papers on different periods and authors of the Salernitan school; see Salerno, eine mittelalterliche Heilund Lehrstelle am Tyrrhenischen Meere, *A.G.M.*, 21:43, 1929. P. CAPPARONI has published some diplomas of Salerno in *R.I.S.*, 3, 1916.

On NURSING in the Middle Ages see H. HAESER: *Geschichte christlicher Krankenpflege und Pflegerschaften* (Berlin, Hertz, 1857); and M. NUTTING and L. L. DOCK: *A History of Nursing* (4 vols., New York and London, Putnam, 1907–12).

CHRISTIAN MEDICINE OF THE MIDDLE AGES has been discussed authoritatively by Sir T. C. ALLBUTT: *Science and Medieval Thought* (London, Clay, 1901); L. C. MACKINNEY: *Early Medieval Medicine with Special Reference to France and Chartres* (Baltimore, Johns Hopkins Press, 1937); J. F. PAYNE: *English Medicine in the Anglo-Saxon Times* (Oxford, Clarendon Press, 1904); A. HARNACK: *Medizinisches aus der ältesten Kirchengeschichte* (Leipzig, 1892); P. DIEPGEN: *Die Theologie und der ärztliche Stand* (Berlin, 1922).

CHAPTER XV

I. On the CULTURAL CURRENTS of this period and the philosophic problems that arose in connection with the progress of medicine, the best reference book is G. SARTON: *Introduction to the History of Science* (3 vols., Washington, Carnegie Institution, 1931), a valuable source of biographical and bibliographical information, with a thorough appreciation of the authors and their work. A survey of the scientific currents is G. F. VON HERTZLING: *Wissenschaftliche Richtungen und philosophische Probleme im dreizehnten Jahrhundert*

(Münch. Akad. d. Wissensch., 1910). Some interesting information, with an over-evaluation of the ecclesiastical influence, however, may be found in J. J. WALSH: *The Thirteenth, Greatest of Centuries* (New York, Catholic Summer School Press, 1924), and in his *The Popes in Science* (New York, 1908). The best study on SIGER and his influence on the Italian schools is P. MANDONNET: *Siger de Brabant et l'averroisme latin au XIIIe siècle* (Friburg [Suisse], Libr. de l'univ., 1899). Noteworthy is G. F. FORT: *Medical Economy during the Middle Ages* (New York, 1883).

II. The origin and early development of the UNIVERSITIES have been dealt with by many historians. The most exhaustive work, which can be regarded as classic, is H. RASH-DALL: *The Universities of Europe in the Middle Ages*, new edition by F. M. Powicke and A. B. Emden (Oxford, Clarendon Press, 1936). It contains a well-documented history of the first universities, their laws and customs, and the life of professors and scholars. For the ancient universities, with a special regard to the French, see S. D'IRSAY: *Histoire des universités françaises et étrangères des origines à nos jours* (2 vols., Paris, Picard, 1933–5).

III. On PIETRO D'ABANO and his work, see S. FERRARI: Per la biografia e per gli scritti di Pietro d'Abano, *R. Acc. d. Lincei, Mem. cl. di sci. mor.*, stor. e fil. ser. 5, 15:69, 1918; B. NARDI: Dante e Pietro d'Abano nella evoluzione del pensiero scientifico medievale, *B.I.S.I.*, 12:65, 1932; and L. THORNDIKE: Manuscripts of the Writings of Peter of Abano, in *B.H.M.*, 15:201, 1944.

On DANTE and medicine see L. GIUFFRÈ: *Dante e le scienze mediche* (Bologna, Zanichelli, 1924); B. NARDI: Dante e Pietro d'Abano, *Nuovo giorn. dant.*, 4:1, 1920; and A. CASTIGLIONI: La medicina ai tempi e nell'opera di Dante, *A.S.S.*, 3:211, 1922.

On the BORGOGNONIS, see M. DELGAIZO: Teodorico dei Borgognoni, *Atti R. Acc. med. chir. di Nap.*, 18:91, 1894; E. PERRENON: *Die Chirurgie des Hugo von Lucca nach den Mitteilungen bei Theodorich* (Berlin, 1899); also L. KARL: Theodoric de l'ordre des prêcheurs et sa chirurgie, *B.S.F.*, 23:150, 1929; and D. GIORDANO: Sulla patria e sulla chirurgia di Frate Teodorico, in his *Scritti e discorsi* (Milano, 1930).

IV. On ANATOMICAL TEACHING in Bologna see G. MARTINOTTI: *L'insegnamento dell'anatomia in Bologna* (Bologna, 1911). Interesting notices on teachers and scholars in Bologna are to be found in G. ZACCAGNINI: *La Vita dei maestri e degli scolari nello Studio di Bologna nei secoli XIII e XIV* (Geneva, 1926). See also A CASTIGLIONI: Bologna in *Ciba Symposia*, 7:5–6, 1945. Good surveys of the beginning of anatomy are C. SINGER: *The Evolution of Anatomy* (New York, Knopf, 1925), and R. VON TOEPLY: *Studien zur Geschichte der Anatomie in Mittelalter* (Leipzig u. Wien, Deuticke, 1898). On Mondino and the other early anatomists of Bologna there are reliable notices in M. MEDICI: *Compendio Storico della scuola medica bolognese* (Bologna, 1857); see also B. VONDERLEGE: *Consilien des M. de L. aus Bologna* (Leipzig, Wurm & Koppe, 1922).

An excellent edition of anatomical texts was published by E. WICKERSHEIMER: *Anatomies de Guido de Vigevano et de Mondino di Luzzi*, critical edition with facsimile and full bibliography (Paris, Droz, 1926).

V. On MEDICAL TEACHING in France and in England some important essays have been published by E. NICAISE: *La Grande Chirurgie de Guy de Chauliac* (Paris, Alcan, 1890), and *La Chirurgie de Maître Henri de Mondeville* (Paris, Alcan, 1893). A good edition of the text with trans. is due to J. L. PAGEL: *Die Chirurgie des Heinrich von Mondeville* (Berlin, Hirschwald, 1892). On English medicine see C. BROECKX: *Traité de médecine pratique de Maître Jan Yperman* (Anvers, Buschmann, 1867); G. PARKER: *The Early History of Surgery in Great Britain* (London, Black, 1920); E. C. VAN LEERSUM: Master Jan Yperman's Cyrurgia, *Janus*, 18:197, 1913. Sir D'Arcy POWER: *De arte phisicali et de chirurgia of Master John Arderne* (London, Bale, 1922) contains an excellent summary of the work of this great surgeon.

On ROGER BACON, a complete bibliography of whom was published by LITTLE on the occasion of the seventh centenary (Oxford, 1914), see W. R. NEWBOLD: *The Cipher of Roger Bacon*, ed. by R. G. KENT (Philadelphia, Univ. of Pennsylvania Press, 1928); *The Opus Major of Roger Bacon* (Philadelphia, Univ. of Pennsylvania Press, 1928); also DE RICCI and WILSON: Census of Medieval and Renaissance Manuscripts in the United States and Canada, 2:1846, 1937. L. A. STRONG, *Science*, 101:608, 1945, credits the "Voynich" manuscript, from which the cipher was derived by Newbolt, to one Anthony Ascham (fl. 1553).

On ARNOLD OF VILLANOVA, see P. DIEPGEN: *Arnold von Villanova als Politiker und Laientheologe* (Berlin u. Leipzig, Rothschild, 1909). On A L B E R T U S M A G N U S, see A. C. A. Schneider: *Die Psychologie Alberts des Grossen* (Münster, Aschendorff, 1903); also L. Choulant: Albertus Magnus in seiner Bedeutung für die Naturwissenschaft, *Janus*, 1:127–60, 1846 (repr. Leipzig, Lorentz, 1931).

VI. The literature of the P L A G U E in the fourteenth century is very rich. The best sources for the history of this terrible epidemic are the contemporary historians. Among the medical books dealing exhaustively with the subject is the classic history by A. Corradi: *Annali delle epidemie occorse in Italia dalle prime memorie fino al 1850* (Bologna, Gamberini, 1865–80), which contains an accurate and reliable record of epidemics. Among recent books the most reliable is G. Sticker: *Abhandlungen aus der Seuchengeschichte und Seuchenlehre* (Giessen, Töpelmann, 1908–10). An important contribution to the history of pestilence and its consequences is L. Thorndike: The Blight of Pestilence on Early Modern Civilization, *Amer. Hist. Rev.*, 32:455, 1927. A complete bibliography of medical and popular treatises on plague was published by K. Sudhoff in *A.G.M.*, 4–11. See also A. C. Klebs and K. Sudhoff: *Die ersten gedruckten Pestschriften* (München, 1926), and R. Crawford: *Plague and Pestilence in Literature and Art* (London, 1944). On U g o B e n z i, see A. Castiglioni: Ugo Benzi da Siena ed il " Trattato circa la conservazione della sanitate," *R.I.S.*, 12:75, 1921, and *Il libro della pestilenza di Giovanni de Albertis da Capodistria (anno 1450)* (Bologna, Licinio Capelli, 1924).

On L E P R O S Y, see A. Hirsch in his *Handbuch der Geographischen und Historischen Pathologie* (Stuttgart, Enke, 1881); English translation from 2nd German ed. by C. Craighton (New Sydenham Soc., 1885). Important information on leper houses is found in C. Mercier: *Leper Houses and Medieval Hospitals* (Fitzpatrick lectures) (London, Lewis, 1915). See also E. Jeanselme: Comment l'Europe au moyen âge se protégea contre la lèpre, *B.S.F.*, 25:1, 1931.

On P U B L I C H E A L T H in the Middle Ages, see L. Kotelmann: *Gesundheitspflege im Mittelalter* (Hamburg u. Leipzig, Voss, 1890).

VII. On medical I N C U N A B U L A one of the best and most reliable books of reference is L. Choulant: *Handbuch der Bücherkunde für die ältere Medizin* (Leipzig, 1841; repr. München, 1926). The excellent book of A. C. Klebs: *Catalogue of Early Herbals* (Lugano, 1925), and his Incunabula scientifica et medica, in *Osiris*, IV, 1937 (repr. in *H. of M.* Series, N. Y. Ac. of Med., 1938), contain an accurate bibliography. See also A. Castiglioni: Herbs and Herbals, in *Ciba Symposia*, 5:5–6, 1943, and A. R. Arber: *Herbals, Their Origin and Evolution* (2nd ed., Cambridge Univ. Press, 1938). H. Peters: *Aus pharmazeutischer Vorzeit in Bild und Wort* (2 vols., Berlin, J. Springer, 1889–91) is richly documented. Charming reading is offered by E. S. Rhode: *The Old English Herbals* (Longmans, Green, 1922).

The Greek herbal of Dioscorides was published with trans. and notes by R. T. Gunther (Oxford Univ. Press, 1934).

Among the early herbalists should be cited R u f i n u s, a Genoese monk and scholar. His herbal, of which a unique exemplar was formerly in the possession of Lord Ashburnham, and is now in the Laurenziana, in Florence, is a handsome illuminated folio, of perhaps the early fourteenth century. It was ended by its author in 1287, and part of it is in thirteenth-century writing. Lynn Thorndike has recently published an excellent edition of this manuscript (Chicago, Univ. of Chicago Press, 1946), making thereby an outstanding contribution to the history of medieval medicine. Another little-known herbalist of the fourteenth century was B e n e d e t t o R i n i o, whose splendid illustrated manuscript is in the Marciana Library in Venice. On this herbal see E. de Toni: Il libro dei semplici di Benedetto Rinio, in *Mem. pont. acc. rom. dei Nuovi Lincei*, ser. II, 5; 171–279, 1919; VII, 275, 398, 1924; VIII, 1, 2, 3–264, 1925.

VIII. On the S U R G E R Y of the fifteenth century consult the encyclopædic work by E. J. Gurlt: *Geschichte der Chirurgie* (Berlin, Hirschwald, 1898), which contains biographical notices and summaries of the works of the most prominent surgeons of that time. For the Bolognese surgeons see M. Medici: *La Scuola di Bologna* (Bologna, 1857). For G. M. F e r r a r i d a G r a d o there is a brilliant study by A. C. Klebs (Zurich, 1924) and a valuable essay by Ferrari: *Une Chaire de médecine au XV siècle* (Thèse de Paris, 1899).

IX. A valuable collection of mediæval P R E S C R I P T I O N S, with notes and comments, is H. E. Sigerist: *Studien und Texte zur frühmittelalterlichen Rezeptliteratur. Stud. z. Gesch. d. Med.* (Leipzig, Barth, 1923). Many important notices on pharmacology and treatment in the fifteenth century are in A. BENEDICENTI: *Malati, medici e farmacisti* (2 vols., Milano, Hoepli, 1925). On balneology, see A. C. KLEBS: Balneology in the Middle Ages, *Trans. Amer. Climat. and Clin. Assn.*, 3, 2:15, 1916, and the interesting paper by G. NOVATI in *Mem. Ist. Lombardo*, ser. 11, 9, 1899.

X. For Italian P H A R M A C Y and its connection with ceramic art, see P. DORVEAUX: *Les Pots de pharmacie* (Toulouse, 1923); A. CASTIGLIONI: Apothecary Jars, *Ciba Symposia*, 6:12, 1945; W. M. MILLEKEN: "Majolica Drug Jars," *Bull. Med. Libr. Assoc.*, 32:3, 1944. The inventory of the pharmacy of S. Maria Novella in Florence was published by A. CORSINI (Florence, 1923). For the costume of the physician in the 14th century see A. CORSINI: Il costume medico d'un tempo, *Illust. med. ital.*, Genova, 2:5, 1920. A very valuable documentary contribution to the history of pharmacy is R. CIASCA: *L'arte dei medici e speziali nella storia e nel commercio fiorentino del secolo XII al XV* (Firenze, Olschki, 1927). On the early development of pharmacy see C. J. S. THOMPSON: *The Mystery and Art of the Apothecary* (London, 1929), and the excellent work by E. KREMERS and G. URDANG: *History of Pharmacy* (Philadelphia, 1940), which contains noteworthy and exhaustive information; also C. H. LA WALL: *Four Thousand Years of Pharmacy* (Philadelphia, Lippincott, 1927).

XI. The P R A C T I C E O F M E D I C I N E in the Middle Ages has been dealt with by L. CHIAPPELLI: Note storiche sull'esercizio professionale medico in Italia nell'alto medio evo, *R.I.S.*, 15:151, 1924; D. RIESMAN: *Medicine in the Middle Ages* (New York, Hoeber, 1935); J. ROGER: *La Vie médicale d'autrefois* (Paris, Baillière, 1907); and J. J. WALSH: *Medieval Medicine* (London, Black, 1920). An interesting survey of medicine in Asia at the time of Marco Polo (1254–1324) is the learned essay by L. OLSCHKI: Medical Matters in Marco Polo's Description of the World, in Suppl. *B.H.M.*, 3 (Baltimore, Johns Hopkins Press, 1944).

CHAPTER XVI

I, II. A N A T O M Y. L E O N A R D O D A V I N C I. The literature on Leonardo is very rich and his work as an anatomist has been published, studied, and commented upon by many authors. Among the most important works are: H. HOPSTOCK: Leonardo as Anatomist, in C. SINGER: *Studies in the History and Method of Science*, Vol. II (Oxford, Clarendon Press, 1921); J. P. McMURRICH: *Leonardo da Vinci, the Anatomist* (Baltimore, Williams & Wilkins, 1930); and A. C. KLEBS: Leonardo da Vinci and His Anatomical Studies, *Bull. Soc. Hist. Med. of Chi.*, 4:66, 1916. A series of remarkable essays on the anatomy of Leonardo have been published by M. HOLL in the *Arch. für Anat. und Physiologie* (Leipzig, 1905–1917). An accurate study of the first Quaderni is in A. and G. FAVARO: A proposito dei tre primi quaderni di anatomia di Leonardo da Vinci, *Atti R. Ist. Veneto d. sc., lett. ed arti*, 73:887, 1913–15. See also G. FAVARO: *Leonardo, i medici e la medicina* (Roma, Maglione e Strini, 1924); *La struttura del cuore nel quarto quaderno di Leonardo* (Venezia, 1915); *Il canone di Leonardo sulle proporzioni del corpo umano* (Venezia, 1917); *Misure e proporzione del corpo umano secondo Leonardo* (Venezia, 1918). The scientific study of the mechanics of the flight of birds was undertaken by Leonardo during his attempts to build a flying machine. The original work was published by T. SABACHNIKOFF, with notes by PIUMATI, French translation by C. RAVAISSON-MOLLIEN (Paris, 1893). The most recent work on Leonardo as anatomist is A. VALLENTIN: *Leonardo da Vinci*, trans. by E. W. DICKES (New York, Viking, 1938); on Leonardo as physiologist see L. BAUMGARTNER in *A.H.M.*, new series, 4:2.

A N D R E A S V E S A L I U S. The bio-bibliography of Vesalius has been published in the work of HARVEY CUSHING: *A Bio-Bibliography of Andreas Vesalius*, ed. by J. F. Fulton (New York, Schuman, 1943), which is the most complete source of information. A fundamental work is the biography by M. ROTH: *Andrea Vesalius Bruxellensis* (Berlin, Reimer, 1892), up to now the best book on the subject. See also F. H. GARRISON: In Defense of Vesalius, *Bull. Soc. Hist. Med. of Chicago*, 4:47, 1916; M. NEUBURGER: Vesal als Gehirnphysiolog, *Med.-chir. Zentralbl.*, 32:198, 1897; L. EDELSTEIN: Andreas Vesalius, the Humanist, *B.H.M.*, 13:1943; W.L. STRAUS, JR., and O. TEMKIN: Some Aspects of the Anatomical Material of Vesalius, *B.H.M.*, 13:1943; E. C. STREETER: Vesalius at the University of Paris, *Yale J. Biol. and Med.*, 16:1943. For the iconography of Vesalius see the exhaustive work of M. H. SPIELMANN:

Iconography of Andreas Vesalius (London, Bale, 1925). See also: A. VESALIUS: *Icones anatomicæ*. History of Medicine series of the Library of the New York Academy of Medicine, no. 3 (New York and Munich, 1934-5).

For the UNIVERSITIES and the great teachers of the Renaissance, see A. CASTIGLIONI: *The Renaissance of Medicine in Italy* (Baltimore, Johns Hopkins Press, 1934); G. FAVARO: Sull'insegnamento anatomico di G. Fabrizio (Venezia, 1921); and *Le tavole di Fabrizio* (Venezia, 1921). On the embryology of FABRICIUS a splendid work was achieved by H. B. ADELMANN: *The Embryological Treatises of Hieronymus Fabricius of Aquapendente* (Cornell Univ. Press, 1943), which contains an exhaustive biography and introduction, a facsimile and translation of the embryological treatises, important notes and commentaries, a complete bibliography, and an excellent index. The work illuminates not only the work of Fabricius but also the whole development of the study of anatomy during this period. See also K. J. FRANKLIN: Valves in the Veins, *Proc. Roy. Soc. Med.* (Sect. Med. Hist.), London, 21:1, 1927, and *De venarum ostiolis (1603) of Fabricius ab Aquapendente*, facsimile edition, with introduction, translation, and notes (Springfield and Baltimore, Thomas, 1933). On EUSTACHIUS, see G. BILANCIONI: Bartolomeo Eustacchi, in his *Veteris vestigia flammæ* (Roma, Casa L. da Vinci, 1922). On G. E. INGRASSIA see I. JACONO: Gianfilippo Ingrassia, *Riforma med.*, 40:422, 1924.

The ANATOMIC ICONOGRAPHY of the Renaissance is dealt with in a masterly manner by J. L. CHOULANT: *Geschichte und Bibliographie der anatomischen Abbildung* (Leipzig, Weigel, 1852), reprinted with preface by M. Frank (Univ. of Chicago Press, 1920). See also C. J. SINGER: *The Evolution of Anatomy* (New York, Knopf, 1925).

III. For the CIRCULATION OF THE BLOOD before Harvey, there is an abundant bibliography. The problem has been thoroughly discussed by C. SINGER: *The Discovery of the Circulation of the Blood* (Classics of Scientific Method) (London, Bell, 1922). Concerning Ibn al-Nafîs see this Bibliography for Chap. xiii. The discussion on the priority of the discovery is still alive. Some of the most important works: G. CERADINI: *La scoperta della circolazione del sangue* in his *Opere* (Milano, Hoepli, 1906); J. C. HEMMETER: The History of the Circulation of the Blood, *Bull. Johns Hopkins Hosp.*, 16:165, 1905; P. L. LADAME: *Michel Servet* (Genève, Jundig, 1912); L. L. MACKALL: Servetus Notes, in *Osler's Anniv. Vol.*, p. 767 (New York, Hoeber, 1919); and *Proc. Roy. Soc. Med.* (Sect. Med. Hist.) 17:35, 1924; H. TOLLIN: *Die Entdeckung des Blutkreislaufs durch Michel Servet* (Jena, Dufft, 1876); and G. A. WILLIAMS: Michael Servetus, Physician and Heretic, *A.H.M.*, 10:287, 1938. For CESALPINO as discoverer of the circulation see V. VIVIANI: *L'iconografia, la vita e le opere di Andrea Cesalpino* (Castiglion Fiorentino, Lovari, 1917); a sharp defence of Cesalpino's priority with rich documentation and quotations from the original is in G. ARCIERI: *La circolazione del sangue scoperta da A. Cesalpino* (Milano, Bocca, 1939; English trans., New York, 1945).

IV. The biography and bibliography of PARACELSUS have been the object of exhaustive studies, especially by K. Sudhoff and his school, and recently by H. E. Sigerist and the Johns Hopkins school. A good biography is K. SUDHOFF: *Paracelsus; ein deutsches Lebensbild aus den Tagen der Renaissance* (Meyers Kleine Handbücher) (Leipzig, 1936). See also A. M. STODDART: *The Life of Paracelsus* (London, Murray, 1911); E. SCHUBERT and K. SUDHOFF: *Paracelsus Forschungen* (Frankfurt, 1887); and J. N. STILLMAN: *Theophrastus Bombast von Hohenheim* (Chicago, 1920). The *Bibliographia Paracelsica*, published in Glasgow, 6 vols., 1877-96, contains many important contributions on Paracelsus and his writing. On the relation between the doctrines of Paracelsus and modern medicine see B. ASCHNER: Paracelsus as a Pioneer of Medical Science, *Aryan Pathol.*, 1:248, 1930, and his translation of Paracelsus' works, *Paracelsus, Sämtliche Werke* (4 vols., Jena, Fischer, 1926-32).

The literature on CARDANO is very rich. His autobiography, *De vita propria liber*, published in 1575, has often been compared with the autobiography of Cellini. It was read, admired or censured as much as the *Confessions* of J. J. Rousseau, and has been translated into English by H. MORLEY (2 vols., London, Chapman & Hall, 1854); by ANNA ROBESON BURR (Boston, Houghton Mifflin, 1909); and by JEAN STONER (New York, Dutton, 1930). An excellent biography with a rich bibliography is: I. ECKMAN: *Jerôme Cardan* (Johns Hopkins Press, 1946).

V. The history of EPIDEMICS during the Renaissance, and chiefly the history of SYPHILIS, have been made the subject of many important studies. Concerning the American origin of syphilis see I. BLOCH: *Der Ursprung der Syphilis* (2 vols., Jena, Fischer, 1901–11). The opposition to the theory of American origin was led by K. SUDHOFF: Über "mal Franzoso" in Italien in der ersten Hälfte des 15. Jahrhunderts, *Verh. d. Ges. deut. Naturf. u. Ärzte*, 83. Vers. 2. Th. pp. 136–8 (Leipzig, Vogel, 1912); *Graphische und typographische Erstlinge der Syphilisliteratur aus den Jahren 1495 und 1496* (Alte Meister der Medizin und Naturkunde, 4.) (München, Kuhn, 1912); and Der Ursprung der Syphilis, *Internat. Congr. Med.*, 1913 (London, 1914), also trans., *Bull. Soc. Med. Hist. of Chicago*, 2:15, 1917. On the same problem see also K. DOHI: Vorwort zu meiner Arbeit: Beiträge zur Geschichte der Syphilis, insbesonders in Ostasien, in *J. of Dermat. and Urol.*, 24:9, 1924; H. U. WILLIAMS: The Origin and Antiquity of Syphilis, *Arch. of Pathol.*, 13:931, 1932; The Origin of Syphilis, *Arch. of Dermat. and Syph.*, 33:783, 1936; E. B. KRUMBHAAR: A Pre-Columbian Peruvian Tibia Exhibiting Syphilitic (?) Periostitis, *A.H.M.*, 38, 1936; U. MANTEGAZZA: *La sifilide alla fine del 400 e nella prima metà del 500* (Pavia, 1933); and M. TRUFFI: La profilassi delle malattie veneree nei primi tempi dell'evo moderno, *Arch. ital. di dermat. e sif.*, 2:3, 1926. An important contribution to this subject is G. VORBERG: *Über den Ursprung der Syphilis* (Stuttgart, Püttmann, 1924). On the Haitian origin of syphilis see R. C. HOLCOMB: *Who Gave the World Syphilis? The Haitian Myth* (New York, Froben Press, 1937). See also *J. Am. Med. Assn.*, 109:156, 1937, and *Mil. Surgeon*, 84:109, 1939. On pre-Columbian syphilis in Europe, see M. GANGOLPHE: Syphilis osseuse préhistorique, *Gaz. méd. de Paris*, 83:349, 1912; P. HILDEBRAND: Syphilis im frühen Mittelalter, *Münch. med. Woch.*, 72:442, 1925; and: Beschreibung eines Falles von Syphilis Congenita durch einen französischen Humanisten des 12. Jahrhunderts, *Med. Klin.*, 20:1451, 1924. The essay of E. JEANSELME: Sur l'origine de la syphilis, *Rass. di studi sess.*, 8:57, 1928, contains case for the American origin.

For the history of the EPIDEMICS in the Renaissance the best source is A. CORRADI: *Annali delle epidemie occorse in Italia delle prime memorie sino al 1850* (6 vols., Bologna, Gamberini, e Parmeggiani, 1865–83); there is excellent summary in V. FOSSEL: *Geschichte der epidemischen Krankheiten*, in M. NEUBERGER and J. PAGEL: *Handb. d. Gesch. d. Med.*, 2:736 (Jena, Fischer, 1903). G. STICKER: *Abhandlungen der Seuchengeschichte und Seuchenlehre* (Giessen, Toepelmann, 1908–10), already cited, is rich in valuable information and has an exhaustive bibliography.

The bibliography on FRACASTORO is very rich and important. An admirable bibliography of the poem *Syphilis* is L. BAUMGARTNER and J. F. FULTON: *A Bibliography of the Poem Syphilis sive Morbus Gallicus by Girolamo Fracastoro* (New Haven, Yale Univ. Press, 1935). The book on *Contagion* was excellently translated by W. C. WRIGHT: *Hieronymi Fracastorii de contagione, libri III* (N.Y.A.M. Hist. of Med. Series, 2) (New York and London, Putnam, 1930). The brilliant paper by W. OSLER: Fracastorius, *Proc. of Charaka Club*, New York, 2:5, 1906, and a masterly study by C. and D. SINGER: The Scientific Position of Girolamo Fracastoro, *A.H.M.*, 1:1, 1917–18, should also be mentioned. See further R. MASSALONGO: Girolamo Fracastoro e la rinascenza della medicina in Italia, *Atti R. Ist. ven. di sc., lett. ed arti*, 74:1, 1914–15.

On defence against the PLAGUE, see E. MORPURGO: *Lo studio di Padova, le epidemie e i contagi durante il governo della Republica Veneta* (Padova, 1922), and the documentary study by D. GIORDANO: Difesa di Venezia contro la peste, *Arch. ital. di sci. med. colon.*, 13:575, 1932. On epidemics see also the original essay of C. F. MAYER: Mignotydea, an Undescribed Epidemiological Monograph of the Cinquecento, Suppl. *B.H.M.*, 3 (Baltimore, Johns Hopkins Press, 1944).

VI. The studies on SURGERY in the Renaissance have centred on AMBROISE PARÉ and his work. There is an excellent bibliography by JANET DOE: *A Bibliography of the Works of Ambroise Paré* (Univ. of Chicago Press, 1937). The *Œuvres complètes de M. Ambroise Paré*, translated by J. F. MALGAIGNE (3 vols., Paris, Baillière, 1840–1), contains a well-documented and very interesting historical introduction. Among recent books, F. R. PACKARD: *Life and Times of Ambroise Paré* (2nd ed., New York, Hoeber, 1926) combines a brilliant biography with important documents and good illustrations. See also S. PAGET: *Ambroise Paré and His Times* (New York and London, Putnam, 1897). A good selection may be found in D. W. SINGER: *Selections from the Works of Ambroise Paré* (London, Bale, 1924).

The most important publication on BERENGARIO is the work of V. PUTTI: *Berengario da Carpi* (Bologna, Cappelli, 1937), with exhaustive documentation, a full bibliography, and a great number of beautiful prints. It is a remarkable historical contribution to the history of surgery of the Renaissance.

On Giovanni DA VIGO see D. GIORDANO: Giovanni da Vigo, *R.I.S.*, 17:21, 1926. On ROESSLIN see D'ARCY POWER: *The Birth of Mankind or The Woman's Book, A Bibliographical Study* (London, 1927). The most important study on TAGLIACOZZI is M. GNUDI and J. P. WEBSTER: *Documenti inediti intorno alla vita di G. Tagliacozzi* (Bologna, 1935), an invaluable collection of documents and notices.

VII. For the teaching of PHARMACOLOGY and the institution of the first botanical gardens see C. FEDELI: *Un nuovo documento sul primo orto botanico Pisano, R.I.S.*, 14:177, 1923, and I. SABBATANI in *Memorie e documenti per la Storia dell'Univ. di Padova*, Vol. I (1922). On Prospero Alpino see P. CAPPARONI: Prosper Alpin, *B.S.F.*, 23:108, 1929.

VIII. The STUDY AND PRACTICE OF MEDICINE in the Renaissance has been the subject of important studies, many of them referred to in the bibliography of the Universities. On the practice of medicine in France the most valuable work is C. A. E. WICKERSHEIMER: *La Médecine et les médecins en France à l'époque de la Renaissance* (2 vols., Paris, Droz, 1936), with a brilliant description of the life of the students and teachers and a rich bibliography. On RABELAIS as physician see A. HEULHARD: *Rabelais, chirurgien* (Paris, Lemerre, 1885); A. F. LE DOUBLE: *Rabelais, anatomiste et physiologiste* (Paris, Léroux, 1899); and E. NOEL: *Rabelais, médecin, écrivain, curé, philosophe* (Paris, Becus, 1880). A good biography of LINACRE was written by Sir W. OSLER: *Thomas Linacre* (Cambridge, Univ. Press, 1908). See also M. BROD: *Reubeni, Fürst der Juden; ein Renaissance Roman* (München, 1925; English trans., New York, Knopf, 1928); and E. FLEG: *Le Juif du Pape* (Paris, Rieder, 1925), about the physician Solomon Molco, inventor of a famous universal remedy and physician of Pope Clement VII. For JOHN CAIUS, founder of Gonville and Caius College, Cambridge, see the edition of his works by E. S. ROBERTS, with a memoir of his life by John VENN (Cambridge Univ. Press, 1912).

The attitude toward psychiatry in this period can be found in G. ZILBOORG: *The Medical Man and the Witch during the Renaissance* (Baltimore, Johns Hopkins Press, 1935).

CHAPTER XVII

I. On the influence of PHILOSOPHICAL CURRENTS on the medicine of this period see J. BARTHÉLMY SAINT-HILAIRE: *Étude sur François Bacon* (Paris, 1900), and A. RIEHL: Logik und Erkenntnistheorie, in *Systematische Philosophie* (Leipzig, 1907); also J. F. FULTON: The Rise of Experimental Methods in *Yale J. of Biol. and Med.*, March 1931.

For DESCARTES the most reliable biography is that by C. ADAM, forming Vol. XII of the *Œuvres de Descartes*, ed. by C. Adam and P. Tannery (13 vols., Paris, 1897-1911), which is the best edition. Concerning the physiology of Descartes see M. FOSTER: *History of Physiology* (London, 1944), and for his psychology, see G. S. BRETT: *History of Psychology* (London, 1921).

For Galileo and his contribution to experimental medicine, see A. FAVARO: Diario del soggiorno di Galileo a Padova 1592-1610, *Memorie e doc. p. la storia d. univ. di Padova* (1921), and *Galileo e lo studio di Padova* (2 vols., Padova, 1883). The most exhaustive book on Galileo and his time is L. OLSCHKI: *Galileo Galilei und seine Zeit* (Halle, Niemeyer, 1927); see also A. CASTIGLIONI: Galileo Galilei and His Influence on the Evolution of Medical Thought, *B.H.M.*, 12:2, 1942. The history of the microscope may be found in I. FISCHER: Das erste Jahrhundert ärztlicher Mikroskopie, *Wien. klin. Woch.*, 39; 1926.

On the ACADEMIES see H. LYONS: *The Royal Society of London: 1660-1940* (Cambridge, 1944); M. ORNSTEIN: *The Role of Scientific Societies in the Seventeenth Century* (Univ. of Chicago Press, 1928); M. MAYLENDER: *Storia delle Accademie d'Italia* (5 vols., Bologna, Cappelli, 1926-30); V. ANTINORI: *Storia dell'Accademia del Cimento* (Roma, 1841).

II. On HARVEY and the discovery of the circulation much has been written. (See also this Bibliography, Chap. xvi, III.) A full bibliography has been published by G. KEYNES: *A Bibliography of the Writings of William Harvey* (Cambridge Univ. Press, 1928), and a further account of his work was published by the Royal College of Physicians in London on the occasion of the tercentenary of his book on circulation. Among the biographies the best are Sir D'ARCY POWER: *William Harvey* (London, Fischer, 1897), and R. B. H. WYATT: *William Harvey* (London, Parsons, and Boston, Small, Maynard, 1924, Roadmaker Series). A facsimile of Harvey's Paduan diploma was published by J. F. PAYNE (London, Royal College of Physicians, 1908). The best edition of Harvey's writings is R. WILLIS: *The Works of William Harvey*, English translation with a biography (London, Sydenham Soc., 1847). For Harvey and his doctrine see J. G. CURTIS: *Harvey's Views on the Use of the Circulation of the Blood* (New York, Columbia Univ. Press, 1915); M. J. P. FLOURENS: *Histoire de la découverte de la circulation du sang* (Paris, Baillière, 2nd ed., 1857); A. MALLOCH: *William Harvey* (New York, Hoeber, 1929); R. HUTCHINSON: *Harvey, the Man, His Method and His Message for Us Today* (Oxford, 1931); J. I. IZQUIERDO: *Harvey, iniciador del método experimental* (Mexico, 1936). See also W. W. HAMBURGER: Contrasting Concepts of the Heart and Circulation in Ancient and Modern Times, *B.H.M.*, 14:2, 1944. On his embryology see T. A. BILIKIEWICZ: *Die Embryologie im Zeitalter des Barock und des Rokoko* (Leipzig, Thieme, 1932); A. W. MEYER: *An Analysis of the De Generatione Animalium* (Stanford Univ. Press, and Oxford Univ. Press, 1936). See also H. R. SPENCER: *William Harvey, Obstetric Physician and Gynæcologist* (London, 1921).

The annual Harveian oration at the Royal College of Physicians in London is generally devoted to an exposition of some part of Harvey's works. Among these orations may be cited W. OSLER: The Growth of Truth (1906); A. CHAPLAIN: Medicine in the Century before Harvey (1922), and C. SINGER: Discovery of the Circulation of the Blood (1923).

III. On the ANATOMISTS of the seventeenth century and the school of Padua see D. BERTELLI: Johann Georg Wirsung, *R. Ist. veneto di scienze lettere ed arti, VII cent. d. univ. di Padova* (Venezia, 1922). On VALSALVA see G. BILANCIONI: La figure e l'opera di Valsalva, *R.I.S.*, 14:319, 1923, and P. M. DAWSON: An Historical Sketch of the Valsalva Experiment in *B.H.M.*, 14:1. On G. ASELLI and his discovery, see C. V. DAREMBERG in his *Histoire des sciences médicales*, Vol. II (Paris, Baillière, 1870); V. DUCCESCHI: I manoscritti di Gaspare Aselli, *A.S.S.*, 3:125, 1922; and V. GABBI: Aselli, Nel terzo centenario dalla scoperta dei vasi chiliferi, *R.I.S.*, 14:31, 1923. On A. SPIGELIUS see G. FAVARO: Contributo alla biografia di Adriano Spigelio, *Atti R. Ist. Veneto*, 852:213, 1925. On CASSERIUS, the best biography is that by G. STERZI: *Giulio Casserio* (Venezia, 1910). On SANTORIO see A. CASTIGLIONI: *La vita e l'opera di Santorio Santorio capodistriano* (Bologna-Trieste, Cappelli, 1920); also *Med. Life*, 38:727–86, 1931; D. GIORDANO: Santorio Santorio, *R.I.S.*, 15:227, 1924. On VAN HELMONT see E. LITTRÉ: Du système de van Helmont, *Journ. hebd. de méd.*, Paris, 6:513, 1830; F. PRESCOTT: Van Helmont on Fermentation, *Arch. für Gesch. d. Math. u. Naturw.*, 12:70, 1929; G. ROMMELLAERE: *Études sur J. B. van Helmont* (Bruxelles, Manceaux, 1868); F. STRUNZ: *Johann Baptist van Helmont* (Wien, 1907). On Franciscus SYLVIUS: Sir M. FOSTER: *Lectures on the History of Physiology* (Cambridge Univ. Press, 1901); S. E. JELLIFFE: Franciscus Sylvius, *Proc. Charaka Club*, New York, 3:14, 1910. On F. REDI: R. COLE: Redi, Francesco, physician, naturalist, poet, *A.H.M.*, 8:347, 1926; A. CORSINI: Sulla vita di Francesco Redi, *R.I.S.*, 13:86, 1922; U. VIVIANI: *Vita, opere, iconografia, vocabolario inedito delle voci aretine e libro inedito dei " Ricordi di Francesco Redi,"* 3 vols. in 2, Coll. di publ. stor. e lett. aretine, 9, 10, e 11 (Arezzo, Viviani, 1924–31).

On the ENGLISH PHYSIOLOGISTS, see the excellent bibliographies of J. F. FULTON: *A Bibliography of Two Oxford Physiologists, Richard Lower, John Mayow* (Oxford Univ. Press, 1936), and *A Bibliography of the Honourable Robert Boyle* (Oxford Univ. Press, 1932; with Addenda, 1934). An important contribution was made by F. GOTCH: *Two Oxford Physiologists* (Oxford, 1908). See also W. S. MIDDLETON: The Medical Aspect of Robert Hooke, *A.H.M.*, 9:227, 1927, and E. T. WITHINGTON: Locke as a Medical Practitioner, *Janus*, 4:393, 457, 527, 579, 1899.

On Marcello MALPIGHI and his work see Sir M. FOSTER: *Lectures in the History of Physiology* (Cambridge Univ. Press, 1901). For biographical and bibliographical information see G. ATTI: *Notizie edite ed inedite della vita e delle opere di Marcello Malpighi e di Lorenzo Bellini* (Bologna, 1847); E. FERRARIO: *Notizie biografiche intorno a Marcello Malpighi* (Milano, Tipogr. Lombardi, 1860); W. G. MACCALLUM: Marcello Malpighi, *Bull. Johns Hopkins Hosp.*, 16:275, 1905; B. W. RICHARDSON: *Marcello Malpighi* (London, Asclepiad, 1893). See also J. DONLEY: A Note on the Last Illness and the Post-mortem Examination of Malpighi, *A.H.M.*, 3:238, 1921. On the discovery of the histology of the kidneys, see J. M. HAYMAN, JR.: Malpighi's "Concerning the Structure of the Kidneys," trans. and introd., *A.H.M.*, 7:242, 1925.

IV. On SYDENHAM, his last work, *Processus Integri*, a sketch of pathology and practice, has been more often republished in England and other countries than any other of his writings. His collected works appeared in an English translation with a biography by G. R. LATHAM (2 vols., London, 1848). See also M. GREENWOOD: Sydenham as an Epidemiologist, *Proc. Roy. Soc. Med.*, London (Sect. Epid. and State Med.), 12:55, 1918–19; J. PAGEL: Zur Erinnerung an Thomas Sydenham, *Deut. med. Woch.*, 15:1068, 1889; J. F. PAYNE: Letters and Fragments of Thomas Sydenham, *Janus*, 3:4, 1898, and *Thomas Sydenham*, Masters of Medicine (New York, Longmans, Green, 1900); D. RIESMAN: *Thomas Sydenham* (New York, Hoeber, 1926); K. SUDHOFF: Thomas Sydenham, *Münch. Med. Woch.*, 71:1322, 1924. A good biography was written by Sir G. NEUMAN: *Thomas Sydenham, Clinician and Reformer of English Medicine* (London, 1924). Selected works have been published by J. D. COMRIE, with a short biography and explanatory note (London, 1922); see also the brilliant paper by L. EDELSTEIN: Sydenham and Cervantes, *B.H.M.*, Suppl. 3, 1944.

V. On the SURGERY of this period the classic book of E. J. GURLT: *Geschichte der Chirurgie* (3 vols., Berlin, Hirschwald, 1898), contains valuable information and an excellent bibliography. See also the learned essay of J. F. MALGAIGNE: Essai sur l'histoire et la philosophie de la chirurgie, *Bull. Ac. Méd.*, Paris, 1846–7. On Zambeccari and splenectomy, see the excellent paper by S. JARCHO: Giuseppe Zambeccari, a 17th-century Pioneer in Experimental Physiology, *B.H.M.*, 9:144–76, 1941.

VI. The history of the obstetrical FORCEPS was told by A. FISCHER: *Über die Anlegung der Kopfzange an den nachfolgenden Kopf* (Marburg, Friedrich, 1877).

VII. LEGAL MEDICINE. The life and work of Codronchi are described in an essay by G. MAZZINI: Battista Codronchi, *R.I.S.*, 14:310, 1923.

VIII. PHARMACOLOGY. On the history of CINCHONA, see C. R. MARKHAM: *A Memoir of the Lady Ana de Osorio, Countess of Chinchon and Vice-Queen of Peru (1629–1639)* (London, Trübner, 1874), and H. ROLLESTON: History of Cinchona and Its Therapeutics, *A.H.M.*, 3:261, 1931. The most exhaustive study of the introduction of cinchona in medicine was written by A. W. HAGGIS: Fundamental Errors in the Early History of Cinchona, *B.H.M.*, 10:3–4, 1941. He asserts that the whole story of the Countess is a legend, that she never introduced the remedy in Europe, because she died before she left the New World, and that the Vice-Regal physician, Juan de Vega, did not return to Spain and consequently neither carried a consignment of the bark nor sold it in Seville. The question of who first introduced cinchona to Europe still lacks an answer. Haggis's paper quotes in detail from many contemporary unpublished documents. A pleasant history of quinine has been written by M. L. DURAN-REYNALS: *The Fever Bark Tree* (New York, Doubleday, 1946).

IX. On B. RAMAZZINI, see A. CASTIGLIONI: B. Ramazzini, *Minerva medica*, 2:449, 1933; L. DEVOTO: Nel 200mo. anniversario della morte di Bernardino Ramazzini, *Lavoro*, 7:395, 1914; J. M. McDONALD: Ramazzini's Dissertations on Rinderpest, *B.H.M.*, 12, 3:1942. Ramazzini's work, *De morbis artificum*, has been excellently translated by W. WRIGHT (Univ. of Chicago Press, 1940). On Ramazzini as founder of industrial hygiene the best source is F. KOELSCH: *Bernardino Ramazzini, der Vater der Gewerbehygiene* (Stuttgart, Enke, 1912). See also A. MAGGIORA: In ricorrenza del II centenario della morte di B. Ramazzini, *R. Acc. di sci. lett. ed arti*, Modena, ser. 2, t. 13, 1918.

On LANCISI: A. BACCHINI: *La vita e le opere di Giovanni Maria Lancisi* (Roma, Sansaini, 1920), and E. MARCHIAFAVA et al.: Nel secondo centenario delle morte di Lancisi, *Giorn. med. milit.*, Roma, 68:543, 1920. A good account of Lancisi's cardiology is M. CALABRESI: Giovanni Maria Lancisi and "*De Subitaneis Mortibus*," *B.H.M.*, Suppl. 3, 1944.

On the PLAGUE of 1630, see J. W. S. JOHNSON: *Storia della peste avvenuta nel Borgo di Busto Arsizio 1630* (Copenhagen, Koppel, 1924), with accurate documentation. For occupational sanitary legislation in Venice, see N. SPADA: *Leggi veneziane sulle industrie chimiche* (Venezia, R. Deput. di storia patria, 1930).

X. On medical TEACHING AND PRACTICE in the seventeenth century see J. LÉVY-VALENSI: *La Médecine et les médecins français au XVII siècle* (Paris, Baillière, 1933), and M. ORNSTEIN: *The Rôle of Scientific Societies in the Seventeenth Century* (3rd ed., Univ. of Chicago Press, 1938). The history of medical JOURNALISM in France has been treated by J. J. A. LABOULBÈNE: Histoire du journalisme médical, 1679–1880, *Gaz. d. Hop.*, 53:1057,

1065, 1073, 1089, 1880; in Italy, by L. Piccioni: *Storia del giornalismo in Italia* (Torino, 1894), and A. Castiglioni: *Albori del giornalismo medico italiano* (Trieste, 1923). For the first medical journal in England, see P. Johnston-Saint: The First English Medical Journal, *Med. Press and Circ.*, 201:117, 1939.

For the physician and medical subjects in the work of REMBRANDT, there is an interesting study by J. B. De Lint: *Rembrandt* (The Hague, Kruseman, 1930).

CHAPTER XVIII

I. On the influence of GERMAN PHILOSOPHY, and especially on LEIBNITZ, reliable information may be found in H. Peters: Leibnitz als Chemiker, *Arch. für d. Gesch. d. Naturw.*, 7:85, 220, 275, 1916–17, and *Leibnitz in Naturwissenschaft und Heilkunde* (Hildesheim, Lax, 1916); and W. Wundt: *Leibnitz, zu seinem 200 jährigen Todestag* (Leipzig, 1917).

II. The work of the SYSTEMATISTS and their doctrine gave rise to a large amount of literature. Some of the most important studies on this subject are A. Lamoine: *Stahl et l'animisme* (Paris, 1858); C. Lasègue: *L'École de Halle* (Paris, Baillière, 1866); and the excellent study by R. Koch: War Georg Ernst Stahl ein selbständiger Denker? *A.G.M.*, 18:20, 1926. A good survey on Hoffmann and his works is J. H. Schulzen: Lebenslauf von F. Hoffmann, in Hoffmann's *Abhandlung von den fürnehmsten Kinderkrankheiten* (Frankfurt und Leipzig, Moeller, 1741). On W. CULLEN, the most reliable source is J. Thompson: *An Account of the Life, Lectures and Writings of William Cullen* (Edinburgh, Blackwood, 1859). A good appreciation of his work is F. Staples: Cullen, His Place in the History of the Progress of Medicine, *New York Med. J.*, 65:689, 1897.

On JOHN BROWN and the Brunonian doctrine see B. Hirschel: *Geschichte des Brown'schen Systems* (Leipzig, 1850), and H. C. Pfaff: *A Treatise on Brown's System of Medicine*, trans. by John Richardson (London, 1802). For Brown's Italian followers see S. de Renzi: *Storia della medicina in Italia* (Napoli, Filiatra Sebezio, 1845), Vol. II, 171–211.

For MESMER, there is a good biography in H. Lehmann: *Mesmerism* (Stuttgart, 1908). See also F. Podmore: *Mesmerism and Christian Science* (Philadelphia, Jacobs, 1909), and the brilliant study by S. Zweig in *Mental Healers* (New York, Viking, 1932). In recent times the doctrine of Mesmer has been the subject of careful studies by modern psychiatrists.

For Emanuel SWEDENBORG, see E. A. G. Kleen: *Swedenborg, en lefnadsskildring* (Stockholm, Sandberg, 1917); O. M. Ramstrom: *Emanuel Swedenborg's Investigations in Natural Science and the Basis for His Statements Concerning the Functions of the Brain* (Univ. of Uppsala, 1910), and the excellent contribution by M. Neuburger: Swedenborg's Beziehungen zur Gehirnphysiologie, *Wien. med. Woch.*, 41:2077, 1901. The literature on HAHNEMANN AND HOMEOPATHY is very rich. The biography by R. W. Hobhouse: *Life of Christian Samuel Hahnemann* (London, Daniel, 1933), may be cited, and R. E. Dudjeon: *Hahnemann, A Biographical Sketch* (London, 1892). See also C. T. Campbell: *Personality of Hahnemann* (Cleveland, 1892), and the brilliant paper by A. Bier: Wie sollen wir uns zu der Homoeopathie stellen? *Münich, med. Woch.*, 72:713, 773, 1925, which was passionately discussed. A recent attractive biography was written by M. Gumpert: *Hahnemann, a Medical Rebel* (New York, Fischer, 1945).

On G. RASORI and his role as physician and politician, see A. Monti: *G. Rasori nella storia della scienza e dell'idea nazionale* (Pavia, 1928); C. Pasetti: Giovanni Rasori (1766–1837), *Osp. Maggiore*, Milano, 3 ser., 6:60, 1918. The history of the doctrine of the systematists is brilliantly exposed in the book of A. Benedicenti: *Malati, medici e farmacisti* (Milan, 1925), Vol. II, Chap. xxi.

III. ANATOMISTS and PATHOLOGISTS. The life and work of JOHN and WILLIAM HUNTER were the subject of many important studies; among them are R. H. Fox: *William Hunter* (London, Lewis, 1901); Samuel D. Gross: *John Hunter and His Pupils* (Philadelphia, Blakiston, 1881); J. R. Mather: *Two Great Scotsmen, the Brothers William and John Hunter* (Glasgow, Maclehose, 1893); S. Paget: *John Hunter* (Masters of Medicine) (London, Longmans, Green, 1898); and G. C. Peachey: *A Memoir of William and John Hunter* (Plymouth, Brendon, 1924). See also J. Foot: *John Hunter* (London, Becket, 1794); D'Arcy Power: *John Hunter, a Martyr to Science* (London, Hunterian Oration, 1925). See also the Annual Hunterian Orations, as listed in the *Surgeon General's Catalogue*. Some new aspects of J. and W. Hunter have been illustrated by J. M. OPPEN-HEIMER: *Everard Home and the Destruction of the John Hunter Manuscripts* and *William Hunter and his Contemporaries* (New York, Schumann, 1946).

For MORGAGNI, see A. CORRADI: *Lettere di Lancisi a Morgagni* (Pavia, 1866); R. VIRCHOW: Morgagni und der anatomische Gedanke, *Atti d. XI cong. med. intern.*, 1:88 (Roma, 1894); F. FALK: *Die pathologische Anatomie und Physiologie des Joh. Bapt. Morgagni, 1682–1771* (Berlin, Hirschwald, 1887); J. A. STEVEN: *Morgagni to Virchow, an Epoch in the History of Medicine* (Glasgow, McDougall, 1905). A memorial volume with many important contributions was published in Siena in 1931. On D. COTUGNO, see D. PACE: Domenico Cotugno, *Riforma med.*, 40:430, 1924, and the book by A. LEVISON: *Cerebrospinal Fluid* (St. Louis). On other anatomists see G. FAVARO: Antonio Scarpa e l'università di Padova, *Illust. med. ital.*, 14:4, 1932; A. FERRANNINI: Domenico Cirillo, *Riforma med.*, 40:443, 1924; T. H. BAST: The Life and Work of Samuel Thomas von Sömmering, *A.H.M.*, 6:36, 1924.

IV. A collection of papers on A. VON HALLER was published on the occasion of the centenary of his death (Bern, 1877). See J. C. HEMMETER: Albrecht von Haller's Scientific, Literary and Poetic Activity, *Bull. Johns Hopkins Hosp.*, 19:65, 1908; H. KRONECKER: Haller Redivivus, *Mitt. d. Naturf. Ges. in Bern*, p. 203, 1902–3, and P. DIEPGEN: Albrecht von Haller und die Geschichte der Medizin, in *Sticker's Festschrift* (Berlin, Springer, 1930).

On SPALLANZANI, see J. L. ALBERT: *Éloges historiques* (Paris, Crapart, 1806); B. CUMMINS: Spallanzani, *Science Prog.*, London, 11:236, 1916; G. PIGHINI: *Viaggi ed escursioni scientifiche di L. Spallanzani* (Bologna, Cappelli, 1929), and F. PRESCOTT: Spallanzani on Spontaneous Generation and Digestion, *Proc. Roy. Soc. Med.*, London (Sect. Med. Hist.), 23:495, 1930. A brilliant biographical study appeared in P. DE KRUIF: *Microbe Hunters* (New York, 1932).

On the evolution of CHEMISTRY in the eighteenth century, see M. BERTHELOT: *La Révolution chimique, Lavoisier* (Paris, Alcan, 1890); A. E. CLARK-KENNEDY: *Stephen Hales, an 18th century Biography* (Cambridge Univ. Press, 1929); P. M. DAWSON: The Biography of Stephen Hales, *Bull. Johns Hopkins Hosp.*, 15:185, 1904; and Sir W. RAMSAY: *Life of Joseph Black* (London, Constable, 1918).

V. CLINICAL MEDICINE. The most exhaustive biography of BOERHAAVE is W. BURTON: *An Account of the Life and Writings of Hermann Boerhaave* (2nd ed., London, Lintot, 1746). An important contribution was made by E. C. VAN LEERSUM: Hermann Boerhaave, *Janus*, 23:193, 1918. See also D. SCHOUTE: *Hermann Boerhaave* (Leiden, 1938). On the occasion of the second centenary of his death a collection of important papers was published under the title: *Memorialia Hermanni Boerhaavi optimi medici* (Haarlem, Bohn, 1939).

On Van Swieten and the VIENNESE SCHOOL the best sources of information are V. KREUZINGER: Zum 150. Todestage Gerhard van Swieten's, *Janus*, 26:177, 1922; E. LEYDEN: Van Swieten und die moderne Klinik, *Verh. d. Ges. deut. Naturf. u. Ärzte*, 66:31, 1894; M. NEUBURGER: Die Versammlungen deutscher Naturforscher und Ärzte in Wien, *Wien. med. Woch.*, 63:2455, 1913; and Anton de Haen als Experimentalforscher, *Wien. med. Presse*, 39:1669, 1898; also *Die Entwicklung der Medizin in Österreich* (Wien und Leipzig, Fromme, 1918). See also H. LEBERT: *Über den Einfluss der Wiener medizinischen Schule des 18ten Jahrhunderts* (Berlin, Hirschwald, 1865).

On AUENBRUGGER, see J. J. WALSH: Auenbrugger, Inventor of Percussion, in *Makers of Modern Medicine* (New York, Fordham Univ. Press, 1907); B. PINCHERLE: Giovanni Malfatti medico di Beethoven e del Duca di Reichstadt, *B.I.S.I.*, 30:30, 1931. On Heberden, see L. CRUMMER: *An Introduction to the Study of Physic by William Heberden* (New York, Hoeber, 1929). On Lettsom see J. J. ABRAHAM: *Lettsom* (London, Heinemann, 1933). Much has been written on Benjamin Rush. A good biography is N. J. GOODMAN: *Benjamin Rush, Physician and Citizen* (Philadelphia, Univ. of Penn. Press, 1934); see also Benjamin Rush number of *Medical Life*, New York, 1929. An important contribution to the biography and bibliography of Rush is G. GMINDER: An Exhibit on the Life and Works of Benjamin Rush, M.D., *B.H.M.*, 19:1, 1946. There is a brilliant chapter on American medicine in W. MAC-MICHAEL: *The Gold-headed Cane*, ed. by W. Munk (London, Murray, 1827; New York, Froben Press, 1932).

For the history of PELLAGRA, the first description was in G. CASAL: *Historia natu-ral y medical del Principado de Asturias* (Madrid, Marsing, 1762), pp. 337–46. Consult also C. L. FARINI: *Sulla pellagra* (Bologna, Nobili, 1839), and G. STRAMBIO: *La pellagra, i pel-lagrologi e la amministrazioni pubbliche; saggi di storia e di critica sanitaria* (Milano, 1790).

Concerning the history of PEDIATRICS, Dr. Ernest CAULFIELD of Hartford, Conn., has written such entertaining essays as: *The Infant Welfare Movement in the Eight-eenth Century* (New York, Hoeber, 1931), *A True History of the Throat Distemper* (New Haven, Beaumont Medical Club, 1939), and *The Hysterical Disturbances in Children during the Salem Witch Trials*. A comprehensive survey of the progress in pediatrics may be found in G. F. STILL: *The History of Pediatrics up to the Eighteenth Century* (London, Milford, 1931).

VI. SURGERY. For the history of SURGERY in this period, a good survey was given by G. FISCHER: *Chirurgie vor hundert Jahren* (Leipzig, Vogel, 1876); English trans. abstr. by G. B. VON KLEIN in *J.A.M.A.*, 28:307, 1897; 30:2, 1898. See also E. PARISET: *Histoire des membres de l'Académie Royale de médecine* (Paris, Dubois, 1850).

VII. For the history of OBSTETRICS a good source is G. BURKHARDT: *Studien sur Geschichte des Hebammenwesens*. (Leipzig, Engelmann, 1912); there is a comprehensive survey in F. LA TORRE: *L'utero attraverso i secoli* (Città di Castello, Unione arti graf., 1917); and E. S. TARNIER: *Conférences historiques faites pendant l'année 1865* (Paris, Germer-Baillière, 1866). On THOMAS YOUNG, see H. GURNEY: *Memoir of the life of Thomas Young*, with a catalogue of his works (London, Arch, 1831).

VIII. For OPHTHALMOLOGY and the operation of the cataract see VAN DUYSE: Michel Brisseau, " le Tournaisien " et le siège de la cataracte, *Arch. d'ophth.*, Paris, 37:385, 1920; M. LAIGNEL-LAVASTINE: Daviel, opérateur de la cataracte, *Aesculape*, 16:14, 1925; G. OVIO: *G. B. Morgagni nella storia dell'oculistica* (Milano, Villardi, 1923); P. PANSIER: La Pratique ophtalmologique de Daviel, *Ann. d'ocul.*, Paris, 134:338, 1905; N. SCALINCI: Antonio Maître-Jean e Michele Brisseau nella determinazione della sede anatomica della cataratta, *R.I.S.*, 12:69, 134, 1921.

IX. PSYCHIATRY and LEGAL MEDICINE. An excellent survey of the history of psychiatry is M. LAIGNEL-LAVASTINE and D. VINCHON: *Les Malades de l'esprit et leurs médecins du XVI au XIX siècles* (Paris, Maloine, 1930). On PINEL, a good biography is C. ARCHARD: Centième Anniversaire de la mort de Pinel, *Clin. et lab.*, 6:81, 1927. See also R. SÉMÉLAIGNE: *Aliénistes et philanthropes. Les Pinel et les Tuke* (Paris, Steinheil, 1912). On CHIARUGI see D. BARDUZZI: Vincenzo Chiarugi, *R.I.S.*, 12:49, 1921.

X. HYGIENE. Of J. HOWARD the best bibliography is L. BAUMGARTNER: *John Howard, a Bibliography* (Baltimore, Johns Hopkins Press, 1939). Of E. JENNER an interesting biography is F. D. DREWITT: *The Note-book of Edward Jenner* (London, Ox-ford Univ. Press, 1931). There is also a good biography by J. BARON: *The Life of Edward Jenner* (London, Colburn, 1827–8). See also the catalogue of the exhibition commemorating the centenary of his death (London, Wellcome Museum, 1923); E. BERTARELLI: *Eduardo Jenner e la scoperta della vaccinazione* (Milano, Ist. sieroterap. Milanese, 1932). On J. P. FRANK see his *Autobiography* (Wien, Schaumburg, 1892); on his outstanding accom-plishments, M. NEUBURGER: Johann Peter Frank und die Neuropathologie, *Wien. klin. Woch.*, 26:627, 1913, and F. E. F. SCHMITZ: *Die Bedeutung Johann Peter Franks für die Entwicklung der socialen Hygiene* (Berlin, Schoetz, 1917). Frank's work: *The People's Misery, Mother of Disease*, was translated and edited with an introduction by H. E. SIGERIST, *B.H.M.*, 9, 1941. On LAVOISIER see E. H. ACKERKNECHT: Metabolism and Respiration from Erasistratos to Lavoisier, *Ciba Symp.*, 6, 1944; and H. METZGER and A. MIELI: Le Rôle de Lavoisier dans l'histoire de la science, *A.S.S.*, 14, 1941.

XI. On WITHERING and the introduction of digitalis, see A. R. CUSHNY: William Withering, *Proc. Roy. Soc. Med.*, London (Sect. Hist. Med.), 8:85, 1915; L. H. RODDIS: *William Withering. The Introduction of Digitalis into Medical Practice* (New York, Hoe-ber, 1936); and the brilliant contribution by J. F. FULTON: Charles Darwin and the History of the Early Use of Digitalis, *Bull. N. Y. Ac. of Med.*, 10:8, 1934. For QUACKS AND QUACK-ERY, see A. CORSINI: *Medici ciarlatani e ciarlatani medici* (Bologna, Zanichelli, 1922).

XII. On GALVANI and his discovery the best source is O. E. J. SEYFFER: *Geschicht-liche Darstellung des Galvanismus* (Stuttgart, 1848). For JOHN MORGAN see W. S. MID-DLETON: John Morgan, Father of Medical Education in North America, *A.H.M.*, 9, 1927;

M. I. Wilburt: *John Morgan, the Founder of the First Medical School and the Originator of Pharmacies in America* (Philadelphia, 1904); J. J. Walsh: *Makers of Modern Medicine* (New York, Fordham Univ., 1907). See also B. Rush: An Account of the Late Dr. John Morgan, *Phila. J. Med. and Phys. Science*, 1:439, 1920; and A. Castiglioni: Il dott. John Morgan da Filadelfia e la sua visita a G. B. Morgagni, *Rass. clin. scient.*, 8, 1934.

An interesting historical survey of MEDICAL LIFE in this period is P. Délaunay: *La Vie médicale aux XVI, XVII et XVIII siècles* (Paris, Le François, 1935). A reliable bibliography on medical historical literature was compiled by E. Heischkel: *Die Medizinhistoriographie im XVIII. Jahrhundert* (Leyde, Brill, 1931).

To the history of AMERICAN MEDICINE in this period an excellent contribution was made with the brilliant book by J. T. Flexner: *Doctors on Horseback* (New York, Viking, 1938). The story of the Pennsylvania Hospital, the oldest independent hospital in the United States, has been written by T. G. Morton: *The History of the Pennsylvania Hospital* (Philadelphia, 1897), and F. R. Packard: *Some Account of the Pennsylvania Hospital* (Philadelphia, 1938). See also J. E. Ransom: The Beginnings of Hospitals in the United States, *B.H.M.*, 13:514–539, 1943.

On SOUTH AMERICAN colonial hospitals, see the interesting essay by C. Martínez Durán: Los Hospitales de America durante la Época Colonial, Suppl. 3, *B.H.M.* (Baltimore, Johns Hopkins Press, 1944). An important chapter of South American medicine was written by C. E. Paz Soldán: Medidas de Seguridad contra la Fiebre Amarilla durante el Virreynato del Perú, *B.H.M.*, Suppl. 3 (Baltimore, Johns Hopkins Press, 1944).

CHAPTER XIX

I. On CHARLES DARWIN's biography the best source is *Life and Letters of Darwin, Including an Autobiographical Chapter*, ed. by his son Francis Darwin (3 vols., London, 1887), and *More Letters* (2 vols., London, 1903). See also T. H. Huxley: Charles Robert Darwin, *Proc. Roy. Soc. Medicine*, I: i–xxxv, 1888; P. B. Poulton: *Darwin and His Theory of Natural Selection* (London, 1896); and V. L. Kellogg: *Darwinism Today* (London, 1906). For the philosophical consideration of Darwinism, see E. Schertel: Schelling und der Entwicklungsgedanke, *Zool. Annalen*, 4:312, 1912, and C. Siegel: *Geschichte der deutschen Naturphilosophie* (Leipzig, 1913).

On BICHAT see R. Blanchard: Sur la tombe de Bichat, *B.S.F.*, Paris, 1:261, 1902, and A. Prieur: La Maison où est mort Bichat, *B.S.F.*, 1:214, 261, 309, etc., 1902. On Charles BELL there is a complete bibliography in *Medical Classics*, October 1936, and an excellent biography by A. Pichot: *The Life and Labours of Sir Charles Bell* (London, Bentley, 1860). See also E. R. Corson: *Sir Charles Bell, the Man and His Work* (Baltimore, 1910). A survey of his anatomical work is given by Sir A. Keith: *An Address on the Position of Sir Charles Bell amongst Anatomists* (London, 1911). On J. Henle see V. Robinson: *The Life of Jacob Henle* (New York, Med. Life Press, 1921).

On the RESURRECTIONISTS, see G. Macgregor: *The History of Burke and Hare, a Fragment from the Criminal Annals of Scotland* (London, Hamilton, 1884); also J. B. Bailey: *The Diary of a Resurrectionist, 1811–1812* (London, 1896).

II. On the progress of anatomy in the ITALIAN SCHOOLS, see G. B. Grassi: *Progressi della biologia* (Roma, 1910). On the outstanding anatomists, G. Bilancioni: Alfonso Corti, *Valsalva*, I: 314, 1925; G. Brueckner: Beiträge zu einer Biographie des Marchese Alfonso Corti, *Arch. f. d. Gesch. d. Naturw.*, 5, 1913, and B. Pincherle: Contributo alla biografia di A. Corti, *Atti, VIII Congr. int. di st. d. med.* (Roma, 1930); also C. A. Torrigiani: Le osservazioni di Atto Tigri, *Valsalva*, 2, 1926; A. Vedrani: Eusebio Valli, in *Gli scienziati italiani* (Roma, 1921), and C. Fedeli: Eusebio Valli, *Riforma med.*, 41:812, 1925.

Many have been struck by the strange fact that, although the MICROSCOPE was extensively used in the seventeenth century for biological study, and was adequate to reveal minute objects like spermatozoa and red blood cells, it played no great role in biology until the first half of the nineteenth century. This was in large measure due to the following optical improvements in the objectives, which changed the inadequate compound microscope of 1800 to the relatively clear, accurate instrument of 1840: in 1807, Herman van Deyl reduced chromatic aberration by combining flint and crown glass (first tried by Chester HALL, 1733); the construction was further improved by V. and C. CHEVALIER (1825–30), who reduced refractile error by placing a layer of Canada balsam between the crown and flint glass, and diminished spherical aberration by the use of several layers of the optical glass. The IMPROVED MICROSCOPE, now truly an instrument of precision, at once began to be important in the study of the cell, and still more so when homogeneous immersion was introduced by Amici (water between lens and object in 1840, oil in 1850). Still further improvements were made by Abbe (apochromats, illuminating system, etc.), Spencer, and others; but the light microscope has not been greatly improved in the past fifty years. Greater resolution (and therefore magnification) was obtained by the use of ultraviolet light (A. Köhler, *Zts. f. Mikr*, 21, 129, 1904) on photographic films, and H. SIEDENTOPF's ultra microscope (useful for size and outline rather than detail); and much greater resolution still by the electron microscope. For theoretical aspects, see *Encyclopædia Britannica*, 11th ed., and P. HARTING: *Das Microskop* (Braunschweig, F. W. Theile, 1859). Simon H. GAGE in *The Microscope* (17 ed., 1941) has a good "Brief History of Lenses and Microscopes." See also E. F. GENUNG: The Development of the Compound Microscope, *B.H.M.*, 12:575–94, 1942.

III. PHYSIOLOGY. A brilliant biography of CLAUDE BERNARD was written by Sir Michael FOSTER: *Claude Bernard* (London, Fisher Unwin, 1899). An accurate biography is J. M. OLMSTEAD: *Claude Bernard, Physiologist* (New York, Harper, 1938). See also J. PISUÑER: *El Pensamiento vivo de Claude Bernard* (Buenos Aires, Losada, 1944), and W. RIESE: Claude Bernard in the Light of Modern Science, *B.H.M.*, 14:281–94, 1943; J. J. IZQUIERDO: *Bernard y su obra:* (Mexico, 1942). On F. MAGENDIE, see the eloquent biography by his pupil C. BERNARD: *François Magendie* (Paris, Baillière, 1856); one may also consult J. P. M. FLOURENS: *Éloge historique de François Magendie* (Paris, Garnier, 1858). A complete bibliography with a correct appreciation of his work is in J. M. OLMSTEAD: *François Magendie, Pioneer in Experimental Physiology and Scientific Medicine* (New York, Schuman's, 1944). The best biography of HELMHOLTZ is E. DU BOIS-REYMOND: *Hermann von Helmholtz* (Leipzig, Veit, 1897); another L. KÖNIGSBERGER: *Hermann von Helmholtz* (Braunschweig, Vieweg, 1902–3); English trans., F. R. WELBY (Masters of Medicine), 1906. An excellent biography of W. BEAUMONT is J. S. MYER: *Life and Letters of William Beaumont* (St. Louis, Mosby, 1912); reprinted with preface by W. OSLER, 1939). See also W. S. MILLER: *William Beaumont, M.D.* (New York, 1933). There is an excellent appreciation by Sir W. OSLER: William Beaumont, a Pioneer American Physiologist, in *J.A.M.A.*, November 12, 1902. An interesting survey of the success of Beaumont's work is G. ROSEN: *The Reception of William Beaumont's Discovery in Europe* (New York, Schuman's, 1943).

On JOHANNES MÜLLER see W. HABERLING: *Johannes Müller . . . ein rheinischer Naturforscher* (Leipzig, Akad. Verlag, 1924), and R. VIRCHOW: *Johannes Müller* (Berlin, Hirschwald, 1858). A masterly review of the history of brain physiology was made by M. NEUBURGER: *Die historische Entwicklung der experimentalen Gehirn- und Rückenmarksphysiologie vor Flourens* (Stuttgart, Enke, 1897).

IV. PATHOLOGY. On A. BASSI see G. B. GRASSI: Agostino Bassi, il procursore, *Difesa sociale*, v. 3 (Roma, 1924), and a very valuable contribution by R. H. MAJOR: Agostino Bassi and the Parasitic Theory of Diseases, in *B.H.M.*, 16:2, 1944. On R. VIRCHOW see Sir W. OSLER: *Rudolf Virchow, the Man and Student* (Boston, Damrell and Upham, 1891), and J. L. STEVEN: *Morgagni to Virchow, an Epoch in the History of Medicine* (Glasgow, MacDougall, 1905). See also W. BECHER: *Rudolf Virchow* (Berlin, Karger, 1891), and the obituaries by F. VON RECKLINGHAUSEN: Nachruf auf Rudolf Virchow, *Arch. f. path. Anat.*, 121:2, 1903, and H. W. G. WALDEYER: Gedächtnisrede auf Rudolf Virchow, *Abhandl. d. kgl. Akad. d. Wissensch.* (Berlin, 1903). A special issue of the *Berl. klin. Woch.*, 38:1033–76, 1901, contained articles by various authors on Virchow and his work on the occasion of his eightieth birthday.

V. On the FRENCH CLINICIANS see P. REIS: *Étude sur Broussais et sur son œuvre* (Paris, Anselm, 1869); H. SAINTIGNON: *Laënnec, sa vie et son œuvre* (thèse de Paris, 1904); W. S. THAYER: On Some Unpublished Letters of Laënnec, *Bull. Johns Hopkins Hosp.*, 31:425, 1920; G. B. WEBB: *René Théophile Hyacinthe Laënnec, a Memoir* (New York, Hoeber, 1928); and J. ROGER: *Les Médecins bretons du XVI au XX siècle* (Paris, Baillière, 1900). On the ENGLISH CLINICIANS: *William Stokes, His Life and Work* (autobiography)

(London, Longmans, Green, 1897); W. S. THAYER: Richard Bright, *Guy's Hosp. Rep.,* 77:253, 1927; Sir W. HALE-WHITE: Thomas Addison, *Guy's Hosp. Rep.,* 76:253-79, 1926.

The history of GUY'S HOSPITAL and its great clinicians has been well written by WILKS, SAMUEL, and BETHANY: *A Biographical History of Guy's Hospital* (London, Ward, 1892), which gives an interesting picture of the splendid development of English clinical medicine. See also B. CHANCE: Dr. Richard Bright, *A.H.M.,* 9:332, 1927. On the AMERICANS see O. JUETTNER: *Daniel Drake and His Followers* (Cincinnati, Harvey Pub. Co., 1909), and C. CALDWELL: *Autobiography* (Philadelphia, Lippincott, 1875).

On the VIENNESE SCHOOL: M. STERNBERG: *Josef Skoda* (Wien, Springer, 1924); and the excellent books by M. NEUBURGER: *Die Entwicklung der Medizin in Österreich* (Wien, Fromme, 1918); *Das alte medizinische Wien* (Wien, Perles, 1921); *Hermann Nothnagel. Leben und Wirken eines deutschen Klinikers* (Wien, Rikola, 1922).

On the ITALIAN SCHOOLS see A. FERRANNINI: M. Semmola e S. Tommasi, in *Riforma med.,* 40:439, 1924; A. GNUDI: M. Bufalini, *R.I.S.,* 17:45, 1926; A. MURRI: *Maurizio Bufalini nel cinquantenario di sua morte* (Bologna, Zanichelli, 1925).

A brilliant paper on TRUDEAU is S. CHALMERS: The Beloved Physician, Edward Livingston Trudeau, *Atlantic Monthly,* 117:87, 1916.

On the school of EDINBURGH the most important sources are: J. B. COMRIE: *A Century of Medicine in the Edinburgh School* (Newcastle, 1935), and B. BRAUNWELL: *The Edinburgh Medical School, 1865-69* (Edinburgh, 1923). See also J. BELL: *Letters on Professional Characters* (Edinburgh, Moer, 1810), and A. L. TURNER: *Sir William Turner, a Chapter in Medical History* (Edinburgh, Blackwood, 1919).

VI. SURGERY. On DUPUYTREN, see A. T. VIDAL DE CASSIS: *Essai historique sur Dupuytren* (Paris, Rouvier, 1835), and L. DELHOUME: *Dupuytren* (3rd ed., Paris, 1835). On LISTER, the most authoritative biography is by R. J. GODLEE: *Lord Lister* (London, Macmillan, 1917). An important contribution was made by G. T. WRENCH: *Lord Lister, His Life and Work* (New York, Stokes, 1913). See also St. Clair THOMSON: A House-surgeon's Memories of Joseph Lister, *A.H.M.,* 2:93, 1919; Sir C. A. BALLANCE: *The Lister Memorial Lecture* (Dundee, D. C. Thomson, 1933); W. W. FORD: *The Bacteriological Work of J. Lister* (New York, 1928); and E. L. GILCREEST: *Lord Lister and the Renaissance of Surgery* (London, 1927). A centenary volume (1827-1927) was edited for the Lister Centenary Committee of the British Medical Association by A. LOGAN TURNER (Edinburgh, Oliver and Boyd, 1927), and an interesting exhibition was prepared by the Wellcome Historical Medical Museum in London (*Catalogue,* London, 1927).

On ITALIAN SURGERY see A. CORRADI: *Della chirurgia in Italia dagli ultimi anni del secolo scorso fino al presente* (Bologna, Gamberini, 1871), and P. DE VECCHI: *Modern Italian Surgery and Old Universities of Italy* (New York, Hoeber, 1921).

Worthy contributions to the history of American surgery were written by S. D. GROSS: *Autobiography . . . with Sketches of His Contemporaries* (2 vols., edited by his sons, Philadelphia, Barrie, 1887), and Surgery, *Am. J. Med. Sci.,* 71:431, 1876.

On the history of GERMAN SURGERY at this time see A. WEINLAND: *Philipp Franz von Walther und seine Bedeutung für die deutsche Chirurgie und Augenheilkunde* (München, Wolf, 1905), and N. PIROGOFF: *Lebensfragen* (Stuttgart, Cotta, 1894).

VII. For the history of OBSTETRICS and GYNÆCOLOGY, especially in Vienna, some important contributions were made by I. FISCHER: Zur Geschichte der operativen Gynaekologie im Altertum, *Ber d. Ges. f Gynäkol. u. Geburtsh.,* 2:177, 1923-4; Die Anfänge der Gynäkologie in Wien, *Wien. klin. Woch.,* 38:601, 1925, and Die jüngere Wiener geburtshilflich-gynäkologische Schule, *Wien. med. Woch.,* 75:1279, 1926; also *Geschichte der Geburtshilfe in Wien* (Leipzig und Wien, Deuticke, 1909). For obstetrics in Italy see A. CORRADI: *Dell'ostetricia in Italia dalla metà del secolo fino al presente* (3 vols., Bologna, Gamberini, 1874), and A. G. MILLET: *De l'obstétrique en Italie* (Paris, Doin, 1882).

The life of McDowell and the history of the first OVARIOTOMY was told by M. Y. RIDENBAUGH: *The Biography of Ephraim McDowell, M.D.* (New York, Webster, 1890), including many articles relating to the subject, with letters from surgeons of different countries addressed to McDowell. See also L. S. McMURTRY: *Ephraim McDowell* (New York, 1909; repr. from *N. Y. Med. J.*).

A good general survey on the obstetrics of this period is in R. DOHRN: *Geschichte der Geburtshilfe der Neuzeit* (Tübingen, Pietzcker, 1903-4).

The autobiography of MARION SIMS, *The Story of My Life*, ed. by H. M. SIMS (New York, Appleton, 1894), contains many important dates and an interesting picture of medical life in Sims's time.

VIII. OPHTHALMOLOGY. For the work of F. C. DONDERS, the best review is that by E. CLARKE: *Problems in the Accommodation and Refraction of the Eye, a Brief Review of the Work of Donders and the Progress Made during the Last Fifty Years* (London, Baillière, 1914). See also J. MOLESCHOTT: *Franciscus Cornelius Donders* (Giessen, Roth, 1888).

The biography of GRAEFE was written by JACOBSOHN (Berlin, 1885). See also the speech by C. SCHWEIGER: *Rede zur Enthüllungsfeier des Graefe-Denkmals am 22. Mai 1882* (Berlin, 1882). On the BELGIAN SCHOOL: F. DE LAPERSONNE: Belgian Ophthalmologists, *Ophth. Congr.*, Brussels, 1925.

IX. OTO-RHINO-LARYNGOLOGY. The history of the bitter priority contest for the invention of the laryngoscope was told by B. FRANKEL: Wem gebührt die Priorität der Erfindung der Laryngoskopie? *Berl. klin. Woch.*, 43:404, 1906; T. VON GYOERY: Die historische Wahrheit in dem Prioritätsstreit Czermak-Türck, *Berl. klin. Woch.*, 43:26, 1906; and R. VON JAKSCH: Dem Andenken Wilhelm Czermaks, *Prager med. Woch.*, 31:571, 1906. On intubation see J. J. WALSH: *Makers of Modern Medicine* (New York, Fordham Univ. Press, 1907). A noteworthy contribution is the work of J. WRIGHT: *History of Laryngology and Rhinology* (Philadelphia and New York, 1914); also K. KASSEL: *Geschichte der Nasenheilkunde* (Würzburg, 1914).

X. The best contributions to the history of DERMATOLOGY and SYPHILOLOGY are: I. BLOCH: Geschichte der Hautkrankheiten in der neueren Zeit, *Handbuch der Gesch. der Medizin*, ed. by M. Neuburger and J. Pagel (Jena, Fischer, 1901–5), III, 393; and J. PROKSCH: *Die Geschichte der venerischen Krankheiten* (2 vols., Bonn, Hanstein, 1895).

XI. PSYCHIATRY and NEUROLOGY. An excellent biography and bibliography of Charcot was published in the *Revue Neurologique*, 1:6, 1925, on the occasion of his centenary (Paris,/1925). A good appreciation of his work is that by B. NAUNYN: Jean Martin Charcot, *Arch. f. exp. Path.*, 33:1, 1893. See also F. DAMRAU: *Pioneers in Neurology* (St. Louis, Dios Chem. Co., 1927).

XII. LEGAL MEDICINE. On legal medicine, see V. JANOVSKY: Die geschichtliche Entwicklung der gerichtlichen Medizin, in *Handb. der gerichtl. Med.* (Tübingen, Laupp, 1881), Vol. I.

XIII. An accurate history of THERAPEUTICS is I. FISCHER: *Zur Geschichte der Therapie* (Wien, Springer, 1925). An important contribution was made by F. C. LEONHARDI: Die Wandlungen der medizinischen Therapie in unserem Jahrhunderte, *Samml. klin. Vortr.*, n. F., 1895, no. 127. The return to the Hippocratic doctrine of the healing power of nature was masterfully dealt with by M. NEUBURGER: *Die Lehre von der Heilkraft der Natur im Wandel der Zeiten* (Stuttgart, Enke, 1926).

XIV. Good summaries of the evolution of PUBLIC HEALTH in this period were made by R. FINKELBURG: Geschichtliche Entwicklung und Organisation der öffentlichen Gesundheitspflege, in *Handb. der Hygiene*, ed. by Weyl., Vol. I (Jena, Fischer, 1893), and M. RUBNER: *Zur Vorgeschichte der modernen Hygiene* (Berlin, Francke, 1905). To the great sanitary awakening are devoted four chapters of C. E. A. WINSLOW's attractive book: *The Conquest of Epidemic Disease* (Princeton, 1943), with an excellent review of the work of Pettenkofer. See also C. VON VOIT: *Max von Pettenkofer zum Gedächtnis* (München, Roth, 1902). H. ZINSSER: *Rats, Lice and History* (Boston, Little, Brown, 1935) is a fascinating book on this subject.

On W. C. GORGAS see M. D. GORGAS and B. J. HENDRICK: *William Crawford Gorgas, His Life and Work* (New York, Doubleday, Page, 1924).

XV. On the HISTORY OF MEDICINE during this period see M. MASTORILLI: Salvatore de Renzi e l'opera sua per la storia della medicina, *R.I.S.*, 10:28, 1919; A. VENEZIANI: *La vita e l'opera di Angelo Camillo de Meis* (Bologna, Zanichelli, 1921); U. VIVIANI: Un Aretino professore di storia della medicina: Carlo Pigli, *R.I.S.*, 9:365, 1918.

Among the early historians of medicine must be cited POLYDORE VERGIL of Urbino, who came to England in 1500 as a Papal appointee to collect Peter's pence and remained there for nearly fifty years. He emerged not only as the first historian of medicine after the advent of printing, but the first widely recognized historian of England, his adopted country.

He was born at Urbino in about 1470. His *De Inventoribus Rerum Libri Tres* was published in Venice in 1499 from the press of Cristoforo de Pensis. In this book he gives the first account of the history of medicine. For his life and work see the excellent study by J. F. FULTON: Polydore Vergil, His Chapters on the History of Physick and His Anglica Historia, *B.H.M.*, Suppl. 3 (Baltimore, Johns Hopkins Press, 1944). Frédéric BÉRARD (1789-1828) wrote an interesting account of the medical school of Montpellier and its doctrine. See, for both biography and bibliography, R. DE SAUSSURE: Frédéric Bérard, historien de la médecine, *B.H.M.*, Suppl. 3 (Baltimore, Johns Hopkins Press, 1944).

For the history of VACCINATION see E. M. CROOKSHANK: *History and Pathology of Vaccination* (2 vols., London, Lewis, 1889), and A. C. KLEBS: The Historic Evolution of Variolation, *Bull. Johns Hopkins Hosp.*, 1913, 24. A valuable bibliographical essay is G. L. ANNAN: An Exhibition of Books on the History of Vaccination, Its Early Advocates and Opponents, *Bull. N. Y. Ac. of Med.*, 17:715, 1941; see also W. H. BARLOW: *A Sketch of the History of Small-pox and Vaccination* (Manchester, 1871).

CHAPTER XX

I. Introduction. Many of the historical books dealing with the history of medicine in this period are listed in the General Bibliography, C. Others will be referred to in the Bibliography of Chapter xxi. We should like to cite here L. LANDOUZY: La Médecine française en ces cinquante dernières années, *Presse méd.*, 23:185, 1915, and G. B. GRASSI: *I progressi della biologia e delle sue applicazioni pratiche conseguiti in Italia nell'ultimo cinquantennio* (Roma, 1911).

II. Excellent summaries of the history of BIOLOGY are C. J. SINGER: *A Short History of Biology* (Oxford, Clarendon Press, 1931), and J. A. THOMSON: *The Science of Life, an Outline of the History of Biology and Its Recent Advances* (Chicago, Stone, 1899). One of the most complete histories of biological doctrines is the classic work of E. RADL: *Geschichte der biologischen Theorien in der Neuzeit* (Leipzig, Engelmann, 1905-13; English trans., London, Oxford Univ. Press, 1930). See also the excellent works by E. NORDENSKIÖLD: *Geschichte der Biologie* (Jena, Fischer, 1926; English trans., New York, Knopf, 1928), and W. A. LOCY: *Biology and Its Makers* (New York, Holt, 1908). On the history of cellular pathology, see F. BOSCH: *Aus der Geschichte der Zellenlehre* (Düsseldorf, Schwann, 1910). An interesting autobiography was written by C. E. VON BAER: *Nachrichten über Leben und Schriften des C. E. von Baer, mitgetheilt von ihm selbst* (St. Petersburg, 1865; 2nd ed., Braunschweig, 1886). Many important references to the evolution of biology are given by E. HAECKEL: *Autobiographie* (Leipzig, 1921), and H. ILTIS: *Gregor Johann Mendel* (Berlin, Springer, 1924). Important notices are to be found in J. HUXLEY: *Evolution, the Modern Synthesis* (New York, Harper, 1943), and J. H. HILL: *Germs and the Man* (New York, Putnam, 1940). For the history of biology in America, see R. T. YOUNG: *Biology in America* (Boston, Badger, 1922).

III. ANATOMY. On the subject of nineteenth-century anatomy an important contribution was made by J. CHAINE: *Histoire de l'anatomie comparative* (Bordeaux, Daguerre, 1925), and G. Honigmann: *Geschichtliche Entwicklung der Medizin* (München, Lehmann, 1925). On the life and works of RAMÓN Y CAJAL, see his autobiography: *Recuerdos de mi vida* (2 vols., Madrid, Fortanet, 1901-17; English trans. by E. Horne Craigie, Philadelphia, American Philosophical Soc., 1937); J. SOBOTTA: Ramón y Cajal, *Münch. med. Woch.*, 54:579, 1907. On J. LEIDY, see H. C. Chapman: Memoir of Joseph Leidy, *Proc. Acad. of Nat. Sci. of Philadelphia*, 43:342, 1891.

IV. PHYSIOLOGY. On the life and works of the great physiologists of this period see J. B. SANDERSON: C. Ludwig and Modern Physiology, *Sci. Progress*, London, 5:1, 1896; G. ROSEN: C. Ludwig and His American Students, *B.H.M.*, 4:1, 1936; T. LEWIS: William Einthoven, *Brit. Med. J.*, 2:664, 1927; A. HERLITZKA: L'opera scientifica di Angelo Mosso, *Arch. di fisiol.*, 9:123, 1911; J. VON KRIES: *Carl Ludwig* (Leipzig, Freiburg, 1895); G. PEACOCK: Life of Thomas Young, in his *Miscellaneous Works*, Vol. I (London, Murray, 1855); R. TIGERSTEDT: *Iwan Petrowitsch Pawlow* (Institut impérial de médecine expérimentale, 1904); Y. C. BROUGHER: William Sharpey, 1802-80, *A. H. M.*, 9:124, 1927.

V. For the progress of BIOCHEMISTRY see R. H. CHITTENDEN: *The Development of Physiological Chemistry in the United States* (New York, Chemical Catalog Co., 1930).

VI. PATHOLOGY. An excellent biography of VIRCHOW is C. POSNER: *Rudolf Virchow* (Berlin, 1891; 2nd ed. Wien, Rikola, 1921). See also K. BLIND: *Personal Recollections of Virchow* (Boston, 1902); Sir W. OSLER: *Rudolf Virchow, the Man and the Student* (Boston, 1891), and the interesting paper by H. G. SCHLUMBÉRGER: Rudolf Virchow, Revolutionist, *A.H.M.*, 4:147, 1942. For the fight against MALARIA see A. CELLI-FRAENTZEL: Malaria-Bekämpfung in der römischen Campagna, *Arch. f. Schiffs- u. Tropen-Hyg.*, 29:675, 1925. On BANTI, see L. CASTALDI: Guido Banti, *Rass. internaz. di clin. e terap.*, Napoli, 6:60, 1925. A good biography of ROKITANSKI and a review of his work are F. R. MENNE: Carl Rokitanski as Pathologist, in *A.H.M.*, 7:379, 1925. On METABOLISM see E. H. ACKERKNECHT: Metabolism and History of Metabolic Diseases, *Ciba Symposia*, 6, 1944, and A. MAGNUS-LEVY: Dietetic in the Preinsulin Era, in *B.H.M.*, Suppl. 3, 1944.

VII. MICROBIOLOGY. An excellent source for the history of BACTERIOLOGY, unfortunately not complete, is F. LOEFFLER: *Vorlesungen über die geschichtliche Entwicklung der Lehre von den Bacterien* (Leipzig, Vogel, 1887). On PASTEUR see the excellent biography by R. VALLERY-RADOT: *La Vie de Pasteur* (Paris, Hachette, 1900; English trans., 2 vols., London, Constable, 1911). On the occasion of Pasteur's centenary, 1922, a special very attractive issue of *L'Illustration*, Paris, was published. See also P. COMPTON: *The Genius of Louis Pasteur* (New York, Macmillan, 1932), and S. PAGET: *Pasteur and after-Pasteur* (London, Black, 1914). The complete history of the studies on rabies was published by J. R. SUZOR: *La Rage* (Paris, Jouve, 1887).

On Robert KOCH and his work see W. W. FORD: The Life and Work of Robert Koch, *Bull. Johns Hopkins Hosp.*, 22:250. Other excellent biographies are those by B. HEYMANN: *Robert Koch* (Leipzig, Akad. Verlag, 1932); E. WEZEL: *Robert Koch* (Berlin, Hirschwald, 1912); and W. BECHER: *Robert Koch* (Berlin, Konitzer, 1891). On E. KLEBS see E. MARCHIAFAVA: Edwin Klebs, *Med. nuova*, Roma, 1914. One of the most attractive medical autobiographies is RONALD ROSS: *Memoirs* (London, Murray, 1923). See also R. L. MEGROZ: *Ronald Ross, Discoverer and Creator* (London, Allén & Unwin, 1931). On H. NOGUCHI see G. ECKSTEIN: *Noguchi* (New York and London, Harper, 1941). On BEHRING see M. VON GRUBER: E. A. von Behring, *Münch. med. Woch.*, 64:1235, 1917. On MANSON an excellent source is P. H. MANSON-BAHR and A. ALCOCK: *The Life and Work of Sir Patrick Manson* (New York, Wood, 1924). An excellent biography of WELCH was written by S. FLEXNER and J. F. FLEXNER: *W. H. Welch and the Heroic Age of American Medicine* (New York, Viking, 1941); see also the volume published on his eightieth birthday (New York, 1930), and the *Account of the Origin and Development of the W. Welch Medical Library at Johns Hopkins University* (Baltimore, Williams & Wilkins, 1929).

VIII. INTERNAL MEDICINE. There is a splendid biography of W. OSLER by H. CUSHING: *Life of William Osler* (2 vols., Oxford, Clarendon Press, 1925), which obtained the Pulitzer Prize and is one of the best and most brilliant of modern medical biographies. See also F. H. GARRISON: Sir William Osler, *Science*, 51:55, 1920. On JAMES MCKENZIE, see R. McN. WILSON: *The Beloved Physician, Sir James McKenzie* (London, Murray, 1926).

Many of the references cited in the chronological list of the discoveries of some microorganisms (especially in the column of present names) are to be found in BERGEY's *Manual of Determinative Bacteriology* (4th ed., Baltimore, Williams & Wilkins, 1934). Other references appear in the appropriate volumes of the British *System of Bacteriology in Relation to Medicine*, by various authors, which also contains a good but brief history in Vol. I (London: His Majesty's Stat. Office, 1929-31).

For the biographies of the ITALIAN CLINICIANS of this period see A. GERRINI: *Guido Baccelli* (Torino, 1916), and the beautiful biography written by his son, A. BACCELLI: *Mio Padre* (Roma, 1924); G. BILANCIONI: Achille de Giovanni, *R.I.S.*, 7:201, 1916; C. GOLGI: Carlo Forlanini, Necrologia, *Rend. R. Ist. lomb. di sci. e lett.*, Milano, 1918; L. KLEINWAECHTER: Arnaldo Cantani, *Janus*, 9:325, 1904; and F. SCHUPPER and C. BADUEL: Pietro Grocco, *Atti d. acc. med.-fis. fiorent.*, Firenze, 29: 1916.

The evolution of the GERMAN SCHOOLS is dealt with in a brilliant essay by MAGNUS-LEVY: The Heroic Age of German Medicine, *B.H.M.*, 14:331-42, 1944. For biographies of the German leaders in clinical medicine see A. GOLDSCHEIDER: Hermann Senator, Gedächtnisrede, *Berl. klin. Woch.*, 48:1961, 1911; A. KUSSMAUL: *Jugenderinnerungen eines alten*

Arztes (Stuttgart, Bonz, 1900); E. VON LEYDEN: *Lebenserinnerungen* (Stuttgart und Leipzig, Dtsch. Verlagsanstalt, 1910); M. NEUBURGER: *Hermann Nothnagel* (Wien und Berlin, Rikola, 1922); and R. VIRCHOW: Zur Erinnerung an L. Traube, *Berl. klin. Woch.*, 13:209, 1876.

Important for the biography and bibliography of FRENCH TEACHERS of this time is *Les Biographies médicales*, published in annual volumes by BUSQUET and GENTY, 1927–40. An excellent study by P. TRIAR: *Bretonneau et ses correspondants* (2 vols., Paris, Alcan, 1892), gives an interesting picture of the French medical school.

For AMERICAN physicians see F. N. THORPE: *William Pepper, M.D., LL.D.* (Philadelphia and London, Lippincott, 1904); and E. G. READ: *Life and Convictions of William Sydney Thayer* (New York, Oxford Univ. Press, 1936). On J. C. WARREN, see E. WARREN: *The Life of John Collin Warren from His Autobiography and Journals* (Boston, Ticknor & Fields, 1860); for NATHAN SMITH, see E. SMITH: *The Life and Letters of Nathan Smith* (New Haven, Yale Univ. Press, 1914); for H. J. BIGELOW and other great American clinicians of that time, a good source of information is H. CLARKE: *A Century of American Medicine* (Philadelphia, Lea, 1876).

IX. A good survey of the recent history of SURGERY may be found in W. A. F. von BRUNN: *Geschichtliche Einführung in die Chirurgie* (Berlin-Wien, Urban u. Schwarzenberg, 1924).

For the history of ANESTHESIA see the bibliography by L. CLENDENING in *Bull. Med. Libr. Ass.*, 33:1, 1945; J. W. SIMPSON: *Account of a New Anesthetic Agent as a Substitute for Sulphuric Ether in Surgery and Midwifery* (Edinburgh, Sutherland & Knox, 1847); F. L. TAYLOR: *Crawford W. Long* (New York, Hoeber, 1928); J. T. GWATHMEY: *Anesthesia* (New York, Appleton, 1914); H. H. YOUNG: Crawford W. Long the Pioneer in Ether Anesthesia, *B.H.M.*, 1:2, 1942. There is a complete historical survey in T. E. KEYS: *The History of Surgical Anesthesia* (New York, Schuman's, 1945). See also: E. S. ELLIS: *Ancient Anodyna and Primitive Anesthesia* (London, Heinemann, 1946); J. F. FULTON, and M. E. STANTON: *The Centennial of Surgical Anesthesia* (New York, Schuman, 1946) and the attractive book by V. ROBINSON: *Victory over Pain* (New York, Schuman, 1946).

For the history of GERMAN SURGERY see H. TILLMANNS: Hundert Jahre Chirurgie, *Allg. Wien. med. Ztg.*, 43:435, 1928; also F. TRENDELENBURG: *Aus heiteren Jugendtagen* (Berlin, Springer, 1924). A good biography of Billroth is J. VON MIKULICZ: Theodor Billroth, *Berl. klin. Woch.*, 31:109, 1894; see also J. C. HEMMETER: *Theodor Billroth, Musical and Surgical Philosopher* (Baltimore, 1900). Billroth's letters (published in Hannover, Hahn, 1899) give a fascinating portrait of his personality. This great surgeon was very much interested in historical studies; see T. BILLROTH: *Historical Studies on the Nature and Treatment of Gunshot Wounds from the 15th Century to the Present Time* (Berlin, Reimer, 1859; trans. by C. P. Rhoads, New Haven, 1933). On Langenbeck many important essays and papers are collected in Vol. C of the *Arch. f. Chirurgie* devoted to him.

The history of FRENCH SURGERY was brilliantly told by J. DE FOURMESTRAUX: *Histoire de la chirurgie française (1790–1920)* (Paris, Masson, 1934). On ITALIAN SURGERY see E. BURCI: La scuola fiorentina chirurgica, *Sperimentale*, 78:644, 1924; E. GUALANDI: La scuola di chirurgia di Bologna, *Studi e mem. per la storia dell'Univ. d. Bologna*, Vol. IV, 1918.

X. On OBSTETRICS and GYNÆCOLOGY see the excellent book of W. J. S. McKAY: *The History of American Gynecology* (New York, 1901); also J. A. RICCI: *The Genealogy of Gynecology* (Philadelphia, 1943), and *One Hundred Years of Gynecology (1800–1900 A.D.)* (Philadelphia, Blakiston, 1945). On CÆSAREAN SECTION: J. H. YOUNG: *The History and Development of the Cæsarean Operation from Earliest Times* (London, 1944). A good biography of SEMMELWEIS is Sir W. SINCLAIR: *Semmelweis, His Life and Doctrine* (Manchester Univ. Press, 1909); also Schürer von WALTHEIM: *Semmelweis, sein Leben und Wirken* (Leipzig, Hartleben, 1905). The literature on OLIVER WENDELL HOLMES and his work is very rich. Among others may be cited Sir W. OSLER: Oliver Wendell Holmes, *Johns Hopkins Hosp. Bull.*, Oct. 1894, and R. FITZ: Oliver Wendell Holmes, *Bull. N. Y. Ac. of Med.*, 1943. Some interesting notes about obstetrics in America are in T. A. EMMETT: *Reminiscences of the Founders of the Woman's Hospital Association* (New York, 1903).

XI. For the history of PEDIATRICS see J. RUHRÄH, ed.: *Pediatrics of the Past* (New York, Hoeber, 1925); A. LEVINSON: Development of Modern Infant Feeding, and Pediatric

Progress in the Last Fifty Years, also an article on Abraham Jacobi, *Med. Life*, 33:443, 1926; see also his *Pioneers in Pediatrics* (New York, Froben Press, 1943). A good biography of A. Jacobi is V. ROBINSON: The Life of A. Jacobi, *Med. Life*, 35:5, 6, 7, 1928.

XII. On the progress of OPHTHALMOLOGY see A. A. HUBBELL: *The Development of Ophthalmology in America 1800–1870* (Chicago, Am. Med. Ass. Press, 1908); A. BADER: *Entwicklung der Augenheilkunde im 18ten und 19ten Jahrh., besonders in der Schweiz* (Basel, Schwabe, 1933); A. SORSBY: *A Short History of Ophthalmology* (London, Bale, 1933).

XIII. In the field of OTORHINOLARYNGOLOGY, the history of ENDOSCOPY has been written by J. GRUENFELD: *Zur Geschichte der Endoskopie und der endoskopischen Apparate* (Wien, Überreuter, 1897), and G. KILLIAN: Zur Geschichte der Endoskopie von den ältesten Zeiten bis Bozzini, *Arch. f. Laryngol. u. Rhinol.*, 23:347, 1915. On OTOLOGY see C. CHAUVEAU: Évolution de la physiologie de l'oreille au cours de ces dernières années, *Arch. int. de laryngologie*, 35:823, 1913. The best and most reliable history of OTOLOGY AND LARYNGOLOGY was written by A. POLITZER: *Geschichte der Ohrenheilkunde* (2 vols., Stuttgart, G. Enke, 1907–13). The section on this period, in which Politzer was the outstanding othologist in Europe, is full of important biographical and bibliographical notices and critical judgments. On CHEVALIER JACKSON, see his *Autobiography* (New York, Macmillan, 1938).

XIV. The history of UROLOGY, with special emphasis on the French school, was brilliantly told by M. W. DESNOS: Histoire de l'urologie, *Encycl. franç. d'urol.* (Vol. I, Paris, Doin, 1914), with splendid prints and excellent portraits.

XV. A good survey of the history of DERMATOLOGY and VENEREOLGY is W. A. PUSEY: *The History of Dermatology* (Springfield, Thomas, 1933). On T. A. Fournier see P. E. BECHET: Alfred Fournier, the Master Syphilologist, *N. Y. State Med. J.*, 1930; and B. B. BAESEN: Alfred Fournier, His Life and Works, *Arch. of Derm. and Syph.*, 1924:10. The contribution of Fournier to the nosography of syphilis was outstanding; see his *Pictorial Atlas of Skin Diseases and Syphilitic Affections* (London, Rebmen, 1895–7).

XVI. On ORTHOPEDICS see E. M. BICK: *History and Source Book of Orthopedic Surgery* (New York, Hosp. for Joint Diseases, 1933).

XVII. STOMATOLOGY and DENTISTRY. Valuable information on the evolution of dentistry in this period may be found in the books quoted in General Bibliography C, dealing with the history of this branch.

XVIII. A history of PSYCHIATRY in the nineteenth century was written by A. KRAEPELIN: Hundert Jahre Psychiatrie, *Zeitschr. f. d. ges. Neurol. u. Psychiat.*, 38:161, 1918, and E. MORSELLI: Cento e più anni di conquiste della psichiatria, *Quaderni*, 7:229, 1920. On Lombroso, see C. FOÀ: O Museu de Psiquiatria e de Antropolitia Criminal Organizado por Cesare Lombroso, Suppl. 3, *B.H.M.* (Baltimore, Johns Hopkins Press, 1944).

XIX. For the history of LEGAL MEDICINE see: S. E. CHAILLÉ: *Origin and Progress of Legal Jurisprudence 1776–1876, a Centennial Address* (Philadelphia, 1876). For the Italian school see F. LEONCINI: Ricordi della scuola fiorentina di medicina legale, *R.I.S.*, 16:237, 1935.

XX. PHARMACOLOGY. On RUDOLF BUCHHEIM, see O. SCHMIEDEBERG: Rudolf Buchheim, *Arch. f. exper. Path.*, 67:1, 1912. For the evolution of PHARMACY in the nineteenth century the best information can be found in the excellent book of E. KREMERS and G. URDANG: *History of Pharmacy* (Philadelphia, Lippincott, 1940).

XXI. On MILITARY MEDICINE there is an important contribution by F. H. GARRISON: *Notes on the History of Military Medicine* (Washington, Ass. of Mil. Surgeons, 1922); see also J. MONÉRY: *Le Musée de Val-de-Grâce* (Paris, Val-de-Grâce, 1923); and the brilliant book by A. CABANÈS: *Chirurgiens et blessés à travers l'histoire* (Paris, Michel, 1918). For W. GORGAS, see his classic paper: *A Few General Directions with Regard to the Destruction of Mosquitoes* (Washington, Govt. Press, 1918). There is a good biography by C. JUDSON: *Soldier Doctor, the Story of William Gorgas* (New York, Scribner, 1942).

XXII. An interesting contribution to the development of PUBLIC HEALTH in America is the address by JOHN SHAW BILLINGS: *Public Health and Municipal Government* (Philadelphia, 1891. Of remarkable historical importance is the essay of M. VON PETTENKOFER: *The Value of Health for a City*, English trans. with introd. by H. E. SIGERIST (Baltimore, Johns Hopkins Press, 1941). For the evolution of public health in Germany see A. FISCHER: *Geschichte des deutschen Gesundheitswesens* (Berlin, Herbig, 1933).

XXIII. On the STUDY AND PRACTICE OF MEDICINE the bibliography is very abundant. Among the many interesting books are W. A. Pusey: *A Doctor in the 1870's and 1880's* (Springfield, Thomas, 1932); S. W. Mitchell: *Doctor and Patient* (Philadelphia, Lippincott, 1888); also *Dr. North and His Friends* (New York, Century Co., 1900). One of the most popular books on this subject is E. G. Liek: *The Doctor's Mission*, which was first published in German and then translated into all languages (English, London, Murray, 1930) arousing a large discussion.

CHAPTER XXI

I. On the ORIENTATION OF MODERN MEDICINE see I. Galdston: *Progress in Medicine* (New York, Knopf, 1940); F. S. Taylor: *The Century of Science* (London, Heinemann, 1941). The relation between social conditions and disease is stressed in B. J. Stern: *Society and Medical Progress* (New York, 1941). A brilliantly written survey on medical advances in the last hundred years is C. D. Haagensen and W. E. Lloyd: *A Hundred Years of Medicine* (2nd ed., New York, Sheridan, 1943). The collection of *Lectures to the Laity*, published annually by the New York Academy of Medicine (1926–45) gives an interesting and lively picture of medical progress, presented in plain form by eminent scientists. Another excellent source of information is C. Singer: *A Short History of Science in the Nineteenth Century* (Oxford, 1941).

II. Among the numerous books dealing with the history of BIOLOGY, especially in recent times, the best sources of information are G. Bohn: *Le Mouvement biologique en Europe* (Paris, Colin, 1921); S. Baglioni: Sviluppo storico della biologia medica in Italia, in *L'Italia e la scienza* (Firenze, Petrucci, 1932); W. E. R. Buddenbrock: *Bilder aus der Geschichte der biologischen Grundprobleme* (Berlin, Borntraeger, 1930); J. G. Crowther: *The Progress of Science, an Account of Recent Fundamental Researches in Physics, Chemistry, and Biology* (London, Paul, 1934).

III. On ANATOMY see F. J. Cole: *History of Comparative Anatomy, from Aristotle to the Eighteenth Century* (New York, Macmillan, 1945), an interesting source for the study of the relation between ancient and modern doctrines.

An excellent historical presentation of the history of EMBRYOLOGY is to be found in R. C. Oppenheimer: The Non-specificity of the Germ Layers, *Quart. Rev. Biol.*, 1940. A good review of experimental embryology, as well as a critical historical survey of morphologic research, is given in J. Needham: *Biochemistry and Morphogenesis* (New York, Macmillan, 1942). See also A. W. Meyer: *The Rise of Embryology* (Stanford Univ. Press, 1939), and D. K. Tertiakow: The Founders of Comparative Embryology, *Priroda*, Leningrad, 29:95, 95–104, 1940. Many important historical notices may be found in L. Aschoff: *Hundert Jahre Zellforschung* (Berlin, 1938).

IV. On the development of PHYSIOLOGY see K. J. Franklin: *A Short History of Physiology* (London, Bale, 1933). J. F. Fulton: *Physiology of the Nervous System* (Oxford Univ. Press, 1944), gives at the beginning of each chapter important historical notes.

V. For the recent progress in BIOCHEMISTRY see P. Wenger: Evolution of Biochemistry, *Mitt. aus dem Geb. der Lebensmittelunters. und Hyg.*, 34:250–62, 1943. A good survey is T. Pryde: *Recent Advances in Biochemistry* (London, Churchill, 1926). Many important notices on recent developments may be found in F. Lieben: *Geschichte der physiologischen Chemie* (Leipzig, Deuticke, 1935).

VI. On the development of PATHOLOGY in this period see G. Hadfield and L. P. Garrod: *Recent Advances in Pathology* (several cumulative editions, London, Churchill, 1942 and earlier); G. Fichera: Estado actual de los estudios sobre el cáncer según la orientación en diversas naciones, *Bol. inst. de med. exper. por el estud. y trat. del cáncer*, Buenos Aires, 1:798, 1924–5. On influenza see E. P. Campbell: The Epidemiology of Influenza Illustrated by Historical Accounts, *B.H.M.*, 13:389–403, 1943.

VII. MICROBIOLOGY. The history of BACTERIOLOGY is well told in W. Bullock: *The History of Bacteriology* (London, Oxford Univ. Press, 1938), which contains important biographical notices. W. W. Ford: *Bacteriology* (New York, Hoeber, 1939), is an excellent volume of the Clio Medica series.

VIII. INTERNAL MEDICINE. A comprehensive survey is L. Brown: *The History of*

Clinical Pulmonary Tuberculosis (Baltimore, Williams & Wilkins, 1941). On INFLUENZA see F. M. BURNET and E. CLARK: *Influenza, a survey of the last fifty years in the light of modern work on the virus of epidemic influenza* (Melbourne, 1942).

IX. SURGERY. On blood TRANSFUSION see G. L. KEYNES: *The History of Blood Transfusion, 1628–1914* (Bristol, England, 1942), and N. H. SBARRA: Historia de la transfusión sanguinea, *An. Fac. med.,* La Plata, 6:269–379, 1940; see also: E. W. REED: Selected Bibliography for a Study in the History of Blood Transfusion, *B. Med. Libr. Ass.,* 30:3, 1924, and J. H. ALCANTARA: A propósito del primer centenario de la transfusión de la sangre in America, *Revista mensual de medicina,* Mexico, 18:2, 3, 1945.

An excellent survey of the history of ABDOMINAL SURGERY is V. Z. COPE: *Pioneers in Acute Abdominal Surgery* (London, H. Milford, 1939). On BRAIN SURGERY, C. A. BALLANCE: *A Glimpse into the History of Surgery of the Brain* (London, Coll. of Surgeons, 1921).

The medico-historical literature on PLASTIC SURGERY is scanty. For earlier periods see E. ZEIS: *Die Literatur und Geschichte der plastischen Chirurgie* (Leipzig, 1863), with a detailed bibliography. Modern aspects are best seen in original articles, or in books such as H. D. GILLIES: *Plastic Surgery of the Face* (Oxford Univ. Press, 1920); and E. LEXER: *Die gesamte Wiederherstellungs-chirurgie* (Berlin, 1931). W. FILATOV's article on the subject first appeared in Russian in *Wiestnik Oftalmologuii,* 4–5, April, May 1917; it was translated in 1923 in *Presse médicale,* 19, 1061, 1923: Opérations plastiques a Tige Ronde. A good survey on ÆSTHETIC SURGERY is W. E. KUNSTLER: Aesthetic Considerations in Surgical Operations from Antiquity to Recent Times, *B.H.M.,* 12:1, pp. 27–69, 1942. For an excellent chronologic review see M. MALTZ: *Evolution of Plastic Surgery* (Philadelphia, Blakiston, 1946).

For the BIOGRAPHY of surgeons see A. REPPLIER: *J. William White* (Boston, Houghton Mifflin, 1919); S. PAGES: *Sir Victor Horsley* (London, Constable, 1919); and *Harvey Cushing, a Biography,* by J. F. FULTON (Springfield, Thomas, 1946), which is splendidly documented and includes an appreciation of the work of the great surgeon, collector, and historian, with beautiful reproductions of his drawings.

For the history of surgical INSTRUMENTS, an interesting and reliable source is C. J. S. THOMPSON: *The History and Evolution of Surgical Instruments* (New York, Schuman's, 1942).

X. A good selection of classic writings on OBSTETRICS AND GYNÆCOLOGY is H. THOMS: *Classic Contributions to Obstetrics and Gynecology* (Springfield, Thomas, 1935). On recent developments see A. W. BOURNE and L. H. W. WILLIAMS: *Recent Advances in Obstetrics and Gynecology* (2nd ed., London, Churchill, 1942); also A. M. CLAYE: *The Evolution of Obstetric Analgesia* (London, 1939).

XI. For recent progress in PEDIATRICS see H. C. CAMERON: Fifty Years of Progress in Pediatrics, *Clin. J.,* 70:113, 1941, and G. F. POWERS: Pediatrics in the Past Quarter Century, *Bull. Vancouver M. A.,* 17:162, 1941. An interesting contribution to the development of modern pediatrics is G. ARÁOZ ALFARO: On Pediatrics in Relation to Social Medicine and Health, in *Bul. Inst. Intern. Amer. de Proteción á la infancia,* 15:365, 1942. The *History of Pediatrics,* by F. H. GARRISON (Philadelphia, 1923), is a brilliant summary of the more important progress in this field.

XII. For the history of OPHTHALMOLOGY see J. HIRSCHBERG: Die Augenheilkunde in der Neuzeit, in GRAEFE-SAEMISCH: *Handb. d. ges. Augenhlk.,* 14: pt. 5:1 (Leipzig, Engelmann, 1915). See also W. M. BRUCKER: *The Story of Optometry* (Minneapolis, 1939).

XIII. For the development of OTOLARYNGOLOGY and RHINOLOGY see G. BILANCIONI: Per la storia della laringoiatria, *R.I.S.,* 11:25, 117, 1920; also G. D. SEARLE: *Medical History of Allergic Rhinitis* (Chicago, Searle, 1945). See also: T. H. BRYAN: The history of Laringology and rhinology and the influence of America (*A.H.M.,* n.s. 5, 151–170: 1933), and D. B. DELAVAN: The origin of Laryngology (*Diplomate,* 9:1937) and T. WRIGHT: *A history of Laringology and Rhinology,* (2nd ed. Philadelphia, Lea and Febiger, 1914).

XIV. UROLOGY. An exhaustive *History of Urology* has been edited by the American Urological Association (2 v. Baltimore, Williams and Wilkins, 1933). See also: T. J. KIRWIN, *Urology, its evolution as a medical specialty* (New York, Oxford Univ. Press, 1932). An interesting contribution to the history of urological instruments was given by O. PASTEAU: Les instruments de chirurgie urinaire en France d'après les documents originaux du XVIme au XXme siècle (Paris, Boulange, 1914).

XV. For the history of DERMATOLOGY AND VENEREOLOGY see E. B. TANTER: Dermatology, its past, its present, its future (*J.A.M.A.* 97, 1931) and J. DARIER: Considérations historiques sur le developpment de la dermatologie (*Ann. derm, typh.*, 7, 1936) also: W. N. GOLDSMITH: *Recent Advances in Dermatology* (London, Churchill, 1936). For EHRLICH and his work two excellent contributions are: A. ASCOLI: Der leitende Gedanke in dem Werke Paul Ehrlich's (*Seuchenbekämpfung* 3, 1925) and the exhaustive biography by M. MARQUARDT: *Paul Ehrlich als Mensch und Arbeiter* (Stuttgart, Enke, 1924).

XVI. For the history of ORTHOPEDICS in this period see A. BLENCKE and H. GOCHT: *Die orthopädische Welt-Literatur, 1903-30, ergänzt, 1931-35* (3 vols., Stuttgart, Enke, 1936-8), and E. G. BICK: *Source Book of Orthopædics* (Baltimore, William & Wilkins, 1937). See also R. B. OSGOOD: *The Evolution of Orthopædic Surgery* (St. Louis, Mosby, 1925).

An excellent book containing a picture of the development of modern orthopedics is Sir A. KEITH: *Menders of the Maimed* (2nd ed., London, Frowde, 1925). On French orthopedics see J. C. FAVREAU: French Orthopedics, *Un. Méd. du Canada*, 73:3077, 1944.

A good biography is G. M. GOODWIN: *Russell A. Hidds, Pioneer in Orthopedic Surgery, 1869-1932* (New York, 1935). See also the biography of R. Jones by F. WATSON: *The Life of Sir Robert Johns* (Baltimore, William Wood, 1934).

XVII. The history of DENTAL DISEASE and treatment from the earliest times up to the nineteenth century is briefly told by K. SUDHOFF in his *Geschichte der Zahnheilkunde* (1921, 1926). See also M. D. K. BREMNER: *The Story of Dentistry* (Brooklyn, 1939), and A. MICHAUD: *Histoire de la prothèse dentaire* (Château-d'Ex, 1939). An interesting contribution to the history of dentistry was made by B. W. WEINBERGER: *Orthodontics* (St. Louis, 1926). C. PROSKAUER has recently reprinted *B.H.M.*, Suppl. 3, 1944, a little-known skit, *Der Bauern Aderlass sampt einem Zahnbrecher* by Hans SACHS, the famous Meistersinger and shoemaker of Nürnberg. He calls attention to its special interest as the only detailed account from the period of the Reformation of the way that the "toothbreaker" (puller) carried on his trade.

XVIII. For the history of PSYCHIATRY see G. ZILBOORG and G. W. HENRY, ed.: *A History of Medical Psychology* (New York, 1941); and G. ZILBOORG, J. K. HALL, and A. G. BUNKER, ed.: *One Hundred Years of American Psychiatry* (New York, Columbia Univ. Press, 1944).

An interesting sketch on the relation between psychiatrists and NEUROSURGEONS was written by H. CUSHING: Psychiatrists, Neurologists, and the Neurosurgeons, *Yale J. Biol. and Med.*, 7:191, 1935.

On PSYCHOANALYSIS see S. FREUD: *The History of the Psychoanalytic Movement*, trans. by A. BRILL (New York, Nerve and Mental Disease Publ. Co., 1917). S. FREUD: *An Autobiographical Sketch*, trans. by J. STRACHEY (New York, 1935), is interesting. A good biography is F. WITTELS: *Sigmund Freud*, trans. by E. and C. BAUL (London, Allen & Unwin, 1924).

On the history of NEUROLOGY see F. DAMRAU: *Pioneers in Neurology* (New York, 1937).

XIX. LEGAL MEDICINE. A good survey of the evolution of legal medicine is A. COUSIN: *Essai sur l'origine de la médecine légale* (Thèse de Paris, 1905, n. 252). See also H. E. G. HILLAIRET: *Étude historique sur la responsibilité médicale* (Lille, Leblanc, 1923). An attractive biography is H. R. OSWALD: *Memoirs of a London Coroner* (London, Paul, 1936). The problem of the coroner system in America has been dealt with by H. S. MARCHAND: *Dr. Watson and Mr. Sherlock Holmes*, in *Landmarks in Medicine* (New York, Appleton, 1939).

XX. PHARMACOLOGY. An interesting survey of some of the latest developments is I. GALDSTON: *Behind the Sulfa Drugs* (New York, 1943). See also J. GRIFFITH: Fifty Years of Progress in Pharmacy, *Merck Rep.*, 50:4-7, 1941. On penicillin see F. B. SOKOLOFF: *The Story of Penicillin* (Chicago, Ziff-Davis, 1945).

For the history of INSULIN see S. HARRIS: *Bantings Miracle: the story of the discovery of insulin* (Philadelphia, Lippincott, 1946) and L. STEVENSON: *Sir Fr. Banting* (Toronto, Ryerson, 1946).

On CHEMOTHERAPY and its development see: A. FLEMING: *Chemotherapy, yesterday and to-morrow* (Cambridge Univ. Press, 1946).

For the history of PHYSIOTHERAPY see J. S. COULTER: *Physical Therapy* (Clio

Medica Series, New York, Hoeber, 1932), and R. J. CYRIAX: A Short History of Mechano-therapeutics in Europe until the Time of Ling, *Janus*, 19:178, 1914.

XXI. For the history of X-RAYS a good source is O. GLASSER: *Wilhelm Conrad Roentgen and the Early History of the Roentgen Rays* (Springfield, Ill., Thomas, 1924). A summary of the latest developments is E. T. PENDERGAST: Developments in Radiology during the Last Fifty Years, *Am. J. Surgery*, 51:225, 1941; see also J. J. KAPLAN: Recent Advances in Radiotherapy, *M. Clin. N. Am.*, 25:803, 1941.

A fascinating biography is EVE CURIE: *Madame Curie* (New York, Doubleday, Doran, 1938).

XXII. The historical literature on MILITARY MEDICINE has increased remarkably during World War II. A comprehensive survey is E. E. HUME: *Victories of Army Medicine: Scientific Accomplishments of the Medical Department of the United States Army* (Philadelphia, Lippincott, 1943). See also A. Q. MAISEL: *Miracles of Military Medicine* (New York, 1943), and an interesting autobiographical book by G. S. SEAGRAVE: *Burma Surgeon* (New York, 1943), a medico-historical best seller.

Important contributions to the subject are I. R. DARNALL: Contribution of the World War to the Advancement of Medicine, *J.A.M.A.*, CXV, 1443–57 (1940); M. GUMPERT: Red Cross in War and Peace, *Ciba Symposia*, 4, 1942; and W. H. TALIAFERRO, ed.: *Medicine and the War*, a series of ten lectures (Chicago, 1944).

A brilliant survey of the evolution of AVIATION MEDICINE is offered by Brig. Gen. E. G. REINARTS in his essay on Aviation Medicine in the Army, *Scient. Monthly*, 19:6, 1944. A bibliography of aviation medicine has been published by J. F. FULTON and C. HOFF (New York, 1944). A brilliant monograph on Paul Bert and his work is E. H. ACKERKNECHT: Paul Bert's Triumph, in *B.H.M.*, Suppl. 3, 1944.

XXIII. The history of NURSING has a rich bibliography. Among the best books are M. GOODNOW: *Nursing History* (2nd ed., Philadelphia, Saunders, 1942), and E. M. JANNESON and M. SEWALA: *Trends in Nursing History* (2nd ed., Philadelphia, Saunders, 1944).

For ARMY NURSES see J. O. FLIKKE: *Nurses in Action: The Story of the Army Nurse Corps* (Philadelphia, Lippincott, 1943). A good biography of Clara Barton is W. W. BARTON: *The Life of Clara Barton, Founder of the American Red Cross* (2 vols., Boston, 1923).

XXIV. The history of PUBLIC HEALTH and its development in the last fifty years may be found in the statistics published by the public health offices of different countries. A general survey of progress in public health is given in C. E. A. WINSLOW: *The Conquest of Epidemic Disease* (New York, 1943). See also G. NEWMAN: *The Rise of Preventive Medicine* (London, 1932). On public health in England good sources are M. G. KAHN: *Public Health and Preventive Medicine* (2 vols., London, 1942); M. MORRIS: *The Story of English Public Health* (London, 1919); and Sir A. NEWSHOLME: *Fifty Years in Public Health* (London, Allen, 1935). The evolution of public health in America has been dealt with by W. S. MANGOLD: *A Study of Sanitation in the United States* (Los Angeles, 1932); SCHIEFFELIN, ed.: *One Hundred and Fifty Years Service to American Health* (New York, 1944); also M. P. RAVENEL: *A Half Century of Public Health* (New York, American Pub. Health Association, 1931).

For the progress in the field of TROPICAL MEDICINE see C. M. WINSLOW: *Ambassadors in White, the Story of American Tropical Medicine* (New York, 1942). The yellow-fever episode is told by A. E. TRUBY: *Memoir of Walter Reed: The Yellow Fever Episode* (New York, 1943). See also H. H. SCOTT: *A History of Tropical Medicine* (2nd ed., New York, 1942). On MALARIA: Contemporary Tendencies in the History of Malariology, *B.H.M.*, 16:4, 1944.

For PUBLIC WELFARE an excellent historical survey is H. E. SIGERIST: *Medicine and Human Welfare* (New Haven, Yale Univ. Press, 1941). A good survey of public welfare in New York State is D. M. SCHNEIDER and A. DEUTSCH: *The History of Public Welfare in New York State, 1867–1940* (Univ. of Chicago Press, 1941). See also G. C. WHIPPLE: *State Sanitation* (2 vols., Harvard Univ. Press, 1917).

On LEPROSY a good historical sketch is A. A. MOORITZ: *A Brief World History of Leprosy* (Honolulu, 1943).

For MENTAL DISEASES in America see A. DEUTSCH: *The Mentally Ill in America* (2nd ed., New York, 1938).

For the future of PREVENTIVE MEDICINE see A. J. STIEGLITZ: *A Future for Preventive Medicine* (N. Y. Academy of Medicine, 1946).

For the development of INDUSTRIAL MEDICINE see E. F. BELLINGHAM: *Comparative Bibliography of Industrial Hygiene, 1900–1943, a selected list* (Washington, U. S. Government Printing Office, 1945).

An excellent review on the GOVERNMENT'S role in medicine is H. S. MUSTARD: *Government in Public Health* (New York, Commonwealth Fund, 1945). See also M. L. ROEMER: Government's Role in American Medicine, *B.II.M.*, 18:2, 1945.

An exhaustive study on the history of HOSPITALISATION in the U.S. is J. T. RICHARDSON: *The origin and development of Hospitalisation in the United States 1890–1940*, (Univ. of Columbia Press, 1945).

On the evolution of public health in SOVIET RUSSIA the best source is H. E. SIGERIST: *Socialized Medicine in the Soviet Union* (New York, Norton, 1937). See also R. MAURER: *Soviet Health Care in Peace and War* (New York, Ass. for Cult. Relations with the Soviet Union, 1937).

XXV. For the HISTORY OF MEDICINE see P. DIEPGEN: Zur Geschichte der Historiographie der Medizin, in *Finke's Festgabe* (Münster i. W., Aschendorff, 1925). On the TEACHING OF MEDICINE: W. OSLER: A Note on the Teaching of History of Medicine, *B.M.J.*, 2:93, 1902; and H. E. SIGERIST: Die Geschichte der Medizin im ak. Unterricht, *Kyklos*, 1:147, 1928; see also A. C. KLEBS: The History of Medicine as a Subject of Teaching and Research, *Bull. Johns Hopkins Hosp.*, January 1914. For the development of medical-historical teaching see F. H. GARRISON: Medical Bibliography and Medical History in the Medical Curriculum, *J.A.M.A.*, January 1929; also H. E. SIGERIST: Medical History in the Medical Schools of the U. S., *B.H.M.*, 7:6–27, 1938, and O. TEMKIN: An Essay on the Usefulness of Medical History for Medicine, *B.H.M.*, 19:1, 1946.

A good bibliography of medico-historical publications in the sixteenth and eighteenth centuries was made by E. HEISCHKEL: *Die Geschichte der Medizin von ihren Anfängen bis zum 16ten Jahrh.* (Leiden, Brill, 1931). There is also the splendid oration by H. CUSHING, *The Doctor and His Books* (Cleveland Med. Libr. Ass., 1926).

Concerning medical libraries a brilliant contribution was made by G. L. ANNAN: Medical Libraries and Medical History, *Bull. N.Y. Ac. of Med.*, 21, 63, 1945; also Rare Books and the History of Medicine, in *Medical Library Practice* (Chicago, 1943).

For further information on the development of the history of medicine, the following sources may be valuable: E. ABBOTT: *Sir William Osler Memorial Volume* (Toronto, Murray, 1926) (see also her *Classified and Annotated Bibliography*, 2nd ed., Montreal, McGill Univ., 1939); G. GARRIELI: A. Favaro e gli studi italiani di storia della scienza, *Isis*, 7:456, 1925; F. H. GARRISON: Prof. Karl Sudhoff and the Institute of Medical History of Leipzig, *Bull. Soc. Med. Hist.*, Chicago, 3:1, 1923; R. S. KAGAN: Professor Max Neuburger, A Biography and Bibliography, *B.H.M.*, 14, 1943; A. MIELI: Stanislao Cannizzaro, storico della scienza, *A.S.S.*, 7:80, 1926, and La storia della scienza in Italia, *A.S.S.*, 7:36, 1926; H. E. SIGERIST: Medical History in the Medical Schools of the U. S., *B.H.M.*, 1938, and The History of the History of Medicine, in *Milestones in Medicine* (New York and London, 1938).

XXVI. An excellent picture of the STUDY AND PRACTICE of medicine is given in a brilliant book by V. G. HEISER: *An American Doctor's Odyssey* (New York, Norton, 1936); see also H. E. SIGERIST: *American Medicine* (New York, Norton, 1934), and R. FITZ: Medicine and the Changing World in *The March of Medicine* (New York, Acad. of Med., 1945). H. CUSHING's books: *Consecratio Medici* (Boston, 1940), and *The Medical Career* (Boston, 1940), are attractive and inspiring reading. The attractive book by H. E. SIGERIST: *The University at the Crossroads* (New York, Schumann, 1946) gives an interesting picture of the actual problems of medical teaching.

On WOMEN PHYSICIANS see E. LOVEJOY: *Women Physicians and Surgeons* (New York, 1940).

On SOCIAL LEGISLATION see H. E. SIGERIST: From Bismarck to Beveridge; Developments and Trends in Social Security Legislation, *B.H.M.*, 13:4, 365–88, 1943; and M. FISHBEIN: Cultural Education of a Physician, *J.A.M.A.*, 119, 1942.

The problem of SPECIALIZATION has been discussed by G. ROSEN: *The Specialization of Medicine with Particular Reference to Ophthalmology* (New York, Froben, 1944).

XXVII. On the orientation of MEDICAL THOUGHT in the twentieth century there is a remarkable number of recent publications. Among them are R. ALLENDY: *Orientation des idées médicales* (Paris, 1930); B. ASCHNER: *Die Krise der Medizin, Konstitutionstherapie als Ausweg* (Stuttgart, Hippokrates Verlag, 1928); P. E. BLEULER: *Das autistisch-undiszi-plinierte Denken in der Medizin und seine Überwindung* (Berlin, Springer, 1922); O. BUMKE: *Eine Krisis der Medizin* (München, Huber, 1929); A. CASTIGLIONI: *Il volto di Ippocrate* (Milano, Unitas, 1926), and *L'orientamento neoippocratico del pensiero medico contemporaneo* (Torino, 1933; English trans., New York, Medical Life Press, 1936); A. P. CAWADIAS: *The Neohippocratic Theory as Basis of Contemporary Medical Thought and Practice* (London, Internat. Soc. of Med. Hydrol., 1938); P. DIEPGEN: Vitalismus und Medizin im Wandel der Zeiten, *Klin. Woch.*, 10:1433, 1931; C. FRUGONI: L'essenza e gli obietti dell'insegnamento clinico, *Policlinico* (sez. prat.), 39:125, 1932; F. GALDI: Genesi ed evoluzione dell'orientamento clinico moderno, *Minerva med.*, 23:156, 1932.

An interesting correlation of the evolution of medicine and the sociological aspect of health and disease is given by H. E. SIGERIST in his attractive book: *Civilization and Disease* (Ithaca, Cornell Univ. Press, 1943); see also: B. J. STERN: *Society and Medical Progress* (Princeton Univ. Press, 1941).

GENERAL BIBLIOGRAPHY

Medico-historical references of general interest are included below under four headings: A, General; B, History of Medicine by Countries; C, The Specialties and Miscellaneous; D, Biographical and Bibliographical. A necessarily incomplete list, in view of the huge literature of value on the history of medicine, the references are intended as a guide to the reader who wishes to know the more important and more easily available works on the general and special aspects of the history of medicine. Non-medical works on history and general culture have not been included.

A. GENERAL

ACKERMANN, J. C. G.: *Institutiones historiæ medicinæ*. Norimbergæ, 1792.

ALLBUTT, SIR THOMAS C.: *The Historical Relations of Medicine and Surgery to the End of the Sixteenth Century*. London and New York, Macmillan, 1905.

ASCHOFF, L., and DIEPGEN, P.: *Kurze Übersichtstabelle zur Geschichte der Medizin*. 3 Aufl., München, Bergmann, 1936.

BAAS, J. H.: *Die geschichtliche Entwicklung des ärztlichen Standes*. Berlin, Wreden, 1896.

——: *Grundriss der Geschichte der Medizin und des heilenden Standes*. Stuttgart, Enke, 1876.

BARTELS, M.: *Die Medizin der Naturvölker*. Leipzig, Grieben, 1893.

BENEDICENTI, A.: *Malati medici e farmacisti*. Milano, Hoepli, 1924, 2nd ed. 1946.

DE BORDEN, T.: *Recherches sur l'histoire de la médecine*. Paris, 1882.

BOUCHUT, J. E.: *Histoire de la médecine et des doctrines médicales*. 2 v. Paris, Germer-Baillière, 1873.

BRUNET, P., and MIELI, A.: *Histoire des sciences. I. Antiquité*. Paris, Payot, 1935.

BUCHNER, E.: *Ärzte und Kurpfuscher*. München, Langen, 1922.

BUCK, A. A.: *The Growth of Medicine from the Earliest Times to 1800*. New Haven, Yale Univ. Press, 1917.

——: *The Dawn of Modern Medizine* (18th and 19th centuries). Yale Univ. Press, 1920.

CAMAC, C. N. B.: *From Imhotep to Harvey*. New York, Hoeber, 1931.

COMRIE, J. D.: *History of Medicine*. Edinburgh, Univ. of Edinburgh, 1910.

CUMSTON, C. G.: *Introduction to the History of Medicine from the Time of the Pharaohs to the End of the 18th Century*. London, K. Paul, 1926.

DANA, C. L.: *The Peaks of Medical History*. New York, Hoeber, 1926.

DANNEMANN, J. F.: *Die Naturwissenchaften in ihrer Entwicklung und ihrem Zusammenhange*. 2 v. Leipzig, Engelmann, 1910–11.

DAREMBERG, C. V.: *Histoire des sciences médicales*. 2 v. Paris, Baillière, 1870.

DIEPGEN, P.: *Geschichte der Medizin*. 5 v. (Sammlung Göschen) Berlin u. Leipzig, 1914–28.

DUMESNIL, R.: *Histoire illustreé de la médecine*. Paris, Plon [1935].

FABER, K.: *Nosography*. 2nd ed. New York, Hoeber, 1930.

FAHRÆUS, R.: *Läkekonstens Historia*, I., Stockholm, Bonnier, 1944.
FOSSEL, V.: *Studien zur Geschichte der Medizin.* Stuttgart, Enke, 1909.
GARRISON, F. H.: *An Introduction to the History of Medicine.* 4th ed. Philadelphia and London, Saunders, 1929.
GUTHRIE, D.: *A History of Medicine.* London, Nelson & Sons, 1945.
HAESER, H.: *Lehrbuch der Geschichte der Medizin.* 3 v. Jena, Dufft, 1875–82.
HAGGAR, E. H. W.: *The Doctor in History.* New Haven, Yale Press, 1934.
HECKER, J. F. C.: *Geschichte der Heilkunde.* 2 v. Berlin, Enslin, 1822–9.
——: *Geschichte der neueren Heilkunde* (18th century). Berlin, Enslin, 1839.
HIRSCH, A.: *Handbuch der historisch-geograph. Pathologie.* 2 Aufl. Stuttgart, Enke, 1881.
HOVORKA, O. VON, and KRONFELD, A.: *Vergleichende Volksmedizin.* 2 v. Stuttgart, Strecker u. Schroeder, 1908–9.
ISENSEE, E.: *Die Geschichte der Medizin und ihrer Hilfswissenschaften.* 4 v. in 6. Berlin, Liebmann, 1840.
KREMERS, E., and URDANG, G.: *History of Pharmacy.* Philadelphia, Lippincott, 1940.
KRONFELD, A.: *Beiträge zur Geschichte der Medizin.* Wien, Perles, 1911.
KRUMBHAAR, E. B., ed.: *Clio Medica* (series on history of medicine). 22 v., New York, Hoeber, 1926–39.
LAIGNEL-LAVASTINE, M.: *Histoire générale de la médecine, de la pharmacie, de l'art dentaire et de l'art vétérinaire* (2 v. already pub.) Paris, Michel, 1936, 1938.
LE CLERC, D.: *Histoire de la médecine.* La Haye, Van der Kloot, 1729.
MAGNUS, H.: *Die Volksmedizin.* Breslau, Abhandl. z. Gesch. d. Med., 1905.
MEUNIER, L.: *Histoire de la médecine.* Paris, Le François, 1924.
MEYER-STEINEG, T., and SUDHOFF, K.: *Geschichte der Medizin.* Jena, Fischer, 3rd ed., 1928.
MIELI, A.: *Manuale di storia della scienza.* Roma, Casa ed. Leonardo da Vinci, 1925.
NEUBURGER, M.: *Geschichte der Medizin.* 2 v. Stuttgart, Enke, 1906–11 (English trans. by E. Playfair. London, Oxford Press, 1910, 1925).
——: *Die Lehre von der Heilkraft der Natur im Wandel der Zeiten.* Stuttgart, Enke, 1926.
OSLER, SIR W.: *The Evolution of Modern Medicine.* New Haven, Yale Press, 1921.
——: *A Concise History of Medicine.* Baltimore, Standard Books, 1919.
PAGEL, J. L.: *Einführung in die Geschichte der Medizin.* 2 v. Berlin, Karger, 1898.
—— and NEUBURGER, M.: *Puschmann's Handbuch der Geschichte der Medizin.* 3 v. Jena, Fischer, 1902–5.
PETERSEN, J.: *Hauptmomente in der geschichtlichen Entwicklung der medizinischen Klinik.* Copenhagen, Host, 1890.
POWER, SIR D'ARCY: *The Foundation of Medical History.* Baltimore, Williams & Wilkins, 1931.
PUCCINOTTI, F.: *Storia della medicina.* 3 v. Livorno, Wagner, 1850–5.
RIESMAN, D.: *Medicine in Modern Society.* Princeton, Princeton Univ. Press, 1939.
ROBINSON, V.: *The Story of Medicine.* New York, Boni, 1931, 2nd ed. New Home Library, 1943.
——: *Syllabus of Medical History.* New York, Froben Press, 1931.
ROGER, J.: *La vie médicale d'autrefois.* Paris, Baillière, 1907.
SARTON, G.: *The History of Science and the New Humanism.* New York, Holt, 1931.
——: *Introduction to the History of Science.* 3 v. Baltimore, Williams & Wilkins, 1927–31.
SCHWALBE, E.: *Vorlesungen über die Geschichte der Medizin.* 3 Aufl., Jena, Fischer, 1919.
SCUDERI, R.: *Introduzione alla storia della medicina antica e moderna.* Napoli, Porcelli, 1794.
SHRYOCK, R. H.: *The Development of Modern Medicine.* Philadelphia, Univ. of Pennsylvania Press, 1936.
SIGERIST, H. E.: *Einführung in die Medizin.* Leipzig, Thieme, 1931 (trans. as *Man and Medicine*, by M. G. Boise, New York, Norton, 1932).
SINGER, C.: *Studies in the History and Method of Science.* 2 v. Oxford, Clarendon Pr., 1917, 1921.
——: *A Short History of Medicine.* Oxford, Univ. Pr., 1928.
SPRENGEL, K.: *Versuch einer pragmatischen Geschichte der Arzneikunde.* 5 v. Halle, Gebauer, 1792–1803.
STUBBS, S. G. B., and BLIGH, E. W.: *Sixty Centuries of Health and Physick.* London, Sampson Low, 1931.

THORNDIKE, L.: *History of Magic and Experimental Science*, 6 v. New York, Macmillan, 1931–41.
WITHINGTON, E. T.: *Medical History from the Earliest Times*. London, Science Press, 1894.
WUNDERLICH, C. A.: *Geschichte der Medizin*. Stuttgart, Ebner, 1859.

B. HISTORY OF MEDICINE BY COUNTRIES

ABBOTT, M. E.: *History of Medicine in the Province of Quebec*. Montreal, McGill, 1931.
ANDEL, M. A. VAN: *Volksgeneeskunst in Nederland*. Leiden, Akademisch Proefschrift, 1909.
ARATA, P.: *L'arte medica nelle iscrizioni latine*. Genova, 1902.
BELTRAN, J. R.: *Historia del Protomedicato de Buenos Aires*. Buenos Aires, El Ateneo, 1937.
BRAMBILLA, G. A.: *Storia delle scoperte fisico-mediche fatte dagli Italiani*. Milano, Imp. Monast. d. S. Ambrogio Maggiore, 1792.
BROECKX, C.: *Histoire de la médecine belge avant le XIXᵉ siècle*. Gand, Hebbelynck, 1837.
CANTON, E.: *Historia de la medicina en el Rio de la Plata*. 4 v. Madrid, Bibl. de hist. Hispano-Amer., 1928.
CARBONELLI, G.: *Commenti sopra alcune miniature e pitture italiane a soggetto medico*. Roma, Centenari, 1918.
CASTALDI, L.: *Una centuria di rivendicazioni mediche italiane*. Milano, Uff. Stampa Medica, 1929.
CASTIGLIONI, A.: *Italian Medicine; trans. by E. B. Krumbhaar*. (Clio Medica.) New York, Hoeber, 1932.
——: *The Renaissance of Medicine in Italy*. Baltimore, Johns Hopkins Press, 1934.
CHARCOT, J. M., RICHER, P. et al.: *Nouvelle Iconographie de la Salpêtrière*. Paris, Delahaye et Lecrosnier, 1888–1918.
COMRIE, J. D.: *History of Scottish Medicine*. 2 v. London, Baillière, 1932.
CURÀTULO, G. E.: *Die Kunst der Juno Lucina in Rom*. Berlin, Hirschwald, 1902.
DAWSON, W. R.: *The Beginnings — Egypt and Assyria*. (Clio Medica.) New York, Hoeber, 1930.
DE PINA GUIMARAES, L. J.: *Histoire de la médecine portugaise*. Porto, Enciclop. Portug., 1934.
DE RENZI, S.: *Storia della medicina in Italia*. 5 v. Napoli, Tip. Filiatra Sebezio, 1845–9.
DE VECCHI, P.: *Modern Italian Surgery*. New York, Hoeber, 1921.
D'HARCOURT, R.: *La Médecine dans l'ancien Pérou*. Paris, Maloine, 1939.
ELGOOD, C.: *Medicine in Persia*. (Clio Medica.) New York, Hoeber, 1934.
FERRANNINI, A.: *Medicina italica*. 2nd ed., Milano, Uff. Stampa Med. Ital., 1935.
FLORES, F. A.: *Historia de la medicina en México*. 3 v. Mexico, Of. Tip. d. l. Secr. de fomento, 1886–8.
FOURMESTRAUX, J. DE: *Histoire de la chirurgie française, 1790–1920*. Paris, Masson, 1934.
FUJIKAWA, Y.: *Geschichte der Medizin in Japan*. Tokyo, 1911 (English trans. by J. Ruhräh, Clio Medica, New York, Hoeber, 1934).
GANTT, W. A. H.: *Russian Medicine*. (Clio Medica.) New York, Hoeber, 1934.
GARCIA DEL REAL, E.: *Historia de la medicina en España*. Madrid, Reus, 1921.
GARZON MACEDA, F.: *La medicina en Córdoba*. Buenos Aires, Giles, 1916–17.
GROSS, S. D.: *History of American Medical Literature*. Philadelphia, Collins, 1876.
GUALINO, L.: *Storia medica dei romani pontefici*. Torino, Edizioni Minerva medica, 1934.
HABERLING, W.: *German Medicine; trans. by J. Freund*. (Clio Medica.) New York, Hoeber, 1934.
HEAGERTY, J. J.: *Four Centuries of Medical History in Canada*. 2 v. Toronto, Macmillan, 1928.
HOWELL, W. B.: *Medicine in Canada*. (Clio Medica.) New York, Hoeber, 1933.
INGERSLEV, J. V. C.: *Danmarks laeger og laegevesen*. 2 v. Kjøbenhavn, Jespersen, 1873.
IONESCU-GOMOIU, V.: *Istoria medicinei si a invatamantului medical in Romania*. Bucarest, Tip. Furnica, 1936.
JEE, SIR BHAGAVAT SINH: *A Short History of Aryan Medical Science*. London, Macmillan, 1896.

BIBLIOGRAPHY

KETTING, G. N. A.: *Bijdrage tot de geschiedenis van de lepra in Nederland.* 'S Gravenhage, Mouton, 1922.

LACHTIN, M. J.: Die Anfänge der russischen Medizin, *Wien. med. Woch.,* 78:1576, 1928.
——: Geschichte der russischen Medizin, 1807–1927, *A.G.M.,* 32:356, 1929.

LAIGNEL-LAVASTINE, M., and MOLINÉRY, M. R.: *French Medicine;* trans. by E. B. Krumbhaar. (Clio Medica.) New York, Hoeber, 1934.

LEMOS, M., JR.: *Historia da medicina em Portugal.* Lisbona, Gomez, 1891.

LEON, L.: La obstetrica en Mexico, Mexico, *Cron. med. Mex.,* 12:40, 71, 89, 141, 197, 1909.

LUND, F. B.: *Greek Medicine.* (Clio Medica.) New York, Hoeber, 1936.

MARTÍNEZ DURÁN, C.: *Las ciencias medicas en Guatemala.* Guatemala, Tip. nacional, 1941.

MEISEN, V.: *Prominent Danish Scientists through the Ages.* Copenhagen, Levin & Munksgaard, 1932.

MOLL, A. A.: *Æsculapius in Latin America.* Philadelphia, Saunders, 1944.

MOORE, N.: *History of the Study of Medicine in the British Isles.* Oxford, Clarendon Press, 1908.

——: *History of St. Bartholomew's Hospital.* 2 v. London, Pearson, 1918.

—— and PAGET, S.: *The Royal Medical and Chirurgical Society of London* (w. Supp. down to 1920). Aberdeen Univ. Press, 1905.

MORRIS, E. W.: *A History of the London Hospital.* London, Arnold, 1910.

MORSE, W. R.: *Chinese Medicine.* (Clio Medica.) New York, Hoeber, 1934.

MORTON, T. G.: *The History of the Pennsylvania Hospital.* Rev. ed., Philadelphia, Times Press House, 1897.

MÜNZ, I.: *Die jüdischen Aerzte im Mittelalter.* Frankfurt, Kauffman, 1922.

MUKHOPADHYAYA, G.: *History of Indian Medicine.* 2 v. Calcutta, Univ. of Calcutta, 1923.

MUMFORD, J. G.: *A Narrative of Medicine in America.* Philadelphia, Lippincott, 1903.

NEUBURGER, M.: *British Medicine and the Vienna School: Contacts and Parallels.* London, Heinemann, 1943.

NORWOOD, W. F.: *Medical Education in the U.S. before the Civil War.* Philadelphia, Univ. Penn. Press, 1944.

OCARANZA, F.: *Historia de la medicina en Mexico.* Mexico City, Farm. Midy., 1934.

O'DONOGHUE, E. G.: *Bridewell Hospital.* London, Lane, 1923.

OGAWA, K.: *History of Japanese Ophthalmology.* Tokyo, 1904.

PACKARD, F. R.: *History of Medicine in the United States.* 2 v. 2nd ed., New York, Hoeber, 1931.

PARSONS, R. P.: *History of Haitian Medicine.* New York, Hoeber, 1930.

PAYNE, J. F.: *English Medicine in the Anglo-Saxon Times.* Oxford, Clarendon Press, 1904.

PAZZINI, A.: *Storia dell'insegnamento medico in Roma.* Bologna, Licinio Capelli, 1935.

PEDRAZZINI, C. U. C.: *La farmacia storica e artistica italiana.* Milano, 1934.

PELLEGRINI, F.: *La medicina militare nel regno di Napoli.* Verona, Cabianca, 1932.

POWER, SIR D'ARCY: *British Medical Societies.* London, Baillière, Tyndall, 1939.
——: *Medicine in the British Isles.* (Clio Medica.) New York, Hoeber, 1930.

RASHDALL, H.: *Medieval England;* ed. by H. W. C. Davis. Oxford, Clarendon Press, 1889.

RICHTER, W. M.: *Geschichte der Medizin in Russland.* 3 v. Moskwa, Wsewolojsky, 1813–19.

RIESMAN, D.: *Story of Medicine in the Middle Ages.* New York, Hoeber, 1935.

SACKLAND, W.: *Sveriges Läkare historia.* Stockholm, 1822–76.

SCHIAFFINO, R.: *Historia de la medicina en Uruguay.* 2 v., Montevideo, Impr. Nacional 1927–37.

SIGERIST, H. E.: *Beiträge zur Geschichte der Medizin in der Schweiz.* Zürich, 1923–4.
——: *Amerika und die Medizin.* Leipzig, Thieme, 1933 engl. New York, Norton, 1934.

SPIVAK and HEILPRIN: Jewish Medicine, in *Jewish Encyclopedia.* New York, 1904.

STONE, E.: *Medicine among the American Indians.* (Clio Medica.) New York, Hoeber, 1932.

SÜHEYL, A.: *Zur Geschichte der Medizin und Hygiene in der Türkei.* Basilea, 1934.

TONER, J. M.: *Contributions to . . . Medical Progress and Medical Education in the United States before and during the War of Independence.* Washington, Gov't Printing Off., 1874.

VALDIZAN, H., and MALDONADO: *La medicina popular peruana.* Lima, Aguirre, 1922.

VIANA, O., and VOZZA, F.: *L'ostetricia e la ginecologia in Italia.* Milano, Soc. ital. di ost. e ginec., 1933.

WALSH, J. J.: *The History of Medicine in New York.* 5 v. New York, Nat'l. Ave. Soc., 1919.
WASHBURN, F. A.: *The Massachusetts General Hospital.* Boston, Houghton Mifflin, 1939.
WECK, W.: *Heilkunde und Volkstum auf Bali.* Stuttgart, Enke, 1937.

C. THE SPECIALTIES AND MISCELLANEOUS

ADAM, H. A.: *Über Geisteskrankheit in alter und neuer Zeit.* Regensb., Rath, 1928.
ALLBUTT, SIR CLIFFORD: *The Historical Relations of Medicine and Surgery to the End of the Sixteenth Century.* London and New York, Macmillan, 1905.
ANDRÉ-POINTIER, L.: *Histoire de la pharmacie.* Paris, Doin, 1900.
BALLANCE, SIR C. A.: *History of the Surgery of the Brain.* London, Macmillan, 1922.
BARCHI, L., ed.: *Medici e naturalisti reggiani.* Reggio Emilia, Rossi, 1935.
BARDEEN, CHARLES R.: Anatomy in America, Madison, *Bull. Univ. Wisconsin,* No. 115, 1905.
BARTHOLINUS, T.: *De medicis poetis dissertatio.* Hafniæ, Paulli, 1669.
BILANCIONI, G.: *Veteris vestigia flammæ, pagine storiche.* Roma, Leonardo da Vinci, 1922.
BILLINGS, J. S.: (Surgery) Introductory chapter in DENNIS, F. S., and BILLINGS, J. S.: *System of Surgery.* Philadelphia, Lea, 1895–96.
BLANCHARD, E. A.-E.: *L'Épigraphie médicale.* Paris, Asselin et Houzeau, 1909–15.
BLOCH, I.: *Der Ursprung der Syphilis.* 2 v. Jena, Fischer, 1901, 1911.
BOKAY, J. VON: *Die Geschichte der Kinderheilkunde,* Berlin, Springer, 1922.
BRUNN, W. VON: *Kurze Geschichte der Chirurgie.* Berlin, Springer, 1928.
BULLOCH, W.: *The History of Bacteriology.* London, Oxford Univ. Press, 1938.
BURCKHARDT, F.: *Zur Geschichte der Chirurgie.* Basel, Reinhardt, 1902.
CABANÈS, A.: *Chirurgiens et blessés à travers l'histoire.* Paris, Michel, 1918.
——: *Dents et dentistes à travers l'histoire.* Paris, Lab. Bottu, n.d.
CASARINI, A.: *La medicina militare nella leggenda e nella storia.* Roma, Giorn. di med. milit., 1929.
CASTIGLIONI, A.: *Storia dell'igiene, in Trattato Italiano d'Igiene.* Torino, Un. tip. ed., 1926.
CELLI, A.: *Storia della malaria nell'agro Romano.* Città di Castello, 1923.
CHAINE, J.: *Histoire de l'anatomie comparative.* Bordeaux, Duguerre, 1925.
CHANCE, B.: *Ophthalmology.* (Clio Medica.) New York, Hoeber, 1939.
CHAUVEAU, C.: *Histoire des maladies du pharynx.* 5 v. Paris, Baillière, 1901–5.
CHIEVITZ, J. H.: *Anatomiens historie.* Kjøbenhavn, Gyldendal, 1904.
CHOULANT, J. L.: *Geschichte und Bibliographie der anatomischen Abbildung.* Leipzig, 1852. (Repr. Chicago, Univ. of Chicago Press, 1920.)
CONCI, G.: *Pagine di storia della farmacia.* Milano, Vittoria, 1934.
CORNER, G. W.: *Anatomy.* (Clio Medica.) New York, Hoeber, 1930.
CORRADI, A.: *Annali delle epidemie occorse in Italia dalle prime memorie fino al 1850.* Bologna, Gamberini, 1865–80.
COULTER, J. S.: *Physical Therapy.* (Clio Medica.) New York, Hoeber, 1932.
CROOKSHANK, E. M.: *History and Pathology of Vaccination.* 2 v. London, Lewis, 1889.
DAMPIER-WHETHAM, W. C. D.: *A History of Science and Its Relations with Philosophy and Religion.* Cambridge and New York, Cambridge Univ. Pr., 1931.
DARMSTÄDTER, L.: *Handbuch zur Geschichte der Naturwissenschaften und der Technik.* Berlin, Springer, 1908.
DESNOS, E.: *Histoire de l'urologie.* Paris, Doin, 1914.
DIEPGEN, P.: *Geschichte der sozialen Medizin.* Leipzig, Barth, 1934.
DISNEY, A. N.: *Origin and Development of the Microscope.* London, Royal Micr. Soc., 1928.
DUVAL, M. M., and CUYER, E.: *Histoire de l'anatomie plastique.* Paris, Picard, 1899.
FASBENDER, H.: *Geschichte der Geburtshilfe.* Jena, Fischer, 1906.
FISCHER, I.: Zur Geschichte der operativen Gynäkologie im Altertum, *Berichte üb. d. ges. Gynäk. u. Geburtshilfe,* 2:177, 1923–4.
FLEMMING, C. F.: *Geschichte der Psychiatrie.* Leipzig, 1859.
FLEXNER, J. T.: *Doctors on Horseback, Pioneers of American Medicine.* New York, Viking, 1937.
FLEXNER, S.: *A Half Century of American Medicine.* Chicago, Lincoln Press, 1937.
FOSTER, SIR MICHAEL: *Lectures on the History of Physiology.* Cambridge Univ. Press, 1901.

FULTON, J. F.: *Physiology*. (Clio Medica.) New York, Hoeber, 1931.
——: *Selected Readings in the History of Physiology*. Baltimore, Thomas, 1930.
GARCIA DEL REAL, E.: *Historia contemporanea de la medicina*. Madrid, Espasa-Calpe, 1934.
GARRISON, F. H.: *Notes on Military Medicine*. Washington, Assoc. Mil. Surg., 1922.
GEIST-JACOBI, G. P.: *Geschichte der Zahnheilkunde*. Tübingen, 1896.
GIORDANO, D.: *Scritti e discorsi pertinenti alla storia della medicina e ad argomenti diversi*. Milano, Riv. di terap. med. e di med. prat., 1930.
GOLDSCHMID, E.: *Entwicklung und Bibliographie der pathologisch-anatomischen Abbildung*. Leipzig, Hiersemann, 1925.
GUERINI, A.: *A History of Dentistry*. Philadelphia and New York, Lea & Febiger, 1909.
GURLT, E. J.: *Geschichte der Chirurgie*. 3 v. Berlin, Hirschwald, 1898.
HADDON, A. C., and QUIGGIN, A. H.: *History of Anthropology*. London and New York, Putnam, 1910.
HAESER, H.: *Geschichte christlicher Krankenpflege und Pflegerschaften*. Berlin, Hertz, 1857.
——: *Übersicht der Geschichte der Chirurgie und des chirurgischen Standes*. Stuttgart, Enke, 1879.
HÄFLIGER, J. A.: *Pharmazeutische Altertumskunde und die Schweizerische Sammlung für historisches Apothekenwesen an der Universität Basel*. Zürich, Buchd. der alten Univ., 1931.
HEMMETER, J. C.: *Master Minds in Medicine*. New York, Medical Life, 1927.
HIMES, N. E.: *Medical History of Contraception*. Baltimore, Williams & Wilkins, 1936.
HIRSCH, M.: Alte und neue Heilkunde im Lichte der Lehre von der inneren Sekretion, in *Handbuch der inn. Sekretion*, v. 1. Leipzig, Kabitzsch, 1926.
HIRSCHBERG, J.: *Geschichte der Augenheilkunde*. 4 v. in 10. Leipzig, Engelmann, 1899–1918.
HOLLAENDER, E.: *Die Medizin in der klassischen Malerei*. 2 Aufl., Stuttgart, Enke, 1913.
——: *Plastik und Medizin*. Stuttgart, Enke, 1912.
——: *Die Karikatur und Satire in der Medizin*. Stuttgart, Enke, 1905.
——: *Wunder, Wundergeburt und Wundergestalten*. Stuttgart, Enke, 1921.
——: *Aeskulap und Venus*. Berlin, Propyl. Verl., 1928.
HOWARD, J.: *An Account of the Principal Lazarettos in Europe*. London, Johnson, 1791.
HUME, E. E.: *Doctors East, Doctors West*. New York, Norton, 1946.
——: *Medals of the U.S. Army Med. Dept*. New York, Am. Numism. Soc., 1942.
ILVENTO, A.: *La tubercolosi attraverso i secoli*. Torino, Un. tip. edit. Torinese, 1933.
JAMESON, E.: *Gynecology and Obstetrics*. (Clio Medica.) New York, Hoeber, 1936.
JONES, W. H. S.: *Malaria and Greek History*. Manchester, Univ. Pr., 1909.
KANNABICH, J. W.: *History of Psychiatry* (in Russian). Moscow, Medizin Staatsveil, 1929.
KASSEL, K.: *Geschichte der Nasenheilkunde*. Würzburg, Kabitzsch, 1914.
KEYS, T. E.: *The History of Surgical Anesthesia*. New York, Schuman's, 1945.
KIRCHHOFF, F. A. T.: Grundriss einer Geschichte der deutschen Irrenpflege, in *Handbuch der Psychiatrie*. Leipzig u. Deuticke, 1912.
KLEBS, A. C.: The Historic Evolution of Variolation, *Bull. Johns Hopkins Hosp.*, 24:69, 1913.
KRUMBHAAR, E. B.: *Pathology*. (Clio Medica.) New York, Hoeber, 1937.
LÄHR, H.: *Die Literatur der Psychiatrie, Neurologie und Psychologie, von 1459–1799*. Berlin, Reimer, 1900.
LA TORRE, F.: *L'utero attraverso i secoli*. Castello, Un. arti graf, 1917.
LA WALL, C. H.: *Four Thousand Years of Pharmacy*. Philadelphia and London, Lippincott, 1927.
LEONARDO, R. A.: *History of Surgery*. New York, Froben Press, 1943.
LEVINSON, A.: *Pioneers of Pediatrics*. New York, Froben Press, 1943.
LEYMAN, C. P.: *History of Veterinary Medicine*. Cambridge, 1898.
LINT, J. G. DE: *Atlas van de geschiedenis de geneeskunde*. (*Anatomie*.) Amsterdam, 1925 (English trans., New York, Hoeber, 1926).
——: *Rembrandt*. The Hague, Kruseman, 1930.
LIPINSKA, M.: *Histoire des femmes médecins*. Paris, Jacques, 1900.
LONG, E. R.: *A History of Pathology*. Baltimore, Williams & Wilkins, 1928.
——: *Selected Readings in Pathology*. Springfield, Thomas, 1929.
LUSK, G.: *Nutrition*. (Clio Medica.) New York, Hoeber, 1933.
MAJOR, R. H.: *Classic Descriptions of Disease*. Springfield, Thomas, 1932. 2nd ed., 1939.

MALGAIGNE, J. F.: *Histoire de la chirurgie en Occident depuis le VIe jusqu'au XVIe siècle.* Paris, Baillière, 1870.

MARCET, W.: *A Contribution to the History of Respiration of Man.* (Croonian Lectures.) London, Churchill, 1897.

MARX, K. F. H.: *Beziehungen der darstellenden Kunst zur Heilkunst.* Göttingen, Dietrichsen, 1861.

MEAD, K. C.: *A History of Women in Medicine.* Haddam, Conn., Haddam Press, 1938.

MÜLLERSHEIM, R.: *Die Wochenstube in der Kunst.* Stuttgart, Enke, 1904.

NEEDHAM, G.: A *History of Embryology.* Cambridge, 1934.

NEWMAN, SIR GEORGE: *The Rise of Preventive Medicine.* Oxford Univ. Press, 1932.

NEWSHOLME, SIR ARTHUR: *The Evolution of Preventive Medicine.* Baltimore, Williams & Wilkins, 1927.

——: *The Story of Modern Preventive Medicine. A Continuation.* Baltimore, Williams & Wilkins, 1929.

NORDENSKIÖLD, E.: *Die Geschichte der Biologie.* Jena, Fischer, 1926.

NUTTING, M. A., and DOCK, L. L.: *A History of Nursing.* 4 v. New York, Putnam, 1907–12.

PANSIER, P.: *Histoire des lunettes.* Paris, Melvine, 1901.

PETERS, H.: *Aus pharmazeutischer Vorzeit.* 2 v. Berlin, 1888–1891 (English trans. by W. Netter, Chicago, Engelhard, 1889).

——: *Der Arzt und die Heilkunst in der deutschen Vergangenheit.* Leipzig, Diederichs, 1900.

PFEIFFER, L., and RULAND, C.: *Pestilentia in nummis.* Tübingen, Laupp, 1882.

PIÉRY, M., and ROSHEM, J.: *Histoire de la tuberculose.* Paris, Doin, 1931.

POLITZER, A.: *Geschichte der Ohrenheilkunde.* 2 v. Stuttgart, Enke, 1907–13.

PREDOEHL, A.: *Zur Geschichte der Tuberkulose.* Hamburg, Voss, 1888.

PROKSCH, J.: *Geschichte der venerischen Krankheiten.* Bonn, Hanstein, 1895.

——: *Die Literatur über die venerischen Krankheiten.* 3 v. Bonn, Hanstein, 1889–1900.

PROSKAUER, C.: *Iconographia odontologica.* Berlin, Meusser, 1926.

PUSCHMANN, T.: *Geschichte der medizinischen Unterrichts.* Leipzig, Veit, 1889.

RADL, W.: *Geschichte der Biologischen Theorien.* 2 Aufl., Leipzig u. Berlin, Engelmann, 1913 (English trans. by E. J. Hatfield, London, Oxford Univ. Press, 1930).

RAVOGLI, A.: History of Dermatology, *Medical Life,* 33:492, 1926.

RICCI, J. V.: *The Genealogy of Gynæcology; History of the Development of Gynæcology throughout the Ages, 2000 B.C.–1800 A.D.* Philadelphia, Blakiston, 1943.

RICHER, P. M. L. P.: *L'Art et la médecine.* Paris, Gaultier, 1903.

RIESMAN, D.: *Medicine in the Middle Ages.* New York, Hoeber, 1935.

ROBINSON, V.: *Pioneers of Birth Control in England and America.* New York, Voluntary Parenthood League, 1919.

——: *Victory over Pain.* New York, Schuman's 1946.

——: *White Caps, the History of Nursing.* Philadelphia, Lippincott, 1946.

ROHDE, E. S.: *The Old English Herbals.* London, Longmans, Green, 1922.

ROLLESTON, SIR H.: *Internal Medicine.* (Clio Medica.) New York, Hoeber, 1930.

——: *The Endocrine Glands in Health and Disease, with an historical review.* London, 1936.

ROLLESTON, J. D.: The History of Scarlet Fever, *Brit. Med. Jr.,* 2:926, 1928.

ROSEN, G.: *The History of Miners' Diseases.* New York, Schuman's, 1943.

RUBNER, M.: *Handbuch der Hygiene. Historische Einleitung.* Leipzig, Hirzel, 1911.

SAITTA, S.: *Il servizio sanitario di guerra attraverso i secoli.* Catania, 1924.

SALVERAGLIO, F.: *Bibliografia della pellagra.* Nuova ed., Pavia, Tip. coop., 1914.

SCHELENZ, H.: *Geschichte der Pharmazie.* Berlin, Springer, 1904.

SCHMIDT, A.: *Drogen und Drogenhandel im Altertum.* Leipzig u. Köln, Gelily, 1924.

SIEBOLD, C. J. VON: *Versuch einer Geschichte der Geburtshilfe.* 3 v. Tübingen, Pietzker, 1901–4.

SIGERIST, H. E.: *Socialized Medicine in the Soviet Union.* New York, Norton, 1937.

——: *Wandlungen des Konstitutionsbegriffes.* Jena, 1928.

SINGER, C. J.: *The Evolution of Anatomy.* New York, Knopf, 1925.

——: *From Magic to Science.* London, Benn, 1928.

SMITH, SIR F.: *The Early History of Veterinary Literature.* 3 v. London, Baillière, 1919–30.

SPENCER, H. R.: *History of British Midwifery.* London, Bale, 1927.

STICKER, G.: *Abhandlungen der Seuchengeschichte.* 2 v. Giessen, Töpelmann, 1908–12.

STILL, G. F.: *The History of Pediatrics*. London, Oxford Univ. Press, 1931.
STORER, H. R.: *Medicina in Nummis*. Boston, Wright & Potter, 1931.
SUDHOFF, K.: *Erstlinge der pädiatrischen Literatur*. München, Münchener Drucke, 1925.
——: Geschichte des Krankenhauswesens, in *Ergebn. d. Krankenhaus-Wesens*, v. 2. Jena, 1913.
——: *Geschichte der Zahnheilkunde*. Leipzig, Barth, 1926.
——: *Katalog der hygienischen Ausstellung*. Dresden, 1911.
TAYLOR, N.: *Quinine: The Story of Cinchona*. New York, Sc. monthly, 1943.
TISCHNER, R.: *Geschichte der Homöopathie*. 2 v. Leipzig, Schwabe, 1932–9.
TRISCA, P.: *Apercu sur l'histoire de la médecine préventive*. Paris, Maloine, 1923.
TRUC, M., and PANSIER, P.: *L'Ophtalmologie à l'école de Montpellier du Xe an XXe siècle*. Paris, Maloine, 1907.
VETH, C.: *Der Arzt in der Karikatur*. Berlin, 1928.
VIEILLARD, C.: *L'Urologie et les médecins urologistes dans la médecine ancienne*. Paris, de Rudeval, 1903.
VIRCHOW, R.: Zur Geschichte des Aussatzes und der Spitäler, *Virch. Arch.*, 18:138, 273, 1860; 19:43, 1860; 20:166, 1861.
WALSH, J. J.: *Catholic Churchmen in Science*. 2 v. Philadelphia, Am. Eccl. Rev., 1906–9.
——: *Mediæval Medicine*, London, Black, 1920.
WEBB, G. B.: *Tuberculosis*. (Clio Medica.) New York, Hoeber, 1936.
WEINBERGER, B. W.: Early Dental Literature, *Bull. Med. Libr. Assn.*, Boston, 26:222, 1938.
WEINDLER, F.: *Geschichte der gynäkologisch-anatomischen Abbildung*. Dresden, Zahn u. Jaensch, 1908.
WIENER, J.: *Geschichte des Mikroskops*. Wien, 1864.
WINCKEL, FRANZ VON: *Handb. d. Geburtshülfe*. 3 Teile. Wiesbaden, Bergman, 1903–7.
WITKOWSKI, G. J. A.: *Histoire des accouchements de tous les peuples*. Paris, Steinheil, 1887.
WOLFF, J.: *Die Lehre von der Krebskrankheit von den ältesten Zeiten bis zur Gegenwart*. 4 v. Jena, Fischer, 1907–28.
WRIGHT, J.: *History of Laryngology and Rhinology*. 2nd ed., Philadelphia, Lea & Febiger, 1914.
ZAMBACO, D. A., pacha: *La Lèpre à travers les siècles*. Paris, 1914.
ZINSSER, H.: *Rats, Lice and History*. Boston, Little, Brown, 1935.

D. BIOGRAPHICAL AND BIBLIOGRAPHICAL

AFFLITTO: *Memorie dagli scrittori del regno di Napoli*. 2 v. Napoli, 1782–4.
BAYLE, A. L., and THILLAYE, A. J.: *Biographie médicale par ordre chronologique d'aprés Dàniel Leclerc, Eloy*, etc. 2 v. in 1. Paris, Délahaye, 1855.
BETTANY, G. T.: *Eminent Doctors, Their Lives and Works*. 2 v. London, Glogg, 1885.
Biographie médicale (par A. and L. Jourdan). 7 v. Paris, Pankoucke, 1820–5.
Biographie universelle ancienne et moderne. 85 v. Paris, Michaud frères et Beck, 1811–62.
BONINO, G. G.: *Biografia medica piemontese*. 2 v. Torino, Bianco, 1824–5.
BRUNET, G.: *Manuel du libraire et de l'amateur de livres*. 6 v. Paris, Didot, 1860–5 (Repr. 1932).
BUSQUET, P., GILBERT, A. and GENTY, M.: *Les Biographies médicales*. 5 v. Paris, Baillière, 1927–38.
CALLISEN, A.: *Medizinisches Schriftstellerlexicon der jetzt lebenden Ärzte*. . . . Copenhagen, Altona, 1830–45.
CAPPARONI, P.: *Profili bibliografici di medici e naturalisti italiani*. 2 v. Roma, Ist. naz. med. farmacol. Serono, 1925–8.
CARBONELLI, G.: *Bibliographia medica pedemontana*. Roma, Centenari, 1914 (1919).
CERVETTO, G.: *Cenni per una storia dei medici veronesi*. Verona, 1834.
CHINCHILLA, A.: *Anales historicos de la medicina en general, y biografico-bibliograficos de la española en particular*. Valencia, Lopez, 1841–8.
CHOULANT, J.: *Bibliotheca medico-historica*. Leipzig, Engelmann, 1842.
——: *Handbuch der Bücherkunde für die ältere Medizin*. Leipzig, Voss, 1828 and 1841 (Repr. München, 1926).

CHOULANT, L.: *Graphische-Incunabeln für Naturgeschichte und Medizin.* Leipzig, Weigel, 1858 (Repr. München, 1924).

DELPRAT, C. C.: De geschiedenis der Nederlandsche geneeskundige tijdschriften 1680–1857, *Nederl. tijdschr. v. geneesk.,* 71:3, 1927.

DEZEIMERIS, J. E., et al.: *Dictionnaire historique de la médecine.* 4 v. Paris, Bechet, 1828–39.

Dictionary of National Biography, ed. by L. Stephen. 63 v. London and New York, Macmillan, 1885–1901.

FANTUZZI, G.: *Notizie sugli scrittori bolognesi.* 9 v. Bologna, d'Aquina, 1781–9.

FISCHER, I.: *Die Eigennamen in der Krankheitsterminologie.* Wien, Perles, 1931.

———: *Biographisches Lexikon der hervorragenden Ärzte der letzten fünfzig Jahre.* 2 v. Berlin u. Wien, Urban, 1932–4.

FOPPENS, J. F.: *Bibliotheca belgica.* 2 v. Bruxelles, P. Foppens, 1739.

GARRISON, F. H.: Revised Student's Check List of Texts Illustrating History of Medicine, *Bull. of Inst. of Hist. of Med.,* 1:333, 1933.

GOLDSTEIN, M.: *Internationale Bibliographie der altägyptischen Medizin.* Berlin-Charlottenburg, M. Goldstein, 1933.

GROSS, S. D.: *Lives of American Physicians and Surgeons in the Nineteenth Century.* Philadelphia, 1861.

GROTE, L. R., ed.: *Die Medizin der Gegenwart in Selbstdarstellungen* (numerous vols., each containing short autobiographies). Leipzig, Meiner, 1923.

GURLT, E., et al.: *Biographisches Lexikon der hervorragenden Ärzte.* 2nd ed., by W. Haberling, 6 v. Berlin u. Wien, Urban u. Schwarzenberg, 1929–35.

GUTTMANN, W.: *Medizinische Terminologie.* 8th ed. Berlin u. Wien, Urban, 1937.

HAESER, H.: *Bibliotheca epidemiographica.* Jena, Mauke, 1843.

HAHN, L.: *Essais de bibliographie médicale.* Paris, Steinheil, 1897.

HALLER, A.: *Bibliotheca anatomica, chirurgica, medica practica.* 8 v. Basileæ, Schweighauser u. Bernae, E. Haller, 1774–8.

HEMMETER, J. C.: *Master Minds in Medicine.* New York, Medical Life Pr., 1927.

HOFF, E. C., and FULTON, J. F.: *A Bibliography of Aviation Medicine.* Springfield, Ill., 1942.

HUTCHINSON, B.: *Biographical Medicine.* 2 v. London, Johnson, 1799.

JOURDAN: *Encyclopédie des sciences médicales.* Paris, 1920–5.

KELLY, H.: *Cyclopedia of American Medical Biography.* Philadelphia and London, Saunders, 1912; 2nd ed., Boston and New York, 1928.

———: *Dictionary of American Medical Biography.* New York, Appleton, 1928.

LAMBERT, S. W., and GOODWIN, G. M.: *Medical Leaders from Hippocrates to Osler.* Indianapolis, Bobbs-Merrill, 1929.

LEVI, M. G.: *Ricordo intorno ai medici veneziani.* Venezia, 1835.

LINDEN, J. A. VAN DER: *De scriptis medicis.* 3rd ed., Amsterdam, Blaev, 1662.

MACMICHAEL, W.: *Lives of British Physicians.* London, Murray, 1830.

——— and MUNK, W.: *The Gold-headed Cane.* London, Murray, 1827 (Repr. New York, Froben Pr., 1932).

MARINI, G. L.: *Degli archiatri pontifici.* 2 v. Roma, Stamp. Pagliarini, 1784.

MAZZETTI, S.: *Repertorio di tutti i professori antichi dell'università di Bologna.* Bologna, Tip. S. Tommaso, 1848.

MEISEN, V.: *Medicinsk Historiske Afhandlinger og Portrætter.* Kœbenhavn, Levin & Munksgaards, 1933.

MIELI, A.: *Bibliografia metodica,* in *A.S.S.,* I, IV, V, VI, 1920, 1923–5.

MOREJON, A. H.: *Historia bibliografica de la medicina española.* 7 v. Madrid, 1842–52.

Osleriana, Bibliotheca, ed. by W. W. Francis, R. H. Hill, and A. Malloch. Oxford, Clarendon Press, 1929. (A résumé that contains much valuable information in Osler's annotations.)

PAGEL, J. L.: *Biographisches Lexicon der hervorragenden Ärzte des XIX. Jahrhunderts.* Berlin u. Wien, Urban u. Schwarzenberg, 1901.

PANELLI, G.: *Memorie degli uomini illustri in medicina del Piceno.* 2 v. Ascoli, Ricci, 1757–8.

PETTIGREW, T. J.: *Medical Portrait Gallery.* 4 v. in 2. London, Fisher, n.d. [1840].

POWER, SIR D'ARCY, ed.: *British Masters of Medicine.* London, Med. Press, 1936.

Quarterly Cumulative Index Medicus. Chicago, Am. Med. Assn., 1916–current.

ROBINSON, V.: *Pathfinders in Medicine.* New York, Medical Life Press, 1929.

ROLLESTON, SIR HUMPHRY: *The Cambridge Medical School. A Biographical History*. Cambridge Univ. Press, 1932.

SAMBUCUS, T.: *Icones veterum aliquot ac recentium medicorum*. Antwerpen, Nederlandsche Boekhandel, 1901 (Repr. of orig. ed. of 1574).

SCHMID, J. F.: *Bibliographie der öffentlichen Hygiene*. Bern, Wyss, 1898–1906.

SIGERIST, H. E.: *Grosse Ärzte. Eine Geschichte der Heilkunde in Lebensbildern*. München, Lehmann, 1932. (Am. ed., *The Great Doctors*. New York, Norton, 1933.)

THATCHER, J.: *American Medical Biography*. 2 v. Boston, Richardson, 1828.

TIPALDO, E. DE: *Biblioteca degli Italiani illustri*. 10 v. Venezia, Tip. di Alvisopoli, 1834–5.

VALDIZAN, H.: *Dicionario de medicina peruana*. Lima, 1923.

VEDOVA, G.: *Biografia degli scrittori padovani*. 2 v. Padova, coi tipi della Minerva, 1832.

WALSH, J. J.: *Makers of Modern Medicine*. New York, Fordham Univ. Press, 1907.

WICKERSHEIMER, C. A. E.: *Dictionnaire biographique des médecins en France au moyen âge*. Paris, Droz, 1936.

——: *La Médecine et les médecins en France à l'époque de la renaissance*. Paris, Maloine, 1906.

INDEX OF SUBJECTS

[i]

INDEX OF NAMES

The dates of birth and death of persons quoted in the text have been given here as exactly and completely as possible. Of many living physicians, editors, and translators, especially of those living abroad, exact information was impossible to obtain.

Printed and bound by CPI Group (UK) Ltd, Croydon, CR0 4YY

23/10/2024

01778268-0003